Differential Diagnosis for PHYSICAL THERAPISTS

Screening for Referral

ELSEVIER

evolve

• To access your Student Resources, visit:

http://evolve.elsevier.com/GoodmanSnyder/differential/

Evolve® Student Learning Resources for *Goodman/Snyder: Differential Diagnosis for Physical Therapists: Screening for Referral* 4th Edition offer the following features:

Student Resources

- **Forms for Practice**
  - A. Screening Summary
  - B. Special Questions to Ask
  - C. Special Forms to Use
  - D. Special Tests to Perform

- **Practice Questions**
  Printable version of those questions from each chapter

- **Weblinks**
  Links to other helpful resources and information

- **Updates**
  Updated periodically with additional information

Differential Diagnosis *for* PHYSICAL THERAPISTS

Screening for Referral

Catherine Cavallaro Goodman, MBA, PT

Medical Multimedia Group
Faculty Affiliate
University of Montana
Missoula, Montana

Teresa E. Kelly Snyder, MN, RN, OCN

Oncology Treatment Area
Montana Cancer Specialists
Missoula, Montana

SAUNDERS

ELSEVIER

SAUNDERS
ELSEVIER

11830 Westline Industrial Drive
St. Louis, Missouri 63146

DIFFERENTIAL DIAGNOSIS FOR PHYSICAL THERAPISTS: SCREENING FOR
REFERRAL

Copyright © 2007 by Saunders, an imprint of Elsevier Inc.

Notice

Knowledge and best practice in this field are constantly changing. As new research and
experience broaden our knowledge, changes in practice, treatment and drug therapy may
become necessary or appropriate. Readers are advised to check the most current information
provided (i) on procedures featured or (ii) by the manufacturer of each product to be
administered, to verify the recommended dose or formula, the method and duration of
administration, and contraindications. It is the responsibility of the practitioner, relying on
their own experience and knowledge of the patient, to make diagnoses, to determine dosages
and the best treatment for each individual patient, and to take all appropriate safety
precautions. To the fullest extent of the law, neither the Publisher nor the Authors assume
any liability for any injury and/or damage to persons or property arising out or related to
any use of the material contained in this book.

The Publisher

Library of Congress Cataloging-in-Publication Data

Goodman, Catherine Cavallaro.
  Differential diagnosis for physical therapists: screening for referral / Catherine
  Cavallaro Goodman, Teresa E. Kelly Snyder.
    p. cm.
  ISBN-13: 978-07216-0619-4   ISBN-10: 0-7216-0619-9
  1. Physical therapy.   2. Diagnosis, Differential.   I. Snyder, Teresa E. Kelly.   II. Title.

RM701.G658 2006
615.8'2—dc22

2006051253

Previous editions copyrighted 2000, 1995, 1990

ISBN-13: 978-0-7216-0619-4

ISBN-10: 0-7216-0619-9

Publishing Director: Linda Duncan
Senior Editor: Kathy Falk
Senior Developmental Editor: Christie M. Hart
Freelance Developmental Editor: Peg Waltner
Publishing Services Manager: Pat Joiner
Project Manager: David Stein
Design Direction: Amy Buxton
Cover and Interior Designer: Sheilah Barrett Carroll

Printed in the United States of America

Last digit is the print number: 9 8 7 6 5 4

Foreword

Catherine Goodman and Teresa Snyder are to be commended for making several important contributions to the role of physical therapists as diagnosticians with this revision of their classic text. The first step in the diagnostic process is to determine if the patient's condition necessitates a referral to a medical doctor. Therefore this book is an invaluable guide because the authors have provided a model that is focused and complete. Although the focus of the text is on identifying the most common conditions that mimic musculoskeletal problems, Goodman and Snyder also note that this is just the first step in the diagnostic process and have made suggestions for future directions. Thus the authors are providing a timely guide to practice and professional development by addressing the issue of terminology associated with diagnosis.

As physical therapy seeks to clarify its professional responsibilities by providing education at the clinical doctoral level, emphasizing diagnostic skills, and providing direct access care, a necessary component is accuracy in communicating these responsibilities. For many years, the issue of appropriate terminology and/or the context in which it is used with regard to diagnosis in physical therapy has been one of confusion. The scope of the confusion is reflected in a variety of editorials,[1-7] textbooks, and advertisements that are inconsistent in their use of differential diagnosis.

Goodman and Snyder have provided a model for approaching this confusion. Appropriately, this book's title, *Differential Diagnosis for Physical Therapists: Screening for Referral*, clarifies that a primary responsibility of the physical therapist is to recognize the possible presence of a medical condition that supersedes or mimics a condition requiring physical therapy treatment. Clarification that differential diagnosis does not mean identifying the specific disease is important in our relationship with physicians and in maintaining our legal scope of practice, as physical therapists assume a larger role in direct access and primary care.[1]

As stated in this text, the first step in the diagnostic process is for the physical therapist to be able to identify medical conditions that are to be referred to the appropriate practitioner. Clearly this is a skill that any physical therapist must be able to demonstrate. Not only does this book provide the necessary information, but also the manner in which the material is presented should enable every reader to achieve a high level of skill. This book is intended to augment both the reader's skill in screening for medical conditions and also his or her skill in navigating the entire diagnostic process. The highly consumer-friendly and engaging format of this book is among the many reasons every student and clinician should include the book in their personal library.

But as Catherine Goodman and Teresa Snyder have so wisely stated in the preface, the primary focus of this book is just the first step in an evaluation that must ultimately lead to a diagnosis that directs physical therapy intervention. To their credit they have also provided an

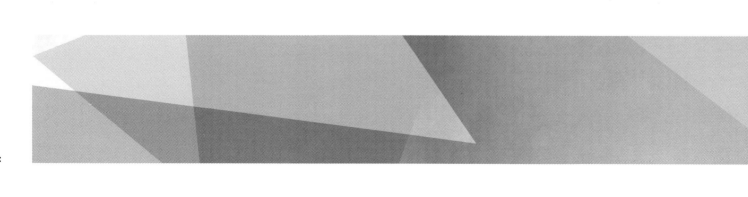

vii

introduction to the next steps in the complete diagnostic process. In keeping with the *Guide to Physical Therapist Practice*, Goodman and Snyder have addressed the importance of the concept of the movement system to physical therapy and thus to another level of differential diagnosis. They have directed our attention to a developing system of diagnoses of movement system impairments. This system requires differentiating among movement system impairment conditions at both the tissue and the movement level and then using this information to establish a diagnosis that directs physical therapy treatment.

In addition to providing information for physical therapists, Goodman and Snyder have also attempted to assist other health professionals in identifying which conditions should be referred to a physical therapist. This effort is another reflection of their prescient recognition of the direction of practice. The examination and diagnostic skills of the physical therapist, whether for ruling out or identifying a medical condition or cogently labeling a movement impairment syndrome, must become the most highly visible aspects of the profession's role in health care.

Historically the profession has mainly been considered one in which the practitioner provided treatment based on the physician's diagnosis. Evaluation, examination, diagnosis, and program planning whether sought by a client, a physician, or another health professional is the necessary direction for the profession if we are to assume our role in health promotion, maintenance, and/or remediation. Exercise, which is the prevailing form of physical therapy treatment, continues to receive increased attention as the most effective form of preventive and restorative care for lifestyle–induced diseases. Yet physical therapists are

not readily consulted for their expertise in developing programs that cannot only address lifestyle–induced diseases but that can also prevent inducing musculoskeletal problems.

An important goal of the profession is to promote recognition that we are the health profession with the expertise to appropriately screen, diagnose, and then develop treatment programs that are safe and effective for individuals with all levels of movement system dysfunction. We are indebted to Catherine Goodman and Teresa Snyder for their contributions to enabling us to achieve this goal.

Shirley Sahrmann, PT, PhD, FAPTA
Professor Physical Therapy, Neurology,
Cell Biology & Physiology
Washington University School of
Medicine—St. Louis, MO

REFERENCES

1. Boissonnault W, Goodman C: Physical therapists as diagnosticians: drawing the line on diagnosing pathology, *J Ortho Sports Phys Ther* 36(6):351-353, 2006.
2. Davenport TE, Kulig K, Resnick C: Diagnosing pathology to decide the appropriateness of physical therapy: what's our role? *J Orthop Sports Phys Ther* 36(1):1-2, 2006.
3. Guccione AA: Physical therapy diagnosis and the relationship between impairments and function, *Phys Ther* 71(7):499-503, 1991.
4. Jette AM: Diagnosis and classification by physical therapists: a special communication, *Phys Ther* 69(11):967-969, 1989.
5. Rose SJ: Physical therapy diagnosis: role and function, *Phys Ther* 69(7):535-537, 1989.
6. Sahrmann SA: Diagnosis by the physical therapist—a prerequisite for treatment: a special communication, *Phys Ther* 1703-1706, 1988.
7. Sahrmann SA: Are physical therapists fulfilling their responsibilities as diagnosticians? *J Ortho Sports Phys Ther* 35(9):556-558, 2005.
8. Zimny NJ: Diagnostic classification and orthopaedic physical therapy practice: what can we learn from medicine? *J Orthop Sports Phys Ther* 34(3):105-111, 2004.

Preface

If you have ever looked in this book hoping for a way to figure out just what is wrong with your client's back or neck or shoulder but did not find the answer, then you understand the need for a title to clarify just what is in here.

The new name, *Differential Diagnosis for Physical Therapists: Screening for Referral*, does not reflect a change in the content of the text so much as it reflects a better understanding of the screening process as the first step in making a diagnosis. Before implementing a plan of care the therapist must confirm (or rule out) the need for physical therapy intervention. We must ask and answer these questions:

- Is this an appropriate physical therapy referral?
- Is there a problem that does not fall into one of the four categories of conditions outlined by the Guide?
- Are there any red flag histories, red flag risk factors, or cluster of red flag signs and/or symptoms?

This text provides students, physical therapist assistants, and physical therapy clinicians with a step-by-step approach to client evaluation that follows the standards for competency established by the American Physical Therapy Association (APTA) related to conducting a screening examination.

In fact, we present a screening model that can be used with each client. By following these steps—Past Medical History, Risk Factor Assessment, Clinical Presentation, Associated Signs and Symptoms, and Review of Systems—the therapist will avoid omitting any critical part of the screening process. With the physical therapy screening interview as a foundation for subjectively evaluating patients and clients, each organ system is reviewed with regard to the most common disorders encountered, particularly those that may mimic primary musculoskeletal problems.

A cognitive processing-reasoning orientation is used throughout the text to encourage students to gather and analyze data, pose and solve problems, infer, hypothesize, and make clinical judgments. Many new case examples have been added. Case examples and case studies are used to integrate screening information and help the therapist make decisions about how and when to treat, refer, or treat AND refer.

The text is divided into three sections: Part 1 introduces the screening interview along with a new chapter on physical assessment for screening with many helpful photographs and illustrations. Another new chapter presents pain types and viscerogenic pain patterns. How and why the organs can refer pain to the musculoskeletal system is explained.

Section 2 presents a systems approach looking at each organ system and the various diseases, illnesses, and conditions that can refer symptoms to the neuromuscular or musculoskeletal system. Red flag histories,

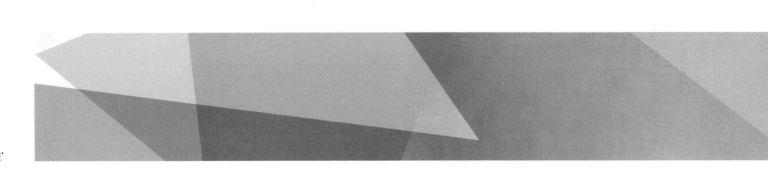

risk factors, clinical presentation, and signs and symptoms are reviewed for each system. As in previous editions, helpful screening clues and guidelines for referral are included in each chapter.

In the third and final section, the last chapter in the previous editions has been expanded into five separate chapters. An individual screening focus is presented based on the various body parts from head to toe.

As always, while screening for medical disease, side effects of medications, or other unrecognized comorbidities, the therapist must still conduct a movement exam to identify the true cause of the pain or symptom(s) should there be a primary neuromuscular or primary musculoskeletal problem. And there are times when therapists are treating patients and/or clients with a movement system impairment who also report signs and symptoms associated with a systemic disease or illness. For many conditions, early detection and referral can reduce morbidity and mortality.

The goal of this text is to provide the therapist (both students and clinicians) with a consistent way to screen for systemic diseases and medical conditions that can mimic neuromusculoskeletal problems. It is not our intent to teach physical therapists how to diagnose pathology or medical conditions, which we consider outside the scope of the physical therapist's practice.

Catherine Cavallaro Goodman, MBA, PT
Teresa E. Kelly Snyder, MN, RN, OCN

Acknowledgments

We never imagined our little book would ever go beyond a first edition. The first edition was a direct result of our experience in the military as nurse (Teresa) and physical therapist (Catherine), although we did not know each other at that time. So to the many men and women of the United States Armed Forces who have worked as independent practitioners and fine-tuned this material, we say thank you.

In addition, special thanks go to the many fine folks (past and present) at Elsevier Science:

Andrew Allen
Louise Beirig
Julie Burchett
Amy Buxton
Linda Duncan
Sue Hontscharik
Christie M. Hart
Kathy Falk
Kathy Macciocca
Jacqui Merrill
RF Schneider, permissions dept.
David Stein
Marion Waldman

Unnamed but appreciated copy editors, production staff, marketing personnel, sales representatives, editorial assistants, and many more we don't even know about! Please consider yourselves appreciated and thanked.

To all the others as well:

Maj. Richard E. Baxter
Nancy Bloom
Bill Boissonnault
Chuck Ciccone
Nancy Ciesla
Brent Dodge
Kenda Fuller
Brant Goode
Janet Hulme
Michael Keith, APTA Governance
Leanne Lenker
Pam Little
Charles L. McGarvey, III
Brian Murphy
Barbara Norton

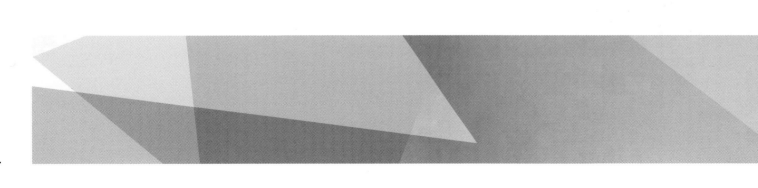

Cindy Pfalzer
Sue Queen
Shirley Sahrmann
Saint Patrick's Hospital and Health Sciences Center, Center for Health Information (Dana Kopp, Ginny Bolten, and Marianne Farr)
University of Montana: Steve Fehrer, Dave Levison, Beth Ikeda
Ken Saladin
Jason Taitch
Steve Tepper

Peg and Doug Waltner
Valerie Wang
Karen Wilson

And to any other family member, friend, or colleague whose name should have been on this list but was inadvertently missed . . . a special hug of thanks.

Catherine Cavallaro Goodman, MBA, PT
Teresa E. Kelly Snyder, MN, RN, OCN

Contents

SECTION THREE
SYSTEMIC ORIGINS OF NEUROMUSCULAR OR
MUSCULOSKELETAL PAIN AND DYSFUNCTION

Differential Diagnosis *for* PHYSICAL THERAPISTS

Screening for Referral

Introduction to the
Screening Process

Introduction to Screening for Referral in Physical Therapy

It is the therapist's responsibility to make sure that each patient/client is an appropriate candidate for physical therapy. In order to be as cost-effective as possible, we must determine what biomechanical or neuromusculoskeletal problem is present and then treat the problem as specifically as possible.

As part of this process, the therapist may need to screen for medical disease. Physical therapists must be able to identify signs and symptoms of systemic disease that can mimic neuromuscular or musculoskeletal (herein referred to as neuromusculoskeletal or NMS) dysfunction. Peptic ulcers, gallbladder disease, liver disease, and myocardial ischemia are only a few examples of systemic diseases that can cause shoulder or back pain. Other diseases can present as primary neck, upper back, hip, sacroiliac, or low back pain and/or symptoms.

Cancer screening is a major part of the overall screening process. Cancer can present as primary neck, shoulder, chest, upper back, hip, groin, pelvic, sacroiliac, or low back pain/symptoms. Whether primary cancer or cancer that has recurred or metastasized, clinical manifestations can mimic NMS dysfunction. The therapist must know how and what to look for to screen for cancer.

The purpose and the scope of this text are not to teach therapists to be medical diagnosticians. The purpose of this text is twofold. The first is to help therapists recognize areas that are beyond the scope of a physical therapist's practice or expertise. The second is to provide a step-by-step method for therapists to identify clients who need a medical (or other) referral or consultation.

As more states move toward direct access and independent practice, physical therapists are increasingly becoming the first contact that patient/clients seek,* particularly for care of musculoskeletal dysfunction. This makes it critical for physical therapists to be well versed in determining when and how referral to a physician (or other appropriate health care professional) is necessary. Each individual case must be reviewed carefully.

Even without direct access, screening is an essential skill because any client can present with red flags requiring reevaluation by a medical specialist. The methods and clinical decision-making model for screening presented in this text remain the same with or without direct access and in all practice settings.

---

* The *Guide to Physical Therapist Practice* (2003) defines *patients* as "individuals who are the recipients of physical therapy care and direct intervention" and *clients* as "individuals who are not necessarily sick or injured but who can benefit from a physical therapist's consultation, professional advice, or prevention services." In this introductory chapter the term patient/client is used in accordance with the patient/client management model as presented in the *Guide.* In all other chapters, the term "client" is used except when referring to hospital in-patient/clients or out-patient/clients.

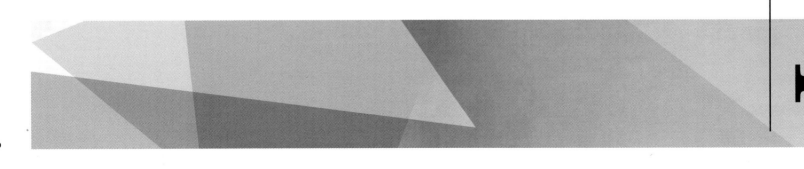

▶ EVIDENCE-BASED PRACTICE

Clinical decisions must be based on the best evidence available. The clinical basis for diagnosis, prognosis, and intervention must come from a valid and reliable body of evidence referred to as *evidence-based practice*. Each therapist must develop the skills necessary to assimilate, evaluate, and make the best use of evidence when screening patient/clients for medical disease.

Evidence-based clinical decision making consistent with the patient/client management model as presented in the *Guide to Physical Therapist Practice*[1] will be the foundation upon which a physical therapist's differential diagnosis is made. Screening for systemic disease or viscerogenic causes of NMS symptoms begins with a well-developed client history and interview.

The foundation for these skills is presented in Chapter 2. In addition, the therapist will rely heavily on clinical presentation and the presence of any associated signs and symptoms to alert him or her to the need for more specific screening questions and tests.

Under evidence-based medicine, relying on a red-flag checklist based on the history has proved to be a very safe way to avoid missing the presence of serious disorders. When serious conditions have been missed, it is not for lack of special investigations but for lack of adequate and thorough attention to clues in the history.[2,3]

Some conditions will be missed even with screening because the condition is early in its presentation and has not progressed enough to be recognizable. In some cases, early recognition makes no difference to the outcome, either because nothing can be done to prevent progression of the condition or there is no adequate treatment available.[2]

▶ STATISTICS

How often does it happen that a systemic or viscerogenic problem masquerades as a neuromuscular or musculoskeletal problem? There are very limited statistics to quantify how often organic disease masquerades or presents as NMS problems. Osteopathic physicians suggest this happens in approximately 1% of cases seen by physical therapists, but there is no data to confirm this estimate.[4,5]

Personal experience suggests this figure would be higher if therapists were screening routinely.

The three key factors that create a need for screening are:
- Side effects of medications
- Comorbidities
- Visceral pain mechanisms

If the medical diagnosis is delayed, then the correct diagnosis is eventually made when

1. The patient/client does not get better with physical therapy intervention,
2. The patient/client gets better then worse, and
3. Other associated signs and symptoms eventually develop.

There are times when a patient/client with NMS complaints is really experiencing the side effects of medications. In fact this is probably the most common source of associated signs and symptoms observed in the clinic. Side effects of medication as a cause of associated signs and symptoms, including joint and muscle pain, will be discussed more completely in Chapter 2. Visceral pain mechanisms are the entire subject of Chapter 3.

As for comorbidities, many patient/clients are affected by other conditions such as depression, diabetes, incontinence, obesity, chemical dependency, hypertension, osteoporosis, and deconditioning, to name just a few. These conditions can contribute to significant morbidity (and mortality) and must be documented as part of the problem list. Physical therapy intervention is often appropriate in affecting outcomes, and/or referral to a more appropriate health care or other professional may be needed.

Finally, consider the fact that some clients with a systemic or viscerogenic origin of NMS symptoms get better with physical therapy intervention. Perhaps there is a placebo effect. Perhaps there is a physiologic effect of movement on the diseased state. The therapist's intervention may exert an influence on the neuroendocrine-immune axis as the body tries to regain homeostasis. You may have experienced this phenomenon yourself when coming down with a cold or symptoms of a virus. You felt much better and even symptom-free after exercising.

Movement, physical activity, and moderate exercise aid the body and boost the immune system,[6-8] but sometimes such measures are unable to prevail, especially if other factors are present such as inadequate hydration, poor nutrition, fatigue, depression, immunosuppression, and stress. In such cases the condition will progress to the point that warning signs and symptoms will be observed or reported and/or the patient/client's condition will deteriorate. The need for medical

BOX 1-1 ▼ Reasons for Medical Screening

- Direct access: Therapist has primary responsibility or first contact.
- Quicker and sicker patient/client base.
- Signed prescription: Clients may obtain a signed prescription for physical/occupational therapy based on similar past complaints of musculoskeletal symptoms without direct physician contact.
- Medical specialization: Medical specialists may fail to recognize underlying systemic disease.
- Disease progression: Early signs and symptoms are difficult to recognize, or symptoms may not be present at the time of medical examination.
- Patient/client disclosure: Client discloses information previously unknown or undisclosed to the physician.
- Client does not report symptoms or concerns to the physician because of forgetfulness, fear, or embarrassment.
- Presence of one or more yellow (caution) or red (warning) flags.

referral or consultation will become much more evident.

▶ REASONS TO SCREEN

There are many reasons why the therapist may need to screen for medical disease. Direct access (see definition and discussion later in this chapter) is only one of those reasons (Box 1-1).

Early detection and referral is the key to prevention of further significant comorbidities or complications. In all practice settings, therapists must know how to recognize systemic disease masquerading as NMS dysfunction. This includes practice by physician referral, independent practice via the direct access model, or as a primary practitioner.

The practice of physical therapy has changed many times since it was first started with the Reconstruction Aides. Clinical practice, as it was shaped by World War I and then World War II, was eclipsed by the polio epidemic in the 1940s and 1950s. With the widespread use of the live, oral polio vaccine in 1963, polio was eradicated in the United States and clinical practice changed again (Fig. 1-1).

Today, most clients seen by therapists have impairments and disabilities that are clearly NMS-related (Fig. 1-2). Most of the time, the client

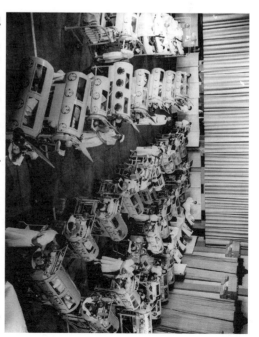

Fig. 1-1 • Patients in iron lungs receive treatment at Rancho Los Amigos during the polio epidemic of the 1940s and 1950s. (Courtesy of Rancho Los Amigos, 2005.)

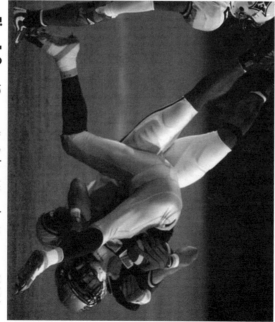

Fig. 1-2 • (Courtesy Jim Baker, Missoula, Montana, 2005.)

history and mechanism of injury point to a known cause of movement dysfunction.

However, therapists practicing in all settings must be able to evaluate a patient/client's complaint knowledgeably and determine whether there are signs and symptoms of a systemic disease or a medical condition that should be evaluated by a more appropriate health care provider. This text endeavors to provide the necessary information that will assist the therapist in making these decisions.

Quicker and Sicker

The aging of America has impacted general health in significant ways. "Quicker and sicker" is a term used to describe patient/clients in the current health care arena (Fig. 1-3).[9] "Quicker" refers to how health care delivery has changed in the last 10 years to combat the rising costs of health care. Hospital inpatient/clients are discharged much faster today than they were even 10 years ago. Outpatient/client surgery is much more common, with same-day discharge for procedures that would have required a 7- to 10-day hospitalization in the recent past. Patient/clients on the medical-surgical wards of most hospitals today would have been in the intensive care unit (ICU) 20 years ago.

Today's health care environment is complex and highly demanding. The therapist must be alert to red flags of systemic disease at all times but especially in those clients who have been given early release from the hospital or transition unit. Warning flags may come in the form of reported symptoms or observed signs. It may be a clinical presentation that does not match the recent history.

"Sicker" refers to the fact that patient/clients in acute care, rehabilitation, or outpatient/client setting with any orthopedic or neurologic problems may have a past medical history of cancer or a current personal history of diabetes, liver disease, thyroid condition, peptic ulcer, and/or other conditions or diseases.

The number of people with at least one chronic disease or disability is reaching epidemic proportions. According to the National Institute on Aging,[10] 79% of adults over 70 have at least one of seven potentially disabling chronic conditions (arthritis, hypertension, heart disease, diabetes, respiratory diseases, stroke, and cancer).[11] The presence of multiple comorbidities emphasizes the need to view the whole patient/client and not just the body part in question.

Signed Prescription

Under direct access, the physical therapist may have primary responsibility or become the first contact for some clients in the health care delivery system. On the other hand, clients may obtain a signed prescription for physical therapy from their primary care physician or other health care provider, based on similar past complaints of musculoskeletal symptoms, without actually seeing the physician or being examined by the physician (Case Example 1-1).

Follow-Up Questions

Always ask a client who provides a signed prescription:

- Did you actually see the physician (chiropractor, dentist, nurse practitioner, physician assistant)?
- Did the doctor (dentist) examine you?

Medical Specialization

Additionally, with the increasing specialization of medicine, clients may be evaluated by a medical specialist who does not immediately recognize the underlying systemic disease, or the specialist may assume that the referring primary care physician has ruled out other causes (Case Example 1-2).

Progression of Time and Disease

In some cases, early signs and symptoms of systemic disease may be difficult or impossible to recognize until the disease has progressed enough to create distressing or noticeable symptoms (Case Example 1-3). In some cases, the patient/client's clinical presentation in the physician's office may

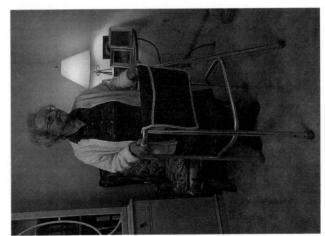

Fig. 1-3 • The aging of America from the "traditionalists" (born before 1946) and the Baby Boom generation ("boomer" born 1946-1964) will result in older adults with multiple comorbidities in the care of the physical therapist. Even with a known orthopedic and/or neurologic impairment, these clients will require a careful screening for the possibility of other problems, side effects from medications, and primary/secondary prevention programs. (From Sorrentino SA: *Mosby's Textbook for Nursing Assistants,* ed 5, St. Louis, 2004, Mosby.)

CASE EXAMPLE 1-1   Physician Visit without Examination

A 60-year-old man retired from his job as the president of a large vocational technical school and called his physician the next day for a long-put-off referral to physical therapy. He arrived at an outpatient orthopedic physical therapy clinic with a signed physician's prescription that said, "Evaluate and Treat."

His primary complaint was left anterior hip and groin pain. This client had a history of three previous total hip replacements (anterior approach, lateral approach, posterior approach) on the right side, performed over the last 10 years.

Based on previous rehabilitation experience, he felt certain that his current symptoms of hip and groin pain could be alleviated by physical therapy.

- Social History: Recently retired as the director of a large vocational rehabilitation agency, married, three grown children

- Past Medical History (PMHx): Three total hip replacements (THRs) to the left hip (anterior, posterior, and lateral approaches) over the last 7 years

  - Open heart surgery 10 years ago
  - Congestive heart failure (CHF) 3 years ago
  - Medications: Lotensin daily, 1 baby aspirin per day, Zocor (20 mg) once a day

- Clinical presentation:

  - Extensive scar tissue around the left hip area with centralized core of round, hard tissue (4 by 6 cm) over the greater trochanter on the left

  - Bilateral pitting edema of the feet and ankles (right greater than left)

  - Positive Thomas (30-degree hip flexion contracture) test for left hip

  - Neurologic screen: Negative but general deconditioning and global decline observed in lower extremity strength

  - Vital signs*:

    Blood pressure (sitting, right arm) 92/58 mm Hg
    Heart rate 86 bpm
    Respirations 22/min
    Pulse oximeter 89%
    Body temperature 97.8° F

The client arrived at the physical therapy clinic with a signed prescription in hand, but when asked if he had actually seen the physician, he explained that he received this prescription after a telephone conversation with his physician.

How Do You Communicate Your Findings and Concerns to the Physician?

It is always a good idea to call and ask for a copy of the physician's dictation or notes. It may be that the doctor is well aware of the client's clinical presentation. Health Insurance Portability and Accountability Act (HIPAA) regulations require the client to sign a disclosure statement before the therapist can gain access to the medical records. To facilitate this process, it is best to have the paperwork requirements completed on the first appointment before the therapist sees the client.

Sometimes a conversation with the physician's office staff is all that is needed. They may be able to look at the client's chart and advise you accordingly. At the same time, in our litigious culture, outlining your concerns or questions almost always obligates the medical office to make a follow-up appointment with the client.

It may be best to provide the client with your written report that he or she can hand carry to the physician's office. Sending a fax, email, or mailed written report may place the information in the chart, but not in the physician's hands at the appropriate time. It is always advised to do both (fax or mail along with a hand-carried copy).

Make your documentation complete, but your communication brief. Thank the physician for the referral. Outline the problem areas (physical therapy diagnosis, impairment classification, and planned intervention). Be brief! The physician is only going to have time to scan what you sent.

Any associated signs and symptoms or red flags can be pointed out as follows:

During my examination, I noted the following:
Bilateral pitting edema of lower extremities
Vital signs:

---

* The blood pressure and pulse measurements are difficult to evaluate given the fact that this client is taking antihypertensive medications. Ace inhibitors and beta-blockers, for example, reduce the heart rate so that the body's normal compensatory mechanisms (e.g., increased stroke volume and therefore increased heart rate) are unable to function in response to the onset of congestive heart failure. Low blood pressure and high pulse rate with higher respiratory rate and mildly diminished oxygen saturation (especially on exertion) must be considered red flags. Auscultation would be in order here. Light crackles in the lung bases might be heard in this case.

CASE EXAMPLE 1-1   Physician Visit without Examination—cont'd

Blood pressure (sitting, right arm) 92/58 mm Hg
Heart rate 86 bpm
Respirations 22/min
Pulse oximeter 89%
Body temperature 97.8° F

Some of these findings seem outside the expected range. Please advise.

Note to the Reader: If possible, highlight this last statement in order to draw the physician's eye to your primary concern.

It is outside the scope of our practice to suggest possible reasons for the client's symptoms (e.g., congestive failure, side effect of medication). Just make note of the findings and let the physician make the medical diagnosis. An open-ended comment such as "Please advise" or question such as "What do you think?" may be all that is required.

Of course, in any collaborative relationship you may find that some physicians ask for your opinion. It is quite permissible to offer the evidence and draw some possible conclusions.

Result: An appropriate physical therapy program of soft tissue mobilization, stretching, and home exercise was initiated. However, the client was returned to his physician for an immediate follow-up appointment. A brief report from the therapist stated the key objective findings and outlined the proposed physical therapy plan. The letter included a short paragraph with the following remarks:

Given the client's sedentary lifestyle, previous history of heart disease, and blood pressure reading today, I would like to recommend a physical conditioning program. Would you please let me know if he is medically stable? Based on your findings, we will begin him in a preaerobic training program here and progress him to a home-based or fitness center program.

CASE EXAMPLE 1-2   Medical Specialization

A 45-year-old long-haul truck driver with bilateral carpal tunnel syndrome was referred for physical therapy by an orthopedic surgeon specializing in hand injuries. During the course of treatment the client mentioned that he was also seeing an acupuncturist for wrist and hand pain. The acupuncturist told the client that, based on his assessment, acupuncture treatment was indicated for liver disease.

Comment: Protein (from food sources or from a gastrointestinal bleed) is normally taken up and detoxified by the liver. Ammonia is produced as a by-product of protein breakdown and then transformed by the liver to urea, glutamine, and asparagine before being excreted by the renal system. When liver dysfunction results in increased serum ammonia and urea levels, peripheral nerve function can be impaired. (See detailed explanation on neurologic symptoms in Chapter 9.)

Result: The therapist continued to treat this client, but knowing that the referring specialist did not routinely screen for systemic causes of carpal tunnel syndrome (or even screen for cervical involvement) combined with the acupuncturist's information, raised a red flag for possible systemic origin of symptoms. A phone call was made to the physician with the following approach:

Say, Mr. Y was in for therapy today. He happened to mention that he is seeing an acupuncturist who told him that his wrist and hand pain is from a liver problem. I recalled seeing some information here at the office about the effect of liver disease on the peripheral nervous system. Since Mr. Y has not improved with our carpal tunnel protocol, would you like to have him come back in for a reevaluation?

Comment: How to respond to each situation will require a certain amount of diplomacy, with consideration given to the individual therapist's relationship with the physician and the physician's openness to direct communication.

It is the physical therapist's responsibility to recognize when a client's presentation falls outside the parameters of a true neuromusculoskeletal condition. Unless prompted by the physician, it is not the therapist's role to suggest a specific medical diagnosis or medical testing procedures.

CASE EXAMPLE 1-3 ▪ Progression of Disease

A 44-year-old woman was referred to the physical therapist with a complaint of right paraspinal/low thoracic back pain. There was no reported history of trauma or assault and no history of repetitive movement. The past medical history was significant for a kidney infection treated 3 weeks ago with antibiotics. The client stated that her follow-up urinalysis was "clear" and the infection resolved.

The physical therapy examination revealed true paraspinal muscle spasm with an acute presentation of limited movement and exquisite pain in the posterior right middle to low back. Spinal accessory motions were tested following application of a cold modality and were found to be mildly restricted in right sidebending and left rotation of the T8-T12 segments. It was the therapist's assessment that this joint motion deficit was still the result of muscle spasm and guarding and not true joint involvement.

Result: After three sessions with the physical therapist in which modalities were used for the acute symptoms, the client was not making observable, reportable, or measurable improvement. Her fourth scheduled appointment was cancelled because of the "flu."

Given the recent history of kidney infection, the lack of expected improvement, and the onset of constitutional symptoms (see Box 1-3), the therapist contacted the client by telephone and suggested that she make a follow-up appointment with her doctor as soon as possible.

As it turned out, this woman's kidney infection had recurred. She recovered from her back sequelae within 24 hours of initiating a second antibiotic treatment. This is not the typical medical picture for a urologically compromised person. Sometimes it is not until the disease progresses that the systemic disorder (masquerading as a musculoskeletal problem) can be clearly differentiated.

Last, sometimes clients do not relay all the necessary or pertinent medical information to their physicians but will confide in the physical therapist. They may feel intimidated, forget, become unwilling or embarrassed, or fail to recognize the significance of the symptoms and neglect to mention important medical details (see Box 1-1).

Knowing that systemic diseases can mimic neuromusculoskeletal dysfunction, the therapist is responsible for identifying as closely as possible what neuromusculoskeletal pathologic condition is present.

The final result should be to treat as specifically as possible. This is done by closely identifying the underlying neuromusculoskeletal pathological condition and the accompanying movement dysfunction, while at the same time investigating the possibility of systemic disease.

This text will help the clinician quickly recognize problems that are beyond the expertise of the physical therapist. The therapist who recognizes hallmark signs and symptoms of systemic disease will know when to refer clients to the appropriate health care practitioner.

Knowing what medical conditions can cause shoulder, back, thorax, pelvic, hip, sacroiliac, and groin pain is essential. Familiarity with risk factors for various diseases, illnesses, and conditions is an important tool for early recognition in the screening process.

Given enough time, a disease process will eventually progress and get worse. Symptoms may become more readily apparent or more easily clustered. In such cases the alert therapist may be the first to ask the patient/client pertinent questions to determine the presence of underlying symptoms requiring medical referral.

The therapist must know what questions to ask clients in order to identify the need for medical referral.

The patient/client history and interview are very different from what the therapist observes when days or weeks separate the two appointments. Holidays, vacations, finances, scheduling conflicts, and so on can put delays between medical examination and diagnosis and that first appointment with the therapist.

Patient/Client Disclosure

Finally, sometimes patient/clients tell the therapist things about their current health and social history unknown or unreported to the physician. The content of these conversations can hold important screening clues to point out a systemic illness or viscerogenic cause of musculoskeletal or neuromuscular impairment.

Yellow or Red Flags

A large part of the screening process is identifying yellow (cautionary) or red (warning) flag histories and signs and symptoms (Box 1-2). A yellow flag is a cautionary or warning symptom that signals "slow down" and think about the need for screening. A red-flag symptom requires immediate attention, either to pursue further screening questions and/or tests, or to make an appropriate referral.

The presence of a single yellow or red flag is not usually cause for immediate medical attention. Each cautionary or warning flag must be viewed in the context of the whole person given the age, gender, past medical history, known risk factors, medication use, and current clinical presentation of that patient/client.

It is time to take a closer look when risk factors for specific diseases are present, when a cluster of three or more red flags are present, or both risk factors and red flags are present at the same time. Clusters of yellow and/or red flags do not always warrant medical referral. Each case is evaluated on its own.

The patient/client's history, presenting pain pattern, and possible associated signs and symptoms must be reviewed along with results from the objective evaluation in making a treatment-versus-referral decision.

Medical conditions can cause pain, dysfunction, and impairment of the

- Back/neck
- Shoulder
- Chest/breast/rib
- Hip/groin
- Sacroiliac (SI)/sacrum/pelvis

For the most part, the organs are located in the central portion of the body and refer symptoms to the nearby major muscles and joints. In general, the back and shoulder represent the primary areas of referred viscerogenic pain patterns. Cases of isolated symptoms will be presented in this text as they occur in clinical practice. Symptoms of any kind that present bilaterally always raise a red flag for concern and further investigation (Case Example 1-4).

Monitoring vital signs is a quick and easy way to screen for medical conditions. Vital signs are discussed more completely in Chapter 4. Asking about the presence of constitutional symptoms is important, especially when there is no known cause. Constitutional symptoms refer to a constellation of signs and symptoms present whenever the patient/client is experiencing a systemic illness. No matter what system is involved, these core signs and symptoms are often present (Box 1-3).

BOX 1-2 ▼ Red Flags

The presence of any one of these symptoms is not usually cause for extreme concern, but should raise a red flag for the alert therapist. The therapist is looking for a pattern that suggests a viscerogenic or systemic origin of pain and/or symptoms. The therapist will proceed with the screening process depending on which symptoms are grouped together. Often the next step is to conduct a risk-factor assessment and look for associated signs and symptoms.

Past Medical History (Personal or Family)

- Personal or family history of cancer
- Recent (last 6 weeks) infection (e.g., mononucleosis, upper respiratory infection (URI), urinary tract infection (UTI), bacterial such as streptococcal or staphylococcal; viral such as measles, hepatitis), especially when followed by neurologic symptoms 1 to 3 weeks later (Guillain-Barré syndrome), joint pain, or back pain
- Recurrent colds or flu with a cyclical pattern; i.e., the client reports that he or she just cannot shake this cold or the flu; it keeps coming back over and over
- Recent history of trauma such as motor vehicle accident or fall (fracture; any age) or minor trauma in older adult with osteopenia/osteoporosis
- History of immunosuppression (e.g., steroids, organ transplant, HIV)
- History of injection drug use (infection)

Risk Factors

Risk factors vary depending on family history, previous personal history, and disease, illness, or condition present. For example, risk factors for heart disease will be different from risk factors for osteoporosis or vestibular or balance problems. As with all decision-making variables, a single risk factor may or may not be significant and must be viewed in context of the whole patient/client presentation. This represents only a partial list of all the possible health risk factors.

BOX 1-2 ▼ Red Flags—cont'd

Substance use/abuse
Tobacco use
Age
Gender
Body Mass Index (BMI)
Exposure to radiation
Alcohol use/abuse
Sedentary lifestyle
Race/ethnicity
Domestic violence
Hysterectomy/oophorectomy
Occupation

Clinical Presentation

No known cause, unknown etiology, insidious onset

Symptoms that are unrelieved by physical therapy intervention is a red flag.

Physical therapy intervention does not change the clinical picture; client may get worse!

Symptoms that get better after physical therapy, but then get worse again is also a red flag identifying the need to screen further

Significant weight loss or gain without effort (more than 10% of the client's body weight in 10 to 21 days)

Gradual, progressive, or cyclical presentation of symptoms (worse/better/worse)

Unrelieved by rest or change in position; no position is comfortable

If relieved by rest, positional change, or application of heat, in time, these relieving factors no longer reduce symptoms

Symptoms seem out of proportion to the injury

Symptoms persist beyond the expected time for that condition

Unable to alter (provoke, reproduce, alleviate, eliminate, aggravate) the symptoms during exam

Does not fit the expected mechanical or neuromusculoskeletal pattern

No discernible pattern of symptoms

A growing mass (painless or painful) is a tumor until proved otherwise; a hematoma should decrease (not increase) in size with time

Postmenopausal vaginal bleeding (bleeding that occurs a year or more after the last period [significance depends on whether the woman is on hormone replacement therapy and which regimen is used])

Bilateral symptoms:

Edema
Numbness, tingling
Skin-pigmentation changes
Clubbing
Nail-bed changes
Skin rash

Change in muscle tone or range of motion (ROM) for individuals with neurologic conditions (e.g., cerebral palsy, spinal-cord injured, traumatic-brain injured, multiple sclerosis)

Pain Pattern

Back or shoulder pain (most common location of referred pain; other areas can be affected as well, but these two areas signal a particular need to take a second look)

Pain accompanied by full and painless range of motion (see Table 3-1)

Pain that is not consistent with emotional or psychologic overlay (e.g., Waddell's test is negative or insignificant; ways to measure this are discussed in Chapter 3); screening tests for emotional overlay are negative

Night pain (constant and intense; see complete description in Chapter 3)

Symptoms (especially pain) are constant and intense (Remember to ask anyone with "constant" pain: Are you having this pain right now?)

Pain made worse by activity and relieved by rest (e.g., intermittent claudication; cardiac: upper quadrant pain with the use of the lower extremities while upper extremities are inactive)

Pain described as throbbing (vascular) knifelike, boring, or deep aching

Pain that is poorly localized

Pattern of coming and going like spasms, colicky

Pain accompanied by signs and symptoms associated with a specific viscera or system (e.g., GI, GU, GYN, cardiac, pulmonary, endocrine)

Change in musculoskeletal symptoms with food intake or medication use (immediately or up to several hours later)

Associated Signs and Symptoms

Recent report of confusion (or increased confusion); this could be a neurologic sign; it could be drug-induced (e.g., NSAIDs) or a sign of infection; usually it is a family member who takes the therapist aside to report this concern

Presence of constitutional symptoms (see Box 1-3) or unusual vital signs (see Discussion, Chapter 4); body temperature of 100° F (37.8° C) usually indicates a serious illness

Proximal muscle weakness, especially if accompanied by change in DTRs (see Fig. 13-3)

Joint pain with skin rashes, nodules (see discussion of systemic causes of joint pain, Chapter 3; see Table 3-6)

Any cluster of signs and symptoms observed during the Review of Systems that are characteristic of a particular organ system (see Box 4-17; Table 13-5)

Unusual menstrual cycle/symptoms; association between menses and symptoms

It is imperative at the end of each interview that the therapist ask the client a question like the following:

• Are there any other symptoms or problems anywhere else in your body that may not seem related to your current problem?

CASE EXAMPLE 1-4 Bilateral Hand Pain

A 69-year-old man presented with pain in both hands that was worse on the left. He described the pain as "deep aching" and reported it interfered with his ability to write. The pain got worse as the day went on.

There was no report of fever, chills, previous infection, new medications, or cancer. The client was unaware that joint pain could be caused by sexually transmitted infections, but said that he was widowed after 50 years of marriage to the same woman and did not think this was a problem.

There was no history of occupational or accidental trauma. The client viewed himself as being in "excellent health." He was not taking any medications or herbal supplements.

Wrist range of motion was limited by stiffness at end ranges in flexion and extension. There was no obvious soft tissue swelling, warmth, or tenderness over or around the joint. A neurologic screening examination was negative for sensory, motor, or reflex changes.

There were no other significant findings from various tests and measures performed. There were no reported signs and symptoms of any kind anywhere else in the muscles, limbs, or general body.

What Are the Red-Flag Signs and Symptoms Here? Should a Medical Referral Be Made? Why or Why Not?

Red Flags

Age

Bilateral symptoms

Lack of other definitive findings

It is difficult to treat as specifically as possible without a clear differential diagnosis. You can treat the symptoms and assess the results before making a medical referral. Improvement in symptoms and motion should be seen within one to three sessions.

However, in light of the red flags, best practice suggests a medical referral to rule out a sys-

temic disorder before initiating treatment. This could be rheumatoid arthritis, osteoarthritis, osteoporosis, the result of a thyroid dysfunction, gout, or other arthritic condition.

How Do You Make this Suggestion to the Client, Especially if He Was Coming to You to Avoid a Doctor's Visit/Fee?

Perhaps something like this would be appropriate:

Mr. J,

You have very few symptoms to base treatment on. When pain or other symptoms are present on both sides, it can be a sign that something more systemic is going on. For anyone over 40 with bilateral symptoms and a lack of other findings, we recommend a medical exam.

Do you have a regular family doctor or primary care physician? It may be helpful to have some X-rays and lab work done before we begin treatment here. Who can I call or send my report to?

Result: X-rays showed significant joint space loss in the radiocarpal joint, as well as sclerosis and cystic changes in the carpal bones. Calcium deposits in the wrist fibrocartilage pointed to a diagnosis of calcium pyrophosphate dihydrate (CPPD) crystal deposition disease (pseudogout).

There was no osteoporosis and no bone erosion present.

Treatment was with oral nonsteroidal antiinflammatory drugs for symptomatic pain relief. There is no evidence that physical therapy intervention can change the course of this disease or even effectively treat the symptoms.

The client opted to return to physical therapy for short-term palliative care during the acute phase.

To read more about this condition, consult the *Primer on the Rheumatic Diseases*, 12th edition. Arthritis Foundation (www.arthritis.org), Atlanta, 2001.

Data from: Raman S, Resnick D: Chronic and increasing bilateral hand pain, *The Journal of Musculoskeletal Medicine* 13(6):58-61, 1996.

BOX 1-3 ▼ Constitutional Symptoms

Fever
Diaphoresis (unexplained perspiration)
Night sweats (can occur during the day)
Nausea
Vomiting
Diarrhea
Pallor
Dizziness/syncope (fainting)
Fatigue
Weight loss

BOX 1-4 ▼ Physical Therapist Role in Disease Prevention

Primary Prevention: Stopping the process(es) that lead to the development of disease(s), illness(es), and other pathologic health conditions through education, risk-factor reduction, and general health promotion.

Secondary Prevention: Early detection of disease(s), illness(es), and other pathologic health conditions through regular screening; this does not prevent the condition but may decrease duration and/or severity of disease and thereby improve the outcome, including improved quality of life.

Tertiary Prevention: Providing ways to limit the degree of disability while improving function in patients/clients with chronic and/or irreversible diseases.

Health Promotion and Wellness: Providing education and support to help patients/clients make choices that will promote health or improved health. The goal of wellness is to give people greater awareness and control in making choices about their own health.

Secondary Prevention involves the regular screening for early detection of disease or other health-threatening conditions such as hypertension, osteoporosis, incontinence, diabetes, or cancer. This does not prevent any of these problems, but improves the outcome. The *Guide* outlines the physical therapist's role in secondary prevention as "decreasing duration of illness, severity of disease, and number of sequelae through early diagnosis and prompt intervention" [p. 33].

Another way to look at this is through the use of screening and surveillance. *Screening* is a method for detecting disease or body dysfunction before an individual would normally seek medical care. Medical screening tests are usually administered to individuals who do not have current symptoms, but who may be at high risk for certain adverse health outcomes.

Surveillance is the analysis of health information to look for problems occurring in the general population, in specific groups, or in the workplace that require targeted prevention. Surveillance often uses screening results from groups of individuals to look for abnormal trends in health status.

▲ SCREENING AND SURVEILLANCE

Therapists can have an active role in both primary and secondary prevention through screening and education. Primary Prevention involves stopping the process(es) that lead to the formation of cancer in the first place (Box 1-4).

According to the *Guide*,[1] physical therapists are involved in primary prevention by "preventing a target condition in a susceptible or potentially susceptible population through such specific measures as general health promotion through risk-factor assessment and risk reduction efforts" [p. 33]. Risk-factor assessment and risk reduction fall under this category.

▲ DIAGNOSIS BY THE PHYSICAL THERAPIST

It is the policy of the American Physical Therapy Association (APTA) that physical therapists shall establish a diagnosis for each patient/client. Prior to making a patient/client management decision, physical therapists shall utilize the diagnostic process in order to establish a diagnosis for the specific conditions in need of the physical therapist's attention.[12]

The diagnostic process requires evaluation of information obtained from the patient/client examination, including the history, systems review, administration of tests, and interpretation of data. Physical therapists use diagnostic labels that identify the impact of a condition on function at the level of the system (especially the movement system) and the level of the whole person.[13]

The physical therapist is qualified to make a diagnosis regarding primary NMS conditions though we must do so in accordance with the state practice act. The profession must continue to develop the concept of movement as a physiologic system and work to get physical therapists recognized as experts in that system.[14]

The concepts around the "diagnostic process" remain part of an evolving definition that will

continue to be discussed and clarified by physical therapists. There has been some discussion that evaluation is a process with diagnosis as the end result.[15] According to the *Guide*, the diagnostic-based practice requires the physical therapist to integrate five elements of patient/client management (Box 1-5) in a manner designed to maximize outcomes (Fig. 1-4).

One of those proposed modifications is in the Elements of Patient/Client Management proposed by the APTA in the *Guide*. Fig. 1-4 does not illustrate all decisions possible.

Boissonnault proposed a fork in the clinical decision-making pathway to show three alternative decisions including

1. Referral/consultation,
2. Diagnose and treat, or
3. Both (Fig. 1-5).[16]

The decision to refer or consult with the physician can also apply to referral to other appropriate health care professionals and/or practitioners (e.g., dentist, chiropractor, nurse practitioner, psychologist).

Definition of Physical Therapy Diagnosis

Diagnosis by the physical therapist is a concept based on the Disablement Model. Whereas the physician makes a medical diagnosis based on the pathologic or pathophysiologic state at the cellular level, diagnosis by the physical therapist is a label

---

BOX 1-5 ▼ Elements of Patient/Client Management

Examination: History, systems review, and tests and measures
Evaluation: Assessment or judgment of the data
Diagnosis: Determined within the scope of practice
Prognosis: Projected outcome
Intervention: Coordination, communication, and documentation of an appropriate treatment plan for the diagnosis based on the previous four elements

Data from *Guide to Physical Therapist Practice*, ed 2 (Revised), Alexandria, Va, 2003, American Physical Therapy Association (APTA).

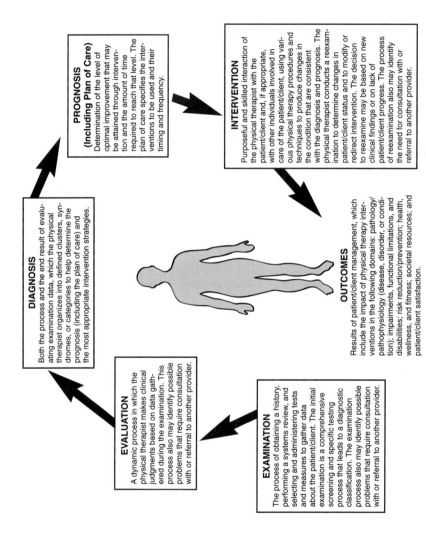

DIAGNOSIS
Both the process and the end result of evaluating examination data, which the physical therapist organizes into defined clusters, syndromes, or categories to help determine the prognosis (including the plan of care) and the most appropriate intervention strategies.

PROGNOSIS (Including Plan of Care)
Determination of the level of optimal improvement that may be attained through intervention and the amount of time required to reach that level. The plan of care specifies the interventions to be used and their timing and frequency.

INTERVENTION
Purposeful and skilled interaction of the physical therapist with the patient/client and, if appropriate, with other individuals involved in care of the patient/client, using various physical therapy procedures and techniques to produce changes in the condition that are consistent with the diagnosis and prognosis. The physical therapist conducts a reexamination to determine changes in patient/client status and to modify or redirect intervention. The decision to reexamine may be based on new clinical findings or on lack of patient/client progress. The process of reexamination also may identify the need for consultation with or referral to another provider.

OUTCOMES
Results of patient/client management, which include the impact of physical therapy interventions in the following domains: pathology/pathophysiology (disease, disorder, or condition); impairments, functional limitations, and disabilities; risk reduction/prevention; health, wellness, and fitness; societal resources; and patient/client satisfaction.

EVALUATION
A dynamic process in which the physical therapist makes clinical judgments based on data gathered during the examination. This process also may identify possible problems that require consultation with or referral to another provider.

EXAMINATION
The process of obtaining a history, performing a systems review, and selecting and administering tests and measures to gather data about the patient/client. The initial examination is a comprehensive screening and specific testing process that leads to a diagnostic classification. The examination process also may identify possible problems that require consultation with or referral to another provider.

Fig. 1-4 ● The elements of patient/client management leading to optimal outcomes. Screening takes place anywhere along this pathway. (Reprinted with permission from *Guide to Physical Therapist Practice*, ed 2 [Revised], 2003, Fig. 1-4, p. 35.)

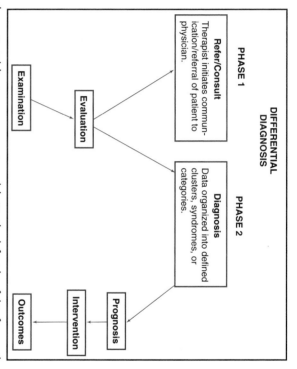

Fig. 1-5 • Modification to the patient/client management model. On the left side of this figure, the therapist starts by collecting data during the examination. Based on the data collected, the evaluation leads to clinical judgments. The current model in the *Guide* gives only one decision-making option, and that is the diagnosis. In this adapted model a fork in the decision-making pathway allows the therapist the opportunity to make one of three alternative decisions as described in the text. This model is more in keeping with recommended clinical practice. (From Boissonnault WG, Umphred DA: Differential diagnosis phase I. In Umphred DA, editors: *Neurological Rehabilitation*, ed 4. St. Louis, 2001, Mosby.)

encompassing a cluster of signs and symptoms commonly associated with a disorder or syndrome or category of impairment, functional limitation, or disability.

It is the decision reached as a result of the diagnostic process, which is the evaluation of information obtained from the patient/client examination.[12] Diagnosis is both the process and the end result of evaluating examination data, which the therapist organizes into defined clusters, syndromes, or categories to help determine the prognosis and the most appropriate intervention strategies.[1]

APTA Vision Sentence for Physical Therapy 2020

By 2020, physical therapy will be provided by physical therapists who are doctors of physical therapy, recognized by consumers and other health care professionals as the practitioners of choice to whom consumers have direct access for the diagnosis of, interventions for, and prevention of impairments, functional limitations, and disabilities related to movement, function, and health.[17]

The vision sentence points out that physical therapists are capable of making a diagnosis and making the determination whether the patient/client can be helped by physical therapy intervention. In an autonomous profession the therapist can decide if physical therapy should be a part of the plan, the entire plan, or not needed at all.

When communicating with physicians, it is helpful to understand the definition of a medical diagnosis and how it differs from a physical therapy diagnosis. The medical diagnosis is traditionally defined as the recognition of disease.

It is the determination of the cause and nature of pathologic conditions. Medical differential diagnosis is the comparison of symptoms of similar diseases and medical diagnostics (laboratory and test procedures performed) so that a correct assessment of the patient/client's actual problem can be made.

A differential diagnosis by the physical therapist is the comparison of neuromusculoskeletal (NMS) signs and symptoms to identify the underlying movement dysfunction so that treatment can be planned as specifically as possible.

One of the APTA goals is that physical therapists will be universally recognized and promoted as the practitioners of choice for persons with conditions that affect movement, function, health, and wellness.[18]

Purpose of the Diagnosis

In simple terms, the purpose of the diagnosis is to:

- Treat as specifically as possible by determining the most appropriate intervention strategy for each patient/client
- Recognize the need for a medical referral

More broadly stated, the purpose of the diagnosis is to guide the physical therapist in determining the most appropriate intervention strategy for each patient/client with a goal of decreasing disability and increasing function. In the event the diagnostic process does not yield an identifiable cluster, disorder, syndrome, or category, intervention may be directed toward the alleviation of symptoms and remediation of impairment, functional limitation, or disability.[12]

Sometimes the patient/client is too acute to examine fully on the first visit. At other times we evaluate problems medically diagnosed as "shoulder pain" or "back pain." When the patient/client is referred with a previously established diagnosis, the physical therapist determines that the clinical findings are consistent with that diagnosis[12] (Case Example 1-5).

Sometimes the screening and diagnostic process identifies a systemic problem as the underlying cause of NMS symptoms. At other times it confirms that the patient/client has a NMS problem after all (Case Example 1-5[19]; see also Case Example 1-7).

Historical Perspective

The idea of physical therapy diagnosis is not a new one. In fact, from its earliest beginnings until now, it has officially been around for at least 20 years. It was first described in the literature by Shirley Sahrmann[20] as the name given to a collection of relevant signs and symptoms associated with the primary dysfunction toward which the physical therapist directs treatment. The dysfunction is identified by the physical therapist based on the information obtained from the history, signs, symptoms, examination, and tests the therapist performs or requests.

CASE EXAMPLE 1-5   Verify Medical Diagnosis

A 31-year-old man was referred to physical therapy by an orthopedic physician. The diagnosis was "shoulder-hand syndrome." This client had been evaluated for this same problem by three other physicians and two physical therapists before arriving at our clinic. Treatment to date had been unsuccessful in alleviating symptoms.

The medical diagnosis itself provided some useful information about the referring physician. "Shoulder-hand syndrome" is an outdated nomenclature previously used to describe reflex sympathetic dystrophy syndrome (RSDS or RSD), now known more accurately as complex regional pain syndrome (CRPS).[19]

Shoulder-hand syndrome was a condition that occurred following a myocardial infarct, or MI (heart attack), usually after prolonged bedrest. This condition has been significantly reduced in incidence by more up-to-date and aggressive cardiac rehabilitation programs. Today CRPS, primarily affecting the limbs, develops after injury or surgery, but it can still occur as a result of a cerebrovascular accident (CVA) or heart attack.

This client's clinical presentation included none of the typical signs and symptoms expected with CRPS, such as skin changes (smooth, shiny, red skin), hair growth pattern (increased dark hair patches or loss of hair), temperature changes (increased or decreased), hyperhidrosis (excessive perspiration), restricted joint motion, and severe pain. The clinical picture appeared consistent with a trigger point of the latissimus dorsi muscle, and, in fact, treatment of the trigger point completely eliminated all symptoms.

Conducting a thorough physical therapy examination to identify the specific underlying cause of symptomatic presentation was essential to the treatment of this case. Treatment approaches for a trigger point differ greatly from intervention protocols for CRPS.

Accepting the medical diagnosis without performing a physical therapy diagnostic evaluation would have resulted in wasted time and unnecessary charges for this client.

The International Association for the Study of Pain replaced the term *RSDS* with *CPRS I* in 1995.[19] Other names given to RSD included neurovascular dystrophy, sympathetic neurovascular dystrophy, algodystrophy, "red-hand disease," Sudeck's atrophy, and causalgia.

In 1984, the APTA House of Delegates (HOD) made a motion that *The physical therapist may establish a diagnosis within the scope of their knowledge, experience, and expertise.* This was further qualified in 1990 when the Education Standards for Accreditation described "Diagnosis" for the first time.

In 1990, teaching and learning content and the skills necessary to determine a diagnosis became a required part of the curriculum standards established then by the Standards for Accreditation for Physical Therapist Educational Program. At that time the therapist's role in developing a diagnosis was described as:

- 3.8.3.18 Engage in the diagnostic process in an efficient manner consistent with the policies and procedures of the practice setting.

- 3.8.3.19 Engage in the diagnostic process to establish differential diagnoses for patient/clients across the lifespan based on evaluation of results of examinations and medical and psychosocial information.

- 3.8.3.20 Take responsibility for communication or discussion of diagnoses or clinical impressions with other practitioners.

In 1995, the HOD amended the 1984 policy to make the definition of *diagnosis* consistent with the (then) upcoming *Guide to Physical Therapist Practice.* The first edition of the *Guide* was published in 1997. It was revised and published as a second edition in 2001; the second edition was revised in 2003.

Classification System

According to Rothstein,[21] in many fields of medicine when a medical diagnosis is made, the pathologic condition is determined and stages and classifications that guide treatment are also named. Although we recognize that the term *diagnosis* relates to a pathologic process, we know that pathologic evidence alone is inadequate to guide the physical therapist.

Physical therapists do not diagnose disease in the sense of identifying a specific organic pathologic condition. However, identified clusters of signs, symptoms, symptom-related behavior, and other data from the patient/client history and other testing can be used to confirm or rule out the presence of a physical therapy problem. These diagnostic clusters can be labeled as *impairment classifications* or *movement dysfunctions* by physical therapists and can guide efficient and effective management of the client.[22]

Within the profession of physical therapy, diagnostic classification systems that direct treatment interventions are being developed based on client prognosis and definable outcomes demonstrated in the literature.[1,23] The *Guide* groups preferred practice patterns into four categories of conditions: musculoskeletal, neuromuscular, cardiovascular/pulmonary, and integumentary. An individual may belong to one or more of these groups or patterns.

▶ DIFFERENTIAL DIAGNOSIS VERSUS SCREENING

If you are already familiar with the term *differential diagnosis* you may be wondering about the new title for this fourth edition. Previous editions were entitled *Differential Diagnosis in Physical Therapy.*

The new name *Differential Diagnosis for Physical Therapists: Screening for Referral* does not reflect a change in the content of the text as much as it reflects a better understanding of the screening process and a more appropriate use of the term "differential diagnosis" to identify and describe the specific movement impairment present.

When the first edition of this text was published the term "physical therapy diagnosis" was not yet commonly used nomenclature. Diagnostic labels were primarily within the domain of the physician. Over the years as our profession has changed and progressed, the concept of diagnosis by the physical therapist has evolved.

A diagnosis by the physical therapist describes the patient/client's primary dysfunction(s). This is done through the classification of a patient/client within a specific practice pattern as outlined in the *Guide.* The diagnostic process begins with the collection of data (examination), proceeds through the organization and interpretation of data (evaluation), and ends in the application of a label (i.e., the diagnosis).[1]

As part of the examination process, the therapist may conduct a screening examination. This is especially true if the diagnostic process does not yield an identifiable movement dysfunction. Throughout the evaluation process, the therapist must ask himself or herself:

- Is this an appropriate physical referral?
- Is there a problem that falls into one of the four categories of conditions described in the *Guide?*
- Is there a history or cluster of signs and/or symptoms that raises a yellow (cautionary) or red (warning) flag?

The presence of risk factors and yellow or red flags alerts the therapist to the need for a screening examination. Once the screening process is

complete and the therapist has confirmed the client is appropriate for physical therapy intervention, then the objective examination continues.

Sometimes in the early presentation, there are no red flags or associated signs and symptoms to suggest an underlying systemic or viscerogenic cause of the client's NMS symptoms or movement dysfunction.

It is not until the disease progresses that the clinical picture changes enough to raise a red flag. This is why the screening process is not necessarily a one-time evaluation. Screening can take place anywhere along the circle represented in Fig. 1-4.

The most likely place screening occurs is during the examination when the therapist obtains the history, performs a systems review, and carries out specific tests and measures. It is here that the client reports constant pain, skin lesions, gastrointestinal problems associated with back pain, digital clubbing, palmar erythema, shoulder pain with stair climbing, or any of the many indicators of systemic disease.

The therapist may hear the client relate new onset of symptoms that were not present during the examination. Such new information may come forth anytime during the episode of care. If the patient/client does not progress in physical therapy or presents with new onset of symptoms unreported before, the screening process may have to be repeated.

Red-flag signs and symptoms may appear for the first time or develop more fully during the course of physical therapy intervention. In some cases, exercise stresses the client's physiology enough to tip the scales. Previously unnoticed, unrecognized, or silent symptoms suddenly present more clearly.

As mentioned, a lack of progress signals the need to conduct a reexamination or to modify/redirect intervention. The process of reexamination may identify the need for consultation with or referral to another health care provider (*Guide*, Figure 1: Intervention, p. 43). The medical doctor is the most likely referral recommendation, but referral to a nurse practitioner, physician assistant, chiropractor, dentist, psychologist, or other appropriate health care professional may be more appropriate at times.

Scope of Practice

A key phrase in the APTA standards of practice is "within the scope of physical therapist practice." Establishing a diagnosis is a professional standard within the scope of a physical therapist practice, but may not be permitted according to the therapist's state practice act (Case Example 1-6).

As we have pointed out repeatedly, mechanical or movement dysfunction can masquerade as an organic problem. Identification of causative factors or etiology by the physical therapist is important in the screening process. By remaining within the scope of our practice the diagnosis by a physical therapist is limited primarily to those pathokinesiologic problems associated with faulty biomechanical or neuromuscular action.

When no apparent movement dysfunction, causative factors, or syndrome can be identified, the therapist may treat symptoms as part of an ongoing diagnostic process. Sometimes even physi-

---

CASE EXAMPLE 1-6   Scope of Practice

A licensed physical therapist volunteered at a high school athletic event and screened an ankle injury. After performing a heel strike test (negative), the PT recommended R.I.C.E. (Rest, Ice, Compression, and Elevation) and follow-up with a medical doctor if the pain persisted.

A complaint was filed 2 years later claiming that the physical therapist violated the state practice act by "... engaging in the practice of physical therapy practice in excess of the scope of physical therapy practice by undertaking to diagnose and prescribe appropriate treatment for an acute athletic injury."

The therapist was placed on probation for 2 years. The case was appealed and amended as it was clearly shown that the therapist was practicing within the legal bounds of the state's practice act. Imagine the impact this had on the individual in the community and as a private practitioner.

Know your state practice act and make sure it allows physical therapists to draw conclusions and make statements about findings of evaluations, i.e., physical therapy diagnosis.

cians use physical therapy as a diagnostic tool, observing the client's response during the episode of care to confirm or rule out medical suspicions.

If, however, the findings remain inconsistent with what is expected for a musculoskeletal or neuromuscular dysfunction and/or the patient/client does not improve with intervention, then referral to an appropriate medical professional may be required. Always keep in mind that the screening process may, in fact, confirm the presence of a musculoskeletal or neuromuscular problem.

The flip side of this concept is that client complaints that cannot be associated with a medical problem should be referred to a physical therapist to identify mechanical problems (Case Example 1-7). Physical therapists have a responsibility to educate the medical community as to the scope of our practice and our role in identifying mechanical problems and movement disorders.

Staying within the scope of physical therapist practice, the therapist communicates with physicians and other health care practitioners to request or recommend further medical evaluation. Whether in a private practice, school or home health setting, acute care hospital, or rehabilitation setting, physical therapists may observe and report important findings outside the realm of NMS disorders that require additional medical evaluation and treatment.

▼ DIRECT ACCESS

Direct access is the right of the public to obtain examination, evaluation, and intervention from a licensed physical therapist without previous examination by, or referral from, a physician, gatekeeper, or other practitioner. In the civilian sector, the need to screen for medical disease was first raised as an issue in response to direct-access leg-

---

CASE EXAMPLE 1-7   Identify Mechanical Problems: Cervical Spine Arthrosis Presenting as Chest Pain

A 42-year-old woman presented with primary chest pain of unknown cause. She was employed as an independent pediatric occupational therapist. She has been seen by numerous medical doctors who have ruled out cardiac, pulmonary, esophageal, upper GI, and breast pathology as underlying etiologies.

Since her symptoms continued to persist, she was sent to physical therapy for an evaluation.

She reported symptoms of chest pain/discomfort across the upper chest rated as a 5 or 6 and sometimes an 8 on a scale from 0 to 10. The pain does not radiate down her arms or up her neck. She cannot bring the symptoms on or make them go away. She cannot point to the pain, but reports it as being more diffuse than localized.

She denies any shortness of breath, but admits to being "out of shape" and hasn't been able to exercise due to a failed bladder neck suspension surgery 2 years ago. She reports fatigue, but states this is not unusual for her with her busy work schedule and home responsibilities.

She has not had any recent infections, no history of cancer or heart disease, and her mammogram and clinical breast exam are up-to-date and normal. She does not smoke or drink, but by her own admission has a "poor diet" due to time pressure, stress, and fatigue.

Final Result: After completing the evaluation with appropriate questions, tests, and measures, a Review of Systems pointed to the cervical spine as the most likely source of this client's symptoms. The jaw and shoulder joint were cleared, although there were signs of shoulder movement dysfunction from a possible impingement syndrome.

After relaying these findings to the client's primary care physician, radiographs of the cervical spine were ordered. Interestingly, despite the thousands of dollars spent on repeated diagnostic work-ups for this client, a simple x-ray had never been taken.

Results showed significant spurring and lipping throughout the cervical spine from early osteoarthritic changes of unknown cause. Cervical spine fusion was recommended and performed for instability in the midcervical region.

The client's chest pain was eliminated and did not return even up to 2 years after the cervical spine fusion. The physical therapist's contribution in pinpointing the location of referred symptoms brought this case to a successful conclusion.

islation. Until direct access, the only therapists performing medical screening were the military PTs.

Before 1957 a physician referral was necessary in all 50 states for a client to be treated by a physical therapist. Direct access was first obtained in Nebraska in 1957, when that state passed a licensure and scope-of-practice law that did not mandate a physician referral for a physical therapist to initiate care.[24]

One of the goals of the American Physical Therapy Association as outlined in the APTA 2020 vision statement is to achieve direct access to physical therapy services for citizens of all 50 states by the year 2020. At the present time, all but a handful of states in the United States permit some form of direct access to allow patient/clients to consult a physical therapist without first being referred by a physician, dentist, or chiropractor. At the time of this publication, 42 states have direct-access laws for physical therapy treatment; 48 have some form of evaluation without referral.

It is possible to have a state direct-access law but a state practice act that forbids therapists from seeing Medicare clients without a referral. A therapist in that state can see privately insured clients without a referral, but not Medicare clients. Passage of the Medicare Patient/Client Access to Physical Therapists Act (PAPTA) will extend direct-access nationwide to all Medicare beneficiaries.

Full, unrestricted direct access is not available in all states with a direct-access law. Various forms of direct access are available on a state-by-state basis. Many direct-access laws are permissive, as opposed to mandatory. This means that consumers are permitted to see therapists without a physician's referral; however, a payer can still require a referral before providing reimbursement for services. Each therapist must be familiar with the practice act and direct-access legislation for the state in which he or she is practicing.

Sometimes states enact a two- or three-tiered restricted or provisional direct-access system. For example, some states' direct-access law only allows evaluation and treatment for therapists who have practiced for 3 years. Some direct-access laws only allow physical therapists to provide services for up to 14 days without physician referral. Other states list up to 30 days as the standard.

There may be additional criteria in place, such as the patient/client must have been referred to physical therapy by a physician within the past 2 years or the therapist must notify the patient/client's identified primary care practitioner no later than 3 days after intervention begins.

In a three tiered–direct access state, three or more requirements must be met before practicing without a physician referral. For example, licensed physical therapists must practice for a specified number of years, complete continuing education courses, and obtain references from two or more physicians before treating clients without a physician referral.

There are other factors that prevent therapists from practicing under full direct-access rights even when granted by state law. For example, some therapists think that the way to avoid malpractice lawsuits is to continue operating under a system of physician referral. Therapists in a private practice driven by physician referral may not want to be placed in a position as competitors of the physicians who serve as a referral source.

Primary Care

Primary care is the coordinated, comprehensive, and personal care provided on a first-contact and continuous basis. It incorporates primary and secondary prevention of chronic disease states, wellness, personal support, education (including communication of information about illness, prevention, and health maintenance), and addresses the personal health care needs of patient/clients within the context of family and community.[25,26]

In the primary care delivery model, the therapist is responsible as a patient/client advocate to see that the patient/client's NMS and other health care needs are identified and prioritized, and a plan of care is established. The primary care model provides the consumer with first point-of-entry access to the physical therapist as the most skilled practitioner for movement system dysfunction. The physical therapist may also serve as a key member of a multidisciplinary primary care team that works together to assist the patient/client in maintaining his or her overall health and fitness.[26]

Through a process of screening, triage, examination, evaluation, referral, intervention, coordination of care, education, and prevention, the therapist prevents or reduces impairments, functional limitations, and disabilities while achieving cost-effective clinical outcomes.[1,27]

Expanded privileges beyond the traditional scope of the physical therapist practice may become part of the standard future physical therapist primary care practice. In addition to the usual privileges included in the scope of the physical therapist practice, the primary care therapist may eventually refer patient/clients to radiology for diagnostic imaging and other diagnostic evalu-

ations. In some settings (e.g., U.S. military) the therapist is already doing this and is credentialed to prescribe analgesic and nonsteroidal antiin-flammatory medications.[28]

Direct Access Versus Primary Care

Direct access is the vehicle by which the patient/client comes to the physical therapist, i.e., directly without first seeing a physician, dentist, chiropractor, or other health care professional. Direct access does not describe the type of practice the therapist is engaging in.

Primary care physical therapy is not a setting but rather describes a philosophy of whole-person care. The therapist is the first point-of-entry into the health care system. After screening and triage, patient/clients who do not have NMS conditions are referred to the appropriate health care spe-cialist for further evaluation.

The primary care therapist is not expected to diagnose conditions that are not neuromuscular or musculoskeletal. However, risk-factor assessment and screening for a broad range of medical condi-tions (e.g., high blood pressure, incontinence, dia-betes, vestibular dysfunction, peripheral vascular disease) is possible and an important part of primary and secondary prevention.

Autonomous Practice

Autonomous is defined as "self-governing," "not controlled by others."[29] Autonomous practice is defined as independent, self-determining profes-sional judgment and action.[30] Autonomous practice for the physical therapist does not mean practice independent of collaborative and collegial commu-nication with other health care team members (Box 1-6).

APTA Vision Statement for Physical Therapy 2020

Physical therapy, by 2020, will be provided by physical therapists who are doctors of physical therapy and who may be board-certified special-ists. Consumers will have direct access to physical therapists in all environments for patient/client management, prevention, and wellness services.

Physical therapists will be practitioners of choice in patient/clients' health networks and will hold all privileges of autonomous practice. Physi-cal therapists may be assisted by physical thera-pist assistants who are educated and licensed to provide physical therapist-directed and supervised components of interventions.[17]

Self-determination means the privilege of making one's own decisions, but only after key

information has been obtained through examina-tion, history, and consultation. The autonomous practitioner independently makes professional decisions based on a distinct or unique body of knowledge. For the physical therapist, that profes-sional expertise is confined to the examination, evaluation, diagnosis, prognosis, and intervention of movement impairments.

Physical therapists have the capability, ability, and responsibility to exercise professional judg-ment within their scope of practice. In this con-text, the therapist must conduct a thorough examination, determine a diagnosis, and recognize when physical therapy is inappropriate, or when physical therapy is appropriate but the client's condition is beyond the therapist's training, expe-rience, or expertise. In such a case, referral is required, but referral may be to a qualified physi-cal therapist who specializes in treating such dis-orders or conditions.[31,32]

Reimbursement Trends

Despite research findings that episodes of care for patient/clients who received physical therapy via

direct access were shorter, included fewer numbers of services, and were less costly than episodes of care initiated through physician referral,[33] many payers still require physician referral.[34]

Direct-access laws give consumers the legal right to seek physical therapy services without a medical referral. These laws do not always make it mandatory that insurance companies, third-party payers (including Medicare/Medicaid), self-insured, or other insurers reimburse the physical therapist without a physician's prescription.

Some state home-health agency license laws require referral for all client care regardless of the payer source. Further legislation and regulation are needed in many states to amend the insurance statues and state agency policies to assure statutory compliance.

This policy, along with large deductibles, poor reimbursement, and failure to authorize needed services has resulted in a trend toward a cash-based, private-pay business. This trend in reimbursement is also referred to as direct contracting, first-party payment, direct consumer services, or direct fee-for-service.[35] In such an environment, decisions can be made based on the good of the clients rather than on cost or volume.

In such circumstances consumers are willing to pay out-of-pocket for physical therapy services, bypassing the need for a medical evaluation unless requested by the physical therapist. A therapist can use a cash-based practice only where direct access has been passed and within the legal parameters of the state practice act.

In any situation where authorization for further intervention by a therapist is not obtained despite the therapist's assessment that further skilled services are needed, the therapist can notify the client and/or the family of their right to an appeal with the agency providing health care coverage.

The client has the right to make informed decisions regarding pursuit of insurance coverage or to make private-pay arrangements. Too many times the insurance coverage ends but the client's needs have not been met. Creative planning and alternate financial arrangements should remain an option discussed and made available.

▶ DECISION-MAKING PROCESS

This text is designed to help students, physical therapist assistants, and physical therapy clinicians screen for medical disease when it is appropriate to do so. But just exactly how is this done? Several guidelines are used in conducting a screening evaluation for any client (Box 1-7).

BOX 1-7 ▼ Guidelines for Decision-Making in the Screening Process

- Past Medical History
- Patient/Client Demographics
  - Age
  - Gender
  - Race/Ethnicity
  - Occupation
- Personal and Family History
  - Risk factors for disease
  - Medical/surgical history
  - Medications (current, recent past)
- Psychosocial
  - Education
  - Family system
  - Culture/religion
- Risk-Factor Assessment
- Clinical Presentation
- Associated Signs and Symptoms of Systemic Diseases
- Review of Systems

By using these decision-making tools, the therapist will be able to identify chief and secondary problems, identify information that is inconsistent with the presenting complaint, identify noncontributory information, generate a working hypothesis regarding possible causes of complaints, and determine whether referral or consultation is indicated.

The screening process is carried out through the client interview and verified during the physical examination. Therapists compare the subjective information (what the client tells us) with the objective findings (what we find during the examination) to identify NMS dysfunction (that which is within the scope of our practice) and to rule out systemic involvement (requiring medical referral). This is the basis for the *evaluation process*.

Given today's time constraints in the clinic, a fast and efficient method of screening is essential. Checklists (see Appendix), special questions to ask (see the end of each chapter; see also Appendix), and the decision-making tools listed in Box 1-7 can guide and streamline the screening process.

If a young, healthy athlete comes in with a sprained ankle and no other associated signs and symptoms there may be no need to screen further. But if that same athlete has an eating disorder, uses anabolic steroids illegally, or is on antidepressants the clinical picture, and possibly the intervention, changes. Risk-factor assessment and

a screening physical examination are the most likely ways to screen more thoroughly.

Or take, for example, an older adult who presents with hip pain of unknown cause. There are two red flags already present (age and insidious onset). As clients age, the past medical history and risk-factor assessment become more important assessment tools. After investigating the clinical presentation, screening would focus on these two elements next.

Or, if after ending the interview by asking, "Are there any symptoms of any kind anywhere else in your body that we have not talked about yet?" the client responds with a list of additional symptoms, it may be best to step back and conduct a Review of Systems.

Past Medical History

Most of history taking is accomplished through the client interview and includes both family and personal history. The client/patient interview is very important because it helps the physical therapist distinguish between problems that he or she can treat and problems that should be referred to a physician (or other appropriate health care professional) for medical diagnosis and intervention.

In fact, the importance of history taking cannot be emphasized enough. Physicians cite a shortage of time as the most common reason to skip the client history, yet history taking is the essential key to a correct diagnosis by the physician (or by the physical therapist).[36]

In Chapter 2, an interviewing process is described that includes concrete and structured tools and techniques for conducting a thorough and informative interview. The use of follow-up questions (FUPs) helps complete the interview. This information establishes a solid basis for the therapist's objective evaluation, assessment, and therefore intervention.

During the screening interview it is always a good idea to use a standard form to complete the personal/family history (see Fig. 2-2). Any form of checklist assures a thorough and consistent approach and spares the therapist from relying on his or her memory.

The types of data generated from a client history are presented in Fig. 2-1. Most often age, race/ethnicity, gender, and occupation (general demographics) are noted. Information about social history, living environment, and health status, functional status, and activity level is often important to the patient/client's clinical presentation and outcomes. Details about the current condition, medical (or other) intervention for the condition,

and use of medications is also gathered and considered in the overall evaluation process.

The presence of any yellow or red flags elicited during the screening interview or observed during the physical examination should prompt the therapist to consider the need for further tests and questions. Many of these signs and symptoms are listed in Appendix A-2.

Psychosocial history may provide insight into the client's clinical presentation and overall needs. Age, gender, race/ethnicity, education, occupation, family system, health habits, living environment, medication use, and medical/surgical history are all part of the client history evaluated in the screening process.

Risk-Factor Assessment

Greater emphasis has been placed on risk-factor assessment in the health care industry recently. Risk-factor assessment is an important part of disease prevention. Knowing the various risk factors for different kinds of diseases, illnesses, and conditions is an important part of the medical screening process.

Therapists can have an active role in both primary and secondary prevention through screening and education. According to the Guide,[1] physical therapists are involved in primary prevention by preventing a target condition in a susceptible or potentially susceptible population through such specific measures as general health promotion efforts.

Educating clients about their risk factors is a key element in risk-factor reduction. Identifying risk factors may guide the therapist in making a medical referral sooner than would otherwise seem necessary.

In primary care, the therapist assesses risk factors, performs screening exams, and establishes interventions to prevent impairment, dysfunction, and disability. For example, does the client have risk factors for osteoporosis, urinary incontinence, cancer, vestibular or balance problems, obesity, cardiovascular disease, and so on? The physical therapist practice can include routine screening for any of these as well as other problems.

Imagine a world where computerized kiosks are available in every mall, doctors' offices, physical therapy clinics, and even local grocery stores. Individuals could enter information regarding age, gender, and personal and family history, and then answer questions to establish individual risk factors. The computer program would take the person's vital signs and identify diseases, illnesses, or conditions to which the individual may be pre-

disposed along with recommended suggestions for ways to prevent each identified problem.

Eventually genetic screening will augment or even replace risk-factor assessment. Virtually every human illness has a hereditary component. The most common problems seen in a physical therapist practice (outside of traumatic injuries) are now believed to have a genetic component, even though the specific gene may not yet be discovered.[37]

Exercise as a successful intervention for many diseases, illness, and conditions will become prescriptive as research shows how much and what kind of exercise can prevent or mediate each problem. There is already a great deal of information on this topic published, and an accompanying need to change the way people think about exercise.

Convincing people to establish lifelong patterns of exercise and physical activity will continue to be a major focus of the health care industry. Therapists can advocate disease prevention, wellness, and promotion of healthy lifestyles by delivering health care services intended to prevent health problems or maintain health and by offering annual wellness screening as part of primary prevention.

Clinical Presentation

Clinical presentation including pain patterns and pain types is the next part of the decision making process. To assist the physical therapist in making a treatment-versus-referral decision, specific pain patterns corresponding to systemic diseases are provided in Chapter 3. Drawings of primary and referred pain patterns are provided in each chapter for quick reference. A summary of key findings associated with systemic illness is listed in Box 1-2.

The presence of any one of these variables is not cause for extreme concern, but should raise a yellow or red flag for the alert therapist. The therapist is looking for a pattern that suggests a viscerogenic or systemic origin of pain and/or symptoms. This pattern will not be consistent with what we might expect to see with the neuromuscular or musculoskeletal systems.

The therapist will proceed with the screening process depending on all findings. Often the next step is to look for associated signs and symptoms. Special follow-up questions are listed in the subjective examination to help the physical therapist determine when these pain patterns are accompanied by associated signs and symptoms that indicate visceral involvement.

Associated Signs and Symptoms of Systemic Diseases

The major focus of this text is the recognition of yellow- or red-flag signs and symptoms either reported by the client subjectively or observed objectively by the physical therapist.

Signs are observable findings detected by the therapist in an objective examination (e.g., unusual skin color, clubbing of the fingers [swelling of the terminal phalanges of the fingers or toes], hematoma [local collection of blood], effusion [fluid]). Signs can be seen, heard, smelled, measured, photographed, shown to someone else, or documented in some other way.

Symptoms are reported indications of disease that are perceived by the client but cannot be observed by someone else. Pain, discomfort, or other complaints such as numbness, tingling, or "creeping" sensations are symptoms that are difficult to quantify but are most often reported as the chief complaint.

Because physical therapists spend a considerable amount of time investigating pain, it is easy to remain focused exclusively on this symptom when clients might otherwise bring to the forefront other important problems.

Thus the physical therapist is encouraged to become accustomed to using the word *symptoms* instead of *pain* when interviewing the client. It is likewise prudent for the physical therapist to refer to symptoms when talking to clients with chronic pain in order to move the focus away from pain.

Instead of asking the client, "How are you today?" try asking:

Follow-Up Questions

- Are you better, same, or worse today?
- What can you do today that you couldn't do yesterday? (or last week/last month).

This approach to questioning progress (or lack of progress) may help you see a systemic pattern sooner than later.

The therapist can identify the presence of associated signs and symptoms by asking the client,

Follow-Up Questions

- Are there any symptoms of any kind anywhere else in your body that we have not talked about yet?
- Alternately: Are there any symptoms or problems anywhere else in your body that may not be related to your current problem?

The patient/client may not see a connection between shoulder pain and blood in the urine from kidney impairment or blood in the stools from chronic nonsteroidal antiinflammatory (NSAID) use. Likewise the patient/client may not think the diarrhea present is associated with the back pain (GI dysfunction).

The client with temporomandibular joint (TMJ) pain from a cardiac source usually has some other associated symptoms, and, in most cases, the client does not see the link. If the therapist does not ask, the client does not offer the extra information.

Each visceral system has a typical set of core signs and symptoms associated with impairment of that system (see Box 4-17). Systemic signs and symptoms that are listed for each condition should serve as a warning to alert the informed physical therapist of the need for further questioning and possible medical referral.

For example, the most common symptoms present with *pulmonary* pathology are cough, shortness of breath and pleural pain. *Liver* impairment is marked by abdominal ascites, right upper quadrant tenderness, jaundice, and skin and nailbed changes. Signs and symptoms associated with *endocrine* pathology may include changes in body or skin temperature, dry mouth, dizziness, weight change, or excessive sweating.

Being aware of signs and symptoms associated with each individual system may help the therapist make an early connection between viscerogenic and/or systemic presentation of NMS problems. The presence of constitutional symptoms is always a red flag that must be evaluated carefully (see Box 1-3).

Systems Review Versus Review of Systems

The Systems Review is defined in the *Guide* as a brief or limited exam of the anatomical and physiological status of the cardiovascular/pulmonary, integumentary, musculoskeletal, and neuromuscular systems. The Systems Review also includes assessment of the client's communication ability, affect, cognition, language, and learning style.

The specific tests and measures for this type of Systems Review are outlined in the *Guide* (Appendix 5, Guidelines for Physical Therapy Documentation, pp. 695-696). As part of this Systems Review, the client's ability to communicate, process information, and any barriers to learning are identified.

The Systems Review looks beyond the primary problem that brought the client to the therapist in the first place. It gives an overview of the "whole person," and guides the therapist in choosing appropriate tests and measures. The Systems Review helps the therapist answer the questions, "What should I do next?" and "What do I need to examine in depth?" It also answers the question, "What don't I need to do?"[38]

In the screening process, a slightly different approach may be needed, perhaps best referred to as a *Review of Systems*. After conducting an interview, performing an assessment of the pain type and/or pain patterns, and reviewing the clinical presentation, the therapist looks for any characteristics of systemic disease. Any identified clusters of associated signs and symptoms are reviewed to search for any indication that the client's problem is outside the scope of a physical therapist's practice.

The Review of Systems as part of the screening process (see discussion, Chapter 4) is a useful tool in recognizing clusters of associated signs and symptoms and the possible need for medical referral. Using this final tool, the therapist steps back and takes a look at the big picture, taking into consideration all of the presenting factors, and looking for any indication that the client's problem is pointing to a potential pattern that will identify the underlying system involved.

The therapist conducts a Review of Systems in the screening process by categorizing all of the complaints and associated signs and symptoms. Once these are listed, compare this list to Box 4-17. Are the signs and symptoms all genitourinary (GU)-related? Gastrointestinal (GI) in nature?

Perhaps the therapist observes dry skin, brittle nails, cold or heat intolerance, excessive hair loss, and realizes these signs could be pointing to an endocrine problem. At the very least the therapist recognizes that the clinical presentation is not something within the musculoskeletal or neuromuscular systems.

If, for example, the client's signs and symptoms fall primarily within the genitourinary group, turn to Chapter 10 and use additional, pertinent screening questions at the end of the chapter. The client's answers to these questions will guide the therapist in making a decision about referral to a physician or other health-care professional.

The physical therapist is not responsible for identifying the specific pathologic disease underlying the clinical signs and symptoms present. However, the alert therapist who classifies groups of signs and symptoms in a review of systems will be more likely to recognize a problem outside the scope of physical therapy practice and make a timely referral.

CASE EXAMPLES AND CASE STUDIES

Case examples and case studies are provided with each chapter to give the therapist a working understanding of how to recognize the need for additional questions. In addition, information is given concerning the type of questions to ask and how to correlate the results with the objective findings.

Cases will be used to integrate screening information in making a physical therapy differential diagnosis and deciding when and how to refer to the physician or other health care professional. Whenever possible, information about when and how to refer a client to the physician is presented.

Each case study is based on actual clinical experiences in a variety of inpatient/client and outpatient/client physical therapy practices to provide reasonable examples of what to expect when the physical therapist is functioning under any of the circumstances listed in Box 1-1.

▶ PHYSICIAN REFERRAL

As previously mentioned, the therapist may treat symptoms as part of an ongoing medical diagnostic process. In other words, sometimes the physician sends a patient/client to physical therapy "to see if it will help." This may be part of the medical differential diagnosis. Medical consultation or referral is required when no apparent movement dysfunction, causative factors, or syndrome can be identified and/or the findings are not consistent with a NMS dysfunction.

Communication with the physician is a key component in the referral process. Phone, email, and fax make this process faster and easier than ever before. Persistence may be required in obtaining enough information to glean what the doctor knows or thinks to avoid sending the very same problem back for his/her consideration. This is especially important when the physician is using physical therapy intervention as part of the medical differential diagnostic process.

The hallmark of professionalism in any health care practitioner is the ability to understand the limits of his or her professional knowledge. The physical therapist, either on reaching the limit of his or her knowledge or on reaching the limits prescribed by the client's condition, should refer the patient/client to the appropriate personnel. In this way the physical therapist will work within the scope of his or her level of skill, knowledge, and practical experience.

Knowing when and how to refer a client to another health care professional is just as important as the initial screening process. Once the therapist recognizes red flag histories, risk factors, signs and symptoms, and/or a clinical presentation that do not fit the expected picture for NMS dysfunction, then this information must be communicated effectively to the appropriate referral source.

Knowing how to refer the client or how to notify the physician of important findings is not always clear. In a direct access or primary care setting, the client may not have a personal or family physician. In an orthopedic setting, the client in rehab for a total hip or total knee may be reporting signs and symptoms of a nonorthopedic condition. Do you send the client back to the referring (orthopedic) physician or refer him or her to the primary care physician?

Suggested Guidelines

When the client has come to physical therapy without a medical referral (i.e., self-referred) and the physical therapist recommends medical follow-up, the patient/client should be referred to the primary care physician if the patient/client has one.

Occasionally, the patient/client indicates that he or she has not contacted a physician, or was treated by a physician (whose name cannot be recalled) a long time ago, or that he or she has just moved to the area and does not have a physician.

In these situations the client can be provided with a list of recommended physicians. It is not necessary to list every physician in the area, but the physical therapist can provide several appropriate choices. Whether or not the client makes an appointment with a medical practitioner, the physical therapist is urged to document subjective and objective findings carefully, as well as the recommendation made for medical follow-up. The therapist should make every effort to get the physical therapy records to the consulting physician.

Before sending a client back to his or her doctor, have someone else (e.g., case manager, physical therapy colleague or mentor, nursing staff if available) double check your findings and discuss your reasons for referral. Recheck your own findings at a second appointment. Are they consistent?

Consider checking with the medical doctor by telephone. Perhaps the physician is aware of the problem, but the therapist does not have the patient/client records and is unaware of this fact. As mentioned it is not uncommon for physicians to

send a client to physical therapy as part of their own differential diagnostic process. For example, they may have tried medications without success and the client does not want surgery or more drugs. The doctor may say, "Let's try physical therapy. If that doesn't change the picture, the next step is. . . ."

As a general rule, try to send the client back to the referring physician. If this does not seem appropriate, call and ask the physician how he or she wants to handle the situation. Describe the problem and ask:

Follow-Up Questions

- Do you want Mr. X/Mrs. Y to check with his/her family doctor . . . or do you prefer to see him/her yourself?

Perhaps an orthopedic client is demonstrating signs and symptoms of depression. This may be a side effect from medications prescribed by another physician (e.g., gynecologist, gastroenterologist). Provide the physician with a list of the observed cluster of signs and symptoms and an open-ended question such as:

Follow-Up Questions

- How do you want to handle this? or How do you want me to handle this?

Do not suggest a medical diagnosis. When providing written documentation, a short paragraph of physical therapy findings and intervention is followed by a list of concerns, perhaps with the following remarks, "These do not seem consistent with a neuromuscular or musculoskeletal problem (choose the most appropriate phrase for the client or name the medical diagnosis e.g., S/P THR)." Then follow-up with one of two questions/comments:

Follow-Up Questions

- What do you think? or Please advise.

Special Considerations

What if the physician refuses to see the client or finds nothing wrong? We recommend being patiently persistent. Sometimes it is necessary to wait until the disease progresses to a point that medical testing can provide a diagnosis. This is unfortunate for the client, but a reality in some cases.

Sometimes it may seem like a good idea to suggest a second opinion. You may want to ask your client:

Follow-Up Questions

- Have you ever thought about getting a second opinion?

It is best not to tell the client what to do. If the client asks you what he or she should do, pose this question:

Follow-Up Questions

- What do you think your options are? or What are your options?

It is perfectly acceptable to provide a list of names (more than one) where the client can get a second opinion. If the client asks which one to see, suggest whoever is closest geographically or with whom he or she can get an appointment as soon as possible.

What do you do if the client's follow-up appointment is scheduled 2 weeks away, and you think immediate medical attention is needed? Call the physician's office and see what is advised: does the physician want to see the client in the office or send him/her to the emergency department?

For example, what if a patient/client with a recent total hip replacement develops chest pain and shortness of breath during exercise? The client also reports a skin rash around the surgical site. This will not wait for 2 weeks. Take the client's vital signs (especially body temperature in case of infection) and report these to the physician. In some cases the need for medical care will be obvious, such as in the case of acute myocardial infarct or if the client collapses.

Documentation and Liability

Documentation is any entry into the patient/client record. Documentation may include consultation reports, initial examination reports, progress notes, flow sheets, checklists, reexamination reports, discharge summaries, and so on.[1] Various forms are available for use in the *Guide to Physical Therapist Practice* to aid in collecting data in a standardized fashion.

The U.S. Department of Health and Human Services (HHS) is taking steps in building a national electronic health care system that will allow patient/clients and health care providers access to their complete medical records anytime and anywhere they are needed, leading to reduced medical errors, improved care, and reduced health care costs. The goal is to have digital health records for most Americans by the year 2014.[39]

Documentation is required at the onset of each episode of physical therapy care and includes the elements described in Box 1-5, Elements of Patient/Client Management. Documentation of the initial episode of physical therapy care includes examination, comprehensive screening, and specific testing leading to a diagnostic classification and/or referral to another practitioner (*Guide* p. 695).[1]

Clients with complex medical histories and multiple comorbidities are increasingly common in a physical therapist's practice. Risk management has become an important consideration for many clients. Documentation and communication must reflect this practice.

Sometimes the therapist will have to be more proactive and assertive in communicating with the client's physician. It may not be enough to suggest or advise the client make a follow-up appointment with his or her doctor. Leaving the decision up to the client is a passive and indirect approach. It does encourage client/consumer responsibility, but may not be in his/her best interest.

In the APTA *Standards of Practice and the Criteria* (HOD 06-00-11-22) it states, "The physical therapy service collaborates with all disciplines as appropriate [Administration of the Physical Therapy Service, Section II, Item J].

And in HOD 06-90-15-28 (*Referral Relationships*) it states, "The physical therapist must refer patient/clients/clients to the referring practitioner or other health care practitioners if symptoms are present for which physical therapy is contraindicated or are indicative of conditions for which treatment is outside the scope of his/her knowledge."[40]

In cases where the seriousness of the condition can affect the client's outcome, the therapist may need to contact the physician directly and describe the problem. If the therapist's assessment is that the client needs medical attention, advising the client to see a medical doctor as soon as possible may not be enough.

Good risk management is a proactive process that includes taking action to minimize negative outcomes. If a client is advised to contact his or her physician and fails to do so, the therapist should call the doctor.[41]

Failure on the part of the therapist to properly report on a client's condition reflects a lack of professional judgment in the management of the client's case. A number of positions and standards of the APTA Board of Directors emphasize the importance of PT communication and collaboration with other health care providers. This is a key to

providing the best possible client care (Case Example 1-8).[42]

HOD 06-97-06-19 (Policy on *Diagnosis by Physical Therapists*) states that, "as the diagnostic process continues, physical therapists may identify findings that should be shared with other health professionals, including referral sources, to ensure optimal patient/client care." Part of this process may require "appropriate follow-up or referral."

Failure to share findings and concerns with the physician or other appropriate health care provider is a failure to enter into a collaborative team approach. Best-practice standards of optimal patient/client care support and encourage interactive exchange.

Prior negative experiences with difficult medical personnel do not exempt the therapist from best practice, which means making every attempt to communicate and document clinical findings and concerns.

The therapist must describe his or her concerns. Using the key phrase "scope of practice" may be helpful. It may be necessary to explain that the symptoms do not match the expected pattern for a musculoskeletal or neuromuscular problem. The problem appears to be outside the scope of a physical therapist's practice . . ., or the problem requires a greater collaborative effort between health care disciplines.

It may be appropriate to make a summary statement regarding key objective findings with a follow-up question for the physician. This may be filed in the client's chart or electronic medical record in the hospital or sent in a letter to the outpatient/client's physician (or other health care provider).

For example, after treatment of a person who has not responded to physical therapy, a report to the physician may include additional information: "Miss Jones reported a skin rash over the backs of her knees 2 weeks before the onset of joint pain and experiences recurrent bouts of sore throat and fever when her knees flare up. These features are not consistent with an athletic injury. Would you please take a look?" (For an additional sample letter, see Fig. 1-6.)

Other useful wording may include "Please advise" or "What do you think?" The therapist does not suggest a medical cause or attempt to diagnose the findings medically. Providing a report and stating that the clinical presentation does not follow a typical neuromuscular or musculoskeletal pattern may be all that is needed.

CASE EXAMPLE 1-8   Failure to Collaborate and Communicate with the Physician

A 43-year-old woman was riding a bicycle when she was struck from behind and thrown to the ground. She was seen at the local walk-in clinic and released with a prescription for painkillers and muscle relaxants. X-rays of her head and neck were unremarkable for obvious injury.

She came to the physical therapy clinic 3 days later with complaints of left shoulder, rib, and wrist pain. There was obvious bruising along the left chest wall and upper abdomen. In fact, the ecchymosis was quite extensive and black in color indicating a large area of blood extravasation into the subcutaneous tissues.

She had no other complaints or problems. Shoulder range of motion was full in all planes, although painful and stiff. Ribs 9, 10, and 11 were painful to palpation but without obvious deformity or derangement.

A neurologic screening exam was negative. The therapist scheduled her for 3 visits over the next 4 days and started her on a program of Codman's exercises, progressing to active shoulder motion. The client experienced progress over the next 5 days and then reported severe back muscle spasms.

The client called the therapist and cancelled her next appointment because she had the flu with fever and vomiting. When she returned, the therapist continued to treat her with active exercise progressing to resistive strengthening. The client's painful shoulder and back symptoms remained the same, but the client reported that she was "less stiff."

Three weeks after the initial accident, the client collapsed at work and had to be transported to the hospital for emergency surgery. Her spleen had been damaged by the initial trauma with a slow bleed that eventually ruptured.

The client filed a lawsuit in which the therapist was named. The complaint against the therapist was that she failed to properly assess the client's condition and failed to refer her to a medical doctor for a condition outside the scope of physical therapy practice.

Did the PT Show Questionable Professional Judgment in the Evaluation and Management of this Case?

There are some obvious red-flag signs and symptoms in this case that went unreported to a

medical doctor. There was no contact with the physician at any time throughout this client's physical therapy episode of care. The physician on-call at the walk-in clinic did not refer the client to physical therapy—she referred herself.

However, the physical therapist did not send the physician any information about the client's self-referral, physical therapy evaluation, or planned treatment.

Subcutaneous blood extravasation is not uncommon after a significant accident or traumatic impact such as this client experienced. The fact that the physician did not know about this and the PT did not report it demonstrates questionable judgment. Left shoulder pain after trauma may be Kehr's sign, indicating blood in the peritoneum (see the discussion in Chapter 18).

The new onset of muscle spasm and unchanging pain levels with treatment are potential red-flag symptoms. Concomitant constitutional symptoms of fever and vomiting are also red flags, even if the client thought it was the flu.

The therapist left herself open to legal action by failing to report symptoms unknown to the physician and failing to report the client's changing condition. At no time did the therapist suggest the client go back to the clinic or see a primary care physician. She did not share her findings with the physician either by phone or in writing.

The therapist exercised questionable professional judgment by failing to communicate and collaborate with the attending physician. She did not screen the client for systemic involvement, based on the erroneous thinking that this was a traumatic event with a clear etiology.

She assumed in a case like this where the client was a self-referral and the physician was a "doc-in-a-box" that she was "on her own." She failed to properly report on the client's condition, failed to follow the APTA's policies governing a physical therapist's interaction with other health care providers, and was legally liable for mismanagement in this case.

Referral. A 32-year-old female university student was referred for physical therapy through the student health service 2 weeks ago. The physician's referral reads: "Possible right oblique abdominis tear/possible right iliopsoas tear." A faculty member screened this woman initially, and the diagnosis was confirmed as being a right oblique abdominal strain.

History. Two months ago, while the client was running her third mile, she felt "severe pain" in the right side of her stomach, which caused her to double over. She felt immediate nausea and had abdominal distension. She cannot relieve the pain by changing the position of her leg. Currently, she still cannot run without pain.

Presenting Symptoms. Pain increases during sit-ups, walking fast, reaching, turning, and bending. Pain is eased by heat and is reduced by activity. Pain in the morning versus evening depends on body position. Once the pain starts, it is intermittent and aches. The client describes the pain as being severe, depending on her body position. She is currently taking aspirin when necessary.

SAMPLE LETTER

Date

John Smith, M.D.
University of Montana Health Service
Eddy Street
Missoula, MT 59812

Re: Jane Doe

Dear Dr. Smith,
Your client, Jane Doe, was evaluated in our clinic on 5/2/06 with the following pertinent findings:

Subjective. She has severe pain in the right lower abdominal quadrant associated with nausea and abdominal distension. Although the onset of symptoms started while the client was running, she denies any precipitating trauma. She describes the course of symptoms as having begun 2 months ago with temporary resolution and now with exacerbation of earlier symptoms. Additionally, she reports chronic fatigue and frequent night sweats.

Objective. Presenting pain is reproduced by resisted hip or trunk flexion with accompanying tenderness/tightness on palpation of the right iliopsoas muscle (compared with the left iliopsoas muscle). There are no implicating neurologic signs or symptoms.

Assessment. A musculoskeletal screening examination is consistent with your diagnosis of a possible iliopsoas or abdominal oblique tear. Jane appears to have a combination of musculoskeletal and systemic symptoms, such as those outlined earlier. Of particular concern are the symptoms of fatigue, night sweats, abdominal distension, nausea, repeated episodes of exacerbation and remission, and severe quality of pain and location (right lower abdominal quadrant). These symptoms appear to be of a systemic nature rather than caused by a musculoskeletal lesion.

Recommendations. I suggest that the client return to you for further medical follow-up to rule out any systemic involvement before the initiation of physical therapy services. I am concerned that my proposed intervention of ultrasound, soft tissue mobilization, and stretching may aggravate an underlying disease process.

I will contact you directly by telephone by the end of the week to discuss these findings and to answer any questions that you may have. Thank you for this interesting referral.

Sincerely,

Catherine C. Goodman, M.B.A., P.T.

Result. This client returned to the physician, who then ordered laboratory tests. After an acute recurrence of the symptoms described earlier, she had exploratory surgery. A diagnosis of a ruptured appendix and peritonitis was determined at surgery. In retrospect, the proposed ultrasound and soft tissue mobilization would have been contraindicated in this situation.

Fig. 1-6 • Sample letter of the physical therapist's findings that is sent to the referring physician.

Guidelines for Immediate Medical Attention

After each chapter in this text, there is a section on Guidelines For Physician Referral. Guidelines for immediate medical attention are provided whenever possible. An overall summary is provided here but specifics for each viscerogenic system and NMS situation should be reviewed in each chapter as well.

For example, immediate medical attention is advised when:

- Client with anginal pain not relieved in 20 minutes with reduced activity and/or administration of nitroglycerin; angina at rest

- Client with angina has nausea, vomiting, profuse sweating
- Client presents with bowel/bladder incontinence and/or saddle anesthesia secondary to cauda equina lesion or cervical spine pain concomitant with urinary incontinence
- Client is in anaphylactic shock (see Chapter 12)
- Client has symptoms of inadequate ventilation or CO_2 retention (see the section on Respiratory Acidosis in Chapter 7)
- Client with diabetes appears confused or lethargic or exhibits changes in mental function (perform fingerstick glucose testing and report findings)
- Client has positive McBurney's point (appendicitis) or rebound tenderness (inflamed peritoneum) (see Chapter 8)
- Sudden worsening of intermittent claudication may be due to thromboembolism and must be reported to the physician immediately
- Throbbing chest, back, or abdominal pain that increases with exertion accompanied by a sensation of a heartbeat when lying down and palpable pulsating abdominal mass may indicate an aneurysm
- Changes in size, shape, tenderness, and consistency of lymph nodes; detection of palpable, fixed, irregular mass in the breast, axilla, or elsewhere, especially in the presence of a previous history of cancer

Guidelines for Physician Referral

Medical attention must be considered when any of the following are present. This list represents a general overview of warning flags or conditions presented throughout this text. More specific recommendations are made in each chapter based on impairment of each individual visceral system.

General Systemic

- Unknown cause
- Lack of significant objective neuromusculoskeletal (NMS) signs and symptoms
- Lack of expected progress with physical therapy intervention
- Development of constitutional symptoms or associated signs and symptoms any time during the episode of care
- Discovery of significant past medical history unknown to physician
- Changes in health status that persist 7 to 10 days beyond expected time period
- Client who is jaundiced and has not been diagnosed or treated

For Women

- Low back, hip, pelvic, groin, or sacroiliac symptoms without known etiologic basis and in the presence of constitutional symptoms
- Symptoms correlated with menses
- Any spontaneous uterine bleeding after menopause
- For pregnant women:
  - Vaginal bleeding
  - Elevated blood pressure
  - Increased Braxton-Hicks (uterine) contractions in a pregnant woman during exercise

Vital Signs (Report These Findings)

- Persistent rise or fall of blood pressure
- Blood pressure elevation in any woman taking birth control pills (should be closely monitored by her physician)
- Pulse amplitude that fades with inspiration and strengthens with expiration
- Pulse increase over 20 BPM lasting more than 3 minutes after rest or changing position
- Difference in pulse pressure (between systolic and diastolic measurements) of more than 40 mm Hg
- Persistent low-grade (or higher) fever, especially associated with constitutional symptoms, most commonly sweats
- Any unexplained fever without other systemic symptoms, especially in the person taking corticosteroids
- See also yellow warning signs presented Box 4-6 and the section on Physician Referral: Vital Signs in Chapter 4

Cardiac

- More than three sublingual nitroglycerin tablets required to gain relief from angina
- Angina continues to increase in intensity after stimulus (e.g., cold, stress, exertion) has been eliminated
- Changes in pattern of angina
- Abnormally severe chest pain
- Anginal pain radiates to jaw/left arm
- Upper back feels abnormally cool, sweaty, or moist to touch
- Client has any doubts about his or her condition
- Palpitation in any person with a history of unexplained sudden death in the family requires medical evaluation; more than six episodes of palpitation in 1 minute or palpitations lasting for hours or occurring in association with pain, shortness of breath, fainting, or severe lightheadedness requires medical evaluation

- Clients who are neurologically unstable as a result of a recent CVA, head trauma, spinal cord injury, or other central nervous system insult often exhibit new arrhythmias during the period of instability; when the client's pulse is monitored, any new arrhythmias noted should be reported to the nursing staff or physician
- Anyone who cannot climb a single flight of stairs without feeling moderately to severely winded or who awakens at night or experiences shortness of breath when lying down should be evaluated by a physician
- Anyone with known cardiac involvement who develops progressively worse dyspnea should notify the physician of these findings
- Fainting (syncope) without any warning period of lightheadedness, dizziness, or nausea may be a sign of heart valve or arrhythmia problems; unexplained syncope in the presence of heart or circulatory problems (or risk factors for heart attack or stroke) should be evaluated by a physician

Cancer

Early warning sign(s) of cancer:
- Seven early warning signs plus two additional signs are pertinent to the physical therapy examination (see Box 13-1)
- All soft tissue lumps that persist or grow, whether painful or painless
- Any woman presenting with chest, breast, axillary, or shoulder pain of unknown etiologic basis, especially in the presence of a positive medical history (self or family) of cancer
- Any man with pelvic, groin, sacroiliac, or low back pain accompanied by sciatica and a history of prostate cancer
- Bone pain, especially on weight-bearing, that persists more than 1 week and is worse at night
- Any unexplained bleeding from any area

Pulmonary

- Shoulder pain aggravated by respiratory movements; have the client hold his or her breath and reassess symptoms; any reduction or elimination of symptoms with breath holding or the Valsalva maneuver suggests pulmonary or cardiac source of symptoms
- Shoulder pain that is aggravated by supine positioning; pain that is worse when lying down and improves when sitting up or leaning forward is often pleuritic in origin (abdominal contents push up against diaphragm and in turn against parietal pleura; see Figs. 4-4 and 4-5)

- Shoulder or chest (thorax) pain that subsides with autosplinting (lying on painful side)
- For the client with asthma: Signs of asthma or abnormal bronchial activity during exercise
- Weak and rapid pulse accompanied by fall in blood pressure (pneumothorax)
- Presence of associated signs and symptoms, such as persistent cough, dyspnea (rest or exertional), or constitutional symptoms (see Box 1-3).

Genitourinary

- Abnormal urinary constituents—for example, change in color, odor, amount, flow of urine
- Any amount of blood in urine
- Cervical spine pain accompanied by urinary incontinence (unless cervical disk protrusion already has been medically diagnosed)

Gastrointestinal

- Back pain and abdominal pain at the same level, especially when accompanied by constitutional symptoms
- Back pain of unknown cause in a person with a history of cancer
- Back pain or shoulder pain in a person taking nonsteroidal antiinflammatory drugs, especially when accompanied by gastrointestinal upset or blood in the stools
- Back or shoulder pain associated with meals or back pain relieved by a bowel movement

Musculoskeletal

- Symptoms that seem out of proportion to the injury or symptoms persisting beyond the expected time for the nature of the injury
- Severe or progressive back pain accompanied by constitutional symptoms, especially fever
- New onset of joint pain following surgery with inflammatory signs (warmth, redness, tenderness, swelling)

Precautions/Contraindications to Therapy

- Uncontrolled chronic heart failure or pulmonary edema
- Active myocarditis
- Resting heart rate 120 or 130 BPM*
- Resting systolic rate 180 to 200 mm Hg*
- Resting diastolic rate 105 to 110 mm Hg*
- Moderate dizziness, near-syncope
- Marked dyspnea
- Unusual fatigue
- Unsteadiness

---

* Unexplained or poorly tolerated by client.

- Irregular pulse with symptoms of dizziness, nausea, or shortness of breath or loss of palpable pulse
- Postoperative posterior calf pain
- For the client with diabetes: Chronically unstable blood sugar levels must be stabilized (fasting target glucose range: 70 to 110 mg/dL; precaution: <100 or >250 mg/dL)

Clues to Screening for Medical Disease

Some therapists suggest a lack of time as an adequate reason to skip the screening process. A few minutes early in the evaluation process may save the client's life. Less dramatically, it may prevent delays in choosing the most appropriate intervention.

Listening for yellow- or red-flag symptoms and observing for red-flag signs can be easily incorporated into everyday practice. It is a matter of listening and looking intentionally. If you do not routinely screen clients for systemic or viscerogenic causes of NMS impairment or dysfunction, then at least pay attention to this red flag:

Red Flag

- Client does not improve with physical therapy intervention or gets worse with treatment.

If someone fails to improve with physical therapy intervention, gets better and then worse, or just gets worse, the treatment protocol may not be in error. Certainly, the first step is to review the selected intervention(s), but also consider the possibility of a systemic or viscerogenic origin of symptoms. Use the screening tools outlined in this chapter to evaluate each individual client (see Box 1-7).

KEY POINTS TO REMEMBER

✔ Systemic diseases can mimic neuromusculoskeletal (NMS) dysfunction.

✔ It is the therapist's responsibility to identify what NMS impairment is present.

✔ There are many reasons for medical screening of the physical therapy client (see Box 1-1).

✔ Screening for medical disease is an ongoing process and does not occur just during the initial evaluation.

✔ The therapist uses several parameters in making the screening decision: client history, risk factors, clinical presentation including pain patterns/pain types, associated signs and symptoms, and Review of Systems. Any red flags in the first three parameters will alert the therapist to the need for a screening examination. In the screening process, a Review of Systems includes identifying clusters of signs and symptoms that may be characteristic of a particular organ system.

✔ The two body parts most commonly affected by visceral pain patterns are the back and the shoulder, although the thorax, pelvis, hip, sacroiliac, and groin can be involved.

✔ The physical therapist is qualified to make a diagnosis regarding primary NMS conditions.

✔ The purpose of the physical therapist's diagnosis, established through the subjective and objective examinations, is to identify as closely as possible the underlying NMS condition. In this way the therapist is screening for medical disease, ruling out the need for medical referral, and treating the physical therapy problem as specifically as possible.

✔ Sometimes in the diagnostic process the symptoms are treated because the client's condition is too acute to evaluate thoroughly. Usually even medically diagnosed problems (e.g., "shoulder pain" or "back pain") are evaluated.

✔ Careful, objective, detailed evaluation of the client with pain is critical for accurate identification of the sources and types of pain (underlying impairment process) and for accurate assessment of treatment effectiveness.[42]

✔ Painful symptoms that are out of proportion to the injury or that are not consistent with objective findings may be a red flag indicating systemic disease. The therapist must be aware of and screen for other possibilities such as physical assault (see the section on Domestic Violence in Chapter 2) and emotional overlay (see Chapter 3).

✔ If the client or the therapist is in doubt, communication with the physician, dentist, family member, or referral source is indicated.

✔ The therapist must be familiar with the practice act for the state in which he or she is practicing. These can be accessed on the APTA website at: http://www.apta.org (search window type in: State Practice Acts).

PRACTICE QUESTIONS

1. The primary purpose of a diagnosis by the physical therapist is
   a. to obtain reimbursement
   b. to guide intervention strategies
   c. to practice within the scope of physical therapy
   d. to meet the established standards for accreditation

2. Direct access is the only reason physical therapists must screen for systemic disease.
   a. true
   b. false

3. A patient/client gives you a written prescription from a physician, chiropractor, or dentist. The first screening question to ask is:
   a. What did the physician (dentist, chiropractor) say is the problem?
   b. Did the physician (dentist, chiropractor) examine you?
   c. When do you go back to see the doctor (dentist, chiropractor)?
   d. How many times per week did the doctor (dentist, chiropractor) suggest you come to therapy?

4. Screening for medical disease takes place:
   a. only during the first interview
   b. just before the client returns to the physician for his/her next appointment
   c. throughout the episode of care
   d. none of the above

5. Physical therapists are qualified to make a diagnosis regarding primary neuromusculoskeletal conditions, but we must do so in accordance with:
   a. the *Guide to the Physical Therapist Practice*
   b. the State Practice Act
   c. the screening process
   d. the SOAP method

6. Medical referral for a problem outside the scope of the physical therapy practice occurs when:
   a. no apparent movement dysfunction exists
   b. no causative factors can be identified
   c. findings are not consistent with neuromuscular or musculoskeletal dysfunction
   d. client presents with suspicious red-flag symptoms
   e. any of the above
   f. none of the above

7. Physical therapy evaluation and intervention may be part of the physician's differential diagnosis.
   a. true
   b. false

8. What is the difference between a yellow- and a red-flag symptom?

9. What are the major decision-making tools used in the screening process?

10. See if you can quickly name 6 to 10 red flags that suggest the need for further screening.

REFERENCES

1. *Guide to Physical Therapist Practice*, ed 2 (Revised), Alexandria, Va, 2003, American Physical Therapy Association.
2. Bogduk N: *Evidence-based clinical guidelines for the management of acute low back pain*, The National Musculoskeletal Medicine Initiative, National Health and Medical Research Council, Nov. 1999.
3. McGuirk B, King W, Govind J, et al: Safety, efficacy, and cost effectiveness of evidence-based guidelines for the management of acute low back pain in primary care, *Spine* 26(23):2615-2622, 2001.
4. Kuchera ML, Philadelphia, Pennsylvania, 2005, Philadelphia College of Osteopathic Medicine.
5. Graham K: Personal communication, 2005.
6. Goodman CC, Kapasi Z: The effect of exercise on the immune system, *Rehabilitation Oncology* 20(1):13-26, 2002.
7. Malm C, Celsing F, Friman G: Immune defense is both stimulated and inhibited by physical activity, *Lakartidningen* 102(11):867-873, 2005.
8. Kohut ML, Senchina DS: Reversing age-associated immunosenescence via exercise, *Exercise Immunology Rev* 10:6-41, 2004.
9. Sinnott M: Challenges 2000: Acute care/hospital clinical practice, *PT Magazine* 8(1):43-46, 2000.
10. National Institute on Aging, Fiscal Year 2004 Justification.
11. National Center for Health Statistics (NCHS), Health, United States, 1999 with health and aging chartbook. Hyattsville, Md, 1999, Figure 41, page 41.
12. American Physical Therapy Association (APTA) House of Delegates (HOD): Diagnosis by physical therapists HOD 06-97-06-19 (Program 32) [Amended HOD 06-95-12-07; HOD 06-94-22-35, Initial HOD 06-84-19-78]. APTA Governance.
13. *A normative model of physical therapist professional education: version 2004*, APTA, 2004, Alexandria, Va.
14. Ellis J: Paving the path to a brighter future. Sahrmann challenges colleagues to move precisely during 29th McMillan lecture at PT '98. *PT Bulletin* 13(29):4-10, 1998.
15. Fosnaught M: A critical look at diagnosis, *PT Magazine* 4(6):48-54, 1996.
16. Boissonnault WG: Differential diagnosis: taking a step back before stepping forward. *PT Magazine* 8(11):45-53, 2000.
17. Vision sentence and vision statement for physical therapy 2020 [Hod 06-00-24-35 (Program 01)].

18. American Physical Therapy Association: Vision 2020, Annual Report 2004. APTA.

19. Raj PP: *Pain medicine: a comprehensive review*, St Louis, 1996, Mosby.

20. Sahrmann S: Diagnosis by the physical therapist—a prerequisite for treatment. A special communication, *Phys Ther* 68:1703-1706, 1988.

21. Rothstein JM: Patient classification, *Phys Ther* 73(4):214-215, 1993.

22. Delitto A, Snyder-Mackler L: The diagnostic process: examples in orthopedic physical therapy, *Phys Ther* 75(3):203-211, 1995.

23. Guccione A: *Diagnosis and diagnosticians: the future in physical therapy. Combined sections meeting*, Dallas, February 13-16, 1997.

24. Moore J: Direct access under Medicare Part B: the time is now! *PT Magazine* 10(2):30-32, 2002.

25. Mulley AG, Goroll AH, editors: *Primary care medicine: office evaluation and management of the adult patient*, ed 4, Philadelphia, 2000, Lippincott, Williams & Wilkins.

26. Murphy B: Personal communication, May 2005.

27. APTA primary care and the role of the physical therapist HOD 06-02-23-46 (Program 32) [Initial HOD 06-95-26-16].

28. Ryan GG, Greathouse D, Matsui I, et al: Introduction to primary care medicine. In Boissonnault WG, editor: *Primary care for the physical therapist*, Philadelphia, 2005, WB Saunders, pp. 3-17.

29. Merriam-Webster On-line Dictionary.

30. Autonomous physical therapist practice: definitions and privileges, *BOD* 03-03-12-28.

31. Schunk C, Thut C: Autonomous practice: issues of risk, *PT Magazine* 11(5):34-40, May 2003.

32. Cooperman J, Lewis DK: A physical therapist's road to referral, *HSPO Risk Advisor, Physical Therapist Edition* 4(2):Summer, 2001.

33. Mitchell IM, de Lissovoy G: A comparison of resource use and cost in direct access versus physician referral episodes of physical therapy, *Phys Ther* 77(1):10-18, 1997.

34. Fosnaught M: Direct access: exploring new opportunities, *PT Magazine* 10(2):58-62, 2002.

35. Johnson LH: Is cash-only reimbursement for you? *PT Magazine* 11(1):35-39, 2003.

36. Gonzalez-Urzelai V, Palacio-Elua L, Lopez-de-Munain J: Routine primary care management of acute low back pain: adherence to clinical guidelines, *Eur Spine J* 12(6):589-594, 2003.

37. Poirot L: Genetic disorders and engineering: implications for physical therapists. *PT Magazine* 13(2):54-60, 2005.

38. Giallonardo L: Guide in action, *PT Magazine* 8(9):76-88, 2000.

39. McGee MK: U.S. Health Department launches plans for electronic health records. Business Technology Network, Information Week.

40. American Physical Therapy Association (APTA). Referral relationships HOD 06-90-15-28.

41. Arriaga R: Stories from the front, Part II: Complex medical history and communication. PT Magazine 11(7):23-25, July 2003.

42. Management of the individual with pain. I. Physiology and evaluation, *PT Magazine* 4(11):54-63, 1996.

Introduction to the Interviewing Process

2

The client interview, including the personal and family history, is the single most important tool in screening for medical disease. The client interview as it is presented here is the first step in the screening process.

Interviewing is an important skill for the clinician to learn. It is generally agreed that 80% of the information needed to clarify the cause of symptoms is given by the client during the interview. This chapter is designed to provide the physical therapist with interviewing guidelines and important questions to ask the client.

Medical practitioners (including nurses, physicians, and therapists) begin the interview by determining the client's chief complaint. The **chief complaint** is usually a symptomatic description by the client (i.e., symptoms reported for which the person is seeking care or advice). The **present illness,** including the chief complaint and other current symptoms, gives a broad, clear account of the symptoms—how they developed and events related to them.

Questioning the client may also assist the therapist in determining whether an injury is in the acute, subacute, or chronic stage. This information guides the clinician in addressing the underlying pathology while providing symptomatic relief for the acute injury, more aggressive intervention for the chronic problem, and a combination of both methods of treatment for the subacute lesion.

The interviewing techniques, interviewing tools, Core Interview, and review of the inpatient hospital record in this chapter will help the therapist determine the location and potential significance of any symptom (including pain).

The interview format provides detailed information regarding the frequency, duration, intensity, length, breadth, depth, and anatomic location as these relate to the client's chief complaint. The physical therapist will later correlate this information with objective findings from the examination to rule out possible systemic origin of symptoms.

The subjective examination may also reveal any contraindications to physical therapy intervention or indications for the kind of intervention that is most likely to be effective. The information obtained from the interview guides the therapist in either referring the client to a physician or planning the physical therapy intervention.

CONCEPTS IN COMMUNICATION

Interviewing is a skill that requires careful nurturing and refinement over time. Even the most experienced health care professional should self-assess and work toward improvement. Taking an accurate medical history can be a challenge. Clients' recollections of their past symptoms, illnesses, and episodes of care are often inconsistent from one inquiry to the next.[1]

Clients may forget, underreport, or combine separate health events into a single memory, a process called *telescoping*. They may even (intentionally or unintentionally) fabricate or falsely recall medical events and symptoms that never occurred. The individual's personality and mental state at the time of the illness or injury may influence their recall abilities.[1]

Adopting a compassionate and caring attitude, monitoring your communication style, and being aware of cultural differences will help ensure a successful interview. Using the tools and techniques presented in this chapter will get you started or help you improve your screening abilities throughout the subjective examination.

Compassion and Caring

Compassion is the desire to identify with or sense something of another's experience and is a precursor of caring. Caring is the concern, empathy, and consideration for the needs and values of others. Interviewing clients and communicating effectively, both verbally and nonverbally, with compassionate caring takes into consideration individual differences and the client's emotional and psychological needs.[2]

Establishing a trusting relationship with the client is essential when conducting a screening interview and examination. The therapist may be asking questions no one else has asked before about body functions, assault, sexual dysfunction, and so on. A client who is comfortable physically and emotionally is more likely to offer complete information regarding personal and family history.

Be aware of your own body language and how it may affect the client. Sit down when obtaining the history and keep an appropriate social distance from the client. Take notes while maintaining adequate eye contact. Lean forward, nod, or encourage the individual occasionally by saying, "Yes, go ahead. I understand."

Silence is also a key feature in the communication and interviewing process. Silent attentiveness gives the client time to think or organize his or her thoughts. The health care professional is often tempted to interrupt during this time, potentially disrupting the client's train of thought. Silence can give the therapist time to observe the client and plan the next question or step.

Communication Styles

Everyone has a slightly different interviewing and communication style. The interviewer may need to adjust his or her personal interviewing style to communicate effectively.

Relying on one interviewing style may not be adequate for all situations.

There are gender-based styles and temperament/personality-based styles of communication for both the therapist and the client. There is a wide range of ethnic identifications, religions, socioeconomic differences, beliefs, and behaviors for both the therapist and the client.

There are cultural differences based on family of origin or country of origin, again for both the therapist and the client. In addition to spoken communication, different cultural groups may have nonverbal, observable differences in communication style. Body language, tone of voice, eye contact, personal space, sense of time, and facial expression are only a few key components of differences in interactive style.[3]

Illiteracy

Throughout the interviewing process and even throughout the episode of care, the therapist must keep in mind that 44 million American adults are illiterate, and an additional 35 million read only at a functional level for social survival. According to the Department of Education, illiteracy is on the rise in the United States.[4]

Functional illiteracy means that although many of these individuals can read up to a fourth-grade level, they need higher levels of literacy to function effectively in society, to find employment, or to be trained for new jobs as the workplace changes.[5]

It is likely that the rates of health illiteracy defined as the inability to read, understand, and respond to health information are much higher. It is a problem that has gone largely unrecognized and unaddressed. Health illiteracy is more than just the inability to read. People who can read may still have great difficulty understanding what they read.

The Institute of Medicine (IOM) estimates nearly half of all American adults (90 million people) demonstrate a low health literacy. They have trouble obtaining, processing, and understanding the basic information and services they need to make appropriate and timely health decisions.

Low health literacy translates into more severe, chronic illnesses, and lower quality of care when care is accessed. There is also a higher rate of health service utilization (e.g., hospitalization, emergency services) among people with limited health literacy.[6]

And it is not just the lower socioeconomic and less-educated population that is affected. Interpreting medical jargon, diagnostic test results, and

understanding pharmaceuticals is a challenge even for many highly educated individuals.

We are living at a time when the amount of health information available to us is almost overwhelming, and yet most Americans would be shocked at the number of their friends and neighbors that (sic) can't understand the instructions on their prescription medications or how to prepare for a simple medical procedure.[7,8]

English as a Second Language (ESL)

The therapist must keep in mind that many people in the United States speak English as a second language, and many of those people do not read English. More than 14 million people age 5 and older in the United States speak English poorly or not at all. Up to 86% of non-English speakers who are illiterate in English are also illiterate in their native language.

In addition, 19.8 million immigrants enter U.S. communities every year. Of these people, 1.7 million who are age 25 and older have less than a fifth-grade education. There is a heavy concentration of persons with low literacy skills among the poor and those who are dependent on public financial support.

Although the percentages of illiterate African American and Hispanic adults are much higher than those of white adults, the actual number of white nonreaders is twice that of African American and Hispanic nonreaders, a fact that dispels the myth that literacy is not a problem among Caucasians.[5]

People who are illiterate cannot read instructions on bottles of prescription medicine or over-the-counter medications. They may not know when a medicine is past the date of safe consumption; nor can they read about allergic risks, warnings to diabetics, or the potential sedative effect of medications.

They cannot read about "the seven warning signs" of cancer or which fasting glucose levels signal a red flag for diabetes. They cannot take online surveys to assess their risk for breast cancer, colon cancer, heart disease, or any other life-threatening condition.

The Physical Therapist's Role

The therapist should be aware of the possibility of any form of illiteracy and watch for risk factors such as age (over 55 years old), education (0-8 years or 9-12 years but without a high school diploma), lower paying jobs, living below the poverty level and/or receiving government assis-tance, and ethnic or racial minority groups (e.g., African American, Hispanic/Latino, Asian).

Health illiteracy can present itself in different ways. In the screening process, the therapist must be careful when having the client fill out medical history forms. The illiterate or functionally illiterate adult may not be able to understand the written details on a health insurance form, accurately complete a Family/Personal History form, or read the details of exercise programs provided by the therapist. The same is true for individuals with learning disabilities and mental impairments.

When given a choice between "yes" and "no" answers to questions, functionally illiterate adults often circle "no" to everything. The therapist should briefly review with each client to verify the accuracy of answers given on any questionnaire or health form.

For example, you may say, "I see you circled 'no' to any health problems in the past. Has anyone in your immediate family (or have you) ever had cancer, diabetes, hypertension . . ." and continue to name some or all of the choices provided. Sometimes, just naming the most common conditions is enough to know the answer is really "no"—or that there may be a problem with literacy.

The IOM has called upon health care providers to take responsibility for providing clear communication and adequate support to facilitate health-promoting actions based on understanding. Their goal is to educate society so that people have the skills they need to obtain, interpret, and use health information appropriately and in meaningful ways.[6]

Therapists should minimize the use of medical terminology. Use simple but not demeaning language to communicate concepts and instructions. Encourage clients to ask questions and confirm knowledge or tactfully correct misunderstandings.[6]

Consider including the following questions:

Follow-Up Questions

- What questions do you have?
- What would you like me to go over?

Resources

There is a pocket guide available to help health care professionals improve communication with clients of different cultural backgrounds. Widely accepted cultural practices of various ethnic groups are included along with descriptions of cultural and language nuances of subcultures within each ethnic group.[9]

Identifying personality style may be helpful for each therapist as a means of improving communi-

cation. Resource materials are available to help with this.[10,11] Types of temperaments and temperament analysis are available.[12] The Myers-Briggs Type Indicator, a widely used questionnaire designed to identify one's personality type, is also available on the Internet at www.myersbriggs.org.

For the experienced clinician, it may be helpful to reevaluate individual interviewing practices. Making an audio or videotape during a client interview can help the therapist recognize interviewing patterns that may need to improve. Watch and/or listen for any of the guidelines listed in Box 2-1.

Texts are available with the complete medical interviewing process described. These resources are helpful not only to give the therapist an understanding of the training physicians receive and methods they use when interviewing clients, but also to provide helpful guidelines when conducting a physical therapy screening or examination interview.[13,14]

The therapist should be aware that under federal civil rights laws and the Medicaid Act, any client with limited English proficiency (LEP) has the right to an interpreter free of charge if the health care provider receives federal funding.

▲ CULTURAL COMPETENCE

Interviewing and communication require a certain level of cultural competence as well. *Culture* refers to integrated patterns of human behavior that include the language, thoughts, communications, actions, customs, beliefs, values, and institutions of racial, ethnic, religious, or social groups.[2,15] Multiculturalism is a term that takes into account that

---

BOX 2-1 ▼ Interviewing Do's and Don'ts

DO's

Do use a sequence of questions that begins with open-ended questions.

Do leave closed-ended questions for the end as clarifying questions.

Do select a private location where confidentiality can be maintained.

Do listen attentively and show it both in your body language and by occasionally making reassuring verbal prompts, such as "I see" or "Go on."

Do ask one question at a time and allow the client to answer the question completely before continuing with the next question.

Do encourage the client to ask questions throughout the interview.

Do listen with the intention of assessing the client's current level of understanding and knowledge of his or her current medical condition.

Do eliminate unnecessary information and speak to the client at his or her level of understanding.

Do correlate signs and symptoms with medical history and objective findings to rule out systemic disease.

Do provide several choices or selections to questions that require a descriptive response.

DONT's

Don't jump to premature conclusions based on the answers to one or two questions. (Correlate all subjective and objective information before consulting with a physician.)

Don't interrupt or take over the conversation when the client is speaking.

Don't destroy helpful open-ended questions with closed-ended follow-up questions before the person has a chance to respond (e.g., How do you feel this morning? Has your pain gone?).

Don't use professional or medical jargon when it is possible to use common language (e.g., don't use the term *myocardial infarct* instead of heart attack).

Don't overreact to information presented. Common overreactions include raised eyebrows, puzzled facial expressions, gasps, or other verbal exclamations such as "Oh, really?" or "Wow!" Less dramatic reactions may include facial expressions or gestures that indicate approval or disapproval, surprise, or sudden interest. These responses may influence what the client does or does not tell you.

Don't use leading questions. Pain is difficult to describe, and it may be easier for the client to agree with a partially correct statement than to attempt to clarify points of discrepancy between your statement and his or her pain experience.

Leading Questions	Better Presentation of Same Questions
Where is your pain?	Do you have any pain associated with your injury?
Does it hurt when you first get out of bed?	If yes, tell me about it. When does your back hurt?
Does the pain radiate down your leg?	Do you have this pain anywhere else?
Do you have pain in your lower back?	Point to the exact location of your pain.

every member of a group or country does not have the same ideals, beliefs, and views.

Cultural competence can be defined as the ability to understand, honor, and respect the beliefs, lifestyles, attitudes, and behaviors of others.[16] Cultural competency goes beyond being "politically correct." As health care professionals, we must develop a deeper sense of understanding of how ethnicity, language, cultural beliefs, and lifestyles affect the interviewing, screening, and healing process.

Minority Groups

The need for culturally competent physical therapy care has come about, in part, because of the rising number of minorities in the United States. Groups other than "white" or "Caucasian" counted as race/ethnicity by the U.S. Census are listed in Box 2-2.

Some minority groups are no longer a "minority" in the United States because of changing demographics. According to the U.S. Census Bureau, 31% of the U.S. population belongs to a racial/ethnic minority group. By the year 2050, Caucasians will represent only 52% of the population (currently at approximately 75%).

Hispanic Americans will comprise nearly a quarter of the American population (currently 12.5% and expected to reach 24% by 2050). African Americans make up 12.5% of the population (as of 1990). This will increase to approximately 15%.

Asian/Pacific Island Americans will make up almost 10% in 2050.[17,18]

Cultural Competence in the Screening Process

Clients from a racial/ethnic background may have unique health care concerns and risk factors. It is important to learn as much as possible about each minority group served (Case Example 2-1). Clients who are members of a cultural minority are more likely to be geographically isolated and/or underserved in the area of health services. Risk-factor assessment is very important, especially if there is no primary care physician involved.

BOX 2-2 ▼ Racial/Ethnic Designations

Some individuals may consider themselves "multiracial" based on the combination of their father and mother's racial background. The categories below are used by the U.S. government for census-taking but do not recognize multiple racial combinations. This grouping was adopted for use by the APTA in the *Guide to Physical Therapist Practice*, ed 2 (Revised), 2003.

American Indian/Alaska Native
Asian
Black/African American
Hispanic or Latino (of any race)
Native Hawaiian/Pacific Islander
White/Caucasian

CASE EXAMPLE 2-1   Cultural Competency

A 25-year-old African American woman who is also a physical therapist came to a physical therapy clinic with severe right knee joint pain. She could not recall any traumatic injury but reported hiking 3 days ago in the Rocky Mountains with her brother. She lives in New York City and just returned yesterday.

A general screening examination revealed the following information:

- Frequent urination for the last 2 days
- Stomach pain (related to stress of visiting family and traveling)
- Fatigue (attributed to busy clinic schedule and social activities)
- Past medical history: Acute pneumonia, age 11
- Nonsmoker, social drinker (1-3 drinks/week)

What Are the Red-Flag Signs/Symptoms? How Do You Handle a Case like This?

- Young age
- African American

With the combination of red flags (change in altitude, increased fatigue, increased urination, and stomach pain) there could be a possible systemic cause, not just life's stressors as attributed by the client. The physical therapist treated the symptoms locally but not aggressively and referred the client immediately to a medical doctor.

Result: The client was subsequently diagnosed with sickle cell anemia. Medical treatment was instituted along with client education and a rehab program for local control of symptoms and a preventive strengthening program.

Communication style may be unique from group to group. For example, Native Americans may not volunteer information, requiring additional questions in the interview or screening process. Courtesy is very important in Asian cultures. Clients may act polite, smiling and nodding, but not really understand the clinician's questions. English as a second language (ESL) may be a factor. The client may not understand the therapist's questions, but will not show his or her confusion and will not ask the therapist to repeat the question.

In addition to the guidelines in Box 2-1, Box 2-3 offers some "Dos" in a cultural context for the physical therapy or screening interview.

BOX 2-3 ▲ Cultural Competency in a Screening Interview

- Wait until the client has finished speaking before interrupting or asking questions
- Allow "wait time" (time gaps) for some cultures (e.g., Native Americans, ESL)
- Be aware that eye contact, body-space boundaries, even handshaking may differ from culture to culture

When Working with an Interpreter:

- Choosing an interpreter is important. A competent medical interpreter is familiar with medical terminology, cultural customs, and the policies of the health care facility in which the client is receiving care
- There may be problems if the interpreter is younger than the client; in some cultures it is considered rude for a younger person to give instructions to an elder
- In some cultures (e.g., Muslim) information about the client's diagnosis and condition are relayed to the head of the household who then makes the decision to share the news with the client or other family members
- Listen to the interpreter but direct your gaze and eye contact to the client (as appropriate; sustained direct eye contact may be considered aggressive behavior in some cultures)
- Watch the client's body language while listening to him or her speak
- Head nodding and smiling do not necessarily mean understanding or agreement; when in doubt, always ask the interpreter to clarify any communication
- Keep comments, instructions, and questions simple and short. Do not expect the interpreter to remember everything you said and relay it exactly as you said it to the client if you do not keep it short and simple
- Avoid using medical terms or professional jargon

Resources

Learning about cultural preferences helps therapists become familiar with factors that could impact the screening process. More information on cultural competency is available to help therapists develop a deeper understanding of culture and cultural differences, especially in health and health care.[3,19,20]

The Health Policy and Administration Section of the APTA has a Cross-Cultural Special Interest Group (SIG) with information available regarding international physical therapy, international health-related issues, and physical therapists working in third world countries or with ethnic groups.[21] The APTA also has a department dedicated to Minority and International Affairs with additional information available online regarding cultural competence.[16]

The U.S. Department of Health and Human Services' Office of Minority Health has published national standards for culturally and linguistically appropriate services (CLAS) in health care. These are available on the Office of Minority Health's Web site (www.omhrc.gov/clas).[22]

Resources on the language and cultural needs of minorities, immigrants, refugees, and other diverse populations seeking health care is available, including strategies for overcoming language and cultural barriers to health care.[23] For more specific information about the Muslim culture, visit The Council on American-Islamic Relations[24] or the Muslim American Society.[25,26] The APTA also offers a wide range of information on cultural competence.[27] The Gay and Lesbian Medical Association (GLMA) offers publications on professional competencies in providing a safe clinical environment for Lesbian-Gay-Bisexual-Transgender-Intersex (LGBTI) health (www.glma.org> clinic on Publications> scroll down to Professional Competency in LGBTI Health).

Information on laws and legal issues affecting minority health care are also available. Best practices in culturally competent health services are provided, including summary recommendations for medical interpreters, written materials, and cultural competency of health professionals.[27]

▲ THE SCREENING INTERVIEW

The therapist will use two main interviewing tools during the screening process. The first is the Family/Personal History form as presented in Fig. 2-2. With the client's responses on this form and/or the client's chief complaint in hand, the interview begins.

The overall client interview is referred to in this text as the Core Interview (see Fig. 2-3). The Core Interview as presented in this chapter gives the therapist a guideline for asking questions about the present illness and chief complaint. Screening questions may be interspersed throughout the Core Interview as seems appropriate, based on each client's answers to questions.

There may be times when additional screening questions are asked at the end of the Core Interview or even on a subsequent date at a follow-up appointment. Specific series of questions related to a single symptom (e.g., dizziness, heart palpitations, night pain) or event (e.g., assault, work history, breast examination) are included throughout the text and compiled in the Appendix for the clinician to use easily.

Interviewing Techniques

An organized interview format assists the therapist in obtaining a complete and accurate database. Using the same outline with each client ensures that all pertinent information related to previous medical history and current medical problem(s) is included. This information is especially important when correlating the subjective data with objective findings from the physical examination.

The most basic skills required for a physical therapy interview include:

- Open-ended questions
- Closed-ended questions
- Funnel sequence or technique
- Paraphrasing technique

Open-Ended and Closed-Ended Questions

Beginning an interview with an *open-ended question* (i.e., questions that elicit more than a one-word response) is advised, even though this gives the client the opportunity to control and direct the interview.

Initiating an interview with the open-ended directive, "Tell me why you are here," can potentially elicit more information in a relatively short (5- to 15-minute) period than a steady stream of

closed-ended questions requiring a "yes" or "no" type of answer (Table 2-1). Moving from the open-ended line of questions to the closed-ended questions is referred to as the *funnel technique* or *funnel sequence*.

Each question format has advantages and limitations. The use of open-ended questions to initiate the interview may allow the client to control the interview (Case Example 2-2), but it can also prevent a false-positive or false-negative response that would otherwise be elicited by starting with closed-ended (yes or no) questions.

False responses elicited by closed-ended questions may develop from the client's attempt to please the health care provider or to comply with what the client believes is the correct response or expectation.

Closed-ended questions tend to be more impersonal and may set an impersonal tone for the relationship between the client and the therapist. These questions are limited by the restrictive nature of the information received so that the client may respond only to the category in question and may omit vital, but seemingly unrelated, information.

Use of the funnel sequence to obtain as much information as possible through the open-ended format first (before moving on to the more restrictive but clarifying "yes" or "no" type of questions at the end) can establish an effective forum for trust between the client and the therapist.

FOLLOW-UP QUESTIONS

The funnel sequence is aided by the use of *follow-up* questions, referred to as *FUPs* in the text. Beginning with one or two open-ended questions in each section, the interviewer may follow up with a series of closed-ended questions, which are listed in the Core Interview presented later in this chapter.

For example, after an open-ended question such as: "How does rest affect the pain or symptoms?" the therapist can follow up with clarifying questions such as:

TABLE 2-1 ▼ Interviewing Techniques

Open-ended questions	Closed-ended questions
1. How does bed rest affect your back pain?	1. Do you have any pain after lying in bed all night?
2. Tell me how you cope with stress and what kinds of stressors you encounter on a daily basis.	2. Are you under any stress?
3. What makes the pain (better) worse?	3. Is the pain relieved by food?
4. How did you sleep last night?	4. Did you sleep well last night?

CASE EXAMPLE 2-2   Monologue

You are interviewing a client for the first time, and she tells you, "The pain in my hip started 12 years ago, when I was a waitress standing on my feet 10 hours a day. It seems to bother me most when I am having premenstrual symptoms.

"My left leg is longer than my right leg, and my hip hurts when the scars from my bunionectomy ache. This pain occurs with any changes in the weather. I have a bleeding ulcer that bothers me, and the pain keeps me awake at night. I dislocated my shoulder 2 years ago, but I can lift weights now without any problems." She continues her monologue, and you feel out of control and unsure how to proceed.

This scenario was taken directly from a clinical experience and represents what we call "an organ recital." In this situation the client provides detailed information regarding all previously experienced illnesses and symptoms, which may or may not be related to the current problem.

How Do You Redirect This Interview?

A client who takes control of the interview by telling the therapist about every ache and pain of every friend and neighbor can be rechanneled effectively by interrupting the client with a polite statement such as:

Follow-Up Questions

- I'm beginning to get an idea of the nature of your problem. Let me ask you some other questions.

At this point the interviewer may begin to use closed-ended questions (i.e., questions requiring the answer to be "yes" or "no") in order to characterize the symptoms more clearly.

Follow-Up Questions

- Are your symptoms aggravated or relieved by any activities? If yes, what?
- How has this problem affected your daily life at work or at home?
- How has it affected your ability to care for yourself without assistance (e.g., dress, bathe, cook, drive)?

PARAPHRASING TECHNIQUE

A useful interviewing skill that can assist in synthesizing and integrating the information obtained during questioning is the *paraphrasing technique*. When using this technique, the interviewer repeats information presented by the client.

This technique can assist in fostering effective, accurate communication between the health care recipient and the health care provider. For example, once a client has responded to the question, "What makes you feel better?" the therapist can paraphrase the reply by saying, "You've told me that the pain is relieved by such and such, is that right? What other activities or treatment brings you relief from your pain or symptoms?"

If the therapist cannot paraphrase what the client has said, or if the meaning of the client's response is unclear, then the therapist can ask for clarification by requesting an example of what the person is saying.

Interviewing Tools

With the emergence of evidence-based practice, therapists are required to identify problems, to quantify symptoms (e.g., pain), and to demonstrate the effectiveness of intervention.

Documenting the effectiveness of intervention is called *outcomes management*. Using standardized tests, functional tools, or questionnaires to relate pain, strength, or range of motion to a quantifiable scale is defined as *outcome measures*. The information obtained from such measures is then compared with the functional outcomes of treatment to assess the effectiveness of those interventions.

In this way therapists are gathering information about the most appropriate treatment progression for a specific diagnosis. Such a database shows the efficacy of physical therapy intervention and provides data for use with insurance companies in requesting reimbursement for service.

Along with impairment-based measures therapists must use reliable and valid functional outcome measures. No single instrument or method of assessment can be considered the best under all circumstances.

Pain assessment is often a central focus of the therapist's interview, so for the clinician interested

in quantifying pain, some way to quantify and describe pain is necessary. There are numerous pain assessment scales designed to determine the quality and location of pain or the percentage of impairment or functional levels associated with pain (see further discussion in Chapter 3).

There are a wide variety of anatomic region, function, or disease-specific assessment tools available. Each test has a specific focus—whether to assess pain levels, level of balance, risk for falls, functional status, disability, quality of life, and so on.

Some tools focus on a particular kind of problem such as activity limitations or disability in people with low back pain (e.g., Oswestry Disability Questionnaire,[28] Quebec Back Pain Disability Scale,[29] Duffy-Rath Questionnaire.[30] The Simple Shoulder Test,[31] and the Disabilities of the Arm, Shoulder, and Hand Questionnaire (DASH)[32] may be used to assess physical function of the shoulder. Nurses often use the PQRST mnemonic to help identify underlying pathology or pain (see Box 3-3).

Other examples of specific tests include the
• Visual Analogue Scale (VAS; see Figure 3-6)
• Verbal Descriptor Scale (see Box 3-1)
• McGill Pain Questionnaire (see Fig. 3-11)
• Pain Impairment Rating Scale (PAIRS)
• Likert Scale
• Alzheimer's Discomfort Rating Scale

A more complete evaluation of client function can be obtained by pairing disease- or region-specific instruments with the Short-Form Health Survey (SF-36 Version 2).[33,34] The SF-36 is a well-established questionnaire used to measure the client's perception of his or her health status. It is a generic measure, as opposed to one that targets a specific age, disease, or treatment group. It includes eight different subscales of functional status that are scored in two general components: physical and mental.

An even shorter survey form (the SF-12 Version 2) contains only 1 page and takes about 2 minutes to complete. There is a Low-Back SF-36 Physical Functioning survey[35] and also a similar general health survey designed for use with children (SF-10 for children). All of these tools are available at: www.sf-36.org/tools/sf36.shtml. To see a sample of the SF-36 v.2 go to www.sf-36.org/demos/SF-36v2.html.

The initial Family/Personal History form (see Fig. 2-2) gives the therapist some idea of the client's previous medical history (personal and family), medical testing, and current general health status. Make a special note of the box inside the form labeled "Therapists." This is for liability purposes. Anyone who has ever completed a deposition for a legal case will agree it is often difficult to remember the details of a case brought to trial years later.

A client may insist that a condition was (or was not) present on the first day of the examination. Without a baseline to document initial findings, this is often difficult, if not, impossible to dispute. The client must sign or initial the form once it is complete. The therapist is advised to sign and date it to verify that the information was discussed with the client.

Resources

The Family/Personal History form presented in this chapter is just one example of a basic intake form. The *Guide to Physical Therapist Practice*[36] provides an excellent template for both inpatient and outpatient histories (see Appendix 6). Other commercially available forms have been developed for a wide range of prescreening assessments.[37]

Therapists may modify the information collected from these examples depending on individual differences in client base and specialty areas served. For example, a hospital or institution accreditation agencies such as Commission on Accreditation of Rehabilitation Facilities (CARF) and the Joint Commission on Accreditation of Health Care Organizations (JCAHO) may require the use of their own forms.

An orthopedic-based facility or a sports-medicine center may want to include questions on the intake form concerning current level of fitness and the use of orthopedic devices used, such as orthotics, splints, or braces. Therapists working with the geriatric population may want more information regarding current medications prescribed or levels of independence in activities of daily living.

The Review of Systems (see Box 4-17; see also Appendix D-5), which provides a helpful chart of signs and symptoms characteristic of each visceral system, can be used along with the Family/Personal History form. The *Guide* also provides both an outpatient and an inpatient documentation template for similar purposes (see *Guide*, Appendix 6).

A teaching tool with practice worksheets is available to help students and clinicians learn how to document findings from the history, systems review, tests and measures, problems statements, and subjective and objective information using both the SOAP note format and the Patient/Client Management model shown in Fig. 1-4.[38]

▲ SUBJECTIVE EXAMINATION

The subjective examination is usually thought of as the "client interview." It is intended to provide a database of information that is important in determining the need for medical referral or the direction for physical therapy intervention. Risk-factor assessment is conducted throughout the subjective and objective examinations.

Key Components of the Subjective Examination

The subjective examination must be conducted in a complete and organized manner. It includes several components, all gathered through the interview process. The order of flow may vary from therapist to therapist and clinic to clinic (Fig. 2-1). The traditional medical interview begins with family/personal history and then addresses the

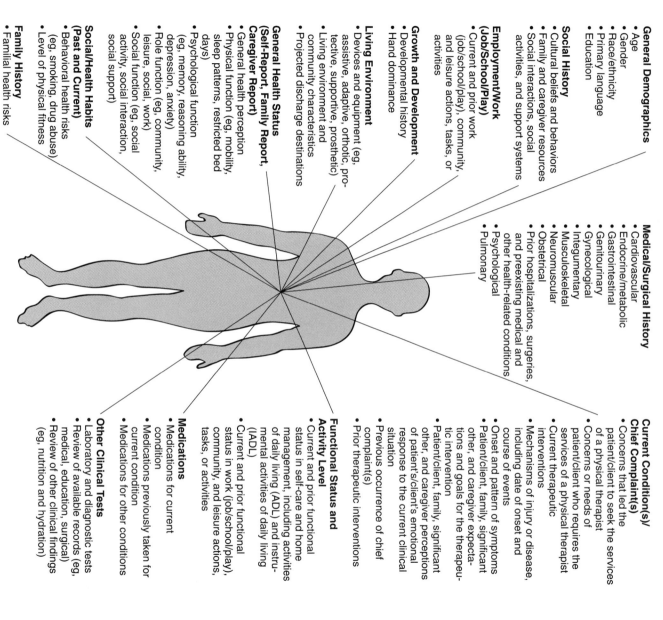

General Demographics
• Age
• Gender
• Race/ethnicity
• Primary language
• Education

Social History
• Cultural beliefs and behaviors
• Family and caregiver resources
• Social interactions, social activities, and support systems

Employment/Work (Job/School/Play)
• Current and prior work (job/school/play), community, and leisure actions, tasks, or activities

Growth and Development
• Developmental history
• Hand dominance

Living Environment
• Devices and equipment (eg, assistive, adaptive, orthotic, protective, supportive, prosthetic)
• Living environment and community characteristics
• Projected discharge destinations

General Health Status (Self-Report, Family Report, Caregiver Report)
• General health perception
• Physical function (eg, mobility, sleep patterns, restricted bed days)
• Psychological function (eg, memory, reasoning ability, depression, anxiety)
• Role function (eg, community, leisure, social, work)
• Social function (eg, social activity, social interaction, social support)

Social/Health Habits (Past and Current)
• Behavioral health risks (eg, smoking, drug abuse)
• Level of physical fitness

Family History
• Familial health risks

Medical/Surgical History
• Cardiovascular
• Endocrine/metabolic
• Gastrointestinal
• Genitourinary
• Gynecological
• Integumentary
• Musculoskeletal
• Neuromuscular
• Obstetrical
• Prior hospitalizations, surgeries, and preexisting medical and other health-related conditions
• Psychological
• Pulmonary

Current Condition(s)/Chief Complaint(s)
• Concerns that led the patient/client to seek the services of a physical therapist
• Concerns or needs of patient/client who requires the services of a physical therapist
• Current therapeutic interventions
• Mechanisms of injury or disease, including date of onset and course of events
• Onset and pattern of symptoms
• Patient/client, family, significant other, and caregiver expectations and goals for the therapeutic intervention
• Patient/client, family, significant other, and caregiver perceptions of patient's/client's emotional response to the current clinical situation
• Previous occurrence of chief complaint(s)
• Prior therapeutic interventions

Functional Status and Activity Level
• Current and prior functional status in self-care and home management, including activities of daily living (ADL) and instrumental activities of daily living (IADL)
• Current and prior functional status in work (job/school/play), community, and leisure actions, tasks, or activities

Medications
• Medications for current condition
• Medications previously taken for current condition
• Medications for other conditions

Other Clinical Tests
• Laboratory and diagnostic tests
• Review of available records (eg, medical, education, surgical)
• Review of other clinical findings (eg, nutrition and hydration)

Fig. 2-1 • Types of data that may be generated from a client history. In this model, data about the visceral systems is reflected in the Medical/Surgical history. The data collected in this portion of the patient/client history is not the same as information collected during the Review of Systems (ROS). It has been recommended that the ROS component be added to this figure.[39] (From *Guide to Physical Therapist Practice,* ed 2 [Revised], 2003.)

chief complaint. Therapists may find it works better to conduct the Core Interview and then ask additional questions after looking over the client's responses on the Family/Personal History form.

In a screening model, the therapist is advised to have the client complete the Family/Personal History form before the client-therapist interview. The therapist then quickly reviews the history form, making mental note of any red-flag histories. This information may be helpful during the subjective and objective portions of the examination. Information gathered will include:

- Family/Personal History (see Fig. 2-2)
  - Age
  - Gender
  - Race and Ethnicity
  - Past Medical History
  - General Health
  - Past Medical and Surgical History
  - Clinical Tests
  - Work and Living Environment
- The Core Interview (see Fig. 2-3)
  - History of Present Illness
    - Chief Complaint
    - Pain and Symptom Assessment
    - Medical Treatment and Medications
    - Current Level of Fitness
    - Sleep-related History
    - Stress (Emotional/Psychologic screen)
    - Final Questions
  - Associated Signs and Symptoms
  - Special Questions
- Review of Systems

Family/Personal History

It is unnecessary and probably impossible to complete the entire subjective examination on the first day. Many clinics or health care facilities use some type of initial intake form before the client's first visit with the therapist.

The Family/Personal History form presented here (Fig. 2-2) is one example of an initial intake form. Throughout the rest of this chapter, the text discussion will follow the order of items on the Family/Personal History form. The reader is encouraged to follow along in the text while referring to the form.

As mentioned, the *Guide* also offers a form for use in an outpatient setting and a separate form for use in an inpatient setting. This component of the subjective examination can elicit valuable data regarding the client's family history of disease and personal lifestyle, including working environment and health habits.

The therapist must keep the client's family history in perspective. Very few people have a clean and unencumbered family history. It would be unusual for a person to say that nobody in the family ever had heart disease, cancer, or some other major health issue.

A check mark in multiple boxes on the history form does not necessarily mean the person will have the same problems. Onset of disease at an early age in a first-generation family member (sibling, child, parent) can be a sign of genetic disorders and is usually considered a red flag. But an aunt who died of colon cancer at age 75 is not as predictive.

A family history brings to light not only shared genetic traits but also shared environment, shared values, shared behavior, and shared culture. Factors such as nutrition, attitudes toward exercise and physical activity, and other modifiable risk factors are usually the focus of primary and secondary prevention.

Resources

The U.S. Department of Health and Human Services has developed a computerized tool to help people learn more about their family health history. "My Family Health Portrait" is available online at: www.hhs.gov/familyhistory/download. html.

The download is free and helps identify common diseases that may run in the family. The therapist can encourage each client to use this tool to create and print out a graphic representation of his or her family's generational health disorders. This information should be shared with the primary health care provider for further screening and evaluation.

The National Library of Medicine also offers a variety of interactive questionnaires, quizzes, and calculations to assess health status: www.nlm.nih.gov/medlineplus/interactivetools.

Follow-Up Questions (FUPs)

Once the client has completed the Family/Personal History intake form, the clinician can then follow up with appropriate questions based on any "yes" selections made by the client. Beware of the client who circles one column of either all "Yeses" or all "Nos." Take the time to carefully review this section with the client. The therapist may want to ask some individual questions whenever illiteracy is suspected or observed.

Each clinical situation requires slight adaptations or alterations to the interview. These modifications, in turn, affect the depth and range of questioning. For example, a client who has pain

FAMILY/PERSONAL HISTORY

Date: _____

Client's Name: _____ DOB: _____ Age: _____

Race/ethnicity: ☐ American Indian/Alaska Native ☐ Asian

☐ Black/African American ☐ Caucasian/white

☐ Hispanic/Latino ☐ Native Hawaiian/Pacific Islander

☐ Multiracial ☐ Other/unknown

Language: ☐ English understood ☐ Interpreter needed ☐ Primary language: _____

Medical Diagnosis: _____

Physician: _____ Date of surgery (if any): _____ Date of onset: _____

Past Medical History

Have you or any immediate family member (parent, sibling, child) ever been told you have:

(Do **NOT** complete) **For the therapist:**

		Relation to Client	Date of Onset	Current Status
Circle one:				
• Allergies	Yes No			
• Angina or chest pain	Yes No			
• Anxiety/Panic attacks	Yes No			
• Arthritis	Yes No			
• Asthma, hay fever, or other breathing problems	Yes No			
• Cancer	Yes No			
• Chemical dependency (alcohol/drugs)	Yes No			
• Cirrhosis/liver disease	Yes No			
• Depression	Yes No			
• Diabetes	Yes No			
• Eating disorder (bulimia, anorexia)	Yes No			
• Headaches	Yes No			
• Heart attack	Yes No			
• Hemophilia/slow healing	Yes No			
• High cholesterol	Yes No			
• Hypertension or high blood pressure	Yes No			
• Kidney disease/stones	Yes No			
• Multiple sclerosis	Yes No			
• Osteoporosis	Yes No			
• Stroke	Yes No			
• Tuberculosis	Yes No			
• Other (please describe)	Yes No			

Therapists: Use this space to record baseline information. This is important in case something changes in the client's status. You are advised to record the date and sign or initial this form for documentation and liability purposes, indicating that you have reviewed this form with the client. You may want to have the client sign and date it as well.

Fig. 2-2 • Sample of a Family/Personal History Form

Personal History

Have you ever had:

• Anemia	Yes	No	• Chronic bronchitis	Yes	No
• Epilepsy/seizures	Yes	No	• Emphysema	Yes	No
• Fibromyalgia/myofascial pain syndrome	Yes	No	• GERD	Yes	No
			• Gout	Yes	No
• Hepatitis/jaundice	Yes	No	• Guillain-Barré Syndrome	Yes	No
• Joint replacement	Yes	No	• Hypoglycemia	Yes	No
• Parkinson's disease	Yes	No	• Peripheral vascular disease	Yes	No
• Polio/postpolio	Yes	No	• Pneumonia	Yes	No
• Shortness of breath	Yes	No	• Prostate problems	Yes	No
• Skin problems	Yes	No	• Rheumatic/scarlet fever	Yes	No
• Urinary incontinence (dribbling, leaking)	Yes	No	• Thyroid problems	Yes	No
• Urinary tract infection	Yes	No	• Ulcer/stomach problems	Yes	No
			• Varicose veins	Yes	No

For women:

History of endometriosis	Yes	No
History of pelvic inflammatory disease	Yes	No
Are you/could you be pregnant?	Yes	No
Any trouble with leaking or dribbling urine?	Yes	No
Number of pregnancies _____	Number of live births _____	
Have you ever had a miscarriage/abortion?	Yes	No

General Health

1. I would rate my health as (circle one):   Excellent   Good   Fair   Poor

2. Are you taking any prescription or over-the-counter medications? Yes No
   If yes, please list:

3. Are you taking any nutritional supplements (any kind, including vitamins)? Yes No

4. Have you had any illnesses within the last 3 weeks (e.g., colds, influenza, bladder or kidney infection)? Yes No
   If yes, have you had this before in the last 3 months? Yes No

5. Have you noticed any lumps or thickening of skin or muscle anywhere on your body? Yes No

6. Do you have any sores that have not healed or any changes in size, shape, or color of a wart or mole? Yes No

7. Have you had any unexplained weight gain or loss in the last month? Yes No

8. Do you smoke or chew tobacco? Yes No
   If yes, how many packs/pipes/pouches/sticks a day? _____
   How many months or years? _____

9. I used to smoke/chew but I quit Yes No
   If yes: pack or amount/day _____   Year quit _____

10. I would like to quit smoking/using tobacco Yes No

11. How much alcohol do you drink in the course of a week? (one drink is equal to 1 beer, 1 glass of wine or 1 shot of hard liquor) _____

12. Do you use recreational or street drugs (marijuana, cocaine, crack, meth, amphetamines, or others)? If yes, what, how much, how often? Yes No

13. How much caffeine do you consume daily (including soft drinks, coffee, tea, or chocolate)? _____

14. Are you on any special diet? Yes No

15. Do you have (or have you recently had) any of these problems:

Fig. 2-2 • cont'd

Medical/Surgical History

☐ Blood in urine, stool, vomit, mucous
☐ Dizziness, fainting, blackouts
☐ Fever, chills, sweats (day or night)
☐ Nausea, vomiting, loss of appetite
☐ Changes in bowel or bladder
☐ Throbbing sensation/pain in belly or anywhere else
☐ Skin rash or other changes

☐ Cough
☐ Dribbling or leaking urine
☐ Heart palpitations or fluttering
☐ Numbness or tingling
☐ Swelling or lumps anywhere
☐ Problems seeing or hearing
☐ Unusual fatigue, drowsiness

☐ Difficulty swallowing/speaking
☐ Memory loss
☐ Confusion
☐ Sudden weakness
☐ Trouble sleeping
☐ None of these

1. Have you ever been treated with chemotherapy, radiation therapy, biotherapy, or brachytherapy (radiation implants)?   Yes   No
   If yes, please describe:

2. Have you had any x-rays, sonograms, computed tomography (CT) scans, or magnetic resonance imaging (MRI) or other imaging done recently?   Yes   No
   If yes, what?   When?   Results?

3. Have you had any laboratory work done recently (urinalysis or blood tests)?   Yes   No
   If yes, what?   When?   Results (if known)?

4. Any other clinical tests?   Yes   No
   Please describe:

5. Please list any operations that you have ever had and the date(s):   Yes   No
   Operation   Date

6. Do you have a pacemaker, transplanted organ, joint replacement, breast implants, or any other implants?   Yes   No
   If yes, please describe:

Work/Living Environment

1. What is your job or occupation?
2. Military service: (When and where):
3. Does your work involve:
   [ ] Prolonged sitting (e.g., desk, computer, driving)
   [ ] Prolonged standing (e.g., equipment operator, sale clerk)
   [ ] Prolonged walking (e.g., mill worker, delivery service)
   [ ] Use of large or small equipment (e.g., telephone, forklift, computer, drill press, cash register)
   [ ] Lifting, bending, twisting, climbing, turning
   [ ] Exposure to chemicals, pesticides, toxins, or gases
   [ ] Other: please describe
   [ ] Not applicable; none of these

4. Do you use any special supports:
   [ ] Back brace, corset
   [ ] Back cushion, neck cushion
   [ ] Other kind of brace or support for any body part
   [ ] None; not applicable

History of falls:

   [ ] In the past year, I have had no falls.
   [ ] I have just started to lose my balance/fall.
   [ ] I fall occasionally.
   [ ] I fall frequently (more than two times during the past 6 months)
   [ ] Certain factors make me cautious (e.g., curbs, ice, stairs, getting in and out of the tub).

I live:

   [ ] Alone [ ] With family, spouse, partner
   [ ] Nursing home [ ] Assisted Living [ ] Other _____

For the physical therapist:

Vital Signs
Resting pulse rate:
Respirations:
Blood pressure: 1st reading   2nd reading

Oral temperature:
Oxygen saturation:

Position: Sitting   Standing   Extremity: Right   Left

Fig. 2-2 • cont'd

associated with a traumatic anterior shoulder dislocation and who has no history of other disease is unlikely to require in-depth questioning to rule out systemic origins of pain.

Conversely, a woman with no history of trauma but with a previous history of breast cancer who is self-referred to the therapist without a previous medical examination and who complains of shoulder pain should be interviewed more thoroughly. The simple question "How will the answers to the questions I am asking permit me to help the client?" can serve as a guide to you.[40]

Continued questioning may occur both during the objective examination and during treatment. In fact, the therapist is encouraged to carry on a continuous dialogue during the objective examination, both as an educational tool (i.e., reporting findings and mentioning possible treatment alternatives) and as a method of reducing any apprehension on the part of the client. This open communication may bring to light other important information.

The client may wonder about the extensiveness of the interview, thinking, for example, "Why is the therapist asking questions about bowel function when my primary concern relates to back pain?"

The therapist may need to make a qualifying statement to the client regarding the need for such detailed information. For example, questions about bowel function to rule out stomach or intestinal involvement (which can refer pain to the back) may seem to be unrelated to the client but make sense when the therapist explains the possible connection between back pain and systemic disease.

Throughout the questioning, record both positive and negative findings in the subjective and objective reports in order to correlate information when making an initial assessment of the client's problem. Efforts should be made to quantify all information by frequency, intensity, duration, and exact location (including length, breadth, depth, and anatomic location).

Age and Aging

Age is the most common primary risk factor for disease, illness, and comorbidities. It is the number one risk factor for cancer. The age of a client is an important variable to consider when evaluating the underlying neuromusculoskeletal pathologic condition and when screening for medical disease.

Age-related changes in metabolism increase the risk for drug accumulation in older adults. Older adults are more sensitive to both the therapeutic and toxic effects of many drugs, especially analgesics.

Functional liver tissue diminishes and hepatic blood flow decreases with aging, thus impairing the liver's capacity to break down and convert drugs. Therefore aging is a risk factor for a wide range of signs and symptoms associated with drug-induced toxicities.

It is helpful to be aware of NMS and systemic conditions that tend to occur during particular decades of life. Signs and symptoms associated with that condition take on greater significance when age is considered. For example, prostate problems usually occur in men after the fourth decade (age 40+). A past medical history of prostate cancer in a 55-year-old man with sciatica of unknown cause should raise the suspicions of the therapist. Table 2-2 provides some of the age-related systemic and neuromusculoskeletal pathologic conditions.

Epidemiologists report that the U.S. population is beginning to age at a rapid pace, with the first baby boomers turning 65 in 2011. Between now and the year 2030, the number of individuals age 65 and older will double, reaching 70.3 million and making up a larger proportion of the entire population (increasing from 13% in 2000 to 20% in 2030).[41]

Of particular interest is the explosive growth expected among adults age 85 and older. This group is at increased risk for disease and disability. Their numbers are expected to grow from 4.3 million in the year 2000 to at least 19.4 million in 2050. As mentioned previously the racial and ethnic makeup of the older population will change dramatically as well, creating a more diverse population of older Americans.[42]

Human aging is best characterized as the progressive constriction of each organ system's homeostatic reserve. This decline, often referred to as "homeostenosis," begins in the third decade and is gradual, linear, and variable among individuals. Each organ system's decline is independent of changes in other organ systems and is influenced by diet, environment, and personal habits.

Dementia increases the risk of falls and fracture. Delirium is a common complication of hip fracture that increases the length of hospital stay and mortality. Older clients take a disproportionate number of medications, predisposing them to adverse drug reactions related to aging changes in pharmacokinetics and pharmacodynamics.[43]

An abrupt change or sudden decline in any system or function is always due to disease and not to "normal aging." In the absence of disease the decline in homeostatic reserve should cause no symptoms and impose no restrictions on activities

TABLE 2-2 ▼ Some Age-Related Medical Conditions

Diagnosis	Gender	Age in (years)
Neuromusculoskeletal		
Guillain-Barré syndrome		Any age; history of infection/alcoholism
Multiple sclerosis		15-50
Rotator cuff degeneration		30+
Spinal stenosis	Men > women	60+
Tietze's syndrome		Before 40, including children
Costochondritis	Women > men	40+
Neurogenic claudication		40-60+
Systemic		
AIDS/HIV	Men > women	20-49
Buerger's disease	Men > women	20-40 (smokers)
Abdominal aortic aneurysm	(hypertensive) Men > women	40-70
Cancer		
Breast cancer	Women > men	45-70 (peak incidence)
Hodgkin's disease	Men > women	20-40, 50-60
Osteoid osteoma (benign)	Men > women	10-20
Pancreatic carcinoma	Men > women	50-70
Skin cancer	Men = women	Rarely before puberty
Gallstones	Women > men	40+
Gout	Men > women	40-59
Gynecologic conditions	Women	20-45 (peak incidence)
Paget's disease	Men > women	60+
Prostatitis	Men	40+
Primary biliary cirrhosis	Women > men	40-60
Reiter's syndrome	Men > women	20-40
Renal tuberculosis	Men > women	20-40
Rheumatic fever	Girls > boys	4-9; 18-30
Shingles		60+
Spontaneous pneumothorax	Men > women	20-40
Systemic backache		45+
Thyroiditis	Women > Men	30-50
Vascular claudication		40-60+

of daily living regardless of age. In short, "old people are sick because they are sick, not because they are old."

The onset of a new disease in older people generally affects the most vulnerable organ system, which often is different from the newly diseased organ system and explains why disease presentation is so atypical in this population. For example, at presentation, less than one fourth of older clients with hyperthyroidism have the classic triad of goiter, tremor, and exophthalmos; more likely symptoms are atrial fibrillation, confusion, depression, syncope, and weakness.

Because the "weakest links" with aging are so often the brain, lower urinary tract, or cardiovascular or musculoskeletal system, a limited number of presenting symptoms predominate no matter what the underlying disease. These include:

- Acute confusion
- Depression
- Falling
- Incontinence
- Syncope

The corollary is equally important: The organ system usually associated with a particular symptom is less likely to be the cause of that symptom in older individuals than in younger ones. For example, acute confusion in older adults is less often due to a new brain lesion, incontinence is less often due to a bladder disorder; falling, to a neuropathy; or syncope, to heart disease.

Gender

In the screening process, gender may be an important issue (Case Example 2-3). To some extent, men and women experience some diseases that are

CASE EXAMPLE 2-3 Gender as a Risk Factor

Clinical Presentation: A 45-year-old woman presents with midthoracic pain that radiates to the interscapular area on the right. There are two red flags recognizable immediately: age and back pain. Gender can be a red flag and should be considered during the evaluation.

Referred pain from the gallbladder is represented in Fig. 9-10 as the light pink areas. If the client had a primary pain pattern with gastrointestinal symptoms, she would have gone to see a medical doctor first.

Physical therapists see clients with referred pain patterns, often before the disease has progressed enough to be accompanied by visceral signs and symptoms. They may come to us from a physician or directly.

Risk-Factor Assessment: Watch for specific risk factors. In this case, look for the five Fs associated with gallstones: fat, fair, forty (or older), female, and flatulent.

Clients with gallbladder disease do not always present this way, but the risk increases with each additional risk factor. Other risk factors for gallbladder disease include:

- Age: increasing incidence with increasing age
- Obesity

- Diabetes mellitus
- Multiparity (multiple pregnancies and births)

Women are at increased risk of gallstones because of their exposure to estrogen. Estrogen increases the hepatic secretion of cholesterol and decreases the secretion of bile acids. Additionally, during pregnancy, the gallbladder empties more slowly, causing stasis and increasing the chances for cholesterol crystals to precipitate.

For any woman over 40 presenting with midthoracic, scapular or right shoulder pain, consider gallbladder disease as a possible underlying etiology. To screen for systemic disease, look for known risk factors and ask about:

Associated Signs and Symptoms: When the disease advances, gastrointestinal distress may be reported. This is why it is always important to ask clients if they are having any symptoms of any kind anywhere else in the body. The report of recurrent nausea, flatulence, and food intolerances points to the gastrointestinal system and a need for medical attention.

---

different from each other. When they have the same disease, the age at onset, clinical presentation, and response to treatment is often different.

MALE GENDER

It may be appropriate to ask some specific gender-based screening questions. A list of gender-based questions is provided in Chapter 14 (see also Appendices B-21 and B-32). Taking a sexual history (see Appendix B-29) may be appropriate at some point during the episode of care.

For example, the presentation of joint pain accompanied by (or a recent history of) skin lesions in an otherwise healthy, young adult raises the suspicion of a sexually transmitted infection (STI). Being able to recognize STIs is helpful in the clinic. The therapist who recognized the client presenting with joint pain of "unknown cause" and also demonstrating signs of an STI may help bring the correct diagnosis to light sooner than later. Chronic

pelvic or low back pain of unknown cause may be linked to incest or sexual assault.

The therapist may need to ask men about prostate health (e.g., history of prostatitis, benign prostatic hypertrophy, prostate cancer) or about a history of testicular cancer. In some cases, a sexual history (see Appendix B-29) may be helpful. Many men with a history of prostate problems are incontinent. Routinely screening for this condition may bring to light the need for intervention.

Men and Osteoporosis In an awkward twist of reverse gender bias, many men are not receiving intervention for osteoporosis. In fact the overall prevalence of osteoporosis among men of all ages remains unknown, with ranges from 20% to 36% reported in the literature.[44] Osteoporosis is prevalent but poorly documented in men in long-term care facilities.[45]

Men have a higher mortality rate after fracture compared with women.[46] Thirty percent of older men who suffer a hip fracture will die within a year

of that fracture—double the rate for older adult women. Only 1.1% of the men brought to the hospital for a serious fracture ever receive a bone density test to evaluate their overall risk. Only 1% to 5% of men discharged from the hospital following hip fracture are treated for osteoporosis. This is compared to 27% or more for women.[47,48]

Keeping this information in mind and watching for risk factors of osteoporosis (see Fig. 11-8) can guide the therapist in recognizing the need to screen for osteoporosis in men and women.

FEMALE GENDER

According to the Health Resources and Services Administration (HRSA), women today are more likely than men to die of heart disease, and women between the ages of 26 and 49 are nearly twice as likely to experience serious mental illness as men in the same age group.[49]

Women have a unique susceptibility to the neurotoxic effects of alcohol. Fewer drinks with less alcohol content have a greater physiologic impact on women compared to men. Women may be at greater risk of alcohol-induced brain injury than men, suggesting medical management of alcoholism in women may require a different approach from that for men.[50]

Sixty-two percent of American women are overweight and 33% are obese. Lung cancer caused an estimated 27% of cancer deaths among women in 2004, followed by breast cancer (15%) and cancer of the colon and rectum (10%).[51]

These are just a few of the many ways that female gender represents a unique risk factor requiring special consideration when assessing the overall individual and when screening for medical disease.

Questions about past pregnancies, births and deliveries, past surgical procedures (including abortions), incontinence, endometriosis, history of sexually transmitted or pelvic inflammatory disease(s), and history of osteoporosis and/or compression fractures are important in the assessment of some female clients (see Appendix B-32). The therapist must use common sense and professional judgment in deciding what questions to ask and which follow-up questions are essential.

Life Cycles For women, it may be pertinent to find out where each woman is in the life cycle (Box 2-4) and correlate this information with age, personal and family history, current health, and the presence of any known risk factors. It may be necessary to ask if the current symptoms occur at the

---

BOX 2-4 ▲ Life Cycles of a Woman

- Premenses (before the start of the monthly menstrual cycle; may include early puberty)
- Reproductive Years (including birth, delivery, miscarriage and/or abortion history; this time period may include puberty)
- Perimenopause (usually begins without obvious symptoms in the mid-30s and continues until symptoms of menopause occur)
- Menopausal (may be natural or surgical menopause, i.e., hysterectomy)
- Postmenopausal (cessation of blood flow associated with menstrual cycle)

---

same time each month in relation to the menstrual cycle (e.g., day 10 to 14 during ovulation or at the end of the cycle during the woman's period).

Each phase in the life cycle is really a process that occurs over a number of years. There are no clear distinctions most of the time as one phase blends gradually into the next one.

Perimenopause is a term that was first coined in the 1990s. It refers to the transitional period from physiologic ovulatory menstrual cycles to eventual ovarian shut down. During the perimenopausal time before cessation of menses, signs and symptoms of hormonal changes may become evident. These can include fatigue, memory problems, weight gain, irritability, sleep disruptions, enteric dysfunction, painful intercourse, and change in libido.

Early stages of physiologic perimenopause can occur when a woman is in her mid-30s. Symptoms may not be as obvious in this group of women; infertility may be the most obvious sign in women who have delayed childbirth.[52]

Menopause is an important developmental event in a woman's life. Menopause means pause or cessation of the monthly, referring to the menstrual cycle. The term has been expanded to include approximately 1½ to 2 years before and after cessation of the menstrual cycle.

Menopause is not a disease but rather a complex sequence of biologic aging events, during which the body makes the transition from fertility to a nonreproductive status. The usual age of menopause is between 48 and 54 years. The average age for menopause is still around 51 years of age, although many women stop their periods much earlier.[53]

The pattern of menstrual cessation varies. It may be abrupt, but more often it occurs over 1 to 2 years. Periodic menstrual flow gradually occurs less frequently, becoming irregular and less in amount. Occasional episodes of profuse bleeding

may be interspersed with episodes of scant bleeding.

Menopause is said to have occurred when there have been no menstrual periods for 12 consecutive months. Postmenopause describes the remaining years of a woman's life when the reproductive and menstrual cycles have ended. *Any spontaneous uterine bleeding after this time is abnormal and is considered a red flag.*

The significance of postmenopausal bleeding depends on whether or not the woman is taking hormone replacement therapy (HRT) and which regimen she is using. Women who are on continuous-combined HRT (estrogen in combination with progestin taken without a break) are likely to have irregular spotting until the endometrium atrophies, which takes about 6 months. Medical referral is advised if bleeding persists or suddenly appears after 6 months without bleeding.

Women on sequential HRT (estrogen taken daily or for 25 days each month with progestin taken for 10 days) normally bleed lightly each time the progestin is stopped. Postmenopausal bleeding in women who are not on HRT always requires a medical evaluation.

Within the past decade, removal of the uterus (hysterectomy) has become a common major surgery in the United States. In fact, more than one third of the women in the United States have hysterectomies. The majority of these women have this operation between the ages of 25 and 44 years.

Removal of the uterus and cervix, even without removal of the ovaries, usually brings on an early menopause (surgical menopause), within 2 years of the operation. Oophorectomy (removal of the ovaries) brings on menopause immediately, regardless of the age of the woman, and early surgical removal of the ovaries (before age 30) doubles the risk of osteoporosis.

Women and Hormone Replacement Therapy For a time, it was enough to find out which women in their menopausal years were taking HRT. It was thought these women were protected against cardiac events, osteoporosis, and hip fractures.

Women who were not on HRT were targeted with information about the increased risk of osteoporosis and hip fractures. Anyone with cardiac risk factors was encouraged to begin taking HRT. Research from the landmark Women's Health Initiative study[54] has shown that HRT is not cardioprotective as was once thought. In fact there is an increase in myocardial infarction (MI) and stroke in healthy women taking HRT along with an increase in breast cancer and blood clots. HRT is associated with a decrease in colorectal cancer and hip fracture.[54]

The next wave of research reported that these findings applied to long-term use, not short-term use to alleviate symptoms. Doctors started prescribing HRT as a short-term intervention to manage symptoms rather than with the intention of replacing naturally diminishing hormones. However, a newer study[55] reported there are only 1- to 2-point differences (scale 0-100) for a large study comparing women taking versus not taking HRT for symptomatic relief. After 3 years, even those slight differences disappeared.

Women and Heart Disease When a 55-year-old woman with a significant family of heart disease comes to the therapist with shoulder, upper back, or jaw pain, it will be necessary to take the time and screen for possible cardiovascular involvement.

For women, gender-linked protection against coronary artery disease ends with menopause. At age 45 years, one in nine women develops heart disease. By age 65 years, this statistic changes to one in three women.[56]

Ten times as many women die of heart disease and stroke as they do of breast cancer (about $\frac{1}{2}$ million every year in the United States for heart disease compared to about 41,000 from breast cancer).[51] More women die of heart disease each year in the United States than the combined deaths from the next seven causes of death in women. In fact more women than men die of heart disease every year.[56,57]

Women under 50 are more than twice as likely to die of heart attacks compared to men in the same age group. Two thirds of women who die suddenly have no previously recognized symptoms. Prodromal symptoms as much as 1 month before

Clinical Signs and Symptoms of

Menopause

- Fatigue and malaise
- Depression, mood swings
- Difficulty concentrating; "brain fog"
- Headache
- Altered sleep pattern (insomnia)
- Hot flashes
- Irregular menses, cessation of menses
- Vaginal dryness, pain during intercourse
- Atrophy of breasts and vaginal tissue
- Pelvic floor relaxation (cystocele/rectocele)
- Urge incontinence

a myocardial infarction go unrecognized (see Table 6-4).

Therapists who recognize age combined with the female gender as a risk factor for heart disease will look for other risk factors and participate in heart disease prevention. See Chapter 6 for further discussion of this topic.

Women and Osteoporosis As health care specialists, therapists have a unique opportunity and responsibility to provide screening and prevention for a variety of diseases and conditions. Osteoporosis is one of those conditions.

To put it into perspective a woman's risk of developing a hip fracture is equal to her combined risk of developing breast, uterine, and ovarian cancer. Women have higher fracture rates than men of the same ethnicity. Caucasian women have higher rates than black women.

Assessment of osteoporosis and associated risk factors along with further discussion of osteoporosis as a condition are discussed in Chapter 11.

RESOURCES

Websites with information about men's health issues are available:

- Medline Plus (www.nlm.nih.gov/medlineplus/menshealthissues.html)
- National Institutes of Health (health.nih.gov/search.asp/25)

Websites with information for health care professionals about women's health issues are also available. The National Health Lung and Blood Institute (NHLBI) offers information about the Women's Health Initiative and heart health care for women (www.nhlbi.nih.gov/health/pubs/pub_slct.htm#women).

Other available websites include:

- FDA Office of Women's Health (www.fda.gov/womens)
- The National Women's Health Information Center (www.4woman.org)
- National Institutes of Health (www.nih.gov/PHTindex.htm)

Race and Ethnicity

The Genome Project dispelled previous ideas of biologic differences based on race. It is now recognized that humans are the same biologically regardless of race or ethnic background.[58,59] In light of these new findings, the focus of research is centered now on cultural differences including religious, social, and economic factors and how these might explain health differences among ethnic groups.

The distinction between the terms "race" and "ethnicity" are not always clear. A child born in Korea but adopted by a Caucasian American family will grow up speaking English, eating American food, and studying U.S. history. Ethnically, the child is American but will be viewed racially by others as Asian.

Epidemiologists and demographic researchers use the term "race" as a sociopolitical way of categorizing a population. As a category, race is used epidemiologically as a medical profiling for risk of disease based on genetically defined differences. Ethnicity looks at geographical origins, cultural differences in diet, and other habits.[60]

An individual's ethnicity is defined by a unique sociocultural heritage that is passed down from generation to generation but can change as the person changes geographical locations or joins a family with different cultural practices. Often the terms are combined and discussed as "racial/ethnic minorities."

Ethnicity is a risk factor for health outcomes. Despite tremendous advances and improved public health in America, noncaucasian racial/ethnic groups listed in Box 2-2 are medically underserved and suffer higher levels of illness, premature death, and disability. These include cancer, heart disease and stroke, diabetes, infant mortality, and HIV and AIDS.[61]

Racial/ethnic minorities living in rural areas may be at greater risk when health care access is limited.[62] For example, Indians living on reservations may benefit from many services for free that might not be available in other areas, while city-dwelling (urban) American Indians are more likely than the general population to die from diabetes, alcohol-related causes, lung cancer, liver disease, pneumonia, and influenza.[63] The therapist must remember to look for these risk factors when conducting a risk-factor assessment.

Black men have a higher risk factor for hypertension and heart disease than white men. Black women have 250% higher incidence with twice the mortality of white women for cervical cancer. Black women are more likely to die of pneumonia, influenza, diabetes, and liver disease. Scientists and epidemiologists ask if this could be the result of socioeconomic factors such as later detection. Perhaps the lack of health insurance prevents adequate screening and surveillance.

Epidemiologists tracking cancer statistics point out that African Americans have the highest mortality and worst survival of any population and the statistics have gotten worse over the last 20 years. Studies have shown that equal treatment yields equal outcomes among individuals with equal disease.[64] Conversely minority status can be

translated into disparities in health care with worse outcomes in many cases for a variety of illnesses.[65]

African American teenagers and young adults are three to four times more likely to be infected with hepatitis B than whites. Asian Americans and Pacific Islanders are twice as likely to be infected with hepatitis B than whites. Of all the cases of tuberculosis reported in the United States over the last 10 years, almost 80% were in racial/ethnic minorities.[61]

Mexican Americans, who make up two thirds of Hispanics, are also the largest minority group in the United States. Stroke prevention and early intervention are important in this group because their risk for stroke is much higher than for non-Hispanic or white adults.

Mexican Americans ages 45 to 59 are twice as likely to suffer a stroke, and those in their 60s and early 70s are 60% more likely to have a stroke. Family history of stroke or transient ischemic attack (TIA) is a warning flag in this population.[66,67]

Other studies are underway to compare ethnic differences among different groups for different diseases (Case Example 2-4).

RESOURCES

For a report on racial and ethnic disparities, see the Institute of Medicine's (IOM) Unequal Treat-

ment, Confronting Racial and Ethnic Disparities in Health Care.[65]

The U.S. National Library of Medicine and the National Institutes of Health offer the latest news on health care issues and other topics related to African Americans.[68] Baylor College of Medicine's Intercultural Cancer Council provides information about cancer and various racial/ethnic groups.[69]

Past Medical and Personal History

It is important to take time with these questions and to ensure that the client understands what is being asked. A "yes" response to any question in this section would require further questioning, correlation to objective findings, and consideration of referral to the client's physician.

For example, a "yes" response to questions on this form directed toward *allergies, asthma,* and *hay fever* should be followed up by asking the client to list the allergies and to list the symptoms that may indicate a manifestation of allergies, asthma, or hay fever. The therapist can then be alert for any signs of respiratory distress or allergic reactions during exercise or with the use of topical agents.

Likewise, clients may indicate the presence of *shortness of breath* with only mild exertion or without exertion, possibly even after waking at night. This condition of breathlessness can be associated with one of many conditions, including

---

heart disease, bronchitis, asthma, obesity, emphysema, dietary deficiencies, pneumonia, and lung cancer.

Some "no" responses may warrant further follow-up. The therapist can screen for diabetes, depression, liver impairment, eating disorders, osteoporosis, hypertension, substance use, incontinence, bladder or prostate problems, and so on. Special questions to ask for many of these conditions are listed in the appendices.

Many of the screening tools for these conditions are self-report questionnaires, which are inexpensive, require little or no formal training, and are less time consuming than formal testing. Knowing the risk factors for various illnesses, diseases, and conditions will help guide the therapist in knowing when to screen for specific problems. Recognizing the signs and symptoms will also alert the therapist to the need for screening.

EATING DISORDERS AND DISORDERED EATING

Eating disorders such as bulimia nervosa, binge eating disorder, and anorexia nervosa are good examples of past or current conditions that can impact the client's health and recovery. The therapist must consider the potential for a negative impact of anorexia on bone mineral density, while also keeping in mind the psychologic risks of exercise (a common intervention for osteopenia) in anyone with an eating disorder.

The first step in screening for eating disorders is to look for risk factors for eating disorders. Female gender, Caucasian/white, perfectionist personality traits, personal or family history of obesity and/or eating disorders, sports or athletic involvement, and history of sexual abuse or other trauma are common risk factors associated with eating disorders.

Distorted body image and disordered eating are probably underreported, especially in male athletes. Athletes participating in sports that use weight classifications such as wrestling and weightlifting are at greater risk for anorexic behaviors such as fasting, fluid restriction, and vomiting.[70]

Researchers have recently described a form of body image disturbance in male bodybuilders and weightlifters referred to as *muscle dysmorphia*. Previously referred to as "reverse anorexia" this disorder is characterized by an intense and excessive preoccupation or dissatisfaction with a perceived defect in appearance, even though the men are usually large and muscular. The goal in disordered eating for this group of men is to increase body weight and size. The use of performance-

enhancing drugs and dietary supplements is common in this group of athletes.[71]

Gay men tend to be more dissatisfied with their body image and may be at greater risk for symptoms of eating disorders compared to heterosexual men.[72] Screening is advised for anyone with risk factors and/or signs and symptoms of eating disorders. Questions to ask may include:

Follow-Up Questions

- Are you satisfied with your eating patterns?
- Do you force yourself to exercise, even when you don't feel well?
- Do you exercise more when you eat more?
- Do you think you will gain weight if you stop exercising for a day or two?
- Do you exercise more than once a day?
- Do you take laxatives, diuretics (water pills), or any other pills as a way to control your weight or shape?
- Do you ever eat in secret? (Secret eating refers to individuals who do not want others to see them eat or see what they eat; they may eat alone or go into the bathroom or closet to conceal their eating)
- Are there days when you don't eat anything?
- Do you ever make yourself throw up after eating as a way to control your weight?

Clinical Signs and Symptoms of Eating Disorders

Physical

- Weight loss or gain
- Skeletal myopathy and weakness
- Chronic fatigue
- Dehydration or rebound water retention
- Broken blood vessels in the eyes from induced vomiting
- Enlarged parotid (salivary) glands (facial swelling) from repeated contact with vomit
- Tooth marks, scratches, scars, or calluses on the backs of hands from inducing vomiting (Russell's sign)
- Discoloration or staining of the teeth from contact with stomach acid
- Irregular or absent menstrual periods; delay of menses onset in young adolescent girls
- Inability to tolerate cold
- Dry skin and hair; brittle nails; hair loss and growth of downy hair (lanugo) all over the body including the face

Continued on p. 58

- Reports of heartburn, abdominal bloating or gas, constipation or diarrhea
- Vital signs: slow heart rate (bradycardia); low blood pressure
- In women/girls: irregular or absent menstrual cycles

Behavioral

- Preoccupation with weight, food, calories, fat grams, dieting, clothing size, body shape
- Mood swings, irritability
- Binging and purging (bulimia) or food restriction (anorexia); frequent visits to the bathroom after eating
- Frequent comments about being "fat" or over-weight despite looking very thin
- Excessive exercise to burn off calories
- Use of diuretics, laxatives, enemas, or other drugs to induce urination, bowel movements, and vomiting (purging)

General Health

Self-assessed health is a strong and independent predictor of mortality and morbidity. People who rate their health as "poor" are four to five times more likely to die than those who rate their health as "excellent."[73,74] Self-assessed health is also a strong predictor of functional limitation.[75]

At least one study has shown similar results between self-assessed health and outcomes after total knee replacement.[76] The therapist should consider it a red flag anytime a client chooses "poor" to describe his or her overall health.

MEDICATIONS

Although the Family/Personal History form includes a question about prescription or over-the-counter (OTC) medications, specific follow-up questions come later in the Core Interview under Medical Treatment and Medications. Further discussion about this topic can be found in that section of this chapter.

It may be helpful to ask the client to bring in any prescribed medications he or she may be taking. In the older adult with multiple comorbidities, it is not uncommon for the client to bring a gallon-sized ziplock bag full of pill bottles. Taking the time to sort through the many prescriptions can be time consuming.

Start by asking the client to make sure each one is a drug that is being taken as prescribed on a regular basis. Make a list for future investigation if the clinical presentation or presence of possible side effects suggests the need for consultation with the pharmacy.

RECENT INFECTIONS

Recent infections such as mononucleosis, hepatitis, or upper respiratory infections may precede the onset of Guillain-Barré syndrome. Recent colds, influenza, or upper respiratory infections may also be an extension of a chronic health pattern of systemic illness.

Further questioning may reveal recurrent influenza-like symptoms associated with headaches and musculoskeletal complaints. These complaints could originate with medical problems, such as endocarditis (a bacterial infection of the heart), bowel obstruction, or pleuropulmonary disorders, which should be ruled out by a physician.

Knowing that the client has had a recent bladder, vaginal, uterine, or kidney infection, or that the client is likely to have such infections, may help explain back pain in the absence of any musculoskeletal findings.

The client may or may not confirm previous back pain associated with previous infections. If there is any doubt, a medical referral is recommended. On the other hand, repeated coughing after a recent upper respiratory infection may cause chest, rib, back, or sacroiliac pain.

SCREENING FOR CANCER

Any "yes" responses to early screening questions for cancer (General Health questions 5, 6, and 7) must be followed up by a physician. An in-depth discussion of screening for cancer is presented in Chapter 13.

Changes in appetite and unexplained weight loss can be associated with cancer, onset of diabetes, hyperthyroidism, depression, or pathologic anorexia (loss of appetite). Weight loss significant for neoplasm would be a 10% loss of total body weight over a 4-week period unrelated to any intentional diet or fasting.

A significant, unexplained weight gain can be caused by congestive heart failure, hypothyroidism, or cancer. The person with back pain who, despite reduced work levels and decreased activity, experiences unexplained weight loss demonstrates a key "red flag" symptom.

Weight gain/loss does not always correlate with appetite. For example, weight gain associated with neoplasm may be accompanied by appetite loss, whereas weight loss associated with hyperthyroidism may be accompanied by increased appetite.

SUBSTANCE ABUSE

Substances refer to any agents taken nonmedically that can alter mood or behavior. Addiction refers to the daily need for the substance in order to function, an inability to stop, and recurrent use when it is harmful physically, socially, and/or psychologically. Addiction is based on physiologic changes associated with drug use but also has psychologic and behavioral components. Individuals who are addicted will use the substance to relieve psychologic symptoms even after physical pain or discomfort is gone.

Dependence is the physiologic dependence on the substance so that withdrawal symptoms emerge when the drug is stopped abruptly. Once a medication is no longer needed, the dosage will have to be tapered down for the client to avoid withdrawal symptoms. *Tolerance* refers to the individual's need for increased amounts of the substance to produce the same effect.

Among the substances most commonly used that cause physiologic responses but are not usually thought of as drugs are alcohol, tobacco, coffee, black tea, and caffeinated carbonated beverages.

Other substances commonly abused include *depressants* such as alcohol, barbiturates (barbs, downers, pink ladies, rainbows, reds, yellows, sleeping pills), *stimulants* such as amphetamines and cocaine (crack, crank, coke, snow, white, lady, blow, rock), *opiates* (heroin), *cannabis derivatives* (marijuana, hashish), and *hallucinogens* (LSD or acid, mescaline, magic mushroom, PCP, angel dust).

More recently *methylenedioxymethamphetamine* (MDMA; also called Ecstasy, hug, beans, love drug), a synthetic, psychoactive drug chemically similar to the stimulant methamphetamine and the hallucinogen mescaline has been reported sold in clubs around the country. It is often given to individuals without their knowledge and used in combination with alcohol and other drugs.

Drug and alcohol addiction is the number one health problem in the United States. Public health officials tell us addictions (especially alcohol) have reached epidemic proportions in this country. Yet, it is largely ignored and often goes untreated.[77,78] Other countries report up to one third of workers use these illegal, psychoactive substances to face up to job strain.[79]

Risk Factors Many teens and adults are at risk for using and abusing various substances (Box 2-5). Often, they are self-medicating the symptoms of a variety of mental illnesses, learning disabilities, and personality disorders. The use of alcohol to self-medicate depression is very common,

especially after a traumatic injury or event in one's life.

Baby boomers (born between 1946 and 1964) with a history of substance use, aging adults (or others) with a history of substance use, sleep disturbances or sleep disorders, and anyone with an anxiety or mood disorder is at increase risk for use and abuse of substances. Think about this in terms of risk-factor assessment.

It is estimated that 50% of all traumatic brain-injured (TBI) cases are alcohol-or drug-related—either by the clients themselves or by the perpetrator of the accident. Some centers estimate this figure to be much higher, around 80%.[80]

The most common alcohol-related trauma patient is not the chronic alcoholic. It is a young man who drinks heavily and often uses drugs at the same time on a casual basis (e.g., once a week or on the weekends).[81]

Signs and Symptoms of Substance Use/Abuse Behavioral and physiologic responses to any of these substances depend on the characteristics of the chemical itself, the route of administration, and the adequacy of the client's circulatory system (Table 2-3).

The physiologic effects and adverse reactions have the additional ability to delay wound healing or the repair of soft tissue injuries. Soft tissue infections such as abscess and cellulitis are common complications of injection drug use (IDU). Affected individuals may present with swelling and tenderness in a muscular area from intramuscular injections. Low-grade fever may be found when taking vital signs.[82]

Screening for Substance Use/Abuse Questions designed to screen for the presence of chemical substance abuse need to become part of the physical therapy assessment. Clients who depend on alcohol and/or other substances require lifestyle intervention. However, direct questions may be offensive to some people, and identifying a person

---

TABLE 2-3 ▼ Physiologic Effects and Adverse Reactions to Substances

Caffeine	Cannabis	Depressants	Narcotics	Stimulants	Tobacco
Examples					
Coffee, espresso Chocolate, some over-the-counter "alert aids" used to stay awake, black tea and other beverages with caffeine (e.g., Red Bull, caffeinated water)	Marijuana, hashish	Alcohol, sedatives/ sleeping pills, barbiturates tranquilizers	Heroin, opium, morphine, codeine	Cocaine and its derivatives, amphetamines, methamphetamine, MDMA (ecstasy)	Cigarettes, cigars, pipe smoking, smokeless tobacco products (chew, snuff)
Effects					
Nervousness Irritability Agitation Sensory disturbances Tachypnea Urinary frequency Sleep disturbances Fatigue Muscle tension Headaches Intestinal disorders Enhances pain perception Heart palpitation Vasoconstriction	Short-term memory loss Sedation Tachycardia Euphoria Increased appetite Relaxed inhibitions Fatigue Paranoia Psychosis Ataxia, tremor	Vasodilation Fatigue Altered pain perception Slurred speech Altered behavior Slow, shallow breathing Clammy skin Coma (overdose)	Euphoria Drowsiness Respiratory depression	Increased alertness Excitation Euphoria Increased pulse rate Increased blood Insomnia Loss of appetite Agitation, increased body temperature, hallucinations, convulsions, death (overdose)	Increased heart rate Vasoconstriction Decreased oxygen to heart Increased risk of thrombosis Loss of appetite Poor wound healing Poor bone grafting Disc degeneration Increased risk of pneumonia Increased risk of cataracts Increased risk of aneurysm Increased risk of cancer

Adapted from Goodman CC, Boissonnault WG, Fuller KS: *Pathology: implications for the physical therapist,* ed 2, Philadelphia, 2003, WB Saunders.

as an alcohol abuser often results in referral to professionals who treat alcoholics, a label that is not accepted in the early stage of this condition.

Because of the controversial nature of interviewing the alcohol- or drug-dependent client, the questions in this section of the Family/Personal History form are suggested as a guideline for interviewing.

After (or possibly instead of) asking questions about use of alcohol, tobacco, caffeine, and other chemical substances, the therapist may want to use a new screening approach that makes no mention of substances but asks about previous trauma. Questions include[83]:

Follow-Up Questions

- Have you had any fractures or dislocations to your bones or joints?
- Have you been injured in a road traffic accident?
- Have you injured your head?
- Have you been in a fight or assault?

These questions are based on the established correlation between trauma and alcohol or other substance use. "Yes" answers to two or more of these questions should be discussed with the physician. It may be best to record the client's answers with a simple + for "yes" or a − for "no" to avoid taking notes during the discussion of sensitive issues.

The RAFFT Questionnaire[84] (Relax, Alone, Friends, Family, Trouble) poses five questions that appear to tap into common themes related to adolescent substance use, such as peer pressure, self-esteem, anxiety, and exposure to friends and family members who are using drugs or alcohol. Similar dynamics may still be present in adult substance users, although their use of drugs and alcohol may become independent from these psychosocial variables.

- **R:** Relax—Do you drink or take drugs to relax, feel better about yourself, or fit in?
- **A:** Alone—Do you ever drink or take drugs while you are alone?
- **F:** Friends—Do any of your closest friends drink or use drugs?
- **F:** Family—Does a close family member have a problem with alcohol or drugs?
- **T:** Trouble—Have you ever gotten into trouble from drinking or taking drugs?

Depending on how the interview has proceeded thus far, the therapist may want to conclude with one final question: "Are there any drugs or substances you take that you haven't mentioned?"

Other screening tools for assessing alcohol abuse are available, as are more complete guidelines for interviewing this population.[14,85]

Resources The American Academy of Pediatrics has published a guide on substance abuse for health care professionals.[86] This resource may help the therapist learn more about identifying, referring, and preventing substance abuse in their clients.

The University of Washington provides a Substance Abuse Screening and Assessments Instruments database to help health care providers find instruments appropriate for their work setting.[87] The database contains information on more than 225 questionnaires and interviews; many have proven clinical utility and research validity, while others are newer instruments that have not yet been thoroughly evaluated.

Many are in the public domain and can be freely downloaded from the Web; others are under copyright and can only be obtained from the copyright holder. The Partnership for a Drug-Free America also provides information on the effects of drugs, alcohol, and other illicit substances available at: www.drugfree.org.

ALCOHOL

Other than tobacco, alcohol is the most dominant addictive agent in the United States. One in 13 adults meets the diagnostic criteria for alcoholism and alcohol abuse defined as[88]:

- More than 14 alcoholic drinks/week (men); more than 4 drinks on any day
- More than 7 alcoholic drinks/week (women); more than 3 drinks on any day

One drink is equal to one 12oz beer, one 5oz glass of wine, or 1.5oz of hard liquor.

Using these definitions, the National Institute on Alcohol Abuse and Alcoholism reports that 2% to 10% of individuals aged 65 years or older are alcoholics. That percentage translates into about 3 million older Americans and 14 million total number of adults in the United States and is likely a gross underestimate.[88]

As the graying of America continues, this figure may escalate, especially as baby boomers, having grown up in an age of alcohol and substance abuse, carry that practice into old age.

Older adults are not the only ones affected. Alcohol consumption is a major contributor to risky behaviors and adverse health outcomes in adolescents and young adults. Motor vehicle accidents, homicides, suicides, and accidental injuries are the four leading causes of death in individuals aged 15 to 20 years, and alcohol plays a substantial role in

many of these events.[89] In addition, the use of alcohol is associated with risky sexual behavior, teen pregnancy, and sexually transmitted diseases (STDs).

Effects of Alcohol Use Excessive alcohol use can cause or contribute to many medical conditions. Alcohol is a toxic drug that is harmful to all body tissues. Certain social and behavioral changes, such as heavy regular consumption, frequent intoxication, concern expressed by others about one's drinking, and alcohol-related accidents, may be early signs of problem drinking and unambiguous signs of dependence risk.[90]

Alcohol has both vasodilatory and depressant effects that may produce fatigue and mental depression or alter the client's perception of pain or symptoms. Alcohol has deleterious effects on the gastrointestinal, hepatic, cardiovascular, hematopoietic, genitourinary, and neuromuscular systems.

Prolonged use of excessive alcohol may affect bone metabolism, resulting in reduced bone formation, disruption of the balance between bone formation and resorption, and incomplete mineralization.[91] Alcoholics are often malnourished, which exacerbates the direct effects of alcohol on bones. Alcohol-induced osteoporosis (the predominant bone condition in most people with cirrhosis) may progress for years without any obvious symptoms.

Regular consumption of alcohol may indirectly perpetuate trigger points through reduced serum and tissue folate levels and because of poor nutrition from eating habits. Ingestion of alcohol reduces the absorption of folic acid, while increasing the body's need for it.[92]

Therapists may also see alcoholic polyneuropathy, alcoholic myopathy, nontraumatic hip osteonecrosis, injuries from falls, and stroke[93] from heavy alcohol use.

Alcohol may interact with prescribed medications to produce various effects, including death. Prolonged drinking changes the way the body processes some common prescription drugs, potentially increasing the adverse effects of medications or impairing or enhancing their effects.

Binge drinking commonly seen on weekends and around holidays can cause atrial fibrillation, a condition referred to as "holiday heart." The affected individual may report dyspnea, palpitations, chest pain, dizziness, fainting or near-fainting and signs of alcohol intoxication. Strenuous physical activity is contraindicated until the cardiac rhythm converts to normal sinus rhythm. Medical evaluation

is required in cases of suspected holiday heart syndrome.[94]

Of additional interest to the therapist is the fact that alcohol diminishes the accumulation of neutrophils necessary for "clean-up" of all foreign material present in inflamed areas. This phenomenon results in delayed wound healing and recovery from inflammatory processes involving tendons, bursae, and joint structures.

Signs and Symptoms of Alcohol Withdrawal The therapist must be alert to any signs or symptoms of alcohol withdrawal. This is especially true in the acute care setting for individuals who are recently hospitalized for a motor vehicle accident or other trauma or the postoperative orthopedic patient (e.g., total hip or total knee patient). Alcohol withdrawal may be a factor in recovery for any orthopedic or neurologic patient (e.g., stroke, total joint, fracture), especially trauma patients.

Early recognition can bring about medical treatment that can reduce the symptoms of withdrawal as well as identify the need for long-term intervention. Withdrawal begins 3 to 36 hours after the last drink. Symptoms of autonomic hyperactivity may include insomnia, general restlessness, agitation, and loss of appetite. Mental confusion, disorientation, and acute fear and anxiety can occur.

Tremors of the hands, feet, and legs may be visible. Symptoms may progress to hyperthermia, delusions, and paranoia called *alcohol hallucinosis* lasting 1 to 5 or more days. Seizures occur in up to one third of affected individuals, usually 12 to 48 hours after the last drink. Five percent have delirium tremens (DTs). This is an acute and sometimes fatal psychotic reaction caused by cessation of excessive intake of alcohol.[95]

Clinical Signs and Symptoms of
Alcohol Withdrawal

- Agitation, irritability
- Headache
- Insomnia
- Anorexia, nausea, vomiting, diarrhea
- Loss of balance, incoordination
- Seizures (occurs 12 to 48 hours after the last drink)
- Delirium tremens (occurs 2 to 3 days after the last drink)
- Motor hyperactivity, tachycardia
- Elevated blood pressure

Screening for Alcohol Abuse In the United States alcohol use/abuse is often considered a

moral problem and may pose an embarrassment for the therapist and/or client when asking questions about alcohol use. Keep in mind the goal is to obtain a complete health history of factors that can affect healing and recovery as well as pose risk factors for future health risk.

Based on the definition of alcohol abuse defined earlier in this section, four broad categories of drinking patterns exist[88]:

1. Abstaining or infrequent drinking (fewer than 12 drinks/year)
2. Drinking within the screening limits
3. Exceeding daily limits, occasionally and frequently
4. Exceeding weekly limits

There is little to no risk of developing an alcohol disorder in categories 1 and 2. Individuals in category 3 have a 7% chance of becoming alcohol dependent whether in the occasional or frequent group. Group 4 have a 1 in 4 or 25% chance of developing alcohol dependence.[88]

There are several tools used to assess a client's history of alcohol use, including the Short Michigan Alcoholism Screening Test (SMAST),[96] the CAGE questionnaire, and a separate list of alcohol-related screening questions (Box 2-6). The CAGE questionnaire helps clients unwilling or unable to recognize a problem with alcohol, although it is possible for a person to answer "no" to all of the CAGE questions and still be drinking heavily and at risk for alcohol dependence. The specificity of this test is high for assessing alcohol abuse pre-traumatic and posttraumatic brain injury.[97]

The AUDIT (Alcohol Use Disorders Identification Test) developed by the World Health Organization to identify persons whose alcohol consumption has become hazardous or harmful to their health is another popular and easy to administer screening tool (Box 2-7).[90]

The AUDIT is designed as a brief, structured interview or self-report survey that can easily be incorporated into a general health interview, lifestyle questionnaire, or medical history. It is a 10-item screening questionnaire with questions on the amount and frequency of drinking, alcohol dependence, and problems caused by alcohol. When presented in this context by a concerned and interested interviewer, few clients will be offended by the questions. Results are most accurate when given in a nonthreatening, friendly environment to a client who is not intoxicated and who has not been drinking.[90]

The experience of the WHO collaborating investigators indicated that AUDIT questions were answered accurately regardless of cultural back-

---

BOX 2-6 ▲ Screening for Excessive Alcohol

CAGE Questionnaire

C: Have you ever thought you should *cut down* on your drinking?
A: Have you ever been *annoyed* by criticism of your drinking?
G: Have you ever felt *guilty* about your drinking?
E: Do you ever have an *eye-opener* (a drink or two) in the morning?

Key

- One "yes" answer suggests a need for discussion and follow-up; taking the survey may help some people in denial to accept that a problem exists
- Two or more "yes" answers indicates a problem with alcohol; intervention likely needed

Alcohol-Related Screening Questions

- Have you had any fractures or dislocations to your bones or joints since your eighteenth birthday?
- Have you been injured in a road traffic accident?
- Have you ever injured your head?
- Have you been in a fight or been hit or punched in the last 6 months?

Key

- "Yes" to two or more questions is a red flag

ground, age, or gender. In fact, many individuals who drank heavily were pleased to find that a health worker was interested in their use of alcohol and the problems associated with it.

The best way to administer the test is to give the client a copy and have him or her fill it out (see Appendix B-1). This is suggested for clients who seem reliable and literate. Alternately, the therapist can interview clients by asking them the questions. Some health care workers use just two questions (one based on research in this area and one from the AUDIT) to quickly screen.

Follow-Up Questions

- How often do you have six or more drinks on one occasion?
  0 = Never 1 = Less than Monthly 2 = Monthly 3 = Weekly 4 = Daily or Almost Daily
- How many drinks containing alcohol do you have each week?
  - More than 14/week for men constitutes a problem
  - More than 7/week for women constitutes a problem

BOX 2-7 ▼ Alcohol Use Disorders Identification Test (AUDIT)

Therapists: This form is available in Appendix B-1 for clinical use. It is also available on-line: www.uml.edu/student-services/counseling/alcdrug/alctest.html.

1) **How often do you have a drink containing alcohol?**
   (0) NEVER   (1) MONTHLY OR LESS   (2) TWO TO FOUR TIMES A MONTH
   (3) TWO TO THREE TIMES A WEEK   (4) FOUR OR MORE TIMES A WEEK

2) **How many drinks containing alcohol do you have on a typical day when you are drinking?**
   (0) 1 OR 2   (1) 3 OR 4   (2) 5 OR 6   (3) 7 OR 8   (4) 10 OR MORE

3) **How often do you have six or more drinks on one occasion?**
   (0) NEVER   (1) LESS THAN MONTHLY   (2) MONTHLY
   (3) WEEKLY   (4) DAILY OR ALMOST DAILY

4) **How often during the last year have you found that you were unable to stop drinking once you had started?**
   (0) NEVER   (1) LESS THAN MONTHLY   (2) MONTHLY
   (3) WEEKLY   (4) DAILY OR ALMOST DAILY

5) **How often during the last year have you failed to do what was normally expected from you because of drinking?**
   (0) NEVER   (1) LESS THAN MONTHLY   (2) MONTHLY
   (3) WEEKLY   (4) DAILY OR ALMOST DAILY

6) **How often during the last year have you needed a first drink in the morning to get going after a heavy drinking session?**
   (0) NEVER   (1) LESS THAN MONTHLY   (2) MONTHLY
   (3) WEEKLY   (4) DAILY OR ALMOST DAILY

7) **How often during the last year have you had a feeling of guilt or remorse after drinking?**
   (0) NEVER   (1) LESS THAN MONTHLY   (2) MONTHLY
   (3) WEEKLY   (4) DAILY OR ALMOST DAILY

8) **How often during the last year have you been unable to remember the night before because you had been drinking?**
   (0) NEVER   (1) LESS THAN MONTHLY   (2) MONTHLY
   (3) WEEKLY   (4) DAILY OR ALMOST DAILY

9) **Have you or someone else been injured as the result of your drinking?**
   (0) NO   (2) YES, BUT NOT IN THE LAST YEAR   (4) YES, DURING THE LAST YEAR

10) **Has a relative, friend, or health professional been concerned about your drinking or suggested you cut down?**
   (0) NO   (2) YES, BUT NOT IN THE LAST YEAR   (4) YES, DURING THE LAST YEAR
   TOTAL SCORE: _____

Key:
The numbers for each response are added up to give a composite score. Scores above 8 warrant an in-depth assessment and may be indicative of an alcohol problem. See options presented to clients in Appendix: AUDIT Questionnaire.

Data from World Health Organization, 1992. Available for clinical use without permission.

When administered during the screening interview, it may be best to use a transition statement such as:

Now I am going to ask you some questions about your use of alcoholic beverages during the past year. Because alcohol use can affect many areas of health (and may interfere with healing and certain medications), it is important for us to know how much you usually drink and whether you have experi- *enced any problems with your drinking. Please try to be as honest and as accurate as you can be.*

Alternately, if the client's breath smells of alcohol, the therapist may want to say more directly:

Follow-Up Questions

• I can smell alcohol on your breath right now. How many drinks have you had today?

As a follow-up to such direct questions, you may want to say:

- Alcohol, tobacco, and caffeine often increase our perception of pain, mask or even increase other symptoms, and delay healing. I would like to ask you to limit as much as possible your use of any of these stimulants. At the very least, it would be better if you didn't drink alcohol before our therapy sessions, so I can see more clearly just what your symptoms are. You may progress and move along more quickly through our plan of care if these substances aren't present in your body.

A helpful final question to ask at the end of this part of the interview may be:

- Are there any other drugs or substances you take that you haven't mentioned?

Follow-Up Questions

- Are there any other drugs or substances you take that you haven't mentioned?

Physical Therapist's Role[95] Incorporating screening questions into conversation during the interview may help to engage individual clients. Honest answers are important to guiding treatment. Reassure clients that all information will remain confidential and will be used only to ensure the safety and effectiveness of the plan of care. Specific interviewing techniques such as normalization, symptom assumption, and transitioning may be helpful.[96,98]

Normalization involves asking a question in a way that lets the person know you find a behavior normal or at least understandable under the circumstances. The therapist might say, "Given the stress you're under, I wonder if you've been drinking more lately?"

Symptom assumption involves phrasing a question that assumes a certain behavior already occurs and the therapist will not be shocked by it. For example, "What kinds of drugs do you use when you're drinking?" or "How much are you drinking?"

Transitioning is a way of using the client's previous answer to start a question such as, "You mentioned your family is upset by your drinking. Have your coworkers expressed similar concern?"[95]

What is the best way to approach alcohol and/or substance use/abuse? Unless the client has a chemical dependency on alcohol, appropriate education may be sufficient for the client experiencing negative effects of alcohol use during the episode of care. Some physicians advocate treating suspected or known excessive alcohol consumption no differently than diabetes, high blood pressure, or poor

vision. We must recognize the distinct and negative physiologic effects each substance or addictive agent can have on the client's physical body, personality, and behavior.

If the client's health is impaired by the use and abuse of substances, then physical therapy intervention may not be effective as long as the person is under the influence of chemicals.

Encourage the client to seek medical attention or let the individual know you would like to discuss this as a medical problem with the physician (Case Example 2-5).

Research shows that the longer people spend in treatment, the more likely they are to recover. A California study by the Rand Corporation showed that for every $1.00 spent on treatment for addictions, $7.00 is saved in social costs.[99] Often the general sentiment in the medical community is that alcoholism and addictions are not treatable. Yet, the national statistics show that one third stay sober after one year. Of the two thirds that relapse, 50% will get well if they go back to treatment.[99]

Alcohol-related trauma patients have a high reinjury rate. Even a brief intervention can reduce this by up to half. A single question or single suggestion from a health care worker can make a difference. It may mean the client will be sober in 2018 instead of in 2035.[100,101]

Physical therapists are not chemical dependency counselors or experts in substance abuse, but armed with a few questions, the therapist can still make a significant difference. Hospitalization or physical therapy intervention for an injury is potentially a teachable moment. Clients with substance abuse problems have worse rehabilitation outcomes, are at increased risk for reinjury or new injuries, and additional comorbidities.

Therapists can actively look for and address substance use/abuse problems in their clients. At the very minimum, therapists can participate in the National Institute on Alcohol Abuse and Alcoholism's National Alcohol Screening Day (www.mentalhealthscreening.org/events/nasd/index.aspx) with a program that includes the CAGE questionnaire, educational materials, and an opportunity to talk with a health care professional about alcohol.

When screening in any setting or circumstance, if a red flag is raised after completing any of the screening questions, the therapist may want to follow-up with:

Follow-Up Questions

- How do you feel about the role of alcohol in your life?

CASE EXAMPLE 2-5   Substance Abuse

A 44-year-old man previously seen in the physical therapy clinic for a fractured calcaneus returns to the same therapist 3 years later because of new onset of midthoracic back pain. There was no known cause or injury associated with the presenting pain. This man had been in the construction business for 30 years and attributed his symptoms to "general wear and tear."

Although there were objective findings to support a musculoskeletal cause of pain, the client also mentioned symptoms of fatigue, stomach upset, insomnia, hand tremors, and headaches. From the previous episode of care, the therapist recalled a history of substantial use of alcohol, tobacco, and caffeine (three six-packs of beer after work each evening, 2 pack/day cigarette habit, 18+ cups of caffeinated coffee during work hours).

The therapist pointed out the potential connection between the client's symptoms and the level of substance use, and the client agreed to "pay more attention to cutting back." After 3 weeks the client returned to work with a reduction of back pain from a level of 8 to a level of 0-3 (intermittent symptoms), depending on the work assignment.

Six weeks later this client returned again with the same symptomatic and clinical presen-

tation. At that time, given the client's age, the insidious onset, the cyclic nature of the symptoms, and significant substance abuse, the therapist recommended a complete physical with a primary care physician.

Medical treatment began with nonsteroidal antiinflammatories (NSAIDs), which caused considerable gastrointestinal upset. The GI symptoms persisted even after the client stopped taking the NSAIDs. Further medical diagnostic testing determined the presence of pancreatic carcinoma. The prognosis was poor, and the client died 6 months later, after extensive medical intervention.

In this case it could be argued that the therapist should have referred the client to a physician immediately because of the history of substance abuse and the presence of additional symptoms. A more thorough screening examination during the first treatment for back pain may have elicited additional red-flag gastrointestinal symptoms (e.g., melena or bloody diarrhea in addition to the stomach upset).

Earlier referral for a physical examination may have resulted in earlier diagnosis and treatment for the cancer. Unfortunately, these clinical situations occur often and are very complex, requiring ongoing screening (as happened here).

• Is there something you want or need to change?

And finally, the APTA recognizes that physical therapists and physical therapist assistants can be adversely affected by alcoholism and other drug addictions. Impaired therapists or assistants should be encouraged to enter into the recovery process. Reentry into the work force should occur when the well-being of the physical therapy practitioner and patient/client are assured.[102]

RECREATIONAL DRUG USE

As with tobacco and alcohol use, recreational or street drug use can lead to or compound already present health problems. Although the Personal/Family Health Form (see Fig. 2-2) asks the question, "Do you use recreational or street drugs?" it is questionable whether the client will answer "yes" to this question.

At some point in the interview the therapist may need to ask these questions directly:

Follow-Up Questions

• Have you ever used "street" drugs such as cocaine, crack, crank, "downers," amphetamines ("uppers"), methamphetamine, or other drugs?
• Have you ever injected drugs?
    • If yes, have you been tested for HIV or hepatitis?

Cocaine and amphetamines affect the cardiovascular system in the same manner as does sympathetic stress. The drugs stimulate the sympathetic nervous system to increase its production of adrenaline. Surging adrenaline causes severe constriction of the arteries, a sharp rise in blood pressure, rapid and irregular heartbeats, and seizures.[103]

Heart rate can accelerate by as much as 60 to 70 beats per minute. In otherwise healthy and fit people, this overload can cause death in minutes, even in first-time cocaine users. In addition, cocaine can cause the aorta to rupture, the lungs to fill with fluid, the heart muscle and its lining to become inflamed, blood clots to form in the veins, and strokes to occur as a result of cerebral hemorrhage.

TOBACCO

Tobacco and tobacco products are known carcinogens. This includes secondhand smoke, pipes, cigars, cigarettes, and chewing (smokeless) tobacco. Tobacco is well documented in its ability to cause vasoconstriction and delay wound healing. More people die from tobacco use than alcohol and all the other addictive agents combined.

As health care providers, the therapist has an important obligation to screen for tobacco use and incorporate smoking cessation education into the physical therapy plan of care whenever possible. The American Cancer Society publishes a chart (and pamphlet for distribution) of the benefits of smoking cessation starting from 20 minutes since the last cigarette until 15 years later.[104] Therapists can encourage the clients to decrease (or eliminate) tobacco use while in treatment.

Client education includes a review of the physiologic effects of tobacco (see Table 2-3). Nicotine in tobacco, whether in the form of chewing tobacco or pipe or cigarette smoking, acts directly on the heart, blood vessels, digestive tract, kidneys, and nervous system.

For the client with respiratory or cardiac problems, nicotine stimulates the already compensated heart to beat faster, narrows the blood vessels, reduces the supply of oxygen to the heart and other organs, and increases the chances of developing blood clots. Narrowing of the blood vessels is also detrimental for anyone with peripheral vascular disease, diabetes, or delayed wound healing.

Smoking markedly increases the need for vitamin C, which is poorly stored in the body. One cigarette can consume 25 mg of vitamin C (one pack would consume 500 mg/day). The capillary fragility associated with low ascorbic acid levels greatly increases the tendency for tissue bleeding, especially at injection sites.[105]

Smoking has been linked with disc degeneration[106,107] and acute lumbar and cervical intervertebral disc herniation.[108,109] Nicotine interacts with cholinergic nicotinic receptors, which leads to increased blood pressure, vasoconstriction, and vascular resistance. These systemic effects of nicotine may cause a disturbance in the normal nutrition of the disc.[106]

The combination of coffee ingestion and smoking raises the blood pressure of hypertensive clients about 15/30 mm Hg for as long as 2 hours. All these effects have a direct impact on the client's ability to exercise and must be considered when the client is starting an exercise program. Careful monitoring of vital signs during exercise is advised.

The commonly used formula to estimate cigarette smoking history is done by taking the number of packs smoked per day multiplied by the number of years smoked. If a person smoked two packs per day for 30 years, this would be a 60-pack year history (two packs per day × 20 years = 60-pack years). A 60-pack year history could also be achieved by smoking three packs of cigarettes per day for 20 years, and so on (Case Example 2-6).

If the client indicates a desire to quit smoking or using tobacco (see Fig. 2-2, General Health: Question 10) the therapist must be prepared to help him or her explore options for smoking cessation. Many hospitals, clinics, and community organizations such as the local chapter of the American Lung Association sponsor annual (or ongoing) smoking cessation programs. Pamphlets and other reading material should be available for any client interested in tobacco cessation. Referral to medical doctors who specialize in smoking cessation may be appropriate for some clients.

CAFFEINE

Caffeine is a substance with specific physiologic (stimulant) effects. Caffeine ingested in toxic amounts has many effects, including nervousness, irritability, agitation, sensory disturbances, tachypnea (rapid breathing), heart palpitations (strong, fast, or irregular heartbeat), nausea, urinary frequency, diarrhea, and fatigue.

The average cup of coffee or tea in the United States is reported to contain between 40 and 150 mg of caffeine; specialty coffees (e.g., espresso) may contain much higher doses. Over-the-counter supplements used to combat fatigue typically contain 100-200 mg caffeine per tablet. Many prescription drugs and over-the-counter analgesics contain between 32 and 200 mg of caffeine.

People who drink 8 to 15 cups of caffeinated beverages per day have been known to have problems with sleep, dizziness, restlessness, headaches, muscle tension, and intestinal disorders. Caffeine may enhance the client's perception of pain. Pain levels can be reduced dramatically by reducing the daily intake of caffeine.

CASE EXAMPLE 2-6 Recognizing Red Flags

A 60-year-old man was referred to physical therapy for weakness in the lower extremities. The client also reports dysesthesia (pain with touch).

Social/work history: single, factory worker, history of alcohol abuse, 60-pack year* history of tobacco use.

Clinically, the client presented with mild weakness in distal muscle groups (left more than right). Over the next 2 weeks, the weakness increased and a left footdrop developed. Now the client presents with weakness of right wrist and finger flexors and extensors.

What Are the Red Flags Presented in this Case? Is Medical Referral Required?

- Age
- Smoking history
- Alcohol use
- Bilateral symptoms
- Progressive neurologic symptoms

Consultation with the physician is certainly advised given the number and type of red flags present, especially the progressive nature of the neurologic symptoms in combination with other key red flags.

* Pack years = # packs/day × number of years. A 60-pack year history could mean 2 packs/day for 30 years or 3 packs/day for 20 years.

In large doses caffeine is a stressor, but the abrupt withdrawal from caffeine can be equally stressful. Withdrawal from caffeine induces a syndrome of headaches, lethargy, fatigue, poor concentration, nausea, impaired psychomotor performance, and emotional instability, which begins within 12 to 24 hours and lasts about 1 week.[110,111] Anyone seeking to break free from caffeine dependence should do so gradually over a week's time or more.

Fatal caffeine overdoses in adults are relatively rare; physiologically toxic doses are measured as more than 250 mg/day or three average cups of caffeinated coffee.[112]

New research suggests that habitual, moderate caffeine intake from coffee and other caffeinated beverages may not represent a health hazard after all and may even be associated with beneficial effects on cardiovascular health.[113]

Other sources of caffeine are tea (black and green), cocoa, chocolate, caffeinated-carbonated beverages, and some drugs, including many over-the-counter medications. Some people also take caffeine in pill form (e.g., Stay Awake, Vivarin). There are even off-label uses of drugs such as Provigil, normally used as an approved therapy for narcolepsy. This unauthorized use is for increasing alertness and cutting short the number of hours required for sleep.

Decaffeinated coffee may not have caffeine in it, but coffee contains several hundred different substances. It has been shown to have specific cardio-vascular effects.[114] Drinking decaf also increases the risk of rheumatoid arthritis among older women.[115]

ASPARTAME

According to the American Dietetic Association (ADA), artificial sweeteners are safe when used in amounts specified by the FDA.[116] Other experts still question the potential toxic effects of these substances.[117-119]

From the author's own clinical experience it appears that some individuals may react to artificial sweeteners and can experience generalized joint pain, myalgias, fatigue, headaches, and other nonspecific symptoms.

For anyone with these symptoms, connective tissue disorders, fibromyalgia, multiple sclerosis, or autoimmune disorders such as systemic lupus erythematosus, it may be helpful to ask about the use of products containing artificial sweeteners.

Follow-Up Questions

- Do you drink diet soda or diet pop or use aspartame, Equal, saccharin, NutraSweet, Splenda or other artificial sweeteners?

If the client uses these products in any amount, the therapist can suggest eliminating them on a trial basis for 30 days. Artificial sweetener-induced symptoms may disappear in some people; effects from use of the new product Splenda have not been reported.

CLIENT CHECKLIST

Screening for medical conditions can be aided by the use of a client checklist of associated signs and symptoms. Any items checked will alert the therapist to the possible need for further questions or tests.

A brief list here of the most common systemic signs and symptoms is one option for screening. It may be preferable to use the Review of Systems checklist (see Box 4-17; see also Appendix D-5).

MEDICAL AND SURGICAL HISTORY

Tests contributing information to the physical therapy assessment may include radiography (x-rays, sonograms), computed tomography (CT) scans, magnetic resonance imaging (MRI), bone scans and other imaging, lumbar puncture analysis, urinalysis, and blood tests. The client's medical records may contain information regarding which tests have been performed and the results of the tests. It may be helpful to question the client directly by asking:

Follow-Up Questions

- What medical test have you had for this condition?
- After giving the client time to respond, the therapist may need to probe further by asking:
- Have you had any x-ray films, sonograms, CT scans, MRIs, or other imaging studies done in the last 2 years?
- Do you recall having any blood tests or urinalyses done?

If the response is affirmative, the therapist will want to know when and where these tests were performed and the results (if known to the client). Knowledge of where the test took place provides the therapist with access to the results (with the client's written permission for disclosure).

Surgical History Previous surgery or surgery related to the client's current symptoms may be indicated on the Family/Personal History form (see Fig. 2-2). Whenever treating a client postoperatively, the therapist should read the surgical report. Look for notes on complications, blood transfusions, and the position of the client during the surgery and the length of time in that position.

Clients in an early postoperative stage (within 3 weeks of surgery) may have stiffness, aching, and musculoskeletal pain unrelated to the diagnosis, which may be attributed to position during the

surgery. Postoperative infections can lie dormant for months. Accompanying constitutional symptoms may be minimal with no sweats, fever, or chills until the infection progresses with worsening of symptoms or significant change in symptoms.

Specific follow-up questions differ from one client to another depending on the type of surgery, age of client, accompanying medical history, and so forth, but it is always helpful to assess how quickly the client recovered from surgery to determine an appropriate pace for physical activity and exercise prescribed during episode of care.

Clinical Tests The therapist will want to examine the available test results as often as possible. Familiarity with the results of these tests, combined with an understanding of the clinical presentation. Knowledge of testing and test results also provides the therapist with some guidelines for suggesting or recommending additional testing for clients who have not had a radiologic workup or other potentially appropriate medical testing.

Laboratory values of interest to therapists are displayed on the inside covers of this book.

WORK/LIVING ENVIRONMENT

Questions related to the client's daily work activities and work environments are included in the Family/Personal History to assist the therapist in planning a program of client education that is consistent with the objective findings and proposed plan of care.

For example, the therapist is alerted to the need for follow-up with a client complaining of back pain who sits for prolonged periods without a back support or cushion. Likewise, a worker involved in bending and twisting who complains of lateral thoracic pain may be describing a muscular strain from repetitive overuse. These work-related questions may help the client report significant data contributing to symptoms that may otherwise have gone undetected.

Questions related to occupation and exposure to toxins such as chemicals or gases are included because well-defined physical (e.g., cumulative trauma disorder) and health problems occur in people engaging in specific occupations.[120] For example pesticide exposure is common among agricultural workers. Asthma and sick building syndrome are reported among office workers. Lung disease is associated with underground mining and silica. There is a higher prevalence of tuberculosis in health care workers compared to the general population.

Each geographic area has its own specific environmental/occupational concerns but overall, the chronic exposure to chemically based products and pesticides has escalated the incidence of environmental allergies and cases of multiple chemical sensitivity. Frequently, these conditions present in a physical therapy setting with nonspecific neuromusculoskeletal manifestations.[121]

Exposure to cleaning products can be an unseen source of problems. Headaches, fatigue, skin lesions, joint arthralgias, myalgias, and connective tissue disorders may be the first signs of a problem. The therapist may be the first person to put the pieces of the puzzle together. Clients who have seen every kind of specialist end up with a diagnosis of fibromyalgia, rheumatoid arthritis, or some other autoimmune disorder and find their way to the physical therapy clinic (Case Example 2-7).

Military service at various periods and associated with specific countries or geographical areas has potential association with known diseases. For example, survivors of the Vietnam War who have been exposed to the defoliant mixtures, including Agent Orange, are at risk for developing soft tissue sarcoma, non-Hodgkin's lymphoma, Hodgkin's disease, and a skin-blistering disease called chloracne.[122]

About 30,000 U.S. soldiers who served in the Gulf War have reported symptoms linked to Gulf War syndrome, including chronic fatigue, headaches, chemical sensitivity, memory loss, joint pain and inflammation, and other fibromyalgia-like musculoskeletal disorders.[123]

Survivors of the Gulf War are nearly twice as likely to develop Amyotrophic Lateral Sclerosis (ALS; Lou Gehrig's disease) than other military personnel. Classic early symptoms include irregular gait and decreased muscular coordination. Other occupational-related illnesses and diseases have been reported (Table 2-4).

When to Screen Taking an environmental, occupational, or military history may be appropriate when a client has a history of asthma, allergies, fibromyalgia, chronic fatigue syndrome, connective tissue or autoimmune disease, or in the presence of other nonspecific disorders.

Conducting a quick survey may be helpful when a client presents with puzzling, nonspecific symptoms including myalgias, arthralgias,

---

CASE EXAMPLE 2-7   Cleaning Products

A 33-year-old dental hygienist came to physical therapy for joint pain in her hands and wrists. In the course of taking a symptom inventory, the therapist discovered that the client had noticed multiple arthralgias and myalgias over the last 6 months.

She reported being allergic to many molds, dusts, foods, and other allergens. She was on a special diet, but had obtained no relief from her symptoms. The doctor, thinking the client was experiencing painful symptoms from repetitive motion, sent her to physical therapy.

A quick occupational survey will include the following questions[120].

- What kind of work do you do?
- Do you think your health problems are related to your work?
- Are your symptoms better or worse when you're at home or at work?
- Do others at work have similar problems?

The client answered "No" to all work-related questions, but later came back and reported that other dental hygienists and dental assistants had noticed some of the same symptoms, although in a much milder form.

None of the other support staff (receptionist, bookkeeper, secretary) had noticed any health problems. The two dentists in the office were not affected either. The strongest red flag came when the client took a 10-day vacation and returned to work symptom-free. Within 24-hours of her return to work, her symptoms had flared up worse than ever.

This is not a case of emotional stress and work avoidance. The women working in the dental cubicles were using a cleaning spray after each dental client to clean and disinfect the area. The support staff was not exposed to it and the dentists only came in after the spray had dissipated. When this was replaced with an effective cleaning agent with only natural ingredients, everyone's symptoms were relieved completely.

TABLE 2-4 ▼ Common Occupational Exposures

Occupation	Exposure
Agriculture	Pesticides, herbicides, insecticides, fertilizers
Industrial	Chemical agents or irritants, fumes, dusts, radiation, loud noises, asbestos, vibration
Health care workers	Tuberculosis, hepatitis
Office workers	Sick building syndrome
Military service	Gulf War syndrome, connective tissue disorders, amyotrophic lateral sclerosis (ALS), non-Hodgkin's lymphoma, soft tissue sarcoma, chloracne (skin blistering)

Follow-Up Questions

- Do you think your health problems are related to your work?
- Do you wear a mask at work?
- Are your symptoms better or worse when you are at home or at work?
  Follow-up if worse at work: Do others at work have similar problems?
  Follow-up if worse at home: Have you done any remodeling at home in the last 6 months?
- Are you now or have you previously been exposed to dusts, fumes, chemicals, radiation, loud noise, tools that vibrate, or a new building/office space?
- Have you ever been exposed to chemical agents or irritants, such as asbestos, asphalt, aniline dyes, benzene, herbicides, fertilizers, wood dust, or others?
- Do others at work have similar problems?
- Have you ever served in any branch of the military?
  If yes, were you ever exposed to dusts, fumes, chemicals, radiation or other substances?

headaches, back pain, sleep disturbance, loss of appetite, loss of sexual interest, or recurrent upper respiratory symptoms.

After determining the client's occupation and depending on the client's chief complaint and accompanying associated signs and symptoms, the therapist may want to ask[120]:

The idea in conducting a work/environmental screening is to look for patterns in the past medical history that might link the current clinical presentation with the reported or observed associated

signs and symptoms. Further follow-up questions are listed in Appendix B-13.

The mnemonic CH²OPD² (Community, Home, Hobbies, Occupation, Personal habits, Diet, and Drugs) can be used as a tool to identify a client's history of exposure to potentially toxic environmental contaminants[124]:

- **Community**   Live near a hazardous waste site or industrial site
- **Home**   Home is more than 40 years old; recent renovations; pesticide use in home, garden, or on pets
  Work with stained glass, oil-based paints, varnishes
- **Hobbies**
- **Occupation**   Air quality at work; exposure to chemicals
- **Personal Habits**   Tobacco use, exposure to secondhand smoke
- **Drugs**   Prescription, over-the-counter drugs, home remedies, illicit drug use

Resources Further suggestions and tools to help health care professionals incorporate environmental history questions can be found online. The Children's Environmental Health Network (www.cehn.org) has an online training manual, Pediatric Environmental Health: Putting It into Practice. Download and review the chapter on environmental history taking.

The Agency for Toxic Substances and Disease Registry (ATSDR) Web site, (www.atsdr.cdc.gov) offers information on specific chemical exposures.

HISTORY OF FALLS

In the United States, falls are the second leading cause of traumatic brain injury (TBI) among persons aged 65 or older[125]. Older adults who fall often sustain more severe head injuries than their younger counterparts. Falls are a major cause of intracranial lesion among older persons because of their greater susceptibility to subdural hematoma[125].

It is reported that approximately one in four Americans in this age category who are living at home will fall during the next year. There is a possibility that older adults are falling even more often than is generally reported[126].

By assessing risk factors (prediction) and offering preventive and protective strategies, the therapist can make a significant difference in the number of fall-related injuries and fractures. There are many ways to look at falls assessment. For the screening process, there are four main categories:

- Well-adult (no falling pattern)
- Just starting to fall
- Falls frequently (more than once every 6 months)
- Fear of falling

Healthy older adults who have no falling patterns may have a fear of falling in specific instances (e.g., getting out of the bath or shower; walking on ice, curbs, or uneven terrain). Fear of falling can be considered a mobility impairment or functional limitation. It restricts the client's ability to perform specific actions, thereby preventing the client from doing the things he or she wants to do. Functionally, this may appear as an inability to take a tub bath, walk on grass unassisted, or even attempt household tasks such as getting up on a sturdy step stool to change a light bulb (Case Example 2-8).

CASE EXAMPLE 2-8 Fracture After a Fall

Case Description: A 67-year-old woman fell and sustained a complete transverse fracture of the left fibula and an incomplete fracture of the tibia. The client reported she lost her footing while walking down four steps at the entrance of her home.

She was immobilized in a plaster cast for 9 weeks. Extended immobilization was required after the fracture because of slow rate of healing secondary to osteopenia/osteoporosis. She was non-weight bearing and ambulated with crutches while her foot was immobilized. Initially this client was referred to physical therapy for range of motion (ROM), strengthening, and gait training.

Client is married and lives with her husband in a single-story home. Her goals were to ambulate independently with a normal gait.

Past Medical History: Type II diabetes, hypertension, osteopenia, and history of alcohol use. Client used tobacco (1½ packs a day for 35 years) but has not smoked for the past 20 years. Client described herself as a "weekend alcoholic," meaning she did not drink during the week but drank six or more beers a day on weekends.

Current medications include tolbutamide, enalapril, hydrochlorothiazide, Fosamax and supplemental calcium, and multivitamin.

Intervention: The client was seen six times before a scheduled surgery interrupted the plan of care. Progress was noted as increased ROM and increased strength through the left lower extremity, except dorsiflexion.

Seven weeks later, the client returned to physical therapy for strengthening and gait training secondary to a "limp" on the left side. She reported that she noticed the limping had increased since she had both her big toenails removed. She also noted increased toe dragging, stumbling, and leg cramps (especially at night). She reported she had decreased her use of alcohol since she fractured her leg because of the pain medications and recently because of fear of falling.

Minimal progress was noted in improving balance or improving strength in the lower extremity. The client felt that her loss of strength could be attributed to inactivity following the foot surgery, even though she reported doing her home exercise program.

Neurologic screening exam was repeated with hyperreflexia observed in the lower extremities, bilaterally. There was a positive Babinski reflex on the left. The findings were reported to the primary care physician who requested that physical therapy continue.

During the next week and a half, the client reported that she fell twice. She also reported that she was "having some twitching in her [left] leg muscles." The client also reported "coughing a lot while [she] was eating; food going down the wrong pipe."

Outcome: The client presented with a referral for weakness and gait abnormality thought to be related to the left fibular fracture and fall that did not respond as expected and, in fact, resulted in further loss of function.

The physician was notified of the client's need for a cane, no improvement in strength, fasciculations in the left lower extremity, and the changes in her neurologic status. The client returned to her primary care provider who then referred her to a neurologist.

Results: Upon examination by the neurologist, the client was diagnosed with amyotrophic lateral sclerosis (ALS). A new physical therapy plan of care was developed based on the new diagnosis.

From Chanoski C: Adapted from case report presented in partial fulfillment of DPT 910, Principles of Differential Diagnosis, Institute for Physical Therapy Education, Widener University, Chester, Pennsylvania, 2005. Used with permission.

Risk Factors for Falls If all other senses and reflexes are intact and muscular strength and coordination are normal, the affected individual can regain balance without falling. Many times, this does not happen. The therapist is a key health care professional to make early identification of adults at increased risk for falls.

With careful questioning, any potential problems with balance may come to light. Such information will alert the therapist to the need for testing static and dynamic balance and to look for potential risk factors and systemic or medical causes of falls (Table 2-5).

All of the variables and risk factors listed in Table 2-5 for falls are important. Older adults may have impaired balance, slower reaction times, and decreased strength, leading to more frequent falls. There are five key areas that are the most common factors in falls among the aging adult population:

- Vision/hearing
- Balance
- Blood pressure regulation
- Medications/substances
- Elder assault

As we age, cervical spinal motion declines, as does peripheral vision. These two factors alone contribute to changes in our vestibular system and the balance mechanism. Macular degeneration, glaucoma, cataracts, or any other visual problems can result in loss of depth perception and even greater loss of visual acuity.

The autonomic nervous system's (ANS) ability to regulate blood pressure is also affected by age. A sudden drop in blood pressure can precipitate a fall. Coronary heart disease, peripheral vascular disease, diabetes mellitus, and blood pressure medications are just a few of the factors that can put additional stress on the regulating function of the ANS.

Lower standing balance, even within normotensive ranges, is an independent predictor of falls in community-dwelling older adults. Older women (65 years old or older) with a history of falls and with lower systolic blood pressure should have more attention paid to the prevention of falls and related accidents.[127]

The subject of balance impairment and falls as it relates to medical conditions and medications is very important in the diagnostic and screening process. Chronic diseases and multiple pathologies are more important predictors of falling than even polypharmacy (use of four or more medications during the same period).[128]

Multiple comorbidities often mean the use of multiple drugs (polypharmacy). These two vari-ables together increase the risk of falls in older adults. Some medications (especially psychotropics such as tranquilizers and antidepressants including amitriptyline, doxepin, Zoloft, Prozac, Paxil, Remeron, Celexa, Wellbutrin) are red flag-risk factors for loss of balance and injuries from falls.

The therapist should watch for clients with chronic conditions who are taking any of these drugs. Anyone with fibromyalgia, depression, cluster migraine headaches, chronic pain, obsessive-compulsive disorders (OCD), panic disorder, and anxiety who is on a psychotropic medication must be monitored carefully for dizziness, drowsiness, and postural orthostatic hypotension (a sudden drop in blood pressure with an increase in pulse rate). In addition, alcohol can interact with many medications, increasing the risk of falling.

It is not uncommon for clients on hypertensive medication (diuretics) to become dehydrated, dizzy, and lose their balance. Postural orthostatic hypotension can (and often does) occur in the aging adult—even in someone taking blood pressure-regulating medications.

Orthostatic hypotension as a risk factor for falls may occur as a result of volume depletion (e.g., diabetes mellitus, sodium or potassium depletion), venous pooling (e.g., pregnancy, varicosities of the legs, immobility following a motor vehicle or cerebrovascular accident), side effects of medications such as antihypertensives, starvation associated with anorexia or cachexia, and sluggish normal regulatory mechanisms associated with anatomic variations or secondary to other conditions such as metabolic disorders or diseases of the central nervous system.

Remember too that falling is a primary symptom of Parkinson's disease. Any time a client reports episodes of dizziness, loss of balance, or a history of falls, further screening and possible medical referral is needed. This is especially true in the presence of other neurologic signs and symptoms such as headache, confusion, depression, irritability, visual changes, weakness, memory loss, and drowsiness or lethargy.

Screening for Risk of Falls Aging adults who have just started to fall or who fall frequently may be fearful of losing their independence by revealing this information even to a therapist. If the client indicates no difficulty with falling, the therapist is encouraged to review this part of the form (see Fig. 2-2) carefully with each older client.

Some potential screening questions may include (see Appendix B-10 for full series of questions):

SBP, Systolic blood pressure.

TABLE 2-5 ▲ Risk Factors For Falls

Age changes	Environmental/living conditions	Pathologic conditions	Medications	Other
Muscle weakness; loss of joint motion (especially lower extremities)	Poor lighting	Vestibular disorders; episodes of dizziness or vertigo from any cause	Antianxiety; benzodiazepines	History of falls
Impaired or abnormal balance	Throw rugs, loose carpet, complex carpet designs	Orthostatic hypotension (especially before breakfast)	Anticonvulsants	Elder abuse/assault
Impaired proprioception or sensation	Cluster of electric wires or cords	Neuropathies	Antidepressants	Nonambulatory status (requiring transfers)
Delayed muscle response/ increased reaction time	Stairs without handrails	Cervical myelopathy	Antihypertensives	
↑ SBP (<140 mm Hg in adults age over 65 years old)	Bathroom without grab bars	Osteoarthritis; rheumatoid arthritis	Antipsychotics	Gait changes (decreased stride length or speed)
Stooped or forward bent posture	Slippery floors (water, urine, floor surface, ice); icy sidewalks, stairs, or streets	Visual or hearing impairment; multifocal eyeglasses; change in perception of color; loss of depth perception; decreased contrast sensitivity	Diuretics	Postural instability; reduced postural control
	Restraints	Cardiovascular disease	Narcotics	Fear of falling
	Footwear, especially slippers	Urinary incontinence	Sedative-hypnotics	Postmenopausal status
	Use of alcohol or other substances	Cognitive impairment; dementia; depression	Phenothiazines	Dehydration from any cause
		Central nervous system disorders (e.g., stroke, Parkinson's disease, multiple sclerosis)	Use of more than four medications (polypharmacy)	
		Osteopenia, osteoporosis		
		Pathologic fractures		
		Any mobility impairments (e.g., amputation, neuropathy, deformity)		

Follow-Up Questions

- Do you have any episodes of dizziness? If yes, does turning over in bed cause (or increase) dizziness?
- Do you have trouble getting in or out of bed without losing your balance?
- Can you/do you get in and out of your tub or shower?
- Do you avoid walking on grass or curbs to avoid falling?
- Have you started taking any new medications, drugs, or pills of any kind?
- Has there been any change in the dosage of your regular medications?

During the Core Interview, the therapist will have an opportunity to ask further questions about the client's Current Level of Fitness (see discussion later in this chapter).

Performance-based tests such as the Functional Reach Test,[129,130] One-Legged Stance Test,[131] Berg Balance Scale (BBS),[132,133] and the Timed "Up and Go" Test (TUGT)[134-136] can help identify functional limitations, though not necessarily the causes, for balance impairment.

Fear of falling can be measured using the Falls Efficacy Scale (FES)[137,138] and the Survey of Activities and Fear of Falling in the Elderly (SAFE) assessment. The Activities-specific Balance Confidence Scale (ABC) can measure balance confidence.[139,140]

No one balance scale best predicts falls risk in older adults. The ABC and FES are highly correlated with each other, meaning they measure similar constructs. These two tests are moderately correlated with the SAFE, indicating they predict differently. It is likely that using more than one scale will help identify individuals who may be at risk and are candidates for an intervention program.[141]

Measuring vital signs and screening for postural orthostatic hypotension is another important tool in predicting falls. Positive test results for any of the tests mentioned require further evaluation, especially in the presence of risk factors predictive of falls.

Resources

As the population of older people in the United States continues to grow, the number of TBIs, fractures, and other injuries secondary to falls also is likely to grow.[125] Therapists are in a unique position to educate people on using strength, flexibility, and endurance activities to help maintain proper posture, improve balance, and prevent falls. The APTA has a Balance and

Falls Kit (Item number PR-294) available to assist the therapist in this area.[142]

National Committee on Aging (NCOA) has partnered with the APTA to provide a Falls Free plan that can help reduce fall dangers for older adults. More information on the plan is accessible at www.healthyagingprograms.org.

VITAL SIGNS

Taking a client's vital signs remains the single easiest, most economical, and fastest way to screen for many systemic illnesses. Dr. James Cyriax, a renowned orthopedic physician, admonishes therapists to always take the body temperature in any client with back pain of unknown cause.[143]

A place to record vital signs is provided at the end of the Family/Personal History form (see Fig. 2-2). The clinician must be proficient in taking vital signs, an important part of the screening process. All the vital signs are important, but the client's temperature and blood pressure have the greatest utility as early screening tools. An in-depth discussion of vital signs as part of the screening physical assessment is presented in Chapter 4.

▲ **CORE INTERVIEW**

Once the therapist reviews the results of the Family/Personal History form and reviews any available medical records for the client, the client interview (referred to as the Core Interview in this text) begins (Fig. 2-3).

Screening questions may be interspersed throughout the Core Interview and/or presented at the end. When to screen depends on the information provided by the client during the interview.

Special questions related to sensitive topics such as sexual history, assault or domestic violence, and substance or alcohol use are often left to the end or even on a separate day after the therapist has established sufficient rapport to broach these topics.

History of Present Illness

Chief Complaint

The history of present illness (often referred to as the chief complaint and other current symptoms) may best be obtained through the use of open-ended questions. This section of the interview is designed to gather information related to the client's reason(s) for seeking clinical treatment.

The following open-ended statements may be appropriate to start an interview:

THE CORE INTERVIEW

HISTORY OF PRESENT ILLNESS

Chief Complaint (Onset)

- Tell me why you are here today.
- Tell me about your injury.

Alternate question: What do you think is causing your problem/pain?

FUPs: How did this injury or illness begin?

- ○ Was your injury or illness associated with a fall, trauma, assault, or repetitive activity (e.g., painting, cleaning, gardening, filing papers, driving)?
- ○ Have you been hit, kicked, or pushed? [For the therapist: See text (Assault) before asking this question.]
- ○ When did the present problem arise and did it occur gradually or suddenly?

Systemic disease: Gradual onset without known cause.

- ○ Have you ever had anything like this before? If yes, when did it occur?
- ○ Describe the situation and the circumstances.
- ○ How many times has this illness occurred? Tell me about each occasion.
- ○ Is there any difference this time from the last episode?
- ○ How much time elapses between episodes?
- ○ Do these episodes occur more or less often than at first?

Systemic disease: May present in a gradual, progressive, cyclical onset: worse, better, worse.

PAIN AND SYMPTOM ASSESSMENT

- Do you have any pain associated with your injury or illness? If yes, tell me about it.

Location

- Show me exactly where your pain is located.

FUPs: Do you have this same pain anywhere else?

- ○ Do you have any other pain or symptoms anywhere else?
- ○ If yes, what causes the pain or symptoms to occur in this other area?

Description

- What does it feel like?

FUPs: Has the pain changed in quality, intensity, frequency, or duration (how long it lasts) since it first began?

Pattern

- Tell me about the pattern of your pain or symptoms.

Alternate question: When does your back/shoulder [name the body part] hurt?

Alternate question: Describe your pain/symptoms from first waking up in the morning to going to bed at night. (See special sleep-related questions that follow.)

FUPs: Have you ever experienced anything like this before?

- ○ If yes, do these episodes occur more or less often than at first?
- ○ How does your pain/symptom(s) change with time?
- ○ Are your symptoms worse in the morning or in the evening?

Frequency

- How often does the pain/symptom(s) occur?

FUPs: Is your pain constant, or does it come and go (intermittent)?

- ○ Are you having this pain now?
- ○ Did you notice these symptoms this morning immediately after awakening?

Duration

- How long does the pain/symptom(s) last?

Systemic disease: Constant.

Fig. 2-3 • Core Interview

Intensity

- On a scale from 0 to 10, with 0 being no pain and 10 being the worst pain you have experienced with this condition, what level of pain do you have right now?

  Alternate question: How strong is your pain?

  1 = Mild

  2 = Moderate

  3 = Severe

  FUPs: Which word describes your pain right now?
  - Which word describes the pain at its worst?
  - Which word describes the least amount of pain?

  Systemic disease: Pain tends to be intense.

Associated Symptoms

- What other symptoms have you had that you can associate with this problem?

  FUPs: Have you experienced any of the following?

  ☐ Blood in urine, stool, vomit, mucous

  ☐ Dizziness, fainting, blackouts

  ☐ Fever, chills, sweats (day or night)

  ☐ Nausea, vomiting, loss of appetite

  ☐ Changes in bowel or bladder

  ☐ Throbbing sensation/pain in belly or anywhere else

  ☐ Skin rash or other changes

  ☐ Headaches

  ☐ Cough   ☐ Difficulty swallowing/speaking

  ☐ Dribbling or leaking urine   ☐ Memory loss

  ☐ Heart palpitations or fluttering ☐ Confusion

  ☐ Numbness or tingling   ☐ Sudden weakness

  ☐ Swelling or lumps anywhere   ☐ Trouble sleeping

  ☐ Problems seeing or hearing

  ☐ Unusual fatigue, drowsiness

  ☐ Joint pain

  Systemic disease: Presence of symptoms bilaterally (e.g., edema, nail bed changes, bilateral weakness, paresthesia, tingling, burning). Determine the frequency, duration, intensity, and pattern of symptoms. Blurred vision, double vision, scotomas (black spots before the eyes), or temporary blindness may indicate early symptoms of multiple sclerosis (MS), cerebral vascular accident (CVA), or other neurologic disorders.

Aggravating Factors

- What kinds of things affect the pain?

  FUPs: What makes your pain/symptoms worse (e.g., eating, exercise, rest, specific positions, excitement, stress)?

Relieving Factors

- What makes it better?

  Systemic disease: Unrelieved by change in position or by rest.

Medical Treatment

  FUPs: Are your symptoms aggravated or relieved by any activities? If yes, what?
  - How does rest affect the pain/symptoms?
  - How has this problem affected your daily life at work or at home?
  - How has it affected your ability to care for yourself without assistance (e.g., dress, bathe, cook, drive)?

MEDICAL TREATMENT AND MEDICATIONS

Medical Treatment

- What medical treatment have you had for this condition?

  FUPs: Have you been treated by a physical therapist for this condition before? If yes:
  - When?
  - Where?
  - How long?
  - What helped?
  - What didn't help?
  - Was there any treatment that made your symptoms worse? If yes, please elaborate.

Medications

- Are you taking any prescription or over-the-counter medications?

  FUPs: If no, you may have to probe further regarding use of laxatives, aspirin, acetaminophen (Tylenol), and so forth. If yes:
  - What medication do you take?
  - How often?

Fig. 2-3 ▪ cont'd

o What dose do you take?

o Why are you taking these medications?

o When was the last time that you took these medications? Have you taken these drugs today?

o Do the medications relieve your pain or symptoms?

o If yes, how soon after you take the medications do you notice an improvement?

o Do you notice any increase in symptoms or perhaps the start of symptoms after taking your medication(s)? (This may occur 30 minutes to 2 hours after ingestion.)

o If prescription drugs, who prescribed them for you?

o How long have you been taking these medications?

o When did your physician last review these medications?

o Are you taking any medications that weren't prescribed for you?

If no, follow-up with: Are you taking any pills given to you by someone else besides your doctor?

CURRENT LEVEL OF FITNESS

• What is your present exercise level?

FUPs: What type of exercise or sports do you participate in?

o How many times do you participate each week (frequency)?

o When did you start this exercise program (duration)?

o How many minutes do you exercise during each session (intensity)?

o Are there any activities that you could do before your injury or illness that you cannot do now? If yes, please describe.

Dyspnea: Do you ever experience any shortness of breath (SOB) or lack of air during any activities (e.g., walking, climbing stairs)?

FUPs: Are you ever short of breath without exercising?

o If yes, how often?

o When does this occur?

o Do you ever wake up at night and feel breathless? If yes, how often?

o When does this occur?

SLEEP-RELATED HISTORY

• Can you get to sleep at night? If no, try to determine whether the reason is due to the sudden decrease in activity and quiet, which causes you to focus on your symptoms.

• Are you able to lie or sleep on the painful side? If yes, the condition may be considered to be chronic, and treatment would be more vigorous than if no, indicating a more acute condition that requires more conservative treatment.

• Are you ever wakened from a deep sleep by pain?

FUPs: If yes, do you awaken because you have rolled onto that side? Yes may indicate a subacute condition requiring a combination of treatment approaches, depending on objective findings.

o Can you get back to sleep?

FUPs: If yes, what do you have to do (if anything) to get back to sleep? (The answer may provide clues for treatment.)

• Have you had any unexplained fevers, night sweats, or unexplained perspiration?

Systemic disease: Fevers and night sweats are characteristic signs of systemic disease.

STRESS

• What major life changes or stresses have you encountered that you would associate with your injury/illness?

Alternate question: What situations in your life are "stressors" for you?

• On a scale from 0 to 10, with 0 being no stress and 10 being the most extreme stress you have ever experienced, in general, what number rating would you give to your stress at this time in your life?

• What number would you assign to your level of stress today?

• Do you ever get short of breath or dizzy or lose coordination with fatigue (anxiety-produced hyperventilation)?

FINAL QUESTION

• Do you wish to tell me anything else about your injury, your health, or your present symptoms that we have not discussed yet?

Alternate question: Is there anything else you think is important about your condition that we haven't discussed yet?

FUPs, Follow-up Questions

Fig. 2-3 • cont'd

Follow-Up Questions

- Tell me how I can help you.
- Tell me why you are here today.
- Tell me about your injury.
- (Alternate) What do you think is causing your problem or pain?

During this initial phase of the interview, allow the client to carefully describe his or her current situation. Follow-up questions and paraphrasing as shown in Fig. 2-3 can be used in conjunction with the primary, open-ended questions.

Pain and Symptom Assessment

The interview naturally begins with an assessment of the chief complaint, usually (but not always) pain. Chapter 3 of this text presents an in-depth discussion of viscerogenic sources of neuromusculoskeletal pain and pain assessment including questions to ask to identify specific characteristics of pain.

For the reader's convenience, a brief summary of these questions is included in the Core Interview (see Fig. 2-3). In addition, the list of questions is included in Appendices B-25 and C-4 for use in the clinic.

Beyond a pain and symptom assessment, the therapist may conduct a screening physical examination as part of the objective assessment (see Chapter 4). Table 4-13 and Boxes 4-14 and 4-15 are helpful tools for this portion of the examination and evaluation.

Insidious Onset

When the client describes an insidious onset or unknown cause, it is important to ask further questions. Did the symptoms develop after a fall, trauma (including assault), or some repetitive activity (such as painting, cleaning, gardening, filing, or driving long distances)?

The client may wrongly attribute the onset of symptoms to a particular activity that is really unrelated to the current symptoms. The alert therapist may recognize a true causative factor. Whenever the client presents with an unknown etiology of injury or impairment or with an apparent cause, always ask yourself these questions:

Follow-Up Questions

- Is it really insidious?
- Is it really caused by such and such (whatever the client told you)?

Trauma

When the symptoms seem out of proportion to the injury, or when the symptoms persist beyond the expected time for that condition, a red flag should be raised in the therapist's mind. Emotional overlay is often the most suspected underlying cause of this clinical presentation. But trauma from assault and undiagnosed cancer can also present with these symptoms.

Even if the client has a known (or perceived) cause for his or her condition, the therapist must be alert for trauma as an etiologic factor. Trauma may be intrinsic (occurring within the body) or extrinsic (external accident or injury, especially assault or domestic violence).

Twenty-five percent of clients with primary malignant tumors of the musculoskeletal system report a prior traumatic episode. Often the trauma or injury brings attention to a preexisting malignant or benign tumor. Whenever a fracture occurs with minimal trauma or involves a transverse fracture line, the physician considers the possibility of a tumor.

INTRINSIC TRAUMA

An example of intrinsic trauma is the unguarded movement that can occur during normal motion. For example, the client who describes reaching to the back of a cupboard while turning his or her head away from the extended arm to reach that last inch or two. He or she may feel a sudden "pop" or twinge in the neck with immediate pain and describe this as the cause of the injury.

Intrinsic trauma can also occur secondary to extrinsic (external) trauma. A motor vehicle accident, assault, fall, or known accident or injury may result in intrinsic trauma to another part of the musculoskeletal system or other organ system. Such intrinsic trauma may be masked by the more critical injury and may become more symptomatic as the primary injury resolves.

Take for example the client who experiences a cervical flexion/extension (whiplash) injury. The initial trauma causes painful head and neck symptoms. When these resolve (with treatment or on their own), the client may notice midthoracic spine pain or rib pain.

The midthoracic pain can occur when the spine fulcrums over the T4-6 area as the head moves forcefully into the extended position during the whiplash injury. In cases like this, the primary injury to the neck is accompanied by a secondary intrinsic injury to the midthoracic spine. The symptoms may go unnoticed until the more painful cervical lesion is treated or healed.

Likewise, if an undisplaced rib fracture occurs during a motor vehicle accident, it may be asymptomatic until the client gets up the first time. Movement or additional trauma may cause the rib to displace, possibly puncturing a lung. These are all examples of intrinsic trauma.

EXTRINSIC TRAUMA

Extrinsic trauma occurs when a force or load external to the body is exerted against the body. Whenever a client presents with NMS dysfunction, the therapist must consider whether this was caused by an accident, injury, or assault.

The therapist must remain aware that some motor vehicle "accidents" may be reported as accidents but are, in fact, the result of domestic violence in which the victim is pushed, shoved, or kicked out of the car or deliberately hit by a vehicle.

ASSAULT

Domestic violence is a serious public health concern that often goes undetected by clinicians. Women (especially those who are pregnant or disabled), children, and older adults are at greatest risk, regardless of race, religion, or socioeconomic status. Early intervention may reduce the risk of future abuse.

It is imperative that physical therapists and physical therapist assistants remain alert to the prevalence of violence in all sectors of society. Therapists are encouraged to participate in education programs on screening, recognition, and treatment of violence and to advocate for people who may be abused or at risk for abuse.[144]

Addressing the possibility of sexual or physical assault/abuse during the interview may not take place until the therapist has established a working relationship with the client. Each question must be presented in a sensitive, respectful manner with observation for nonverbal cues.

Although some interviewing guidelines are presented here, questioning clients about abuse is a complex issue with important effects on the outcome of rehabilitation. All therapists are encouraged to familiarize themselves with the information available for screening and intervening in this important area of clinical practice.

Generally, the term *abuse* encompasses the terms physical abuse, mental abuse, sexual abuse, neglect, self-neglect, and exploitation (Box 2-8). *Assault* is by definition any physical, sexual, or psychologic attack. This includes verbal, emotional, and economic abuse. *Domestic violence (DV)* or *Intimate partner violence* (IPV) is a pattern of coercive behaviors perpetrated by a current or former intimate partner that may include physical, sexual, and/or psychologic assaults.[145]

Violence against women is more prevalent and dangerous than violence against men,[146] but men can be in an abusive relationship with a parent or partner (male or female).[147,148] For the sake of simplicity, the terms "she" and "her" are used in this section, but this could also be "he" and "his."

BOX 2-8 ▼ Definitions of Abuse

Abuse—Infliction of physical or mental injury, or the deprivation of food, shelter, clothing, or services needed to maintain physical or mental health

Sexual abuse—Sexual assault, sexual intercourse without consent, indecent exposure, deviate sexual conduct, or incest; adult using a child for sexual gratification without physical contact is considered sexual abuse

Neglect—Failure to provide food, shelter, clothing, or help with daily activities needed to maintain physical or mental well-being; client often displays signs of poor hygiene, hunger, or inappropriate clothing

Material exploitation—Unreasonable use of a person, power of attorney, guardianship, or personal trust to obtain control of the ownership, use, benefit, or possession of the person's money, assets, or property by means of deception, duress, menace, fraud, undue influence, or intimidation

Mental abuse—Impairment of a person's intellectual or psychologic functioning or well-being

Emotional abuse—Anguish inflicted through threats, intimidation, humiliation, and/or isolation; belittling, embarrassing, blaming, rejecting behaviors from adult toward child; withholding love, affection, approval

Physical abuse—Physical injury resulting in pain, impairment, or bodily injury of any bodily organ or function, permanent or temporary disfigurement, or death

Self-neglect—Individual is not physically or mentally able to obtain and perform the daily activities of life to avoid physical or mental injury

Data from: Smith L, Putnam DB: The abuse of vulnerable adults. Montana State Bar. *The Montana Lawyer* magazine, June/July 2001. Available at http://www.montanabar.org/montanalawyer/junejuly2001/elderabuse.html. Accessed July 5, 2005.

Intimate partner assault may be more prevalent against gay men than against heterosexual men.[149] Many men have been the victims of sexual abuse as children or teenagers.

Child abuse includes neglect and maltreatment that includes physical, sexual, and emotional abuse. Failure to provide for the child's basic physical, emotional, or educational needs is considered neglect even if it is not a willful act on the part of the parent, guardian, or caretaker.[142]

Screening for Assault or Domestic Violence

As health care providers, therapists have an important role in helping to identify cases of domestic violence and abuse. Routinely incorporating screening questions about domestic violence into history taking only takes a few minutes and is advised in all settings. When interviewing the client it is often best to use some other word besides "assault."

Many people who have been physically struck, pushed, or kicked do not consider the action an assault, especially if someone they know inflicts it. The therapist may want to preface any general screening questions about domestic violence and screening questions can be prefaced with one of the following lead-ins:

Follow-Up Questions

- Abuse in the home is so common today we now ask all our clients:
- Are you threatened or hurt at home or in a relationship with anyone?
- Do you feel safe at home?
- Many people are in abusive relationships but are afraid to say so. We ask everyone about this now.
- FUP: Has this ever happened to you?
- We are required to ask everyone we see about domestic violence. Many of the people I treat tell me they are in difficult, hurtful, sometimes even violent relationships. Is this your situation?
- Is anyone from a previous relationship making you feel unsafe now?
- Alternate: Are your symptoms today caused by someone kicking, hitting, pushing, choking, throwing, or punching you?
- Alternate: I'm concerned someone hurting you may have caused your symptoms. Has anyone been hurting you in any way?
- FUP: Is there anything else you would like to tell me about your situation?

Indirect Questions[142]

- I see you have a bruise here. It looks like it's healing well. How did it happen?
- Are you having problems with your partner?
- Have you ever gotten hurt in a fight?
- You seem concerned about your partner. Can you tell me more about that?
- Does your partner keep you from coming to therapy or seeing family and friends?

Follow-Up Questions[142] Follow-up questions will depend on the client's initial response. The timing of these personal questions can be very delicate. A private area for interviewing is best at a time when the client is alone (including no children, friends, or other family members). The following may be helpful:

Follow-Up Questions

- May I ask you a few more questions?
- If yes, has anyone ever touched you against your will?
- How old were you when it started? When it stopped?
- Have you ever told anyone about this?

Follow-Up Questions

- *Client is offended*
  I'm sorry to offend you. Many people need help but are afraid to ask.

- *Client denies abuse*
  Response: I know sometimes people are afraid or embarrassed to say they've been hit. If you are ever hurt by anyone, it's safe to tell me about it.

- *Client says "Yes"*
  Listen, believe, document if possible. Take photographs if the client will allow it. If the client does not want to get help at this time, offer to give her/him the photos for future use or to keep them on file should the victim change his/her mind. See documentation guidelines. Provide information about local resources. During the interview (and subsequent episode of care), watch out for any of the risk factors and red

Follow-Up Questions

- Have you been kicked, hit, pushed, choked, punched or otherwise hurt by someone in the last year?
- Do you feel safe in your current relationship?

A quick three-question screening tool is positive for partner violence if even one question is answered "yes"[150]:

BOX 2-9 ▼ Risk Factors and Red Flags for Domestic Violence

- Women with disabilities
- Cognitively impaired adult
- Chronically ill and dependent adult (especially adults over age 75)
- Chronic pain clients
- Physical and/or sexual abuse history (men and women)
- Daily headache
- Previous history of many injuries and accidents (including multiple motor vehicle accidents)
- Somatic disorders
  - Injury seems inconsistent with client's explanation; injury in a child that is not consistent with the child's developmental level
  - Injury takes much longer to heal than expected
- Pelvic floor problems
  - Incontinence
  - Infertility
  - Pain
- Recurrent unwanted pregnancies
- History of alcohol abuse in male partner

---

flags for violence (Box 2-9) or any of the clinical signs and symptoms listed in this section. The physical therapist should not turn away from signs of physical or sexual abuse.

In attempting to address such a sensitive issue, the therapist must make sure that the client will not be endangered by intervention. Physical therapists who are not trained to be counselors should be careful about offering advice to those believed to have sustained abuse (or even those who have admitted abuse).

The best course of action may be to document all observations and, when necessary or appropriate, to communicate those documented observations to the referring or family physician. When an abused individual asks for help or direction, the therapist must always be prepared to provide information about available community resources.

In considering the possibility of assault as the underlying cause of any trauma, the therapist should be aware of cultural differences and how these compare with behaviors that suggest excessive partner control. For example:

- Abusive partner rarely lets the client come to the appointment alone (partner control)

BOX 2-10 ▼ Warning Signs of Elder Abuse

- Multiple trips to the emergency department
- Depression
- "Falls"/fractures
- Bruising/suspicious sores
- Malnutrition/weight loss
- Pressure ulcers
- Changing physicians/therapists often
- Confusion attributed to dementia

- Collectivist cultures (group-oriented) often come to the clinic with several family members; such behavior is a cultural norm
- Noncompliance/missed appointments (could be either one)

ELDER ABUSE

Health care professionals are becoming more aware of elder abuse as a problem. Last year, more than 5 million cases of elder abuse were reported. It is estimated that 84% of elder abuse and neglect is never reported. The National Center on Elder Abuse (NCEA) has more information (www.elderabusecenter.org).

The therapist must be alert at all times for elder abuse. Skin tears, bruises, and pressure ulcers are not always predictable signs of aging or immobility. During the screening process, watch for warning signs of elder abuse (Box 2-10).

CLINICAL SIGNS AND SYMPTOMS

Physical injuries caused by battering are most likely to occur in a central pattern (i.e., head, neck, chest/breast, abdomen). Clothes, hats, or hair easily hides injuries to these areas, but they are frequently observable by the therapist in a clinical setting that requires changing into a gown or similar treatment attire.

Assessment of cutaneous manifestations of abuse is discussed in greater detail in this text in Chapter 4. The therapist should follow guidelines provided when documenting the nature (e.g., cut, puncture, burn, bruise, bite), location, and detailed description of any injuries. The therapist must be aware of Mongolian spots, which can be mistaken for bruising from child abuse in certain population groups (see Fig. 4-23).

Other medical disorders in adults such as cardiovascular,[151] gastrointestinal, endocrine,[152] respiratory, gynecologic, and neurologic problems may be linked to childhood sexual or physical abuse.[153-156]

Clinical Signs and Symptoms of Domestic Violence

Physical Cues

- Bruises, black eyes, malnutrition, fractures in various stages of healing
- Skin problems (e.g., eczema, sores that do not heal, burns); see Chapter 4
- Chronic or migraine headaches
- Diffuse pain, vague or nonspecific symptoms
- Chronic or multiple injuries in various stages of healing
- Vision and hearing loss
- Chronic low back, sacral, or pelvic pain
- Temporomandibular joint (TMJ) pain
- Dysphagia (difficulty swallowing) and easy gagging
- Gastrointestinal disorders
- Patchy hair loss, redness, or swelling over the scalp from violent hair pulling
- Easily startled, flinching when approached

Social Cues

- Continually missing appointments
- Bringing all the children to a clinic appointment
- Spouse, companion, or partner always accompanying client
- Changing physicians often
- Multiple trips to the emergency department
- Multiple car accidents

Psychologic Cues

- Anorexia/bulimia
- Panic attacks, nightmares, phobias
- Hypervigilance, tendency to startle easily or be very guarded
- Substance abuse
- Depression, anxiety, insomnia
- Self-mutilation or suicide attempts
- Multiple personality disorders
- Mistrust of authority figures
- Demanding, angry, distrustful of health care provider

WORKPLACE VIOLENCE

Workers in the health care profession are at risk for workplace violence in the form of physical assault and aggressive acts. Threats or gestures used to intimidate or threaten are considered assault. Aggressive acts include verbal or physical actions aimed at creating fear in another person. Any unwelcome physical contact from another person is battery. Any form of workplace violence can be perpetrated by a co-worker, member of a co-worker's family, by a client, or a member of the client's family.[157]

Predicting violence is very difficult, making this occupational hazard one that must be approached through preventative measures rather than relying on individual staff responses or behavior. Institutional policies must be implemented to protect health care workers and provide a safe working environment.[158]

Clients with a mental disorder and history of substance abuse have the highest probability of violent behavior. Adverse drug reactions can lead to violent behavior, as well as conditions that impair judgment or cause confusion, such as alcohol- or HIV-induced encephalopathy, trauma (especially head trauma), seizure disorders, and senility.[157]

Therapists must be alert for risk factors (e.g., dependence on drugs or alcohol, depression, signs of paranoia) and behavioral patterns that may lead to violence (e.g., aggression toward others, blaming others, threats of harm toward others) and immediately report any suspicious incidents or individuals.[157]

THE PHYSICAL THERAPIST'S ROLE

Providing referral to community agencies is perhaps the most important step a health care provider can offer any client who is the victim of abuse, assault, or domestic violence of any kind. Experts report that the best approach to addressing abuse is a combined law enforcement and public health effort.

Any health care professional who asks these kinds of screening questions, must be prepared to respond. Having information and phone numbers available is imperative for the client who is interested. Each therapist must know what reporting requirements are in place in the state in which he or she is practicing (Case Example 2-9).

The therapist should avoid assuming the role of "rescuer," but rather, recognize domestic violence, offer a plan of care and intervention for injuries, assess the client's safety, and offer information regarding support services. The therapist should provide help at the pace the client can handle. Reporting a situation of domestic violence can put the victim at risk.

The client usually knows how to stay safe and when to leave. Whether leaving or staying, it is a complex process of decision-making influenced by shame, guilt, finances, religious beliefs, children, depression, perceptions, and realities. The therapist does not have to be an expert to help someone

CASE EXAMPLE 2-9 Elder Abuse

An 80-year-old female (Mrs. Smith) was referred to home health by her family doctor for an assessment following a mild cerebrovascular accident (CVA). She was living with her 53-year-old divorced daughter (Susan). The daughter works full-time to support herself, her mother, and three teenaged children.

The CVA occurred 3 weeks ago. She was hospitalized for 10 days during which time she had daily physical and occupational therapy. She has residual left-sided weakness.

Home health nursing staff notes that she has been having short-term memory problems in the last week. When the therapist arrived at the home, the doors were open, the stove was on with the stove door open, and Mrs. Smith was in front of the television set. She was wearing a nightgown with urine and feces on it. She was not wearing her hearing aid, glasses, or false teeth.

Mrs. Smith did not respond to the therapist or seem surprised that someone was there. While helping her change into clean clothes, the therapist noticed a large bruise on her left thigh and another one on the opposite upper arm. She did not answer any of the therapist's questions, but talked about her daughter constantly. She repeatedly said, "Susan is mean to me."

How Should the Therapist Respond in this Situation?

Physical therapists do have a role in prevention, assessment, and intervention in cases of abuse and neglect. Keeping a nonjudgmental attitude is helpful.

Assessment: Examination and Evaluation

1. Attempt to obtain a detailed history.
2. Conduct a thorough physical exam. Look for warning signs of pressure ulcers, burns, bruises, or other signs suggesting force.

Include a cognitive and neurologic assessment. Document findings with careful notes, drawings, and photographs whenever possible.

Intervention: Focus on Providing the Client with Safety and the Family with Support and Resources

1. Contact the case manager or nurse assigned to Mrs. Smith.
2. Contact the daughter before calling the county's Adult Protective Services (APS).
3. Team up with the nurse if possible to assess the situation and help the daughter obtain help.
4. When meeting with the daughter, acknowledge the stress the family has been under. Offer the family reassurance that the home health staff's role is to help Mrs. Smith get the best care possible.
5. Let the daughter know what her options are but acknowledge the need to call APS (if required by law).
6. Educate the family and prevent abuse by counseling them to avoid isolation at home. Stay involved in other outside activities (e.g., church/synagogue, school, hobbies, friends).
7. Encourage the family to recognize their limits and seek help when and where it is available.

Result: APS referred Mrs. Smith to an adult day health care program covered by Medicaid. She receives her medications, two meals, and programming with other adults during the day while her daughter works.

The daughter received counseling to help cope with her mother's declining health and loss of mental faculties. She also joined an Alzheimer's "36-hour/day" support group. Respite care was arranged through the adult day care program once every 6 weeks.

who is a victim of domestic violence. Identifying the problem for the first time and listening is an important first step.

During intervention procedures the therapist must be aware that hands-on techniques such as pushing, pulling, stretching, compressing, touching, and rubbing may impact a client with a history of abuse in a negative way. Behaviors such as persistence in cajoling, cheerleading, and demanding compliance meant as encouragement on the part of the therapist may further victimize the individual.[159]

Reporting Abuse The law is clear in all U.S. states regarding abuse of a minor (under age 18 years) (Box 2-11):

BOX 2-11 ▼ Reporting Child Abuse

- The law requires professionals to report suspected child abuse and neglect.
- The therapist must know the reporting guidelines for the state in which he or she is practicing.
- Know who to contact in your local child protective service agency and police department.
- The duty to report findings only requires a reasonable suspicion that abuse has occurred, not certainty.[160]
- A professional who delays reporting until doubt is eliminated is in violation of the reporting law.
- The decision about maltreatment is left up to investigating officials, not the reporting professional.

Data from Mudd SS, Findlay JS: The cutaneous manifestations and common mimickers of physical child abuse, *J Pediatr Health Care* 18(3):123-129, 2004.

When a professional has reasonable cause to suspect, as a result of information received in a professional capacity, that a child is abused or neglected, the matter is to be reported promptly to the department of public health and human services or its local affiliate.[160]

Guidelines for reporting abuse in adults are not always so clear. Some states require health care professionals to notify law enforcement officials when they have treated any individual for an injury that resulted from a domestic assault. There is much debate over such laws as many domestic violence advocate agencies fear mandated police involvement will discourage injured clients from seeking help. Fear of retaliation may prevent abused persons from seeking needed health care because of required law enforcement involvement. The therapist should be familiar with state laws or statutes regarding domestic violence for the geographic area in which he or she is practicing. The Elder Justice Act of 2003 requires reporting of neglect or assault in long-term care facilities in all 50 U.S. states. The National Center on Elder Abuse (NCEA) has more information (www.elderabusecenter.org).

Documentation. Most state laws also provide for the taking of photographs of visible trauma on a child without parental consent. Written permission must be obtained to photograph adults. Always offer to document the evidence of injury.

Even if the client does not want a record of the injury on file, he or she may be persuaded to keep a personal copy for future use if a decision is made to file charges or prosecute at a later time. Polaroid and digital cameras make this easy to accomplish with certainty that the photographs clearly show the extent of the injury or injuries.

The therapist must remember to date and sign the photograph. Record the client's name and injury location on the photograph. Include the client's face in at least one photograph for positive identification. Include a detailed description (type, size, location, depth) and how the injury/injuries occurred.

Record the client's own words regarding the assault and the assailant. For example, "Ms. Jones states, 'My partner Doug struck me in the head and knocked me down.'" Identifying the presumed assailant in the medical record may help the client pursue legal help.[161]

RESOURCES

Consult your local directory for information about adult and child protection services, state elder abuse hotlines, shelters for the battered, or other community services available in your area. For national information, contact:

- National Domestic Violence Hotline. Available 24 hours/day with information on shelters, legal advocacy and assistance, and social service programs. Available at: www.ndvh.org or 1-800-799-SAFE (1-800-799-7233).
- Family Violence Prevention Fund. Updates on legislation related to family violence, information on the latest tools and research on prevention of violence against women and children. Posters, displays, safety cards, and educational pamphlets for use in a health care setting are also available at: http://endabuse.org/ or 1-415-252-8900.
- U.S. Department of Justice. Office on Violence Against Women provides lists of state hotlines, coalitions against domestic violence, and advocacy groups (www.ojp.usdoj.gov/vawo).
- Elder Care Locator. Information on senior services. The service links those who need assistance with state and local area agencies on aging and community-based organizations that serve older adults and their caregivers www.eldercare.gov/Eldercare/Public/Home.asp or 1-800-677-1116.
- U.S. Department of Health and Human Services Administration for Children and Families. Provides fact sheets, laws and policies regarding minors, and phone numbers for reporting abuse.

Available at: www.acf.dhhs.gov/programs/cb/ or 1-800-4-A-CHILD (1-800-422-4453).

Specific Web sites devoted to just men, just women, or any other specific group are available. Anyone interested can go to www.google.com and type in key words of interest.

There are a number of articles and books regarding abuse written for the health care specialist and some directed toward the physical therapist (see Bibliography, this chapter). The APTA offers three publications related to domestic violence, available online at www.apta.org (click on Areas of Interest>Publications):

- Guidelines for Recognizing and Providing Care for Victims of Child Abuse (2005)
- Guidelines for Recognizing and Providing Care for Victims of Domestic Abuse (2005)
- Guidelines for Recognizing and Providing Care for Victims of Elder Abuse (2000)

Medical Treatment and Medications

Medical Treatment

Medical treatment includes any intervention performed by a physician (family practitioner or specialist), dentist, physician's assistant, nurse, nurse practitioner, physical therapist, or occupational therapist. The client may also include chiropractic treatment when answering the question:

Follow-Up Questions

- What medical treatment have you had for this condition?
- Alternate: What treatment have you had for this condition? (allows the client to report any and all modes of treatment including complementary and alternative medicine)

In addition to eliciting information regarding specific treatment performed by the medical community, follow-up questions relate to previous physical therapy treatment:

Follow-Up Questions

- Have you been treated by a physical therapist for this condition before?
- If yes, when, where, and for how long?
- What helped and what didn't help?
- Was there any treatment that made your symptoms worse? If yes, please describe.

Knowing the client's response to previous types of treatment techniques may assist the therapist in determining an appropriate treatment protocol

for the current chief complaint. For example, previously successful treatment intervention described may provide a basis for initial treatment until the therapist can fully assess the objective data and consider all potential types of treatments.

Medications

Medication use, especially with polypharmacy, is important information. Side effects of medications can present as an impairment of the integumentary, musculoskeletal, cardiovascular/pulmonary, or neuromuscular system. Medications may be the most common or most likely cause of systemically induced neuromusculoskeletal signs and symptoms.

Medications (either prescription or over-the-counter) may or may not be listed on the Family/Personal History form at all facilities. Even when a medical history form is used, it may be necessary to probe further regarding the use of over-the-counter preparations such as aspirin, acetaminophen (Tylenol), ibuprofen (e.g., Advil, Motrin), laxatives, antihistamines, antacids, and decongestants or other drugs that can alter the client's symptoms.

RISK FACTORS FOR ADVERSE DRUG REACTIONS

Pharmacokinetics (the processes that affect drug movement in the body) represent the biggest risk factor for adverse drug reactions (ADRs). Absorption, distribution, metabolism, and excretion are the main components of pharmacokinetics affected by age, size, polypharmacy, and other risk factors listed in Box 2-12.

BOX 2-12 ▼ Risk Factors for Adverse Drug Reactions (ADRs)

- Age (over 65, but especially over 75)
- Small physical size or stature (decrease in lean body mass)
- Gender (men and women respond differently to different drugs)
- Polypharmacy (taking several drugs at once; duplicate or dual medications)
- Organ impairment and dysfunction (e.g., renal or hepatic insufficiency)
- Concomitant alcohol consumption
- Concomitant use of certain nutraceuticals
- Previous history of ADRs
- Mental deterioration or dementia (unintentional repeated dosage)
- Racial/ethnic variations

Once again ethnic background is a risk factor to consider. Herbal and home remedies may be used by clients based on their ethnic, spiritual, or cultural orientation. Alternative healers may be consulted for all kinds of conditions from diabetes to depression to cancer. Home remedies can be harmful or interact with some medications.

Some racial groups respond differently to medications. Effectiveness and toxicity can vary among racial and ethnic groups. Differences in metabolic rate, clinical drug responses, and side effects of many medications such as antihistamines, analgesics, cardiovascular agents, psychotropic drugs, and central nervous system agents have been documented. Genetic factors also play a significant role.[162,163]

Women metabolize drugs differently throughout the month as influenced by hormonal changes associated with menses. Researchers are investigating the differences in drug metabolism in women who are premenopausal versus postmenopausal.[164]

Clients receiving home healthcare are at increased risk for medication errors such as uncontrolled hypertension despite medication, confusion or falls while on psychotropic medications, or improper use of medications deemed dangerous to the older adult such as muscle relaxants. Nearly one third of home health clients are misusing their medications as well.[165]

POTENTIAL DRUG SIDE EFFECTS

Doctors are well aware that drugs have side effects. They may even fully expect their patients to experience some of these side effects. The goal is to obtain maximum benefit from the drug's actions with the minimum amount of side effects. These are referred to as "tolerable" side effects.

The most common side effects of medications are constipation, nausea, and sedation. Adverse events such as falls, anorexia, fatigue, cognitive impairment, urinary incontinence, and constipation can occur.[43]

Medications can mask signs and symptoms or produce signs and symptoms that are seemingly unrelated to the client's current medical problem. For example, long-term use of steroids resulting in side effects such as proximal muscle weakness, tissue edema, and increased pain threshold may alter objective findings during the examination of the client.

A detailed description of gastrointestinal (GI) disturbances and other side effects caused by nonsteroidal antiinflammatory drugs (NSAIDs) resulting in back, shoulder, or scapular pain is presented in Chapter 8. Every therapist should be very familiar with these.

Physiologic or biologic differences can result in different responses and side effects to drugs. Race, gender, age, weight, metabolism, and for women, the menstrual cycle can impact drug metabolism and effects. In the aging population, drug side effects can occur even with low doses that usually produce no side effects in younger populations. Older people, especially those who are taking multiple drugs, are two or three times more likely than young to middle-aged adults to have adverse drug reactions.

Seventy-five percent of all older clients take OTC medications that may cause confusion, cause or contribute to additional symptoms, and interact with other medications. Sometimes the client is receiving the same drug under different brand names, increasing the likelihood of drug-induced confusion. Watch for the four *D*s associated with OTC drug use:

- Dizziness
- Drowsiness
- Depression
- Visual disturbance

Because many older people do not consider these "drugs" worth mentioning (i.e., over-the-counter drugs "don't count"), it is important to ask specifically about OTC drug use. Additionally, drug abuse and alcoholism are more common in older people than is generally recognized, especially in depressed clients. Screening for substance use in conjunction with medication use may be important for some clients.

Common medications in the clinic that produce other signs and symptoms include:

- Skin reactions, noninflammatory joint pain (antibiotics; see Fig. 4-11)
- Muscle weakness/cramping (diuretics)
- Muscle hyperactivity (caffeine and medications with caffeine)
- Back and/or shoulder pain (NSAIDs; retroperitoneal bleeding)
- Hip pain from femoral head necrosis (corticosteroids)
- Gait disturbances (Thorazine/tranquilizers)
- Movement disorders (anticholinergics, antipsychotics, antidepressants)
- Hormonal contraceptives (elevated blood pressure)
- Gastrointestinal symptoms (nausea, indigestion, abdominal pain, melena)

This is just a partial listing, but gives an idea why paying attention to medications and potential side effects is important in the screening process.

Not all, but some medications (e.g., antibiotics, antihypertensives, and antidepressants) must be taken as prescribed in order to obtain pharmacologic efficacy.

NONSTEROIDAL ANTIINFLAMMATORY DRUGS (NSAIDs)

Nonsteroidal antiinflammatory drugs (NSAIDs) are a group of drugs that are useful in the symptomatic treatment of inflammation; some appear to be more useful as analgesics. Over-the-counter (OTC) nonsteroidal antiinflammatory (NSAID) drugs are listed in Table 8-3. NSAIDs are commonly used postoperatively for discomfort; for painful musculoskeletal conditions, especially among the older adult population; and in the treatment of inflammatory rheumatic diseases.

The incidence of adverse reactions to NSAIDs is low—complications develop in about 2% to 4% of NSAID users each year.[166] However, 30 to 40 million Americans are regular users of NSAIDs. The widespread use of readily available OTC NSAIDs results in a large number of people being affected. It is estimated that approximately 80% of outpatient orthopedic clients are taking NSAIDs. Many are taking dual NSAIDs (combination of NSAIDs and aspirin) or duplicate NSAIDs (two or more agents from the same class).[167]

Side Effects of NSAIDs NSAIDs have a tendency to produce adverse effects on multiple-organ systems, with the greatest damage to the gastrointestinal tract.[168] GI impairment can be seen as subclinical erosions of the mucosa or more seriously, as ulceration with life-threatening bleeding and perforation. People with NSAID-induced GI impairment can be asymptomatic until the condition is advanced. NSAID-related gastropathy causes thousands of hospitalizations and deaths annually.

For those who are symptomatic, the most common side effects of NSAIDs are stomach upset and pain, possibly leading to ulceration. GI ulceration occurs in 15% to 30% of adults using NSAIDS[169]; physical therapists are seeing a large percentage of these people. NSAID use among surgical patients can cause postoperative complications such as wound hematoma, upper GI tract bleeding, hypotension, and impaired bone or tendon healing.[170]

NSAIDS are also potent renal vasoconstrictors and may cause increased blood pressure and peripheral edema. Clients with hypertension or congestive heart failure are at risk for renal complications, especially those using diuretics or ACE inhibitors.[171] NSAID use may be associated with confusion and memory loss in the older adult.[172]

People with coronary artery disease taking NSAIDs may also be at slight increased risk for a myocardial event during times of increased myocardial oxygen demand (e.g., exercise, fever).

Older adults taking NSAIDs and antihypertensive agents must be monitored carefully. Regardless of the NSAID chosen, it is important to check blood pressure when exercise is initiated and periodically afterwards.

Clinical Signs and Symptoms of

NSAID Complications

* May be asymptomatic
* May cause confusion and memory loss in the older adult

Gastrointestinal

* Indigestion, heartburn, epigastric or abdominal pain
* Esophagitis, dysphagia, odynophagia
* Nausea
* Unexplained fatigue lasting more than 1 or 2 weeks
* Ulcers (gastric, duodenal), perforations, bleeding
* Melena

Renal

* Polyuria, nocturia
* Nausea, pallor
* Edema, dehydration
* Muscle weakness, restless legs syndrome

Integumentary

* Pruritus (symptom of renal impairment)
* Delayed wound healing
* Skin reaction to light (photodermatitis)

Cardiovascular/Pulmonary

* Elevated blood pressure
* Peripheral edema
* Asthma attacks in individuals with asthma

Musculoskeletal

* Increased symptoms after taking the medication
* Symptoms linked with ingestion of food (increased or decreased depending on location of GI ulcer)
* Midthoracic back, shoulder, or scapular pain
* Neuromuscular
* Muscle weakness (sign of renal impairment)
* Restless legs syndrome (sign of renal impairment)
* Paresthesias (sign of renal impairment)

Screening for Risk Factors and Effects of NSAIDs

Screening for risk factors is as important as looking for clinical manifestations of NSAID-induced complications. High-risk individuals are older with a history of ulcers and any coexisting diseases that increase the potential for GI bleeding. Anyone receiving treatment with multiple NSAIDs is at increased risk, especially if the dosage is high and/or includes aspirin.

As with any risk-factor assessment, we must know what to look for before we can recognize signs of impending trouble. In the case of NSAID use, back and/or shoulder pain can be the first symptom of impairment in its clinical presentation.

Any client with this presentation in the presence of the risk factors listed in Box 2-13 raises a red flag of suspicion.[173] Look for the presence of associated GI distress such as indigestion, heartburn, nausea, unexplained chronic fatigue, and/or melena (tarry, sticky, black or dark stools from oxidized blood in the GI tract) (Case Example 2-10). A scoring system to estimate the risk of GI problems in clients with rheumatoid arthritis who are also taking NSAIDs is presented in Table 2-6 (Case Example 2-11).

Correlate increased musculoskeletal symptoms after taking medications. Expect to see a decrease (not an increase) in painful symptoms after taking

---

BOX 2-13 ▼ Risk Factors for NSAID Gastropathy

Back, shoulder, neck, or scapular pain in any client taking NSAIDs in the presence of the following risk factors for NSAID-induced gastropathy raises a red flag of suspicion:

- Age (65 years and older)
- History of peptic ulcer disease, GI disease, or rheumatoid arthritis
- Tobacco or alcohol use
- NSAIDs combined with oral corticosteroid use
- NSAIDs combined with anticoagulants (blood thinners; even when used for cardioprotection at a lower dose, e.g., 81 to 325 mg aspirin/day, especially for those already at increased risk)[173]
- NSAIDs combined with selective serotonin reuptake inhibitors (SSRIs; antidepressants such as Prozac, Zoloft, Celexa, Paxil)
- Chronic use of NSAIDs (duration: 3 months or more)
- Higher doses of NSAIDs, including the use of more than one NSAID (dual or duplicate use)
- Concomitant infection with *Helicobacter pylori* (under investigation)
- Use of acid suppressants (e.g., H_2-receptor antagonists, antacids); these agents may mask the warning symptoms of more serious GI complications, leaving the client unaware of ongoing damage

---

CASE EXAMPLE 2-10   Assessing for NSAID Complications

A 72-year-old orthopedic outpatient presented 4 weeks status post (S/P) left total knee replacement (TKR). She did not attain 90 degrees of knee flexion and continued to walk with a stiff leg. Her orthopedic surgeon sent her to physical therapy for additional rehabilitation.

Past Medical History: The client reports generalized osteoarthritis. She had a left shoulder replacement 18 months ago with very slow recovery and still does not have full shoulder ROM. She has a long-standing hearing impairment of 60 years and lost her left eye to macular degeneration 2 years ago.

Reported drug use: Darvocet for pain 3x/day. Vioxx daily for arthritis (this drug was later removed from the market). She also took Feldene when her shoulder bothered her and daily ibuprofen.

The client walks with a bilateral Trendelenburg gait and drags her left leg using a wheeled walker. Her current symptoms include: left knee and shoulder pain, intermittent dizziness, sleep disturbance, finger/hand swelling in the afternoons, and early morning nausea.

How Do You Assess for NSAID Complications?

1. First, review Box 2-14 for any risk factors:
   Shoulder pain
   Age: 65 years old or older (72 years old)
   Ask about tobacco and alcohol use
   Nausea: ask about the presence of other GI symptoms and previous history of peptic ulcer disease
   Ask about use of corticosteroids, anticoagulants, antidepressants, and acid suppressants
2. Ask about the timing of symptoms in relation to taking her Vioxx, Feldene, and ibuprofen (i.e., see if her shoulder pain is worse 30 minutes to 2 hours after taking the NSAIDs)
3. Take blood pressure
4. Observe for peripheral edema

TABLE 2-6 ▼ Is Your Client at Risk for NSAID-Induced Gastropathy?

This scoring system allows clinicians to estimate the risk of GI problems in clients with rheumatoid arthritis who are also taking NSAIDs. Risk is equal to the sum of:

Age in years	× 2 =
History of NSAID symptoms e.g., upper abdominal pain, bloating, nausea, heartburn, loss of appetite, vomiting	+ 50 points
* ARA class (see below)	add 0, 10, 20 or 30 based on class 1-4
† NSAID dose (fraction of maximum recommended)	× 15
If currently using prednisone	add 40 points
TOTAL SCORE	

* American Rheumatism Association (ARA) Functional Class

+0 points for class 1 (normal)
+10 points for ARA class 2 (adequate)
+20 points for ARA class 3 (limited)
+30 points for ARA class 4 (unable)

ARA Criteria for Classification of Functional Status in Rheumatoid Arthritis:

Class 1 Completely able to perform usual ADLs (self-care, vocational, avocational)
Class 2 Able to perform usual self-care and vocational activities, but limited in avocational activities
Class 3 Able to perform usual self-care activities, but limited in vocational and avocational activities
Class 4 Limited in ability to perform usual self-care, vocational, and avocational activities

† NSAID dose used in this formulation is the fraction of the manufacturer's highest recommended dose. The manufacturer's highest recommended dose on the package insert is given a value of 1.00. The dose of each individual is then normalized to this dose. For example, the value 1.03 indicates the client is taking 103% of the manufacturer's highest recommended dose. Most often, clients are taking the highest dose recommended. They receive a 1.0. Anyone taking less will have a fraction percentage less than 1.0. Anyone taking more than the highest dose recommended will have a fraction percentage greater than 1.0. See Case Example 2-11.

Risk Calculation: To determine the risk (%) of hospitalization or death caused by GI complications over the next 12 months, use the TOTAL SCORE in the following formula:

Risk %/year = [TOTAL SCORE − 100] ÷ 40

Risk percentage is the likelihood of a GI event leading to hospitalization or death over the next 12 months for the person with rheumatoid arthritis on NSAIDs. Higher Total Scores yield greater predictive risk. The risk ranges from 0.0 (low risk) to 5.0 (high risk).

Data from Fries JF, Williams CA, Bloch DA, et al: Nonsteroidal anti-inflammatory drug-associated gastropathy: incidence and risk factor models. *Amer J Med* 91(3):213-222, 1991.

CASE EXAMPLE 2-11   Risk Calculation for NSAID-Induced Gastropathy

A 66-year-old woman with a history of rheumatoid arthritis (class 3) has been referred to physical therapy after three metacarpal-phalangeal (MCP) joint replacements.

Although her doctor has recommended maximum dosage of ibuprofen (800 mg tid; 2400 mg), she is really only taking 1600/day. She says this is all she needs to control her symptoms. She was taking prednisone before the surgery, but tapered herself off and has not resumed its use.

She has been hospitalized 3 times in the past 6 years for gastrointestinal (GI) problems related to NSAID use, but does not have any apparent GI symptoms at this time.

Use the following model to calculate her risk for serious problems with NSAID use:

Age in years	66 × 2 =	132
History of NSAID symptoms, e.g., abdominal pain, bloating, nausea	+50 points	50
ARA class	add 0, 10, 20 or 30 based on class 1-4	20
NSAID dose (fraction of maximum recommended)	1600/2400 × 15 (0.67 × 15)	10
If currently using prednisone	add 40 points	0
TOTAL Score		212

Risk/year = [Total score − 100] ÷ 40
Risk/year = [212 − 100] ÷ 40
Risk/year = 112 ÷ 40 = 2.80

The scores range from 0.0 (very low risk) to 5.0 (very high risk). A predictive risk of 2.8 is moderately high. This client should be reminded to report GI distress to her doctor immediately. Periodic screening for GI gastropathy is indicated with early referral if warranted.

analgesics or NSAIDs. Ask about any change in pain or symptoms (increase or decrease) after eating (anywhere from 30 minutes to 2 hours later).

Ingestion of food should have no effect on the musculoskeletal tissues, so any change in symptoms that can be consistently linked with food raises a red flag, especially for the client with known GI problems or taking NSAIDs.

The peak effect for NSAIDs when used as an *analgesic* varies from product to product. For example, peak analgesic effect of aspirin is 2 hours, whereas the peak for naproxen sodium (Aleve) is 2 to 4 hours (compared to acetaminophen, which peaks in 30 to 60 minutes). Therefore, the symptoms may occur at varying lengths of time after ingestion of food or drink. It is best to find out the peak time for each antiinflammatory taken by the client and note if maximal relief of symptoms occurs in association with that time.

The time to impact *underlying tissue impairment* also varies by individual and severity of impairment. There is a big difference between 220 mg (OTC) and 500 mg (by prescription) of naproxen sodium. For example, 220 mg may appear to "do nothing" in the client's subjective assessment (opinion) after a week's dosing.

What most adults do not know is that it takes more than 24 to 48 hours to build up a high enough level in the body to impact inflammatory symptoms. The person may start adding more drugs before an effective level has been reached in the body. Five hundred milligrams (500 mg) can impact tissue in a shorter time, especially with an acute event or flare-up; this is one reason why doctors sometimes dispense prescription NSAIDs instead of just using the lower dosage OTC drugs.

Older adults taking NSAIDs and antihypertensive agents must be monitored carefully. Regardless of the NSAID chosen, it is important to check blood pressure when exercise is initiated and periodically afterwards.

Ask about muscle weakness, unusual fatigue, restless legs syndrome, polyuria, nocturia, or pruritus (signs and symptoms of renal failure). Watch for increased blood pressure and peripheral edema (perform a visual inspection of the feet and ankles). Document and report any significant findings.

Women who take nonaspirin NSAIDs or acetaminophen (Tylenol) are twice as likely to develop high blood pressure. This refers to chronic use (more than 22 days/month). There is not a proven cause-effect relationship, but a statistical link exists between the two.[174]

ACETAMINOPHEN

Acetaminophen, the active ingredient in Tylenol and other over-the-counter and prescription pain relievers and cold medicines, is an analgesic (pain reliever) and antipyretic (fever reducer) but not an antiinflammatory agent. Acetaminophen is effective in the treatment of mild to moderate pain and is generally well tolerated by all age groups.

It is the analgesic least likely to cause GI bleeding, but taken in large doses over time, it can cause liver toxicity, especially when used with vitamin C or alcohol. Women are more quickly affected than men at lower levels of alcohol consumption.

Individuals at increased risk for problems associated with using acetaminophen are those with a history of alcohol use/abuse, anyone with a history of liver disease (e.g., cirrhosis, hepatitis), and anyone who has attempted suicide using an overdose of this medication.[175]

Some medications (e.g., phenytoin, isoniazid) taken in conjunction with acetaminophen can trigger liver toxicity. The effects of oral anticoagulants may be potentiated by chronic ingestion of large doses of acetaminophen.[176]

Clients with acetaminophen toxicity may be asymptomatic or have anorexia, mild nausea, and vomiting. The therapist may ask about right upper abdominal quadrant tenderness, jaundice, and other signs and symptoms of liver impairment (e.g., liver palms, asterixis, carpal tunnel syndrome, spider angiomas); see Discussion, Chapter 9.

CORTICOSTEROIDS

Corticosteroids are often confused with the singular word "steroids." There are three types or classes of steroids:

1. Anabolic-androgenic steroids such as testosterone, estrogen, and progesterone,
2. Mineralocorticoids responsible for maintaining body electrolytes, and
3. Glucocorticoids, which suppress inflammatory processes within the body.

All three types are naturally occurring hormones produced by the adrenal cortex; synthetic equivalents can be prescribed as medication. Illegal use of a synthetic derivative of testosterone is a concern with athletes.

Corticosteroids used to control pain and reduce inflammation are associated with significant side effects even when given for a short time. Administration may be by local injection (e.g., into a joint), transdermal (skin patch), or systemic (inhalers or pill form).

Side effects of *local injection* (catabolic glucocorticoids) may include soft tissue atrophy, changes in skin pigmentation, accelerated joint destruction, and tendon rupture, but it poses no problem with liver, kidney, or cardiovascular function. *Transdermal* corticosteroids have similar side effects. The incidence of skin-related changes is slightly higher than with local injection, whereas the incidence of joint problems is slightly lower.

Systemic corticosteroids are associated with GI problems, psychologic problems, and hip avascular necrosis. Physician referral is required for marked loss of hip motion and referred pain to the groin in a client on long-term systemic corticosteroids.

Long-term use can lead to immunosuppression, osteoporosis, and other endocrine-metabolic abnormalities. Therapists working with athletes may need to screen for nonmedical (illegal) use of anabolic steroids. Visually observe for signs and symptoms associated with anabolic steroid use. Monitor behavior and blood pressure.

Clinical Signs and Symptoms of
Anabolic Steroid Use

* Rapid weight gain
* Elevated blood pressure (BP)
* Peripheral edema associated with increased BP
* Acne on face and upper body
* Muscular hypertrophy
* Stretch marks around trunk
* Abdominal pain, diarrhea
* Needle marks in large muscle groups
* Personality changes (aggression, mood swings, "roid" rages)
* Bladder irritation, urinary frequency, urinary tract infections
* Sleep apnea, insomnia

OPIOIDS

Opioids such as codeine, morphine, tramadol, hydrocodone, or oxycodone are safe when used as directed. They do not cause kidney, liver, or stomach impairments and have few drug interactions. Side effects can include nausea, constipation, and dry mouth. The client may also experience impaired balance and drowsiness or dizziness, which can increase the risk of falls.

Addiction (physical or psychologic dependence) is often a concern raised by clients and family members alike. Addiction to opioids is uncommon in individuals with no history of substance abuse. Adults over age 60 are often good candidates for use of opioid medications. They obtain greater pain

control with lower doses and develop less tolerance than younger adults.[177]

Long-term use can create a physical dependence. For this reason opioids are monitored carefully and withdrawn or stopped gradually to avoid withdrawal symptoms. Psychologic dependence tends to occur when opioids are used in excessive amounts and often does not develop until after the expected time for pain relief has passed.

HORMONAL CONTRACEPTIVES

Some women use birth control pills to prevent pregnancy while others take them to control their menstrual cycle and/or manage premenstrual and menstrual symptoms, including excessive and painful bleeding.

Originally, birth control pills contained as much as 20% more estrogen than the amount present in the low-dose, third-generation oral contraceptives available today. Women taking the newer hormonal contraceptives (whether in pill, injectable, or patch form) have a slightly increased risk of high blood pressure, which returns to normal shortly after the hormone is discontinued.

Age over 35, smoking, hypertension, obesity, bleeding disorders, major surgery with prolonged immobilization, and diabetes are risk factors for blood clots (venous thromboembolism, not arterial), heart attacks, and strokes in women taking hormonal contraceptives.[178] Adolescents using the injectable contraceptive Depo-Provera (DMPA) are at risk for bone loss.[179]

Anyone taking hormonal contraception of any kind, but especially premenopausal cardiac clients, must be monitored by taking vital signs, especially blood pressure during physical activity and exercise. Assessing for risk factors is an important part of the plan of care for this group of individuals.

Any woman on combined oral contraceptives (estrogen and progesterin) reporting break-through bleeding should be advised to see her doctor.

ANTIBIOTICS

Skin reactions (see Fig. 4-11) and noninflammatory joint pain (see Box 3-4) are two of the most common side effects of antibiotics seen in a therapist's practice. Often these symptoms are delayed and occur up to 6 weeks after the client has finished taking the drug.

Fluoroquinolones, a class of antibiotics used to treat urinary tract infections; upper respiratory tract infections; infectious diarrhea; gynecologic infections; and skin, soft tissue, bone and joint

infections are known to cause tendinopathies ranging from tendonitis to tendon rupture.

Commonly prescribed fluoroquinolones end in the suffix—*oxacin* and include ciprofloxacin, enoxacin, levofloxacin, norfloxacin, and pefloxacin. Although tendon injury has been reported with most fluoroquinolones, most of the fluoroquinolone-induced tendinopathies of the Achilles tendon are due to ciprofloxacin. The concomitant use of corticosteroids and fluoroquinolones in older adults are the major risk factors for developing musculoskeletal toxicities.[180,181]

Other common side effects include headache, fatigue, GI disturbance (nausea, vomiting, diarrhea), arthralgia (joint pain, inflammation, and stiffness), and neck, back, or chest pain. Symptoms may occur as early as 2 hours after the first dose and as late as 6 months after treatment has ended[182] (Case Example 2-12).

NUTRACEUTICALS

Nutraceuticals are natural products (usually made from plant substances) that do not require a prescription to purchase. They are often sold at health food stores, nutrition or vitamin stores, through private distributors, or on the Internet. Nutraceuticals consist of herbs, vitamins, minerals, antioxidants, and other natural supplements.

The use of herbal and other supplements has increased dramatically in the last decade. Exposure to individual herbal ingredients may continue to rise as more of them are added to mainstream multivitamin products and advertised as cancer and chronic disease preventatives.[183]

CASE EXAMPLE 2-12   Fluoroquinolone-Induced Tendinopathy

A 57-year-old retired army colonel (male) presented to an outpatient physical therapy clinic with a report of swelling and pain in both ankles.

Symptoms started in the left ankle 4 days ago. Then the right ankle and foot became swollen. Ankle dorsiflexion and weight bearing made it worse. Staying off the foot made it better.

Past Medical History:
• Prostatitis diagnosed and treated 2 months ago with antibiotics; placed on levofloxacin 11 days ago when urinary symptoms recurred
• Chronic benign prostatic hypertrophy
• Gastroesophageal reflux (GERD)
• Hypertension

Current medications:
• Omeprazole (Prilosec)
• Lisinopril (Prinivil, Zestril)
• Enteric-coated aspirin
• Tamsulosin (Flomax)
• Levofloxacin (Levaquin)

Clinical Presentation:
• Moderate swelling of both ankles; malleoli diminished visually by 50%
• No lymphadenopathy (cervical, axillary, inguinal)
• Fullness of both Achilles tendons with pitting edema of the feet extending to just above the ankles, bilaterally
• No nodularity behind either Achilles tendon

• Ankle joint tender to minimal palpation; reproduced when Achilles tendons are palpated
• ROM: normal subtalar and plantar flexion of the ankle; dorsiflexion to neutral (limited by pain); inversion and eversion WNL and pain-free; unable to squat due to painfully limited ROM
• Neuro screen: negative
• Knee screen: no apparent problems in either knee

Associated Signs and Symptoms: The client reports fever and chills the day before the ankle started swelling, but this has gone away now. Urinary symptoms have resolved. Reports no other signs or symptoms anywhere else in his body.

Vital signs:
• Blood pressure   128/74 mm Hg taken seated in the left arm
• Heart rate   78 BPM
• Respiratory rate   14 breaths per minute
• Temperature   99.0° F (client states "normal" for him is 98.6° F)

Red Flags:
• Age
• Bilateral swelling

What Are the Red-Flag Signs and Symptoms Here? Should a Medical Referral Be Made? Why or Why Not?

CASE EXAMPLE 2-12   Fluoroquinolone-Induced Tendinopathy—cont'd

- Recent history of new medication (levofloxacin) known to cause tendon problems in some cases
- Constitutional symptoms × 1 day; presence of low-grade fever at the time of the initial evaluation

A cluster of red flags like this suggests medical referral would be a good idea before initiating intervention. If there is an inflammatory process going on, early diagnosis and medical treatment can minimize damage to the joint.

If there is a medical problem it is not likely to be life-threatening, so theoretically the therapist could treat symptomatically for three to five sessions and then evaluate the results. Medical referral could be made at that time if symptoms remain unchanged by treatment. If this option is chosen, the client's vital signs must be monitored closely.

Decision: The client was referred to his primary care physician with the following request (use of minimal highlighting can be very effective as demonstrated below):

Date

Dr. Smith,

This client came to our clinic with a report of bilateral ankle swelling. I observed the following findings:

Moderate swelling of both ankles; malleoli diminished visually by 50%

No lymphadenopathy (cervical, axillary, inguinal)

Fullness of both Achilles tendons with pitting edema of the feet extending to just above the ankles, bilaterally

No nodularity behind either Achilles tendon

Ankle joint tender to minimal palpation; reproduced when Achilles tendons are palpated

ROM: normal subtalar and plantar flexion of the ankle; dorsiflexion to neutral (limited by pain); inversion and eversion WNL and pain-free; unable to squat due to painfully limited ROM

Neuro screen: negative

Knee screen: no apparent problems in either knee

Associated Signs and Symptoms:

The client reports fever and chills the day before the ankle started swelling, but this went away by the time he came to physical therapy. Urinary symptoms also had resolved. The client reported no other signs or symptoms anywhere else in his body.

Vital signs:

Blood pressure	128/74 mm Hg taken seated in the left arm
Heart Rate	78 BPM
Respiratory rate	14 breaths per minute
Temperature	99.0° F (client states "normal" for him is 98.6° F)

I'm concerned by the following cluster of red flags:

Age

Bilateral swelling

Recent history of new medication (levofloxacin)

Constitutional symptoms × 1 day; presence of low-grade fever at the time of the initial evaluation

I would like to request a medical evaluation before beginning any physical therapy intervention. I would appreciate a copy of your report and any recommendations you may have if physical therapy is appropriate.

Thank you. Best regards,

Result: The client was diagnosed (x-rays and diagnostic lab work) with levofloxacin-induced bilateral Achilles tendonitis. Medical treatment included nonsteroidal antiinflammatory medications (NSAIDs), rest, and discontinuation of the levofloxacin.

Symptoms resolved completely within 7 days with full motion and function of both ankles and feet. There was no need for physical therapy intervention. Client was discharged from any further PT involvement for this episode of care.

Recommended Reading: Greene BL: Physical therapist management of fluoroquinolone-Induced Achilles tendinopathy, *Physical Therapy* 82(12):1224-1231, 2002.

Data from McKinley BT, Oglesby RJ: A 57-Year-Old Male Retired Colonel with Acute Ankle Swelling. *Military Medicine* 169(3):254-256, 2004.

These products may be produced with all natural ingredients, but this does not mean they do not cause problems, complications, and side effects. When combined with certain food items or taken with some prescription drugs, nutraceuticals can have potentially serious complications.

Herbal and home remedies may be used by clients based on their ethnic, spiritual, or cultural orientation. Alternative healers may be consulted for all kinds of conditions from diabetes to depression to cancer. Home remedies and nutraceuticals can be harmful when combined with some medications.

The therapist should ask clients about and document their use of nutraceuticals and dietary supplements. In a survey of surgical patients more than 1 in 3 adults had taken an herb that had effects on coagulation, blood pressure, cardiovascular function, sedation, and electrolytes or diuresis within 2 weeks of the scheduled surgery. As many as 70% of these individuals failed to disclose this use during the preoperative assessment.[184]

A pharmacist can help in comparing signs and symptoms present with possible side effects and drug-drug or drug-nutraceutical interactions. Mayo Clinic offers a list of herbal supplements that should not be taken in combination with certain types of medications (www.mayoclinic.com/invoke.cfm?id=SA00039).

THE PHYSICAL THERAPIST'S ROLE

For every client the therapist is strongly encouraged to take the time to look up indications for use and possible side effects of prescribed medications. Drug reference guidebooks that are updated and published every year are available in hospital and clinic libraries or pharmacies. Pharmacists are also invaluable sources of drug information. Web sites with useful drug information are included in the next section (see Resources).

Distinguishing drug-related signs and symptoms from disease-related symptoms may require careful observation and consultation with family members or other health professionals to see whether these signs tend to increase following each dose.[185] This information may come to light by asking the question:

Follow-Up Questions

• Do you notice any increase in symptoms, or perhaps the start of symptoms, after taking your medications? (This may occur 30 minutes to 2 hours after taking the drug.)

Because clients are more likely now than ever before to change physicians or practitioners during an episode of care, the therapist has an important role in education and screening. The therapist can alert individuals to watch for any red flags in their drug regimen. Clients with both hypertension and a condition requiring NSAID therapy should be closely monitored and advised to make sure the prescribing practitioner is aware of both conditions.

The therapist may find it necessary to reeducate the client regarding the importance of taking medications as prescribed, whether on a daily or other regular basis. In the case of antihypertensive medication, the therapist should ask whether the client has taken the medication today as prescribed.

It is not unusual to hear a client report, "I take my blood pressure pills when I feel my heart starting to pound." The same situation may occur with clients taking antiinflammatory drugs, antibiotics, or any other medications that must be taken consistently for a specified period to be effective. Always ask the client if he or she is taking the prescription every day or just as needed. Make sure this is with the physician's knowledge and approval.

Clients may be taking medications that were not prescribed for them, taking medications inappropriately, or not taking prescribed medications without notifying the doctor. Appropriate FUPs include the following:

Follow-Up Questions

• Why are you taking these medications?
• When was the last time that you took these medications?
• Have you taken these drugs today?
• Do the medications relieve your pain or symptoms?
  If yes, how soon after you take the medications do you notice an improvement?
• If prescription drugs, who prescribed this medication for you?
• How long have you been taking these medications?
• When did your physician last review these medications?
• Are you taking any medications that weren't prescribed for you?
  If no, follow-up with: Are you taking any pills given to you by someone else besides your doctor?

Many people who take prescribed medications cannot recall the name of the drug or tell you why they are taking it. It is essential to know whether

the client has taken OTC or prescription medication before the physical therapy examination or intervention because the symptomatic relief or possible side effects may alter the objective findings.

Similarly, when appropriate, treatment can be scheduled to correspond with the time of day when clients obtain maximal relief from their medications. Finally, the therapist may be the first one to recognize a problem with medication or dosage. Bringing this to the attention of the doctor is a valuable service to the client.

RESOURCES

Many resources are available to help the therapist identify potential side effects of medications, especially in the presence of polypharmacy with the possibility of drug interactions.

Find a local pharmacist willing to answer questions about medications. The pharmacist can let the therapist know when associated signs and symptoms may be drug-related. Always bring this to the physician's attention. It may be that the "burden of tolerable side effects" is worth the benefit, but often, the dosage can be adjusted or an alternative drug can be tried.

Several favorite resources include *Mosby's Nursing Drug Handbook*, published each year by Elsevier Science (Mosby, St. Louis), *The People's Pharmacy Guide to Home and Herbal Remedies*,[186] *PDR for Herbal Medicines ed 3*,[187] and *Pharmacology in Rehabilitation*.[188]

A helpful general guide regarding potentially inappropriate medications for older adults called the Beers' list has been published and revised. This list along with detailed information about each class of drug is available online at: www.dcri.duke.edu/ccge/curtis/beers.html.

Easy-to-use Web sites for helpful pharmacologic information include:

- MedicineNet (www.medicinenet.com)
- University of Montana Drug Information Service (DIS) (www.umt.edu/druginfo or by phone: 1-800-501-5491)
- RxList: The Internet Drug Index (www.rxlist.com)
- DrugDigest (www.drugdigest.com; allows therapist to look for side effects of drug combinations)
- National Council on Patient Information and Education: BeMedWise. Advice on use of over-the-counter medications. Available at www.bemedwise.org.

Current Level of Fitness

An assessment of current physical activity and level of fitness (or level just before the onset of the current problem) can provide additional necessary information relating to the origin of the client's symptom complex.

The level of fitness can be a valuable indicator of potential response to treatment based on the client's motivation (i.e., those who are more physically active and healthy seem to be more motivated to return to that level of fitness through disciplined self-rehabilitation).

It is important to know what type of exercise or sports activity the client participates in, the number of times per week (frequency) that this activity is performed, the length (duration) of each exercise or sports session, as well as how long the client has been exercising (weeks, months, years), and the level of difficulty of each exercise session (intensity). It is very important to ask:

Follow-Up Questions

- Since the onset of symptoms, are there any activities that you can no longer accomplish?

The client should give a description of these activities, including how physical activities have been affected by the symptoms. Follow-up questions include:

Follow-Up Questions

- Do you ever experience shortness of breath or lack of air during any activities (e.g., walking, climbing stairs)?
- Are you ever short of breath without exercising?
- Are you ever awakened at night breathless? If yes, how often and when does this occur?

If the Family/Personal History form is not used, it may be helpful to ask some of the questions shown in Fig. 2-2: Work/Living Environment or History of Falls. For example, assessing the history of falls with older people is essential. One third of community-dwelling older adults and a higher proportion of institutionalized older people fall annually. Aside from the serious injuries that may result, a debilitating "fear of falling" may cause many older adults to reduce their activity level and restrict their social life. This is one area that is often treatable and even preventable with physical therapy.

Older persons who are in bed for prolonged periods are at risk for secondary complications, including pressure ulcers, urinary tract infections, pulmonary infections and/or infarcts, congestive

heart failure, osteoporosis, and compression fractures. See previous discussion in this chapter (History of Falls) for more information.

Sleep-Related History

Sleep patterns are valuable indicators of underlying physiologic and psychologic disease processes. The primary function of sleep is believed to be the restoration of body function. When the quality of this restorative sleep is decreased, the body and mind cannot perform at optimal levels.

Physical problems that result in pain, increased urination, shortness of breath, changes in body temperature, perspiration, or side effects of medications are just a few causes of sleep disruption. Any factor precipitating sleep deprivation can contribute to an increase in the frequency, intensity, or duration of a client's symptoms.

For example, fevers and night sweats are characteristic signs of systemic disease. Night sweats occur as a result of a gradual increase in body temperature followed by a sudden drop in temperature. This change in body temperature can be related to pathologic changes in immunologic, neurologic, or endocrine function.

Be aware that many people, especially women, experience sweats associated with menopause, poor room ventilation, or too many clothes and covers used at night. Sweats can also occur in the neutropenic client after chemotherapy or as a side effect of other medications such as some antidepressants, sedatives or tranquilizers, and some analgesics.

Anyone reporting night sweats of a systemic origin must be asked if the same phenomenon occurs during the waking hours. Sweats (present day and night) can be associated with medical problems such as tuberculosis, autoimmune diseases, and malignancies.[189]

An isolated experience of sweats is not as significant as intermittent but consistent sweats in the presence of risk factors for any of these conditions or in the presence of other constitutional symptoms (see Box 1-3). Assess vital signs in the client reporting sweats, especially when other symptoms are present and/or the client reports back or shoulder pain of unknown cause.

Certain neurologic lesions may produce local changes in sweating associated with nerve distribution. For example, a client with a spinal cord tumor may report changes in skin temperature above and below the level of the tumor. At presentation, any client with a history of either night sweats or fevers should be referred to the primary physician. This is especially true for clients with back pain or multiple joint pain without traumatic origin.

Pain at night is usually perceived as being more intense because of the lack of outside distraction when the person lies quietly without activity. The sudden quiet surroundings and lack of external activity create an increased perception of pain that is a major disrupter of sleep.

It is very important to ask the client about pain during the night. Is the person able to get to sleep? If not, the pain may be a primary focus and may become continuously intense so that falling asleep is a problem.

Follow-Up Questions

- Does a change in body position affect the level of pain?

If a change in position can increase or decrease the level of pain, it is likely to be a musculoskeletal problem. If, however, the client is awakened from a deep sleep by pain in any location that is unrelated to physical trauma and is unaffected by a change in position, this may be an ominous sign of serious systemic disease, particularly cancer.

Follow-Up Questions

- If you wake up because of pain, is it because you rolled onto that side?
- Can you get back to sleep?
- If yes, what do you have to do (if anything) to get back to sleep? (This answer may provide clues for treatment.)

Many other factors (primarily environmental and psychologic) are associated with sleep disturbance, but a good, basic assessment of the main characteristics of physically related disturbances in sleep pattern can provide valuable information related to treatment or referral decisions. The McGill Home Recording Card (Fig. 3-7) is a helpful tool for evaluating sleep patterns.

Stress (See Also Chapter 3)

By using the interviewing tools and techniques described in this chapter, the therapist can communicate a willingness to consider all aspects of illness, whether biologic or psychologic. Client self-disclosure is unlikely if there is no trust in the health professional, if there is fear of a lack of confidentiality, or if a sense of disinterest is noted.

Most symptoms (pain included) are aggravated by unresolved emotional or psychologic stress. Prolonged stress may gradually lead to physiologic

changes. Stress may result in depression, anxiety disorders, and behavioral consequences (e.g., smoking, alcohol and substance abuse, and accident proneness).

The effects of emotional stress may be increased by physiologic changes brought on by the use of medications or poor diet and health habits (e.g., cigarette smoking or ingestion of caffeine in any form). As part of the Core Interview, the therapist may assess the client's subjective report of stress by asking:

Follow-Up Questions

- What major life changes or stresses have you encountered that you would associate with your injury/illness?
- Alternate: What situations in your life are "stressors" for you?
- It may be helpful to quantify the stress by asking the client:
- On a scale from 0 to 10, with 0 being no stress and 10 being the most extreme stress you have ever experienced, what number rating would you give your stress in general at this time in your life?
- What number would you give your stress level today?

Emotions such as fear and anxiety are common reactions to illness and treatment intervention and may increase the client's awareness of pain and symptoms. These emotions may cause autonomic (branch of nervous system not subject to voluntary control) distress manifested in such symptoms as pallor, restlessness, muscular tension, perspiration, stomach pain, diarrhea or constipation, or headaches.

It may be helpful to screen for anxiety-provoked hyperventilation by asking:

Follow-Up Questions

- Do you ever get short of breath or dizzy or lose coordination when you are fatigued?

After the objective evaluation has been completed, the therapist can often provide some relief of emotionally amplified symptoms by explaining the cause of pain, outlining a plan of care, and providing a realistic prognosis for improvement. This may not be possible if the client demonstrates signs of hysterical symptoms or conversion symptoms (see Discussion in Chapter 3).

Whether the client's symptoms are systemic or caused by an emotional/psychologic overlay, if the client does not respond to treatment, it may be necessary to notify the physician that there is not a satisfactory explanation for the client's complaints. Further medical evaluation may be indicated at that time.

Final Questions

It is always a good idea to finalize the interview by reviewing the findings and paraphrasing what the client has reported. Use the answers from the Core Interview to recall specifics about the location, frequency, intensity, and duration of the symptoms. Mention what makes it better or worse.

Recap the medical and surgical history including current illnesses, diseases, or other medical conditions; recent or past surgeries; recent or current medications; recent infections; and anything else of importance brought out by the interview process.

It is always appropriate to end the interview with a few final questions such as:

Follow-Up Questions

- Are there any other symptoms of any kind anywhere else in your body that we haven't discussed yet?
- Is there anything else you think is important about your condition that we have not discussed yet?
- Is there anything else you think I should know?

If you have not asked any questions about assault or partner abuse, this may be the appropriate time to screen for domestic violence.

Special Questions for Women

Gynecologic disorders can refer pain to the low back, hip, pelvis, groin, or sacroiliac joint Any woman having pain or symptoms in any one or more of these areas should be screened for possible systemic diseases. The need to screen for systemic disease is essential when there is no known cause of the pain or symptoms.

Any woman with a positive family/personal history of cancer should be screened for medical disease even if the current symptoms can be attributed to a known neuromusculoskeletal cause.

Chapter 14 has a list of special questions to ask women (see also Appendix B-32). The therapist will not need to ask every woman each question listed but should take into consideration the data from the Family/Personal History form, Core Interview, and clinical presentation when choosing appropriate FUPs.

Special Questions for Men

Men describing symptoms related to the groin, low back, hip, or sacroiliac joint may have prostate or urologic involvement. A positive response to any or all of the questions in Appendix B-21 must be evaluated further. Answers to these questions correlated with family history, the presence of risk factors, clinical presentation, and any red flags will guide the therapist in making a decision regarding treatment versus referral.

▲ HOSPITAL INPATIENT INFORMATION

Medical Record

Treatment of hospital or nursing home inpatients requires a slightly different interview (or information-gathering) format. Reviewing the patient's medical record for information will assist the therapist in developing a safe and effective plan of care.

Important information to look for might include:

• Age
• Medical diagnosis
• Surgery report
• Physician's/nursing notes
• Associated or additional problems relevant to physical therapy
• Medications
• Restrictions
• Laboratory results
• Vital signs

An evaluation of the patient's medical status in conjunction with age and diagnosis can provide valuable guidelines for the plan of care.

If the patient has had recent surgery, the physician's report should be scanned for preoperative and postoperative orders (in some cases there is a separate physician's orders book or link to click on if the medical records are in an electronic format). Read the operative report whenever available. Look for any of the following information:

• Was the patient treated preoperatively with physical therapy for gait, strength, range of motion, or other objective assessments?
• Were there any unrelated preoperative conditions?
• Was the surgery invasive, a closed procedure via arthroscopy, fluoroscopy, or other means of imaging, or virtual by means of computerized technology?
• How long was the operative procedure?
• How much fluid and/or blood products were given?

• What position was the patient placed in during the procedure?

Fluid received during surgery may affect arterial oxygenation, leaving the person breathless with minimal exertion and experiencing early muscle fatigue. Prolonged time in any one position can result in residual musculoskeletal complaints.

The surgical position for men and for women during laparoscopy (examination of the peritoneal cavity) may place patients at increased risk for thrombophlebitis because of the decreased blood flow to the legs during surgery.

Other valuable information that may be contained in the physician's report may include:

• What are the current short-term and long-term medical treatment plans?
• Are there any known or listed contraindications to physical therapy intervention?
• Does the patient have any weight-bearing limitations?

Associated or additional problems to the primary diagnosis may be found within the record (e.g., diabetes, heart disease, peripheral vascular disease, or respiratory involvement). The physical therapist should look for any of these conditions in order to modify exercise accordingly and to watch for any related signs and symptoms that might affect the exercise program:

• Are there complaints of any kind that may affect exercise (e.g., shortness of breath [dyspnea], heart palpitations, rapid heart rate [tachycardial], fatigue, fever, or anemia)?

If the patient has diabetes, the therapist should ask:

• What are the current blood glucose levels and recent A1C levels?
• When is insulin administered? Avoiding peak insulin levels in planning exercise schedules is discussed more completely in Chapter 11. Other questions related to medications can follow the Core Interview outline with appropriate follow-up questions:

• Is the patient receiving oxygen or receiving fluids/medications through an intravenous line?
• If the patient is receiving oxygen, will he or she need increased oxygen levels before, during, or following physical therapy? What level(s)? Does the patient have chronic obstructive pulmonary disease (COPD) with restrictions on oxygen use?
• Are there any dietary or fluid restrictions?
• If so, check with the nursing staff to determine the full limitations. For example:

- Are ice chips or wet washcloths permissible?
- How many ounces or milliliters of fluid are allowed during therapy?
- Where should this amount be recorded?

Laboratory values and vital signs should be reviewed. For example:

- Is the patient anemic?
- Is the patient's blood pressure stable?

Anemic patients may demonstrate an increased normal resting pulse rate that should be monitored during exercise. Patients with unstable blood pressure may require initial standing with a tilt table or monitoring of the blood pressure before, during, and after treatment. Check the nursing record for pulse rate at rest and blood pressure to use as a guide when taking vital signs in the clinic or at the patient's bedside.

Nursing Assessment

After reading the patient's chart, check with the nursing staff to determine the nursing assessment of the individual patient. The essential components of the nursing assessment that are of value to the therapist may include:

- Medical status
- Pain
- Physical status
- Patient orientation
- Discharge plans

The nursing staff are usually intimately aware of the patient's current medical and physical status. If pain is a factor:

- What is the nursing assessment of this patient's pain level and pain tolerance?

Pain tolerance is relative to the medications received by the patient, the number of days after surgery or after injury, fatigue, previous history of substance abuse or chemical addiction, and the patient's personality.

To assess the patient's physical status, ask the nursing staff:

- Has the patient been up at all yet?
- If yes, how long has the patient been sitting, standing, or walking?
- How far has the patient walked?
- How much assistance does the patient require?

Ask about the patient's orientation:

- Is the patient oriented to time, place, and person? In other words, does the patient know the date and the approximate time, where he or she is, and who he or she is? Treatment plans may be altered by the patient's awareness; for example, a home program may be impossible without family compliance.
- Are there any known or expected discharge plans?

- If yes, what are these plans and when is the target date for discharge?

Cooperation between nurses and therapists is an important part of the multidisciplinary approach in planning the patient's plan of care. The questions to ask and factors to consider provide the therapist with the basic information needed to carry out an objective examination and to plan the intervention. Each individual patient's situation may require that the therapist obtain additional pertinent information (Box 2-14).

▶ PHYSICIAN REFERRAL

The therapist will be using the questions presented in this chapter to identify symptoms of possible systemic origin. The therapist can screen for medical disease and decide if referral to the physician (or other appropriate health care professional) is indicated by correlating the client's answers with family/personal history, vital signs, and objective findings from the physical examination.

For example, consider the client with a chief complaint of back pain who circles "yes" on the Family/Personal History form, indicating a history of ulcers or stomach problems. Obtaining further information at the first appointment by using Special Questions to Ask is necessary so that a decision regarding treatment or referral can be made immediately.

This treatment-versus-referral decision is further clarified as the interview, and other objective evaluation procedures continue. Thus if further questioning fails to show any association of back pain with gastrointestinal symptoms, and the objective findings from the back evaluation point to a true musculoskeletal lesion, medical referral is unnecessary and the physical therapy intervention can begin.

This information is not designed to make a medical diagnosis, but rather to perform an accurate assessment of pain and systemic symptoms that can mimic or occur simultaneously with a musculoskeletal problem.

Guidelines for Physician Referral

As part of the Review of Systems, correlate *history* with *patterns of pain* and any *unusual findings* that may indicate systemic disease. The therapist can use the decision-making tools discussed in Chapter 1 (see Box 1-7) to make a decision regarding treatment versus referral.

Some of the specific indications for physician referral mentioned in this chapter include the following:

BOX 2-14 ▼ Hospital Inpatient Information

Medical Record

- **Patient Age**
- **Medical Diagnosis**
- **Surgery:** Did the patient have surgery? What was the surgery for?

FUPs:
- Was the patient seen by a physical therapist preoperatively?
- Were there any unrelated preoperative conditions?
- Was the surgery invasive, a closed procedure via arthroscopy, fluoroscopy, or other means of imaging, or virtual by means of computerized technology?
- How long was the procedure? Were there any surgical complications?
- How much fluid and/or blood products were given?
- What position was the patient placed in and for how long?

Physician's report
- What are the short-term and long-term medical treatment plans?
- Are there precautions or contraindications for treatment?
- Are there weight-bearing limitations?
- **Associated or additional problems,** such as diabetes, heart disease, peripheral vascular disease, respiratory involvement

FUPs:
- Are there precautions or contraindications of any kind that may affect exercise?
- If diabetic, what are the current blood glucose levels (normal range: 70 to 100 mg/dl)?
- When is insulin administered? (Use this to avoid the peak insulin levels in planning an exercise schedule.)
- **Medications** (what, when received, what for, potential side effects)

FUPs:
- Is the patient receiving oxygen or receiving fluids/medications through an intravenous line?
- **Restrictions:** Are there any dietary or fluid restrictions?

- Spontaneous postmenopausal bleeding
- A growing mass, whether painful or painless
- Persistent rise or fall in blood pressure
- Hip, sacroiliac, pelvic, groin, or low back pain in a woman without traumatic etiologic complex who reports fever, night sweats, or an association between menses and symptoms

FUPs:
- If yes, check with the nursing staff to determine the patient's full limitation.
- Are ice chips or a wet washcloth permissible?
- How many ounces or milliliters of fluid are allowed during therapy?

- **Laboratory values:** Hematocrit/hemoglobin level (see inside cover for normal values and significance of these tests); exercise tolerance test results if available for cardiac patient; pulmonary function test (PFT) to determine severity of pulmonary problem; arterial blood gas (ABG) levels to determine the need for supplemental oxygen during exercise
- **Vital signs:** Is the blood pressure stable?

FUPs:
- If no, consider initiating standing with a tilt table or monitoring the blood pressure before, during, and after treatment.

Nursing Assessment
- **Medical status:** What is the patient's current medical status?
- **Pain:** What is the nursing assessment of this patient's pain level and pain tolerance?
- **Physical status:** Has the patient been up at all yet?

FUPs:
- If yes, is the patient sitting, standing, or walking? How long and (if walking) what distance, and how much assistance is required?
- **Patient orientation:** Is the patient oriented to time, place, and person? (Does the patient know the date and the approximate time, where he or she is, and who he or she is?)
- **Discharge plans:** Are there any known or expected discharge plans?

FUPs:
- If yes, what are these plans and when will the patient be discharged?
- **Final question:** Is there anything else that I should know before exercising the patient?

- Marked loss of hip motion and referred pain to the groin in a client on long-term systemic corticosteroids
- A positive family/personal history of breast cancer in a woman with chest, back, or shoulder pain of unknown cause
- Elevated blood pressure in any woman taking birth control pills; this should be closely monitored by her physician

✔ KEY POINTS TO REMEMBER

✓ The process of screening for medical disease before establishing a diagnosis by the physical therapist and plan of care requires a broad range of knowledge.

✓ Throughout the screening process, a medical diagnosis is not the goal. The therapist is screening to make sure that the client does indeed have a primary NMS problem within the scope of a physical therapist practice.

✓ The screening steps begin with the client interview, but screening does not end there. Screening questions may be needed throughout the episode of care. This is especially true when progression of disease results in a changing clinical presentation, perhaps with the onset of new symptoms or new red flags after the treatment intervention has been initiated.

✓ The client history is the first and most basic skill needed for screening. Most of the information needed to determine the cause of symptoms is contained within the subjective assessment (interview process).

✓ The Family/Personal History form can be used as the first tool to screen clients for medical disease. Any "yes" responses should be followed up with appropriate questions. The therapist is strongly encouraged to review the form with the client, entering the date and his or her own initials. This form can be used as a document of baseline information.

✓ Screening examinations (interview and vital signs) should be completed for any person experiencing back, shoulder, scapular, hip, groin, or sacroiliac symptoms of unknown cause. The presence of constitutional symptoms will almost always warrant a physician's referral but definitely requires further follow-up questions in making that determination.

✓ It may be necessary to explain the need to ask such detailed questions about organ systems seemingly unrelated to the musculoskeletal symptoms.

✓ Not every question provided in the lists offered in this text needs to be asked; the therapist can scan the list

and ask the appropriate questions based on the individual circumstances.

✓ When screening for domestic violence, sexual dysfunction, incontinence, or other conditions, it is important to explain that a standard set of questions is asked and that some may not apply.

✓ With the older client, a limited number of presenting symptoms often predominate—no matter what the underlying disease is—including acute confusion, depression, falling, incontinence, and syncope.

✓ A recent history of any infection (bladder, uterine, kidney, vaginal, upper respiratory), mononucleosis, influenza, or colds may be an extension of a chronic health pattern or systemic illness.

✓ The use of fluoroquinolones (antibiotic) has been linked with tendinopathies, especially in older adults who are also taking corticosteroids.

✓ Reports of dizziness, loss of balance, or a history of falls require further screening, especially in the presence of other neurologic signs and symptoms such as headache, confusion, depression, irritability, visual changes, weakness, memory loss, and drowsiness or lethargy.

✓ Special Questions for Women and Special Questions for Men are available to screen for gynecologic or urologic involvement for any woman or man with back, shoulder, hip, groin, or sacroiliac symptoms of unknown origin at presentation.

✓ Consider the possibility of physical/sexual assault or abuse in anyone with an unknown cause of symptoms, clients who take much longer to heal than expected, or any combination of physical, social, or psychologic cues listed.

✓ In screening for systemic origin of symptoms, review the subjective information in light of the objective findings. Compare the client's *history* with *clinical presentation* and look for any *associated signs and symptoms*.

CASE STUDY*

REFERRAL

A 28-year-old white man was referred to physical therapy with a medical diagnosis of progressive idiopathic Raynaud's syndrome of the bilateral upper extremities. He had this condition for the last 4 years.

The client was examined by numerous physicians, including an orthopedic specialist. The client had complete numbness and cyanosis of the right second, third, fourth, and fifth digits on contact with even a mild decrease in temperature.

He reported that his symptoms had progressed to the extent that they appear within seconds if he picks up a glass of cold water. This man works almost entirely outside, often in cold weather, and uses saws and other power equipment. The numbness has created a very unsafe job situation.

The client received a gunshot wound in a hunting accident 6 years ago. The bullet entered the posterior left thoracic region, lateral to the lateral border of the scapula, and came out through the anterior lateral superior chest wall. He says that he feels as if his shoulders are constantly rolled forward. He reports no cervical, shoulder, or elbow pain or injury.

PHYSICAL THERAPY INTERVIEW

Note that not all of these questions would necessarily be presented to the client because his answers may determine the next question and may eliminate some questions.

Tell me why you are here today. (Open-ended question)

PAIN

- Do you have any pain associated with your past gunshot wound? If yes, describe your pain.
  FUPs: Give the client a chance to answer and prompt only if necessary with suggested adjectives such as "Is your pain sharp, dull, boring, or burning?" or "Show me on your body where you have pain."

  To pursue this line of questioning, if appropriate:
  FUPs: What makes your pain better or worse?
  What is your pain like when you first get up in the morning, during the day, and in the evening?
- Is your pain constant or does it come and go?
- On a scale from 0 to 10, with zero being no pain and 10 being the worst pain you have ever expe-

rienced with this problem, what level of pain would you say that you have right now?

- Do you have any other pain or symptoms that are not related to your old injury?
- If yes, pursue as above to find out about the onset of pain, etc.
- You indicated that you have numbness in your right hand. How long does this last?
  FUPs: Besides picking up a glass of cold water, what else brings it on?
  How long have you had this problem?
- You told me that this numbness has progressed over time. How fast has this happened?
- Do you ever have similar symptoms in your left hand?

ASSOCIATED SYMPTOMS

Even though this client has been seen by numerous physicians, it is important to ask appropriate questions to rule out a systemic origin of current symptoms, especially if there has been a recent change in the symptoms or presentation of symptoms bilaterally. For example:

- What other symptoms have you had that you can associate with this problem?
- In addition to the numbness, have you had any of the following?
  - Tingling
  - Burning
  - Weakness
  - Vomiting

  - Nausea
  - Dizziness
  - Difficulty with swallowing
  - Heart palpitations or fluttering
  - Unexplained sweating or night sweats
  - Problems with your vision

  - Hoarseness

  - Difficulty with breathing
- How well do you sleep at night? (Open-ended question)
- Do you have trouble sleeping at night? (Closed-ended question)
- Does the pain awaken you out of a sound sleep? Can you sleep on either side comfortably?

MEDICATIONS

- Are you taking any medications? If yes, and the person does not volunteer the information, probe further:
  What medications?
  Why are you taking this medication?
  When did you last take the medication?

* Adapted from Bailey W, Northwestern Physical Therapy Services, Inc. Titusville, Pennsylvania.

CASE STUDY*—cont'd

Do you think the medication is easing the symptoms or helping in any way?

Have you noticed any side effects? If yes, what are these effects?

PREVIOUS MEDICAL TREATMENT

- Have you had any recent medical tests, such as x-ray examination, MRI, or CT scan? If yes, find out the results.
- Tell me about your gunshot wound. Were you treated immediately?
- Did you have any surgery at that time or since then? If yes, pursue details with regard to what type of surgery and where and when it occurred.
- Did you have physical therapy at any time after your accident? If yes, relate when, for how long, with whom, what was done, did it help?
- Have you had any other kind of treatment for this injury (e.g., acupuncture, chiropractic, osteopathic, naturopathic, and so on)?

ACTIVITIES OF DAILY LIVING (ADLs)

- Are you right-handed?
- How do your symptoms affect your ability to do your job or work around the house?
- How do your symptoms affect caring for yourself (e.g., showering, shaving, other ADLs such as eating or writing)?

FINAL QUESTION

- Is there anything else you feel that I should know concerning your injury, your health, or your present situation that I have not asked about?

  Note: If this client had been a woman, the interview would have included questions about breast pain and the date when she was last screened for cancer (cervical and breast) by a physician.

PRACTICE QUESTIONS

1. What is the effect of NSAIDs (e.g., naprosyn, motrin, anaprox, ibuprofen) on blood pressure?
   a. No effect
   b. Increases blood pressure
   c. Decreases blood pressure
2. Most of the information needed to determine the cause of symptoms is contained in the:
   a. Subjective examination
   b. Family/Personal History Form
   c. Objective information
   d. All of the above
   e. a and c
3. With what final question should you always end your interview?
4. A risk factor for NSAID-related gastropathy is the use of:
   a. Antibiotics
   b. Antidepressants
   c. Antihypertensives
   d. Antihistamines
5. After interviewing a new client, you summarize what she has told you by saying, "You told me you are here because of right neck and shoulder pain that began 5 years ago as a result of a car accident. You also have a 'pins and needles' sensation in your third and fourth fingers but no other symptoms at this time. You have noticed a considerable decrease in your grip strength, and you would like to be able to pick up a pot of coffee without fear of spilling it."

PRACTICE QUESTIONS—cont'd

This is an example of:

a. An open-ended question

b. A funnel technique

c. A paraphrasing technique

d. None of the above

6. Screening for alcohol use would be appropriate when the client reports a history of accidents.

a. True

b. False

7. What is the significance of night sweats?

a. A sign of systemic disease

b. Side effect of chemotherapy or other medications

c. Poor ventilation while sleeping

d. All of the above

e. None of the above

8. Spontaneous uterine bleeding after 12 consecutive months without menstrual bleeding requires medical referral.

a. True

b. False

9. Which of the following are red flags to consider when screening for systemic or viscerogenic causes of neuromuscular and musculoskeletal signs and symptoms:

a. Fever, night sweats, dizziness

b. Symptoms are out of proportion to the injury

c. Insidious onset

d. No position is comfortable

e. All of the above

10. A 52-year-old man with low back pain and sciatica on the left side has been referred to you by his family physician. He has had a discectomy and laminectomy on two separate occasions about 5 to 7 years ago. No imaging studies have been performed (e.g., x-ray examination or MRI) since that time. What follow-up questions should you ask to screen for medical disease?

11. You should assess clients who are receiving NSAIDs for which physiologic effect associated with increased risk of hypertension?

a. Decreased heart rate

b. Increased diuresis

c. Slowed peristalsis

d. Water retention

12. Instruct clients with a history of hypertension and arthritis to:

a. Limit physical activity and exercise

b. Avoid over-the-counter medications

c. Inform their primary care provider of both conditions

d. Drink plenty of fluids to avoid edema

13. Alcohol screening tools should be:

a. Used with every client sometime during the episode of care

b. Brief, easy to administer, and nonthreatening

c. Deferred when the client has been drinking or has the smell of alcohol on the breath

d. Conducted with one other family member present as a witness

REFERENCES

1. Barsky AJ: Forgetting, fabricating, and telescoping: the instability of the medical history, *Arch Intern Med* 162(9):981-984, 2002.

2. *A Normative Model of Physical Therapist Professional Education: Version 2004,* American Physical Therapy Association, Alexandria, VA, 2004.

3. Leavitt RL: Developing cultural competence in a multicultural world, Part II, *PT Magazine* 11(1):56-70, 2003.

4. National Adult Literacy Survey (NALS), May 2005, National Center for Education Statistics. Available at: http://nces.ed.gov/naal/faq/faqresults.asp. Accessed on May 26, 2005.

5. Adult Literacy Service. *Facts on literacy in America.* Available at: http://indianriver.fl.us/living/services/als/facts.html. Accessed May 26, 2005.

6. Nielsen-Bohlman L, Panzer AM, Kindig DA, editors: *Health literacy: A prescription to end confusion,* Washington, D.C., 2004, National Academies Press.

7. William H. Mahood, MD, president of the American Medical Association Foundation, the philanthropic arm of the AMA. www.amaassn.org/scipubs/amnews/pick_00/hlse0320.htm

8. National Adult Literacy Agency (NALA). Resource Room. Available at: http://www.nala.ie/. Accessed July 19, 2005.

9. Matthews-Juarez P, Weinberg AD: *Cultural competence in cancer care: A health professional's passport,* Houston, 2004, Baylor College of Medicine Intercultural Cancer Council. Available by calling 1-713-798-4617.

10. Berens LV, et al: *The guide for facilitating the self-discovery process,* Huntington Beach, 2000, Temperament Research Institute.

11. Berens LV, Nardi D: *The 16 personality types: Descriptions for self-discovery,* Huntington Beach, 1999, Telos Publications.

12. Keirsey D: *Please understand me II,* Del Mar, 1998, Prometheus Nemesis Book Company.

13. Cole SA, Bird J: *The medical interview: The three-function approach,* ed 2 St. Louis, 2000, Mosby-Year Book.

14. Coulehan JL, Block MR: *The medical interview: Mastering skills for clinical practice,* ed 4 , Philadelphia, 2001, F.A. Davis.

15. *Assuring cultural competence in health care: Recommendations for national standards and an outcomes-focused research agenda,* Office of Minority Health, Public Health Service, U.S. Department of Health and Human Services, 1999.

16. APTA: *Advocacy: Minority and international affairs.* Available at: http://www.apta.org/AM/Template.cfm?Section=Advocacy&Template=/TaggedPage/TaggedPageDisplay.cfm&TPLID=181&ContentID=18510. Click on left sided Advocacy menu <Minority Affairs> Cultural Competence. Accessed July 29, 2005.

17. U.S. Census Bureau: *United States Census 2000,* American Fact Finder. Available: www.census.gov/. Accessed May 26, 2005.

18. U.S. Census Bureau: *United States Census 2000,* USA Quick Facts. Available: http://quickfacts.census.gov/qfd/. Accessed May 26, 2005.

19. Bonder B, Martin L, Miracle A: Culture in clinical care, Clifton Park, 2001, Delmar Learning.

20. Leavitt RL: Developing cultural competence in a multicultural world, Part I, *PT Magazine* 10(12):36-48, 2002.

21. American Physical Therapy Association. Health and Policy Administration Section. Cross-Cultural & International Special Interest Group (SIG). Available at: http://www.aptasoa.org/sigs/cultural/index.cfm. Accessed July 21, 2005.

22. Office of Minority Health (OMH): *Assuring cultural competence in health care: recommendations for national standards and an outcomes-focused research agenda.* Available at: www.omhrc.gov/clas. Accessed May 30, 2005.

23. Diversity Rx: *Multicultural best practices overview.* Available at: www.diversityrx.org. Accessed May 26, 2005.

24. The Council on American-Islamic Relations (CAIR). Available at: www.cair-net.org. Accessed June 1, 2005.

25. The Muslim American Society (MAS). Available at: www.masnet.org. Accessed June 1, 2005.

26. Siddiqui H: Healthcare barriers for Muslim Americans, *Hemaware* 9(1):18-20, 2004.

27. American Physical Therapy Association: *Tips on how to increase cultural competency.* Available at www.apta.org. Type in Search box: Cultural Competency. Accessed July 30, 2005.

28. Fairbank JC, Couper J, Davies JB, et al: The Oswestry Low Back Pain Disability Questionnaire, *Physiotherapy* 66:271-273, 1980.

29. Kopec JA, Esdaile JM, Abrahamowicz M, et al: The Quebec Back Pain Disability Scale. Measurement properties, *Spine* 20:341-352, 1995.

30. Ventre J, Schenk RJ: Validity of the Duffy-Rath Questionnaire, *Orthopaedic Practice* 17(1):22-28, 2005.

31. Lippitt SB, Harryman DT, Matsen FA: A practical tool for evaluating function: The Simple Shoulder Test. In Matsen FA, Hawkins RJ, Fu FH, editors: *The shoulder: A balance of mobility and stability.* Rosemont, 1993, American Academy of Orthopaedic Surgeons.

32. Hudak PL, Amadio PC, Bombardier C: Development of an upper extremity outcome measure: The DASH (disabilities of the arm, shoulder, and hand), The Upper Extremity Collaborative Group (UECG) *Am J Ind Med* 29:602-608, 1996. Erratum 30:372, 1996.

33. Ware JE, Sherbourne CD: The MOS 36-Item Short Form Health Survey (SF-36): I. Conceptual framework and item selection. *Med Care* 30:473-489, 1992.

34. Ware JE: SF-36 Health Survey update. *Spine* 25(24):3130-3139, 2000.

35. Wright BD, Linacre JM, editors: *Rasch measurement transactions. Part 2. Reasonable Mean-Square Fit Values,* Chicago, 1996, MESA Press.

36. *Guide to physical therapist practice,* ed 2 (Revised), Alexandria, 2003, American Physical Therapy Association.

37. Performance Physio Ltd: Pre-assessment therapy questionnaires. Available at: http://www.mystudiosoft.com/. Accessed June 23, 2005. Mention of these products does not constitute commercial endorsement. No financial benefit was gained by providing this reference.

38. Kettenbach G: *Writing SOAP notes with patient/client management formats,* Philadelphia, 2003, FA Davis.

39. Boissonnault WG: Differential diagnosis: Taking a step back before stepping forward, *PT Magazine* 8(11):45-53, 2000.

40. Wolf GA Jr: *Collecting data from patients,* Baltimore, 1977, University Park Press.

41. Federal Interagency Forum on Aging Related Statistics. *Older Americans 2000: Key indicators of well-being.* 2000.

42. National Institute on Aging. Fiscal Year 2004 Justification. Available at: http://www.nia.nih.gov/NR/rdonlyres/AB6D3C00-0D14-4E60-B067-F95B3AD38245/0/fy2004_justification.pdf. Accessed May 30, 2004.

43. Potter JF: The older orthopaedic patient. General considerations, *Clin Ortho Rel Res* 425:44-49, 2004.

44. Richy F, Gourlay ML, Garrett J, et al: Osteoporosis prevalence in men varies by the normative reference, *J Clin Densitom* 7(2):127-133, 2004.

45. Elliott ME, Drinka PJ, Krause P, et al: Osteoporosis assessment strategies for male nursing home residents. *Maturitas* 48(3):225-233, 2004.

46. Ringe JD, Faber H, Farahmand P, et al: Efficacy of risedronate in men with primary and secondary osteoporosis: Results of a 1-year study. *Rheumatol Int* 26(5):427-431, 2006.

47. Kiebzak GM, Beinart GA, Perser K, et al. Undertreatment of osteoporosis in men with hip fracture, *Arch Intern Med* 162:2217-2222, 2002.

48. Feldstein AC, Nichols G, Orwoll E, et al: The near absence of osteoporosis treatment in older men with fractures. *Osteoporos Int* June 1, 2005.

49. Health Resources and Services Administration (HRSA): *Women's health USA data book,* Rockville, 2004, United States Department of Health and Human Services. Available at www.hrsa.gov/ Accessed June 28, 2005.

50. Prendergast MA: Do women possess a unique susceptibility to the neurotoxic effects of alcohol? *J Am Med Womens Assoc* 59(3):225-227, 2004.

51. Jemal A, Murray T, Ward E, et al: Cancer statistics, 2005, *CA Cancer Journal Clin* 55(1):10-30, 2005.

52. Baird DT, Collins J, Egozcue J, et al: Fertility and ageing, *Hum Reprod Update*11(3):261-276, 2005.

53. Moore M: *The only menopause guide you'll need,* ed 2. Baltimore, Johns Hopkins Press Health Book, 2004, Johns Hopkins University Press.

54. Rossouw JE, Anderson GL, Prentice RL, et al: Risks and benefits of estrogen plus progestin in healthy postmenopausal women: Principal results from the Women's Health Initiative randomized controlled trial, *JAMA* 288(3):321-333, 2002.

55. Grady, D: Postmenopausal hormones—therapy for symptoms only, *NEJM* 348(19): 1835-1837, 2003.

56. U.S. Department of Health and Human Services, Health Resources and Services Administration: *New Statistical Guide to Women's Health.* Available at: www.hrsa.gov/. Accessed July 23, 2005.

57. Mosca L, Appel LJ, Benjamin EJ, et al: Evidence-based guidelines for cardiovascular disease prevention in women. American Heart Association Guidelines, *Circulation* 109:672-693, 2004.

58. National Human Genome Research Institute: Educational Resources. Available at: www.nhgri.nih.gov. Accessed July 20, 2005.

59. Nature, International Weekly Journal of Science: The Human Genome. Available at: www.nature.com/genomics. Accessed July 20, 2005.

60. Brawley OW: Some perspective on black-white cancer statistics, *Cancer Journal for Clinicians* 52(6):322-325, 2002.

61. Fowler K: PTs confront minority health and health disparities, *PT Magazine* 12(5):42-47, 2004.

62. Probst JC, Moore CG, Glover SH, et al: The compounding effects of race/ethnicity and rurality on health, *Am J Public Health* 94(10):1695-1703, 2004.

63. Urban Indian Health Institute. Health status of urban American Indians, 2004. Available at: http://www.uihi.org/. Accessed May 30, 2005.

64. Bach PB, Schrag D, Brawley OW: Survival of blacks and whites after a cancer diagnosis, *JAMA* 287:2106-2113, 2002.

65. Smedley B, Stith A, Nelson A, editors: *Unequal treatment—confronting racial and ethnic disparities in health care*, Washington, DC, 2002, National Academy Press.

66. Morgenstern LB, Smith MA, Lisabeth LD, et al: Excess stroke in Mexican Americans compared with non-Hispanic whites, *Am J Epidemiol* 160(4):376-383, 2004.

67. Lisabeth LD, Kardia SL, Smith MA, et al: Family history of stroke among Mexican-American and non-Hispanic white patients with stroke and TIA: Implications for the feasibility and design of stroke genetics research, *Neuroepidemiology* 24(1-2):96-102, 2005.

68. U.S. National Library of Medicine and the National Institutes of Health. African-American Health. Available at: www.nlm.nih.gov/medlineplus/africanamericanhealth.html May 2005. Accessed May 30, 2005.

69. Intercultural Cancer Council (ICC). Cancer fact sheets. Available at: http://iccnetwork.org/cancerfacts/. Accessed June 1, 2005.

70. Beals KA: Disordered eating and body-image disturbances in male athletes, *Health & Fitness*, ACSM, March/April 2003.

71. Beals KA: *Disordered eating among athletes. A comprehensive guide for health professionals*, Champaign, IL, 2004, Human Kinetics.

72. Kaminski PL, Chapman BP, Haynes SD, et al: Body image, eating behaviors, and attitudes toward exercise among gay and straight men, *Eat Behav* 6(3):179-187, 2005.

73. Long MJ, Marshall BS: The relationship between self-assessed health status, mortality, service use, and cost in a managed care setting, *Health Care Manage Rev* 4:20-27, 1999.

74. Gold DT, Burchett BM, Shipp KM, et al: Factors associated with self-rated health in patients with Paget's disease of bone, *J Bone Miner Res* 14 (Suppl 2):99-102, 1999.

75. Idler EL, Russell LB, Davis D: Survival, functional limitations, and self-rated health in the NHANES I Epidemiologic Follow-up Study 1992: First national health and nutrition examination survey, *Am J Epidemiol* 9:874-883, 2000.

76. Long MJ, McQueen DA, Bangalore VG, et al: Using self-assessed health to predict patient outcomes after total knee replacement, *Clin Ortho Rel Res* 434:189-192, 2005.

77. Storr CL, Trinkoff AM, Anthony JC: Job strain and non-medical drug use, *Drug Alcohol Depend.* 55(1-2): 45-51, 1999.

78. National Institute on Drug Abuse (NIDA). NIDA Info-Facts: Nationwide trends. Available at: http://www.nida.nih.gov/infofacts/nationtrends.html. Accessed June14, 2005.

79. Lapeyre-Mestre M, Sulem P, Niezborala M, et al: Taking drugs in the working environment: A study in a sample of 2106 workers in the Toulouse metropolitan area, *Therapie* 59(6):615-623, 2004.

80. Kolakowsky-Hayner SA: Pre-injury substance abuse among persons with brain injury and persons with spinal cord injury, *Brain Inj* 13(8):571-581, 1999.

81. Bleicher J: Personal communication, 2003.

82. Soft-tissue infections among injection drug users, *MMWR* 50(19):381-384, 2001.

83. Clark T, McKenna LS, Jewell MJ: Physical therapists' recognition of battered women in clinical settings, *Phys Ther* 76(1): 12-19, 1996.

84. Bastiaens L, Francis G, Lewis K: The RAFFT as a screening tool for adolescent substance use disorders, *Am J Addict* 9:10-16, 2000.

85. Goodman CC, Boissonnault WG: *Pathology: implications for the physical therapist*, ed 2, Philadelphia, 2003, WB Saunders.

86. Center for Advanced Health Studies: *Substance abuse. A guide for health professionals*, ed 2, Glendive, 2001, American Academy of Pediatrics.

87. University of Washington Alcohol and Drug Abuse Institute (ADAI). Available at: http://adai.washington.edu/instruments/. Accessed July 8, 2005.

88. National Institute on Alcohol Abuse and Alcoholism (NIAAA). Alcohol Alert. Publications. Available at http://www.niaaa.nih.gov/. Accessed June 15, 2006.

89. Cook RL, Chung T, Kelly TM, et al: Alcohol screening in young persons attending a sexually transmitted disease clinic, *J Gen Intern Med* 20(1):1-6, 2005. Available on-line at: www.medscape.com/viewarticle/500027.

90. Babor TF, de la Fuente JR, Saunders J, et al: AUDIT (The Alcohol Use Disorders Identification Test): Guidelines for use in primary health care, 1992, World Health Organization. Available: http://whqlibdoc.who.int/hq/1992/WHO_PSA_92.4.pdf. Accessed June 15, 2005.

91. Shapira D: Alcohol abuse and osteoporosis, *Semin Arthritis Rheum* 19(6): 371-376, 1990.

92. Simons DG, Travell JG, Simons LS: *Myofascial pain and dysfunction. The trigger point manual. Volume 1. Upper half of body*, Baltimore, 1999, Williams & Wilkins.

93. Mukamal KJ, Ascherio A, Mittleman MA, et al: Alcohol and risk for ischemic stroke in men: The role of drinking patterns and usual beverage, *Ann Intern Med* 142(1):11-19, 2005.

94. Pittman HJ: Recognizing "holiday heart" syndrome, *Nursing 2004* 34(12):32cc6-32cc7, 2004.

95. Henderson-Martin B: No more surprises: Screening patients for alcohol abuse, *Nursing 2000* 100(9):26-32, 2000.

96. Selzer ML: A self-administered Short Michigan Alcoholism Screening Test (SMAST), *J Stud Alcohol* 36(1):117-126, 1975.

97. Ashman TA, Schwartz ME, Cantor JB, et al: Screening for substance abuse in individuals with traumatic brain injury, *Brain Inj* 18(2):191-202, 2004.

98. Carlat DJ: The psychiatric review of symptoms: A screening tool for family physicians, *Am Fam Physician* 58(7):1617-1624, 1998.

99. Sturm R, Stein B, Zhang W, et al: Alcoholism treatment in managed private sector plans. How are carve-out arrangements affecting costs and utilization? *Recent Dev Alcohol* 15:271-84, 2001.

100. Dunn C: Hazardous drinking by trauma patients during the year after injury, *J Trauma* 54(4):707-712, 2003.

101. Gentilello LM: Alcohol interventions in a trauma center as a means of reducing the risk of injury recurrence, *Ann Surg* 230(4):473-483, 1999.

102. American Physical Therapy Association (APTA): Substance Abuse HOD 06-93-25-49 (Program 32, Practice Department), June 2003.

103. Majid PA, Cheirif JB, Rokey R, et al: Does cocaine cause coronary vasospasm in chronic cocaine abusers? A study of coronary and systemic hemodynamics, *Clin Cardiol* 15(4): 253-258, 1992.

104. American Cancer Society (ACS): *Health benefits over time.* Available at: www.cancer.org [In the search box, type in: When Smokers Quit]. Accessed June 21, 2005.

105. Travell JG, Simons DG: *Myofascial pain and dysfunction: The trigger point manual: The lower extremities*, vol 2, Baltimore, 1992, Williams & Wilkins.

106. Kim KS, Yoon ST, Park JS, et al: Inhibition of proteoglycan and type II collagen synthesis of disc nucleus cells by nicotine, *J Neurosurg: Spine* 99(3 Suppl):291-297, 2003.

107. Akmal M, Kesani A, Anand B, et al: Effect of nicotine on spinal disc cells: A cellular mechanism for disc degeneration, *Spine* 29(5):568-575, 2004.

108. Frymoyer JW, Pope MH, Clements JH, et al: Risk factors in low back pain, *J Bone Joint Surg* 65-A: 213-218, 1983.

109. Holm S, Nachemson A: Nutrition of the intervertebral disc: acute effects of cigarette smoking. An experimental animal study, *Upsala J Med Sci* 83: 91-98, 1998.

110. Hughes JR, Oliveto AH, Helzer JE, et al: Should caffeine abuse, dependence, or withdrawal be added to DSM-IV and ICD-10? *Am J Psychiatry* 149(1): 33-40, 1992.

111. Hughes JR, Oliveto AH, Liguori A, et al: Endorsement of DSM-IV dependence criteria among caffeine users, *Drug Alcohol Depend* 52(2): 99-107, 1998.

112. Kerrigan S, Lindsey T: Fatal caffeine overdose. *Forensic Sci Int* 153(1):67-69, 2005. Epub ahead of print, May 31, 2005.

113. Sudano I, Binggeli C, Spieker L: Cardiovascular effects of coffee: Is it a risk factor? *Prog Cardiovasc Nurs* 20(2):65-69, 2005.

114. Corti R, et al: Coffee acutely increases sympathetic nerve activity and blood pressure independently of caffeine content: Role of habitual versus nonhabitual drinking, *Circulation* 106(23):2935-2940, 2002.

115. Mikuls TR, Cerhan JR, Criswell LA, et al: Coffee, tea, and caffeine consumption and risk of rheumatoid arthritis: Results from the Iowa Women's Health Study, *Arthritis Rheum* 46(1):83-91, 2002.

116. Position of the American Dietetic Association (ADA): Use of nutritive and nonnutritive sweeteners, *J Amer Dietetic Assoc*104(2):255-275, 2004. Available at: http://www.eatright.org/

117. Blaylock R: *Excitotoxins: The taste that kills*, Albuquerque, 1996, Health Press.

118. Roberts HJ: *Aspartame disease: The ignored epidemic*, West Palm Beach, 1995, Sunshine Sentinel Press.

119. Roberts HJ: *Defense against Alzheimer's disease*, Palm Beach, 2001, Sunshine Sentinel Press.

120. Newman LS: Occupational illness, *N Engl J Med* 333: 1128-1134, 1995.

121. Radetsky P: *Allergic to the twentieth century: The explosion in environmental allergies*, Boston, 1997, Little, Brown.

122. Frumkin H: Agent orange and cancer: An overview for clinicians, *Cancer J Clin* 53(4):245-255, 2003.

123. Veterans Health Administration (VHA): Gulf War Illnesses. Available at: www.va.gov/gulfwar/. Accessed July 1, 2005

124. Marshall L, Weir E, Abelsohn A, et al: Identifying and managing adverse environmental health effects: Taking an exposure history. *Canadian Medical Association Journal* 166(8):1049-1054, 2002 (www.cmaj.ca/cgi/reprint/166/8/1049.pdf).

125. Cross J, Trent R: Public health and aging: Nonfatal fall-related traumatic brain injury among older adults, *MMWR* 52(13):276-278, 2003.

126. Boulgarides LK, McGinty SM, Willett JA, et al: Use of clinical and impairment-based tests to predict falls by community-dwelling older adults. *Physical Therapy* 83(4):328-339, 2003.

127. Kario K, Tobin JN, Wolfson LI, et al: Lower standing systolic blood pressure as a predictor of falls in the elderly: A community-based prospective study, *J Am Coll Cardiol* 38(1):246-252, 2001.

128. Lawlor DA, Patel R, Ebrahim S: Association between falls in elderly women and chronic diseases and drug use: Cross sectional study, *BMJ* 327(7417):712-717.

129. Weiner D, Duncan P, Chandler J, et al: Functional reach: A marker of physical frailty, *Journal of the American Geriatrics Society* 40(3):203-207, 1992.

130. Newton R: Validity of the multi-directional reach test: A practical measure for limits of stability in older adults, *Journal of Gerontological and Biological Science and Medicine* 56(4):M248-M252, 2001.

131. Vellas BJ, Wayne S, Romero L, et al: One-leg balance is an important predictor of injurious falls in older persons, *J Amer Geriatr Sco.* 45:735-738, 1997.

132. Berg K, Wood-Dauphinee S, Williams JI, Gayton D: Measuring balance in the elderly: Preliminary development of an instrument, *Physiotherapy Canada* 41:304-311, 1989.

133. Berg K, Wood-Dauphinee S, Williams JI, Maki, B: Measuring balance in the elderly: Validation of an instrument. *Can. J. Pub. Health* 83(Supplement 2):S7-11, 1992.

134. Mathias SM, Nayak U, Isaacs B: Balance in elderly patients: The "Get-Up and Go Test," *Archives of Physical & Medical Rehabilitation* 67:387-389, 1986.

135. Podsiadlo D, Richardson S: The timed "Up & Go": A test of basic functional mobility for frail elderly persons, *J Am Geriatr Soc* 39:142-148, 1991.

136. Thompson M, Medley A: Performance of community dwelling elderly on the timed up and go test, *Physical and Occupational Therapy in Geriatrics* 13(3):17-30, 1995.

137. Tinetti ME, Mendes de Leon CF, Doucette JT, et al: Fear of falling and fall-related efficacy in relationship to functioning among community-living elders, *J Gerontol* 49:M140-147, 1984.

138. Tinetti ME, Richman D, Powell LE: Falls efficacy as a measure of fear of falling, *J Gerontol* 45:P239-P243, 1990.

139. Powell LE, Myers AM: The Activities-Specific Balance Confidence (ABC) Scale, *J Gerontol A Biol Sci Med Sci* 50:M28-M34, 1995.

140. Myers AM, Fletcher PC, Myers AH: Discriminative and evaluative properties of the Activities-specific Balance Confidence Scale, *J Gerontol* 53:M287-294, 1998.

141. Hotchkiss A, Fisher A, Robertson R, et al: Convergent and predictive validity of three scales to falls in the elderly, *Am J Occup Ther* 58(1):100-3, Jan-Feb 2004.

142. American Physical Therapy Association (APTA): Guidelines for recognizing and providing care for victims of domestic abuse, 1997. Available at: www.apta.org [1-800-999-2782, ext. 3395. Accessed June 6, 2005.

143. Cyriax JH: *Textbook of orthopedic medicine*, Philadelphia, 1998, W.B. Saunders.

144. American Physical Therapy Association (APTA): *New position on family violence outlinesphysical therapy role*, Alexandria, 2005, APTA.

145. Ketter P: Physical therapists need to know how to deal with domestic violence issues, *PT Bulletin* 12(31): 6-7, 1997.

146. Janssen PA, Nicholls TL, Kumar RA, et al: Of mice and men: Will the intersection of social science and genetics create new approaches for intimate partner violence? *J Interpers Violence* 20(1):61-71, 2005.

147. Goldberg WG, Tomlanovich MC: Domestic violence victims in the emergency department, *JAMA* 251:3259-3264, 1984.

148. George MJ: A victimization survey of female perpetrated assaults in the United Kingdom, *Aggressive Behavior* 25:67-79, 1999.

149. Owen SS, Burke TW: An exploration of prevalence of domestic violence in same sex relationships, *Psychol Rep* 95(1):129-132, 2004.

150. Feldhaus K: Accuracy of 3 brief screening questions for detecting partner violence in the emergency department, *JAMA* 277(17):1357-1361, 1997.

151. Dong M, Giles WH, Felitti VJ, et al: Insights into causal pathways for ischemic heart disease: Adverse childhood experiences study, *Circulation* 110(13):1761-1766, 2004.

152. Friedman MJ, Wang, S, Jalowiec JE, et al: Thyroid hormone alterations among women with posttraumatic stress disorder due to childhood sexual abuse, *Biol Psychiatry* 57(10):1186-1192, 2005.

153. Sachs-Ericsson N, Blazer D, Plant EA, et al: Childhood sexual and physical abuse and the 1-year prevalence of medical problems in the National Comorbidity Survey, *Health Psychol* 24(1):32-40, 2005.

154. Cunningham J: Childhood sexual abuse and medical complaints in adult women, *J of Interpersonal Violence* 3:131-144, 1988.

155. Drossman DA: Sexual and physical abuse in women with functional or organic gastrointestinal disorders, *Annals of Internal Medicine* 113:828-833, 1990.

156. Felitti VJ: Long-term medical consequences of incest, rape, and molestation, *Southern Medical J* 843:328-331, 1991.

157. Keely BR: Could your patient—or colleague—become violent? *Nursing* 2002 32(12):32cc1-32cc5, 2002.

158. Doody L: Defusing workplace violence, *Nursing* 2003 33(8):32hn1-32hn3, 2003.

159. Kimmel D: Association of physical abuse and chronic pain explored, *ADVANCE for Physical Therapists*, February 17, 1997.

160. Myers JE, Berliner L, Briere J, et al: *The APSAC handbook on child maltreatment*, Thousand Oaks, 2002, Sage Publications.

161. Feldhaus KM: Fighting domestic violence: An intervention plan, *J Musculoskel Med* 18(4):197-204, 2001.

162. Burroughs VJ, Maxey RW, Levy RA: Racial and ethnic differences in response to medicines, *J Natl Med Assoc* 94(10Suppl):1-26, 2002.

163. Morrison A, Levy R: Toward individualized pharmaceutical care of East Asians: The value of genetic testing for polymorphisms in drug-metabolizing genes, *Pharmacogenomics* 5(6):673-689, 2004.

164. Gandhi M, Aweeka F, Greenblatt RM, et al: Sex differences in pharmacokinetics and pharmacodynamics, *Annu Rev Pharmacol Toxicol* 44:499-523, 2004.

165. Meredith S, Feldman PH, Frey D, et al: Possible medication errors in home healthcare patients, *J Am GeriatrSoc* 49(6):719-724, 2001.

166. Food and Drug Administration (FDA): Center for Drug Education and Research: NSAIDs. Available at: www.fda.gov. Posted June 15, 2005. Accessed June 17, 2005.

167. Boissonnault WG, Meek PD: Risk factors for antiinflammatory drug or aspirin induced GI complications in individuals receiving outpatient physical therapy services, *J Ortho Sports Phys Ther* 32(10):510-517, 2002.

168. Biederman RE: Pharmacology in rehabilitation: Nonsteroidal anti-inflammatory agents, *JOSPT* 35(6):356-367, 2005.

169. Lefkowith JB: Cyclooxygenase-2 specificity and its clinical implications, *Am J Med* 106:43S-50S, 1999.

170. Reuben SS: Issues in perioperative use of NSAIDs, *J Musculoskel Med* 22(6):281-282, 2005.

171. Huerta C: Nonsteroidal antiinflammatory drugs and risk of acute renal failure in the general population, *Am J Kidney Dis* 45(3):531-539, 2005.

172. Goldstein JL: Personal communication, 2004.

173. Cryer B: Gastrointestinal safety of low-dose aspirin, *Am J Manag Care* 8(22 Suppl):S701-708, 2002.

174. Curhan GC, Willett WC, Rosner B: Frequency of analgesic use and risk of hypertension in younger women, *Archives of Internal Medicine* 162(19):2204-2208, 2002.

175. Schiodt FV, Rochling FA: Acetaminophen toxicity in an urban country hospital, *NEJM* 337(16):1112-1117, 1997.

176. Acello B: Administering acetaminophen safely, *Nursing* 2003 33(11):18, 2003.

177. Buntin-Mushock C, Phillip L, Moriyama K: Agedependent opioid escalation in chronic pain patients, *Anesth Analg* 100(6):1740-1745, 2005.

178. Burkman R, Schlesselman JJ, Zieman M: Safety concerns and health benefits associated with oral contraception, *Am J Obstet Gynecol* 190(4 Suppl):S5-22, 2004.

179. Barclay L, Lie D: Bone loss from Depot Medroxyprogesterone acetate may be reversible, *Arch Pediatr Adolesc Med* 159:139-144, 2005.

180. Filippucci E, Farina A, Bartolucci F, et al: Levofloxacininduced bilateral rupture of the Achilles tendon: Clinical and sonographic findings, *Rheumatiso* 55(4):267-269, 2003.

181. Melhus A: Fluoroquinolones and tendon disorders, *Expert Opin Saf* 4(2):299-309, 2005.

182. Khaliq Y, Zhanel GG: Fluoroquinolone-associated tendinopathy: A critical review of the literature, *Clin Infect Dis* 36(11):1404-1410, 2003.

183. Kelly JP, Kaufman DW, Kelley K, et al: Recent trends in use of herbal and other natural products, *Arch Intern Med* 165(3):281-286, 2005.

184. Trapskin P, Smith KM: Herbal medications in the perioperative orthopedic surgery patient, *Orthopedics* 27(8):819-822, 2004.

185. Ciccone CD: Geriatric pharmacology. In Guccione AA, editor: *Geriatric physical therapy*, St. Louis, 1993, Mosby.

186. Graedon J, Graedon T: *The people's pharmacy guide to home and herbal remedies*, New York, 2002, St. Martin's Press.

187. Gruenwald G: *PDR for herbal medicines*, ed 3, Stamford, 2004, Thomson Healthcare.

188. Ciccone CD: *Pharmacology in rehabilitation*, ed 3, Philadelphia, 2002, FA Davis.

189. Mold JW, Roberts M, Aboshady HM: Prevalence and predictors of nigh sweats, day sweats, and hot flashes in older primary care patients, *Ann Fam Med* 2(5):391-397, 2004.

BIBLIOGRAPHY

Clark RJ et al: Physical therapists' recognition of battered women in clinical settings, *Physical Therapy* 76(1):12-19, 1996.

Dalton A: Family violence: Recognizing the signs, offering help, *PT Magazine* 13(1):34-40, 2005.

Ganley AL: A trainer's manual for health care providers Published by Family Violence Prevention Fund, 1998. Available at http://endabuse.org/ or 1-415-252-8900.

Johnson C: Handling the hurt: Physical therapy and domestic violence, *PT Magazine* 5(1):52-64, 1997.

Neufeld B: SAFE Questions: Overcoming barriers to the detection of domestic violence, *American Family Physician* 53(8):2575-2580, 1996.

Rosenblatt DE et al: Reporting the mistreatment of older adults: The role of physicians, *Journal of the American Geriatrics Society* 44(1):65-70, 1996.

Schachter CL, Stalker CA, Teram E: Toward sensitive practice: Issues for physical therapists working with survivors of childhood sexual abuse, *Physical Therapy* 79(3):248-261, 1999.

Warshaw C: Improving the health care response to domestic violence: A resource manual for health care providers, ed 2, Pennsylvania Coalition Against Domestic Violence, 1998. Available at: www.pcadv.org

Pain Types and Viscerogenic Pain Patterns

Pain is often the primary symptom in many physical therapy practices. Pain assessment is a key feature in the physical therapy interview. Pain is now recognized as the "fifth vital sign"[1] along with blood pressure, temperature, heart rate, and respiration.

Recognizing pain patterns that are characteristic of systemic disease is a necessary step in the screening process. Understanding how and when diseased organs can refer pain to the neuromusculoskeletal (NMS) system helps the therapist identify suspicious pain patterns.

This chapter includes a detailed overview of pain patterns that can be used as a foundation for all the organ systems presented. Information will include a discussion of pain types in general and viscerogenic pain patterns specifically.

Each section discusses specific pain patterns characteristic of disease entities that can mimic pain from musculoskeletal or neuromuscular disorders. In the clinical decision-making process the therapist will evaluate information regarding the location, referral pattern, description, frequency, intensity, and duration of systemic pain in combination with knowledge of associated symptoms and relieving and aggravating factors.

This information is then compared with presenting features of primary musculoskeletal lesions that have similar patterns of presentation. Pain patterns of the chest, back, shoulder, scapula, pelvis, hip, groin, and sacroiliac joint are the most common sites of referred pain from a systemic disease process. These patterns are discussed in greater detail later in this text (see Chapters 14 to 18).

A large component in the screening process is being able to recognize the client demonstrating a significant emotional overlay. Pain patterns from cancer can be very similar to what we have traditionally identified as psychogenic or emotional sources of pain. It is important to know how to differentiate between these two sources of painful symptoms. To help identify psychogenic sources of pain, discussions of conversion symptoms, symptom magnification, and illness behavior are also included in this chapter.

▶ MECHANISMS OF REFERRED VISCERAL PAIN

The neurology of visceral pain is not understood at this time. Proposed models are based on what is known about the somatic sensory system. Scientists have not found actual nerve fibers and specific nociceptors in organs. We do know the afferent supply to internal organs is in close proximity to blood vessels along a path similar to the sympathetic nervous system.[2]

Viscerosensory fibers ascend the anterolateral system to the thalamus with fibers projecting to several regions of the brain. These regions encode the site of origin of visceral pain, although they do it poorly because of low

receptor density, large overlapping receptive fields, and extensive convergence in the ascending pathway. Thus, the cortex cannot distinguish where the pain messages originate from.[3,4]

Studies show there may be multiple mechanisms operating at different sites to produce the sensation we refer to as "pain." The same symptom can be produced by different mechanisms and a single mechanism may cause different symptoms.[5]

In the case of referred pain patterns of viscera there are three separate phenomena to consider. These are:

• Embryologic development
• Multisegmental innervation
• Direct pressure and shared pathways

Embryologic Development

Each system has a bit of its own uniqueness in how pain is referred. For example the viscera in the abdomen comprise a large percentage of all the organs we have to consider. When a person gives a history of abdominal pain, the location of the pain may not be directly over the involved organ (Fig. 3-1).

Functional magnetic resonance imaging (fMRI) and other neuroimaging methods have shown activation of the inferolateral postcentral gyrus by visceral pain so the brain has a role in visceral patterns.[6,7] However, it is likely that embryologic development has the primary role in referred pain patterns for the viscera.

Pain is referred to a site where the organ was located in fetal development. Although the organ migrates during fetal development, its nerves persist in referring sensations from the former location.

Organs such as the kidneys, liver, and intestines begin forming by 3 weeks when the fetus is still less than the size of a raisin. By day 19, the notochord forming the spinal column has closed and by day 21, the heart begins to beat.

Embryologically, the chest is part of the gut. In other words, they are formed from the same tissue in utero. This explains symptoms of intrathoracic organ pathology frequently being referred to the abdomen as a viscero-viscero reflex. For example, it is not unusual for disorders of thoracic viscera such as pneumonia or pleuritis to refer pain that is perceived in the abdomen instead of the chest.[2]

Although the heart muscle starts out embryologically as a cranial structure, the pericardium around the heart is formed from gut tissue. This explains why myocardial infarction or pericarditis can also refer pain to the abdomen.[2]

Another example of how embryologic development impacts the viscera and the soma, consider

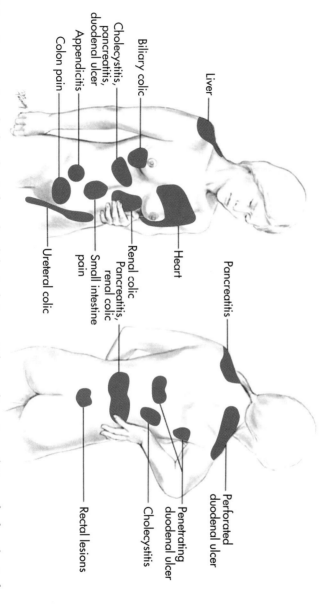

Fig. 3-1 • Common sites of referred pain from the abdominal viscera. When a client gives a history of referred pain from the viscera, the pain's location may not be directly over the impaired organ. Visceral embryologic development is the mechanism of the referred pain pattern. Pain is referred to the site where the organ was located in fetal development. (From Jarvis C: *Physical examination and health assessment*, Philadelphia, 1992, WB Saunders.)

the ear and the kidney. These two structures have the same shape since they come from the same embryologic tissue (otorenal axis of the mesenchyme) and are formed at the same time (Fig. 3-2).

When a child is born with any anomaly of the ear(s) or even a missing ear, the medical staff knows to look for possible similar changes or absence of the kidney on the same side.

A thorough understanding of fetal embryology is not really necessary in order to recognize red flag signs and symptoms of visceral origin. Knowing that it is one of several mechanisms by which the visceral referred pain patterns occur is a helpful start.

However, the more you know about embryologic development of the viscera, the faster you will recognize somatic pain patterns caused by visceral dysfunction. Likewise, the more you know about anatomy, the origins of anatomy, its innervations, and the underlying neurophysiology, the better able you will be to identify the potential structures involved.

This will lead you more quickly to specific screening questions to ask. The manual therapist will especially benefit from a keen understanding of embryologic tissue derivations. An appreciation of embryology will help the therapist localize the problem vertically.

▶ MULTISEGMENTAL INNERVATION

Multisegmental innervation is the second mechanism used to explain pain patterns of a viscerogenic source (Fig. 3-3). The autonomic nervous system (ANS) is part of the peripheral nervous system. As shown in this diagram, the viscera have multisegmental innervations. The multiple levels of innervation of the heart, bronchi, stomach, kidneys, intestines, and bladder are demonstrated clearly.

Pain of a visceral origin can be referred to the corresponding somatic areas. The example of cardiac pain is a good one. Cardiac pain is not felt in the heart, but is referred to areas supplied by the corresponding spinal nerves.

Instead of actual physical heart pain, cardiac pain can occur in any structure innervated by C3 to T4 such as the jaw, neck, upper trapezius, shoulder, and arm. Pain of cardiac and diaphragmatic origin is often experienced in the shoulder, in particular, because the C5 spinal segment supplies the heart, respiratory diaphragm, and shoulder.

Direct Pressure and Shared Pathways

A third and final mechanism by which the viscera refer pain to the soma is the concept of direct pressure and shared pathways (Fig. 3-4). As shown in this illustration, many of the viscera are near the respiratory diaphragm. Any pathologic process that can inflame, infect, or obstruct the organs can bring them in contact with the respiratory diaphragm.

Anything that impinges the *central diaphragm* can refer pain to the *shoulder* and anything that impinges the *peripheral diaphragm* can refer pain to the *ipsilateral costal margins and/or lumbar region* (Fig. 3-5).

This mechanism of referred pain through shared pathways occurs as a result of ganglions from each neural system gathering and sharing information through the cord to the plexuses. The visceral organs are innervated through the autonomic nervous system. The ganglions bring in good information from around the body. The nerve plexuses decide how to respond to this information (what to do) and give the body fine, local control over responses.

Plexuses originate in the neck, thorax, diaphragm, and abdomen, terminating in the pelvis. The brachial plexus supplies the upper neck and shoulder while the phrenic nerve innervates the respiratory diaphragm. More distally, the celiac plexus supplies the stomach and intestines. The neurologic supply of the plexuses is from

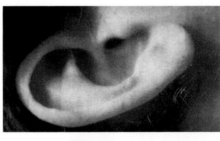

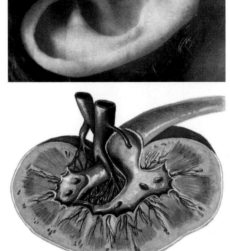

Fig. 3-2 • The ear and the kidney have the same shape since they are formed at the same time and from the same embryologic tissue (otorenal axis of the mesenchyme). This is just one example of how fetal development influences form and function. When a child is born with a deformed or missing ear, the medical staff looks for a similarly deformed or missing kidney on the same side. (From Anderson KN: *Mosby's medical, nursing & allied health dictionary*, ed 5, St. Louis, 1988, Mosby; A-39; and from Seidel HM, Ball JW, Dains JE, et al: *Mosby's physical examination handbook*, St. Louis, 2003, Mosby.)

A

B

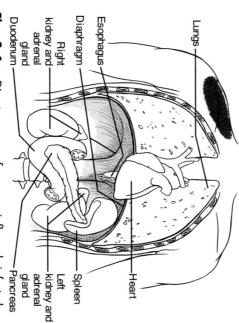

Fig. 3-4 • Direct pressure from any inflamed, infected, or obstructed organ in contact with the respiratory diaphragm can refer pain to the ipsilateral shoulder. Note the location of each of the viscera. The spleen is tucked up under the diaphragm on the left side so any impairment of the spleen can cause left shoulder pain. The tail of the pancreas can come in contact with the diaphragm on the left side potentially causing referred pain to the left shoulder. The head of the pancreas can impinge the right side of the diaphragm causing referred pain to the right side. The gallbladder (not shown) is located up under the liver on the right side with corresponding right referred shoulder pain possible. Other organs that can come in contact with the diaphragm in this way include the heart and the kidneys.

Lungs
Esophagus
Diaphragm
Right kidney and adrenal gland
Duodenum
Heart
Spleen
Left kidney and adrenal gland
Pancreas

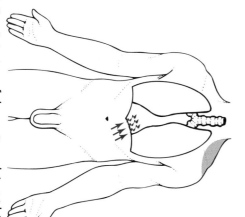

Fig. 3-5 • Irritation of the peritoneal (outside) or pleural (inside) surface of the central area of the respiratory diaphragm can refer sharp pain to the upper trapezius muscle, neck, and supraclavicular fossa. The pain pattern is ipsilateral to the area of irritation. Irritation of the peripheral portion of the diaphragm can refer sharp pain to the costal margins and lumbar region (not shown).

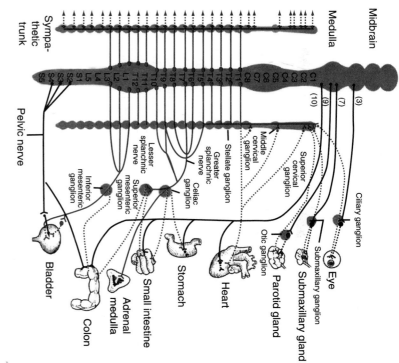

Fig. 3-3 • Sympathetic and parasympathetic divisions of the autonomic nervous system. The visceral afferent fibers mediating pain travel with the sympathetic nerves, except for those from the pelvic organs, which follow the parasympathetics of the pelvic nerve. Major visceral organs have multisegmental innervations overlapping innervations of somatic structures. Visceral pain can be referred to the corresponding somatic area because sensory fibers for the viscera and somatic structures enter the spinal cord at the same levels converging on the same neurons. (From Anderson KN: *Mosby's medical, nursing & allied health dictionary,* ed 5, St. Louis, 1998, Mosby.)

Midbrain
Medulla
Sympathetic trunk
Pelvic nerve

— Sympathetic
— Parasympathetic
== Postganglionic fibers

Middle cervical ganglion
Stellate ganglion
Greater splanchnic nerve
Lesser splanchnic nerve
Superior cervical ganglion
Celiac ganglion
Superior mesenteric ganglion
Inferior mesenteric ganglion
Otic ganglion
Ciliary ganglion
Submaxillary ganglion
Eye
Submaxillary gland
Parotid gland
Heart
Stomach
Small intestine
Adrenal medulla
Colon
Bladder

parasympathetic fibers from the vagus and pelvic splanchnic nerves.[2]

The plexuses work independently of each other, but not independently of the ganglia. The ganglia collect information derived from both the parasympathetic and the sympathetic fibers. The ganglia deliver this information to the plexuses; it is the plexuses that provide fine, local control in each of the organ systems.[2]

For example, the lower portion of the heart is in contact with the center of the diaphragm. The spleen on the left side of the body is tucked up under the dome of the diaphragm. The kidneys (on either side) and the pancreas in the center are in easy reach of some portion of the diaphragm.

The body of the pancreas is in the center of the human body. The tail rests on the left side of the body. If an infection, inflammation, or tumor or other obstruction distends the pancreas, it can put pressure on the central part of the diaphragm.

Since the phrenic nerve (C3-5) innervates the central zone of the diaphragm as well as part of the pericardium, the gallbladder, and the pancreas, the client with impairment of these viscera can present with signs and symptoms in any of the somatic areas supplied by C3-5 (e.g., shoulder).

In other words, the person can experience symptoms in the areas innervated by the same nerve pathways. So a problem affecting the pancreas can look like a heart problem, a gallbladder problem, or a mid-back/scapular or shoulder problem.

Most often, clients with pancreatic disease present with the primary pain pattern associated with the pancreas (i.e., left epigastric pain or pain just below the xiphoid process). The somatic presentation of referred pancreatic pain to the shoulder or back is uncommon, but it is the unexpected, referred pain patterns that we see in a physical or occupational therapy practice.

Another example of this same phenomenon occurs with peritonitis or gallbladder inflammation. These conditions can irritate the phrenic endings in the central part of the diaphragmatic peritoneum. The client can experience referred shoulder pain due to the root origin shared in common by the phrenic and supraclavicular nerves.

Not only is it true that any structure that touches the diaphragm can refer pain to the shoulder, but even structures adjacent to or in contact with the diaphragm in utero can do the same. Keep in mind there has to be some impairment of that structure (e.g., obstruction, distention, inflammation) for this to occur (Case Example 3-1).

ASSESSMENT OF PAIN AND SYMPTOMS

The interviewing techniques and specific questions for pain assessment are outlined in this section. The information gathered during the interview and examination provides a description of the client that is clear, accurate, and comprehensive. The therapist should keep in mind cultural rules and differences in pain perception, intensity, and responses to pain found among various ethnic groups.[8]

Measuring pain and assessing pain are two separate issues. A measurement assigns a number or value to give dimension to pain intensity.[9] A comprehensive pain assessment includes a detailed health history, physical exam, medication history (including nonprescription drug use and complementary and alternative therapies), assessment of functional status, and consideration of psychosocial-spiritual factors.[10]

The portion of the core interview regarding a client's perception of pain is a critical factor in the evaluation of signs and symptoms. Questions about pain must be understood by the client and should be presented in a nonjudgmental manner. A record form may be helpful to standardize pain assessment with each client (Fig. 3-6).

To elicit a complete description of symptoms from the client, the physical therapist may wish to use a term other than *pain*. For example, referring to the client's *symptoms* or using descriptors such as *hurt* or *sore* may be more helpful with some individuals. Burning, tightness, heaviness, discomfort, and aching are just a few examples of other possible word choices. The use of alternative words to describe a client's symptoms may also aid in refocusing attention away from pain and toward improvement of functional abilities.

If the client has completed the McGill Pain Questionnaire (see discussion of McGill Pain Questionnaire in this chapter),[11] the physical therapist may choose the most appropriate alternative word selected by the client from the list to refer to the symptoms (see Table 3-1).

Pain Assessment in the Older Adult

Pain is an accepted part of the aging process but we must be careful to take the reports of pain from older persons as serious and very real and not discount the symptoms as part of aging. Well over half the older adults in the United States report chronic joint symptoms.[12] We are likely to see pain more often as a key feature among older adults as our population continues to age.

CASE EXAMPLE 3-1   Mechanism of Referred Pain

A 72-year-old woman has come to physical therapy for rehabilitation after cutting her hand and having a flexor tendon repair. She uses a walker to ambulate, reports being short of breath "her whole life," and takes the following prescription and over-the-counter medications:

Feldene
Vioxx*
Ativan
Glucosamine
Ibuprofen "on bad days"
Furosemide

And one other big pill once a week on Sunday "for my bones"

During the course of evaluating and treating her hand, she reports constant, aching pain in her right shoulder and a sharp, tingling, burning sensation behind her armpit (also on the right side). She does not have any associated bowel or bladder signs and symptoms, but reports excessive fatigue "since the day I was born."

You suspect the combination of Feldene and Ibuprofen along with long-term use of Vioxx may be a problem.

What is the most likely mechanism of pain: embryologic development, multisegmental innervation of the stomach and duodenum, or direct pressure on the diaphragm?

Even though Vioxx is a Cox-2 inhibitor and less likely to cause problems, gastritis and GI bleeding are still possible, especially with chronic long-term use of multiple nonsteroidal antiinflammatory drugs (NSAIDs).

Retroperitoneal bleeding from peptic ulcer can cause referred pain to the back at the level of the lesion (T6 to T10) or right shoulder and/or upper trapezius pain. Shoulder pain may be accompanied by sudomotor changes such as burning, gnawing, or cramping pain along the lateral border of the scapula. The scapular pain can occur alone as the only symptom.

Side effects of NSAIDs can also include fatigue, anxiety, depression, paresthesia, fluid retention, tinnitus, nausea, vomiting, dry mouth, and bleeding from the nose, mouth, or under the skin. If peritoneal bleeding is the cause of her symptoms, *the mechanism of pain is blood in the posterior abdominal cavity irritating the diaphragm through direct pressure.*

Be sure to take the client's vital signs and observe for significant changes in blood pressure and pulse. Poor wound healing and edema (sacral, pedal, hands) may be present. Ask if the same doctor prescribed each medication and if her physician (or physicians) knows which medications she is taking. It is possible that her medications have not been checked or coordinated from before her hospitalization to the present time.

* Removed from the market by Merck & Co., Inc. in 2004 due to reports of increased risk of cardiovascular events.

The American Geriatrics Society reports the use of over-the-counter analgesic medications for pain, aching, and discomfort is common in older adults along with routine use of prescription drugs. Many older adults have taken these medications for 6 months or more.[13]

Older adults may avoid giving an accurate assessment of their pain. Some may expect pain with aging or fear that talking about pain will lead to expensive tests or medications with unwanted side effects. Fear of losing one's independence may lead others to underreport pain symptoms.

Sensory and cognitive impairment in older, frail adults makes communication and pain assessment more difficult.[13] The client may still be able to report pain levels reliably using the visual ana-

logue scales in the early stages of dementia. Improving an older adult's ability to report pain may be as simple as making sure the client has his or her glasses and hearing aid.

The Verbal Descriptor Scale (VDS) (Box 3-1) may be the most sensitive and reliable among older adults, including those with mild to moderate cognitive impairment.[14] But these and other pain scales rely on the client's ability to understand the scale and communicate a response. As dementia progresses, these abilities are lost as well.

A client with Alzheimer's type dementia loses short-term memory and cannot always identify the source of recent painful stimuli.[15,16] The Alzheimer's Discomfort Rating Scale may be more helpful for older adults who are unable to

Pain Assessment Record Form

Client's name:

Physician's diagnosis: _____   Date: _____   Physical therapist's diagnosis: _____

Medications: _____

Onset of pain (circle one): Was there an:

Accident   Injury   Trauma (violence)   Specific activity

If yes, describe:

Characteristics of pain/symptoms:
Location (Show me exactly where your pain/symptom is located):

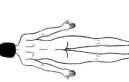

||||| Numbness
  Severe pain
  Moderate pain
→ Shooting pain

Do you have any pain or symptoms anywhere else?   Yes   No

Description (If yes, what does it feel like):

Circle any other words that describe the client's symptoms:

Knifelike	Dull	Aching	Other (describe):
Boring	Burning	Throbbing	
Heaviness	Discomfort	Sharp	
Stinging	Tingling	Stabbing	

Frequency (circle one):   Constant   Intermittent (comes and goes)

If constant: Do you have this pain right now?   Yes   No

If intermittent: How often is the pain present (circle all that apply):

Hourly   Once/daily   Twice/daily   Unpredictable   Other (please describe): _____

Intensity: *Numeric Rating Scale* and the *Faces Pain Scale*

Instructions: On a scale from 0 to 10 with zero meaning 'No pain' and 10 for 'Unbearable pain,' how would you rate your pain right now?

Pain Assessment Scale

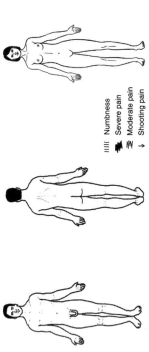

0 1 2 3 4 5 6 7 8 9 10 10+
None Mild Nagging Miserable Intense Unbearable

Alternately: Point to the face that best shows how much pain you are having right now.

Intensity: *Visual Analog Scale*

Instructions: On the line below, put a mark (or point to) the place on the line between 'Pain free' and 'Worst possible pain' that best describes/shows how much pain you are having right now.

Pain Free _____ Worst Possible Pain

Fig. 3-6 • Pain Assessment Record Form. Use this form to complete the pain history and obtain a description of the pain pattern. The form is printed in the Appendix for your use. This form may be copied and used without permission. (From Carlsson AM: Assessment of chronic pain. I. Aspects of the reliability and validity of the visual analogue scale, *Pain* 16(1):87-101, 1983. Used with permission.)

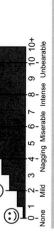

Duration:

How long does your pain (name the symptom) last?

Aggravating factors (What makes it worse?)	**Relieving factors** (What makes it better?)

Pattern

Has the pain changed since it first began? Yes No

If yes, please explain:

What is your pain/symptom like from morning (am) to evening (pm)?

Circle one: Worse in the morning Worse midday/afternoon Worse at night

Circle one: Gradually getting better Gradually getting worse Staying the same

Circle all that apply:

Present upon waking up Keeps me from falling asleep Wakes me up at night

Therapist: Record any details or description about night pain. See also Appendix for *Screening Questions for Night Pain* when appropriate:

Associated symptoms (What other symptoms have you had with this problem?)

Circle any words the client uses to describe his/her symptoms. If the client says there are no other symptoms ask about the presence of any of the following:

Burning	Difficulty breathing	Shortness of breath	Cough
Skin rash (or other lesions)	Change in bowel/bladder	Difficulty swallowing	Painful swallowing
Dizziness	Heart palpitations	Hoarseness	Nausea/vomiting
Diarrhea	Constipation	Bleeding of any kind	Sweats
Numbness	Problems with vision	Tingling	Weakness
Joint pain	Weight loss/gain	Other:_____	

Final question: Are there any other pain or symptoms of any kind anywhere else in your body that we have not talked about yet?

For the therapist:

Follow up questions can include:

Are there any positions that make it feel better? Worse?

How does rest affect the pain/symptoms?

How does activity affect the pain/symptoms?

How has this problem affected your daily life at work or at home?

Has this problem affected your ability to care for yourself without assistance (e.g. dress, bathe, cook, drive)?

Has this problem affected your sexual function or activity?

Therapist's evaluation:

Can you reproduce the pain by squeezing or palpating the symptomatic area?

Does resisted motion reproduce the pain/symptoms?

Is the client taking NSAIDs? Experiencing increased symptoms after taking NSAIDs?

If taking NSAIDs, is the client at risk for peptic ulcer? Check all that apply:

☐ Age>65 years ☐ History of peptic ulcer disease or GI disease

☐ Smoking, alcohol use ☐ Oral corticosteroid use

☐ Anticoagulation or use of other anticoagulants (even when used for heart patients at a lower dose, e.g., 81 to 325 mg aspirin/day)

☐ Renal complications in clients with hypertension or congestive heart failure (CHF) or who use diuretics or ACE inhibitors

☐ NSAIDs combined with selective serotonin reuptake inhibitors (SSRIs; antidepressants such as Prozac, Zoloft, Celexa, Paxil)

☐ Use of acid suppressants (e.g., H_2-receptor antagonists, antacids)

Other areas to consider:

• Sleep quality
• Correlation of symptoms with peak effect of medications (dosage, time of day)
• Evaluation of joint pain (see Appendix: Screening Questions for Joint Pain)
• Bowel/bladder habits
• Depression or anxiety screening score
• For women: correlation of symptoms with menstrual cycle

Fig. 3-6 • cont'd

BOX 3-1 ▼ Verbal Descriptor Scale (VDS)

Directions: Show the scale to your client. Read the descriptors and ask the client to point to the one that best matches his or her pain (achiness, soreness, or discomfort) today. Give the client at least 30 seconds to respond. A verbal reply is acceptable. It is best if the client is sitting upright facing the interviewer. Provide the client with good lighting, his or her eyeglasses, and/or hearing aid(s) if appropriate.

TODAY I HAVE:

0 = NO PAIN
1 = SLIGHT PAIN
2 = MILD PAIN
3 = MODERATE PAIN
4 = SEVERE PAIN
5 = EXTREME PAIN
6 = PAIN AS BAD AS IT CAN BE

BOX 3-2 ▼ Symptoms of Pain in Clients with Cognitive Impairment

- Verbal comments such as ouch or stop
- Nonverbal vocalizations (e.g., moans, signs, gasps)
- Facial grimacing or frowning
- Audible breathing independent of vocalization (labored, short or long periods of hyperventilation)
- Agitation or increased confusion
- Unable to be consoled or distracted
- Bracing or holding onto furniture
- Decreased mobility
- Lying very still; refusing to move
- Clutching the painful area
- Resisting care provided by others; striking out; pushing others away
- Sleep disturbance
- Weight loss
- Depression

communicate their pain.[17] The therapist records the frequency, intensity, and duration of the client's discomfort based on the presence of noisy breathing, facial expressions, and overall body language. Another tool under investigation for Pain Assessment in Advanced Dementia is the PAINAD scale. The PAINAD is a simple, valid, and reliable instrument for measurement of pain in noncommunicative clients developed by the same author as the Alzheimer's Discomfort Rating Scale.[18]

Facial grimacing, nonverbal vocalization such as moans, sighs, or gasps, and verbal comments (e.g., ouch, stop) are the most frequent behaviors among cognitively impaired older adults during painful movement (Box 3-2). Bracing, holding onto furniture, or clutching the painful area are other behavioral indicators of pain. Alternately, the client may resist care by others or stay very still to guard against pain caused by movement.[19]

Untreated pain in an older adult with advanced dementia can lead to secondary problems such as sleep disturbances, weight loss, dehydration, and depression. Pain may be manifested as agitation and increased confusion.[15]

Older adults are more likely than younger adults to have what is referred to as atypical acute pain. For example, silent acute myocardial infarction (MI) occurs more often in the older adult than in the middle-aged to early senior adult. Likewise, the older adult is more likely to experience appendicitis without any abdominal or pelvic pain.[20]

Pain Assessment in the Young Child

Many infants and children are unable to report pain. Even so the therapist should not underesti-

mate or prematurely conclude that a young client is unable to answer any questions about pain. Even some clients (both children and adults) with substantial cognitive impairment may be able to use pain-rating scales when explained carefully.[21]

The Faces Pain Scale (FACES or FPS) for children (see Fig. 3-6) was first presented in the 1980s.[22] It has since been revised (FPS-R)[23] and presented concurrently by other researchers with similar assessment measures.[24]

Most of the pilot work for the FPS was done informally with children from preschool through young school age. Researchers have used the FPS scale with adults, especially the elderly, and have had successful results. Advantages of the cartoon type FPS scale are that it avoids gender, age, and racial biases.[25]

Research shows that use of the word "hurt" rather than pain is understood by children as young as 3 years old.[26,27] Use of a word such as "owie" or "ouchie" by a child to describe pain is an acceptable substitute.[25] Assessing pain intensity with the FPS scale is fast and easy. The child looks at the faces, the therapist or parent uses the simple words to describe the expression, and the corresponding number is used to record the score.

A review of multiple other measures of self-report is also available[9] as well as a review of pain measures used in children by age including neonates.[28]

When using a rating scale is not possible, the therapist may have to rely on the parent or care-

giver's report and/or other measures of pain in children with cognitive or communication impairments and physical disabilities. Look for telltale behavior such as lack of cooperation, withdrawal, acting out, distractibility, or seeking comfort. Altered sleep patterns, vocalizations, and eating patterns provide additional clues.

In very young children and infants, the Child Facial Coding System (CFCS) and the Neonatal Facial Coding System (NFCS) can be used as behavioral measures of pain intensity.[29,30]

Facial actions and movements such as brow bulge, eye squeeze, mouth position, and chin quiver are coded and scored as pain responses. This tool has been revised and tested as valid and reliable for use post-operatively in children ages 0 to 18 months following major abdominal or thoracic surgery.[31]

Vital signs should be documented, but not relied upon, as the sole determinant of pain (or absence of pain) in infants or young children. The pediatric therapist may want to investigate other pain measures available for neonates and infants.[32,33]

Characteristics of Pain

It is very important to identify how the client's description of pain as a symptom relates to sources and types of pain discussed in this chapter. Many characteristics of pain can be elicited from the client during the Core Interview to help define the source or type of pain in question. These characteristics include:

- Location
- Description
- Intensity
- Duration
- Frequency and Duration
- Pattern

Other additional components are related to factors that aggravate the pain, factors that relieve the pain, and other symptoms that may occur in association with the pain. Specific questions are included in this section for each descriptive component. Keep in mind that an increase in frequency, intensity, or duration of symptoms over time can indicate systemic disease.

Location of Pain

Questions related to the location of pain focus the client's description as precisely as possible. An opening statement might be as follows:

Follow-Up Questions

- Show me exactly where your pain is located. Follow up questions may include

- Do you have any other pain or symptoms anywhere else?
- If yes, what causes the pain or symptoms to occur in this other area?

If the client points to a small, localized area and the pain does not spread, the cause is likely to be a superficial lesion and is probably not severe. If the client points to a small, localized area but the pain does spread, this is more likely to be a diffuse, segmental, referred pain that may originate in the viscera or deep somatic structure.

The character and location of pain can change and the client may have several pains at once so repeated pain assessment may be needed.

Description of Pain

To assist the physical therapist in obtaining a clear description of pain sensation, pose the question:

Follow-Up Questions

- What does it feel like? After giving the client time to reply, offer some additional choices in potential descriptors. You may want to ask: Is your pain/Are your symptoms:

Knifelike	Dull
Boring	Burning
Throbbing	Prickly
Deep aching	Sharp

Follow-up questions may include:
- Has the pain changed in quality since it first began?
- Changed in intensity?
- Changed in duration (how long it lasts)?

When a client describes the pain as knifelike, boring, colicky, coming in waves, or a deep aching feeling, this description should be a signal to the physical therapist to consider the possibility of a systemic origin of symptoms. Dull, somatic pain of an aching nature can be differentiated from the aching pain of a muscular lesion by squeezing or by pressing the muscle overlying the area of pain. Resisting motion of the limb may also reproduce aching of muscular origin that has no connection to deep somatic aching.

Intensity of Pain

The level or intensity of the pain is an extremely important, but difficult, component to assess in the overall pain profile. Psychologic factors may play a role in the different ratings of pain intensity measured between African Americans and Caucasians. African Americans tend to rate pain as more

unpleasant and more intense than whites, possibly indicating a stronger link between emotions and pain behavior for African Americans compared with Caucasians.[34]

The same difference is observed between women and men.[35,36] Likewise, pain intensity is reported as less when the affected individual has some means of social or emotional support.[37]

Assist the client with this evaluation by providing a rating scale. You may use one or more of these scales, depending on the clinical presentation of each client (see Fig. 3-6). Show the pain scale to your client. Ask the client to choose a number and/or a face that best describes his or her current pain level. You can use this scale to quantify symptoms other than pain such as stiffness, pressure, soreness, discomfort, cramping, aching, numbness, tingling, and so on. Always use the same scale for each follow-up assessment.

The Visual Analog Scale (VAS)[38,39] allows the client to choose a point along a 10-centimeter (100 mm) horizontal line (see Fig. 3-6). The left end represents "No pain" and the right end represents "Pain as bad as it could possibly be" or "Worst Possible Pain." This same scale can be presented in a vertical orientation for the client who must remain supine and cannot sit up for the assessment. "No pain" is placed at the bottom and "Worst pain" is put at the top.

The VAS scale is easily combined with the numeric rating scale with possible values ranging from 0 (no pain) to 10 (worst imaginable pain). It can be used to assess current pain, worst pain in the preceding 24 hours, least pain in the past 24 hours, or any combination the clinician finds useful.

The numerical rating scale (NRS) (see Fig. 3-6) allows the client to rate the pain intensity on a scale from 0 (no pain) to 10 (the worst pain imaginable). This is probably the most commonly used pain rating scale in both the inpatient and outpatient settings. It is a simple and valid method of measuring pain.

Although the scale was tested and standardized using 0 to 10, the plus is used for clients who indicate the pain is "off the scale" or "higher than a 10." Some health care professionals prefer to describe 10 as "worst pain experienced with this condition" to avoid needing a higher number than 10.

This scale is especially helpful for children or cognitively impaired clients. In general, even adults without cognitive impairments may prefer to use this scale.

An alternative method provides a scale of 1 to 5 with word descriptions for each number[11] and asks:

- How strong is your pain?
  1 = Mild
  2 = Discomforting
  3 = Distressing
  4 = Horrible
  5 = Excruciating

This scale for measuring the intensity of pain can be used to establish a baseline measure of pain for future reference. A client who describes the pain as "excruciating" (or a 5 on the scale) during the initial interview may question the value of therapy when several weeks later there is no subjective report of improvement.

A quick check of intensity by using this scale often reveals a decrease in the number assigned to pain levels. This can be compared with the initial rating, thus providing the client with assurance and encouragement in the rehabilitation process. A quick assessment using this method can be made by asking:

- How strong is your pain?
  1 = Mild
  2 = Moderate
  3 = Severe

The description of intensity is highly subjective. What might be described as "mild" for one person could be "horrible" for another person. Careful assessment of the person's nonverbal behavior (e.g., ease of movement, facial grimacing, guarding movements) and correlation of the person's personality with his or her perception of the pain may help to clarify the description of the intensity of the pain. Pain of an intense, unrelenting (constant) nature is often associated with systemic disease.

The 36-Item Short-Form Health Survey discussed in Chapter 2 includes an assessment of bodily pain along with a general measure of health-related quality of life. Nurses often use the PQRST mnemonic to help identify underlying pathology or pain (Box 3-3).

Frequency and Duration of Pain

The frequency of occurrence is related closely to the pattern of the pain, and the client should be asked how often the symptoms occur and whether the pain is constant or intermittent. Duration of pain is a part of this description.

BOX 3-3 ▼ Nursing Assessment of Pain (PQRST)

Provocation and palliation. What causes the pain and what makes it better or worse?

Quality of pain. What type of pain is present (aching, burning, sharp)?

Region and radiation. Where is the pain located? Does it radiate to other parts of the body?

Severity on a scale from 0 to 10. Does the pain interfere with daily activities, mood, function?

Timing. Did the pain come on suddenly or gradually? Is it constant or does it come and go (intermittent)? How often does it occur? How long does it last? Does it come on at the same time of the day or night?

Follow-Up Questions

- How long do the symptoms last?

  For example, pain related to systemic disease has been shown to be a *constant* rather than an *intermittent* type of pain experience. Clients who indicate that the pain is constant should be asked:

- Do you have this pain right now?
- Did you notice these symptoms this morning immediately when you woke up?

Further responses may reveal that the pain is perceived as being constant but in fact is not actually present consistently and/or can be reduced with rest or change in position, which are characteristics more common with pain of musculoskeletal origin.

Pattern of Pain

After listening to the client describe all the characteristics of his or her pain or symptoms, the therapist may recognize a vascular, neurogenic, musculoskeletal (including spondylogenic), emotional, or visceral pattern (Table 3-1).

The following sequence of questions may be helpful in further assessing the pattern of pain, especially how the symptoms may change with time.

Follow-Up Questions

- Tell me about the pattern of your pain/symptoms.
- *Alternate question:* When does your back/shoulder (name the involved body part) hurt?

TABLE 3-1 ▼ Recognizing Pain Patterns

Vascular	Neurogenic	Musculoskeletal	Emotional
Throbbing	Sharp	Aching	Tiring
Pounding	Crushing	Sore	Miserable
Pulsing	Pinching	Heavy	Vicious
Beating	Burning	Hurting	Agonizing
	Hot	Dull	Nauseating
	Searing	Cramping	Frightful
	Itchy	Deep	Piercing
	Stinging		Dreadful
	Pulling		Punishing
	Jumping		Torturing
	Shooting		Killing
	Pricking		Unbearable
	Gnawing		Annoying
	Electrical		Cruel
			Sickening
			Exhausting

From Melzack R: The McGill Pain Questionnaire: major properties and scoring methods, *Pain* 1:277, 1975.

- *Alternate question:* Describe your pain/symptoms from first waking up in the morning to going to bed at night. (See special sleep-related questions that follow.)

Follow-up questions may include:

- Have you ever experienced anything like this before?
- If yes, do these episodes occur more or less often than at first?
- How does your pain/symptom(s) change with time?
- Are your symptoms worse in the morning or evening?

The pattern of pain associated with systemic disease is often a progressive pattern with a cyclical onset (i.e., the client describes symptoms as being alternately worse, better, and worse over a period of months). When there is back pain, this pattern differs from the sudden sequestration of a discogenic lesion that appears with a pattern of increasingly worse symptoms followed by a sudden cessation of all symptoms. Such involvement of the disk occurs without the cyclical return of symptoms weeks or months later, which is more typical of a systemic disorder.

If the client appears to be unsure of the pattern of symptoms or has "avoided paying any attention" to this component of pain description, it may be useful to keep a record at home assisting the client to take note of the symptoms for 24 hours. A chart such as the McGill Home Recording Card[11]

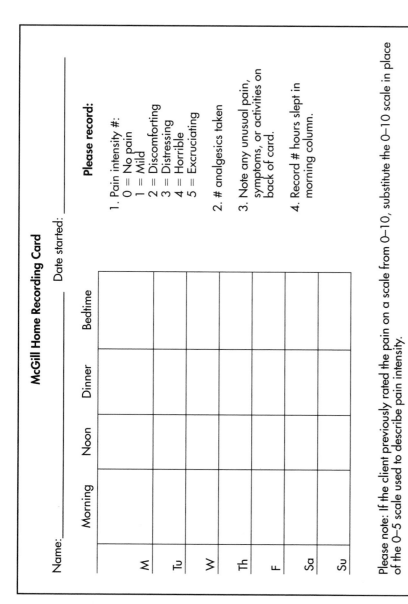

Fig. 3-7 • McGill Home Recording Card. When assessing constant pain, have the client complete this form for 24 to 48 hours. Pay attention to the client who describes a loss of sleep but who is not awake enough to record missed or interrupted sleep. This may help the physician in differentiating between a sleep disorder and sleep disturbance. You may want to ask the client to record sexual activity as a measure of function and pain levels. It is not necessary to record details, just when the client perceived him or herself as being sexually active. (From Melzack R: The McGill Pain Questionnaire: major properties and scoring methods, *Pain* 1:298, 1975.)

(Fig. 3-7) may help the client outline the existing pattern of the pain and can be used later in the episode of care to assist the therapist in detecting any change in symptoms or function.

Medications can alter the pain pattern or characteristics of painful symptoms. Find out how well the client's current medications reduce, control, or relieve pain. Ask how often medications are needed for breakthrough pain.

When using any of the pain rating scales, record the use of any medications that can alter or reduce pain or symptoms such as antiinflammatories or analgesics. At the same time remember to look for side effects or adverse reactions to any drugs or drug combinations.

Watch for clients taking nonsteroidal antiinflammatory drugs (NSAIDs) who experience an increase in shoulder, neck, or back pain several hours after taking the medication. Normally, one would expect symptom relief from NSAIDs so any

increase in symptoms is a red flag for possible peptic ulcer.

A client frequently will comment that the pain or symptoms have not changed despite 2 or 3 weeks of physical therapy intervention. This information can be discouraging to both client and therapist; however, when the symptoms are reviewed, a decrease in pain, increase in function, reduced need for medications, or other significant improvement in the pattern of symptoms may be seen.

The improvement is usually gradual and is best documented through the use of a baseline of pain activity established at an early stage in the episode of care by using a record such as the Home Recording Card (or other pain rating scale).

However, if no improvement in symptoms or function can be demonstrated, the therapist must again consider a systemic origin of symptoms. Repeating screening questions for medical disease is encouraged throughout the episode of care even

if such questions were included in the intake interview.

Because of the progressive nature of systemic involvement, the client may not have noticed any constitutional symptoms at the start of the physical therapy intervention that may now be present. Constitutional symptoms (see Box 1-3) affect the whole body and are characteristic of systemic disease or illness.

Aggravating and Relieving Factors

A series of questions addressing aggravating and relieving factors must be included such as:

Follow-Up Questions

- What brings your pain (symptoms) on?
- What kinds of things make your pain (symptoms) worse (e.g., eating, exercise, rest, specific positions, excitement, stress)?
  To assess relieving factors, ask:
- What makes the pain better?
  Follow-up questions include:
- How does rest affect the pain/symptoms?
- Are your symptoms aggravated or relieved by any activities?
- If yes, what?
- How has this problem affected your daily life at work or at home?

- How has this problem affected your ability to care for yourself without assistance (e.g., dress, bathe, cook, drive)?

The McGill Pain Questionnaire also provides a chart (Fig. 3-8) that may be useful in determining the presence of relieving or aggravating factors.

Systemic pain tends to be relieved minimally, relieved only temporarily, or unrelieved by change in position or by rest. However, musculoskeletal pain is *often* relieved both by a change of position and by rest.

Associated Symptoms

These symptoms may occur alone or in conjunction with the pain of systemic disease. The client may or may not associate these additional symptoms with the chief complaint. The physical therapist may ask:

Follow-Up Questions

- What other symptoms have you had that you can associate with this problem?
  If the client denies any additional symptoms, follow up this question with a series of possibilities such as:

Burning	Heart palpitations	Numbness/ Tingling

Fig. 3-8 • Factors aggravating and relieving pain. (From Melzack R: The McGill Pain Questionnaire: major properties and scoring methods, *Pain* 1:277, 1975.)

Indicate a plus (+) for aggravating factors or a minus (−) for relieving factors.

Liquor		Sleep/rest
Stimulants (e.g., caffeine)		Lying down
Eating		Distraction (e.g., television)
Heat		Urination/defecation
Cold		Tension/stress
Weather changes		Loud noises
Massage		Going to work
Pressure		Intercourse
No movement		Mild exercise
Movement		Fatigue
Sitting		Standing

Difficulty in breathing
Difficulty in swallowing
Dizziness
Hoarseness
Nausea
Night sweats
Problems with vision
Vomiting
Weakness

Whenever the client says "yes" to such associated symptoms, check for the presence of these symptoms bilaterally. Additionally, bilateral weakness, either proximally or distally, should serve as a red flag possibly indicative of more than a musculoskeletal lesion.

Blurred vision, double vision, scotomas (black spots before the eyes), or temporary blindness may indicate early symptoms of multiple sclerosis or may possibly be warning signs of an impending cerebrovascular accident. The presence of any associated symptoms, such as those mentioned here, would require contact with the physician to confirm the physician's knowledge of these symptoms.

In summary, careful, sensitive, and thorough questioning regarding the multifaceted experience of pain can elicit essential information necessary when making a decision regarding treatment or referral. The use of pain assessment tools such as

Fig. 3-6 and Table 3-2 may facilitate clear and accurate descriptions of this critical symptom.

▶ SOURCES OF PAIN

Between the twentieth and twenty-first centuries the science of clinical pain assessment and management made a significant paradigm shift from an empirical approach to one that is based on identifying and understanding the actual mechanisms involved in the pathogenesis of pain.

The implications of this are immense as we move from classifying pain on the basis of disease, duration, and body part or anatomy to a mechanism-based classification. In this approach the major goal of assessment is to identify the pathophysiological mechanism of the pain and use this information to plan appropriate intervention.[5,40]

Physical therapists frequently see clients whose primary complaint is pain, which often leads to a loss of function. However, focusing on sources of pain does not always help us to identify the causes of tissue irritation.

The most effective physical therapy diagnosis will define the syndrome and address the causes of pain rather than just identifying the sources of

TABLE 3-2 ▼ Comparison of Systemic versus Musculoskeletal Pain Patterns

	Systemic pain	Musculoskeletal pain

Onset	• Recent, sudden
	• Does not present as observed for years without progression of symptoms
		• May be sudden or gradual, depending on the history
		  • **Sudden:** Usually associated with acute overload stress, traumatic event, repetitive motion; can occur as a side effect of some medications (e.g., statins)
		  • **Gradual:** Secondary to chronic overload of the affected part; may be present off and on for years

Description	• Knifelike quality of stabbing from the inside out, boring, deep aching • Cutting, gnawing • Throbbing • Bone pain • Unilateral or bilateral	• Local tenderness to pressure is present • Achy, cramping pain • May be stiff after prolonged rest, but pain level decreases • Usually unilateral
Intensity	• Related to the degree of noxious stimuli; usually unrelated to presence of anxiety • Dull to severe • Mild to severe	• May be mild to severe • May depend on the person's anxiety level—the level of pain may increase in a client fearful of a "serious" condition
Duration	• Constant, no change, awakens the person at night	• May be constant but is more likely to be intermittent, depending on the activity or the position • Duration can be modified by rest or change in position

TABLE 3-2 ▼ Comparison of Systemic versus Musculoskeletal Pain Patterns—cont'd

	Systemic pain	Musculoskeletal pain
Pattern	• Although constant, may come in waves • Gradually progressive, cyclic • Night pain 　○ Location: chest/shoulder 　○ Accompanied by shortness of breath, wheezing 　○ Eating alters symptoms 　○ Sitting up relieves symptoms (decreases venous return to the heart: possible pulmonary or cardiovascular etiology) • Symptoms unrelieved by rest or change in position • Migratory arthralgias: Pain/symptoms last for 1 week in one joint, then resolve and appear in another joint	• Restriction of active/passive/accessory movement(s) observed • One or more particular movements "catch" the client and aggravate the pain
Aggravating Factors	• Cannot alter, provoke, alleviate, eliminate, aggravate the symptoms • Organ Dependent (Examples): 　○ Esophagus—eating or swallowing affects symptoms 　○ GI—peristalsis (eating) affects symptoms 　○ Heart—cold, exertion, stress, heavy meal (especially when combined) bring on symptoms	• Altered by movement; pain may become worse with movement or some myalgia decreases with movement
Relieving Factors	• Organ Dependent (Examples): 　○ Gallbladder—leaning forward may reduce symptoms 　○ Kidney—leaning to the affected side may reduce symptoms 　○ Pancreas—sitting upright or leaning forward may reduce symptoms	• Symptoms reduced or relieved by rest or change in position • Muscle pain is relieved by short periods of rest without resulting stiffness, except in the case of fibromyalgia; stiffness may be present in older adults • Stretching • Heat, cold
Associated Signs and Symptoms	• Fever, chills • Night sweats • Unusual vital signs • Warning signs of cancer (see Chapter 13) • GI symptoms: Nausea, vomiting, anorexia, unexplained weight loss, diarrhea, constipation • Early satiety (feeling full after eating) • Bilateral symptoms (e.g., paresthesias, weakness, edema, nail bed changes, skin rash) • Painless weakness of muscles: More often proximal but may occur distally • Dyspnea (breathlessness at rest or after mild exertion) • Diaphoresis (excessive perspiration) • Headaches, dizziness, fainting • Visual disturbances • Skin lesions, rashes, or itching that the client may not associate with the musculoskeletal symptoms • Bowel/bladder symptoms 　○ Hematuria (blood in the urine) 　○ Nocturia 　○ Urgency (sudden need to urinate) 　○ Frequency 　○ Melena (blood in feces) 　○ Fecal or urinary incontinence 　○ Bowel smears	• Usually none, although stimulation of trigger points may cause sweating, nausea, blanching

pain.[41] Usually, a careful assessment of pain behavior is invaluable in determining the nature and extent of the underlying pathology.

The clinical evaluation of pain usually involves identification of the primary disease/etiological factor(s) considered responsible for producing or initiating the pain. The client is placed within a broad pain category usually labeled as nociceptive (e.g., pinprick), inflammatory (e.g., tissue injury), or neuropathic pain (see Table 3-4).[5]

We further classify the pain by identifying the anatomical distribution, quality, and intensity of the pain. Such an approach allows for physical therapy interventions for each identified mechanism involved.

From a screening perspective we look at the possible *sources* of pain and *types* of pain. When listening to the client's description of pain, consider these possible sources of pain (Table 3-3):

- Cutaneous
- Somatic
- Visceral
- Neuropathic
- Referred

Cutaneous Sources of Pain

Cutaneous pain (related to the skin) includes superficial somatic structures located in the skin and subcutaneous tissue. The pain is well localized as the client can point directly to the area that "hurts." Pain from a cutaneous source can usually be localized with one finger. Skin pain or tenderness can be associated with referred pain from the viscera or referred from deep somatic structures.

Impairment of any organ can result in sudomotor changes that present as trophic changes such as itching, dysesthesia, skin temperature changes, or dry skin. The difficulty is that biomechanical dysfunction can also result in these same changes, which is why a careful evaluation of soft tissue structures along with a screening exam for systemic disease is required.

Cutaneous pain perception varies from person to person and is not always a reliable indicator of pathologic etiology. These differences in pain perception may be associated with different pain mechanisms. For example, differences in cutaneous pain perception exist based on gender and ethnicity. There may be differences in opioid activity and baroreceptor-regulated pain systems between the sexes to account for these variations.[35]

Somatic Sources of Pain

Somatic pain can be superficial or deep. Somatic pain is labeled according to its source as deep

---

TABLE 3-3 ▼ Sources of Pain, Pain Types, and Pain Patterns

Sources	Types	Characteristics/patterns
Cutaneous	Myofascial pain	Client describes:
Deep somatic	• Muscle tension	• Location/onset
Visceral	• Muscle spasm	• Description
Neuropathic	• Muscle trauma	• Intensity
Referred	• Muscle deficiency (weakness and stiffness)	• Duration
	• Trigger points (TrPs)	• Frequency
	Joint pain	
	• Drug-induced	Therapist recognizes the pattern
	• Chemical exposure	• Vascular
	• Inflammatory bowel disease	• Neurogenic
	• Septic arthritis	• Musculoskeletal/spondylotic
	• Reactive arthritis	• Visceral
	Radicular pain	• Emotional
	Arterial, pleural, tracheal	
	Gastrointestinal pain	
	Pain at rest	
	Night pain	
	Pain with activity	
	Diffuse pain	
	Chronic pain	

somatic, somatovisceral, somatoemotional (also referred to as psychosomatic), or viscerosomatic.

Most of what the therapist treats is part of the somatic system whether we call that the neuromuscular system, the musculoskeletal system or the neuromusculoskeletal (NMS) system. When psychologic disorders present as somatic dysfunction, we refer to these conditions as psychophysiologic disorders.

Psychophysiologic disorders, including somatoform disorders are discussed in detail elsewhere.[42-44] *Superficial somatic* structures involve the skin, superficial fasciae, tendons sheaths, and periosteum. *Deep somatic pain* comes from pathologic conditions of the periosteum and cancellous (spongy) bone, nerves, muscles, tendons, ligaments, and blood vessels. Deep somatic structures also include deep fasciae and joint capsules. When we talk about the "psycho-somatic" response, we refer to the mind-*body* connection.

Deep somatic pain is poorly localized and may be referred to the body surface, becoming cutaneous (spongy) pain. It can be associated with an autonomic phenomenon, such as sweating, pallor, or changes in pulse and blood pressure, and is commonly accompanied by a subjective feeling of nausea and faintness.

Pain associated with deep somatic lesions follows patterns that relate to the embryologic development of the musculoskeletal system. This explains why such pain may not be perceived directly over the involved organ (see Fig. 3-1).

Parietal pain (related to the wall of the chest or abdominal cavity) is also considered deep somatic. The visceral pleura (the membrane enveloping the organs) is insensitive to pain, but the parietal pleura is well supplied with pain nerve endings. For this reason it is possible for a client to have extensive visceral disease (e.g., heart, lungs) without pain until the disease progresses enough to involve the parietal pleura.

Somatoemotional or *psychosomatic* sources of pain occur when emotional or psychologic distress produces physical symptoms either for a relatively brief period or with recurrent and multiple physical manifestations spanning many months or years. The person affected by the latter may be referred to as a somatizer, and the condition is called a somatization disorder.

Two different approaches to somatization have been proposed. One method treats somatization as a phenomenon that is secondary to psychological distress. This is called *presenting somatization.* The second defines somatization as a primary event characterized by the presence of medically

unexplained symptoms. This model is called *functional somatization.*[45]

Alternately, there are *viscerosomatic* sources of pain when visceral structures affect the somatic musculature, such as the reflex spasm and rigidity of the abdominal muscles in response to the inflammation of acute appendicitis or the pectoral trigger point associated with an acute myocardial infarction. These visible and palpable changes in the tension of skin and subcutaneous and other connective tissues that are segmentally related to visceral pathologic processes are referred to as connective tissue zones or reflex zones.[46]

Somatovisceral pain occurs when a myalgic condition causes functional disturbance of the underlying viscera, such as the trigger points of the abdominal muscles causing diarrhea, vomiting, or excessive burping (Case Example 3-2).

Visceral Sources of Pain

Visceral sources of pain include the internal organs and the heart muscle. This source of pain includes all body organs located in the trunk or abdomen, such as those of the respiratory, digestive, urogenital, and endocrine systems, as well as the spleen, the heart, and the great vessels.

Visceral pain is not well localized for two reasons:

1. Innervation of the viscera is multisegmental
2. There are few nerve receptors in these structures (see Fig. 3-3).

The pain tends to be poorly localized and diffuse. Visceral pain is well known for its ability to produce referred pain (i.e., pain perceived in an area other than the site of the stimuli). Referred pain occurs because visceral fibers synapse at the level of the spinal cord close to fibers supplying specific somatic structures. In other words, visceral pain corresponds to dermatomes from which the organ receives its innervations, which may be the same innervations for somatic structures.

For example, the heart is innervated by the C3-T4 spinal nerves. Pain of a cardiac source can affect any part of the soma (body) also innervated by these levels. This is one reason why someone having a heart attack can experience jaw, neck, shoulder, mid-back, arm or chest pain and accounts for the many and varied clinical pictures of myocardial infarction (see Fig. 6-9).

More specifically, the pericardium (sac around the entire heart) is adjacent to the diaphragm. Pain of cardiac and diaphragmatic origin is often experienced in the shoulder because the C5-6

CASE EXAMPLE 3-2   Somatic Disorder Mimicking Visceral Disease

A 61-year-old woman reported left shoulder pain for the last 3 weeks. The pain radiates down the arm in the pattern of an ulnar nerve distribution. She had no known injury, trauma, or repetitive motion to account for the new onset of symptoms. She denied any constitutional symptoms (nausea, vomiting, unexplained sweating, or sweats). There was no reported shortness of breath.

Pain was described as "gripping" and occurred most often at night, sometimes waking her up from sleep. Physical activity, motion, and exertion did not bring on, reproduce, or make her symptoms worse.

After completing the interview and screening examination, what final question should always be asked every client?

- Do you have any other pain or symptoms of any kind anywhere else in your body?

Result: In response to this question, the client reported left-sided chest pain that radi-

ated to her nipple and then into her left shoulder and down the arm. Palpation of the chest wall musculature revealed a trigger point (TrP) of the pectoralis major muscle. This trigger point was responsible for the chest and breast pain.

Further palpation reproduced a TrP of the left subclavius muscle, which was causing the woman's left arm pain. Releasing the trigger points eliminated all of the woman's symptoms. **Should you make a medical referral for this client?**

Yes, referral should be made to rule out a viscerosomatic reflex causing the TrPs. A clinical breast exam (CBE) and mammography may be appropriate depending on client's history and when she had her last CBE and mammogram.

The client saw a cardiologist. Her echocardiogram and stress tests were negative. She was diagnosed with pseudocardiac disease secondary to a myofascial pain disorder.

From Murphy DR: *Myofascial pain and pseudocardiac disease,* Posted on-line April 22, 2004 [www.chiroweb.com].

---

spinal segment (innervation for the shoulder) also supplies the heart and the diaphragm.

Other examples of organ innervations and their corresponding sensory overlap are as follows:[2]

- Sensory fibers to the heart and lungs enter the spinal cord from T1 to T4 (this may extend to T6).
- Sensory fibers to the gallbladder, bile ducts, and stomach enter the spinal cord at the level of the T7-8 dorsal roots (i.e., the greater splanchnic nerve).
- The peritoneal covering of the gallbladder and/or the central zone of the diaphragm are innervated by the phrenic nerve originating from the C3-5 (phrenic nerve) levels of the spinal cord.
- The phrenic nerve (C3-5) also innervates portions of the pericardium.
- Sensory fibers to the duodenum enter the cord at the T9-10 levels.
- Sensory fibers to the appendix enter the cord at the T10 level (i.e., the lesser splanchnic nerve).
- Sensory fibers to the renal/ureter system enter the cord at the L1-2 level (i.e., the splanchnic nerve).

As mentioned earlier, diseases of internal organs can be accompanied by cutaneous hypersensitivity to touch, pressure, and temperature. This viscerocutaneous reflex occurs during the acute phase of the disease and disappears with its recovery.

The skin areas affected are innervated by the same cord segments as for the involved viscera; they are referred to as Head's zones.[46] Anytime a client presents with somatic symptoms also innervated by any of these levels, we must consider the possibility of a visceral origin.

Keep in mind that when it comes to visceral pain, the viscera have few nerve endings. The visceral pleura are insensitive to pain. It is not until the organ capsule (deep somatic structure) is stretched (e.g., by a tumor or inflammation) that pain is perceived and possibly localized. This is why changes can occur within the organs without painful symptoms to warn the person. It is not until the organ is inflamed or distended enough from infection or obstruction to impinge nearby structures or the lining of the chest or abdominal cavity that pain is felt.

The neurology of visceral pain is not well understood. There is not a known central processing

system unique to visceral pain. Scientists are currently using various theories without proven facts.

For example, exact nerve fibers and specific nociceptors have not been identified in organs. It is known that the afferent supply to internal organs follows a path similar to that of the sympathetic nervous system, often in close proximity to blood vessels.[2] The origins of embryology explain far more of the visceral pain patterns than anything else (see discussion, this chapter).

In the early stage of visceral disease, sympathetic reflexes arising from afferent impulses of the internal viscera can be expressed first as sensory, motor, and/or trophic changes in the skin, subcutaneous tissues, and/or muscles. As mentioned earlier, this may present as itching, dysesthesia, skin temperature changes, or dry skin. The viscera do not perceive pain, but the sensory side is trying to get the message out that something is wrong by creating sympathetic sudomotor changes.

It appears that there is no specific group of spinal neurons that respond only to visceral inputs. Since messages from the soma and viscera come into the cord at the same level (and sometimes visceral afferents converge over several segments of the spinal cord), the nervous system has trouble deciding: Is it somatic or visceral? It sends efferent information back out to the plexus for change or reaction, but the input results in an unclear impulse at the cord level.

The body may get skin or somatic responses such as muscle pain or aching periosteum or it may tell a viscus innervated at the same level to do something it can do (e.g., the stomach increases its acid content). This also explains how sympathetic signals from the liver to the spinal cord can result in itching or other sudomotor responses in the area embryologically related to the liver.[2]

This somatization of visceral pain is why we must know the visceral pain patterns and the spinal versus visceral innervations. We examine one (somatic) while screening for the other (visceral).

Because the somatic and visceral afferent messages enter at the same level, it is possible to get **somatic-somatic** reflex responses (e.g., a bruise on the leg causes knee pain), **somato-visceral** reflex responses (e.g., a biomechanical dysfunction of the 10th rib can cause gallbladder changes), or **viscero-somatic** reflex responses (e.g., gallbladder impairment can result in a sore 10th rib; pelvic floor dysfunction can lead to incontinence; heart attack causes arm or jaw pain). These are actually all referred pain patterns originating in the soma or viscera.

A more in-depth discussion of the visceral-somatic response is available.[47] A visceral-somatic response can occur when biochemical changes associated with visceral disease affect somatic structures innervated by the same spinal nerves.

Prior to her death, Dr. Janet Travell[47] was researching how often people with anginal pain are really experiencing residual pectoralis major trigger points (TrPs) caused by previous episodes of angina or myocardial infarction. This is another example of the viscero-somatic response mentioned.

A **viscero-viscero** reflex occurs when pain or dysfunction in one organ causes symptoms in another organ. For example, the client presents with chest pain and has an extensive cardiac workup with normal findings. The client may be told "it's not in your heart, so don't worry about it."

The problem may really be the gallbladder. Because the gallbladder originates from the same tissue embryologically as the heart, gallbladder impairment can cause cardiac changes in addition to shoulder pain from its contact with the diaphragm. This presentation is then confused with cardiac pathology.[2]

On the other hand, the doctor may do a gallbladder workup and find nothing. The chest pain could be coming from arthritic changes in the cervical spine. This occurs because the cervical spine and heart share common sensory pathways from C3 to the spinal cord.

Information from the cardiac plexus and brachial plexus enter the cord at the same level. The nervous system is not able to identify who sent the message, just what level it came from. It responds as best it can, based on the information present, sometimes resulting in the wrong symptoms for the problem at hand.

Pain and symptoms of a visceral source are usually accompanied by an autonomic nervous system (ANS) response such as change in vital signs, unexplained perspiration (diaphoresis), and/or skin pallor. Signs and symptoms associated with the involved organ system may also be present. We call these *associated signs and symptoms*. They are red flags in the screening process.

Neuropathic Pain

Neuropathic or neurogenic pain results from damage to or pathophysiologic changes of the peripheral or central nervous system.[48] Neuropathic pain can occur as a result of injury or destruction to the peripheral nerves, pathways in the spinal cord, or neurons located in the brain.

Neuropathic pain can be acute or chronic depending on the timeframe.

This type of pain is not elicited by the stimulation of nociceptors or kinesthetic pathways as a result of tissue damage, but rather by malfunction of the nervous system itself.[46] Disruptions in the transmission of afferent and efferent impulses in the periphery, spinal cord, and brain can give rise to alterations in sensory modalities (e.g., touch, pressure, temperature), and sometimes motor dysfunction.

It can be drug-induced, metabolic based, or brought on by trauma to the sensory neurons or pathways in either the peripheral or central nervous system. It appears to be idiosyncratic; not all individuals with the same lesion will have pain.[49] Some examples are listed in Table 3-4.

It is usually described as sharp, shooting, burning, tingling, or producing an electric shock sensation. The pain is steady or evoked by some stimulus that is not normally considered noxious (e.g., light touch, cold). Some affected individuals report aching pain. There is no muscle spasm in neurogenic pain.[46]

Neuropathic pain is not alleviated by opiates or narcotics, although local anesthesia can provide temporary relief. Medications used to treat neuropathic pain include antidepressants, anticonvulsants, antispasmodics, adrenergics, and anesthetics. Many clients have a combination of neuropathic and somatic pain making it more difficult to identify the underlying pathology.

Referred Pain

By definition, referred pain is felt in an area far from the site of the lesion, but supplied by the same or adjacent neural segments. Referred pain occurs by way of shared central pathways for afferent neurons and can originate from any cutaneous, somatic, or visceral source.

Referred pain can occur alone or with accompanying deep somatic or visceral pain. When caused by an underlying visceral or systemic disease, visceral pain usually precedes the development of referred musculoskeletal pain. However, the client may not remember or mention this previous pain pattern . . . and the therapist has not asked about the presence of any other symptoms.

Referred pain is usually well localized (i.e., the person can point directly to the area that hurts), but it does not have sharply defined borders. It can spread or radiate from its point of origin. Local tenderness is present in the tissue of the referred pain area, but there is no objective sensory deficit. Referred pain is often accompanied by muscle hypertonus over the referred area of pain.

Visceral disorders can refer pain to somatic tissue (see Table 3-7). On the other hand, as mentioned in the last topic on visceral sources of pain, some somatic impairments can refer pain to visceral locations or mimic known visceral pain patterns. Finding the original source of referred pain can be quite a challenge (Case Example 3-3).

Always ask one or both of these two questions in your pain interview as part of the screening process:

TABLE 3-4 ▼ Causes of Neuropathic Pain

Central neuropathic pain	Peripheral neuropathic pain
Multiple sclerosis	Trigeminal neuralgia (Tic douloureux)
Headache (migraine)	Poorly controlled diabetes mellitus (metabolic induced)
Stroke	Vincristine (Oncovin) (drug-induced; used in cancer treatment)
Traumatic brain injury (TBI)	Isoniazid (INH) (drug-induced; used to treat tuberculosis)
Parkinson's disease	Amputation (trauma)
Spinal cord injury (incomplete)	Crush injury/brachial avulsion (trauma)
	Herpes Zoster (Shingles, postherpetic neuralgia)
	Complex regional pain syndrome (CRPS2, causalgia)
	Nerve compression syndromes (e.g., carpel tunnel syndrome, thoracic outlet syndrome)
	Paraneoplastic neuropathy (cancer-induced)
	Cancer (tumor infiltration/compression of the nerve)
	Liver or biliary impairment (e.g., liver cancer, cirrhosis, primary biliary cirrhosis)
	Leprosy
	Congenital neuropathy (e.g., porphyria)
	Guillain-Barré Syndrome

CASE EXAMPLE 3-3 Type of Pain and Possible Cause

A 44-year-old woman has come to physical therapy with reports of neck, jaw, and chest pain when using her arms overhead. She describes the pain as sharp and "hurting." It is not always consistent. Sometimes she has it; sometimes she does not. Her job as the owner of a window coverings business requires frequent, long periods of time with her arms overhead.

A) Would you classify this as cutaneous, somatic, visceral, neuropathic, or referred pain?

B) What are some possible causes and how can you differentiate neuromusculoskeletal from systemic?

A) The client has not mentioned the skin hurting or pointed to a specific area to suggest a cutaneous source of pain. It could be referred pain, but we do not know yet if it is referred from the neuromusculoskeletal system (neck, ribs, shoulder) or from the viscera (given the description, most likely cardiac).

Without further information, we can say it is somatic or referred visceral pain. We can describe it as radiating since it starts in the neck and affects a wide area above and below that. No defined dermatomes have been identified to suggest a neuropathic cause, so this must be evaluated more carefully.

B) This could be a pain pattern associated with *thoracic outlet syndrome* (TOS) because the lower cervical plexus can innervate as far down as the nipple line. This can be differentiated when performing tests and measures for TOS.

Since TOS can impact the neuro- or vascular bundle, it is important to measure blood pressure in both arms and compare them for a possible vascular component.

Onset of *anginal pain* occurs in some people with the use of arms overhead. To discern if this may be a cardiac problem, have the client use the lower extremities to exercise without using the arms (e.g., stairs, stationary bike).

Onset of symptoms from a cardiac origin usually has a lag effect. In other words, symptoms do not start until 5 to 10 minutes after the activity has started. It is not immediate as it might be when using impaired muscles. If the symptoms are reproduced 3 to 5 or 10 minutes after the lower extremity activity, consider a cardiac cause. Look for signs and symptoms associated with cardiac impairment. Ask about a personal/family history of heart disease.

At age 44, she may be perimenopausal (unless she has had a hysterectomy, which brings on surgical menopause) and still on the young side for cardiac cause of upper quadrant symptoms. Still, it is possible and would have to be ruled out by a physician if you are unable to find a NMS cause of symptoms.

Chest pain can have a *wide range of causes* including trigger points, anabolic steroid or cocaine use, breast disease, premenstrual symptoms, assault or trauma, lactation problems, scar tissue from breast augmentation or reduction, and so on. See further discussion, Chapter 17.

Follow-Up Questions

- Are you having any pain anywhere else in your body?
- Are you having symptoms of any other kind that may or may not be related to your main problem?

Differentiating Sources of Pain[2]

How do we differentiate somatic sources of pain from visceral sources? It can be very difficult to make this distinction. That is one reason why clients end up in physical therapy even though there is a viscerogenic source of the pain and/or symptomatic presentation.

The superficial and deep somatic structures are innervated unilaterally via the spinal nerves, whereas the viscera are innervated bilaterally through the autonomic nervous system via visceral afferents. The quality of superficial somatic pain tends to be sharp and more localized. It is mediated by large myelinated fibers, which have a low threshold for stimulation and a fast conduction time. This is designed to protect the structures by signaling a problem right away.

Deep somatic pain is more likely to be a dull or deep aching that responds to rest or a non-weight-bearing position. Deep somatic pain is often poorly localized (transmission via small unmyelinated fibers) and can be referred from some other site.

Pain of a deep somatic nature increases after movement. Sometimes the client can find a comfortable spot, but after moving the extremity or joint, cannot find that comfortable spot again. This is in contrast to visceral pain, which usually is not reproduced with movement, but rather, tends to hurt all the time or with all movements.[2]

Pain from a visceral source can also be dull and aching, but usually does not feel better after rest or recumbency. Keep in mind pathologic processes occurring within somatic structures (e.g., metastasis, primary tumor, infection) may produce localized pain that can be mechanically irritated. This is why movement in general (rather than specific motions) can make it worse. Back pain from metastasis to the spine can become quite severe before any radiologic changes are seen.[2]

Visceral diseases of the abdomen and pelvis are more likely to refer pain to the back, whereas intrathoracic disease refers pain to the shoulder(s). Visceral pain rarely occurs without associated signs and symptoms, although the client may not recognize the correlation. Careful questioning will usually elicit a systemic pattern of symptoms.

Back or shoulder range of motion is usually full and painless in the presence of visceral pain, especially in the early stages of disease. When the painful stimulus increases or persists over time, muscle splinting and guarding can result in subsequent changes in biomechanical patterns, making it more difficult to recognize the systemic origin of musculoskeletal dysfunction.

▼ TYPES OF PAIN

Although there are five sources of most physiologic pain (from a medical screening perspective), many types of pain exist within these categories (see Table 3-3).

When orienting to pain from these main sources, it may be helpful to consider some specific types of pain patterns. Not all pain types can be discussed here, but some of the most commonly encountered are included.

Myofascial Pain

Myalgia, or muscle pain, can be a symptom of an underlying systemic disorder. Cancer, renal failure, hepatic disease, and endocrine disorders are only a few possible systemic sources of muscle involvement.

For example, muscle weakness, atrophy, myalgia, and fatigue that persist despite rest may be early manifestations of thyroid or parathyroid disease, acromegaly, diabetes, Cushing's syndrome, or osteomalacia.

Myalgia can be present in anxiety and depressive disorders. Muscle weakness and myalgia can occur as a side effect of drugs. Prolonged use of systemic corticosteroids and immunosuppressive drugs has known adverse effects on the musculoskeletal system including degenerative myopathy with muscle wasting and tendon rupture.

Infective endocarditis caused by acute bacterial infection can present with myalgias and no other manifestation of endocarditis. The early onset of joint pain and myalgia as the first sign of endocarditis is more likely if the person is older and has had a previously diagnosed heart murmur. Joint pain (arthralgia) often accompanies myalgia and the client is diagnosed with rheumatoid arthritis.

Polymyalgia rheumatica (PR; literally "pain in many muscles") is a disorder marked by diffuse pain and stiffness that primarily affects muscles of the shoulder and pelvic girdles.

With PR symptoms are vague and difficult to diagnose resulting in delay in medical treatment. The person may wake up one morning with muscle pain and stiffness for no apparent reason or the symptoms may come on gradually over several days or weeks. Adults over age 50 are affected most often (white women have the highest incidence); most cases occur after age 70.[50]

Temporal arteritis occurs in 25% of all cases of PR. Watch for headache, visual changes (blurred or double vision), intermittent jaw pain (claudication), and cranial nerve involvement. The temporal artery may be prominent and painful to touch and the temporal pulse absent.

From a screening point of view, there are many types of muscle-related pain such as tension, spasm, weakness, trauma, inflammation, infection, neurologic impairment, and trigger points (see Table 3-3).[51] The clinical presentation most common with systemic disease is presented here.

Muscle Tension

Muscle tension, or sustained muscle tone, occurs when prolonged muscular contraction or co-contraction results in local ischemia, increased cellular metabolites, and subsequent pain. Ischemia as a factor in muscle pain remains controversial. Interruption of blood flow in a resting extremity does not cause pain unless the muscle contracts during the ischemic condition.[52]

Muscle tension also can occur with physical stress and fatigue. Muscle tension and the subsequent ischemia may occur as a result of faulty ergonomics, prolonged work positions (e.g., as with

computer or telephone operators), or repetitive motion.

Take for example the person sitting at a keyboard for hours each day. Constant typing with muscle co-contraction does not allow for the normal contract-relax sequence. Muscle ischemia results in greater release of Substance P, a pain neurotransmitter (neuropeptide).

Increased Substance P levels increase pain sensitivity. Increased pain perception results in more muscle spasm as a splinting or protective guarding mechanism. And so the pain-spasm cycle is perpetuated. This is a somatic-somatic response.

Muscle tension from a visceral-somatic response can occur when pain from a visceral source results in increased muscle tension and even muscle spasm. For example, the pain from any inflammatory or infectious process affecting the abdomen (e.g., appendicitis, diverticulitis, pelvic inflammatory disease) can cause increased tension in the abdominal muscles.

Given enough time and combined with overuse and repetitive use or infectious or inflammatory disease, muscle tension can turn into muscle spasm. When opposing muscles such as the flexors and extensors contract together for long periods of time (called co-contraction), muscle tension and then muscle spasm can occur.

Muscle Spasm

Muscle spasm is a sudden involuntary contraction of a muscle or group of muscles, usually occurring as a result of overuse or injury of the adjoining neuromusculoskeletal or musculotendinous attachments. A person with a painful musculoskeletal problem may also have a varying degree of reflex muscle spasm to protect the joint(s) involved (a somatic-somatic response). A client with painful visceral disease can have muscle spasm of the overlying musculature (a viscero-somatic response).

Spasm pain cannot be attributed to transient increased muscle tension because the intramuscular pressure is insufficiently elevated. Pain with muscle spasm may occur from prolonged contraction under an ischemic situation. An increase in the partial pressure of oxygen has been documented inside the muscle in spasm under these circumstances.[53]

Muscle Trauma

Muscle trauma can occur with acute trauma, burns, crush injuries, or unaccustomed intensity or duration of muscle contraction, especially eccentric contractions. Muscle pain occurs as broken fibers leak potassium into the interstitial fluid. Blood extravasation results from damaged blood vessels, setting off a cascade of chemical reactions within the muscle.[52]

When disintegration of muscle tissue occurs with release of their contents (e.g., oxygen-transporting pigment myoglobin) into the blood stream, a potentially fatal muscle toxicity called rhabdomyolysis can occur. Risk factors and clinical signs and symptoms are listed in Table 3-5. Immediate medical attention is required (Case Example 3-4).

Muscle Deficiency

Muscle deficiency (weakness and stiffness) is a common problem as we age. Connective tissue changes may occur as small amounts of fibrinogen (produced in the liver and normally converted to fibrin to serve as a clotting factor) leak from the vasculature into the intracellular spaces, adhering to cellular structures.

The resulting microfibrinous adhesions among the cells of muscle and fascia cause increased muscular stiffness. Activity and movement normally break these adhesions; however, with the aging process, production of fewer and less efficient macrophages combined with immobility for any reason result in reduced lysis of these adhesions.[54]

Other possible causes of aggravated stiffness include increased collagen fibers from reduced collagen turnover, increased cross-links of aged collagen fibers, changes in the mechanical properties of connective tissues, and structural and functional changes in the collagen protein. Tendons and ligaments also have less water content, resulting in increased stiffness.[55]

When muscular stiffness occurs as a result of aging, increased physical activity and movement can reduce associated muscular pain. As part of the diagnostic evaluation, consider a general conditioning program for the older adult reporting generalized muscle pain. Even ten minutes a day on a stationary bike, treadmill or in an aquatics program can bring dramatic and fast relief of painful symptoms when caused by muscle deficiency.

Proximal muscle weakness accompanied by change in one or more deep tendon reflexes is a red flag sign of cancer or neurologic impairment. In the presence of a past medical history of cancer, further screening is advised with possible medical referral required depending on the outcome of the examination/evaluation.

Trigger Points

Trigger points (TrPs; sometimes referred to as myofascial trigger points or MTrPs) are

TABLE 3-5 ▼ Risk Factors for Rhabdomyolysis

Risk factors for rhabdomyolysis	Examples	Signs and symptoms
Trauma	Crush injury Electric shock Severe burns Extended mobility	Profound muscle weakness Pain Swelling Stiffness and cramping Associated Signs and Symptoms: • Reddish-brown urine (myoglobin) • Decreased urine output • Malaise • Fever • Sinus tachycardia • Nausea, vomiting • Agitation, confusion
Extreme Muscular Activity	Strenuous exercise Status epilepticus Severe dystonia	
Toxic Effects	Ethanol Ethylene glycol Isopropanol Methanol Heroin Barbiturates Methadone Cocaine Amphetamines Ecstasy (street drug) Carbon monoxide Snake venom Tetanus	
Metabolic Abnormalities	Hypothyroidism Hyperthyroidism Diabetic ketoacidosis	
Medication-induced	Inadvertent intravenous (IV) infiltration (e.g., amphotericin B, azathioprine, cyclosporine) Cholesterol-lowering statins (e.g., Zocor, Lipitor, Crestor)	

Data from Fort CW: How to combat 3 deadly trauma complications, *Nursing2003* 33(5):58-64, 2003.

hyperirritable spots within a taut band of skeletal muscle or in the fascia. There is often a history of immobility (e.g., cast immobilization after fracture or injury), prolonged or vigorous activity such as bending or lifting, or forceful abdominal breathing such as occurs with marathon running.

TrPs are reproduced with palpation or resisted motions. When pressing on the TrP you may elicit a "jump sign." Some people say the jump sign is a local twitch response of muscle fibers to trigger point stimulation, but this is an erroneous use of the term.[47]

The *jump sign* is a general pain response as the client physically withdraws from the pressure on the point and may even cry out or wince in pain. The *local twitch response* is the visible contraction of tense muscle fibers in response to stimulation.

When trigger points are compressed, local tenderness with possible referred pain results. In other words, pain that arises from the trigger point is felt at a distance, often remote from its source.

The referred pain pattern is characteristic and specific for every muscle. Knowing the trigger point

CASE EXAMPLE 3-4 Military Rhabdomyolysis

A 20-year-old soldier reported to the military physical therapy clinic with bilateral shoulder pain and weakness. He was unable to perform his regular duties due to these symptoms. He attributed this to doing many push-ups during physical training 2 days ago.

When asked if there were any other symptoms of any kind to report, the client said that he noticed his urine was a dark color yesterday (the day after the push-up exercises).

The soldier had shoulder active range of motion to 90 degrees accompanied by an abnormal scapulohumeral rhythm with excessive scapular elevation on both sides. Passive shoulder range of motion was full but painful. Elbow active and passive range of motion were also restricted to 90 degrees of flexion second to pain in the triceps muscles.

The client was too painful to handle manual muscle testing with pain on palpation to the pectoral, triceps, and infraspinatus muscles, bilaterally. The rotator cuff tendon appeared to be intact.

What are the red flags in this case?

- Bilateral symptoms (pain and weakness)
- Age (for cancer, too young [under 25 years old] or too old [over 50] is a red flag sign)
- Change in urine color

Result: The soldier had actually done hundreds of different types of push-ups including regular, wide-arm, and diamond push-ups. Although the soldier was not in any apparent distress, laboratory studies were ordered. Serum CK level was measured as 9600 U/L (normal range: 55-170 U/L).

The results were consistent with acute exertional rhabdomyolysis (AED) and the soldier was hospitalized. Early recognition of a potentially serious problem may have prevented serious complications possible with this condition.

Physical therapy intervention for muscle soreness without adequate hydration could have led to acute renal failure. He returned to physical therapy for a recovery program following hospitalization.

Data from Baxter RE, Moore JH: Diagnosis and treatment of acute exertional rhabdomyolysis, J Orthop Sports Phys Ther 33(3):104-108, 2003.

locations and their referred pain patterns is helpful. By knowing the pain patterns, you can go to the site of origin and confirm (or rule out) the presence of the TrP. The distribution of referred trigger point pain rarely coincides entirely with the distribution of a peripheral nerve or dermatomal segment.[47]

In the screening process, TrPs must be eliminated to rule out systemic pathology as a cause of muscle pain. Beware when your client fails to respond to trigger point therapy. Consider this situation a yellow flag. It is *not* necessarily a red flag suggesting the need for screening for systemic or other causes of muscle pain. Muscle recovery from trigger points is not always so simple.

Muscles with active trigger points fatigue faster and recover more slowly. They show more abnormal neural circuit dysfunction. The pain and spasm of trigger points may not be relieved until the aberrant circuits are corrected.[56]

Any compromise of muscle energy metabolism such as occurs with endocrine or cancer-related disorders can aggravate and perpetuate trigger points making successful intervention a more challenging and lengthy process.

Remember, too, that visceral disease can create tender points. For those who understand the Jones' Strain/Counterstrain concept, some of the Jones' points might happen to fall in the same area as viscerogenic tender point, but the two are not the same points. A careful evaluation is required to differentiate between Jones' points and viscerogenic tender points.

Travell's trigger points (TrPs) can also produce visceral symptoms without actual organ impairment or disease. This is an example of a somatovisceral response. For example, the client may have an abdominal muscle TrP, but the history is one of upset stomach or chest (cardiac) pain. It is possible to have both tender points and TrPs when the underlying cause is visceral disease.

Pain and dysfunction of myofascial tissues is the subject of several texts to which the reader is referred for more information.[47,57,58]

Joint Pain

Noninflammatory joint pain (no redness, no warmth, no swelling) of unknown etiology can be caused by a wide range of pathologic conditions (Box 3-4). Fibromyalgia, leukemia, sexually transmitted infections, artificial sweeteners,[59-61] Crohn's disease (also known as regional enteritis), and infectious arthritis are all possible causes of joint pain.

Joint pain in the presence of fatigue may be a red flag for anxiety, depression, or cancer. The client history and screening interview may help the therapist find the true cause of joint pain. Look for risk factors for any of the listed conditions and review the client's recent activities.

When comparing joint pain associated with systemic versus musculoskeletal causes, one of the major differences is in the area of associated signs and symptoms (Table 3-6). Joint pain of a systemic or visceral origin usually has additional signs or symptoms present. The client may not realize there is a connection, or the condition may not have progressed enough for associated signs and symptoms to develop.

The therapist also evaluates joint pain over a 24-hour period. Joint pain from a systemic cause is more likely to be constant and present with all movements. Rest may help at first but over time even this relieving factor will not alter the symptoms. This is in comparison to the client with osteoarthritis (OA), who often feels better after rest (though stiffness may remain). Morning joint pain associated with OA is less than joint pain at the end of the day after using the joint(s) all day.

On the other hand, muscle pain may be worse in the morning and gradually improves as the client stretches and moves about during the day. The Pain Assessment Record Form (see Fig. 3-6) includes an assessment of these differences across a 24-hour span as part of the "Pattern."

The therapist can use the specific screening questions for joint pain to assess any joint pain of unknown cause or with an unusual presentation or history. Joint pain and symptoms that do not fit the expected pattern for injury, overuse, or aging can be screened using a few important questions (Box 3-5).

Drug-Induced

Joint pain as an allergic response, sometimes referred to as "serum sickness" can occur up to 6 weeks after taking a prescription drug (especially antibiotics). Joint pain is also a potential side effect of statins (e.g., Lipitor, Zocor). These are cholesterol-lowering agents.

Noninflammatory joint pain is typical of a delayed allergic reaction. The client may report fever, skin rash, and fatigue that go away when the drug is stopped.

Chemical Exposure

Likewise, delayed reactions can occur as a result of occupational or environmental chemical exposure. A work and/or military history may be required for anyone presenting with joint or muscle pain or symptoms of unknown cause. These clients can be mislabeled with a diagnosis of autoimmune disease or fibromyalgia. The alert therapist may recognize and report clues to help the client obtain a more accurate diagnosis.

Inflammatory Bowel Disease (IBD)

Ulcerative colitis (UC) and regional enteritis (Crohn's disease; CD) are accompanied by an arthritic component and skin rash in about 25% of all people affected by this inflammatory bowel condition.

BOX 3-4 ▼ Systemic Causes of Joint Pain

Infectious and noninfectious systemic causes of joint pain can include, but are not limited to:

- Allergic reactions (e.g., medications such as antibiotics)
- Side effect of other medications such as statins, prolonged use of corticosteroids, aromatase inhibitors
- Delayed reaction to chemicals or environmental factors
- Sexually transmitted infections (STIs) (e.g., HIV, syphilis, chlamydia, gonorrhea)
- Infectious arthritis
- Infective endocarditis
- Recent dental surgery
- Lyme disease
- Rheumatoid arthritis
- Other autoimmune disorders (e.g., systemic lupus erythematosus, mixed connective tissue disease, scleroderma, polymyositis)
- Leukemia
- Tuberculosis
- Acute rheumatic fever
- Chronic liver disease (hepatic osteodystrophy affecting wrists and ankles; hepatitis causing arthralgias)
- Inflammatory bowel disease (e.g., Crohn's disease or regional enteritis)
- Anxiety or depression (major depressive disorder)
- Fibromyalgia
- Artificial sweeteners

TABLE 3-6 ▼ Joint Pain: Systemic or Musculoskeletal?

	Systemic	Musculoskeletal
Clinical Presentation	Awakens at night Deep aching, throbbing Reduced by pressure* Constant or waves/spasm Cyclical, progressive symptoms	Decreases with rest Sharp Reduced by change in position Reduced or eliminated when stressful action is stopped Restriction of A/PROM Restriction of accessory motions 1 or more movements "catch," reproducing or aggravating pain/symptoms Repetitive motions Arthritis Static postures (prolonged) Trauma (including domestic violence)
Past Medical History	Recent history of infection: Hepatitis, bacterial infection from staphylococcus or streptococcus (e.g., cellulitis), mononucleosis, measles, URI, UTI, gonorrhea, osteomyelitis, cellulitis History of bone fracture, joint replacement or arthroscopy History of human bite Sore throat, headache with fever in the last 3 weeks or family/household member with recently diagnosed strep throat Skin rash (infection, medications) Recent medications (last 6 weeks); any drug but especially statins (cholesterol lowering) and antibiotics History of injection drug use/abuse History of allergic reactions Presence of extensor surface nodules History of GI symptoms Recent history of enteric or venereal infection or new sexual contact (e.g., Reiter's)	
Associated Signs and Symptoms	Jaundice Migratory arthralgias Skin rash/lesions Nodules (extensor surfaces) Fatigue Weight loss Low grade fever Proximal muscle weakness Presence of GI symptoms Cyclic, progressive symptoms Suspicious or aberrant lymph nodes	Usually none Check for trigger points Trigger points may be accompanied by some minimal ANS phenomenon (e.g., nausea, sweating)

URI, Upper respiratory infection; *UTI,* urinary tract infection; *GI,* gastrointestinal; *ANS,* autonomic nervous system; *A/PROM,* active/passive range of motion.

* This is actually a cutaneous or somatic response because the pressure provides a counter irritant; it does not really affect the viscera directly.

The person may have a known diagnosis of IBD, but may not know that new onset of joint symptoms can be part of this condition. The client interview should have brought out the personal history of either UC or CD. See the discussion of IBD in Chapter 8.

Peripheral joint disease associated with IBD involves the large joints, most often a single hip or knee. Joint symptoms often occur simultaneously with UC, but less often at the same time as CD. Ankylosing spondylitis (AS) is also possible with either form of IBD.

BOX 3-5 ▼ Screening Questions for Joint Pain

- Please describe the pattern of pain/symptoms from when you wake up in the morning to when you go to sleep at night.
- Do you have any symptoms of any kind anywhere else in your body? (You may have to explain these symptoms don't have to relate to the joint pain; if the client has no other symptoms, offer a short list including constitutional symptoms, heart palpitations, unusual fatigue, nail or skin changes, sores or lesions anywhere but especially in the mouth or on the genitals, and so forth.)
- Have you ever had
  Cancer of any kind
  Leukemia
  Crohn's disease (regional enteritis)
  Sexually transmitted infection (you may have to prompt with specific diseases such as chlamydia, genital herpes, genital warts, gonorrhea or "the clap," syphilis, Reiter's Syndrome, HIV)
  Fibromyalgia
  Joint replacement or arthroscopic surgery of any kind
- Have you recently (last 6 weeks) had any:
  Fractures
  Bites (human, animal)
  Antibiotics or other medications
  Infections [you may have to prompt with specific infections such as strep throat, mononucleosis, urinary tract, upper respiratory (cold or flu), gastrointestinal, hepatitis]
  Skin rashes or other skin changes
- Do you drink diet soda/pop or use aspartame, Equal, or NutraSweet? (If the client uses these products in any amount, suggest eliminating

them on a trial basis for 30 days; artificial sweetener-induced symptoms may disappear in some people; effects from use of the new product Splenda have not been reported.)

To the therapist: You may have to conduct an environmental or work history (occupation, military, exposure to chemicals) to identify a delayed reaction.

Quick Survey

- What kind of work do you do?
- Do you think your health problems are related to your work?
- Are your symptoms better or worse when you're at home or at work?
- Follow up if worse at work: Do others at work have similar problems?
- Have you been exposed to dusts, fumes, chemicals, radiation, or loud noise?
  Follow up: It may be necessary to ask additional questions based on past history, symptoms, and risk factors present.
- Do you live near a hazardous waste site or any industrial facilities that give off chemical odors or fumes?
- Do you live in a home built more than 40 years ago? Have you done renovations or remodeling?
- Do you use pesticides in your home, on your garden, or on your pets?
- What is your source of drinking water?
- Chronology of jobs (type of industry, type of job, years worked)
- How new is the building you are working in?
- Exposure survey (protective equipment used, exposure to dust, radiation, chemicals, biologic hazards, physical hazards)

As with typical AS, symptoms affect the low back, sacrum, or sacroiliac joint first. The most common symptoms are intermittent low-back pain with decreased low back motion. The course of AS associated with IBD is the same as without the bowel component.

Joint problems usually respond to medical treatment of the underlying bowel disease but in some cases require separate management. Interventions for the musculoskeletal involvement follow the usual protocols for each area affected.

Arthritis

Joint pain (either inflammatory or noninflammatory) can be associated with a wide range of systemic causes including bacterial or viral infection, trauma, and sexually transmitted diseases. There

is usually a positive history or other associated signs and symptoms to help the therapist identify the need for medical referral.

INFECTIOUS ARTHRITIS

Joint pain can be a *local* response to an infection. This is called infectious, septic, or bacterial arthritis. Invading microorganisms cause inflammation of the synovial membrane with release of cytokines (e.g., tumor necrosis factor, interleukin-1) and proteases. The end result can be cartilage destruction even after eradicating the offending organism.[62]

Bacteria can find its way to the joint via the bloodstream (most common) by:

- Direct inoculation (e.g., surgery, arthroscopy, intra-articular corticosteroid injection, central line placement, total joint replacement)

- Penetrating wound (e.g., human bite or fracture)
- Direct extension (e.g., osteomyelitis, cellulitis, diverticulitis, abscess)

Staphylococcus aureus, streptococci, and *gonococci* are the most common infectious causes. A connection between infection and arthritis has been established in Lyme disease. Arthritis can be the first sign of infective endocarditis.[63] Viruses, mycobacteria, fungal agents, and Lyme disease are other causes.[62]

Viral infections such as hepatitis B, rubella (after vaccination), and Fifth's (viral) disease can be accompanied by arthralgias and arthritis sometimes called *viral arthritis.* Joint symptoms appear during the prodromal state of hepatitis (prior to the clinical onset of jaundice).

Sexually transmitted (infectious) diseases (STIs/STDs) are often accompanied by joint pain and symptoms called *gonococcal arthritis.* Joint pain accompanied by skin lesions at the joint or elsewhere may be a sign of sexually transmitted infections.

In the case of STI/STDs with joint involvement, skin lesions over or near a joint have a typical appearance with a central black eschar or scab-like appearance surrounded by an area of erythema (Fig. 3-9). Alternately, the skin lesion may have a hemorrhagic base with a pustule in the center.

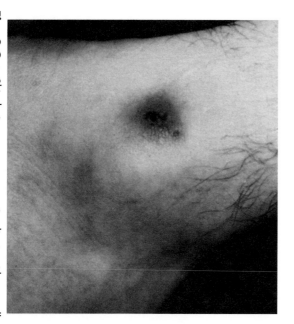

Fig. 3-9 • Skin lesions are common in clients with sexually transmitted infections. The lesion here has occurred in a man with disseminated gonococcal infection presenting as (gonococcal) arthritis in the ankle joint. The typical central black eschar area surrounded by a base of erythema is shown. The skin lesion persisted for 5 to 7 days and healed quickly with antibiotic treatment. (From Williams RC: Infection and arthritis: how are they related? *J Musculoskel Med* 10(6):38-51, 1993; Fig. 1A, p 39.)

Fever and arthritic-like symptoms are usually present (Fig. 3-10).

Anyone with HIV may develop unusual rheumatologic disorders. Diffuse body aches and pain without joint arthritis are common among clients with HIV. (See further discussion on human immunodeficiency syndrome [HIV], in Chapter 12.)

Other forms of arthritis such as systemic lupus erythematosus (SLE), scleroderma, polymyositis, and mixed connective tissue disease may have an infectious-based link but the connection has never been proven definitively.

Infectious (septic) arthritis should be suspected in an individual with persistent joint pain and inflammation occurring in the course of an illness of unclear origin or in the course of a well-documented infection such as pneumococcal pneumonia, staphylococcal sepsis, or urosepsis.

Major risk factors include age (older than 80 years), diabetes mellitus, intravenous drug use, indwelling catheters, immunocompromised condition, rheumatoid arthritis, or osteoarthritis.[62] Look for a history of preexisting joint damage due to bone trauma (e.g., fracture) or degenerative joint disease.

Other predisposing factors are listed in Box 3-6. Infectious arthritis is a rare complication of anterior cruciate ligament (ACL) reconstruction using contaminated bone-tendon-bone allografts.[64,65] Infections in prosthetic joints can occur years after the implant is inserted. Indwelling catheters and urinary tract infections are major risk factors for seeding to prosthetic joints.[55]

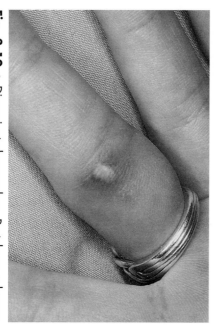

Fig. 3-10 • Disseminated gonorrhea. Pustule on a hemorrhagic base. The typical client presents with fever, arthritis, and scattered lesions as show. Cultures from the lesions are often negative. The therapist should always use standard precautions. Medical referral is required. (From Callen JP, Paller AS, Greer KE et al: *Color atlas of dermatology,* ed 2, Philadelphia, 2000, WB Saunders; Fig. 6-5, p 148.)

history of infection of any kind. Ask about a recent (last 6 weeks) skin lesions or rashes of any kind anywhere on the body, urinary tract infection, or respiratory infection.

Take the client's temperature and ask about recent episodes of fever, sweats, or other constitutional symptoms. Palpate for residual lymphadenopathy. Early diagnosis and intervention are essential to limit joint destruction and preserve function. Diagnosis can be difficult. The physician must differentiate infectious/septic arthritis from reactive arthritis (Case Example 3-5).

Clinical Signs and Symptoms of

Infectious Arthritis

- Fever (low-grade or high), chills, malaise
- Recurrent sore throat
- Lymphadenopathy
- Persistent joint pain
- Single painful swollen joint (knee, hip, ankle, elbow, shoulder)*
- Multiple joint involvement (often migratory)*
- Pain on weight bearing
- Back pain (infective endocarditis)
- Skin lesions (characteristic of the specific underlying infection)
- Conjunctivitis, uveitis
- Other musculoskeletal symptoms depending on the specific underlying infection
  - Myalgias
  - Tenosynovitis (especially wrist and ankle extensor tendon sheaths)
- Elevated C-reactive protein and sedimentation rate

* The particular joint or joints involved and associated signs and symptoms will vary from client to client and are dependent upon the underlying infectious cause. For example, joint involvement with Lyme disease presents differently from Reiter's syndrome or Hepatitis B.

REACTIVE ARTHRITIS

Reactive arthritis is sometimes used synonymously with Reiter's syndrome, a triad of non-gonococcal urethritis, conjunctivitis, and multiple joint involvement of inflammatory arthritis (oligoarthropathy). However, joint symptoms can occur 1 to 4 weeks after either a gastrointestinal (GI) or genitourinary (GU) infection.

The most common GI infections associated with reactive arthritis include *Salmonella*, *Shigella*, and *Campylobacter*, which occur in men and women equally. Reactive arthritis from sexually acquired urethritis is caused by *Chlamydia* or *Ureaplasma* and affects only men.

BOX 3-6 ▼ Risk Factors for Infectious Arthritis

- History of:
  - Previous surgery, especially arthroscopy for joint repair or replacement
  - Human bite, tick bite (Lyme's disease), fracture, central line placement
  - Direct, penetrating trauma
  - Infection of any kind (e.g., osteomyelitis, cellulitis, diverticulitis, abscess (located anywhere), hepatitis A or B, *Staphylococcus aureus*, *streptococcus pneumoniae*, gonococci, urinary tract, or respiratory tract infection)
  - Rheumatoid arthritis, systemic lupus erythematosus, scleroderma, or mixed connective tissue disease
  - Diabetes mellitus
  - Sarcoidosis (inflammatory pulmonary condition can affect knees, PIP joints, wrists, elbows)
  - Sexually active, young adult
  - Injection drug user
  - Chronic joint damage (e.g., rheumatoid arthritis, gout)
  - Previous infection of joint prosthesis
  - Recent immunization
  - Increasing age
  - Indwelling catheter (especially in the client with a prosthetic joint)
  - Malnutrition, skin breakdown
  - Immunosuppression or immunocompromise (e.g., renal failure, steroid treatment, organ transplantation, chemotherapy)

Watch for joint symptoms in the presence of skin rash, low-grade fever, and lymphadenopathy. The rash may appear and disappear before the joint symptoms. Joints may be mildly to severely involved. Fingers, knees, shoulders, and ankles are affected most often (bilaterally). Inflammation is nonerosive, suggestive of rheumatoid arthritis.

Often one joint is involved (knee or hip), but sometimes two or more are also symptomatic depending on the underlying pathologic mechanism.[50] Symptoms can range from mild to severe. Joint destruction can be rapid so immediate medical referral is required. Once treated (antibiotics, joint aspiration), the postinfectious inflammation may last for weeks.[66]

With infectious arthritis, the client may be unable to bear weight on the joint. Usually, there is an acute arthritic presentation and the client has a fever (often low-grade in older adults or in anyone who is immunosuppressed).

Medical referral is important for the client with joint pain with no known cause and a recent

CASE EXAMPLE 3-5 Septic Arthritis

A 62-year-old man presented in physical therapy with left wrist pain. There was no redness, warmth, or swelling. Active motion was mildly limited by pain. Passive motion could not be tested because of pain.

All other clinical tests were negative. Neuro screen was negative. Past medical history includes hypertension and non-insulin-dependent diabetes mellitus controlled by diet and exercise.

The client denied any history of fever, skin rashes, or other lesions. He reported a recent trip to Haiti (his native country) 3 weeks ago.

How do you screen this client for systemic-induced joint pain?

- Review Box 3-6 (Risk Factors for Infectious Arthritis). Besides diabetes, what other risk factors are present? Ask the client about any that apply. Compile a list to review during the Review of Systems.

- Ask the client: Are there any other symptoms of any kind anywhere else in your body?

- Use the client's answer while reviewing *Clinical Signs and Symptoms of Infectious Arthritis* for any signs and symptoms of infectious arthritis.

- Review Box 3-5 (Screening Questions for Joint Pain). Are there any further questions from this list appropriate for the screening process?

- Assess the joints above and below (e.g., elbow, shoulder, neck). Assess for trigger points. Using the information obtained from these steps, look at past medical history, clinical pres-

entation, and associated signs and symptoms. What are the red flags? Review the **Clues To Screening for Viscerogenic Pain Patterns** and **Guidelines for Physician Referral** in this chapter.

Based on your findings, decide whether to treat and re-evaluate or make a medical referral now.

Result: In this case the therapist did not find enough red flags or suspicious findings to warrant immediate referral. Treatment intervention was initiated. The client missed three appointments because of the "flu." When he returned, his wrist pain was completely gone, but he was reporting left knee pain. There was mild effusion and warmth on both sides of the knee joint. The client stated that he still had some occasional diarrhea from his bout with the flu.

The therapist recognized some additional red flags including ongoing gastrointestinal (GI) symptoms attributed by the client to the flu and new onset of inflammatory joint pain. The therapist decided to take the client's vital signs and found he was febrile (100° F).

Given his recent travel history, migratory noninflammatory and inflammatory arthralgias, and ongoing constitutional symptoms, the client was referred to his medical doctor. Lab tests resulted in a physician's diagnosis of joint sepsis with hematogenous seeding to the wrist and knee; possible osteomyelitis. Probable cause: Exposure to pathogens in contaminated water or soil during his stay in Haiti.

The joint is not septic (infected), but rather, aseptic (without infection). Affected joints are often at a site remote from the primary infection. Often only one joint is involved (knee, ankle, foot, distal interphalangeal joint), but two or more can be affected.

Reactive arthritis often causes inflammation along tendons or where tendons attach to the bone resulting in persistent pain from plantar fasciitis and sacroiliitis. Nail bed changes can include onycholysis (fingers or toes).

Anyone with joint pain of unknown cause who presents with a skin rash, lesions on the genitals, or recent history of infection (especially GI or GU;

usually within the last 1 to 3 weeks) must be referred to a health care clinic or medical doctor for further evaluation.

Radicular Pain

Radicular pain results from direct irritation of axons of a spinal nerve or neurons in the dorsal root ganglion and is experienced in the musculoskeletal system in a dermatome, sclerotome, or myotome.

Radicular, radiating, and referred pain are not the same things, although a client can have radicular pain that radiates. Radiating means the pain spreads or fans out from the originating point of pain.

Whereas radicular pain is caused by nerve root compression, referred pain results from activation of nociceptive free nerve endings (nociceptors) of the nervous system in somatic or visceral tissue. The physiologic basis for referred pain is convergence of afferent neurons onto common neurons within the central nervous system.

As mentioned previously, the central nervous system may not be able to distinguish which part of the body is responsible for the input into these common neurons so, for example, ischemia of the heart results in shoulder pain, one of several somatic areas innervated by the same neural segments as the heart.[67]

Differentiating between radicular (pain from the peripheral nervous system) and referred pain from the autonomic nervous system can be difficult. Both can start at one point and radiate outwards. Both can cause pain distal to the site of pathology.

Referred pain occurs most often far away from the site of pathologic origin of symptoms, whereas radicular pain does not skip myotomes, dermatomes, or sclerotomes associated with the affected peripheral nerves.

For example, cardiac pain may be described as beginning retrosternally (behind the sternum) and radiating to the left shoulder and down the inner side of the left arm. This radiating referred pain is generated via the pathways of the ANS but follows the somatic pattern of ulnar nerve distribution. It is not radicular pain from direct irritation of a spinal nerve of the peripheral nervous system but rather referred pain from shared pathways in the spinal cord.

Ischemic cardiac pain does not cause arm pain, hand pain, or pain in somatic areas other than those innervated at the C3 to T4 spinal levels of the autonomic nervous system. Similarly, gallbladder pain may be felt to originate in the right upper abdomen and to radiate to the angle of the scapula. These are the somatic areas innervated by the same level of the autonomic nervous system as the involved viscera mentioned.

Physical disease can localize pain in dermatomal or myotomal patterns. More often the therapist sees a client who describes pain that does not match a dermatomal or myotomal pattern. This is neither referred visceral pain from ANS involvement nor irritation of a spinal nerve. For example, the client who describes whole leg pain or whole leg numbness may be experiencing *inappropriate illness behavior.*

Inappropriate illness behavior is recognized clinically as illness behavior that is out of proportion to the underlying physical disease and is related more to associated psychologic disturbances than to actual physical disease.[68] This behavioral component to pain is discussed in the section on Screening For Systemic Versus Psychogenic Symptoms.

Arterial, Pleural, and Tracheal Pain

Pain arising from arteries, as with arteritis (inflammation of an artery), migraine, and vascular headaches, increases with systolic impulse so that any process associated with increased systolic pressure, such as exercise, fever, alcohol consumption, or bending over, may intensify the already throbbing pain.

Pain from the pleura, as well as from the trachea, correlates with respiratory movements. Look for associated signs and symptoms of the cardiac or pulmonary systems. Listen for a description of pain that is "throbbing" (vascular) or sharp and increased with respiratory movements such as breathing, laughing, or coughing.

Palpation and resisted movements will not reproduce the symptoms, which may get worse with recumbency, especially at night or while sleeping.

Gastrointestinal Pain

Pain arising from the gastrointestinal tract tends to increase with peristaltic activity, particularly if there is any obstruction to forward progress of the food bolus. The pain increases with ingestion and may lessen with fasting or after emptying the involved segment (vomiting or bowel movement).

On the other hand, pain may occur secondary to the effect of gastric acid on the esophagus, stomach, or duodenum. This pain is relieved by the presence of food or by other neutralizing material in the stomach, and the pain is intensified when the stomach is empty and secreting acid. In these cases it is important to ask the client about the effect of eating on musculoskeletal pain. Does the pain increase, decrease, or stay the same immediately after eating and 1 to 3 hours later?

When hollow viscera, such as the liver, kidneys, spleen, and pancreas, are distended, body positions or movements that increase intraabdominal pressure may intensify the pain, whereas positions that reduce pressure or support the structure may ease the pain.

For example, the client with an acutely distended gallbladder may slightly flex the trunk. With pain arising from a tense, swollen kidney (or distended renal pelvis), the client flexes the trunk and tilts toward the involved side; with pancreatic

pain, the client may sit up and lean forward or lie down with the knees drawn up to the chest.

Pain at Rest

Pain at rest may arise from ischemia in a wide variety of tissue (e.g., vascular disease or tumor growth). The acute onset of severe unilateral extremity involvement accompanied by the "five Ps"—pain, pallor, pulselessness, paresthesia, and paralysis—signifies acute arterial occlusion (peripheral vascular disease [PVD]). Pain in this situation is usually described by the client as burning or shooting and may be accompanied by paresthesia.

Pain related to ischemia of the skin and subcutaneous tissues is characterized by the client as burning and boring. All these occlusive causes of pain are usually worse at night and are relieved to some degree by dangling the affected leg over the side of the bed and by frequent massaging of the extremity.

Pain at rest secondary to neoplasm occurs usually at night. Although neoplasms are highly vascularized (a process called angiogenesis), the host organ's vascular supply and nutrients may be compromised simultaneously, causing ischemia of the local tissue. The pain awakens the client from sleep and prevents the person from going back to sleep, despite all efforts to do so. See the next section on Night Pain.

The client may describe pain noted on weight-bearing or bone pain that may be mild and intermittent in the initial stages, becoming progressively more severe and more constant. A series of questions to identify the underlying cause of night pain is presented later in this chapter.

Night Pain

Whenever you take a pain history, an evaluation of night pain is important (Box 3-7). As therapists, we are always gauging pain responses to identify where the client might be on the continuum from acute to subacute to chronic. This information helps guide our treatment plan and intervention.

For example, the client who cannot even lie on the involved side is probably fairly acute. Pain modulation is the first order of business. Modalities and cryotherapy may be most effective here. On the other hand, the client who can roll onto the involved side and stay there for 30 minutes to an hour may be more in the subacute phase. A combination of modalities, hands-on treatment, and exercise may be warranted.

The client who can lie on the involved side for up to two hours is more likely in the chronic phase

---

When screening someone with night pain for the possibility of a systemic or cancerous condition, some possible questions are:

- Tell me about the pattern of your symptoms at night (open-ended question).
- Can you lie on that side? For how long?
- (Alternate question): Does it wake you up when you roll onto that side?
- How are you feeling in general when you wake up?
- Follow-up question: Do you have any other symptoms when the pain wakes you up? Give the client time to answer before prompting with choices such as coughing, wheezing, shortness of breath, nausea, need to go to the bathroom, night sweats.

   Always ask the client reporting night pain of any kind (not just bone pain) the following screening questions:

- What makes it better/worse?
- What happens to your pain when you sit up? [Upright posture reduces venous return to the heart; decreased pain when sitting up may indicate a cardiopulmonary cause].

   How does taking aspirin affect your pain/symptoms? (Disproportionate pain relief can occur using aspirin in the presence of bone cancer.)

- How does eating or drinking affect your pain/symptoms (for shoulder, neck, back, hip, pelvic pain/symptoms; GI system)?
- Does taking an antacid such as Tums change your pain/symptoms? (Some women with pain of a cardiac nature experience pain relief much like men do with nitroglycerin; remember this would be a woman who is postmenopausal, possibly with a personal and/or family history of heart disease—check vital signs!)

---

of the musculoskeletal condition. Tissue ischemia brings on painful symptoms after prolonged static positioning. A more aggressive approach can usually be taken in these cases. These comments all apply to pain of a neuromusculoskeletal (NMS) origin.

Night Pain and Cancer

Pain at night is a classic red flag symptom of cancer, but it does not mean that all pain at night is caused by cancer. For example, the person who lies down at night and has not even fallen asleep who reports increased pain may just be experiencing the first moment in the day without

distractions. Suddenly, his or her focus is on nothing but the pain, so the client may report the pain is much worse at night.

Bone pain at night is the most highly suspicious symptom, especially in the presence of a previous history of cancer. Neoplasms are highly vascularized at the expense of the host. This produces local ischemia and pain.

In the case of bone pain (deep pain; pain on weight bearing), perform a heel strike test. This is done by applying a percussive vertical force with the heel of your hand through the heel of the client's foot in a non-weightbearing (supine) position. Reproduction of painful symptoms is positive and highly suspicious of a bone fracture or stress reaction.[69]

Keep in mind for the older adult that pain on weight bearing may be a symptom of a hip fracture. It is not uncommon for an older adult to fall, have hip pain, and the X-rays are initially negative. If the pain persists, new X-rays or additional imaging may be needed. MRIs are extremely sensitive for a femoral neck fracture very early after the fracture. MRI may miss a pubic rami fracture, requiring Single Photon Emission Computerized Tomography (SPECT) bone scan to rule out an occult fracture in a client who has fallen and is still having hip pain.

In a physically capable client, clear the hip, knee, and ankle by asking the client to assume a full squat position. You may also ask him or her to hop on the involved side. These tests are used to screen for pubic ramus or hip stress fractures (reactions). Stress reactions or stress fractures are discussed in Chapter 16.

Pain with Activity

Pain with activity is common with neuromusculoskeletal pathology. Mechanical and postural factors are common. Pain with activity from a systemic or disease process is most often caused by vascular compromise. In this context activity pain of the upper quadrant is known as angina when the heart muscle is compromised and intermittent vascular claudication in the case of peripheral vascular compromise (lower quadrant).

Pain from an ischemic muscle (including heart muscle) builds up with the use of the muscle and subsides with rest. Thus there is a direct relationship between the degree of circulatory insufficiency and muscle work.

In other words, the interval between the beginning of muscle contraction and the onset of pain depends on how long it takes for hypoxic products of muscle metabolism to accumulate and exceed the threshold of receptor response. This means with vascular-induced pain there is usually a delay or lag time between the beginning of activity and the onset of symptoms.

The client complains that a certain distance walked, a certain level of increased physical activity, or a fixed amount of usage of the extremity brings on the pain. When a vascular pathologic condition causes ischemic muscular pain, the location of the pain depends on the location of the vascular pathologic source. This is discussed in greater detail later in this text (see the section on Arterial Disease in Chapter 6).

The timing of symptom onset offers the therapist valuable screening clues when determining when symptoms are caused by musculoskeletal impairment or by vascular compromise.

Look for immediate pain or symptoms (especially when these can be reproduced with palpation, resistance to movement, and/or a change in position) versus symptoms 5 to 10 minutes after activity begins. Further investigate for the presence of other signs and symptoms associated with cardiac impairment, appropriate risk factors, and positive personal and/or family history.

Diffuse Pain

Diffuse pain that characterizes some diseases of the nervous system and viscera may be difficult to distinguish from the equally diffuse pain so often caused by lesions of the moving parts.

Most clients in this category are those with obscure pain in the trunk, especially when the symptoms are felt only anteriorly.[70] The distinction between visceral pain and pain caused by lesions of the vertebral column may be difficult to make and will require a medical diagnosis.

Chronic Pain

Chronic pain persists past the expected physiologic time of healing. This may be less than 1 month or, more often, longer than 6 months. An underlying pathology is no longer identifiable and may never have been present.[71] The International Association for the Study of Pain has fixed 3 months as the most convenient point of division between acute and chronic pain.[72]

There are some who suggest 6 weeks is a better cut-off point in terms of clinical progress. Any longer than that and the client is at increased risk for chronic pain and behavioral consequences of that pain.[73,74]

Chronic pain syndrome is characterized by a constellation of life changes that produce altered

behavior in the individual and persist even after the cause of the pain has been eradicated. This syndrome is a complex multidimensional phenomenon that requires a focus toward maximizing functional abilities rather than treatment of pain.

With chronic pain, the approach is to assess how the pain has affected the person. Physical therapy intervention can be directed toward decreasing the client's emotional response to pain or developing skills to cope with stress and other changes that impair quality of life.

In acute pain the pain is proportional and appropriate to the problem and is treated as a symptom. In the chronic pain syndrome uncontrolled and prolonged pain alters both the peripheral and central nervous systems through processes of neural plasticity and central sensitization and thus pain becomes a disease itself.[75]

Each person may have a unique response to pain called a neuromatrix or neurosignature. The neuromatrix is initially determined through genetics and early sensory development. Later, life experiences related to pain and coping shape the neural patterns. Each person develops individual perceptual and behavioral responses to pain that are unique to that person.[76]

The person's description of chronic pain often is not well defined and is poorly localized; objective findings are not identified. The person's verbal description of the pain may contain words associated with emotional overlay (see Table 3-1). This is in contrast to the predominance of sensory descriptors associated with acute pain.[71] It may be helpful to ask the client or caregiver to maintain a pain log (see Figs. 3-7 and 3-8).

This should include entries for pain intensity and its relationship to activities or intervention. Clients can be reevaluated regularly for improvement, deterioration, or complications, using the same scales that were used for the initial evaluation.

Always keep in mind that painful symptoms out of proportion to the injury or that are not consistent with the objective findings may be a red flag indicating systemic disease. Pain can be triggered by bodily malfunction or severe illness.

In some cases of chronic pain, a diagnosis is finally made (e.g., spinal stenosis or thyroiditis) and the intervention is specific, not merely pain management. More often, identifying the cause of chronic pain is unsuccessful.

Research evidence has implicated psychologic factors as a key factor in chronic pain. Cognitive processes such as thoughts, beliefs, and expectations are important in understanding chronic pain, adaptation to chronic pain, response to intervention, and disability.[77]

The therapist should be aware that chronic pain can be associated with physical and/or sexual abuse in both men and women. (See discussion of Assault in Chapter 2.) The abuse may be part of the childhood history and/or a continuing part of the adult experience.

Fear-Avoidance Behavior

Fear-avoidance behavior can also be a part of disability from chronic pain. The Fear-Avoidance Model of Exaggerated Pain Perception (FAMEPP) was first introduced in the early 1980s.[78;79] The concept is based on studies that show a person's fear of pain (not physical impairments) is the most important factor in how he or she responds to low back pain.

Fear of pain commonly leads to avoiding physical or social activities. Screening for fear-avoidance behavior can be done using the Fear Avoidance Beliefs Questionnaire (Table 3-7).[80] Elevated fear-avoidance beliefs are not indicative of a red flag for serious medical pathology. They are indicative of someone who has a poorer prognosis for rehabilitation. They are more accurately labeled a "yellow flag" indicating psychosocial involvement and provide insight into the prognosis. Such a yellow flag signals the need to modify intervention[81] and consider the need for referral to a psychologist or behavioral counselor.

When the client shows signs of fear-avoidance beliefs, then the therapist's management approach should include education that addresses the client's fear and avoidance behavior, and should consider a graded approach to therapeutic exercise.[82]

The therapist can teach clients about the difference between pain and tissue injury. Chronic ongoing pain does not mean continued tissue injury is taking place. This common misconception can result in movement avoidance behaviors.

There are no known "cut-off" scores for referral to a specialist.[81;82] Some researchers categorize FABQ scores into "high" and "low" based on the physical activity scale (score range 0-24). Less than 15 is a "low" score (low risk for elevated fear-avoidance beliefs) and more than 15 is "high."

Higher numbers indicate increased levels of fear-avoidance beliefs. The distinction between these two categories is minor and arbitrary. It may be best to consider the scores as a continuum rather than dividing them into low or high.[81;82] A cut-off score for the work scale indicative of having a decreased chance of returning to work has been

TABLE 3-7 ▼ Fear-Avoidance Beliefs Questionnaire (FABQ)

Here are some of the things other patients have told us about their pain. For each statement please circle any number from 0 to 6 to say how much physical activities such as bending, walking, or driving affect or would affect your back pain.

	Completely disagree		Unsure		Completely agree	
1. My pain was caused by physical activity	0	1	2	3	4	5	6
2. Physical activity makes my pain worse	0	1	2	3	4	5	6
3. Physical activity might harm my back	0	1	2	3	4	5	6
4. I should not do physical activities which (might) make my pain worse	0	1	2	3	4	5	6
5. I cannot do physical activities which (might) make my pain worse	0	1	2	3	4	5	6

The following statements are about how your normal work affects or would affect your back pain.

	Completely disagree		Unsure		Completely agree	
6. My pain was caused by my work or by an accident at work	0	1	2	3	4	5	6
7. My work aggravated my pain	0	1	2	3	4	5	6
8. I have a claim for compensation for my pain	0	1	2	3	4	5	6
9. My work is too heavy for me	0	1	2	3	4	5	6
10. My work makes or would make my pain worse	0	1	2	3	4	5	6
11. My work might harm my back	0	1	2	3	4	5	6
12. I should not do my normal work with my present pain	0	1	2	3	4	5	6
13. I cannot do my normal work with my present pain	0	1	2	3	4	5	6
14. I cannot do my normal work until my pain is treated	0	1	2	3	4	5	6
15. I do not think I will be back to my normal work	0	1	2	3	4	5	6
16. I do not think that I will ever be able to go back to that work	0	1	2	3	4	5	6

The Fear-Avoidance Beliefs Questionnaire (FABQ) is used to quantify the level of fear of pain and beliefs clients with low back pain have about the need to avoid movements or activities that might cause pain. The FABQ has 16 items, each scored from 0 to 6, with higher numbers indicating increased levels of fear avoidance beliefs. There are 2 subscales: a 7-item work subscale (Sum of items 6, 7, 9, 10, 11, 12, and 15; score range = 0-42) and a 4-item physical activity subscale (Sum of items 2, 3, 4, and 5; score range = 0-24). The FABQ work subscale is associated with current and future disability and work loss in patients with acute and chronic LBP.
From Waddell G, Somerville D, Henderson I, et al: Fear-avoidance beliefs questionnaire (FABQ) and the role of fear avoidance beliefs in chronic low back pain and disability, *Pain* 52:157-158, 1993.

proposed. The work subscale of the Fear-Avoidance Beliefs Questionnaire is the strongest predictor of work status. There is a greater likelihood of return-to-work for scores less than 30 and less likelihood of return-to-work or increased risk of prolonged work restrictions for scores greater than 34.[83]

Examination of fear-avoidance beliefs may serve as a useful screening tool for identifying clients who are at risk for prolonged work restrictions. Caution is advised when interpreting and applying the results of the FABQ work subscale to individual clients. This screening tool may be a better predictor of low risk for prolonged work restrictions. The work subscale may be less effective in identifying clients at high risk for prolonged work restrictions.[83]

Differentiating Chronic Pain from Systemic Disease

Sometimes a chronic pain syndrome can be differentiated from a systemic disease by the nature and description of the pain. Chronic pain is usually dull and persistent. The chronic pain syndrome is characterized by multiple complaints, excessive preoccupation with pain, and, frequently, excessive drug use. With chronic pain, there is usually a history of some precipitating injury or event.

Systemic disease is more acute with a recent onset. It is often described as sharp, colicky, knife-like, and/or deep. Look for concomitant constitutional symptoms, any red flags in the personal or family history, and/or any known risk factors. Ask about the presence of associated signs and symp-

toms characteristic of a particular organ or body system (e.g., GI, GU, respiratory, gynecologic).

Because pain has an affective component, chronic pain can cause anxiety, depression, and anger. The amount of pain perceived can change with alterations in environmental reinforcers (e.g., increasing as the time to return to work draws near, decreasing when no one is watching). For more information and assessment tools, see the discussions related to anxiety and depression in this chapter.

Secondary gain may be a factor in perpetuating the problem. This may be primarily financial, but social and family benefits, such as increased attention or avoidance of unpleasant activities or work situations, may be factors (see later discussion of behavior responses to injury/illness).

Aging and Chronic Pain

Chronic pain in older adults is very common. One in five older Americans is taking analgesic medications regularly. Many take prescription pain medications for more than 6 months.[84]

Older adults are more likely to suffer from arthritis, bone and joint disorders, back problems, and other chronic conditions. Pain is the single most common problem for which aging adults seek medical care.

At the same time older adults have been observed to present with unusually painless manifestations of common illnesses such as myocardial infarction, acute abdomen, and infections.[85-87]

To address the special needs of older adults, the American Geriatrics Society (AGS) has developed specific recommendations for assessment and management of chronic pain (Box 3-8).[88]

COMPARISON OF SYSTEMIC VERSUS MUSCULOSKELETAL PAIN PATTERNS

Table 3-2 provides a comparison of the clinical signs and symptoms of systemic pain versus musculoskeletal pain using the typical categories described earlier. The therapist must be very familiar with the information contained within this table. Even with these guidelines to follow, the therapist's job is a challenging one.

In the orthopedic setting, physical therapists are very aware that pain can be referred above and below a joint. So, for example, when examining a shoulder problem, the therapist always considers the neck and elbow as potential NMS sources of shoulder pain and dysfunction.

Table 3-8 reflects what is known about referred pain patterns for the musculoskeletal system. Sites for referred pain from a visceral pain mechanism are listed. Lower cervical and upper thoracic impairment can refer pain to the interscapular and posterior shoulder areas.

BOX 3-8 ▲ AGS Recommendations for Chronic Pain Assessment in the Geriatric Population

- All older clients should be assessed for signs of chronic pain.
- Use alternate words for pain when screening older clients (e.g., burning, discomfort, aching, sore, heavy, tight).
- Contact caregiver for pain assessment in adults with cognitive or language impairments
- Clients with cognitive or language impairments should be observed for nonverbal pain behaviors, recent changes in function, and vocalizations to suggest pain (e.g., irritability, agitation, withdrawal, gait changes, tone changes, nonverbal but vocal utterances such as groaning, crying, or moaning)
- Follow AGS guidelines for comprehensive pain assessment including

  Medical history

  Medication history including current and previously used prescription and over-the-counter drugs as well as any nutraceuticals (natural products, "remedies")

  Physical examination

  Review pertinent laboratory results and diagnostic tests (look for clues to the sequence of events leading to present pain complaint)

  Assess characteristics of pain (frequency, intensity, duration, pattern, description, aggravating and relieving factors); use a standard pain scale such as the visual analogue scale (see Fig. 3-6)
- Observe neuromuscular system for:

  Neurologic impairments

  Weakness

  Hyperalgesia; hyperpathia (exaggerated response to pain stimulus)

  Allodynia (skin pain to non-noxious stimulus)

  Numbness, paresthesia

  Tenderness, trigger points

  Inflammation

  Deformity
- Pain that affects function or quality of life should be included in the medical problem list

Data from American Geriatrics Society (AGS) Panel on Chronic Pain in Older Persons. Clinical practice guidelines, *JAGS* 46:635-651, 1998.

TABLE 3-8 ▼ Common Patterns of Pain Referral

Pain mechanism	Lesion site	Referral site
Somatic	C7, T1-5 vertebrae	Interscapular area, posterior shoulder
	Shoulder	Neck, upper back
	L1, L2 vertebrae	Sacroiliac joint and hip
	Hip joint	SI and knee
	Pharynx	Ipsilateral ear
	TMJ	Head, neck, heart
Visceral	Diaphragmatic irritation	Shoulder, lumbar spine
	Heart	Shoulder, neck, upper back, TMJ
	Urothelial tract	Back, inguinal region, anterior thigh, and genitalia
	Pancreas, Liver, Spleen, Gallbladder	Shoulder, midthoracic or low back
	Peritoneal or abdominal cavity (inflammatory or infectious process)	Hip pain from abscess of psoas or obturator muscle
Neuropathic	Nerve or plexus	Anywhere in distribution of a peripheral nerve
	Nerve root	Anywhere in corresponding dermatome
	Central nervous system	Anywhere in region of body innervated by damaged structure

Likewise, shoulder impairment can refer pain to the neck and upper back, while any condition affecting the upper lumbar spine can refer pain and symptoms to the sacroiliac (SI) joint and hip. When examining the hip region, the therapist always considers the possibility of an underlying SI or knee joint impairment and so on.

If the client presents with the typical or primary referred pain pattern, he or she will likely end up in a physician's office. A secondary or referred pain pattern can be very deceiving. The therapist may not be able to identify the underlying pathology (in fact, it is not required), but it is imperative to recognize when the clinical presentation does not fit the expected pattern for NMS impairment.

A few additional comments about systemic versus musculoskeletal pain patterns are important. First, it is unlikely that the client with back, hip, SI, or shoulder pain that has been present for the last 5 to 10 years is demonstrating a viscerogenic cause of symptoms. In such a case, systemic origins are suspected only if there is a sudden or recent change in the clinical presentation and/or the client develops constitutional symptoms or signs and symptoms commonly associated with an organ system.

Secondly, note the word descriptors used with pain of a systemic nature: knifelike, boring, deep, throbbing. Pay attention any time someone uses these particular words to describe the symptoms. Third, observe the client's reaction to the information you provide. Often, someone with a NMS

problem gains immediate and intense pain relief just from the examination provided and evaluation offered. The reason? A reduction in the anxiety level.

Many people have a need for high control. Pain throws us in a state of fear and anxiety and a perceived loss of control. Knowing what the problem is and having a plan of action can reduce the amplification of symptoms for someone with soft tissue involvement when there is an underlying psychologic component such as anxiety.

On the other hand, someone with cancer pain, viscerogenic origin of symptoms or systemic illness of some kind will not obtain relief from or reduction of pain with reassurance. Signs and symptoms of anxiety are presented later in this chapter.

Fourth, aggravating and relieving factors associated with NMS impairment often have to do with change in position or a change (increased or decreased) in activity levels. There is usually some way the therapist can alter, provoke, alleviate, eliminate, or aggravate symptoms of a NMS origin.

Pain with activity is immediate when there is involvement of the NMS system. There may be a delayed increase in symptoms after the initiation of activity with a systemic (vascular) cause.

For the orthopedic or manual therapist, be aware that an upslip of the innominate that does not reduce may be a visceral-somatic reflex. It could be a visceral ligamentous problem. If the

problem can be corrected with muscle energy techniques or other manual therapy intervention, but by the end of the treatment session or by the next day, the correction is gone and the upslip is back, then look for a possible visceral source as the cause.[2]

If you can reduce the upslip, but it does not hold during the treatment session, then look for the source of the problem at a lower level. It can even be a crossover pattern from the pelvis on the other side.[2]

Aggravating and relieving factors associated with systemic pain are organ dependent and based on visceral function. For example, chest pain, neck pain or upper back pain from a problem with the esophagus will likely get worse when the client is swallowing or eating.

Back, shoulder, pelvic, or sacral pain that is made better or worse by eating, passing gas, or having a bowel movement is a red flag. Painful symptoms that start 3 to 5 minutes after initiating an activity and go away when the client stops the activity suggest pain of a vascular nature. This is especially true when the client uses the word "throbbing," which is a descriptor of a vascular origin.

Clients presenting with vascular-induced musculoskeletal complaints are not likely to come to the therapist with a report of cardiac-related chest pain. Rather, the therapist must be alert for the man over age 50 or postmenopausal woman with a significant family history of heart disease, who is borderline hypertensive. New onset or reproduction of back, neck, TMJ, shoulder, or arm pain brought on by exertion with arms raised overhead or by starting a new exercise program is a red flag.

Leaning forward or assuming a hands and knees position sometimes lessens gallbladder pain. This position moves the distended or inflamed gallbladder out away from its position under the liver. Leaning or side bending toward the painful side sometimes ameliorates kidney pain. Again, for some people, this may move the kidney enough to take the pressure off during early onset of an infectious or inflammatory process.

Finally, notice the long list of potential signs and symptoms associated with systemic conditions (see Table 3-2; see Box 4-18). At the same time, note the *lack* of associated signs and symptoms listed on the musculoskeletal side of the table. Except for the possibility of some autonomic nervous system responses with the stimulation of trigger points, there are no comparable constitutional or systemic signs and symptoms associated with the NMS system.

CHARACTERISTICS OF VISCEROGENIC PAIN

There are some characteristics of viscerogenic pain that can occur regardless of which organ system is involved. Any of these by itself is cause for suspicion and careful listening and watching. They often occur together in clusters of two or three. Watch for any of the following components of the pain pattern.

Gradual, Progressive, and Cyclical Pain Patterns

Gradual, progressive, and cyclical pain patterns are characteristic of viscerogenic disease. The one time this pain pattern occurs in an orthopedic situation is with the client who has low back pain of a discogenic origin. The client is given the appropriate intervention and begins to do his/her exercise program. The symptoms improve and the client completes a full weekend of gardening, 18 holes of golf, or other excessive activity.

The activity aggravates the condition and the symptoms return worse than before. The client returns to the clinic, gets firm reminders by the therapist regarding guidelines for physical activity, and is sent out once again with the appropriate exercise program. The "cooperate—get better—then overdo" cycle may recur until the client completes the rehabilitation process and obtains relief from symptoms and return of function.

This pattern can mimic the gradual, progressive, and cyclical pain pattern normally associated with underlying organic pathology. The difference between a NMS pattern of pain and symptoms and a visceral pattern is the NMS problem gradually improves over time whereas the systemic condition gets worse.

Of course, beware of the client with discogenic back and leg pain who suddenly returns to the clinic completely symptom free. There is always the risk of disc herniation and sequestration when the nucleus detaches and becomes a loose body that may enter the spinal canal. In the case of a "miraculous cure" from disc herniation, be sure to ask about the onset of any new symptoms, especially changes in bowel and bladder function.

Constant Pain

Pain that is constant and intense should raise a red flag. There is a logical and important first question to ask anyone who says the pain is "constant." Can you think what this question might be?

Follow-Up Questions

• Do you have that pain right now?

It is surprising how often the client will answer 'No' to this question. While it is true that pain of a NMS origin can be constant, it is also true there is usually some way to modulate it up or down. The client often has one or two positions that make it better (or worse).

Constant, intense pain in a client with a previous personal history of cancer and/or in the presence of other associated signs and symptoms raises a red flag. You may want to use the McGill Home Recording Card to assess the presence of true constant pain (see Fig. 3-7).

It is not necessary to have the client complete an entire week's pain log to assess constant pain. A 24- to 48-hour time period is sufficient. Use the recording scale on the right indicating pain intensity and medications taken (prescription and over-the-counter).

Under item number 3, include sexual activity. The particulars are not necessary, just some indication that the client was sexually active. The client defines "sexually active" for him or herself, whether this just touching and holding or complete coitus. This is another useful indicator of pain levels and functional activity.

Remember to offer clients a clear explanation for any questions asked concerning sexual activity, sexual function, or sexual history. There is no way to know when someone will be offended or claim sexual harassment. It is in your own interest to behave in the most professional manner possible.

There should be no hint of sexual innuendo or humor injected into any of your conversations with clients at any time. The line of sexual impropriety lies where the complainant draws it and includes appearances of misbehavior. This perception differs broadly from client to client.[2]

Finally, the number of hours slept is helpful information. Someone who reports sleepless nights may not actually be awake, but rather, may be experiencing a sleep disturbance. Cancer pain wakes the client up from a sound sleep. An actual record of being awake and up for hours at night or awakened repeatedly is significant (Case example 3-6). See the discussion on Night Pain earlier in this chapter.

Physical Therapy Intervention "Fails"

If a client does not get better with physical therapy intervention, do not immediately doubt yourself.

The lack of progression in treatment could very well be a red flag symptom. If the client reports improvement in the early intervention phase, but later takes a turn for the worse, it may be a red flag. Take the time to step back, reevaluate the client and your intervention, and screen if you have not already done so (or screen again if you have).

If painful, tender, or sore points (e.g., Trigger points, Jones' points, acupuncture/acupressure points/Shiatsu) are eliminated with intervention then return quickly (by the end of the individual session), suspect visceral pathology. If a tender point comes back later (several days or weeks), you may not be holding it long enough.[2]

Bone Pain and Aspirin

There is one odd clinical situation you should be familiar with; not because you are likely to see it, but because the physicians may use this scenario to test your screening knowledge. Before the advent of non-aspirin pain relievers, a major red flag was always the disproportionate relief of bone pain from cancer with a simple aspirin.

The client who reported such a phenomenon was suspected of having osteoid osteoma and a medical work-up would be ordered. The mechanism behind this is explained by the fact that salicylates in the aspirin inhibit the pain-inducing prostaglandins produced by the bone tumor.

When conversing with a physician, it is not necessary for the therapist to identify the specific underlying pathology as a bone tumor. Such a conclusion is outside the scope of a physical therapist's practice.

However, recognizing a sign of something that does not fit the expected mechanical or NMS pattern *is* within the scope of our practice and that is what the therapist can emphasize when communicating with medical doctors. Understanding this concept and being able to explain it in medical terms can enhance communication with the physician.

Pain Does Not Fit the Expected Pattern

In a primary care practice or under direct access, the therapist may see a client reporting back, hip, or sacroiliac pain of systemic or visceral origin early on in its development. In these cases, during early screening, the client often presents with full and pain free range of motion. Only after pain has been present long enough to cause splinting and guarding, does the client exhibit biomechanical changes (Box 3-9).

CASE EXAMPLE 3-6 Constant Night Pain

A 33-year-old man with left shoulder pain reports "constant pain at night." After asking all the appropriate screening questions related to night pain and constant pain, you see the following pattern:

Shoulder pain that is made worse by lying down whether it is at night or during the day. There are no increased pulmonary or breathing problems at night when lying down. Pain is described as a "deep aching." The client cannot find a comfortable position and moves from bed to couch to chair to bed all night long.

He injured his arm 6 months ago in a basketball game when he fell and landed on that shoulder. Symptoms have been gradually getting worse and nothing he does makes it go away. He reports a small amount of relief if he puts a rolled towel under his armpit.

He is not taking any medication, has no significant personal or family history for cancer, kidney, heart, or stomach disease and has no other symptoms of any kind.

Do you need to screen any further for systemic origin of symptoms? Probably not, even though there are what look like red flags:

Constant pain
Deep aching
Symptoms beyond the expected time for physiologic healing
No position is comfortable

Once you complete the objective tests and measures, you will have a better idea if further questions are needed. Although his pain is "constant" and occurs at night, it looks like it may be positional.

An injury 6 months ago with continued symptoms falls into the category of "symptoms persist beyond the expected time for physiologic healing." His description of not being able to find a position of comfort is a possible example of "no position is comfortable."

Given the mechanism of injury and position of mild improvement (towel roll under the arm), it may be more likely that a soft tissue tear is present and physiologic healing has not been possible.

Referral to a physician (or returning the client to the referring physician) may not be necessary just yet. Some clients do not want surgery and opt for a rehabilitation approach. Make sure you have all the information from the primary care physician if there is one involved. Your rehabilitation protocol will depend on a specific diagnosis (e.g., torn rotator cuff, labral tear, impingement syndrome).

If the client does not respond to physical therapy intervention, reevaluation (possibly including a screening component) is warranted with physician referral considered at that time.

BOX 3-9 ▼ Range of Motion Changes with Systemic Disease

- **Early screening:** Full and pain free ROM
- **Late screening:** Biomechanical response to pain results in changes associated with splinting and guarding

---

▶

SCREENING FOR EMOTIONAL AND PSYCHOLOGIC OVERLAY

Pain, emotions, and pain behavior are all integral parts of the pain experience. There is no disease, illness, or state of pain without an accompanying psychologic component.[2] This does not mean the client's pain is not real or does not exist on a physical level. In fact, clients with behavioral changes

may also have significant underlying injury.[89] Physical pain and emotional changes are two sides of the same coin.[90]

Pain is not just a physical sensation that passes up to consciousness and then produces secondary emotional effects. Rather, the neurophysiology of pain and emotions are closely linked throughout the higher levels of the CNS. Sensory and emotional changes occur simultaneously and influence each other.[73]

The sensory discriminative component of pain is primarily physiologic in nature and occurs as a result of nociceptive stimulation in the presence of organic pathology. The motivational-affective dimension of pain is psychologic in nature subject to the underlying principles of emotional behavior.[78]

The therapist's practice often includes clients with personality disorders, malingering, or other

psychophysiologic disorder. Psychophysiologic disorders (also known as *psychosomatic* disorders) are any conditions in which the physical symptoms may be caused or made worse by psychologic factors.

Recognizing somatic signs of any psychophysiologic disorder is part of the screening process. Behavioral, psychologic, or medical treatment may be indicated. Psychophysiologic disorders are generally characterized by subjective complaints that exceed objective findings, symptom development in the presence of psychosocial stresses, and physical symptoms involving one or more organ systems. It is the last variable that can confuse the therapist when trying to screen for medical disease.

It is impossible to discuss the broad range of psychophysiologic disorders that comprise a large portion of the physical therapy caseload in a screening text of this kind. The therapist is strongly encouraged to become familiar with the *Diagnostic and Statistical Manual-IV*[42] to understand the psychologic factors affecting the successful outcome of rehabilitation.

However, recognizing clusters of signs and symptoms characteristic of the psychologic component of illness is very important in the screening process. Likewise, the therapist will want to become familiar with nonorganic signs indicative of psychologic factors.[91-93]

Three key psychologic components have important significance in the pain response of many people:

- Anxiety
- Depression
- Panic Disorder

Anxiety, Depression, and Panic Disorder

Psychologic factors such as emotional stress and conflicts leading to anxiety, depression, and panic disorder play an important role in the client's experience of physical symptoms. In the past, physical symptoms caused or exacerbated by psychologic variables were labeled psychosomatic.

Today the interconnections between the mind, the immune system, the hormonal system, the nervous system, and the physical body have led us to view psychosomatic disorders as psychophysiologic disorders.

There is considerable overlap, shared symptoms, and interaction between these emotions. They are all part of the normal human response to pain and stress[73] and occur often in clients with serious or chronic health conditions. Intervention is not always needed. However, strong emotions experienced over a long period of time can become harmful if excessive.

Depression and anxiety often present with somatic symptoms that may resolve with effective treatment of these disorders. Diagnosis of these conditions is made by a medical doctor or trained mental health professional. The therapist can describe the symptoms and relay that information to the appropriate agency or individual when making a referral.

Anxiety

Anyone who feels excessive anxiety may have a generalized anxiety disorder with excessive and unrealistic worry about day-to-day issues that can last months and even longer.

Anxiety amplifies physical symptoms. It is like the amplifier ("amp") on a sound system. It does not change the sound; it just increases the power to make it louder. The tendency to amplify a broad range of bodily sensations may be an important factor in experiencing, reporting, and functioning with an acute and relatively mild medical illness.[94]

Keep in mind the known effect of anxiety on the *intensity* of pain of a musculoskeletal versus systemic origin. Defining the problem, offering reassurance, and outlining a plan of action with expected outcomes can reduce painful symptoms amplified by anxiety. It does not ameliorate pain of a systemic nature.[95]

Musculoskeletal complaints such as sore muscles, back pain, headache, or fatigue can result from anxiety-caused tension or heightened sensitivity to pain. Anxiety increases muscle tension, thereby reducing blood flow and oxygen to the tissues, resulting in a buildup of cellular metabolites.

Somatic symptoms are diagnostic for several anxiety disorders, including panic disorder, agoraphobia (fear of open places, especially fear of being alone or of being in public places) and other phobias (irrational fears), obsessive-compulsive disorder (OCD), post-traumatic stress disorder (PTSD), and generalized anxiety disorders.

Anxious persons have a reduced ability to tolerate painful stimulation, noticing it more or interpreting it as more significant than do nonanxious persons. This leads to further complaining about pain and to more disability and pain behavior such as limping, grimacing, or medication seeking.

To complicate matters more, persons with an organic illness sometimes develop anxiety known as *adjustment disorder with anxious mood*. Additionally, the advent of a known organic condition, such as a pulmonary embolus or chronic obstruc-

tive pulmonary disease (COPD), can cause an agoraphobia-like syndrome in older persons, especially if the client views the condition as unpredictable, variable, and disabling.

According to C. Everett Koop, the former U.S. Surgeon General, 80% to 90% of all people seen in a family practice clinic are suffering from illnesses caused by anxiety and stress. Emotional problems amplify physical symptoms such as ulcerative colitis, peptic ulcers, or allergies. Although allergies may be inherited, anxiety amplifies or exaggerates the symptoms. Symptoms may appear as physical, behavioral, cognitive, or psychologic (Table 3-9).

The Beck Anxiety Inventory (BAI) quickly assesses the presence and severity of client anxiety in adolescents and adults ages 17 and older. It was designed to reduce the overlap between depression and anxiety scales by measuring anxiety symptoms shared minimally with those of depression.

The BAI consists of 21 items, each scored on a four-point scale between 0 and 3, for a total score ranging from 0 to 63. Higher scores indicate higher levels of anxiety. The BAI is reported to have good reliability for clients with various psychiatric diagnoses.[96,97]

Both physiological and cognitive components of anxiety are addressed in the 21 items describing subjective, somatic, or panic-related symptoms. The BAI differentiates between anxious and nonanxious groups in a variety of clinical settings and is appropriate for all adult mental health populations.

Depression

Once defined as a deep and unrelenting sadness lasting 2 weeks or more, depression is no longer viewed in such simplistic terms. As an understanding of this condition has evolved, scientists have come to speak of *the depressive illnesses*. This term gives a better idea of the breadth of the disorder, encompassing several conditions including depression, dysthymia, bipolar disorder, and seasonal affective disorders (SAD).

Although these conditions can differ from individual to individual, each includes some of the symptoms listed. Often the classic signs of depression are not as easy to recognize in people older

TABLE 3-9 ▼ Symptoms of Anxiety

Physical	Behavioral	Cognitive	Psychologic
Increased sighing respirations	Hyperalertness	Fear of losing mind	Phobias
Increased blood pressure	Irritability	Fear of losing control	Obsessive-compulsive behavior
Tachycardia	Uncertainty		
Shortness of breath	Apprehension		
Dizziness	Difficulty with memory or		
Lump in throat	concentration		
Muscle tension	Sleep disturbance		
Dry mouth			
Diarrhea			
Nausea			
Clammy hands			
Profuse sweating			
Restlessness, pacing, irritability, difficulty concentrating			
Chest pain*			
Headache			
Low back pain			
Myalgia (muscle pain, tension, or tenderness)			
Arthralgia (joint pain)			
Abdominal (stomach) distress			
Irritable bowel syndrome (IBS)			

* Chest pain associated with anxiety accounts for more than half of all emergency department admissions for chest pain. The pain is substernal, a dull ache that does not radiate and is not aggravated by respiratory movements but is associated with hyperventilation and claustrophobia. See Chapter 17 for further discussion of chest pain triggered by anxiety.

than 65, and many people attribute such symptoms simply to "getting older" and ignore them.

Anyone can be affected by depression at any time. There are, in fact, many underlying physical and medical causes of depression (Box 3-10), including medications used for Parkinson's disease, arthritis, cancer, hypertension, and heart disease (Box 3-11). The therapist should be familiar with these.

For example, anxiety and depressive disorders occur at a higher rate in clients with chronic obstructive pulmonary disease (COPD).[98] There is also a link between depression and heart risks in women. Depressed, but otherwise healthy, postmenopausal women face a 50% higher risk of dying from heart disease than women who are not depressed.[99]

People with chronic pain have three times the average risk of developing depression or anxiety

---

BOX 3-11 ▼ Drugs Commonly Associated with Depression

- Anti-anxiety medications (e.g., Valium, Xanax)
- Illegal drugs (e.g., cocaine, crack)
- Antihypertensive drugs (e.g., beta blockers, anti-adrenergics)
- Cardiovascular medications (e.g., digitoxin, digoxin)
- Antineoplastic agents (e.g., vinblastine)
- Opiate analgesics (e.g., morphine, Demerol, Darvon)
- Anticonvulsants (e.g., Dilantin, Phenobarbital)
- Corticosteroids (e.g., Prednisone, cortisone)
- Alcohol
- Hormone replacement therapy and oral contraceptives

For a complete list of drugs that can cause depression see: Wolfe, S: *List of drugs that cause depression*, Public Citizen's Health Research Group, Washington, DC, 2004 http://www.worstpills.org/public/aalist.cfm?aa=73&drug_order=1

BOX 3-10 ▼ Physical Conditions Commonly Associated with Depression

Cardiovascular
Atherosclerosis
Hypertension
Myocardial infarction
Angioplasty or bypass surgery

Central Nervous System
Parkinson's disease
Huntington's disease
Cerebral arteriosclerosis
Stroke
Alzheimer's disease
Temporal lobe epilepsy
Postconcussion injury
Multiple sclerosis
Miscellaneous focal lesions

Endocrine, Metabolic
Hyperthyroidism
Hypothyroidism
Addison's disease
Cushing's disease
Hypoglycemia
Hyperglycemia
Hyperparathyroidism
Hyponatremia
Diabetes mellitus
Pregnancy (post-partum)

Viral
Acquired immunodeficiency syndrome
Hepatitis

Pneumonia
Influenza

Nutritional
Folic acid deficiency
Vitamin B_6 deficiency
Vitamin B_{12} deficiency

Immune
Fibromyalgia
Chronic fatigue syndrome
Systemic Lupus Erythematosus
Sjögren's syndrome
Rheumatoid arthritis
Immunosuppression (e.g., corticosteroid treatment)

Cancer
Pancreatic
Bronchogenic
Renal
Ovarian

Miscellaneous
Pancreatitis
Sarcoidosis
Syphilis
Porphyria
Corticosteroid treatment

From Goodman CC: Biopsychosocial-Spiritual Concepts Related to Health Care. In Goodman CC, Boissonnault WG, Fuller K: *Pathology: implications for the physical therapist*, ed 2, Philadelphia, 2003, WB Saunders; p 54.

and clients who are depressed have three times the average risk of developing chronic pain.[100]

Almost 500 million people are suffering from mental disorders today. One in four families has at least one member with a mental disorder at any point in time. And these numbers are on the increase. Depressive disorders are the fourth leading cause of disease and disability. Public health prognosticators predict that by 2020, clinical depression will be the leading cause of medical disability on earth. Adolescents are increasingly affected by depression.[101]

The reasons for the increased incidence are speculative at best. Rapid cultural change around the world, worldwide poverty, and the aging of the world's population (the incidence of depression and dementia increases with age) have been put forth by researchers as possibilities.[102-104]

Others suggest better treatment of the symptoms has resulted in fewer suicides.[105] Researchers think that genes may play a role in a person's risk of developing depression.[106-108] In earlier times, adults who had this genetic link may have committed suicide before bearing children and passing the gene on. Today, with better treatment and greater longevity, people with major depressive disorders may unwittingly pass the disease on to their children.[109]

New insights on depression have led scientists to see clinical depression as a biologic disease possibly originating in the brain with multiple visceral involvements (Table 3-10). One error in medical treatment has been to recognize and treat the client's esophagitis, palpitations, irritable bowel, heart disease, asthma, chronic low back pain without seeing the real underlying impairment of

TABLE 3-10 ▼ Systemic Effects of Depression

System	Sign or symptom
General (multiple system cross over)	Persistent fatigue Insomnia, sleep disturbance See clinical signs and symptoms of depression (text)
Cardiovascular	Chest pain • Associated with myocardial infarction • Can be atypical chest pain that is not associated with coronary artery disease Palpitations Ventricular tachycardia
Gastrointestinal	Irritable bowel syndrome Esophageal dysmotility Nonulcer dyspepsia Functional abdominal pain (heartburn)
Neurologic (often symmetrical and nonanatomic)	Paresthesia Dizziness Difficulty concentrating and making decisions; problems with memory
Musculoskeletal	Weakness Fibromyalgia (or other unexplained rheumatic pain) Myofascial pain syndrome Chronic back pain
Immune	Multiple allergies Chemical hypersensitivity Autoimmune disorders Recurrent or resistant infections
Dysregulation	Autonomic instability • Temperature intolerance • Blood pressure changes Hormonal dysregulation (e.g., amenorrhea)
Other	Migraine and tension headaches Shortness of breath associated with asthma or not clearly explained Anxiety or panic disorder

Data From: Smith NL: *The effects of depression and anxiety on medical illness*, University of Utah, School of Medicine, Stress Medicine Clinic, Sandy, Utah, 2002.

the central nervous system (CNS dysregulation: depression) leading to these dysfunctions.[105,110,111]

A medical diagnosis is necessary because several known physical causes of depression are reversible if treated (e.g., thyroid disorders, vitamin B_{12} deficiency, medications [especially sedatives], some hypertensives, and H_2 blockers for stomach problems]. About half of clients with panic disorder will have an episode of clinical depression during their lives.

Depression is not a normal part of the aging process, but it is a normal response to pain or disability and may influence the client's ability to cope. Whereas anxiety is more apparent in acute pain episodes, depression occurs more often in clients with chronic pain.

The therapist may want to screen for psychosocial factors, such as depression that influences physical rehabilitation outcomes, especially when a client demonstrates acute pain that persists for more than 6 to 8 weeks. Screening is also important because depression is an indicator of poor prognosis.[112]

In the primary care setting, the physical therapist has a key role in identifying comorbidities that may have an impact on physical therapy intervention. Depression has been clearly identified as a factor that delays recovery for clients with low back pain. The longer depression is undetected,

the greater the likelihood of prolonged physical therapy intervention and increased disability.[112,113]

Tests such as the Beck Depression Inventory II (BDI-II),[114-116] the Zung Depression Scale,[117] or the Geriatric Depression Scale (short form) (Table 3-11) can be administered by a physical therapist to obtain baseline information that may be useful in determining the need for a medical referral. These tests do not require interpretation that is out of the scope of physical therapist practice.

The short form of the BDI, the most widely used instrument for measuring depression, takes five minutes to complete, and is also used to monitor therapeutic progress. The BDI consists of questions that are noninvasive and straightforward in presentation.

The Beck Depression Inventory Second Edition (BDI-II) is a 21-item self-report instrument intended to assess the existence and severity of symptoms of depression in adults and adolescents 13 years of age and older and as listed in the American Psychiatric Association's *Diagnostic and Statistical Manual of Mental Disorders*, Fourth Edition (DSM-IV; 1994).[42]

When presented with the BDI-II, a client is asked to consider each statement as it relates to the way they have felt for the past 2 weeks, to more accurately correspond to the DSM-IV criteria. The authors warn against the use of this instrument as

---

TABLE 3-11 ▼ Geriatric Depression Scale (Short Form)

For each question, choose the answer that best describes how you felt over the past week.

1. Are you basically satisfied with your life?	Yes/NO
2. Have you dropped many of your activities and interests?	YES/No
3. Do you feel that your life is empty?	YES/No
4. Do you often get bored?	YES/No
5. Are you in good spirits most of the time?	Yes/NO
6. Are you afraid that something bad is going to happen to you?	YES/No
7. Do you feel happy most of the time?	Yes/NO
8. Do you often feel helpless?	YES/No
9. Do you prefer to stay at home, rather than going out and doing new things?	YES/No
10. Do you feel you have more problems with memory than most people?	YES/No
11. Do you think it is wonderful to be alive now?	Yes/NO
12. Do you feel pretty worthless the way you are now?	YES/No
13. Do you feel full of energy?	Yes/NO
14. Do you feel that your situation is hopeless?	YES/No
15. Do you think that most people are better off than you are?	YES/No

NOTE: The scale is scored as follows: 1 point for each response in capital letters. A score of 0 to 5 is normal; a score above 5 suggests depression and warrants a follow-up interview; a score above 10 almost always indicates depression.
Used with permission from Sheikh JI, Yesavage JA. Geriatric Depression Scale (GDS): recent evidence and development of a shorter version, *Clin Gerontol* 5:165-173, 1986.

a sole diagnostic measure, because depressive symptoms may be part of other primary diagnostic disorders (see Box 3-10).

In the acute care setting, the therapist may see results of the BDI-II for Medical Patients in the medical record. This seven-item self-report measure of depression in adolescents and adults reflects the cognitive and affective symptoms of depression, while excluding somatic and performance symptoms that might be attributable to other conditions. It is a quick and effective way to assess depression in populations with biological, medical, alcohol, and/or substance abuse problems.

The Beck Scales for anxiety, depression, or suicide can help identify clients from ages 13 to 80 with depressive, anxious, or suicidal tendencies even in populations with overlapping physical and/or medical problems.

The Beck Scales have been developed and validated to assist health care professionals in making focused and reliable client evaluations. Test results can be the first step in recognizing and appropriately treating an affective disorder. These are copyrighted materials and can be obtained directly from The Psychological Corporation now under the new name of Harcourt Assessment.[118]

If the resultant scores for any of these assessment tools suggest clinical depression, psychologic referral is not always necessary. Intervention outcome can be monitored closely and if progress is not made, the therapist may want to review this outcome with the client and discuss the need to communicate this information to the physician. Depression can be treated effectively with a combination of therapies, including exercise, proper nutrition, antidepressants, and psychotherapy.

SYMPTOMS OF DEPRESSION

About one-third of the clinically depressed clients treated do not feel sad or blue. Instead, they report somatic symptoms such as fatigue, joint pain, headaches, or chronic back pain (or any chronic, recurrent pain present in multiple places).

Eighty to 90% of the most common gastrointestinal disorders (e.g., esophageal motility disorder, nonulcer dyspepsia, irritable bowel syndrome) are associated with depressive or anxiety disorders.[111-119]

Some scientists think the problem is over-response of the enteric system to stimuli. The gut senses stimuli too early, receives too much of a

signal, and responds with too much of a reaction. Serotonin levels are low and substance P levels are too high when, in fact, these two neurotransmitters are supposed to work together to modulate the GI response.[120,121]

Other researchers propose that one of the mechanisms underlying chronic disorders associated with depression such as irritable bowel syndrome and fibromyalgia is an increased activation of brain regions concerned with the processing and modulation of visceral and somatic afferent information, particularly in the subregions of the anterior cingulate cortex (ACC).[122]

Another red flag for depression is any condition associated with smooth muscle spasm such as asthma, irritable or overactive bladder, Raynaud's disease, and hypertension. Neurologic symptoms with no apparent cause such as paresthesias, dizziness, and weakness may actually be symptoms of depression. This is particularly true if the neurologic symptoms are symmetrical or not anatomic.[105]

Clinical Signs and Symptoms of
Depression (See Also Table 3-10)

- Persistent sadness, low mood, or feelings of emptiness
- Frequent or unexplained crying spells
- A sense of hopelessness
- Feelings of guilt or worthlessness
- Problems in sleeping
- Loss of interest or pleasure in ordinary activities or loss of libido
- Fatigue or decreased energy
- Appetite loss (or overeating)
- Difficulty in concentrating, remembering, and making decisions
- Irritability
- Persistent joint pain
- Headache
- Chronic back pain
- Bilateral neurologic symptoms of unknown cause (e.g., numbness, dizziness, weakness)
- Thoughts of death or suicide
- Pacing and fidgeting
- Chest pain and palpitations

Modified from Hendrix ML: Understanding panic disorder. Washington, DC, U.S. Department of Health and Human Services, National Institutes of Health, January 1993.

CASE EXAMPLE 3-7   Post-Total Knee Replacement

A 71-year-old woman has been referred for home health following a left total knee replacement. Her surgery was 6 weeks ago and she has had severe pain, swelling, and loss of motion. She has had numerous previous surgeries including right shoulder arthroplasty, removal of the right eye (macular degeneration), rotator cuff repair on the left, hysterectomy, two caesarian sections, and several inner ear surgeries. In all, she proudly tells you she has had 21 operations in 21 years.

Her family tells you she is taking Percocet prescribed by the orthopedic surgeon and Darvon left over from a previous surgery. They estimate she takes at least 10 to 12 pills every-day. They are concerned because she complains of constant pain and sleeps 18 hours a day.

They want you to "do something."

What is the appropriate response in this situation?

As part of the evaluation process, you will be gathering more information about your client's functional level, mental status, and assessing her pain more thoroughly. Take some time to listen to the client's pain description and concerns. Find out what her goals are and what would help her to reach those goals.

Consider using the McGill Pain Question-naire to assess for emotional overlay. With a long

history of medical care she may be dependent on the attention she gets for each operation. Addiction to pain relieving drugs can occur, but it is more likely that she has become dependent on them because of a cycle of pain-spasm-inactivity-pain-spasm, and so on.

Physical therapy intervention may help reduce some of this and change around her pain pattern.

Depression may be a key factor in this case. Review the possible signs and symptoms of depression with the client. It may not be neces-sary to tell the client ahead of time that these signs and symptoms are typical of depression. Read the list and ask her to let you know if she is experiencing any of them. See how many she reports at this time. Afterwards, ask her if she may be depressed and see how she responds to the question.

Medical referral for review of her medications and possible psychologic evaluation may be in her best interest. You may want to contact the doctor with your concerns and/or suggest the family report their concerns as well.

Keep in mind exercise is a key intervention strategy for depression. As the therapist, you may be able to "do something" by including a general conditioning program in addition to her specific knee exercises.

DRUGS, DEPRESSION, OR DEMENTIA?

The older adult often presents with such a mixed clinical presentation, it is difficult to know what is a primary musculoskeletal problem and what could be caused by drugs or depression (Case Example 3-7). Family members confuse signs and symptoms of depression with dementia and often ask the therapist for a differentiation.

Depression and dementia share some common traits, but there are differences. A medical diagno-sis is needed to make the differentiation. The ther-apist may be able to provide observational clues by noting any of the following[123]:

- Mental function: declines more rapidly with depression
- Disorientation: present only in dementia
- Difficulty concentrating: depression
- Difficulty with short-term memory: dementia
- Writing, speaking, and motor impairments: dementia
- Memory loss: people with depression notice and comment; people with dementia are indifferent to the changes

Panic Disorder

Persons with panic disorder have episodes of sudden, unprovoked feelings of terror or impend-ing doom with associated physical symptoms, such as racing or pounding heartbeat, breathlessness, nausea, sweating, and dizziness. During an attack people may fear that they are gravely ill, going to die, or going crazy.

The fear of another attack can itself become debilitating so that these individuals avoid situa-tions and places that they believe will trigger the episodes, thus affecting their work, their relation-ships, and their ability to take care of everyday tasks.

Initial panic attacks may occur when people are under considerable stress, for example, an overload

of work or from loss of a family member or close friend. The attacks may follow surgery, a serious accident, illness, or childbirth. Excessive consumption of caffeine or use of cocaine, other stimulant drugs, or medicines containing caffeine or stimulants used in treating asthma can also trigger panic attacks.[124]

The symptoms of a panic attack can mimic those of other medical conditions, such as respiratory or heart problems. Anxiety or panic is a leading cause of chest pain mimicking a heart attack. Residual sore muscles are a consistent finding after the panic attack and can also occur in individuals with social phobias. People suffering from these attacks may be afraid or embarrassed to report their symptoms to the physician.

The alert therapist may recognize the need for a medical referral. A combination of antidepressants known as selective serotonin reuptake inhibitors (SSRIs) combined with cognitive behavioral therapy (CBT) has been proven effective in controlling symptoms.

Panic disorder is characterized by period of sudden, unprovoked, intense anxiety with associated physical symptoms lasting a few minutes up to a few hours. Dizziness, paresthesias, headaches, and palpitations are common.

Pain perception involves a sensory component (pain sensation) and an emotional reaction referred to as the sensory-discriminative and motivational-affective dimensions, respectively.[125]

Clinical Signs and Symptoms of Panic Disorder

- Racing or pounding heartbeat
- Chest pains and/or palpitations
- Dizziness, lightheadedness, nausea
- Headaches
- Difficulty in breathing
- Bilateral numbness or tingling in nose, cheeks, lips, fingers, toes
- Sweats or chills
- Hand wringing
- Dreamlike sensations or perceptual distortions
- Sense of terror
- Extreme fear of losing control
- Fear of dying

Modified from Hendrix ML: Understanding panic disorder. Washington, DC, U.S. Department of Health and Human Services, National Institutes of Health, 1993. For more information, contact the National Institute of Mental Health: 1-800-64-PANIC.

Psychoneuroimmunology

When it comes to pain assessment, sources of pain, mechanisms of pain, and links between the mind and body, it is impossible to leave out a discussion of a new area of research and study called *psychoneuroimmunology* (PNI). PNI is the study of the interactions among behavior, neural, endocrine, enteric (digestive), and immune system function.

PNI explains the influence of the nervous system on the immune and inflammatory responses, and how the immune system communicates with the neuro-endocrine systems. The immune system can activate sensory nerves and the central nervous system by releasing proinflammatory cytokines, creating an exaggerated pain response.[126]

Further, there is a unique integration of the hypothalamic-pituitary-adrenal axis and the neuro-endocrine-enteric axis. This is accomplished on a biologic basis, a discovery first made in the late 1990s. Physiologically adaptive processes occur as a result of these biochemically based mind-body connections and likely impact the perception of pain and memory of pain.

Researchers at the National Institute of Health (NIH) made a groundbreaking discovery when the biologic basis for emotions (neuropeptides and their receptors) was identified. This new understanding of the interconnections between the mind and body goes far beyond our former understanding of the psychosomatic response in illness, disease, or injury.[127]

Neuropeptides are chemical messengers that move through the blood stream to every cell in the body. These information molecules take messages throughout the body to every cell and organ system. For example, the digestive (enteric) system and the neurologic system communicate with the immune system via these neuropeptides. These three systems can exchange information and influence one another's actions.

More than 30 different classes of neuropeptides have been identified. Every one of these messengers is found in the enteric nervous system of the gut. The constant presence of these neurotransmitters and neuromodulators in the bowel suggests that emotional expression of active coping generates a balance in the neuropeptide-receptor network and physiologic healing beginning in the GI system.

The identification of biologic carriers of emotions has also led to an understanding of a concept well known to physical therapists but previously unnamed: cellular memories.[128-131] Many health

care professionals have seen the emotional and psychological response of a hands-on approach. Concepts labeled as cranio-sacral, unwinding, myofascial release, and soft tissue mobilization are based (in part) with this in mind.

These new discoveries help substantiate the idea that cells containing memories are shuttled through the body and brain via chemical messengers. The biologic basis of emotions and memories helps explain how soft tissues respond to emotions; indeed, the soft tissue structures may even contain emotions by way of neuropeptides.

Perhaps this can explain why two people can experience a car accident and whiplash (flexion-extension) or other injury. One recovers without any problems, while the other develops chronic pain that is resistant to any intervention. The focus of research on behavioral approaches combined with our hands-on intervention may bring a better understanding of what works and why.

Other researchers investigating neuropathic pain see a link between memory and pain. Studies looking at the physical similarities between the way a memory is formed and the way pain becomes persistent and chronic support such a link.[132]

Researchers suggest when somatic pain persists beyond the expected time of healing the pain no longer originates in the tissue that was damaged. Pain begins in the central nervous system instead. The experience changes the nervous system. The memory of pain recurs again and again in the CNS.[132]

The nervous system transmits pain signals efficiently and small pain signals may be amplified until the sensation of pain is out of proportion to what is expected for the injury. Pain amplification occurs in the spinal cord. Spinal cord cells called *glia* become activated, releasing a variety of chemical substances that cause pain messages to become amplified.[133]

Other researchers have reported the discovery of a protein that allows nerve cells to communicate and thereby enhance perceptions of chronic pain. The results reinforce the notion that the basic process that leads to memory formation may be the same as the process that causes chronic pain.[134]

Along these same lines, other researchers have shown a communication network between the immune system and the brain. Pain phenomena are actually modulated by immune function. Proinflammatory cytokines (e.g., tumor necrosis factor [TNF], interleukin-1 [IL-1], interleukin-6 [IL-6]) released by activated immune cells signal the brain by both blood-borne and neural routes, leading to alterations in neural activity.[135]

The cytokines in the brain interfere with cognitive function and memory; the cytokines within the spinal cord exaggerate fatigue and pain. By signaling the central nervous system, these proinflammatory cytokines create exaggerated pain as well as an entire constellation of physiologic, hormonal, and behavioral changes referred to as the *sickness response*.[136,137]

In essence immune processes work well when directed against pathogens or cancer cells. When directed against peripheral nerves, dorsal nerve ganglia, or the dorsal roots in the spinal cord, the immune system attacks the nerves, resulting in extreme pain.

Such exaggerated pain states occur with infection, inflammation, or trauma of the skin, peripheral nerves, and central nervous system. The neuro-immune link may help explain the exaggerated pain state associated with conditions such as chronic fatigue syndrome and fibromyalgia.

With this new understanding that all peripheral nerves and neurons are affected by immune and glial activation, intervention to modify pain will likely change in the near future.[126,138]

SCREENING FOR SYSTEMIC VERSUS PSYCHOGENIC SYMPTOMS

Screening for emotional or psychologic overlay has a place in our examination and evaluation process. Recognizing that this emotion-induced somatic pain response has a scientific basis may help us find better ways to alter or eliminate it.

The key in screening for systemic versus psychogenic basis of symptoms is to identify the client with a significant emotional or psychologic component influencing the pain experience. Whether to refer the client for further psychologic evaluation and treatment or just modify the physical therapy plan of care is left up to the therapist's clinical judgment.

In all cases of pain, watch for the client who reports any of the following red flag symptoms:

- Symptoms are out of proportion to the injury.
- Symptoms persist beyond the expected time for physiologic healing.
- No position is comfortable.

These symptoms reflect both the possibility of an emotional or psychologic overlay as well as the pos-

sibility of a more serious underlying systemic disorder (including cancer). In this next section, we will look at ways to screen for emotional content, keeping in mind what has already been said about anxiety, depression, and panic disorder.

Three Screening Tools

There are three tools that can be used quickly and easily to help screen for emotional overlay in painful symptoms (Box 3-12). The client may or may not be aware that he or she is, in fact, exaggerating pain responses or experiencing pain associated with emotional or psychologic overlay.

This discussion does not endorse physical therapists' practicing as psychologists, which is outside the scope of our expertise and experience. It merely recognizes that, in treating the whole client, not only the physical but also the psychologic, emotional, and spiritual needs of that person will be represented in his or her magnitude of symptoms, length of recovery time, response to pain, and responsibility for recovery.

McGill Pain Questionnaire

The McGill Pain Questionnaire (MPQ) from McGill University in Canada is a well-known and commonly used tool in assessing chronic pain. The MPQ is designed to measure the subjective pain experience in a quantitative form. It is considered a good baseline for assessing pain and has both high reliability and validity in younger adults. It has not been tested specifically with older adults.

The MPQ consists primarily of two major classes of word descriptors, sensory and affective (emotional), and can be used to specify the subjective pain experience. It also contains an intensity scale and other items to determine the properties of pain experience.

There is a shorter version, which some clinicians find more practical for routine use.[139,140] It can be used for both assessment and ongoing monitoring for any condition. However, for screening purposes outlined here, the format of the original McGill Questionnaire may work best (Fig. 3-11).

BOX 3-12 ▼ Screening Tools for Emotional Overlay

- McGill Pain Questionnaire
- Symptom Magnification and Illness Behavior
- Waddell's Nonorganic Signs

The original form of the MPQ with all its affective word descriptors to help clients describe their pain gives results that help the therapist identify the source of the pain: vascular (visceral), neurogenic (somatic), musculoskeletal (somatic), or emotional (psycho-somatic) (see Table 3-1).

When administering this portion of the questionnaire, the therapist reads the list of words in each box. The client is to choose the *one* word that best describes his or her pain. If no word in the box matches, the box is left blank. The words in each box are listed in order of ascending (rank order) intensity.

For example, in the first box, the words begin with "flickering" and "quivering" and gradually progress to "beating" and "pounding." Beating and pounding are considered much more intense than flickering and quivering. Word descriptors included in Group 1 reflect characteristics of pain of a vascular disorder. Knowing this information can be very helpful as the therapist continues the examination and evaluation of the client.

Groups 2 through 8 are words used to describe pain of a neurogenic origin. Group 9 reflects the musculoskeletal system and groups 10 through 20 are all the words a client might use to describe pain in emotional terms (e.g., torturing, killing, vicious, agonizing).

After completing the questionnaire with the client, add up the total number of checks. According to the key, choosing up to eight words to describe the pain is within normal limits. Selecting more than 10 is a red flag for emotional or psychologic overlay, especially when the word selections come from groups 10 through 20.

Illness Behavior Syndrome and Symptom Magnification

Pain in the absence of an identified source of disease or pathologic condition may elicit a behavioral response from the client that is now labeled *illness behavior syndrome*. Illness behavior is what people say and do to show they are ill or perceive themselves as sick or in pain. It does not mean there is nothing wrong with the person. Illness behavior expresses and communicates the severity of pain and physical impairment.[73]

This syndrome has been identified most often in people with chronic pain. Its expression depends on what and how the client thinks about his or her symptoms/illness. Components of this syndrome include

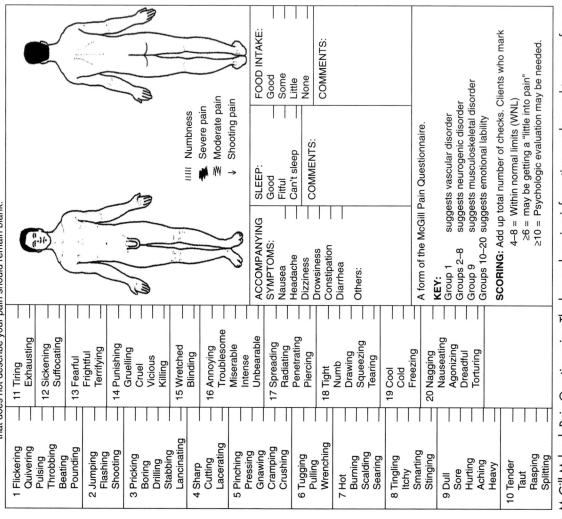

Fig. 3-11 • McGill-Melzack Pain Questionnaire. The key and scoring information can be used to screen for emotional overlay or to identify a specific somatic or visceral source of pain. Instructions are provided in the text. (From Melzack R: The McGill pain questionnaire: major properties and scoring methods, *Pain* 1:277-299, 1975. Used with permission, International Association for the Study of Pain.)

- Dramatization of complaints, leading to overtreatment and overmedication
- Progressive dysfunction, leading to decreased physical activity and often compounding preexisting musculoskeletal or circulatory dysfunction
- Drug misuse

- Progressive dependency on others, including health care professionals, leading to overuse of the health care system
- Income disability, in which the person's illness behavior is perpetuated by financial gain[71] *Symptom magnification syndrome (SMS)* is another term used to describe the phenomenon of

illness behavior; conscious symptom magnification is referred to as *malingering*, whereas unconscious symptom magnification is labeled *illness behavior*.

The term symptom magnification was first coined by Leonard N. Matheson, PhD* in 1977 to describe clients whose symptoms have reinforced their behavior; that is, the symptoms have become the predominant force in the client's function rather than the physiologic phenomenon of the injury determining the outcome.

By definition, SMS is a self-destructive, socially reinforced behavioral response pattern consisting of reports or displays of symptoms that function to control the life of the sufferer.[141-143] The symptoms rather than the physiologic phenomenon of the injury determine the outcome/function.

The affected person acts as if the future cannot be controlled because of the presence of symptoms. All present limitations are blamed on the symptoms: "My (back) pain won't let me . . . ." The client may exaggerate limitations beyond those that seem reasonable in relation to the injury, apply minimal effort on maximal performance tasks, and overreact to physical loading during objective examination.

It is important for physical therapists to recognize that we often contribute to SMS by focusing on the relief of symptoms, especially pain, as the goal of therapy. Reducing pain is an acceptable goal for some types of clients, but for those who experience pain after the injuries have healed, the focus should be restoration, or at least improvement, of function.

In these situations, instead of asking whether the client's symptoms are "better, the same, or worse," it may be more appropriate to inquire about functional outcomes; for example, what can the client accomplish at home that she or he was unable to attempt at the beginning of treatment, last week, or even yesterday.

Conscious or unconscious? Can a physical therapist determine when a client is consciously or unconsciously symptom magnifying? Is it within the scope of the physical therapist's practice to use the label 'malingerer' without a psychologist or psychiatrist's diagnosis of such first?

Some therapists suggest there is a need to keep to what can be measured objectively. Health care professionals have not learned yet how to read someone's mind to determine his/her motivation.[144]

* Director, ERIC Human Performance Laboratory, Washington University School of Medicine, St. Louis, Missouri.

Keep in mind the goal is to screen for a psychologic or emotional component to the client's clinical presentation. The key to achieving this goal is to use objective test measures whenever possible. In this way, the therapist obtains the guidance needed for referral versus modification of the physical therapy intervention.

Compiling a list of nonorganic or behavioral signs and identifying how the client is reacting to pain may be all that is needed. Signs of illness behavior may point the therapist in the direction of more careful management of the psychosocial and behavioral aspects of the client's illness.[89]

Waddell's Nonorganic Signs

Waddell et al[145] identified five nonorganic signs and seven nonanatomic or behavioral descriptions of symptoms (Table 3-12). Each of the nonorganic signs is determined by using one or two of the tests listed. These tests are used to assess a client's pain behavior and detect abnormal illness behavior. The literature supports that these signs may be present in 10% of clients with acute low back pain, but are found most often in people with chronic low back pain.

A score of three or more positive signs places the client in the category of *nonmovement dysfunction*. This person is said to have a clinical pattern of nonmechanical, pain-focused behavior. This type of score is predictive of poor outcome and associated with delayed return-to-work or not working.

One or two positive signs is a low Waddell's score and does not classify the client with a nonmovement dysfunction. The value of these nonorganic signs as predictors for return to work for clients with low back pain has been investigated.[146] Less than two is a good prognosticator of return to work. The results of how this study might affect practice are available.[147]

A positive finding for nonorganic signs does not suggest an absence of pain but rather a behavioral response to pain (see discussion of symptom magnification syndrome). It does not confirm malingering or illness behavior. Neither do these signs imply the non-existence of physical pathology.

Waddell and associates[90,145] have given us a tool that can help us identify early in the rehabilitation process those who need more than just mechanical or physical treatment intervention. Other evaluation tools are available (e.g., Oswestry Back Pain Disability Questionnaire, Roland-Morris Disability Questionnaire). A psychologic evaluation and possibly behavioral therapy or psychologic counseling may be needed as an adjunct to physical therapy.[148]

TABLE 3-12 ▼ Waddell's Nonorganic Signs and Behavioral Symptoms

Test	Signs	Nonanatomic or behavioral description of symptoms
Tenderness	*Superficial*—the client's skin is tender to light pinch over a wide area of lumbar skin; unable to localize to one structure *Nonanatomic*—deep tenderness felt over a wide area, not localized to one structure	(1) Pain at the tip of the tailbone (2) Whole leg pain from the groin down to below the knee in a stocking pattern (not dermatomal or sclerotomal) [intermittent] (3) Whole leg numbness or whole leg "going dead" [intermittent] (4) Whole leg giving way or collapsing (intermittent); client maintains upright position (5) Constant pain for years on end without relief (6) Unable to tolerate any treatment; reaction or side effects to every intervention (7) Emergency admission to hospital for back pain without precipitating traumatic event
Simulation tests	*Axial loading*—light vertical loading over client's skull in the standing position reproduces lumbar (not cervical) spine pain *Acetabular rotation*—lumbosacral pain from upper trunk rotation; back pain reported when the pelvis and shoulders are passively rotated in the same plane as the client stands; this is considered to be a positive test if pain is reported within the first 30 degrees	
Distraction tests	*Straight-leg-raise* (SLR) discrepancy—marked improvement of SLR when client is distracted as compared with formal testing; different response to SLR in supine (worse) compared to sitting (better) when both tests should have the same result in the presence of organic pathology *Double leg raise*—when both legs are raised after straight leg raising, the organic response would be a greater degree of double leg raising; clients with a nonorganic component demonstrate less double leg raise as compared with the single leg raise	
Regional disturbances	*Weakness*—cogwheeling or giving way of many muscle groups that cannot be explained on a neurologic basis *Sensory disturbance*—diminished sensation fitting a "stocking" rather than a dermatomal pattern	
Overreaction	Disproportionate verbalization, facial expression, muscle tension, and tremor, collapsing, or sweating. Client may exhibit any of the following behaviors during the physical examination: guarding, bracing, rubbing, sighing, clenching teeth, or grimacing	

Adapted from Karas R, McIntosh G, Hall H, et al: The relationship between nonorganic signs and centralization of symptoms in the prediction of return to work for patients with low back pain, *Phys Ther* 77(4):354-360, 1997.

Conversion Symptoms

Whereas SMS is a behavioral, learned, inappropriate *behavior*, conversion is a psychodynamic phenomenon and quite rare in the chronically disabled population.

Conversion is a physical expression of an unconscious psychologic conflict, such as an event (e.g., loss of a loved one) or a problem in the person's work or personal life. The conversion may provide a solution to the conflict or a way to express "forbidden" feelings. It may be a means of enacting the sick role to avoid responsibilities, or it may be a reflection of behaviors learned in childhood.[11]

Diagnosis of a conversion syndrome is difficult and often requires the diagnostic and evaluative input of the physical therapist. Presentation always includes a motor and/or sensory component that cannot be explained by a known medical or neuromusculoskeletal condition.

The clinical presentation is often mistaken for an organic disorder such as multiple sclerosis, systemic lupus erythematosus, myasthenia gravis, or idiopathic dystonias. At presentation, when a client has an unusual limp or bizarre gait pattern that cannot be explained by functional anatomy, family members may be interviewed to assess changes in the client's gait and whether this alteration in movement pattern is present consistently.

The physical therapist can look for a change in the wear pattern of the client's shoes to decide if this alteration in gait has been long-standing. During manual muscle testing, true weakness results in smooth "giving way" of a muscle group; in hysterical weakness the muscle "breaks" in a series of jerks.

Often the results of muscle testing are not consistent with functional abilities observed. For example, the person cannot raise the arm overhead during testing but has no difficulty dressing, or the lower extremity appears flaccid during recumbency but the person can walk on the heels and toes when standing.

The physical therapist should carefully evaluate and document all sensory and motor changes. Conversion symptoms are less likely to follow any dermatome, myotome, or sclerotome patterns.

Clinical Signs and Symptoms of
Conversion

- Sudden, acute onset
- Lack of concern about the symptoms
- Unexplainable motor or sensory function impairment

Motor

- Impaired coordination or balance and/or bizarre gait pattern
- Paralysis or localized weakness
- Loss of voice, difficulty swallowing, or sensation of a lump in the throat
- Urinary retention

Sensory

- Altered touch or pain sensation (paresthesia or dysesthesia)
- Visual changes (double vision, blindness, black spots in visual field)
- Hearing loss (mild to profound deafness)
- Hallucinations
- Seizures or convulsions
- Absence of significant laboratory findings
- Electrodiagnostic testing within normal limits
- Deep tendon reflexes within normal limits

Screening Questions for Psychogenic Source of Symptoms

Besides observing for signs and symptoms of psychophysiologic disorders, the therapist can ask a few screening questions (Box 3-13). The client may be aware of the symptoms, but does not know that these problems can be caused by depression, anxiety, or panic disorder.

Medical treatment for physiopsychologic disorders can and should be augmented with exercise. Physical activity and exercise has a known benefit in the management of mild-to-moderate

---

BOX 3-13 ▼ Screening Questions for Psychogenic Source of Symptoms

- Do you have trouble sleeping at night?
- Do you have trouble focusing during the day?
- Do you worry about finances, work, or life in general?
- Do you feel a sense of dread or worry without cause?
- Do you ever feel happy?
- Do you have a fear of being in groups of people? Fear of flying? Public speaking?
- Do you have a racing heart, unexplained dizziness, or unexpected tingling in your face or fingers?
- Do you wake up in the morning with your jaw clenched or feeling sore muscles and joints?
- Are you irritable or jumpy most of the time?

Data from Davidson J, Dreher H: *The anxiety book: developing strength in the face of fear*, New York, 2003, Penguin Putnam.

psychologic disorders, especially depression and anxiety. Aerobic exercise or strength training have both been shown effective in moderating the symptoms of these conditions.[149-152]

Patience is a vital tool for therapists when working with clients who are having difficulty adjusting to the stress of illness and disability or the client who has a psychologic disorder. The therapist must develop personal coping mechanisms when working with clients who have chronic illnesses or psychologic disturbances.

Recognizing clients whose symptoms are the direct result of organic dysfunction helps us in coping with clients who are hostile, ungrateful, noncompliant, negative, or adversarial. Whenever possible, involve a psychiatrist, psychologist, or counselor as part of the management team. This approach will benefit the client as well as the health care staff.

▶ PHYSICIAN REFERRAL

Guidelines for Immediate Physician Referral

- Immediate medical attention is required for anyone with risk factors for and clinical signs and symptoms of rhabdomyolysis (see Table 3-5).
- Clients reporting a disproportionate relief of bone pain with a simple aspirin may have bone cancer. This red flag requires immediate medical referral in the presence of a personal history of cancer of any kind.
- Joint pain with no known cause and a recent history of infection of any kind. Ask about recent (last 6 weeks) skin lesions or rashes of any kind anywhere on the body, urinary tract infection, or respiratory infection. Take the client's temperature and ask about recent episodes of fever, sweats, or other constitutional symptoms. Palpate for residual lymphadenopathy. Early diagnosis and treatment are essential to limit joint destruction and preserve function.[62]

Guidelines for Physician Referral Required

- Proximal muscle weakness accompanied by change in one or more deep tendon reflexes in the presence of a previous history of cancer.
- The physician should be notified of anyone with joint pain of unknown cause who presents with recent or current skin rash or recent history of infection (hepatitis, mononucleosis, urinary

tract infection, upper respiratory infection, sexually transmitted infection, streptococcus).

- A team approach to fibromyalgia requires medical evaluation and management as part of the intervention strategy. Therapists should refer clients suspected with fibromyalgia for further medical follow up.
- Diffuse pain that characterizes some diseases of the nervous system and viscera may be difficult to distinguish from the equally diffuse pain so often caused by lesions of the moving parts. The distinction between visceral pain and pain caused by lesions of the vertebral column may be difficult to make and may require a medical diagnosis.
- The therapist may screen for signs and symptoms of anxiety, depression, and panic disorder. These conditions are often present with somatic symptoms that may resolve with effective intervention. The therapist can describe the symptoms and relay that information to the appropriate agency or individual when making a referral. Diagnosis is made by a medical doctor or trained mental health professional.
- Clients with new onset of back, neck, TMJ, shoulder, or arm pain brought on by a new exercise program or by exertion with the arms raised overhead should be screened for signs and symptoms of cardiovascular impairment. This is especially important if the symptoms are described as "throbbing" and start after a brief time of exercise (3 to 5 up to 10 minutes) and diminish or go away quickly with rest. Look for significant risk factors for cardiovascular involvement. Check vital signs. Refer for medical evaluation if indicated.
- Persistent pain on weight bearing or bone pain at night especially in the older adult with risk factors such as osteoporosis, postural hypotension leading to falls, or previous history of cancer.

Clues to Screening for Viscerogenic Sources of Pain

We know systemic illness and pathologic conditions affecting the viscera can mimic NMS dysfunction. The therapist who knows pain patterns and types of viscerogenic pain can sort through the client's description of pain and recognize when something does not fit the expected pattern for NMS problems.

We must keep in mind that pain from a disease process or viscerogenic source is often a late symptom rather than a reliable danger signal. For

this reason the therapist must remain alert to other signs and symptoms that may be present but unaccounted for.

In this chapter pain types possible with viscerogenic conditions have been presented along with three mechanisms by which viscera refer pain to the body (soma.) Characteristics of systemic pain compared to musculoskeletal pain are presented, including a closer look at joint pain.

Pain with the following features raises a red flag to alert the therapist of the need to take a closer look:

- Pain of unknown cause
- Pain that persists beyond the expected time for physiologic healing
- Pain that is out of proportion to the injury
- Pain that is unrelieved by rest or change in position
- Pain pattern does not fit the expected clinical presentation for a neuromuscular or musculoskeletal impairment
- Pain that cannot be altered, aggravated, provoked, reduced, eliminated, or alleviated
- There are some positions of comfort for various organs (e.g., leaning forward for the gallbladder or side bending for the kidney), but with progression of disease the client will obtain less and less relief of symptoms over time
- Pain, symptoms, or dysfunction are not improved or altered by physical therapy intervention
- Pain that is poorly localized
- Pain accompanied by signs and symptoms associated with a specific viscera (e.g., GI, GU, GYN, cardiac, pulmonary, endocrine)
- Pain that is constant and intense no matter what position is tried and despite rest, eating or abstaining from food; a previous history of cancer in this client is an even greater red flag necessitating further evaluation
- Pain (especially intense bone pain) that is disproportionately relieved by aspirin
- Listen to the client's choice of words to describe pain. Systemic or viscerogenic pain can be described as deep, sharp, boring, knifelike, stabbing, throbbing, colicky, or intermittent (comes and goes in waves)
- Pain accompanied by full and normal range of motion
- Pain that is made worse 3 to 5 minutes after initiating an activity and relieved by rest (possible symptom of vascular impairment) versus pain that goes away with activity (symptom of musculoskeletal involvement); listen for the word

descriptor "throbbing" to describe pain of a vascular nature

- Pain is a relatively new phenomenon and not a pattern that has been present over several years' time
- Constitutional symptoms in the presence of pain
- Pain that is not consistent with emotional or psychologic overlay
- When in doubt, conduct a screening exam for emotional overlay. Observe the client for signs and symptoms of anxiety, depression, and/or panic disorder. In the absence of systemic illness or disease and/or in the presence of suspicious psychologic symptoms, psychologic evaluation may be needed.
- Pain in the absence of any positive Waddell's signs (i.e., Waddell's test is negative or insignificant)
- Manual therapy to correct an upslip is not successful and the problem has returned by the end of the session or by the next day; consider a somato-visceral problem or visceral ligamentous problem.
- If painful, tender or sore points (e.g., Trigger points, Jones' points, acupuncture/acupressure points/Shiatsu) are eliminated with intervention then return quickly (by the end of the treatment session), suspect visceral pathology. If a tender point comes back later (several days or weeks), the clinician may not be holding it long enough[2]
- Back, neck, TMJ, shoulder, or arm pain brought on by exertion with the arms raised overhead may be suggestive of a cardiac problem. This is especially true in the postmenopausal woman or man over age 50 with a significant family history of heart disease and/or in the presence of hypertension.
- Back, shoulder, pelvic, or sacral pain that is made better or worse by eating, passing gas, or having a bowel movement
- Night pain (especially bone pain) that awakens the client from a sound sleep several hours after falling asleep; this is even more serious if the client is unable to get back to sleep after changing position, taking pain relievers, or eating or drinking something
- Joint pain preceded or accompanied by skin lesions (e.g., rash or nodules), following antibiotics or statins, or recent infection of any kind (e.g., gastrointestinal, pulmonary, genitourinary); check for signs and symptoms associated with any of these systems based on recent client history

- Clients can have more than one problem or pathology present at one time; it is possible to for a client to have both a visceral AND a mechanical problem[2]
- Remember Osler's Rule of Age*: Under age 60, most clients' symptoms are related to one problem, but over 60, it is rarely just one problem[2]

* Physicians often rely on ad hoc rules of thumb, or "heuristics," to guide them. These are often referred to as Osler's Rules. Sir William Osler, MD (1849-1919) promoted the idea that good medical science follows from gathering evidence by directly observing patients.

- A careful general history and physical examination is still the most important screening tool; never assume this was done by the referring physician or other staff from the referring agency[2]
- Visceral problems are unlikely to cause muscle weakness, reflex changes, or objective sensory deficits (exceptions include endocrine disease and paraneoplastic syndromes associated with cancer). If pain is referred from the viscera to the soma, challenging the somatic structure by stretching, contracting, or palpating will *not* reproduce the symptoms. For example, if a muscle is not sore when squeezed or contracted, the muscle is not the source of the pain.[2]

🔖 KEY POINTS TO REMEMBER

✓ Pain of a visceral origin can be referred to the corresponding somatic areas. The mechanisms of referred visceral pain patterns are not fully known. Information in this chapter is based on proposed models from what is known about the somatic sensory system.

✓ Recognizing pain patterns that are characteristic of systemic disease is a necessary step in the screening process. Understanding how and when diseased organs can refer pain to the neuromusculoskeletal (NMS) system helps the therapist identify suspicious pain patterns.

✓ At least three mechanisms contribute to referred pain patterns of the viscera (embryologic development, multisegmental innervation, direct pressure, and shared pathways). Being familiar with each one may help the therapist quickly identify pain patterns of a visceral source.

✓ The therapist should keep in mind cultural rules and differences in pain perception, intensity, and responses to pain found among various ethnic groups.

✓ Pain patterns of the chest, back, shoulder, scapula, pelvis, hip, groin, and sacroiliac joint are the most common sites of referred pain from a systemic disease process.

✓ Visceral diseases of the abdomen and pelvis are more likely to refer pain to the back, whereas intrathoracic disease refers pain to the shoulder(s). Visceral pain rarely occurs without associated signs and symptoms, although the client may not recognize the correlation. Careful questioning will usually elicit a systemic pattern of symptoms.

✓ A comprehensive pain assessment includes a detailed health history, physical exam, medication history (including nonprescription drug use and complementary

and alternative therapies), assessment of functional status, and consideration of psychosocial-spiritual factors. Assessment tools vary from the very young to the very old.

✓ Careful, sensitive, and thorough questioning regarding the multifaceted experience of pain can elicit essential information necessary when making a decision regarding treatment or referral. The use of pain assessment tools such as Fig. 3-6 and Table 3-2 may facilitate clear and accurate descriptions of this critical symptom.

✓ The client describes the characteristics of pain (location, frequency, intensity, duration, description). It is up to the therapist to recognize sources and types of pain and to know the pain patterns of a viscerogenic origin.

✓ Choose alternative words to "pain" when discussing the client's symptoms in order to get a complete understanding of the clinical presentation.

✓ Specific screening questions for joint pain are used to assess any joint pain of unknown cause, joint pain with an unusual presentation or history, or joint pain which does not fit the expected pattern for injury, overuse, or aging (Box 3-5).

✓ It is important to know how to differentiate psychogenic and psychosomatic origins of painful symptoms from systemic origins, including signs and symptoms of cancer.

✓ Pain described as constant or present at night, awakening the client from sleep must be evaluated thoroughly. When assessing constant and/or night pain, the therapist must know how to differentiate the characteristics of acute versus chronic pain associated with a neuromusculoskeletal problem from a viscerogenic or systemic presentation.

SUBJECTIVE EXAMINATION

Special Questions to Ask

Pain Assessment

Location of pain

Show me exactly where your pain is located.

Follow up questions may include:

- Do you have any other pain or symptoms any-where else?
- *If yes*, what causes the pain or symptoms to occur in this other area?

Description of pain

What does it feel like?

After giving the client time to reply, offer some additional choices in potential descriptors. You may want to ask: Is your pain/Are your symptoms

Knifelike   Dull
Boring   Burning
Throbbing   Prickly
Deep aching   Sharp

Follow up questions may include:

- Has the pain changed in quality since it first began?
- Changed in intensity?
- Changed in duration (how long it lasts)?

Frequency and duration of pain

How long do the symptoms last?

Clients who indicate that the pain is constant should be asked:

- Do you have this pain right now?
- Did you notice these symptoms this morning immediately when you woke up?

Pattern of pain

Tell me about the pattern of your pain/symptoms.

- *Alternate question:* When does your back/shoulder (name the involved body part) hurt?
- *Alternate question:* Describe your pain/ symptoms from first waking up in the morning to going to bed at night. (See special sleep-related questions that follow.)

Follow up questions may include:

- Have you ever experienced anything like this before?
- *If yes*, do these episodes occur more or less often than at first?
- How does your pain/symptom(s) change with time?
- Are your symptoms worse in the morning or evening?

Aggravating and Relieving Factors

- What brings your pain (symptoms) on?
- What kinds of things make your pain (symptoms) worse (e.g., eating, exercise, rest, specific positions, excitement, stress)?
  To assess relieving factors, ask:
- What makes the pain better?
  Follow up questions include:
- How does rest affect the pain/symptoms?
- Are your symptoms aggravated or relieved by any activities?
  - *If yes*, what?
- How has this problem affected your daily life at work or at home?
- How has this problem affected your ability to care for yourself without assistance (e.g., dress, bathe, cook, drive)?

Associated Symptoms

- What other symptoms have you had that you can associate with this problem?
  If the client denies any additional symptoms, follow up this question with a series of possibilities such as:

Burning   Heart   Numbness/
Difficulty in   palpitations   Tingling
breathing   Hoarseness   Problems with
Difficulty in   Nausea   vision
swallowing   Night sweats   Vomiting
Dizziness   Weakness

- Are you having any pain anywhere else in your body?
  Alternately: Are you having symptoms of any other kind that may or may not be related to your main problem?

Anxiety/Depression (See Table 3-11)

- Have you been under a lot of stress lately?
- Are you having some trouble coping with life in general and/or life's tensions?
- Do you feel exhausted or overwhelmed mentally or physically?
- Does your mind go blank or do you have trouble concentrating?
- Do you have trouble sleeping at night (e.g., difficulty getting to sleep, staying asleep, restless sleep, feel exhausted upon awakening)? Focusing during the day?
- Do you worry about finances, work, or life in general?
- Do you get any enjoyment in life?

SUBJECTIVE EXAMINATION—cont'd

- Do you feel keyed up or restless? Irritable and jumpy? On edge most of the time?
- Do you have a general sense of dread or unknown fears?
- Do you have any of these symptoms: a racing heart, dizziness, tingling, muscle or joint pains?

For the Asian client:

- Do you feel you are having any imbalance of yin and yang?
- Is your chi (internal energy) low?
- Do you believe it is your destiny to have this condition or your destiny not to have this condition (fatalism versus well-being approach to illness)?

Joint Pain (See Box 3-5)

Night Pain (See Box 3-7)

Psychogenic Source of Symptoms (See Box 3-13)

CASE STUDY*

REFERRAL

A 44-year old male was referred to physical therapy with a report of right-sided thoracic pain.

Past Medical History: The client reported a 20-pack year smoking history (one-pack per day for 20 years) and denied the use of alcohol or drugs. There was no other significant past medical history reported. He had a sedentary job.

The client's symptoms began following chiropractic intervention to relieve left-sided lower extremity radiating pain. Within 6 to 8 hours after the chiropractor manipulated the client's thoracic spine, he reported sharp shooting pain on the right side of the upper thoracic spine at T4. The pain radiated laterally under the right axilla into the anterior chest. He also reported tension and tightness along the same thoracic level and moderate discomfort during inspiration. There was no history of thoracic pain prior to the upper thoracic manipulation by the chiropractor.

The client saw his primary care physician who referred him to physical therapy for treatment. No imaging studies were done prior to physical therapy referral. The client rated the pain as a constant 10/10 on the Numeric Rating Scale (NRS) during sitting activities at work. He also reported pain waking him at night.

The client was unable to complete a full day at work without onset of thoracic discomfort; pain was aggravated by prolonged sitting.

EVALUATION

The client was described as slender in build (ectomorph body type) with forward head and shoulders and kyphotic posturing as observed in the upright and sitting positions. There were no significant signs of inflammation or superficial tissue changes observed or palpated in the thoracic spine region. There was palpable tenderness at approximately the T4 costotransverse joint and along the corresponding rib.

* Leanne Lenker, DPT. This case was part of an internship experience at St. Luke's Outpatient Clinic, Allentown, PA under the supervision of Jeff Bays, MSPT (Clinical Instructor). Dr. Lenker is a graduate of the University of St. Augustine for Health Sciences program in St. Augustine, Florida. Used with permission, 2005.

CASE STUDY*—cont'd

A full orthopedic evaluation was conducted to determine the biomechanical and soft tissue dysfunction that produced the client's signs and symptoms. Active and passive motion and intersegmental mobility were tested. Findings were consistent with a physical therapy diagnosis of hypomobile costotransverse joint at level T4.

This was further evidenced by pain at the posterior costovertebral joint with radiating pain laterally into the chest wall. Pain was increased on inspiration. Patient had a smoker's cough, but reported no other associated signs or symptoms of any kind. See the Pain Assessment Record Form that follows.

RESULT

The client obtained gradual relief from painful symptoms after 8 treatment sessions of stretches and costotransverse joint mobilization (grade 4, non-thrust progressive oscillations at the end of the available range). Pain was reduced from 10/10 to 3/10 and instances of night pain had decreased. The client could sit at work with only mild discomfort, which he could correct with stretching.

The client's thoracic pain returned on the 10th and 11th treatment sessions. He attributed this to increased stressors at work and long work hours. Night pain and pain with respiratory movements (inhalation) increased again.

Red flags in this case included:
- Age over 40
- History of smoking (20 pack years)
- Symptoms persisting beyond the expected time for physiologic healing
- Pain out of proportion to the injury
- Recurring symptoms (failure to respond to physical therapy intervention)
- Pain is constant and intense; night pain

The client was returned to his primary care physician for further diagnostic studies and later diagnosed with metastatic lung cancer.

SUMMARY

Working with clients several times a week allows the therapist to monitor their symptoms and the effectiveness of interventions. This case study shows the importance of reassessment and awareness of red flags that would lead a practitioner to suspect the symptoms may be pathologic.

Pain Assessment Record Form

Date: 10/05/06

Client's name: #21022

Physician's diagnosis: *Back pain*

Physical therapist's diagnosis:
Hypomobile costotransverse joint at T4 level

Medications: _pain medication (specifics unknown)_

Onset of pain (circle one) Was there an:

Accident   Injury   Specific activity

If yes, describe:
Chiropractor manipulated the thoracic spine; 6-8 hours later the client had shooting pain as shown below
Date of injury: 2 weeks ago (09/21/06)

(Trauma)/violence — circled

Characteristics of pain/symptoms:

Location (Show me exactly where your pain/symptom is located):

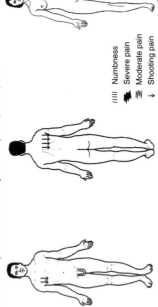

||||| Numbness
ЖЖ Severe pain
ЖЖ Moderate pain
→ Shooting pain

Sharp shooting pain
Right side of upper thoracic spine at T4
Pain radiates laterally under the ®axilla into the anterior chest

Do you have any pain or symptoms anywhere else?   Yes   (No)

Description (If yes, what does it feel like):
Tension and tightness along the same thoracic level

Circle any other words that describe the client's symptoms:

Knifelike	Dull	Aching	Other (describe):
Boring	Burning	Throbbing	
Heaviness	Discomfort	(Sharp)	
Stinging	Tingling	(Stabbing) "shooting"	

Frequency (circle one):

If constant: Do you have this pain right now?   (Constant)   Intermittent (comes and goes)

(Yes)   No

If intermittent: How often is the pain present (circle all that apply):

Hourly   Once/daily   Twice/daily   Unpredictable   Other(please describe):

Intensity: *Numeric Rating Scale* and the *Faces Pain Scale*

Instructions: On a scale from 0 to 10 with zero meaning 'No pain' and 10 for 'Unbearable pain,' how would you rate your pain right now?

Pain Assessment Scale

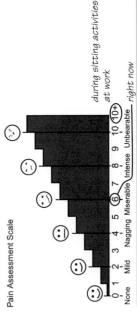

0   1   2   3   4   5   6   7   8   9   10   10+
None Mild Nagging Miserable Intense Unbearable

during sitting activities
at work
right now

Alternately: Point to the face that best shows how much pain you are having right now.

Intensity: *Visual Analog Scale*

Instructions: On the line below, put a mark (or point to) the place on the line between 'Pain free' and 'Worst possible pain' that best describes/shows how much pain you are having right now.

Pain Free _____ Worst Possible Pain

Duration:

How long does your pain (name the symptom) last? *all the time; intensity varies but always present*

Aggravating factors (What makes it worse?)

Prolonged positions, especially sitting
Inhalation

Relieving factors (What makes it better?)

Pattern

Has the pain changed since it first began?   Yes   (No)

If yes, please explain:

What is your pain/symptom like from morning (am) to evening (pm)?

Pain is work/position-related and gets worse after sitting at work; better at home in the evening then much worse at night after several hours sleeping

| **Circle one:** | Worse in the morning | Worse midday/afternoon | (Worse at night) |
| **Circle one:** | Gradually getting better | Gradually getting worse | (Staying the same) |

Circle all that apply:

Present upon waking up   Keeps me from falling asleep   (Wakes me up at night)

Therapist: Record any details or description about night pain. See also Appendix for *Screening Questions for Night Pain* when appropriate:

Associated symptoms (What other symptoms have you had with this problem?)

Circle any words the client uses to describe his/her symptoms. If the client says there are no other symptoms ask about the presence of any of the following:

Burning	(Difficulty breathing)	Shortness of breath	Cough
Skin rash (or other lesions)	Change in bowel/bladder	Difficulty swallowing	Painful swallowing
Dizziness	Heart palpitations	Hoarseness	Nausea/vomiting
Diarrhea	Constipation	Bleeding of any kind	Sweats
Numbness	Problems with vision	Tingling	Weakness
Joint pain	Weight loss/gain	Other:	

Final question: Are there any other pain or symptoms of any kind anywhere else in your body that we have not talked about yet? *No*

For the therapist:

Follow up questions can include:

Are there any positions that make it feel better? Worse?

How does rest affect the pain/symptoms?

How does activity affect the pain/symptoms?

How has this problem affected your daily life at work or at home?

Has this problem affected your ability to care for yourself without assistance (e.g. dress, bathe, cook, drive)?

Has this problem affected your sexual function or activity?

Therapist's evaluation:

Can you reproduce the pain by squeezing or palpating the symptomatic area?

Does resisted motion reproduce the pain/symptoms?

Is the client taking NSAIDs? Experiencing increased symptoms after taking NSAIDs?

If taking NSAIDs, is the client at risk for peptic ulcer? Check all that apply:

☐ Age>65 years   ☐ History of peptic ulcer disease or GI disease

☐ Smoking, alcohol use   ☐ Oral corticosteroid use

☐ Anticoagulation or use of other anticoagulants (even when used for heart patients at a lower dose, e.g., 81 to 325 mg aspirin/day)

☐ Renal complications in clients with hypertension or congestive heart failure (CHF) or who use diuretics or ACE inhibitors

☐ NSAIDs combined with selective serotonin reuptake inhibitors (SSRIs; antidepressants such as Prozac, Zoloft, Celexa, Paxil)

☐ Use of acid suppressants (e.g., H_2-receptor antagonists, antacids)

Other areas to consider:

- Sleep quality
- Correlation of symptoms with peak effect of medications (dosage, time of day)
- Evaluation of joint pain (see Appendix: Screening Questions for Joint Pain)
- Bowel/bladder habits
- Depression or anxiety screening score
- For women: correlation of symptoms with menstrual cycle

PRACTICE QUESTIONS

1. What is the best follow up question for someone who tells you that the pain is constant?
   a. Can you use one finger to point to the pain location?
   b. Do you have that pain right now?
   c. Does the pain wake you up at night after you have fallen asleep?
   d. Is there anything that makes the pain better or worse?

2. A 52-year old woman with shoulder pain tells you that she has pain at night that awakens her. After asking a series of follow up questions, you are able to determine that she had trouble falling asleep because her pain increases when she goes to bed. Once she falls asleep, she wakes up as soon as she rolls onto that side. What is the most likely explanation for this pain behavior?
   a. Minimal distractions heighten a person's awareness of musculoskeletal discomfort.
   b. This is a systemic pattern that is associated with a neoplasm.
   c. It is impossible to tell.
   d. This represents a chronic clinical presentation of a musculoskeletal problem.

3. Referred pain patterns associated with impairment of the spleen can produce musculoskeletal symptoms in:
   a. The left shoulder
   b. The right shoulder
   c. The mid- or upper back, scapular, and right shoulder areas
   d. The thorax, scapulae, right, or left shoulder

4. Associated signs and symptoms are a major red flag for pain of a systemic or visceral origin compared to musculoskeletal pain.
   a. True
   b. False

5. Words used to describe neurogenic pain often include:
   a. Throbbing, pounding, beating
   b. Crushing, shooting, pricking
   c. Aching, heavy, sore
   d. Agonizing, piercing, unbearable

6. Pain (especially intense bone pain) that is disproportionately relieved by aspirin can be a symptom of:
   a. Neoplasm
   b. Assault or trauma
   c. Drug dependence
   d. Fracture

7. Joint pain can be a reactive, delayed, or allergic response to:
   a. Medications
   b. Chemicals
   c. Infections
   d. Artificial sweeteners
   e. All of the above

8. Bone pain associated with neoplasm is characterized by:
   a. Increases with weight bearing
   b. Negative heel strike
   c. Relieved by Tums or other antacid in women
   d. Goes away after eating

9. Pain of a viscerogenic nature is not relieved by a change in position.
   a. True
   b. False

10. Referred pain from the viscera can occur alone, but is usually preceded by visceral pain when an organ is involved.
    a. True
    b. False

11. A 48-year old man presented with low back pain of unknown cause. He works as a carpenter and says he is very active, has workrelated mishaps (accidents and falls), and engages in repetitive motions of all kinds using his arms, back, and legs. The pain is intense when he has it, but it seems to come and go. He is not sure if eating makes the pain better or worse. He has lost his appetite because of the pain. After conducting an examination including a screening exam, the clinical presentation does not match the expected pattern for a musculoskeletal or neuromuscular problem. You refer him to a physician for medical testing. You find out later he had pancreatitis. What is the most likely explanation for this pain pattern?
    a. Toxic waste products from the pancreas are released into the intestines causing irritation of the retroperitoneal space.
    b. Rupture of the pancreas causes internal bleeding and referred pain called Kehr's sign.
    c. The pancreas and low back structures are formed from the same embryologic tissue in the mesoderm
    d. Obstruction, irritation, or inflammation of the body of the pancreas distends the pancreas, thus applying pressure on the central respiratory diaphragm

REFERENCES

1. Flaherty JH: Who's taking your fifth vital sign? *J Gerontol A Biol Sci Med Sci* 56:M397-399, 2001.

2. Rex L: *Evaluation and treatment of somatovisceral dysfunction of the gastrointestinal system*, Edmonds, WA, 2004, URSA Foundation.

3. Haines DE: *Fundamental neuroscience*, ed 2, Philadelphia, 2002, Churchill Livingstone.

4. Saladin KS: Personal communication, Distinguished Professor of Biology, Georgia College and State University, Milledgeville, Georgia, 2004.

5. Woolf CJ, Decosterd I: Implications of recent advances in the understanding of pain pathophysiology for the assessment of pain in patients, *Pain Suppl* 6:S141-147, Aug 1999.

6. Strigio I: Differentiation of visceral and cutaneous pain in the human brain, *J Neurophysiol* 89:3294-3303. Available at http://jn.physiology.org/cgi/content/abstract/89/6/3294

7. Aziz Q: Functional neuroimaging of visceral sensation, *J Clin Neurophysiol* 17:604-612. Available at: http://www.ncbi.nlm.nih.gov/entrez/query.fcgi?cmd=Retrieve&db=PubMed&listuids=11151978&dopt=Abstract

8. Leavitt RL: Developing cultural competence in a multicultural world. Part II, *PT Magazine* 11(1):56-70, 2003.

9. O'Rourke D: The measurement of pain in infants, children, and adolescents: from policy to practice, *Physical Therapy* 84(6):560-570, 2004.

10. Wentz JD: Assessing pain at the end of life, *Nursing2003* 33(8):22, 2003.

11. Melzack R: The McGill Pain Questionnaire: major properties and scoring methods, *Pain* 1:277, 1975.

12. Leveille SG: Musculoskeletal aging, *Curr Opin Rheumatol* 16(2):114-118, 2004.

13. American Geriatrics Society Panel on Persistent Pain in Older Persons (revised guideline), *Journal of the American Geriatrics Society* 50(Suppl 6):205-224, 2002.

14. Herr KA, Spratt K, Mobily PR, et al: Pain intensity assessment in older adults: use of experimental pain to compare psychometric properties and usability of selected pain scales with younger adults, *Clin J Pain* 20(4):207-219, 2004.

15. Lane P: Assessing pain in patients with advanced dementia, *Nursing2004* 34(8):17, 2004.

16. D'Arcy Y: Assessing pain in patients who can't communicate, *Nursing2004* 34(10):27, 2004.

17. Hurley AC: Assessment of discomfort in advanced Alzheimer patients, *Res Nurs Health* 15(5):369-377, 1992.

18. Warden V, Hurley AC, Volicer L: Development and psychometric evaluation of the Pain Assessment in Advanced Dementia (PAINAD) scale, *J Am Med Dir Assoc* 4(1):9-15, 2003.

19. Feldt K: The checklist of nonverbal pain indicators (CNPI), *Pain Manag Nurs* 1(1):13-21, 2000.

20. Pasero C, Reed BA, McCaffery M: Pain in the elderly. In McCaffery M, Pasero C: *Pain: clinical manual*, ed 2, St. Louis, 1999, Mosby; pp 674-710.

21. Ferrell BA: Pain in cognitively impaired nursing home patients, *J Pain Symptom Manage* 10(8):591-598, 1995.

22. Wong D, Baker C: Pain in children: comparison of assessment scales, *Pediatr Nurs* 14(1):9-17, 1988.

23. Hicks CL, von Baeyer CL, Spafford PA, et al: The Faces Pain Scale-Revised: toward a common metric in pediatric pain measurement, *Pain* 93:173-183, 2001.

24. Bieri D: The Faces Pain Scale for the self-assessment of the severity of pain experienced by children: development, initial validation, and preliminary investigation for the ratio scale properties, *Pain* 41(2):139-150, 1990.

25. Wong on Web. FACES *Pain Rating Scale*, Elsevier Health Science Information, 2004. Available at: http://www3.us.elsevierhealth.com/WOW/faces.html, 2004.

26. Baker-Lefkowicz A, Keller V, Wong DL, et al: Young children's pain rating using the FACES Pain Rating Scale with original vs abbreviated word instructions, unpublished, 1996.

27. von Baeyer CL, Hicks CL: Support for a common metric for pediatric pain intensity scales, *Pain Res Manage* 4(2):157-160, 2000.

28. Ramelet AS, Abu-Saad HH, Rees N et al: The challenges of pain measurement in critically ill young children: a comprehensive review, *Aust Crit Care* 17(1):33-45, 2004.

29. Grunau RE, Craig KD: Pain expression in neonates: facial action and cry, *Pain* 28:395-410, 1987.

30. Grunau RE, Oberlander T, Holsti L, et al: Bedside application of the Neonatal Facial Coding System in pain assessment of premature neonates, *Pain* 76:277-286, 1998.

31. Peters JW, Koot HM, Grunau RE, et al: Neonatal Facial Coding System for assessing postoperative pain in infants: item reduction is valid and feasible, *Clin J Pain* 19(6):353-363, 2003.

32. Stevens B: Pain in infants. In McCaffery M, Pasero C, editors: *Pain: clinical manual*, ed 2, St. Louis, 1999, Mosby; pp 626-673.

33. McGrath PA, Gillespie J: Pain assessment in children and adolescents. In Turk DC, Melzack R, editors: *Handbook of pain assessment*, ed 2, New York, 2001, Guilford Press; pp 97-118.

34. Riley JL 3rd, Wade JB, Myers CD, et al: Racial/ethnic differences in the experience of chronic pain, *Pain* 100(3):291-298, 2002.

35. Sheffield D, Biles PL, Orom H, et al: Race and sex differences in cutaneous pain perception, *Psychosom Med* 62(4):517-523, 2000.

36. Unruh AM, Ritchie J, Merskey H: Does gender affect appraisal of pain and pain coping strategies? *Clin J Pain* 15(1):31-40, 1999.

37. Brown JL, Sheffield D, Leary MR, et al: Social support and experimental pain, *Psychosom Med* 65(2):276-283, 2003.

38. Huskinson EC: Measurement of pain, *Lancet* 2:1127-1131, 1974.

39. Carlsson AM: Assessment of chronic pain: aspects of the reliability and validity of the visual analog scale, *Pain* 16:87-101, 1983.

40. Dworkin RH, Nagasako EM, Galer BS: Assessment of neuropathic pain. In Turk DC, Melzack R, editors: *Handbook of pain assessment*, ed 2, New York, 2001, Guilford Press; pp 519-548.

41. Sahrmann S: *Diagnosis and diagnosticians: the future in physical therapy*, Combined Sections Meeting, Dallas, February 13-16, 1997. Available at www.apta.org.

42. American Psychiatric Association (APA): *Diagnostic and statistical manual of mental disorders (DSM-IV-TR)*, Washington, DC, 1994, APA.

43. Goodman CC, Boissonnault WG, Fuller K: *Pathology: implications for the physical therapist*, ed 2, Philadelphia, 2003, WB Saunders.

44. Morrison J: *DSM-IV made easy: the clinician's guide to diagnosis*, New York, 1995, Guilford. Also available from the author at: http://mysite.verizon.net/res7oqx1/index.html [Email: morrison94@usa.net].

45. De Gucht V, Fischler M: Somatization: a critical review of conceptual and methodological issues, *Psychosomatics* 43:1-9, 2002.

46. Wells PE, Frampton V, Bowsher D: *Pain management by physical therapy*, ed 2, Oxford, 1994, Butterworth-Heinemann.

47. Simons D, Travell J: *Myofascial pain and dysfunction: the trigger point manual*, ed 2, Vol 1 and 2, Baltimore, 1999, Williams and Wilkins.

48. Bennett GF: Neuropathic pain. In Wall PD, Melzack R, editors: *Textbook of pain*, ed 3, New York, 1994, Churchill Livingstone; pp 201-224.

49. Tasker RR: Spinal cord injury and central pain. In Aronoff GM, editor: *Evaluation and treatment of chronic pain*, ed 3, Philadelphia, 1999, Lippincott, Williams & Wilkins; pp 131-146.

50. Pachas WN: Joint pains and associated disorders. In Aronoff GM, editor: *Evaluation and treatment of chronic pain*, ed 3, Philadelphia, 1999, Lippincott Williams and Wilkins; pp 201-215.

51. Kraus H: Muscle deficiency. In Rachlin ES, editor: *Myofascial pain and fibromyalgia*, St. Louis, 1994, Mosby.

52. Cailliet R: *Low back pain syndrome*, ed 5, Philadelphia, 1995, FA Davis.

53. Emre M, Mathies H: *Muscle spasms and pain*, Park Ridge, Illinois, 1988, Parthenon.

54. Sinnott M: Assessing musculoskeletal changes in the geriatric population, American Physical Therapy Association Combined Sections Meeting, February 3-7, 1993.

55. Potter JF: The older orthopaedic patient. General considerations, *Clin Orthop Rel Res* 425:44-49, 2004.

56. Headley BJ: *When movement hurts: a self-help manual for treating trigger points.* Innovative Systems, 1997. (Barbara Headley, MS, PT, EMS, director, and CEO of Headley Systems, Colorado, www.360wd.com/headleysystems/home.html).

57. Kostopoulos D, Rizopoulos K: The *manual of trigger point and myofascial therapy*, Thorofare, NJ, 2001, Slack.

58. Rachlin ES, Rachlin IS, editors: *Myofascial pain and fibromyalgia: trigger point management*, ed 2, St. Louis, 2002, Mosby.

59. Blaylock RL: *Excitotoxins: the taste that kills*, New Mexico, 1996, Health Press. Available on-line: www.directtextbook.com/publisher/health-press-nm or http://www.russellblaylockmd.com/.

60. Roberts HJ: *Aspartame disease: the ignored epidemic*, West Palm Beach, Fl, 1995, Sunshine Sentinel Press.

61. Roberts HJ: *Defense against Alzheimer's disease*, West Palm Beach, Fl, 2001, Sunshine Sentinel Press.

62. Issa NC, Thompson RL: Diagnosing and managing septic arthritis: a practical approach, *J Musculoskel Med* 20(2):70-75, 2003.

63. Sapico FL, Liquete JA, Sarma RJ: Bone and joint infections in patients with infective endocarditis: review of a 4-year experience, *Clin Infect Dis* 22:783-787, 1996.

64. Lutz B: Septic arthritis following anterior cruciate ligament reconstruction using tendon allografts–Florida and Louisiana, 2000, *MMWR* 50(48):1081-1083, 2001.

65. Pola E: Onset of Berger disease after *Staphylococcus aureus* infection: septic arthritis after anterior cruciate ligament reconstruction, *Arthroscopy* 19(4):E29, 2003.

66. Kumar S, Cowdery JS: Managing acute monarthritis in primary care practice, *J Musculoskel Med* 21(9):465-472, 2004.

67. Bonica J: *The management of pain*, ed 2, Vol 1, Philadelphia, 1990, Lea & Febiger.

68. Waddell G, Bircher, M, Finlayson D, et al: Symptoms and signs: physical disease or illness behaviour? *BMJ* 289:739-741, 1984.

69. Ozburn MS, Nichols JW: Pubic ramus and adductor insertion stress fractures in female basic trainees, Mil Med 146(5):332-334, 1981.

70. Cyriax J: *Textbook of orthopaedic medicine*, ed 8, Vol 1, London, 1982, Baillière.

71. Management of the individual with pain: Part 1–physiology and evaluation, *PT Magazine* 4(11):54-63, 1996.

72. Merskey H, Bogduk N: *Classification of chronic pain*, ed 2, Seattle, 1994, International Association for the Study of Pain.

73. Waddell G: *The back pain revolution*, ed 2, Philadelphia, 2004, Churchill Livingstone.

74. Hellsing AL, Linton SJ, Kälvemark M: A prospective study of patients with acute back and neck pain in Sweden, *Physical Therapy* 74(2):116-128, 1994.

75. Turk DC, Melzack R, editors: *Handbook of pain assessment*, ed 2, New York, 2001, Guilford Press.

76. Melzack R: From the gate to the neuromatrix, *Pain* 6(suppl 6):S121-126, 1999.

77. Turk DC: Understanding pain sufferers: the role of cognitive processes, *Spine J* 4(1):1-7, 2004.

78. Lethem J, Slade PD, Troup JDG, et al: Outline of a fear-avoidance model of exaggerated pain perception. I, *Behav Res Ther.* 21(4):401-408, 1983.

79. Slade PD, Troup JDG, Lethem J, et al: The fear-avoidance model of exaggerated pain perception. II, *Behav Res Ther* 21(4):409-416, 1983.

80. Waddell G, Somerville D, Henderson I, et al: A fear avoidance beliefs questionnaire (FABQ) and the role of fear avoidance beliefs in chronic low back pain and disability, *Pain* 52:157-168, 1993.

81. George SZ: Personal communication, May 2004.

82. George SZ, Bialosky JE, Fritz JM: Physical therapist management of a patient with acute low back pain and elevated fear-avoidance beliefs, *Physical Therapy* 84(6):538-549, 2004.

83. Fritz JM, George SZ: Identifying psychosocial variables in patients with acute work-related low back pain. The importance of fear-avoidance beliefs, *Physical Therapy* 82(10):973-983, 2002.

84. Cooner E, Amorosi S: The study of pain and older Americans, New York, 1997, Louis Harris and Associates (Harris Opinion Poll).

85. Barsky AJ, Hochstrasser B, Coles NA, et al: Silent myocardial ischemia: Is the person or the event silent? *JAMA* 364:1132-1135, 1990.

86. Kauvar DR: The geriatric acute abdomen, *Clin Geriatr Med* 9:547-558, 1993.

87. Norman DC, Toledo SD: Infections in elderly persons: an altered clinical presentation, *Clin Geriatr Med* 8:713-719, 1992.

88. AGS Panel on Chronic Pain in Older Persons: The management of chronic pain in older persons, *J Am Geriatr Soc* 46:635-651, 1998.

89. Connelly C: Managing low back pain and psychosocial overlie, *J Musculoskel Med* 21(8):409-419, 2004.

90. Main CJ, Waddell G: Behavioral responses to examination: a reappraisal of the interpretation of "nonorganic signs," *Spine* 23(21): 2367-2371, 1998.

91. Scalzitti DA: Screening for psychological factors in patients with low back problems: Waddell's nonorganic signs, *Phys Ther* 77(3):306-312, 1997.

92. Teasell RW, Shapiro AP: Strategic-behavioral intervention in the treatment of chronic nonorganic motor disorders, *Am J Phys Med Rehab* 73(1):44-50, 1994.

93. Waddell G: Symptoms and signs: physical disease or illness behavior? *BMJ* 289:739-741, 1984.

94. Barsky AJ, Goodson JD, Lane RS, et al: The amplification of somatic symptoms, *Psychosom Med* 50(5):510-519, 1988.

95. Turk DC: Understanding pain sufferers: the role of cognitive processes, *Spine J* 4:1-7, 2004.

96. Beck AT, Epstein N, Brown G, et al: An inventory for measuring clinical anxiety: psychometric properties, *J Consult Clin Psych* 56:893-897, 1988.

97. Steer RA, Beck AT: Beck anxiety inventory. In Zalaquett CP, Wood RJ, editors: *Evaluating stress: a book of resources*, Lanham, MD, 1997, Scarecrow Press.

98. Brenes GA: Anxiety and chronic obstructive pulmonary disease: prevalence, impact, and treatment, *Psychosom Med* 65(6):963-970, 2003.

99. Wassertheil-Smoller S, Shumaker S, Ockene J, et al: Depression and cardiovascular sequelae in postmenopausal women. The Women's Health Initiative (WHI), *Arch Intern Med* 164(3):289-298, 2004.

100. Miller MC: Depression and pain, *Harvard Mental Health* 21(3):4, 2004.

101. World Health Organization (WHO): 2004. www.who.int [type in Depression in search window].

102. Andrade L, Caraveo-Anduaga JJ, Berglund P, et al: The epidemiology of major depressive episodes: results from the International Consortium of Psychiatric Epidemiology (ICPE) surveys, *International J Methods Psychiatr Research* 12(3):165, 2003.

103. Abe T: Increased incidence of depression and its socio-cultural background in Japan, *Seishin Shinkeigaku Zasshi* 105(1):36-42, 2003.

104. Kessler RC: Epidemiology of women and depression, *J Affect Disord* 74(1):5-13, 2003.

105. Smith NL: *The effects of depression and anxiety on medical illness*, University of Utah, Stress Medicine Clinic, Sandy, Utah, 2002.

106. Corsico A, McGuffin P: Psychiatric genetics: recent advances and clinical implications, *Epidemiol Psychiatr Soc* 10(4):253-259, 2001.

107. Lotrich FE, Pollock BG: Meta-analysis of serotonin transporter polymorphisms and affective disorders, *Psychiatr Genet* 14(3):121-129, 2004.

108. Lee MS, Lee HY, Lee HJ, et al: Serotonin transporter promoter gene polymorphism and long-term outcome of antidepressant treatment, *Psychiatr Genet* 14(2):111-115, 2004.

109. McGuffin P, Marusic A, Farmer A: What can psychiatric genetics offer suicidology? *Crisis* 22(2):61-65, 2001.

110. Lespérance F, Jaffe AS: Beyond the blues: understanding the link between coronary artery disease and depression. Retrieved June 15, 2006, from *http://www.medscape.com/viewarticle/423461*

111. Lydiard RB: Irritable bowel syndrome, anxiety, and depression. What are the links? *J Clin Psychiatry* 62(Suppl 8):38-45, 2001.

112. Haggman S, Maher CG, Refshauge KM: Screening for symptoms of depression by physical therapists managing low back pain, *Physical Therapy* 84(12):1157-1166, 2004.

113. Sartorius N, Ustun T, Lecrubier Y, et al: Depression comorbid with anxiety: results from the WHO study on psychological disorders in primary health care, *Br J Psychiatry* 168:38-40, 1996.

114. Beck AT, Ward CH, Mendelson M, et al: An inventory for measuring depression, *Arch Gen Psychiatry* 4:561-571, 1961.

115. C de C Williams A, Richardson PH: What does the BDI measure in chronic pain? *Pain* 55:259-266, 1993.

116. Yesavage JA: The geriatric depression scale, *J Psychiatr Res* 17(1):37-49, 1983.

117. Zung WWK: A self-rating depression scale, *Arch Gen Psychiatry* 12:63-70, 1965.

118. Harcourt Assessment (formerly The Psychological Corporation): *The Beck scales*, San Antonio, 2004.

119. Garakani A, Win T, Virk S, et al: Comorbidity of irritable bowel syndrome in psychiatric patients: a review, *Am J Ther* 10(1):61-67, 2003.

120. Campo JV, Dahl RE, Williamson DE, et al: Gastrointestinal distress to serotonergic challenge: a risk marker for emotional disorder? *J Am Acad Child Adolesc Psychiatry* 42(10):1221-1226, 2003.

121. Salt WB: *Irritable bowel syndrome and the mind-body/brain-gut connection*, Columbus, Ohio, 1997, Parkview.

122. Chang L, Berman S, Mayer EA, et al: Brain responses to visceral and somatic stimuli in patients with irritable bowel syndrome with and without fibromyalgia, *Am J Gastroenterol* 98(6):1354-1361, 2003.

123. Miller MC: Understanding depression. A special health report from Harvard Medical School, Boston, 2003.

124. Hendrix ML: *Understanding panic disorder*, Washington, DC, 1993, National Institutes of Health.

125. Melzack R, Dennis SG: Neurophysiologic foundations of pain. In Sternbach RA, editor: *The psychology of pain*, New York, 1978, Raven Press; pp 1-26.

126. Wieseler-Frank J, Maier SF, Watkins LR: Glial activation and pathological pain, *Neurochem Int* 45(2-3):389-395, 2004.

127. Pert C: *Molecules of emotion. The science behind mind-body medicine*, New York, 1998, Simon and Schuster.

128. Knaster, M: Remembering through the body, *Massage Therapy Journal* 33(1):46-59, 1994.

129. Pearsall P: *The heart's code: new findings about cellular memories and their role in the mind/body/spirit connection*, New York, 1998, Broadway Books (Random House).

130. van der Kolk BA: The body keeps the score: memory and the evolving psychobiology of posttraumatic stress, *Harvard Review of Psychiatry* 1(5):253-265, 1994.

131. Van Meeteren NLU, et al: Psychoneuroendocrinology and its relevance for physical therapy [Abstract], *Physical Therapy* 81(5):A66, 2001.

132. Yang J: UniSci International Science News, posted July 30, 2001 [http://unisci.com/], source: University of Rochester Medical Center, Rochester, NY, 2001.

133. Watkins LR, Milligan ED, Maier SF: Glial proinflammatory cytokines mediate exaggerated pain states; implications for clinical pain, *Adv Exp Med Biol* 521:1-21, 2003.

134. Wu CM, Lin MW, Cheng JT, et al: Regulated, electroporation-mediated delivery of pro-opiomelanocortin gene suppresses chronic constriction injury-induced neuropathic pain in rats, *Gene Ther* 11(11):933-940, 2004.

135. Maier SF, Watkins LR: Immune-to-central nervous system communication and its role in modulating pain and cognition: implications for cancer and cancer treatment, *Brain Behav Immun* 17(Suppl 1):S125-131, 2003.

136. Watkins LR, Maier SF: The pain of being sick: implications of immune-to-brain communication for understanding pain, *Annu Rev Psychol* 51:29-57, 2000.

137. Watkins LR, Maier SF: Beyond neurons: evidence that immune and glial cells contribute to pathological pain states, *Physiol Rev* 82(4):981-1011, 2002.

138. Holguin A, O'Connor KA, Biedenkapp J, et al: HIV-1 gp120 stimulates proinflammatory cytokine-mediated pain facilitation via activation of nitric oxide synthase-I (nNOS), *Pain* 110(3):517-530, 2004.

139. Melzack R: The short-form McGill Pain Questionnaire, *Pain* 30:191-197, 1987.

140. Melzack R, Katz J: The McGill Pain Questionnaire: appraisal and current status. In Turk DC, Melzack R, editors: *Handbook of pain assessment*, ed 2, New York, 2001, Guilford Press; pp 35-52.

141. Matheson LN: Work capacity evaluation: systematic approach to industrial rehabilitation, Anaheim, CA, 1986, Employment and Rehabilitation Institute of California.

142. Matheson LN: *Symptom magnification casebook*, Anaheim, CA, 1987, Employment and Rehabilitation Institute of California.

143. Matheson LN: Symptom magnification syndrome structured interview: rationale and procedure, *J Occup Rehab* 1(1):43-56, 1991.

144. Olney C: Matter of semantics (letter to the editor), *ADVANCE for Physical Therapists & PT Assistants* 12(15):5, 2001.

145. Waddell G, McCulloch JA, Kummer E, et al: Nonorganic physical signs in low back pain, *Spine* 5(2):117-125, 1980.

146. Karas R, McIntosh G, Hall H, et al: The relationship between nonorganic signs and centralization of symptoms in the prediction of return to work for patients with low back pain, *Phys Ther* 77(4):354-360, 1997.

147. Rothstein JM, Erhard RE, Nicholson GG, et al: Conference, *Phys Ther* 77(4):361-369, 1997.

148. Rothstein JM: Unnecessary adversaries (editorial), *Physical Therapy* 77(4):352, 1997.
149. Goodwin RD: Association between physical activity and mental disorders among adults in the United States, *Prev Med* 36:698-703, 2003.
150. Lawlor DA, Hopker SW: The effectiveness of exercise as an intervention in the management of depression: systematic review and meta-regression analysis of randomized controlled trials, *BMJ* 322:1-8, 2001.
151. Dunn AL, Trivedi MH, Kampert JB, et al: The DOSE study: a clinical trial to examine efficacy and dose response of exercise as treatment for depression, *Control Clin Trials* 23:584-603, 2002.
152. Dowd SM, Vickers KS, Krahn D: Exercise for depression: physical activity boosts the power of medications and psychotherapy, *Psychiatry Online* 3(6): June 2004.

In the medical model, clients are often assessed from head to toe. The doctor, physician assistant, nurse, or nurse practitioner starts with inspection, followed by percussion and palpation, and finally by auscultation.

In a screening assessment, the therapist may not need to perform a complete head-to-toe physical assessment. If the initial observations, client history, screening questions, and screening tests are negative, move on to the next step. A thorough examination may not be necessary. In most situations, it is advised to assess one system above and below the area of complaint.

When screening for systemic origins of clinical signs and symptoms, the therapist first scans the area(s) that directly relate to the client's history and clinical presentation. For example, a shoulder problem can be caused by a problem in the stomach, heart, liver/biliary, lungs, spleen, kidneys, and ovaries (ectopic pregnancy). Only the physical assessment tests related to these areas would be assessed. And these often can be narrowed down by the client's history, gender, age, presence of risk factors, and associated signs and symptoms linked to a specific system.

More specifically, consider the postmenopausal woman with primary family history of heart disease who presents with shoulder pain that occurs three to four minutes after starting an activity and is accompanied by unexplained perspiration. This individual should be assessed for cardiac involvement. Or think about the 45-year old mother of five children who presents with scapular pain that is worse after she eats. A cardiac assessment may not be as important as a scan for signs and symptoms associated with the gallbladder or biliary system.

Documentation of physical findings is important. From a legal standpoint, if you did not document it, you did not assess it. Look for changes from the expected norm as well as changes for the client's baseline measurements. Use simple and clear documentation that can be understood and used by others. As much as possible, record both normal and abnormal findings for each client.[1] Keep in mind the client's cultural and educational background, beliefs, values, and previous experiences can influence his or her response to questions.

Finally, screening and ongoing physical assessment is often a part of an exercise evaluation, especially for the client with one or more serious health concerns. Listening to the heart and lung sounds before initiating an exercise program may bring to light any contraindications to exercise. A compromised cardiopulmonary system may make it impossible and even dangerous for the client to sustain prescribed exercise levels.

▼ GENERAL SURVEY

Physical assessment begins the moment you meet the client as you observe body size and type, facial expressions, evaluate self-care, and note anything unusual in appearance or presentation. Keep in mind (as discussed

in Chapter 2) that cultural factors may dictate how the client presents himself (e.g., avoiding eye contact when answering questions, hiding or exaggerating signs of pain).

A few pieces of equipment in a small kit within easy reach can make the screening exam faster and easier (Box 4-1). Using the same pattern in screening each time will help the therapist avoid missing important screening clues.

As the therapist makes a general survey of each client, it is also possible to evaluate posture, movement patterns and gait, balance, and coordination. For more involved clients the first impression may be based on level of consciousness, respiratory and vascular function, or nutritional status.

In an acute care or trauma setting the therapist may be using vital signs and the ABCDE (airway, breathing, circulation, disability, exposure) method of quick assessment. A common strategy for history taking in the trauma unit is the mnemonic: AMPLE: **A**llergies, **M**edications, **P**ast medical history, **L**ast meal, and **E**vents of injury.

In any setting, knowing the client's personal health history will also help guide and direct which components of the physical examination to include. We are not just screening for medical disease masquerading as neuromusculoskeletal (NMS) problems. Many physical illnesses, diseases, and medical conditions directly impact the NMS system and must be taken into account. For example inspection of the integument, limb inspection, and screening of the peripheral vascular

system is important for someone at risk for lymphedema.

Neurologic function, balance, reflexes, and peripheral circulation become important when screening a client with diabetes mellitus. Peripheral neuropathy is common in this population group, often making walking more difficult and increasing risk of other problems developing.

Therapists in all settings but especially primary care therapists can use a screening physical assessment to provide education toward primary prevention as well as intervention and management of current dysfunctions and disabilities.

Mental Status

Level of consciousness, orientation, and ability to communicate are all part of the assessment of a client's mental status. Orientation refers to the client's ability to answer correctly questions about time, place, and person. A healthy individual with normal mental status will be alert, speak coherently, and be aware of the date, day, and time of day.

The therapist must be aware of any factor that can affect a client's current mental status. Shock, head injury, stroke, medications, age, and the use of substances and/or alcohol (see discussion, Chapter 2) can cause impaired consciousness.

Other factors affecting mental status may include malnutrition, exposure to chemicals, and hypo- or hyperthermia. Depression and anxiety (see discussion, Chapter 3) also can affect a client's functioning, mood, memory, ability to concentrate, judgment, and thought processes. Educational and socioeconomic background along with communication skills (e.g., English as a second language, aphasia) can affect mental status and function.

In a hospital, transition unit, or extended care facility, mental status is often evaluated and documented by the social worker or nursing service. It is always a good idea to review the client's chart or electronic record regarding this information before beginning a physical therapy evaluation.

It is not uncommon for older adults to experience a change in mental status or go through a stage of confusion after a general anesthetic. Physicians may refer to this as iatrogenic delirium or anesthesia-induced dementia. The cause of deterioration in mental ability is unknown. In some cases dementia appears to be triggered by the shock to the body of anesthesia and surgery.[2,3] It may be a passing phase with complete recovery by the client, although this can take weeks to months.

Several scales are used to assess level of consciousness, performance, and disability. The

BOX 4-1 ▼ Contents of a Screening Examination Kit
• Stethoscope
• Sphygmomanometer
• Thermometer
• Pulse oximeter
• Reflex hammer
• Penlight
• Safety pin or sharp object (tongue depressor broken in half gives sharp and dull sides)
• Cotton-tipped swab or cotton ball
• 2 test tubes
• Familiar objects (e.g., paper clip, coin, marble)
• Tuning fork (128 Hz)
• Watch with ability to count seconds
• Gloves for palpation of skin lesions
• Ruler or plastic tape measure to measure wound dimensions, skin lesions, leg length
• Goniometer

TABLE 4-1 ▼ Karnofsky Performance Scale (Rating in %)

Score	Description
100	Normal, no complaints; no evidence of disease
90	Able to carry on normal activities; minor signs or symptoms of disease
80	Normal activity with effort; some signs or symptoms of disease
70	Cares for self, unable to carry on normal activity or to do active work
60	Requires occasional assistance, but able to care for most of own personal needs
50	Requires considerable assistance and frequent medical care
40	Disabled; requires special care and assistance
30	Severely disabled; hospitalization indicated though death not imminent
20	Very ill; hospitalization required; active supportive treatment necessary
10	Failing rapidly; moribund
0	Dead

Glasgow Outcome Scale[4,5] describes patients/clients on a 5-point scale from good recovery (1) to death (5). Vegetative state, severe disability, and moderate disability are included in the continuum. This and other scales and clinical assessment tools are not part of the screening assessment but are available on-line for use by health care professionals.[6]

The Karnofsky Performance Scale (KPS; Table 4-1) is used widely to quantify functional status in a wide variety of individuals, but especially among those with cancer. It can be used to compare effectiveness of intervention and to assess individual prognosis. The lower the Karnofsky score, the worse the prognosis for survival.

The most practical performance scale for use in any rehabilitation setting for most clients is the ECOG Performance Status Scale (Table 4-2). Researchers and health care professionals use these scales and criteria to assess how an individual's disease is progressing, assess how the disease affects the daily living abilities of the client, and to determine appropriate treatment and prognosis.

Any observed change in level of consciousness, orientation, judgment, communication or speech pattern, or memory should be documented no matter what scale is used. The therapist may be the first to notice increased lethargy, slowed motor responses, or disorientation or confusion. Confusion is not a normal change with aging and must be reported and documented. Confusion

TABLE 4-2 ▼ ECOG Performance Status Scale

Grade	Level of activity
0	Fully active, able to carry on all pre-disease performance without restriction (Karnofsky 90-100%)
1	Restricted in physically strenuous activity but ambulatory and able to carry out work of a light or sedentary nature, e.g., light house work, office work (Karnofsky 70-80%)
2	Ambulatory and capable of all self-care but unable to carry out any work activities. Up and about more than 50% of waking hours (Karnofsky 50-60%)
3	Capable of only limited self-care, confined to bed or chair more than 50% of waking hours (Karnofsky 30-40%)
4	Completely disabled. Cannot carry on any self-care. Totally confined to bed or chair (Karnofsky 10-20%)
5	Dead (Karnofsky 0%)

The Karnofsky Performance Scale allows individuals to be classified according to functional impairment. The lower the score, the worse the prognosis for survival for most serious illnesses.
ECOG, Eastern Cooperative Oncology Group.
From Oken MM, Creech RH, Tormey DC, et al: Toxicity and response criteria of the Eastern Cooperative Oncology Group, *Am J Clin Oncol* 5:649-655, 1982. Available at: www.ecog.org/general/perf_stat.html.

is often associated with various systemic conditions (Table 4-3). Increased confusion in a client with any form of dementia can be a symptom of infection (e.g., pneumonia, urinary tract infection), electrolyte imbalance, or delirium. Likewise a sudden change in muscle tone (usually increased tone) in the client with a neurologic disorder (adult or child) can signal an infectious process.

Nutritional Status

Nutrition is an important part of growth and development and recovery from infection, illness, wounds, and surgery. Clients can exhibit signs of malnutrition or overnutrition (obesity).

Clinical Signs and Symptoms of Undernutrition or Malnutrition

- Muscle wasting
- Alopecia (hair loss)
- Dermatitis; dry, flaking skin
- Chapped lips, lesions at corners of mouth
- Brittle nails
- Abdominal distension
- Decreased physical activity/energy level; fatigue, lethargy
- Peripheral edema
- Bruising

TABLE 4-3 ▼ Systemic Conditions Associated with Confusional States

System	Impairment/Condition
Endocrine	Hypothyroidism, hyperthyroidism Perimenopause, menopause
Metabolic	Severe anemia Fluid and/or electrolyte imbalances; dehydration Wilson's disease (copper disorder) Porphyria (inherited disorder)
Immune/Infectious	Acquired Immunodeficiency Syndrome (AIDS) Cerebral amebiasis, toxoplasmosis, or malaria Fungal or tuberculosis meningitis Lyme disease Neurosyphilis
Cardiovascular	Congestive heart failure (CHF)
Cerebrovascular	Cerebral insufficiency (TIA, CVA) Postanoxic encephalopathy
Pulmonary	Chronic obstructive pulmonary disease (COPD) Hypercapnia ($\uparrow$ CO$_2$) Hypoxemia ($\downarrow$ arterial O$_2$)
Renal	Renal failure, uremia Urinary tract infection
Neurologic	Encephalopathy (hepatic, hypertensive) Head trauma Cancer Cerebrovascular accident (CVA; stroke)
Other	Chronic drug and/or alcohol use Medication (e.g., anticonvulsants, antidepressants, antiemetics, antihistamines, antipsychotics, benzodiazepines, narcotics, sedative-hypnotics, Zantac, Tagamet) Postoperative Severe anemia Cancer metastasized to the brain Sarcoidosis Sleep apnea Vasculitis (e.g., SLE) Vitamin deficiencies (B-12, folate, niacin, thiamine) Whipple's disease (severe intestinal disorder)

Modified from Dains JE, Baumann LC, Scheibel P: *Advanced health assessment & clinical diagnosis in primary care*, ed 2, St. Louis, 2003, Mosby; p 425.

TIA, Transient ischemic attack; *CVA*, cerebrovascular accident; stroke; *SLE*, systemic lupus erythematosus.

Be aware in the health history of any risk factors for nutritional deficiencies (Box 4-2). Remember that some medications can cause appetite changes and that psychosocial factors such as depression, eating disorders, drug or alcohol addictions, and economic variables can affect nutritional status.

It may be necessary to determine the client's ideal body weight by calculating the body mass index (BMI).[7,8] Several websites are available to help anyone make this calculation. There is a separate website for children and teens sponsored by the National Center for Chronic Disease Prevention and Health Promotion.[9]

Whenever nutritional deficiencies are suspected, notify the physician and/or request a referral to a registered dietitian.

Body and Breath Odors

Odors may provide some significant clues to overall health status. For example, a fruity (sweet) breath odor (detectable by some, but not by all health care professionals) may be a symptom of diabetic ketoacidosis. Bad breath (halitosis) can be a

BOX 4-2 ▼ Risk Factors for Nutritional Deficiency

- Economic status
- Living alone
- Older age (metabolic rate slows in older adults; altered sense of taste and smell affects appetite)
- Depression, anxiety
- Eating disorders
- Lactose intolerance (common in Mexican Americans, African Americans, Asians, Native Americans)
- Alcohol/drug addiction
- Chronic diarrhea
- Nausea
- Gastrointestinal impairment (e.g., bowel resection, gastric bypass, pancreatitis, Crohn's disease, pernicious anemia)
- Chronic endocrine or metabolic disorders (e.g., diabetes mellitus, celiac sprue)
- Liver disease
- Dialysis
- Medications (e.g., captopril, chemotherapy, steroids, insulin, lithium) including over-the-counter drugs (e.g., laxatives)
- Chronic disability affecting ADLs (e.g., problems with balance, mobility, food preparation)
- Burns
- Difficulty chewing or swallowing (dental problems, stroke or other neurologic impairment)

symptom of dental decay, lung abscess, throat or sinus infection, or gastrointestinal disturbances from food intolerances, *H. pylori* bacteria, or bowel obstruction. Keep in mind that ethnic foods and alcohol can affect breath and body odor.

Clients who are incontinent (bowel or bladder) may smell of urine, ammonia, or feces. It is important to ask the client about any unusual odors. It may be best to offer an introductory explanation with some follow-up questions:

[If you suspect urinary incontinence]: Are you having any trouble with leaking urine or making it to the bathroom on time? (Ask appropriate follow-up questions about cause, frequency, severity, triggers, and so on; see Appendix B-5).

[If you suspect fecal incontinence]: Do you have trouble getting to the toilet on time for a bowel movement?

Do you have trouble wiping yourself clean after a bowel movement? (Ask appropriate follow-up questions about cause, frequency, severity, triggers, and so on).

[If you detect breath odor]: I notice an unusual smell on your breath. Do you know what might be causing this? (Ask appropriate follow-up questions depending on the type of smell you perceive; you may have to conduct an alcohol screening survey [see Chapter 2 or Appendices B-1 and B-2]).

Follow-Up Questions

Mrs. Smith, as part of a physical therapy exam we always look at our client's overall health and general physical condition. Do you have any other health concerns besides your shoulder/back (Therapist: name the involved body part)?

Are you being treated by anyone for any other problems? [Wait for a response but add prompts as needed: chiropractor? acupuncturist? naturopath?]

Vital Signs

The need for therapists to assess vital signs, especially pulse and blood pressure is increasing.[10] Without the benefit of laboratory values, physical assessment becomes much more important. Vital signs, observations, and reported associated signs and symptoms are among the best screening tools available to the therapist.

Vital sign assessment is an important tool because high blood pressure is a serious concern in the United States. Many people are unaware they have high BP. Often primary orthopedic clients have secondary cardiovascular disease.[11]

Physical therapists practicing in a primary care setting will especially need to know when and how to assess vital signs. The *Guide to the Physical Therapist Practice*[12] recommends that heart rate (pulse) and blood pressure measurements be included in the examination of new clients. Exercise professionals are strongly encouraged to measure blood pressure during each visit.[13]

Taking a client's vital signs remains the single easiest, most economical, and fastest way to screen for many systemic illnesses. All the vital signs are important (Box 4-3); temperature and blood pressure have the greatest utility as early screening tools for systemic illness or disease, while pulse, blood pressure, and oxygen saturation level offer valuable information about the cardiovascular/pulmonary systems.

As an aside comment: using vital signs is an easy, yet effective way to document outcomes. In today's evidence-based practice, the therapist can

use something as simple as pulse or blood pressure to document changes that occur with intervention. For example, if ambulating with a client results in no change in ease of ambulation, speed, or distance, consider taking blood pressure, pulse, and oxygen (O_2) saturation levels before and after each session. Improvement in O_2 saturation levels or faster return to normal of heart rate after exercise are just two examples of how vital signs can become an important part of outcomes documentation.

Assessment of baseline vital signs should be a part of the initial data collected so that correlations and comparisons with future values are available when necessary. The therapist compares measurements taken against normal values and also compares future measurements to the baseline units to identify significant changes (normalizing values or moving toward abnormal findings) for each client.

Normal ranges of values for the vital signs are provided for the therapist's convenience. However, these ranges can be exceeded by a client and still represent normal for that person. Keep in mind that many factors can affect vital signs, especially pulse and blood pressure (Table 4-4). It is the unusual vital sign in combination with other signs and symptoms, medications, and medical status that gives clinical meaning to the pulse rate, blood pressure, and temperature.

BOX 4-3 ▼ Vital Signs

- Pulse (heart rate)
- Blood pressure
- Core body temperature (oral or ear)
- Respirations
- Pulse oximetry (O_2 saturation)
- Skin temperature—digits (thermister)*
- Pain (now called the 5th vital sign; see Chapter 3 for assessment)

* The thermister is a handheld device used to measure skin temperature (fingertips, hand). Similar tools are available as part of some biofeedback equipment. Using skin temperature is an excellent tool for teaching clients how to modulate the autonomic nervous system, a technique called *physiologic quieting*.®

This tool is commercially available with a guided relaxation tape [www.phoenixpub.com; 1-800-549-8371]. It can be a useful intervention with clients who have chronic fatigue syndrome, fibromyalgia, Raynaud's phenomenon or disease, and peripheral vascular disease. Results can be measured using all the vital signs, but especially by measuring and recording changes in skin temperature.

TABLE 4-4 ▼ Factors Affecting Pulse and Blood Pressure

Pulse	Blood pressure*
Age	Age
Anemia	Alcohol
Autonomic dysfunction (diabetes, spinal cord injury)	Anxiety
Caffeine	Blood vessel size
Cardiac muscle dysfunction	Blood viscosity
Conditioned/deconditioned state	Caffeine
Dehydration (decreased blood volume increases heart rate)	Cocaine and cocaine derivatives
Exercise	Diet
Fear	Distended urinary bladder
Fever, heat	Force of heart contraction
Hyperthyroidism	Living at higher altitudes
Infection	Medications
Medications	Ace inhibitors (lowers pressure)
Antidysrhythmic (slows rate)	Adrenergic inhibitors (lowers pressure)
Atropine (increases rate)	Beta blockers (lowers pressure)
Beta blocker (slows rate)	Diuretics (lowers pressure)
Digitalis (slows rate)	Narcotic analgesics (lowers pressure)
Sleep disorders or sleep deprivation	Nicotine
Stress (emotional or psychologic)	Pain
	Time of recent meal (increases SBP)

* Conditions such as chronic kidney disease, renovascular disorders, primary aldosteronism, and coarctation of the aorta are identifiable causes of elevated blood pressure. Chronic over training in athletes, use of steroids and/or nonsteroidal antiinflammatory drugs (NSAIDs), and large increases in muscle mass can also contribute to hypertension.²⁶ Treatment for hypertension, dehydration, heart failure, heart attack, arrhythmias, anaphylaxis, shock (from severe infection, stroke, anaphylaxis, major trauma), and advanced diabetes can cause low blood pressure.

From Goodman CC, Boissonnault WG, and Fuller K: *Pathology: implications for the physical therapist*, ed 2, Philadelphia, 2003, WB Saunders.

Pulse Rate

The pulse reveals important information about the client's heart rate and heart rhythm. A resting pulse rate (normal range: 60 to 100 beats/min), taken at the carotid artery or radial artery pulse point, should be available for comparison with the pulse rate taken during treatment or after exercise.

It is recommended that the pulse always be checked in two places in older adults and in anyone with diabetes (Fig. 4-1). Pulse strength (amplitude) can be graded as

0 Absent, not palpable
1+ Pulse diminished, barely palpable
2+ Easily palpable, normal

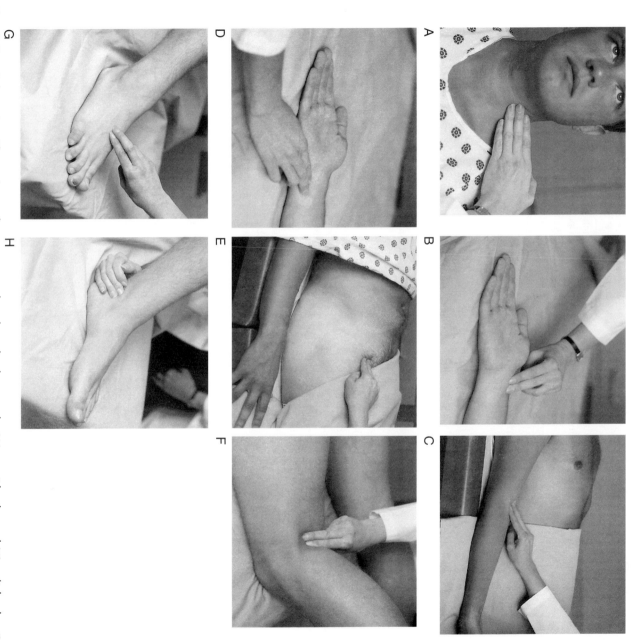

Fig. 4-1 • Pulse points. The easiest and most commonly palpated pulses are the (A) carotid pulse and (B) radial pulse. Other pulse points include: (C) brachial pulse, (D) ulnar pulse, (E) femoral pulse, (F) popliteal pulse (knee slightly flexed), (G) dorsalis pedis, and (H) posterior tibial. The anterior tibial pulse becomes the dorsalis pedis and is palpable where the artery lies close to the skin on the dorsum of the foot. Peripheral pulses are more difficult to palpate in older adults and anyone with peripheral vascular disease. (From Potter PA, Weilitz PB: *Pocket guide to health assessment*, ed 5, St. Louis, 2003, Mosby.)

3+ Full pulse, increased strength
4+ Bounding, too strong to obliterate

Keep in mind that measuring the pulse is not the same as measuring the heart rate. A true measure of heart rate requires measuring the electrical impulses of the heart. A rate above 100 beats per minute indicates tachycardia; below 60 beats per minute indicates bradycardia.

Pulse amplitude (weak or bounding quality of the pulse) gives an indication of the circulating blood volume and the strength of left ventricle ejection. Normally, the pulse increases slightly with inspiration and decreases with expiration. Pulse amplitude that fades with inspiration instead of strengthening and strengthens with expiration instead of fading is *paradoxic* and should be reported to the physician. Paradoxical pulse occurs most commonly in clients with chronic obstructive pulmonary disease (COPD), but is also observed in clients with constrictive pericarditis.[14]

A pulse increase with activity of more than 20 beats per minute lasting for more than 3 minutes after rest or changing position should also be reported. Other pulse abnormalities are listed in Box 4-4.

The resting pulse may be higher than normal with fever, anemia, infections, some medications, hyperthyroidism, anxiety, or pain. A low pulse rate (below 60 bpm) is not uncommon among trained athletes. Medications, such as beta-blockers and calcium channel blockers, can also prevent the normal rise in pulse rate that usually occurs during exercise. In such cases the therapist must monitor rates of perceived exertion (RPE) instead of pulse rate.

When taking the resting pulse or pulse during exercise, some clinicians measure the pulse for 15

seconds and multiply by 4 to get the rate per minute. For a quick assessment, measure for 6 seconds and add a zero. A 6-second pulse count can result in an error of 10 beats per minute if a one-beat error is made in counting. For screening purposes, it is always best to palpate the pulse for a full minute. Longer pulse counts give greater accuracy and provide more time for detection of some dysrhythmias (Box 4-5).[13]

BOX 4-4 ▼ Pulse Abnormalities

- Weak pulse beats alternating with strong beats
- Weak, thready pulse
- Bounding pulse (throbbing pulse followed by sudden collapse or decrease in the force of the pulse)
- Two quick beats followed by a pause (no pulse)
- Irregular rhythm (interval between beats is not equal)
- Pulse amplitude decreases with inspiration/increases with expiration
- Pulse rate too fast (greater than 100 bpm; tachycardia)
- Pulse rate too slow (less than 60 bpm; bradycardia)

BOX 4-5 ▼ Tips on Palpating Pulses

- Assess each pulse for strength and equality.
- Expect to palpate 60 to 90 pulses per minute at all pulse sites.
- Normal pulse is 2+ and equal bilaterally (see scale in text).
- Apply gentle pressure; pulses are easily obliterated in some people.
- Popliteal pulse requires deeper palpation.
- Normal veins are flat; pulsations are not visible. Flat veins in supine that become distended in sitting may indicate heart disease.
- Pulses should be the same from side to side and should not change with inspiration, expiration, or change in position.
- Pulses tend to diminish with age; distal pulses are not palpable in many older adults.
- If pulses are diminished or absent, listen for a bruit to detect arterial narrowing.
- Pedal pulses can be congenitally absent; the client may or may not know if absent pulse at this pulse site is normal or a change in pulse pressure.
- In the case of diminished or absent pulses observe the client for other changes (e.g., skin temperature, texture, color, hair loss, change in toenails); ask about pain in calf or leg with walking that goes away with rest (intermittent claudication; PVD).
- Carotid pulse: Assess in the seated position; have client turn the head slightly toward the side being palpated. Palpate along the medial edge of the sternocleidomastoid muscle (see Fig. 4-1). Palpate one carotid artery at a time; apply light pressure; deep palpation can stimulate carotid sinus with a sudden drop in heart rate and blood pressure.
- Femoral pulse: Femoral artery is palpable below the inguinal ligament midway between the anterior superior iliac spine (ASIS) and the symphysis pubis. It can be difficult to assess in the obese client; place fingertips of both hands on either side of the pulse site; femoral pulse should be as strong (if not stronger) than radial pulse.
- Posterior tibial pulse: Foot must be relaxed with ankle in slight planter flexion (see Fig. 4-1).

Respirations

Try to assess the client's breathing without drawing attention to what is being done. This measure can be taken right after counting the pulse while still holding the client's wrist.

Count respirations for 1 minute unless respirations are unlabored and regular in which case the count can be taken for 30 seconds and multiplied by 2. The rise and fall of the chest equals 1 cycle.

The normal rate is between 12 and 20 breaths per minute. Observe rate, excursion, effort, and pattern. Note any use of accessory muscles and whether breathing is silent or noisy. Watch for puffed cheeks, pursed lips, nasal flaring, or asymmetrical chest expansion. Changes in the rate, depth, effort, or pattern of a client's respirations can be early signs of neurologic, pulmonary, or cardiovascular impairment.

Pulse Oximetry

Oxygen saturation on hemoglobin (SaO_2) and pulse rate can be measured simultaneously using pulse oximetry. This is a noninvasive, photoelectric device with a sensor that can be attached to a finger, the bridge of the nose, toe, or ear lobe. Digital readings are less accurate with clients who are anemic, undergoing chemotherapy, or who use fingernail polish or nail acrylics. In such cases, attach the sensor to one of the other accessible body parts.

The sensor probe emits red and infrared light, which is transmitted to the capillaries. When in contact with the skin, the probe measures transmitted light passing through the vascular bed and detects the relative amount of color absorbed by the arterial blood. The SaO_2 level is calculated from this information.

The normal SaO_2 range is 95 to 100 percent. The exception to this normal range is for clients with a history of tobacco use and/or chronic obstructive pulmonary disease (COPD). Many individuals with COPD tend to retain carbon dioxide and can become apneic if the oxygen levels are too high. For this reason, oxygen saturation levels are normally kept lower for this population.

Increased CO_2 levels trigger the brain to increase the respiratory rate. If the client with COPD is on oxygen and the O_2 levels get too high, the respiratory system is depressed. Monitoring respiratory rate, level of oxygen administered by nasal canula, and oxygen saturation levels is very important in this client population.

Any condition that restricts blood flow (including cold hands) can result in inaccurate SaO_2 readings. Relaxation and physiologic quieting techniques can be used to help restore more normal temperatures in the distal extremities. A handheld device such as the Thermister[15] can be used by the client to improve peripheral circulation. Do not apply a pulse oximetry sensor to an extremity with an automatic blood pressure cuff.[16]

SaO_2 levels can be affected also by positioning because positioning can impact a person's ability to breathe. Upright sitting in individuals with low muscle tone or kyphosis can cause forward flexion of the thoracic spine compromising oxygen intake. Tilting the person back slightly can open the trunk, ease ventilation, and improve SaO_2 levels.[17] Using SaO_2 levels may be a good way to document outcomes of positioning programs for clients with impaired ventilation.

In addition to oxygen saturation levels, assess other vital signs, skin and nail bed color and tissue perfusion, mental status, breath sounds, and respiratory pattern for all clients using pulse oximetry. If the client cannot talk easily whether at rest or while exercising, oxygen saturation levels are likely to be inadequate.

Blood Pressure

Blood pressure (BP) is the measurement of pressure in an artery at the peak of systole (contraction of the left ventricle) and during diastole (when the heart is at rest after closure of the aortic valve, which prevents blood from flowing back to the heart chambers). The measurement (in mm Hg) is listed as:

Systolic (contraction phase)
Diastolic (relaxation phase)

Blood pressure depends on many factors; the normal range differs slightly with age and varies greatly among individuals (see Table 4-4). Normal systolic blood pressure (SBP) ranges from 100 to 120 mm Hg, and diastolic blood pressure (DBP) ranges from 60 to 80 mm Hg. Highly trained athletes may have much lower values. Target ranges for blood pressure are listed in Table 4-5 and Box 4-6.

ASSESSING BLOOD PRESSURE

The blood pressure should be taken in the same arm and in the same position (supine or sitting) each time it is measured. The baseline BP values can be recorded on the Family/Personal History form (see Fig. 2-2).

Cuff size is important and requires the bladder width-to-length be at least 1:2. BP measurements are overestimated with a cuff that is too small.

TABLE 4-5 ▼ Classification of Blood Pressure

	Systolic blood pressure	Diastolic blood pressure
For Adults*		
Normal	<120 mm Hg	<80 mm Hg
Prehypertension	120-139	80-89
Stage 1 Hypertension	140-159	90-99
Stage 2 Hypertension	≥160	≥100
For Children and Adolescents†		
Normal	<90th percentile; 50th percentile is the midpoint of the normal range	
Prehypertension	90th-95th percentile or if BP is greater than 120/80 (even if this figure is <90th percentile)	
Stage 1 Hypertension	95th-99th percentile + 5 mm Hg	
Stage 2 Hypertension	>99th percentile + 5 mm Hg	

The relationship between blood pressure (BP) and risk of coronary vascular disease (CVD) events is continuous, consistent, and independent of other risk factors. The higher the BP, the greater the chance of heart attack, heart failure, stroke, and kidney disease.
For individuals 40 to 70 years of age, each 20 mm Hg incremental increase in systolic BP (SBP) or 10 mm Hg in diastolic BP (DBP) doubles the risk of CVD across the entire BP range from 115/75 to 185/115 mm Hg.
* From *The Seventh Report of the Joint National Committee on Prevention, Detection, Evaluation, and Treatment of High Blood Pressure,* NIH Publication No. 03-5233, May 2003. National Heart, Lung, and Blood Institute (NHLBI) www.nhlbi.nih.gov/.
† From National Heart, Lung, and Blood Institute (NHLBI): Fourth Report on the Diagnosis, Evaluation, and Treatment of High Blood Pressure in Children and Adolescents, *Pediatrics* 114(2):555-576, August 2004.

BOX 4-6 ▼ Guidelines for Blood Pressure in a Physical Therapist's Practice

Consider the following as yellow (warning) flags that require closer monitoring and possible medical referral:

- SBP greater than 120 mm Hg and/or DBP greater than 80 mm Hg, especially in the presence of significant risk factors (age, medications, personal or family history)
- Decrease in DBP below 70 mm Hg in adults age 75 or older (risk factor for Alzheimer's)
- Persistent rise or fall in blood pressure over time (at least 3 consecutive readings over 2 weeks), especially in a client taking NSAIDs (check for edema) or any woman taking birth control pills (should be closely monitored by physician)
- Steady fall in blood pressure over several years in adult over 75 (risk factor for Alzheimer's)
- Lower standing SBP (less than 140 mm Hg) in adults over age 65 with a history of falls (increased risk for falls)
- A difference in pulse pressure greater than 40 mm Hg
- More than 10 mm Hg difference (SBP or DBP) from side to side (upper extremities)
- Approaching or more than 40 mm Hg difference (SBP or DBP) from side to side (lower extremities)
- BP in lower extremities is lower than in the upper extremities
- DBP increases more than 10 mm Hg during activity or exercise
- SBP does not rise as workload increases; SBP falls as workload increases
- SBP exceeds 200 mm Hg during exercise or physical activity; DBP exceeds 100 mm Hg during exercise or physical activity; these values represent the upper limits and may be too high for the client's age, general health, and overall condition.
- Blood pressure changes in the presence of other warning signs such as first-time onset or unstable angina, dizziness, nausea, pallor, extreme diaphoresis
- Sudden fall in blood pressure (more than 10 to 15 mm Hg SBP) or more than 10 mm Hg DBP with concomitant rise (10% to 20% increase) in pulse (orthostatic hypotension); watch for postural hypotension in hypertensive clients, especially anyone taking diuretics (decreased fluid volume/dehydration)

BP, Blood pressure; *SBP,* systolic blood pressure; *DBP,* diastolic blood pressure; *NSAIDs,* nonsteroidal antiinflammatory drugs.

They are less likely to be underestimated by a cuff that is too large, so if a cuff is too small, go to the next size up.[18]

Do not apply the blood pressure cuff above an intravenous (IV) line where fluids are infusing or an arteriovenous (AV) shunt, on the same side where breast or axillary surgery has been performed, or when the arm or hand have been traumatized or diseased. Until research data supports a change, it is recommended that clients who have undergone axillary node dissection (ALND) avoid having blood pressure measurements taken on the affected side.

Although it is recommended that anyone who has had bilateral axillary node dissection should have BP measurements taken in the leg; this is not standard clinical practice across the United States.[19] Leg pressures can be difficult to assess and inaccurate.

Some oncology staff advise taking BPs in the arm with the least amount of nodal dissection. Technique in measuring blood pressure is a key factor in measuring blood pressure in all clients but especially those with ALND (Box 4-7).

A common mistake is to pump the blood pressure cuff up until the systolic measurement is

---

BOX 4-7 ▼ Assessing Blood Pressure (BP)

- Client should avoid tobacco and caffeine for 30 minutes before BP reading; let the client sit quietly for a few minutes; this can help offset the physical exertion of moving to the exam room or the emotional stress of being with a health care professional (white-coat hypertension). The client should be seated comfortably in a chair with the back and arm supported, legs uncrossed, and not talking.

- Assess for factors that can affect BP (see Table 4-4).

- Position the arm extended in a forward direction (sitting) at the heart's level or parallel to the body (supine); avoid using an arm with a fistula, intravenous or arterial line, or with a previous history of lymph node biopsy or breast or axillary surgery.

- Wrap the cuff around the client's upper arm (place over bare skin) 1 inch (2.5 cm) above the antecubital fossa (inside of the elbow); cuff size is critical to accurate measurement. The length of the bladder cuff should encircle at least 80% of the upper arm. The width of the cuff should be about 40% of the upper arm circumference. BP measurement errors are usually worse in cuffs that are too small compared to those that are too big.

- Slide your finger under the cuff to make sure it is not too tight.

- Close the valve on the rubber bulb.

- Place the stethoscope (diaphragm or bell side) over the brachial artery at the elbow; you may hear the low-pitched Korotkoff sounds more clearly using the bell.

- Inflate the cuff 30 to 40 mm Hg above SBP (inflate until you no longer hear a pulse sound and then inflate 30 mm more); record the measurement at the disappearance of sound as the SBP.

- Slowly release the valve on the bulb (deflate at a rate of 2 to 3 mm Hg/second); listen for the first Korotkoff sound (2 consecutive beats signals the systolic reading) and the last Korotkoff sound (diastolic reading).

- If you are new to blood pressure assessment or if the blood pressure is elevated, check the blood pressure twice. Wait one minute and retest. Some sources say to wait at least 2 minutes before retaking BP on the same arm but this is not always done in the typical clinical setting.

- Record date, time of day, client position, extremity measured (arm or leg, left or right), and results for each reading.

- As soon as the blood begins to flow through the artery again, Korotkoff's sounds are heard. The first sounds are tapping sounds that gradually increase in intensity. The initial tapping sound that is heard for at least 2 consecutive beats is recorded as *systolic blood pressure* (SBP).

- The first phase of sound may be followed by a momentary disappearance of sounds that can last from 30 to 40 mm Hg as the needle descends. Following this temporary absence of sound, there are murmuring or swishing sounds (second Korotkoff sound). As deflation of the cuff continues, the sounds become sharper and louder. These sounds represent phase 3. During phase 4, the sounds become muffled rather abruptly and then are followed by silence, which represents phase 5. Phase 5 (the fifth Korotkoff sound or K5), the point at which sounds disappear, is most often used as the *diastolic blood pressure* (DBP).

From American Heart Association Updates Recommendations for Blood Pressure Measurements. Available at: http://www.americanheart.org. Accessed March 2, 2005.

200 mm Hg and then take too long to lower the pressure or to repeat the measurement a second time without waiting. Repeating the blood pressure without a one-minute wait time can damage the blood vessel and set up an inflammatory response.[20] This poor technique is to be avoided, especially in clients at risk for lymphedema or who already have lymphedema.

Take the BP twice at least a minute apart in both arms. If both measurements are within 5 mm Hg of each other, record this as the resting (baseline) measurement. If not, wait one minute and take the BP a third time. Monitor the BP in the arm with the highest measurements.[14]

For clients who have had a mastectomy without ALND (i.e., prophylactic mastectomy), blood pressure can be measured in either arm. These recommendations are to be followed for life.[21]

Until automated blood pressure devices are improved enough to ensure valid and reliable measurements, the blood pressure response to exercise in all clients should be taken manually with a blood pressure cuff (sphygmomanometer) and a stethoscope.[22]

It is advised to invest in the purchase of a well-made, reliable stethoscope. Older models with tubing long enough to put the earpieces in your ears and still place the bell in a lab coat pocket should be replaced. Tubing should be no more than 50 to 60 cm (12 to 15 inches) and 4 mm in diameter. Longer and wider tubing can distort transmitted sounds.[23]

For the student or clinician learning to take vital signs, it may be easier to hear the blood pressure (tapping; Korotkoff) sounds in adults using the left arm because of the closer proximity to the left ventricle. Arm position does make a difference in BP readings. BP measurements are up to 10 percent higher when the elbow is at a right angle to the body with the elbow flexed at heart level. The preferred position is seated with the arms parallel and extended in a forward direction (if supine, then parallel to the body).[24]

It is more accurate to evaluate consecutive blood pressure readings over time rather than using an isolated measurement for reporting blood pressure abnormalities. Blood pressure also should be correlated with any related diet or medication.

Before reporting abnormal blood pressure readings, measure both sides for comparison, remeasure both sides, and have another health professional check the readings. Correlate blood pressure measurements with other vital signs, and screen for associated signs and symptoms such as pallor, fatigue, perspiration, and/or palpitations. A persistent rise or fall in blood pressure requires medical attention and possible intervention.

PULSE PRESSURE

The difference between the systolic and diastolic pressure readings (SBP minus DBP) is called *pulse pressure*. A widened pulse pressure often results from stiffening of the aorta secondary to atherosclerosis. Stroke volume or ventricular pressure (i.e., systolic BP) will increase. A BP of 150/80 would not be uncommon in a situation like this.

Widening of the pulse pressure is linked to a significantly higher risk of stroke and heart failure after the sixth decade. Some medications increase pulse pressure by lowering diastolic pressure more than systolic.[25]

Pulse pressure generally increases in direct proportion to the intensity of exercise as the SBP increases and DBP stays about the same.[26] A difference of more than 40 mm Hg is abnormal and should be reported.

VARIATIONS IN BLOOD PRESSURE

There can be some normal variation in systolic blood pressure from side to side (right extremity compared to left extremity). This is usually no more than 5 to 10 mm Hg DBP or SBP (arms) and 10 to 40 mm Hg SBP (legs). A difference of 10 mm Hg or more in either systolic or diastolic measurements from one extremity to the other may be an indication of vascular problems (look for associated symptoms; in the upper extremity test for thoracic outlet syndrome).

Normally the SBP in the legs is 10 to 20 percent higher than the brachial artery pressure in the arms. BP readings that are lower in the legs as compared with the arms are considered abnormal and should prompt a medical referral for assessment of peripheral vascular disease.[21]

With a change in position (supine to sitting), the normal fluctuation of blood pressure and heart rate increases slightly (about 5 mm Hg for systolic and diastolic pressures and 5 to 10 beats per minute in heart rate).

Systolic pressure increases with age and with exertion in a linear progression. If systolic pressure does not rise as workload increases, or if this pressure falls, it may be an indication that the functional reserve capacity of the heart has been exceeded.

The deconditioned, menopausal woman with coronary heart disease (CHD) requires careful monitoring, especially in the presence of a personal or family history of heart disease and myocardial

infarct (personal or family) or sudden death in a family member.

On the other hand, women of reproductive age taking birth control pills may be at increased risk for hypertension, heart attack, or stroke. The risk of a cardiovascular event is very low with today's low-dose oral contraceptives. However, smoking, hypertension, obesity, undiagnosed cardiac anomalies, and diabetes are factors that increase a woman's risk for cardiovascular events. Any woman using oral contraceptives who presents with consistently elevated blood pressure values must be advised to see her physician for close monitoring and follow-up.[27,28]

The left ventricle becomes less elastic and more noncompliant as we age. The same amount of blood still fills the ventricle, but the pumping mechanism is less effective. The body compensates to maintain homeostasis by increasing the blood pressure. Blood pressure values greater than 120 mm Hg (systolic) and more than 80 mm Hg (diastolic) are treated with lifestyle modifications first, then medication.

BLOOD PRESSURE CHANGES WITH EXERCISE

As mentioned, the SBP increases with increasing levels of activity and exercise in a linear fashion. In a healthy adult under conditions of minimal to moderate exercise, look for normal change (increase) in systolic BP of 20 mm Hg or more.

The ACSM suggests the normal SBP response to incremental exercise is a progressive rise, typically 10 + 2 mm Hg for each metabolic equivalent (MET) where 1 MET = 3.5 ml O_2/kg/min. Expect to see a 40-50 mm change in systolic BP with intense exercise (again, this is in the healthy adult). These values are less likely with cardiac clients and well-conditioned athletes.

Diastolic should be the same side to side with less than 10 mm Hg difference observed. DBP generally remains the same or decreases slightly during progressive exercise.[26]

In an exercise-testing situation, the ACSM recommends stopping the test if the SBP exceeds 260 mm Hg.[26] In a clinical setting without the benefit of cardiac monitoring, exercise or activity should be reduced or stopped if the systolic pressure exceeds 200 mm Hg.

This is a general guideline that can be changed according to the client's age, general health, use of cardiac medications, and other risk factors. Diastolic blood pressure increases during upper extremity exercise or isometric exercise involving any muscle group. Activity or exercise should be monitored closely, decreased, or halted if the diastolic pressure exceeds 100 mm Hg.

This is a general (conservative) guideline when exercising a client without the benefit of cardiac testing (e.g., EKG). This stop-point is based on the ACSM guideline to stop exercise testing at 115 mm Hg DBP. Other sources suggest activity should be decreased or stopped if the DBP exceeds 130 mm Hg.[29]

Other warning signs to moderate or stop exercising include the onset of angina, dyspnea, and heart palpitations. Monitor the client for other signs and symptoms such as fever, dizziness, nausea/vomiting, pallor, extreme diaphoresis, muscular cramping or weakness, and incoordination. Always honor the client's desire to slow down or stop.

HYPERTENSION (see further discussion on hypertension in Chapter 6)

In recent years an unexpected increase in illness and death caused by hypertension has prompted the National Institutes of Health (NIH) to issue new guidelines for more effective blood pressure control. More than one in four Americans has high blood pressure, increasing their risk for heart and kidney disease and stroke.[30]

In adults hypertension is a systolic pressure above 140 mm Hg or a diastolic pressure above 90 mm Hg. Consistent BP measurements between 120 and 139 (systolic) and between 90 and 99 diastolic is classified as pre-hypertensive. The overall goal of treating clients with hypertension is to prevent morbidity and mortality associated with high blood pressure. The specific objective is to achieve and maintain arterial blood pressure below 120/80 mm Hg, if possible (Box 4-8).[22]

The older adult taking nonsteroidal antiinflammatory medications is at risk for increased blood pressure because these drugs are potent renal vasoconstrictors. Monitor blood pressure carefully in these clients and look for sacral and lower extremity edema. Document and report these findings to the physician. Use the risk factor analysis for NSAIDs presented in Chapter 2 (see Box 2-14).

Always beware of white-coat hypertension, a clinical condition in which the client has elevated BP levels when measured in a clinic setting by a health care professional. In such cases, BP measurements are consistently normal outside of a clinical setting.

White-coat hypertension occurs in 15 to 20% of adults with stage I hypertension. It is more common in older adults; antihypertensive treatment in this group may reduce office BP but may not affect ambulatory BP.

At-home BP measurements can help identify adults with white-coat hypertension, ambulatory hypertension, and individuals who do not experience the usual nocturnal drop in BP (decrease of 15 mm Hg), which is a risk factor for cardiovascular events.[31] Excessive morning BP surge is a predictor of stroke in older adults with known hypertension and is also a red flag sign.[32] Medical referral is indicated in any of these situations.

Hypertension in African Americans Nearly 40 percent of African Americans suffer from heart disease and 13 percent have diabetes. Hypertension contributes to these conditions or makes them worse. African Americans are significantly more likely to die of high blood pressure than the general public because current treatment strategies have been unsuccessful.[33,34]

Guidelines for treating high blood pressure in African Americans have been issued by the International Society on Hypertension in Blacks (ISHIB).[35] The ISHIB recommends a blood pressure target of less than 130/80 mm Hg for African Americans with blood pressure screening for all African American adults and early prevention for anyone in the pre-hypertensive range. Aggressive treatment for hypertension is advised using drug combinations.[34]

The therapist can incorporate blood pressure screening into any evaluation for clients with ethnic risk factors. Any client of any ethnic background with risk factors for hypertension should also be screened (see Box 6-6).

Hypertension in Children and Adolescents[36] Up to 3 percent of children under age 18 also have hypertension. New guidelines for children and adolescents are based on *recently revised child height percentiles.* Any child with readings above the 95th percentile for gender, age, and height on three separate occasions is considered to have hypertension. The 50th percentile has been added to the tables to provide the clinician with the BP level at the midpoint of the normal range.

Under the new guidelines, children whose readings fall between the 90th and 95th percentile are now considered to have pre-hypertension. Earlier guidelines called this category "high normal."

The long-term health risks for hypertensive children and adolescents can be substantial; therefore, it is important that elevated blood pressure is

---

BOX 4-8 ▼ Guidelines For Hypertension and Management

The Seventh Report of the Joint National Committee on Prevention, Detection, Evaluation, and Treatment of High Blood Pressure provides a new guideline for hypertension prevention and management. The following are the report's key messages:

- In persons older than 50 years, systolic blood pressure greater than 140 mm Hg is a much more important cardiovascular disease (CVD) risk factor than diastolic blood pressure. Elevated systolic pressure raises the risk of heart attacks, congestive heart failure, dementia, end-stage kidney disease, and cardiovascular mortality.

- The risk of CVD beginning at 115/75 mm Hg doubles with each increment of 20/10 mm Hg; individuals who are normotensive at age 55 have a 90% lifetime risk for developing hypertension.

- Individuals with a systolic blood pressure of 120-139 mm Hg or a diastolic blood pressure of 80-89 mm Hg should be considered as prehypertensive and require health-promoting lifestyle modifications to prevent CVD.

- Thiazide-type diuretics should be used in drug treatment for most clients with uncomplicated hypertension, either alone or combined with drugs from other classes. Certain high-risk conditions are compelling indications for the initial use of other antihypertensive drug classes (angiotensin converting enzyme inhibitors, angiotensin receptor blockers, beta-blockers, calcium channel blockers).

- Most clients with hypertension will require two or more antihypertensive medications to achieve goal blood pressure (less than 140/90 mm Hg, or less than 130/80 mm Hg for clients with diabetes or chronic kidney disease).

- If blood pressure is more than 20/10 mm Hg above goal blood pressure, consideration should be given to initiating therapy with two agents, one of which usually should be a thiazide-type diuretic.

- The most effective therapy prescribed by the most careful clinician will control hypertension only if clients are motivated. Motivation improves when clients have positive experiences with, and trust in, the clinician.

Source: The Seventh Report of the Joint National Committee on Prevention, Detection, Evaluation, and Treatment of High Blood Pressure. NIH Publication No. 03-5233, May 2003. National Heart, Lung, and Blood Institute (NHLBI) *www.nhlbi.nih.gov/*.

recognized early and measures taken to reduce risks and optimize health outcomes.[36]

Children ages 3 to 18 seen in any medical setting should have the BP measured at least once during each health care episode. The preferred method is auscultation with a blood pressure cuff and stethoscope. Correct measurement requires a cuff that is appropriate to the size of the child's upper arm.

The right arm is preferred with children for comparison with standard tables and in the possible event there is a coarctation of the aorta (see Fig. 6-6), which can lead to a false low reading in the left arm.[37]

Preparation of the child can affect the BP level as much as technique. The child should be seated with feet and back supported. The right arm should be supported parallel to the floor with the cubital fossa at heart level.[38,39] Children can be affected by white-coat hypertension as much as adults. Follow the same guidelines for adults as presented in Box 4-7.

HYPOTENSION

Hypotension is a systolic pressure below 90 mm Hg or a diastolic pressure below 60 mm Hg. A blood pressure level that is borderline low for one person may be normal for another. When the blood pressure is too low, there is inadequate blood flow to the heart, brain, and other vital organs.

The most important factor in hypotension is how the blood pressure changes from the normal condition. Most normal blood pressures are in the range of 90/60 mm Hg to 120/80 mm Hg, but a significant change, even as little as 20 mm Hg, can cause problems for some people.

Lower standing SBP (less than 140 mm Hg) even within the normotensive range is an independent predictor of loss of balance and falls in adults over age 65.[40] Diastolic BP does not appear to be related to falls. Older adult women with lower standing SBP and a history of falls are at greatest risk. The therapist has an important role in educating clients with these risk factors in preventing falls and related accidents. See discussion in Chapter 2 related to taking a history of falls.

In older adults a decrease in BP may be an early warning sign of Alzheimer's disease. Diastolic blood pressure below 70 or declines in systolic pressure equal to or greater than 15 mm Hg over a period of 3 years raises the risk of dementia in adults 75 or older. For each 10-point drop in pressure, the risk of dementia increases by 20%.[41,42]

It is unclear if the steady drop in blood pressure during the 3 years before a dementia diagnosis is a cause or effect of dementia as reduced blood flow to the brain accelerates the development of dementia. Perhaps brain cell degeneration characteristic of dementia damages parts of the brain that regulate blood pressure.[41]

POSTURAL ORTHOSTATIC HYPOTENSION

A common cause of low blood pressure is orthostatic hypotension (OH), defined as a sudden drop in blood pressure when changing positions, usually moving from supine to an upright position.

Physiologic responses of the sympathetic nervous system decline with aging putting them at greater risk for OH. Older adults are prone to falls from a combination of OH and antihypertensive medications. Volume depletion and autonomic dysfunction are the most common causes of OH (see Table 2-5).

Postural orthostatic hypotension is more accurately defined as a decrease in systolic blood pressure of at least 20 mm Hg or decrease in diastolic pressure of at least 10 mm Hg and a 10 to 20 percent increase in pulse rate. Changes must be noted in both the blood pressure and the pulse rate with change in position (supine to sitting; sitting to standing) (Box 4-9; Case Example 4-1).[31]

The client should lie supine 2 to 3 minutes prior to BP and pulse check. At least a 1-minute wait is recommended after each subsequent position change before taking the BP and pulse. Standing postural orthostatic hypotension is measured after 3 to 5 minutes of quiet standing. Food ingestion, time of day, age, and hydration can impact this form of hypotension, as can a history of Parkinsonism, diabetes, or multiple myeloma.[30]

Throughout the procedure assess the client for signs and symptoms of hypotension, including dizziness, light-headedness, pallor, diaphoresis, or syncope (or arrhythmias if using a cardiac monitor). Assist the client to a seated or supine position if any of these symptoms develop and report the results. Do not test the client in the standing position if signs and symptoms of hypotension occur while sitting.

Gravitational effects on the circulatory system can cause a 10 mm Hg drop in SBP when a person changes position from supine to sitting to standing. This drop usually occurs without symptoms as the body quickly compensates to ensure there is no reduction in cardiac output.

In clients on prolonged bed rest or on antihypertensive drug therapy, there may be either no reflexive increase in heart rate or a sluggish vasomotor response. These clients may experience

BOX 4-9   ▼   Postural Orthostatic Hypotension

For a diagnosis of Postural Orthostatic Hypotension, the client must have:

- Decrease of 10 to 15 mm Hg of systolic pressure

  AND/OR

- Increase of 10 mm Hg (or more) diastolic blood pressure

  AND

- 10% to 20% increase in pulse rate

These changes occur with change in position (supine to upright sitting, sit to stand). Another measurement after 1 to 5 minutes of standing may identify orthostatic hypotension missed by earlier readings.

Monitor the client carefully since fainting is a possible risk with low blood pressure, especially when combined with the dehydrating effects of diuretics. Oncology patients receiving chemotherapy who are hypotensive are also at risk for dizziness and loss of balance during the repeated BP measurement in the standing position.

This repetition is useful in the older adult (65 years old or older). Waiting to repeat the BP measurements reveals a client's inability to regulate blood pressure after a change in position. The presence of low blood pressure after a prolonged time is a red flag finding. Be sure to check pulse rate.[14]

CASE EXAMPLE 4-1   Vital Signs

A 74-year-old retired homemaker had a total hip replacement (THR) 2 days ago. She remains as an inpatient with complications related to congestive heart failure. She has a previous medical history of gallbladder removal 20 years ago, total hysterectomy 30 years ago, and surgically induced menopause with subsequent onset of hypertension.

Her medications include intravenous furosemide (Lasix), digoxin, and potassium replacement.

During the initial physical therapy intervention, the client complained of muscle cramping and headache but was able to complete the entire exercise protocol. Blood pressure was 100/76 mm Hg. Systolic measurement dropped to 90 mm Hg when the client moved from supine to standing. Pulse rate was 56 bpm with a pattern of irregular beats. Pulse rate did not change with postural change. Platelet count was 98,000 cells/mm³ when it was measured yesterday.

What is the significance of her vital signs? How would you use vital sign monitoring in a patient like this?

Nurses will be monitoring the patient's signs and symptoms closely. Read the chart to stay up with what everyone else knows about Mrs. S. and/or has observed. Read the physician's notes to see what, if any, medical intervention has been ordered based on laboratory values (e.g., platelet levels) or vital signs (e.g., changes in medication).

Do not hesitate to discuss concerns and observations with the nursing staff. This helps them know you are aware of the medical side of care,

but also gives you some perspective from the nursing side. What do they see as significant? What requires immediate medical attention?

Be sure to report anything observed, but not already recorded in the chart such as muscle cramping, headache, irregular heartbeat with bradycardia, low pulse, and orthostatic hypotension.

Bradycardia is one of the first signs of digitalis toxicity. In some hospitals, a pulse less than 60 bpm in an adult would mean withholding the next dose of digoxin and necessitate physician contact. The protocol may be different from institution to institution.

In this case, report and document:

1. Irregular heart beat with bradycardia (a possible sign of digoxin/digitalis toxicity)
2. Muscle cramping (possible side effect of Lasix) and headache (possible side effect of Digoxin)
3. Always chart vital signs; her blood pressure was not too unusual and pulse rate did not change with position change (probably because of medications) so she does not have medically defined orthostatic hypotension.

The response of vital signs to exercise must be monitored carefully and charted; monitor vital signs throughout intervention. Record the time it takes for the client's vital signs to return to normal after exercise or treatment. This can be used as a means of documenting measurable outcomes. Mrs. S. may not ambulate any further or faster in the afternoon compared with the morning, but her vital signs may reflect closer to normal values and a faster return to homeostasis as a measurable outcome.

larger drops in blood pressure and often experience lightheadedness.

Other clients at risk for postural orthostatic hypotension include those who have just donated blood, anyone with autonomic nervous system disease or dysfunction, and post-operative patients. Other risk factors for orthostatic hypotension in aging adults include hypovolemia associated with dehydration, and the overuse of diuretics, anticholinergic medications, antiemetics, and various over-the-counter cough/cold preparations.

Core Body Temperature

Normal body temperature is not a specific number but a range of values that depends on factors such as the time of day, age, medical status, medication use, activity level, or presence of infection. Oral body temperature ranges from 36° to 37.5° C (96.8° to 99.5° F), with an average of 37° C (98.6° F) (Table 4-6). Hypothermic core temperature is defined as less than 35° C (95° F).

Older adults (over age 65) are less likely to have a fever so the predictive value of taking the body temperature is less. They are more likely to develop hypothermia than young adults. There is a tendency among the aging population to develop an increase in temperature on hospital admission or in response to any change in homeostasis. However, some persons with infectious disease remain afebrile, especially the immunocompromised, those with chronic renal disease, alcoholics, and older adults. Unexplained fever in adolescents may be a manifestation of drug abuse or endocarditis.

Postoperative fever is common and may be from an infectious or noninfectious cause. Medical evaluation is needed to make this determination. In the home health setting wound infection, abscess formation, or peritonitis may appear as a hectic fever pattern 3 to 4 days postoperatively with increases and declines of body temperature but no return to

TABLE 4-6 ▼ Core Body Temperature

Oral	96.8° to 99.5° F (36° to 37.5° C)
Rectal	97.3° to 100.2° F (36.3° to 37.9° C)
Tympanic membrane	97.2° to 100° F (36.2° to 37.8° C)

Body temperature below 95° F. (35° C) is a sign of hypothermia.
Body temperature varies throughout the day (lowest in early morning, highest in late afternoon).
Body temperature varies over the lifespan (decreases with age).

baseline (normal). Such a situation would warrant telephone consultation with the physician's office nurse.

Any client who has back, shoulder, hip, sacroiliac, or groin pain of unknown cause must have a temperature reading taken. Temperature should also be assessed for any client who has constitutional symptoms (see Box 1-3), especially night sweats (gradual increase followed by a sudden drop in body temperature), pain, or symptoms of unknown etiologic basis and for clients who have not been medically screened by a physician. Ask about the presence of other signs and symptoms of infection.

When measuring body temperature, the therapist should ask if the person's normal temperature differs from 37° C (98.6° F). A persistent elevation of temperature over time is a red flag sign; a single measurement may not be sufficient to cause concern.

It is also important to ask whether the client has taken aspirin (or other nonsteroidal antiinflammatory drugs [NSAIDs]) or acetaminophen (Tylenol) to reduce the fever, which might mask an underlying problem. Clients taking dopamine blockers such as Thorazine, Mellaril, or less commonly used Navane for schizophrenia have a lowered "normal" temperature (around 96 degrees). Anyone who is chronically immunosuppressed (such as an organ transplant recipient or person being treated with chemotherapy and any older adult) may have an infection without elevation of temperature.

When using a tympanic membrane (ear) thermometer, perform a gentle ear tug to straighten the ear canal. In a child, pull the ear straight back; in an adult, pull it slightly upward and backward. While holding the ear in this position, use a small rotation movement to insert the probe gently and slowly.[43]

The probe must penetrate at least one-third of the external ear canal to prevent air temperature from affecting the reading. Aim the probe toward the tympanic membrane where it will indirectly measure core body temperature by taking infrared temperature readings of the tympanic membrane (eardrum).[43]

Temperatures can vary from side to side, so record which ear was used and try to use the same ear each time the temperature is recorded. For the client with hearing aid(s), take the temperature in the ear without an aid. Or, if hearing aids are present in both ears, remove one hearing aid and wait 20 minutes before measuring that side. The presence of excessive earwax will prevent an accurate reading.

Newer handheld digital forehead thermometers are noninvasive and provide accurate body temperatures. They are quick and easy to use. The forehead plastic temperature strip (forehead thermometer, fever strip) and the pacifier thermometer for children are not accurate methods to take a temperature.

The therapist should use discretionary caution with any client who has a fever. Exercise with a fever stresses the cardiopulmonary system, which may be further complicated by dehydration. Severe dehydration can occur from vomiting, diarrhea, medications (e.g., diuretics), or heat exhaustion.

Clinical Signs and Symptoms of

Dehydration

Mild

- Thirst
- Dry mouth, dry lips

Moderate

- Very dry mouth, cracked lips
- Sunken eyes, sunken fontanel (infants)
- Poor skin turgor (see Fig. 4-4)
- Postural hypotension
- Headache

Severe

- All signs of moderate dehydration
- Rapid, weak pulse (more than 100 bpm at rest)
- Rapid breathing
- Confusion, lethargy, irritability
- Cold hands and feet
- Unable to cry or urinate

Clients at greatest risk of dehydration include post-operative patients, aging adults, and athletes. Severe fluid volume deficit can cause vascular collapse and shock. Clients at risk of shock include burn or trauma patients, clients in anaphylactic shock or diabetic ketoacidosis, and individuals experiencing severe blood loss.

Clinical Signs and Symptoms of

Shock

Stage 1 (early stage)

- Restlessness, anxiety, hyperalert
- Listless, lack of interest in play (children)
- Tachycardia
- Increased respiratory rate, shallow breathing, frequent sighs
- Rapid, bounding pulse (not weak)
- Distended neck veins
- Skin warm and flushed
- Thirst, nausea, vomiting

Stage 2

- Confusion, lack of focused eye contact (vacant look)
- Abrupt changes in affect or behavior
- No crying or excessive, unexplained crying in infant
- Cold, clammy skin, profuse sweating, chills
- Weak pulses (not bounding)
- Hypotension (low blood pressure), dizziness, fainting
- Collapsed neck veins
- Weak or absent peripheral pulses
- Muscle tension

Stage 3 (late stage)

- Cyanosis (blue lips, gray skin)
- Dull eyes, dilated pupils
- Loss of bowel or bladder control
- Change in level of consciousness

TECHNIQUES OF PHYSICAL EXAMINATION

There are four simple techniques used in the medical physical examination: inspection, palpation, percussion, and auscultation. Percussion and some auscultation techniques require advanced clinical skill and are beyond the scope of a screening examination.

Throughout any screening examination the therapist also assesses function of the integument, musculoskeletal, neuromuscular, and cardiopulmonary systems. Assessment techniques are relatively simple; it is using the finding that is more difficult. The saying, "What one knows, one sees" underscores the idea that knowledge of physical assessment techniques and experience in performing these are extremely important and come from practice.

Inspection

Good lighting and good exposure are essential. Always compare one side to the other. Assess for abnormalities in all of the following:

Texture	Tenderness
Size	Shape, contour, symmetry
Position, alignment	Mobility or movement
Color	Location

The therapist should try to follow the same pattern every time to decrease the chances of missing an assessment parameter and to increase accuracy and thoroughness.

Palpation

Palpation is used to discriminate between textures, dimensions, consistencies, and temperature. It is used to define things that are inspected and to reveal things that cannot be inspected. Textures are best detected using the fingertips, whereas dimension or contours are detected using several fingers, the entire hand, or both hands, depending on the area being examined.

Inspection and palpation are often performed at the same time. Muscle tension interferes with palpation so the client must be positioned and draped appropriately in a room with adequate lighting and temperature.

Assess skin temperature with both hands at the same time. The back of the therapist's hands sense temperature best because of the thin layer of skin. Use the palm or heel of the hand to assess for vibration. The finger pads are best to assess texture, size, shape, position, pulsation, consistency, and turgor. Heavy or continued pressure dulls the examiner's palpatory skill and sensation.

Light palpation is used first, looking for areas of tenderness followed by deep palpation to examine organs or look for masses and elicit deep pain. Light palpation (skin is depressed up to $\frac{1}{2}$ inch) is also used to assess texture, temperature, moisture, pulsations, vibrations, and superficial lesions. Deep palpation is used for assessing abdominal structures. During deep palpation enough pressure is used to depress the skin up to 1 inch. Tender or painful areas are assessed last while carefully observing the client's face for signs of discomfort.

Percussion

Percussion (tapping) is used to determine the size, shape, and density of tissue using sound created by vibration. Percussion can also detect the presence of fluid or air in a body cavity such as the abdominal cavity. Most percussive techniques are beyond the scope of a screening examination and are not discussed in detail.

Percussion can be done directly over the client's skin using the fingertip of the examiner's index finger. Indirect percussion is performed by placing the middle finger of the examiner's nondominant hand firmly against the client's skin then striking above or below the interphalangeal joint with the pad of the middle finger of the dominant hand. The palm and fingers stay off the skin during indirect percussion. Blunt percussion using the ulnar surface of the hand or fist to strike the body surface (directly or indirectly) detects pain from infection or inflammation (see Fig. 4-50).

The examiner must be careful not to dampen the sound by dull percussing (sharp percussion is needed), holding a finger too loosely on the body surface, or resting the hand on the body surface. Percussive sounds lie on a continuum from tympany to flat based on density of tissue.

Auscultation

Some sounds of the body can be heard with the unaided ear; others must be heard by auscultation using a stethoscope. The bell side of the stethoscope is used to listen to low-pitched sounds such as heart murmurs and blood pressure (although the diaphragm can also be used for BP).

Pressing too hard on the skin can obliterate sounds. The diaphragm side of the stethoscope is used to listen to high-pitched sounds such as normal heart sounds, bowel sounds, and friction rubs. Avoid holding either side of the stethoscope with the thumb to avoid hearing your own pulse.

Auscultation usually follows inspection, palpation, and percussion (when percussion is performed). The one exception is during examination of the abdomen, which should be assessed in this order: inspection, auscultation, percussion, then palpation as percussion and palpation can affect findings on auscultation.

Besides measuring blood pressure, auscultation can be used to listen for breath sounds, heart sounds, bowel sounds, and abnormal sounds in the blood vessels called bruits. Bruits are abnormal blowing or swishing sounds heard on auscultation of narrowed or obstructed arteries. Bruits with both systolic and diastolic components suggest the turbulent blood flow of partial arterial occlusion possible with aneurysm or vessel constriction. All large arteries in the neck, abdomen, and limbs can be examined for bruits.

A medical assessment (e.g., physician, nurse, physician assistant) may routinely include auscultation of the temporal and carotid arteries and jugular vein in the head and neck as well as vascular sounds in the abdomen (e.g., aorta, iliac, femoral, and renal arteries). The therapist is more likely to assess for bruits when the client's history (e.g., age over 65, history of coronary artery disease), clinical presentation (e.g., neck, back, abdominal, or flank pain), and associated signs and symptoms (e.g., syncopal episodes, signs and symptoms of peripheral vascular disease) warrant additional physical assessment.

The results from inspection, percussion (when appropriate), and palpation should always be correlated with the client's history, risk factors, clinical presentation, and any associated signs and symptoms before making the decision regarding medical referral.

▶ INTEGUMENTARY SCREENING EXAMINATION

When screening for systemic disease, the therapist must increase attention to what is observable on the outside, primarily the skin and nail beds. Changes in the skin and nail beds may be the first sign of inflammatory, infectious, and immunologic disorders and can occur with involvement of a variety of organs.

For example, dermatitis can occur 6 to 8 weeks before primary signs and symptoms of pulmonary malignancy develop. Clubbing of the fingers can occur quickly in various acute illnesses and conditions. Skin, hair, and nail bed changes are common with endocrine disorders. Renal disease, rheumatic disease, and autoimmune diseases are all accompanied by skin and nail bed changes in many physical therapy clients.

When assessing skin conditions of any kind, even benign lesions such as psoriasis (Fig. 4-2) or eczema, the therapist always should use standard precautions because any disruption of the skin increases the risk of infection. Chronic skin conditions of this type may have new, more effective treatment available. In such cases, the therapist may be able to guide the uninformed client to obtain updated medical treatment.

Consider all findings in relation to the client's age, ethnicity, occupation, and general health. The presence of skin lesions may point to a problem with the integumentary system or may be an integumentary response to a systemic problem.

For example, pruritus is the most common manifestation of dermatologic disease, but is also a symptom of underlying systemic disease in up to 50% of individuals with generalized itching.[44] In both situations skin rash is a common accompanying sign. The most common visceral system causing pruritus is the hepatic system. Look for other associated signs and symptoms of liver or gallbladder impairment such as liver flap (asterixis), carpal tunnel syndrome, liver palms (palmar erythema), and spider angiomas (see Fig. 9-3).

At the same time, be aware that pruritus, or itch, is very common among aging adults. The natural attrition of glands that moisturize the skin combined with the effects of sun exposure, medications, excessive bathing, and harsh soaps can result in dry, irritable skin.[45]

Some clients may describe formication, also referred to as a tactile hallucination, the sensation of ants crawling on the skin, sometimes described as an itching, prickling, or crawling feeling.. The most common cause is menopause, but chronic drug or alchohol use can also cause formication. Some schizophrenics also experience formication. As one of the many side effects of crystal methamphetamine addiction, formication is also referred to as speed bumps, meth sores, and crank bugs.

The therapist may see scratch marks or even broken skin where the sufferer has scratched violently. Open, red (often bleeding) sores appear most commonly on the face and arms but can be anywhere on the body. These lesions can become inflamed, swollen, and pus-filled in the presence of a *Staphylococcus* infection. Left untreated, pathogens can enter the blood stream causing dangerous sepsis or deeper abscess. There is no cure but medical evaluation is needed; topical treatment and cryotherapy can help and antibiotic treatment is needed when there is infection.

New onset of skin lesions especially in children should be medically evaluated (Fig. 4-3). Many conditions in adults and children can be treated effectively; some, but not all, can be cured.

Skin Assessment

With the possible exception of a dermatologist, the therapist sees more skin than anyone else in the health care system. Clients are more likely to point out skin lesions or ask the therapist about lumps and bumps. It is important to have a working

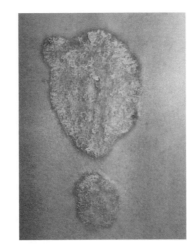

Fig. 4-2 • Psoriasis. A common chronic skin disorder characterized by red patches covered by thick, dry silvery scales that are the result of excessive build-up of epithelial cells. Lesions often come and go and can be anywhere on the body, but are most common on extensor surfaces, bony prominences, scalp, ears, and genitals. Arthritis of the small joints of the hands often accompanies the skin disease (psoriatic arthritis). (From Lookingbill DP, Marks JG: *Principles of dermatology*, ed 2, Philadelphia, 1993, WB Saunders.)

knowledge of benign versus pathologic skin lesions and know when to refer appropriately.

The hands, arms, feet, and legs can be assessed throughout the physical examination for changes in texture, color, temperature, clubbing, circulation including capillary filling, and edema (Box 4-10). Abnormal texture changes include shiny, stiff, coarse, dry, or scaly skin.

Skin mobility and turgor are affected by the fluid status of the client. Dehydration and aging reduce skin turgor (Fig. 4-4) and edema decreases skin mobility. The therapist should be aware of medications that cause skin to become sensitive to sunlight. The most commonly prescribed medications linked with photosensitivity are listed in Box 4-11.

Chronically ill or hospitalized patients should be examined frequently for signs of skin breakdown. Check all pressure points including the ears, sacrum, scapulae, shoulders, area over the greater trochanters, heels, malleoli, and the back of the head. Document staging of any pressure ulcers (Table 4-7).

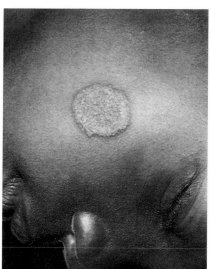

Fig. 4-3 ▲ Tinea corporis or ringworm of the body presents anywhere on the body in adult or children, but more commonly on the chest, abdomen, back of arms, face, and dorsum of the feet. The circular lesions with clear centers can form singly or in clusters and represent a fungal infection that is both contagious and treatable. Tinea pedis (not shown), also known as ringworm of the feet or "athlete's foot" occurs most often between the toes, but also along the sides of the feet and the soles (easily spread and treatable). (From Hurwitz S: *Clinical pediatric dermatology: a textbook of skin disorders of childhood and adolescence,* ed 2, Philadelphia, 1993, WB Saunders.)

BOX 4-10 ▼ Examining a Skin Lesion or Mass

Record observations about any skin lesion or mass using the mnemonic:

5 Students and 5 Teachers around the CAMPFIRE:

- **Site** (location, single vs. multiple)
- **Size**
- **Shape**
- **Spider angiomas** (pregnancy, alcoholism; see Figs. 9-3 and 9-4)
- **Surface** (smooth, rough, indurated, scratches, scarring; see Fig. 4-7), hair growth/loss, bruising [violence, hemophilia, liver damage, thrombocytopenia])
- **Tenderness** or pain
- **Texture**
- **Turgor** (hydration)
- **Temperature**
- **Transillumination** (shine flashlight through it from the side and from the top)
- **Consistency** (soft, spongy, hard), **Color**, **Circulation**
- **Appearance of the client**
- **Mobility** (move the lump in 2 directions: side-to-side and up-down; contract muscle and repeat test)

  Bone: lump is immobile
  Muscle: contraction decreases mobility of the lump
  Subcutaneous: skin moves over lump
  Skin: lump moves with skin

From http://www.clinicalexam.com/pda/g_ref_mass_examination.htm.

- **Pulsation** (place 2 fingers on mass: are fingers pushed in the same direction or apart from each other?)
- **Fluctuation** (does the mass contain fluid: place 2 fingers in V-shape on either side of lump, tap center of lump with index finger of the opposite hand; fingers move if lump is fluid-filled)
- **Irreducibility**
  Compressible: mass goes away or decreases with pressure, but comes back when pressure is released
  Reducible: mass goes away and only comes back with cough or change in position
- **Regional lymph nodes** (examine nearest lymph nodes); **Rash** (e.g., dermatitis, shingles, drug reaction)
- **Edge** (clearly defined, poorly defined, symmetric, asymmetric), **Edema**

If a lesion is present, assess for:

- Associated signs and symptoms (e.g., bleeding, pruritus, fever, joint pain)
- When did the lesion(s) first appear?
- Is it changing over time? How (increasing, decreasing)?
- Were there any known or suspected triggers? (e.g., perfumes, soaps, or cosmetics; medications; environmental/sunlight exposure (includes vectors such as ticks, spiders, scabies, fleas); diet; psychologic or emotional factors)
- A military history may be important.

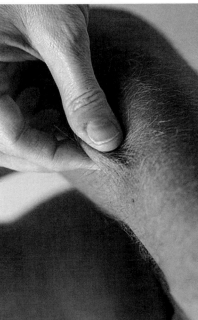

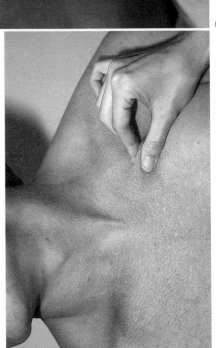

A

B

Fig. 4-4 • To check skin turgor (elasticity or resiliency), gently pinch the skin between your thumb and forefinger, lifting it up slightly, then release. Skin turgor can be tested on the forehead, sternum, beneath the clavicle (**A**), and over the extensor surface of the arm (**B**) or hand. Expect to see the skin lift up easily and return to place quickly. The test is positive for decreased turgor (often caused by dehydration) when the pinched skin remains lifted 5 or more seconds after release and returns to normal very slowly. (**A**, From Seidel HM: *Mosby's guide to physical examination,* ed 4, St. Louis, 1999, Mosby. **B**, From Seidel HM, Ball JW, Dains JE: *Mosby's physical examination handbook,* ed 3, St. Louis, 2003, Mosby.)

TABLE 4-7 ▼ Staging of Pressure Ulcers*

Stage I: Skin changes observable (↑ or ↓ temperature, tissue consistency), sensation (pain, itching)

Stage II: Epidermis and dermis layers are damaged (partial-thickness); ulcer is superficial and presents as an abrasion, blister, or shallow crater

Stage III: Damage through to subcutaneous tissue (full-thickness skin loss); does not extend through fascia; appears as a deep crater

Stage IV: Involvement of muscle, bone, tendon, joint capsule or other supporting structures (full-thickness tissue loss)

*Staging does not indicate the process of wound healing. The National Pressure Ulcer Advisory Panel (NPUAP) also provides the Pressure Ulcer Scale for Healing (PUSH Tool) as a quick, reliable tool to monitor the change in pressure ulcer status over time. Available online at: http://www.npuap.org/push3-0.html.
From U.S. Department of Health and Human Services: *Pressure ulcers in adults: prediction and prevention.* Clinical practice guideline no. 3. AHCPR publication no. 92-0047, Rockville, MD, 1992.

BOX 4-11 ▼ Most Common Medications Causing Photosensitivity

- Ciprofloxacin (antibiotic)
- Doxycycline (antibiotic)
- Furosemide (diuretic)
- Glipizide (hypoglycemic)
- Glyburide (hypoglycemic)
- Ibuprofen (NSAID)
- Ketoprofen (NSAID)
- Naproxen (NSAID)
- Sulfonamides (wide range of antibiotics)
- Tetracycline (antibiotic)
- 5-Fluorouracil (cytotoxic drug)

NSAID, Nonsteroidal anti-inflammatory drug.
From Bergamo BM, Elmets CA: Drug-induced photosensitivity. eMedicine available at:
http://www.emedicine.com/DERM/topic108.htm. Posted October 27, 2004. Accessed March 2005.

The staging system developed by NPUAP is an anatomical description of tissue destruction or wound depth designed for use only with pressure ulcers or wounds created by pressure. While it is essential to have this information, it is also very important to document other wound characteristics such as size, drainage, and granulation tissue, to make the wound assessment complete.

Coordinate with nursing staff to remove prostheses, restraints, and dressings to look beneath them. Anyone with an intravenous line, catheter, or other insertion sites must be examined for signs of infiltration (e.g., pus, erythema), phlebitis, and tape burns.

Observe for signs of edema. Edema is an accumulation of fluid in the interstitial spaces. The potential location of edema helps identify the potential cause. Bilateral edema of the legs may be seen in clients with heart failure or with chronic venous insufficiency.

Abdominal and leg edema can be seen in clients with heart disease, cirrhosis of the liver (or other liver impairment), and protein malnutrition.

Edema may also be noted in dependent areas, such as the sacrum, when a person is confined to bed. Localized edema in one extremity may be the result of venous obstruction (thrombosis) or lymphatic blockage of the extremity (lymphedema).

Vascular changes of an affected extremity may include paresthesia, muscle fatigue and discomfort, or cyanosis with numbness, pain, coolness (poikilothermy), and loss of hair from a reduced blood supply (Box 4-12). Capillary filling of the fingers and toes is an indicator of peripheral circulation. Perform a capillary refill test by pressing down on the nail bed and releasing. Observe first for blanching (whitening) followed by return of color within 3 seconds after release of pressure (normal response).

Change in Skin Color

Skin color changes can occur with a variety of illnesses and systemic conditions. Clients may notice a change in their skin color before anyone else does so be sure and ask about it. Look for pallor; increased or decreased pigmentation; yellow, green, or red skin color; and cyanosis.

Color changes are often observed first in the fingernails, lips, mucous membranes, conjunctiva of the eye, and in dark-skinned people the palms and soles.

Skin changes associated with impairment of the hepatic system include jaundice, pallor, and orange or green skin.

In some situations jaundice may be the first and only manifestation of disease. It is first noticeable

---

BOX 4-12 ▲ Peripheral Vascular Assessment

Inspection

Compare extremities side to side:
Size
Symmetry
Skin (see Box 4-10)
Nail beds
Color
Hair growth
Sensation

Palpation

Pulses (see Fig. 4-1)
Upper Quadrant
Carotid
Brachial
Radial
Ulnar
Lower Quadrant
Femoral
Popliteal
Dorsalis pedis
Posterior tibial

Characteristics of Pulses

Rate
Rhythm
Strength (Amplitude)
• +4 = bounding
• +3 = full, increased
• +2 = normal
• +1 = diminished, weak
• 0 = absent
Check for symmetry (compare right to left)
Compare UE to LE

Arterial Insufficiency of Extremities

Pulses   Decreased or absent
Color   Pale on elevation
     Dusky rubor on dependency
Temperature   Cool/cold
Edema   None
Skin   Shiny, thin pale skin; thick nails;
     hair loss
     Ulcers on toes
Sensation   Pain: increased with exercise
     (claudication) or leg elevation;
     relieved by dependent dangling
     position
     Paresthesias

Venous Insufficiency of Extremities

Pulses   Normal arterial pulses
Color   Pink to cyanotic
     Brown pigment at ankles
Temperature   Warm
Edema   Present
Skin   Discolored, scaly (eczema or stasis
     dermatitis)
     Ulcers on ankles, toes, fingers
     Varicose veins
Sensation   Pain: increased with standing or
     sitting; relieved with elevation or
     support hose

Special (Quick Screening) Tests

Capillary refill time (fingers and toes)
Arterial-Brachial Index (ABI)
Rubor on dependency
Allen test

in the sclera of the eye as a yellow hue when bilirubin level reaches 2 to 3mg/dl. Dark skinned persons may have a normal yellow color to the outer sclera. Jaundice involves the whole sclera up to the iris.

When the bilirubin level reaches 5 to 6mg/dl, the skin becomes yellow. Other skin and nail bed changes associated with liver disease include palmar erythema (see Fig. 9-5), spider angiomas (see Figs. 9-3 and 9-4), and nails of Terry (see Fig. 9-6; see further discussion in Chapter 9).

A bluish cast to skin color can occur with cyanosis when oxygen levels are reduced in the arterial blood (central cyanosis) or when blood is oxygenated normally but blood flow is decreased and slow (peripheral cyanosis). Cyanosis is first observed in the hands and feet, lips, and nose as a pale, blue change in color. The client may report numbness or tingling in these areas.

Central cyanosis is caused by advanced lung disease, congestive heart disease, and abnormal hemoglobin. Peripheral cyanosis occurs with congestive heart failure (decreased blood flow), venous obstruction, anxiety, and cold environment.

Rubor (dusky redness) is a common finding in peripheral vascular disease as a result of arterial insufficiency. When the legs are raised above the level of the heart, pallor of the feet and lower legs develops quickly (usually within 1 minute). When the same client sits up and dangles the feet down, the skin returns to a pink color quickly (usually in about 10 to 15 seconds). A minute later the pallor is replaced by rubor, usually accompanied by pain and diminished pulses. Skin is cool to the touch and trophic changes may be seen (e.g., hair loss over the foot and toes, thick nails, thin skin).

Diffuse hyperpigmentation can occur with Addison's disease, sarcoidosis, pregnancy, leukemia, hemochromatosis, celiac sprue (malabsorption syndrome), scleroderma, and chronic renal failure.

This presents as patchy tan to brown spots most often but may occur as yellow-brown or yellow to tan with scleroderma and renal failure. Any area of the body can be affected, although pigmentation changes in pregnancy tend to affect just the face (melasma or the mask of pregnancy).

Assessing Dark Skin

Clients with dark skin may require a slightly different approach to skin assessment than the Caucasian population. Observe for any obvious changes in the palms of the hands and soles of the feet; tongue, lips, and gums in the mouth; and in the sclera and conjunctiva of the eyes.

Pallor may present as a yellow or ashen-gray due to an absence of the normally present underlying red tones in the skin. The palms and the soles show changes more clearly than the skin. Skin rashes may present as a change in skin texture so palpating for changes is important. Edema can be palpated as "tightness" and darker skin may appear lighter. Inflammation may be perceived as a change in skin temperature instead of redness or erythema of the skin.

Jaundice may appear first in the sclera but can be confused for the normal yellow pigmentation of dark-skinned clients. Be aware that the normal oral mucosa (gums, borders of the tongue, and lining of the cheeks) of dark-skinned individuals may appear freckled.

Petechiae are easier to see when present over areas of skin with lighter pigmentation such as the abdomen, gluteal area, and volar aspect of the forearm. Petechiae and ecchymosis (bruising) can be differentiated from erythema by applying pressure over the involved area. Pressure will cause erythema to blanch, whereas the skin will not change in the presence of petechiae or ecchymosis.

Examining a Mass or Skin Lesion

When examining a skin lesion or mass of any kind, follow the guidelines provided earlier in Box 4-10. In addition, the American Cancer Society (ACS) and the Skin Cancer Foundation advocate using the following ABCD's to assess skin lesions for cancer detection (Fig. 4-5):

A—Asymmetry
B—Border
C—Color
D—Diameter

Round, symmetrical skin lesions such as common moles, freckles, and birthmarks are considered "normal." If an existing mole or other skin lesion starts to change and a line drawn down the middle shows two different halves, medical evaluation is needed.

Common moles and other "normal" skin changes usually have smooth, even borders or edges. Malignant melanomas, the most deadly form of skin cancer, have uneven, notched borders.

Benign moles, freckles, "liver spots," and other benign skin changes are usually a single color (most often a single shade of brown or tan) (Fig. 4-6). A single lesion with more than one shade of black, brown, or blue may be a sign of malignant melanoma.

Even though some of us have moles we think are embarrassingly large, the average mole is really

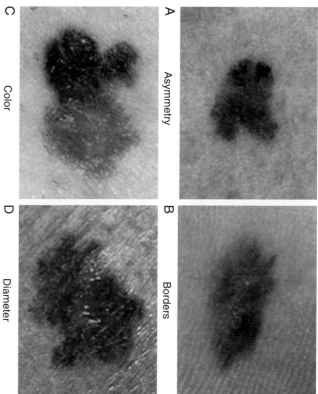

Fig. 4-5 ● Common characteristics associated with early melanomas are described and shown in this photo. **A,** Asymmetry: a line drawn through the middle does not produce matching halves. **B,** Borders are uneven, fuzzy, or have notched or scalloped edges. **C,** Color changes occur with shades of brown, black, tan or other colors present at the same time. **D,** Diameter is greater than the width of a pencil eraser. (From Dermik Laboratories [www.dermnet.com], 2005. Used with permission.)

A   Asymmetry   B   Borders

C   Color   D   Diameter

note of how long the client has had the lesion, if it has changed in the last 6 weeks to 6 months, and whether it has been medically evaluated. Always ask appropriate follow-up questions with this assessment:

Follow Up Questions

- How long have you had this?
- Has it changed in the last 6 weeks to 6 months?
- Has your doctor seen it?
- Does it itch, hurt, feel sore, or burn?
- Does anyone else in your household have anything like this?
- Have you taken any new medications (prescribed or over-the-counter) in the last 6 weeks?
- Have you traveled somewhere new in the last month?
- Have you been exposed to anything in the last month that could cause this? (Consider exposure due to occupational, environmental, and hobby interests.)
- Do you have any other skin changes anywhere else on your body?
- Have you had a fever or sweats in the last 2 weeks?
- Are you having any trouble breathing or swallowing?
- Have you had any other symptoms of any kind anywhere else in your body?

less than ¼ of an inch (about the size of a pencil eraser). Anything larger than this should be inspected carefully.

The Skin Cancer Foundation (www.skincancer.org) has many public education materials available to help the therapist identify suspicious skin lesions. In addition to their website, they have posters, brochures, videos, and other materials available for use in the clinic. It is highly recommended that these types of education materials be available in waiting rooms as part of a nationwide primary prevention program.

Other websites (www.skincheck.com [Skin Cancer Education Foundation]; www.medicine.usyd.edu.au/melanoma/ [The Melanoma Foundation of the University of Sydney Australia]) provide additional photos of suspicious lesions with more screening guidelines. Dermik Laboratories offers an excellent encyclopedia of many categories of skin, finger, and nail bed lesions (www.dermnet.com). The therapist must become as familiar as possible with what suspicious skin aberrations may look like in order to refer as early as possible.

Remember to evaluate risk factors when screening for skin cancer. The average lifetime risk of developing melanoma (Caucasians) is 1 in 70. This has increased from 1 in 90 just in the last two decades. Your risk is much higher if you have any of the risk factors listed in Box 13-2.

For all lesions, masses, or aberrant tissue, observe or palpate for heat, induration, scarring, or discharge. Use the mnemonic in Box 4-10. Make

or discoloration must be noted (photographed if possible).

Start by asking the client if he or she has noticed any changes in the scar. Continue by asking:

Follow Up Questions

- Would you have any objections if I looked at (or examined) the scar tissue?

If the client declines or refuses, be sure to follow up with counsel to perform self-inspection and report any changes to the physician.

In Fig. 4-8, the small scab and granular tissue forming above the scar represent red flags of suspicious local recurrence. Even if the client suggests this is from "picking" at the scar, a medical evaluation is well advised.

The therapist has a responsibility to report these findings to the appropriate health care professional and make every effort to ensure client/patient compliance with follow up.

Common Skin Lesions

Vitiligo

A lack of pigmentation from melanocyte destruction (vitiligo) (Fig. 4-9) can be hereditary and have no significance or it can be caused by conditions such as hyperthyroidism, stomach cancer, pernicious anemia, diabetes mellitus, or autoimmune diseases.

Lesions can occur anywhere on the body but tend to develop in sun-exposed areas, body folds, and around body openings. Intraarticular steroid injections can cause temporary loss of pigmentation at the injection site. Anyone with any kind of skin type and skin color can be affected by vitiligo.

Café-au-lait

Café-au-lait (coffee with milk) spots describe the light-brown macules (flat lesion, different in color) on the skin as shown in Fig. 4-10. This benign skin condition may be associated with Albright's syndrome or a hereditary disorder called neurofibromatosis. The diagnosis is considered when a child presents with five or more of these skin lesions or if any single patch is greater than 1.5 cm in diameter.

Skin Rash

There are many possible causes of skin rash including viruses (e.g., chicken pox, measles, Fifth disease, shingles), systemic conditions (e.g., meningitis, lupus, hives), parasites (e.g., lice, scabies), and reactions to chemicals.

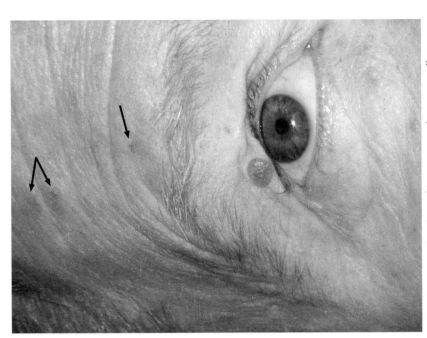

Fig. 4-6 • *Seborrheic keratosis,* a benign well-circumscribed, raised, tan to black lesion often presents on the face, neck, chest, or upper back. This lesion represents a build-up of keratin, the primary component of the epidermis. There is a family tendency to develop these lesions. The more serious lesions are the red patches located on this client's forehead (see arrows), a pre-cancerous lesion called *actinic keratosis,* the result of chronic sun exposure. These lesions have a "sandpaper" feel when palpated. Medical treatment is needed for this premalignant lesion. (Courtesy Catherine C. Goodman, 2005. Used with permission.)

How you ask is just as important as *what* you say. Do not frighten people by first telling them you always screen for skin cancer. It may be better to introduce the subject by saying that as health care professionals, therapists are trained to observe many body parts including the skin, joints, posture, and so on. You notice the client has an unusual mole (or rash . . . or whatever you have observed) and you wonder if this is something that has been there for years. Has it changed in the last six weeks to six months? Has the client ever shown it to the doctor?

Assess Surgical Scars

It is always a good idea to look at surgical scars (Fig. 4-7), especially sites of local cancer removal. Any suspicious scab or tissue granulation, redness,

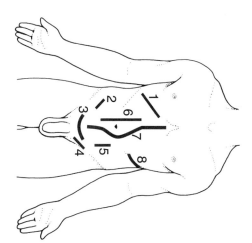

1. Cholecystectomy; a subcostal incision, when made on the right, provides exposure of the gallbladder and common bile duct; used on the left for splenectomy
2. Appendectomy, sometimes called McBurney's or Gridiron incision
3. Transverse suprapubic incision for hysterectomy and other pelvic surgeries
4. Inguinal hernia repair (herniorrhaphy or hernioplasty)
5. Anterior rectal resection (left paramedian incision)
6. Incision through the right flank (right paramedian); called laparotomy or celiotomy; sometimes used to biopsy the liver
7. Midline laparotomy
8. Nephrectomy (removal of the kidney) or other renal surgery

Fig. 4-7 • Abdominal surgical scars. Not shown: puncture sites for laparoscopy, usually close to the umbilicus and one or two other sites.

A common cause of skin rash seen in a physical therapy practice is medications, especially antibiotics (Fig. 4-11). The reaction may occur immediately or there may be a delayed reaction of hours up to 6 to 8 weeks after the drug is stopped.

Skin rash can also occur before visceral malignancy of many kinds. Watch for skin rash or hives in someone who has never had hives before, especially if there has been no contact with medications, new foods, new detergents or perfumes, or travel.

Hemorrhagic Rash

Hemorrhagic rash requires medical evaluation. A hemorrhagic rash occurs when small capillaries under the skin start to bleed forming tiny blood spots under the skin (petechiae). The petechiae increase over time as bleeding continues.

This type of rash does not fade under pressure with continued bleeding. Press a clear see-through drinking glass against the skin. Rashes from allergies or viral infections are more likely to fade and the skin will become white or pale. During later stages of hemorrhagic bleeding the rash does not

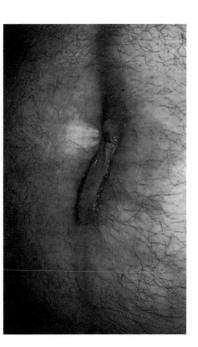

Fig. 4-8 • Squamous cell carcinoma in scar. Always ask to see and examine scars from previous surgeries, especially when there has been a history of any kind of cancer, including skin cancer. Even in this black and white photo, you can see many skin changes to suggest the need for medical evaluation. Look to the far right of the raised scar tissue. You will see a normal, smooth scar. This is what the entire scar should look like. In this photo there is a horizontal line of granulation along the upper edge of the scar as well as a scabbed over area in the middle of the raised scar. There is also a change in skin color on either side of the scar. (From Swartz MH: *Textbook of physical diagnosis,* ed 4, Philadelphia, 2001, WB Saunders.)

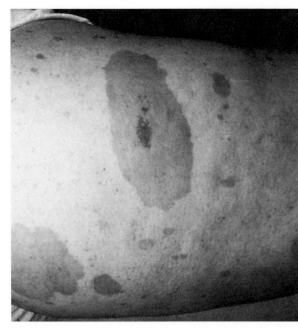

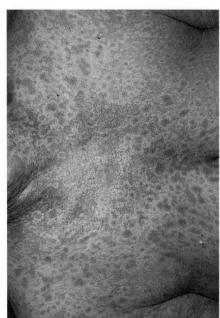

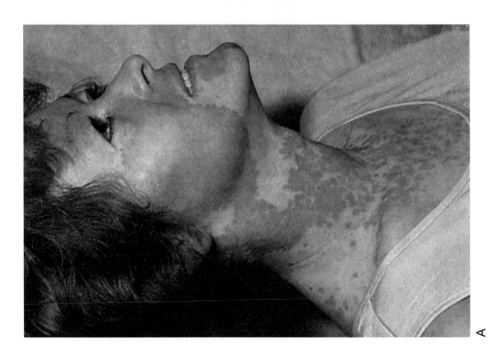

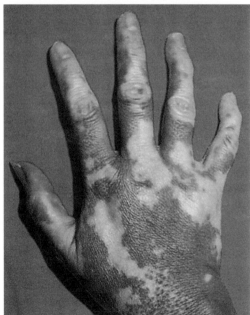

Fig. 4-10 • Café-au-lait patches of varying sizes in a client with neurofibromatosis. Occasional (less than 5) of these tan macules is not significant and can occur normally. Patches 1.5 cm in diameter or larger raise the suspicion of underlying pathology even if there is only one present. (From Epstein O, Perkin GD, deBono DP et al: *Clinical examination.* London, 1992, Gower Medical Publishing. Used with permission, Elsevier Science.)

Fig. 4-11 • Skin rash (reactive erythema) caused by a drug reaction to phenobarbital. Hypersensitivity reactions to drugs is most common with antibiotics (especially penicillin), sulfonamides ("sulfa drugs," antiinfectives), and phenobarbital as shown here. (From Callen JP, Paller AS, Greer KE, et al: *Color atlas of dermatology,* ed 2, Philadelphia, 2000, WB Saunders.)

Fig. 4-9 • Vitiligo. **A,** Woman who developed vitiligo at age 40 with no known cause or known precipitating triggers. **B,** Vitiligo of the hands in a Caucasian male diagnosed with hyperthyroidism. (**A,** From Swartz MH: *Textbook of physical diagnosis,* ed 4, Philadelphia, 2001, WB Saunders. **B,** From Lookingbill DP, Marks JG: *Principles of dermatology,* ed 2, Philadelphia, 1993, WB Saunders.)

fade or become pale with the pressure test; this test is not as reliable during early onset of hemorrhage. Left untreated, hemorrhagic spots may become bruises and then large red-purple areas of blood. Pressure on a bruise will not cause it to blanch.

Dermatitis

Dermatitis (sometimes referred to as eczema) is characterized by skin that is red, brown, or gray; sore; itchy; and sometimes swollen. The skin can develop blisters and weeping sores. Skin changes, especially in the presence of open lesions, puts the client at increased risk of infection. In chronic dermatitis, the skin can become thick and leathery.

There are different types of dermatitis diagnosed on the basis of medical history, etiology (if known), and presenting signs and symptoms. Contributing factors include stress, allergies, genetics, infection, and environmental irritants. For example, contact dermatitis occurs when the skin reacts to something it has come into contact with such as soap, perfume, metals in jewelry, and plants (e.g., poison ivy or oak).

Dyshidrotic dermatitis can affect skin that gets wet frequently. It presents as small, itchy bumps on the sides of the fingers or toes and progresses to a rash. Atopic dermatitis often accompanies asthma or hay fever. It appears to affect genetically predisposed clients who are hypersensitive to environmental allergens. This type of dermatitis can affect any part of the body, but often involves the skin inside the elbow and on the back of the knees.

Rosacea

Rosacea is a chronic facial skin disorder seen most often in adults between the ages of 30 and 60 years. It can cause a facial rash easily mistaken for the butterfly rash associated with lupus. Features include erythema, flushing, telangiectasia, papules, and pustules affecting the cheeks and nose of the face. An enlarged nose is often present and the condition progressively gets worse (Fig. 4-12).

Rosacea can be controlled with dermatologic or other medical treatment in some cases. Recent studies suggest rosacea may be linked to gastrointestinal disease caused by the *Helicobacter pylori* bacteria.[46-48] Such cases may respond favorably to antibiotics. Medical referral is needed for an accurate diagnosis.

Thrombocytopenia

Decrease in platelet levels can result in thrombocytopenia, a bleeding disorder characterized by petechiae (tiny purple or red spots), multiple bruises, and hemorrhage into the tissues (Fig. 4-13). Joint bleeds, nose and gum bleeds, excessive

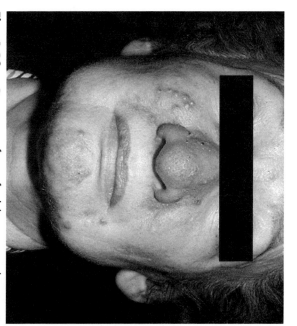

Fig. 4-12 • Rosacea, a form of adult acne may be associated with *Helicobacter pylori*; medical evaluation and treatment is needed to rule out this possibility. (Courtesy of the University of Iowa Virtual Hospital. Copyright protected material used with permission of the authors and the University of Iowa's Virtual Hospital; www.vh.org/adult/provider/dermatology/PietteDermatology/BlackTray/33Rosacea.html.)

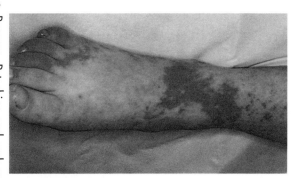

Fig. 4-13 • Purpura. Petechiae and ecchymoses are seen in this flat macular hemorrhage from thrombocytopenia (platelet level less than $100,000\ mm^3$). This condition also occurs in older adults as blood leaks from capillaries in response to minor trauma. It can occur in fair-skinned people with skin damage from a lifetime of exposure to ultraviolet radiation. Exposure to UVB and UVA rays can cause permanent damage to the structural collagen that supports the walls of the skin's blood vessels. Combined with thinning of the skin that occurs with aging, radiation-impaired blood vessels are more likely to rupture with minor trauma. (From Hurwitz S: *Clinical pediatric dermatology: a textbook of skin disorders of childhood and adolescence*, ed 2, Philadelphia, 1993, WB Saunders.)

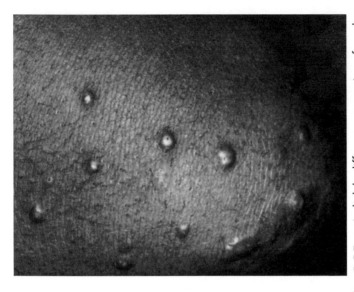

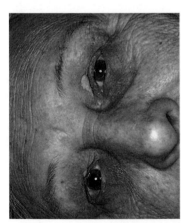

Fig. 4-14 • Xanthelasma. Soft, raised yellow plaques also known as xanthomas commonly occur with aging and may be a sign of high cholesterol levels. Shown here on the eyelid, these benign lesions also occur on the extensor surfaces of tendons, especially in the hands, elbows, and knees. They may have no pathologic significance but they often appear in association with disorders of lipid metabolism. (From Albert DM, Jakobiec FA: *Principles and practice of ophthalmology*, Vol 3, Philadelphia, 1994, WB Saunders.)

menstruation, and melena (dark, tarry, sticky stools from oxidized blood in the GI tract) can occur with thrombocytopenia.

There are many causes of thrombocytopenia. In a physical therapy practice the most common causes seen are bone marrow failure from radiation treatment, leukemia, or metastatic cancer; cytotoxic agents used in chemotherapy; and drug-induced platelet reduction, especially among adults with rheumatoid arthritis treated with gold or inflammatory conditions treated with aspirin or other NSAIDs.

Post-operative thrombocytopenia can be heparin-induced for patients receiving intravenous heparin. Watch for limb ischemia, cyanosis of fingers or toes, signs and symptoms of a stroke, heart attack, or pulmonary embolus. (See further discussion on Thrombocytopenia in Chapter 5.)

Xanthomas

Xanthomas are benign fatty fibrous yellow plaques, nodules, or tumors that develop in the subcutaneous layer of skin (Fig. 4-14), often around tendons. The lesion is characterized by the intracellular accumulation of cholesterol and cholesterol esters.

These are seen most often associated with disorders of lipid metabolism, primary biliary cirrhosis, and uncontrolled diabetes (Fig. 4-15). They may have no pathologic significance but can occur in association with malignancy such as leukemia, lymphoma, or myeloma. Xanthomas require a medical referral if they have not been evaluated

Fig. 4-15 • A slightly different presentation of xanthomas, this time associated with poorly controlled diabetes mellitus. Although the lesion is considered "benign" the presence of these skin lesions in anyone with diabetes signals the need for immediate medical attention. The therapist also plays a key role in client education and the development of an appropriate exercise program to bring blood glucose levels under adequate control. (From Callen JP, Jorizzo J, Greer KE, et al: *Dermatological signs of internal disease*, Philadelphia, 1988, WB Saunders.)

by a physician. When associated with diabetes, these nodules will resolve with adequate glucose control.

The therapist has an important role in education and prescriptive exercise for the client with xanthomas from poorly controlled diabetes. Gaining control of glucose levels using the three keys of intervention (diet, exercise, and insulin or oral hypoglycemic medication) is essential and requires a team management approach.

Rheumatologic Diseases

Skin lesions are often the first sign of an underlying rheumatic disease (Box 4-13). In fact, the skin has been called a "map to rheumatic diseases." The butterfly rash over the nose and cheeks associated with lupus erythematosus can be seen in the acute (systemic) phase, whereas discoid lesions are more common with chronic integumentary form of lupus (Fig. 4-16).[49]

Dermatomyosites often have a heliotrope rash and/or Gottron papules. Scleroderma is

Fig. 4-16 • Skin lesions associated with discoid lupus erythematosus. These disk-shaped lesions look like warts or squamous cell carcinoma. A medical examination is needed to make the definitive differential diagnosis. (From Callen JP, Jorizzo J, Greer KE, et al: *Dermatological signs of internal disease*, Philadelphia, 1988, WB Saunders.)

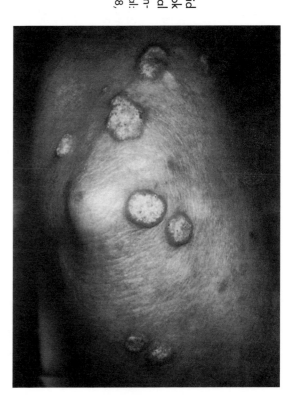

---

accompanied by many skin changes; pitting of the nails is common with psoriatic arthritis. Skin and nail bed changes are common with some sexually transmitted diseases that also have a rheumatologic component (see Figs. 3-10, 4-18, and 4-19).[50]

Steroid Skin

Steroid skin is the name given when bruising or ecchymosis occurs as a result of chronic use of topical or systemic corticosteroids (Fig. 4-17). In the case of topical steroid creams, this is a red flag that pain is not under control and medical attention for an underlying (probably inflammatory) condition is needed.

Whenever signs and symptoms of chronic corticosteroids are seen, a medical evaluation may be

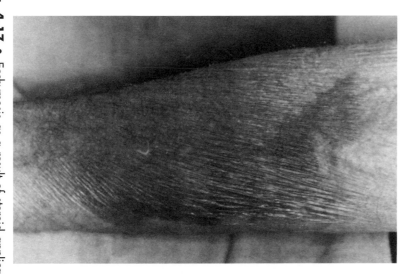

Fig. 4-17 • Ecchymosis as a result of steroid application. Also note the cutaneous atrophy produced by topical steroids. This skin condition is referred to as "steroid skin" when associated with chronic oral or topical steroid use. Medical referral may be needed for better pain control. (From Callen JP, Jorizzo J, Greer KE, et al: *Dermatological signs of internal disease*, Philadelphia, 1988, WB Saunders.)

needed to review medical management of the problem. In the case of steroid corticosteroid use, ask if the physician has seen (or knows about) the signs and symptoms and how long it has been since medications have been reviewed. The multiple side effects of chronic corticosteroid use are discussed in association with Cushing's syndrome (see Chapter 11).

Erythema Chronicum Migrans

One or more erythema migrans rash may occur with Lyme disease. There is no one prominent rash. The rash varies in size and shape and may have purple, red, or bruised-looking rings. The rash may appear as a solid red expanding rash or blotch, or as a central red spot surrounded by clear skin that is ringed by an expanding red rash. It may be smooth or bumpy to the touch and it may itch or ooze. The Lyme Disease Foundation provides a photo gallery of possible rashes associated with Lyme disease.[50]

This rash, which develops in most people with Lyme disease, appears most often 1 to 2 weeks after the disease is transmitted (via tick bite) and may persist for 3 to 5 weeks. It usually is not painful or itchy but may be warm to the touch. The bull's-eye rash may be more difficult to see on darker-skinned people. A dark, bruise-like appearance is more common in those cases. Other symptoms are listed in Chapter 12.

Effects of Radiation

Radiation for the treatment of some cancers has some specific effects on the skin. Pigment producing cells can be affected by either low dose radiation causing hyperpigmentation or by high dose radiation resulting in depigmentation (vitiligo). Pigmentation changes can be localized or generalized.[51]

Radiation recall reaction can occur months later as a post-irradiation effect. The physiologic response is much like overexposure to the sun with erythema of the skin in the same pattern as the radiation exposure without evidence of disease progression at that site. It is usually precipitated by some external stimuli or event such as exposure to the sun, infection, or stress.

Radiation recall is also more likely to occur when an individual receives certain chemotherapies (e.g., cyclophosphamide, paclitaxel, doxorubicin, gemcitabine) after radiation.[52,53] The chemotherapy causes the previously radiated area to become inflamed and irritated.

Radiation dermatitis and X-ray keratosis, separate from radiation recall, are terms used to describe acute (expected) skin irritation caused by radiation at the time of radiation.

Skin changes can also occur as a long-term effect of radiation exposure. Radiation levels administered to oncology patients even 10 years ago were much higher than today's current treatment regimes. Always look at previous radiation sites for evidence of long-term effects.

Sexually Transmitted Infections

Sexually transmitted diseases (STDs), also known as sexually transmitted infections (STIs) are often accompanied by skin and/or nail bed lesions and joint pain. Being able to recognize STIs is helpful in the clinic. Someone presenting with joint pain of "unknown cause" and also demonstrating signs of a STI (see Fig. 3-10) may help bring the correct diagnosis to light sooner than later.

Around the world, STIs pose a major health problem. In 1970 there were two major STIs; today there are 25. The prevalence of STIs is rapidly increasing to epidemic proportions in the United States. Two-thirds of all STIs occur in people 25 years of age or younger.[54,55]

STIs have been positively identified as a risk factor for cancer. Not all STIs are linked with cancer, but studies have confirmed that human papilloma virus (HPV) is the primary cause of cervical cancer (Fig. 4-18).[56] HPV is the leading viral STI in the U.S. More than 70 types of HPV have been identified; 23 infect the cervix, 13 types are associated with cancer (men and women). Infection with one of these viruses does not predict cancer, but the risk of cancer is increased.

Syphilis is on the rise again with the number of cases doubled in the last few years among gay and bisexual men suggesting an erosion of safe sex practices.[57,58] It is highly contagious, spread from person to person by direct contact with a syphilis sore on the body of an infected person. Sores occur at the site of infection, mainly on the external genitals, vagina, anus, or rectum. Sores can also occur on the lips and in the mouth.

Transmission occurs during vaginal, anal, or oral sex. An infected pregnant woman can also pass the disease to her unborn child. Syphilis cannot be spread by contact with toilet seats, doorknobs, swimming pools, hot tubs, bathtubs, shared clothing, or eating utensils.

In the first stage of syphilis, a syphilis chancre may appear (Fig. 4-19) at the site of inoculation (usually the genitals, anus, or mouth). The chancre occurs 4 weeks after initial infection and is often

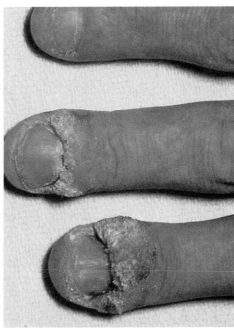

Fig. 4-18 • Common warts of the hands caused by human papilloma virus (nonsexual transmission). The virus can be transmitted through sexual contact and is a precursor to cancer of the cervix. Genital warts do not typically occur by autoinoculation from the hands. In other words, warts on the fingers caused by HPV are probably NOT transmitted from finger to genitals. They occur with contact of someone else's genital warts. Warts on the fingers caused by sexually transmitted HPV do not transmit the STI to the therapist if the therapist shakes hands with the client or touches the warts. However, standard precautions are always recommended whenever skin lesions of any kind are present. For a summary of Standard Precautions, see Goodman et al., 2003.[56] (From Parkin JM, Peters BS: *Differential diagnosis in AIDs,* London, 1991, Mosby-Wolfe.)

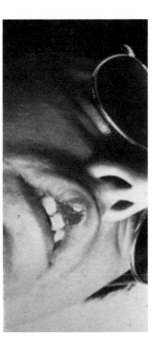

Fig. 4-19 • The first stage (primary syphilis) is marked by a very infectious sore, called a chancre. The chancre is usually small, firm, round with well-demarcated edges, and painless. It appears at the spot where the bacteria entered the body. Chancres last 1 to 5 weeks and heal on their own. (Courtesy Pfizer Laboratories Division, Pfizer Inc, New York, New York. From "A close look at venereal disease." A slide presentation produced as a public service. Pfizer Laboratories, New York, New York, date unknown. Permission granted 2004.)

not noticed in women when present in the genitalia. The chancre is often accompanied by lymphadenopathy.

Without treatment, the chancre is often not noticed in women when present in the genitalia. The appearance of these skin lesions occurs after the primary chancre disappears. During this time the risk of human

Without treatment, the spread of the bacteria through the blood causes the second stage

A
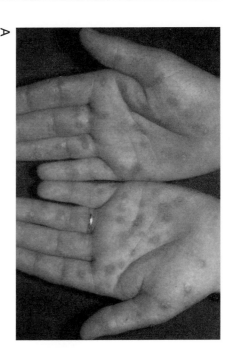

B
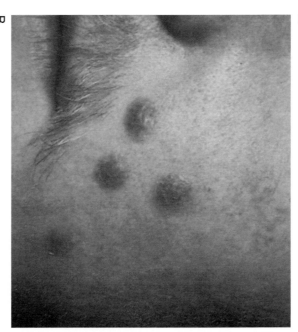

Fig. 4-20 • Maculopapular rash associated with secondary syphilis appears as pink, dusky, brownish-red or coppery, indurated, oval or round lesion with a raised border. These are referred to as "copper penny" spots. The lesions do not bleed and are usually painless. They usually appear scattered on the palms **(A)** or the bottom of the feet (not shown), but may also present on the face **(B).** The second stage begins 2 weeks to 6 months after the initial chancre disappears. The client may report joint pain with general flu-like symptoms (e.g., headache, sore throat, swollen glands, muscle aches, fatigue). Patchy hair loss may be described or observed. (From Mir MA: *Atlas of clinical diagnosis,* London, 1995, WB Saunders; p 198.)

(secondary syphilis). Therapists may also see lesions associated with secondary syphilis (Fig. 4-20).

The client may report or present with a characteristic rash that can appear all over the body, most often on the palms and soles. The appearance of these skin lesions occurs after the primary chancre disappears. During this time the risk of human

immunodeficiency virus (HIV) transmission from unsafe sexual practices is increased twofold to fivefold.

Syphilis can be tested for with a blood test and treated successfully with antibiotics. Left untreated, tertiary (late stage) syphilis can cause paralysis, blindness, personality changes or dementia, and damage to internal organs and joints. The therapist can facilitate early detection and treatment through immediate medical referral. See further discussion on Infectious Causes of Pelvic Pain in Chapter 15 including special questions to ask concerning sexual activity and STIs.

HERPES VIRUS

Several herpes viruses are accompanied by characteristic skin lesions. Herpes simplex virus (HSV) 1 and 2 are the most common. Most people have been exposed at an early age and already have immunity. In fact, four out of five Americans harbor HSV-1. Due to the universal distribution of these viruses, most individuals have developed immunity by the ages of 1 to 2 years.

The HSV 1 and HSV 2 viruses are virtually identical, sharing approximately 50% of their DNA. Both types infect the body's mucosal surfaces, usually the mouth or genitals, and then establish latency in the nervous system.[59] Both can cause skin and nail bed changes.

Cold sores caused by HSV 1 (also known as recurrent herpes labialis; "fever blister") are found on the lip or the skin near the mouth. HSV 1 usually establishes latency in the trigeminal ganglion, a collection of nerve cells near the ear. HSV 1 generally only infects areas above the waistline and occurs when oral secretions or mucous membranes infected with HSV come in contact with a break in the skin (e.g., torn cuticle, skin abrasion).

HSV-1 can be transmitted to the genital area during oral sex. In fact, HSV-1 can be transmitted oral-to-oral, oral-to-genital, anal-to-genital and oral-to-anal. HSV-1 actually predominates for oral transmission, while a second herpesvirus (genital herpes; HSV-2) is more often transmitted sexually.

HSV 2, also known as "genital herpes" can cause cold sores but usually does not; rather, it is more likely to infect body tissues below the waistline as it resides in the sacral ganglion at the base of the spine.

Most HSV 1 and 2 infections are not a major health threat in most people but slowing the spread of genital herpes is important. The virus is more of a social problem than a medical one. The exception is that genital lesions from herpes can make it easier for a person to become infected with other viruses, including the human immunodeficiency virus (HIV), which increases the risk of developing autoimmune deficiency syndrome (AIDS).

Nonmedical treatment with over-the-counter products is now available for cold sores. Outbreaks of genital herpes can be effectively treated with medications but these do not "cure" the virus. HSV-1 is also the cause of herpes whitlow, an infection of the finger and "wrestler's herpes," a herpes infection on the chest or face.

Herpetic Whitlow Herpetic whitlow, an intense painful infection of the terminal phalanx of the fingers is caused by HSV 1 (60%) and HSV 2 (40%). The thumb and index fingers are most commonly involved. There may be a history of fever or malaise several days before symptoms occur in the fingers.

Common initial symptoms of infection include tingling pain or tenderness of the affected digit, followed by throbbing pain, swelling, and redness. Fluid-filled vesicles form, which eventually crust over ending the contagious period. The client with red streaks down the arm and lymphadenopathy may have a secondary infection. Take the client's vital signs (especially body temperature) and report all findings to the physician.[60]

As in other herpes infections, viral inoculation of the host occurs through exposure to infected body fluids via a break in the skin, such as a paper cut or a torn cuticle. Autoinoculation can occur in anyone with other herpes infections such as genital herpes. It is an occupational risk among health care workers exposed to infected oropharyngeal secretions of clients, easily prevented by using standard precautions.[61]

Herpes Zoster Varicella-zoster virus or VZV (herpes zoster or "shingles") is another herpes virus with skin lesions characteristic of the condition. VZV is caused by the same virus that causes chickenpox. After an attack of chickenpox, the virus lies dormant in the nerve tissue, usually the dorsal root ganglion. If the virus is reactivated the virus can reappear in the form of shingles.

Shingles is an outbreak of a rash or blisters (vesicles with an erythematosus base) on the skin that may be associated with severe pain (Fig. 4-21). The pain is associated with the involved nerve root and associated dermatome and generally presents on one side of the body or face in a pattern characteristic for the involved site (Fig. 4-22). Early signs of shingles include burning or shooting pain and tingling or itching. The rash or blisters are present anywhere from 1 to 14 days.

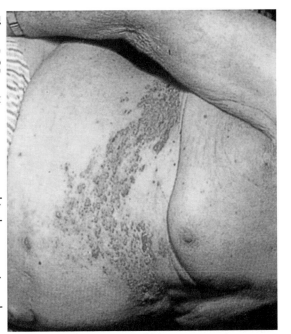

Fig. 4-21 • Herpes zoster or shingles appearing along spinal nerve dermatome in an older adult. Affected individuals report itching, burning, tingling, or shooting pain that can be intolerable. (From Bryant RA: *Acute and chronic wounds: nursing management*, St. Louis, 1992, Mosby.)

has healed. PHN can be very debilitating. Early intervention within the first 72 hours of onset with anti-retroviral medications may diminish or eliminate PHN. Early identification and intervention is very important to outcomes.

Adults with shingles are infectious to anyone who has not had chickenpox. Anyone who has had chickenpox can develop shingles when immuno-compromised. Other risk factors for VZV include age (young or old), and immunocompromise from HIV infection, chemotherapy or radiation treatment, transplant recipients, aging, and stress. It is highly recommended that health care professionals with no immunity to varicella-zoster receive the varicella vaccine. Therapists who have never had chickenpox (and especially women of childbearing age who have not had the chickenpox) should be tested for immune status.

Cutaneous Manifestations of Abuse

Signs of child abuse or domestic violence in adults may be seen as skin lesions. Cigarette burns leave a punched out ulceration with dry, purple crusts (see www.dermatlas.org). Splash marks or scald lines from thermal (hot water) burns occur most often on the buttocks and distal extremities.[62] Bruising from squeezing and shaking involving the mid-portion of the upper arms is a suspicious sign.

Accidental bruising in young children is common; the therapist should watch for nonacci-dental bruising found in atypical areas such as the buttocks, hands, and trunk or in a child who is not yet biped (up on two feet) and cruising (walking along furniture or holding an object while taking steps). To make an accurate assessment, it is important to differentiate between inflicted cutaneous injuries and mimickers of physical abuse.

For example, infants with bruising may be demonstrating early signs of bleeding disorders.[62] Mongolian spots can also be mistaken for bruising from child abuse (see next section). The therapist is advised to take digital or Polaroid photos of any suspicious lesions in children under the age of 18. Document the date and provide a detailed description.

The law requires that professionals report suspected child abuse and neglect to the appropriate authorities. It is not up to the health care professional to determine child abuse has occurred, this is left up to investigating officials. See other guidelines regarding child abuse and domestic violence in Chapter 2. Understanding the reporting guidelines helps direct practitioners in their decision making.[62]

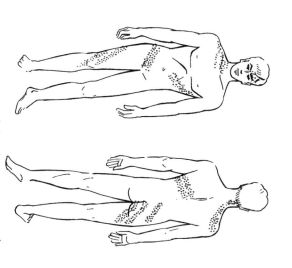

Fig. 4-22 • Symptoms of shingles appear on only one side of the body, usually on the torso or face. Most often, the lesions are visible externally. In unusual cases clients report the same symptoms internally along the dermatome but without a corresponding external skin lesion. (From Malasanos L, Barkauskas V, Stoltenberg-Allen K: *Health assessment*, ed 4, St. Louis, 1990, Mosby.)

Complications of shingles involving cranial nerves include hearing and vision loss. Postherpetic neuralgia (PHN) can also occur, a condition in which the pain from shingles persists for months, sometimes years, after the shingles rash

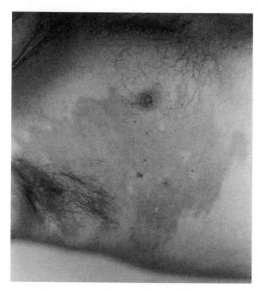

Fig. 4-24 ● Metastatic carcinoma presenting as a cellulitic skin rash on the anterior chest wall as a result of carcinoma of the lung. This rash can be red, tan, or brown with a flat or raised appearance. When associated with a paraneoplastic syndrome it may appear far from the site of the primary cancer. (From Callen JP, Jorizzo J, Greer KE, et al: *Dermatological signs of internal disease*, Philadelphia, 1988, WB Saunders.)

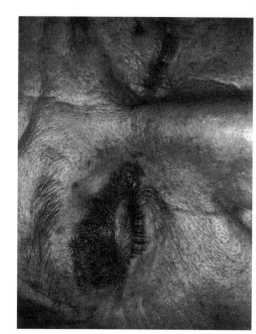

Fig. 4-25 ● Pinch purpura in an individual with multiple myeloma caused by amyloidosis of the skin. The purpura shown here is a recent skin change for this client. (From Callen JP, Jorizzo J, Greer KE, et al: *Dermatological signs of internal disease*, ed 2, Philadelphia, 1995, WB Saunders.)

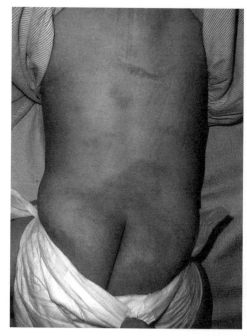

Fig. 4-23 ● Mongolian spots (congenital dermal melanocytosis). Mongolian spots are common among people of Asian, East Indian, Native American, Inuit, African, and Latino or Hispanic heritage. They are also present in about one in ten fair-skinned infants. Bluish gray to deep brown to black skin markings, they often appear on the base of the spine, on the buttocks and back and even sometimes on the shoulders, ankles, or wrists. Mongolian spots may cover a large area of the back. When the melanocytes are close to the surface, they look deep brown. The deeper they are in the skin, the more bluish they look, often mistaken for signs of child abuse. These spots "fade" with age as the child grows and usually disappear by age 5. (Courtesy Dr. Dubin Pavel, 2004.)

MONGOLIAN SPOTS

Discoloration of the skin in newborn infants called Mongolian spots (Fig. 4-23) can be mistaken for signs of child abuse. The Mongolian spot is a congenital, developmental condition exclusively involving the skin and is very common in children of Asian, African, Indian, Native American, Eskimo, Polynesian, or Hispanic origins.

These benign pigmentation changes appear as flat dark blue or black areas and come in a variety of sizes, shapes, and colors. The skin changes result from entrapment of melanocytes (skin cells containing melanin, the normal pigment of the skin) during their migration from the neural crest into the epidermis.

Cancer-Related Skin Lesions

When screening for primary skin cancer, keep in mind there are other cancer-related skin lesions to watch out for as well. For example, skin rash can present as an early sign of a paraneoplastic syndrome before other manifestations of cancer or cancer recurrence (Fig. 4-24). See further discussion of paraneoplastic syndromes in Chapter 13.

Pinch purpura, a purplish, brown or red discoloration of the skin can be mistaken by the therapist for a birthmark or port wine stain (Fig. 4-25). Using the question "How long have you had this?" can help differentiate between something the person has had his or her entire life and a suspicious skin lesion or recent change in the integument.

When purpura causes a raised and palpable skin lesion, it is called *palpable purpura*. The palpable hemorrhages are caused by red blood cells extravasated (escaped) from damaged vessels into the dermis.

This type of purpura can be associated with cutaneous vasculitis, pulmonary-renal syndrome, or drug reaction. The lower extremities are affected most often.

Many older adults assume this is a "normal" sign of aging (and in fact, purpura does occur more often in aging adults; see Fig. 4-13); they do not see a physician when it first appears. Early detection and referral is always the key to a better prognosis. In asking the three important questions, the therapist plays an instrumental part in the cancer screening process.

A client with a past medical history of cancer now presenting with a suspicious skin lesion (Fig. 4-26) that has not been evaluated by the physician must be advised to have this evaluated as soon as possible. We must be aware of how to present this recommendation to the client. There is a need to avoid frightening the client while conveying the importance of early diagnosis of any unusual skin lesions.

Kaposi's Sarcoma

Kaposi's sarcoma is a form of skin cancer common in older Jewish men of Mediterranean descent that presents with a wide range of appearance. A gallery of photos can be seen by doing a Google search of "Kaposi's sarcoma." [Go to www.Google.com and type in the words: Kaposi's sarcoma, then click on the word 'Images' on the Google page). It is not contagious to touch and does not usually cause death or disfigurement.

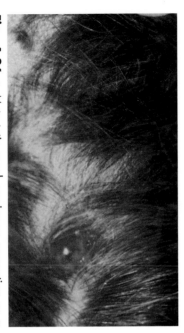

Fig. 4-26 • Metastatic renal carcinoma presenting as a nodule in the scalp. Observing any skin lesions no matter what part of the body the therapist is examining must be followed by the three assessment questions listed in the text. (From Callen JP, Jorizzo J, Greer KE, et al: *Dermatological signs of internal disease*, Philadelphia, 1988, WB Saunders.)

More recently, Kaposi's sarcoma has presented as an opportunistic disease in adults with HIV/AIDS. With the more successful treatment of AIDS with antiretroviral agents, opportunistic diseases such as Kaposi's sarcoma are on the decline.

Even though this skin lesion will not transmit skin cancer or the human immunodeficiency virus, the therapist is always advised to use standard precautions with anyone who has skin lesions of any type.

Lymphomas

Round patches of reddish-brown skin with hair loss over the area are lymphomas, a type of neoplasm of lymphoid tissue (Fig. 4-27). The most common forms of lymphoma are Hodgkin's disease and non-Hodgkin's lymphoma (NHL).

Typically, the appearance of a painless, enlarged lymph node or skin lesion of this type is followed by weakness, fever, and weight loss. A history of chronic immunosuppression (e.g., anti-rejection drugs for organ transplants, chronic use of immunosuppressant drugs for inflammatory or autoimmune diseases, cancer treatment) in the presence of this clinical presentation is a major red flag.

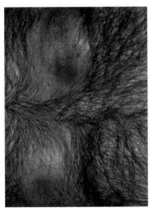

Fig. 4-27 • Lymphomas seen here just below the nipples on the chest of an adult male arise in individuals who are chronically immunosuppressed for any reason. (From Conant MA: The link between HIV and skin malignancies, *The Skin Cancer Foundation Journal*, Vol XII, 1994.)

▼ NAIL BED ASSESSMENT

As with assessment of the skin, nail beds (fingers and toes) should be evaluated for color, shape, thickness, texture, and the presence of lesions (Box 4-14). Systemic changes affect both fingernails and toenails, but the signs are typically more prominent in the faster-growing fingernails.[63]

The normal nail consists of three parts: the nail bed, the nail plate, and the cuticle (Fig. 4-28). The nail bed is highly vascularized and gives the nail

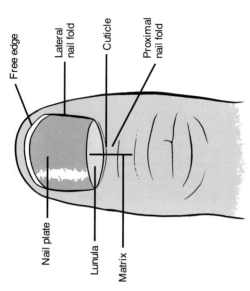

Free edge
Lateral nail fold
Cuticle
Proximal nail fold
Nail plate
Lunula
Matrix

Fig. 4-28 • Normal nail structure. The nail matrix forms the nail plate and begins about 5 mm to 8 mm beneath the proximal nail fold and extends distally to the edge of the lunula, where the nail bed begins. The lunula (half-moon) is the exposed part of the nail matrix, distal to the proximal nail fold; it is not always visible.

Many individual variations in color, texture, and grooming of the nails are influenced by factors unrelated to disease, such as occupation, chronic use of nail polish or acrylics, or exposure to chemical dyes and detergents. Longitudinal lines of darker color (pigment) may be seen in the normal nails of clients with darker skin.

In assessing the older adult, minor variations associated with the aging process may be observed (e.g., gradual thickening of the nail plate, appearance of longitudinal ridges, yellowish-gray discoloration).

In the normal individual, pressing or blanching the nail bed of a finger or toe produces a whitening effect; when pressure is released, a return of color should occur within 3 seconds. If the capillary refill time exceeds 3 seconds, the lack of circulation may be due to arterial insufficiency from atherosclerosis or spasm.

Nail Bed Changes

Some of the more common nail bed changes seen in a physical therapy practice are included in this chapter. With any nail or skin condition, ask if the nails have always been like this or if any changes have occurred in the last 6 weeks to 6 months. Referral may not be needed if the physician is aware of the new onset of nail bed changes. Ask about the presence of other signs and symptoms consistent with any of the conditions listed here that can cause any of these nail bed changes.

BOX 4-14 ▼ Hand and Nail Bed Assessment

Observe The Hands For:

- Palmar erythema (see Fig. 9-5)
- Tremor (e.g., liver flap or asterixis; see Fig. 9-7)
- Pallor of palmar creases (anemia, GI malabsorption)
- Palmar xanthomas (lipid deposits on palms of hands; hyperlipidemia, diabetes)
- Turgor (lift skin on back of hands; hydration status; see Fig 4-4)
- Edema

Observe The Fingers and Toenails For:

- Color (capillary refill time, Nails of Terry: see Fig. 9-6)
- Shape and curvature
- Clubbing:
  Crohn's or Cardiac/cyanosis
  Lung (cancer, hypoxia, cystic fibrosis)
  Ulcerative colitis
  Biliary cirrhosis
  Present at birth (harmless)
  Neoplasm
  GI involvement
- Nicotine stains
- Splinter hemorrhages (see Fig. 4-32)
- Leukonychia (whitening of nail plate with bands, lines, or white spots; inherited or acquired from malnutrition from eating disorders, alcoholism, or cancer treatment; myocardial infarction, renal failure, poison, anxiety)
- Koilonychia ("spoon nails;" see Fig. 4-30); congenital or hereditary, iron-deficiency anemia, thyroid problem, syphilis, rheumatic fever)
- Beau's lines (see Fig. 4-31); decreased production of the nail by the matrix caused by acute illness or systemic insult such as chemotherapy for cancer; recent myocardial infarction, chronic alcohol abuse, or eating disorders. This can also occur in isolated nail beds from local trauma
- Adhesion to the nail bed. Look for onycholysis (loosening of nail plate from distal edge inward; Grave's disease, psoriasis, reactive arthritis, obsessive compulsive behavior: "nail pickers")
- Pitting (psoriasis, eczema, alopecia areata)
- Thinning/thickening

---

its pink color. The hard nail is formed at the proximal end (the matrix). About one-fourth of the nail is covered by skin known as the proximal nail fold. The cuticle seals and protects the space between the proximal fold and the nail plate.[63]

Again, as with visual inspection of the skin, this section of the text is only a cursory look at the most common nail bed changes. Many more are not included here. A well-rounded library should include at least one text with color plates and photos of various nail bed changes.[64-68] This is not to help the therapist diagnose a medical problem, but rather provides background information, which can be used in the referral decision-making process.

Onycholysis

Onycholysis, a painless loosening of the nail plate, occurs from the distal edge inward (Fig. 4-29). Fingers and toes may both be affected as a consequence of dermatologic conditions such as dermatitis, fungal disease, lichen planus, and psoriasis. Systemic diseases associated with onycholysis include myeloma, neoplasia, Graves' disease, anemia, and reactive arthritis.[69]

Medications such as tetracycline, fluoroquinolones, anticancer drugs, nonsteroidal antiinflammatories, psoralens, retinoids, zidovudine, and quinine can cause photo-onycholysis (toes and fingers can cause photo-onycholysis (toes must be exposed to the sun for the condition to occur).[69]

Local causes from chemical, physical, cosmetic, or traumatic sources can bring on this condition. In the case of trauma, a limited number of nails are affected. For example, in clients with onycholysis as a result of nervous or obsessive-compulsive behaviors, only one or two nails are targeted. The individual picks around the edges until the nail is

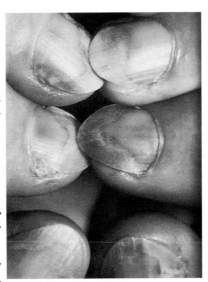

Fig. 4-29 • Onycholysis. Loosening of the nail plate, usually from the tip of the nail, progressing inward and from the edge of the nail moving inward. Possible causes include Graves' disease, psoriasis, reactive arthritis, and obsessive-compulsive behaviors (nail pickers). (From Arndt KA, Wintroub BU, Robinson JK, et al: *Primary care dermatology*, Philadelphia, 1997, WB Saunders.)

raised and separated from the nail bed. When there is an underlying systemic disorder, it is more common to see all the nail plates affected.

Koilonychia

Koilonychia or "spoon nails" may be a congenital or hereditary trait and as such is considered "normal" for that individual. These are thin, depressed nails with lateral edges tilted upward, forming a concave profile (Fig. 4-30).

Koilonychia can occur as a result of hypochromic anemia, iron deficiency (with or without anemia), poorly controlled diabetes of more than 15 years duration, chemical irritants, local injury, developmental abnormality, or psoriasis. It can also be an outward sign of thyroid problems, syphilis, and rheumatic fever.

Beau's Lines

Beau's lines are transverse grooves or ridges across the nail plate as a result of a decreased or interrupted production of the nail by the matrix (Fig. 4-31). The cause is usually an acute illness or systemic insult such as chemotherapy for cancer. Other common conditions associated with Beau's lines are poor peripheral circulation, eating disorders, cirrhosis associated with chronic alcohol use, and recent myocardial infarction (MI).

Since the nails grow at an approximate rate of 3mm/month, the date of the initial onset of illness or disease can be estimated by the location of the line. The dent appears first at the cuticle and moves forward as the nail grows. Measure the distance (in millimeters) from the dent to the cuticle and add 3 to account for the distance from the cuticle to the matrix. This is the number of weeks ago the person first had the problem.

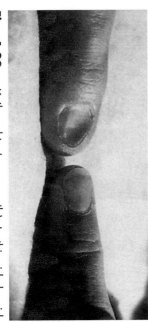

Fig. 4-30 • Koilonychia (spoon nails). In this side-by-side view, the affected nail bed is on the left and the normal nail on the right. With a spoon nail, the rounded indentation would hold a drop or several drops of water, hence the name. (From Swartz MH: *Textbook of physical diagnosis*, ed 4, Philadelphia, 2001, WB Saunders.)

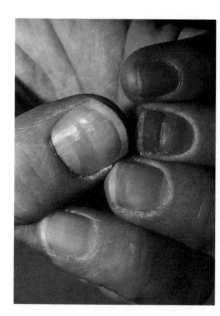

Fig. 4-31 • Beau's lines or grooves across the nail plate. A depression across the nail extends down to the nail bed. This occurs with shock, illness, malnutrition, or trauma severe enough to impair nail formation, such as acute illness, prolonged fever, or chemotherapy. A dent appears first at the cuticle and moves forward as the nail grows. All nails can be involved, but with local trauma, only the involved nail will be affected. This photo shows a client post-insult after full recovery. At the time of the illness, nails loss is obvious often with change in nailbed color such as occurs with chemotherapy. (From Callen JP, Greer KE, Hood AF, et al: *Color atlas of dermatology*, Philadelphia, 1994, WB Saunders.)

Beau's lines are temporary until the impaired nail formation is corrected (if and when the individual returns to normal health). These lines can also occur as a result of local trauma to the hand or fingers.

In the case of an injury, the dent may be permanent. Hand therapists see this condition most often. If it is not the result of a recent injury, the client may be able to remember sustaining an injury years ago.

Splinter Hemorrhages

Splinter hemorrhages may be the sign of a silent myocardial infarct (MI) or the client may have a known history of MI. These red-brown linear streaks (Fig. 4-32) can also signal other systemic conditions such as bacterial endocarditis, vasculitis, or renal failure.

In a hospital setting, they are not uncommon in the cardiac care unit (CCU) or other intensive care unit (ICU). In such a case, the therapist may just take note of the nail bed changes and correlate it with the pathologic insult probably already a part of the medical record.

When present in only one or two nail beds, local trauma may be linked to the nail bed changes. Asking the client about recent trauma or injury to the hand or fingers may bring this to light.

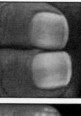
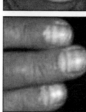
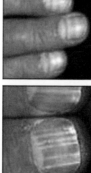

Splinter hemorrhages

Fig. 4-32 • Splinter hemorrhages. These red-brown streaks, embolic lesions, occur with subacute bacterial endocarditis, sepsis, rheumatoid arthritis, vitamin C deficiency, or hematologic neoplasm. They can occur from local trauma in which case only the injured nail beds will have the telltale streak. Splinter hemorrhages also may be a nonspecific sign. (From Jarvis C: *Physical examination and health assessment*, Philadelphia, 2004, WB Saunders.)

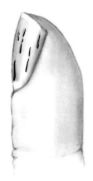

Fig. 4-33 • Leukonychia, acquired or inherited white discoloration in the nail. There is a wide range of possibilities in the clinical presentation of leukonychia. Spots, vertical lines, horizontal lines, and even full nail bed changes can occur on individual nail beds of the fingers and/or toes. One or more nails may be affected. (Courtesy Radek Klubal, MD, Consultant in Allergy and Clinical Immunology, Dermatology and Pediatrics, Prague, Czech Republic, 2005. Used with permission.)

Whenever splinter hemorrhages are observed in the nails, visually inspect both hands and the toenails as well. If the client cannot recall any recent illness, look for a possible cardiac history or cardiac risk factors. In the case of cardiac risk factors with no known cardiac history, proper medical follow up and diagnosis is essential in the event the client has had a silent MI.

Leukonychia

Leukonychia or white nail syndrome is characterized by dots or lines of white that progress to the free edge of the nail as the nail grows (Fig. 4-33). White nails can be congenital, but more often, it is acquired in association with hypocalcemia, severe hypochromic anemia, Hodgkin's disease, renal failure, malnutrition from eating disorders, myocardial infarction, leprosy, hepatic cirrhosis, and arsenic poisoning.

Acquired leukonychia is caused by a disturbance to the nail matrix. Repeated trauma such as

keyboard punching is a more recently described acquired cause of this condition.[70] When the entire nail plate is white, the condition is called leukonychia totalis (Case Example 4-2).

Paronychia

Paronychia (not shown) is an infection of the fold of skin at the margin of a nail. There is an obvious red, swollen site of inflammation that is tender or painful. This may be acute as with a bacterial infection or chronic in association with an occupationally induced fungal infection referred to as "wet work" from having the hands submerged in water for long periods of time.

The client may also give a history of finger exposure to chemical irritants, acrylic nails or nail glue, or sculpted nails. Paronychia of one or more fingers is not uncommon in people who pick, bite, or suck their nails. Health care professionals with these nervous habits working in a clinical setting (especially hospitals) are at increased risk for parony-chia from infection with bacteria such as

Streptococcus or *Staphylococcus*. Green coloration of the nail may indicate *Pseudomonas* infection.

Paronychia infections may spread to the pulp space of the finger developing a painful felon (an infection with localized abscess). Untreated infection can spread to the deep spaces of the hand and beyond.

It is especially important to recognize any nail bed irregularity because it may be a clue to malignancy. Likewise, anyone with diabetes mellitus, immunocompromise, or history of steroids and retroviral use are at increased risk for paronychia formation. Early identification and medical referral are imperative to avoid more serious consequences.

Clubbing

Clubbing of the fingers (Fig. 4-34) and toes usually results from chronic oxygen deprivation in these tissue beds. It is most often observed in clients with advanced chronic obstructive pulmonary disease, congenital heart defects, and cor pulmonale but

---

A 24-year-old male (Caucasian) was seen in physical therapy for a work-related back injury. When asked the final interview questions,

• Are there any other symptoms of any kind anywhere else in your body?

• Is there anything else about your condition that we have not discussed yet?

The client showed the therapist his nails and asked what could be the cause of the white discoloration in all the nail beds.

He reported the nails seem to grow out from time to time. There was tenderness along the sides of the nails and at the distal edge of the nails. It was obvious the nails were bitten and there were several nails that were red and swollen. The client admitted to picking at his nails when he was nervous. He was observed tapping his nails on the table repeatedly during the exam. No changes of any kind were observed in the feet.

Past medical history was negative for any significant health problems. He was not taking any medications, over-the-counter drugs, or using recreational drugs. He did not smoke and denied

the use of alcohol. His job as a supervisor in a machine shop did not require the mechanical use of his hands. He was not exposed to any unusual chemicals or solvents at work.

Result: When asked, "How long have you had this?" the client reported for 2 years. When asked, "Have your nails changed in the last six weeks to six months?" the answer was, "Yes, the condition seems to come and go." When asked, "Has your doctor seen these changes?" the client did not think so.

The therapist did not know what was causing the nail bed changes and suggested the client ask his physician about the condition at his next appointment. The physician also observed the client repeatedly tapping his nails and performed a screening exam for anxiety.

The nail bed condition was diagnosed as leukonychia from repeated microtrauma to the nail matrix. The patient was referred to psychiatry to manage the observed anxiety symptoms. The nails returned to normal in about 3 months (90 to 100 days) after the client stopped tapping, restoring normal growth to the nail matrix.

From Maino Kimberly, Stashower ME: Traumatic transverse leukonychia, *SKINmed* 3(1):53-55, 2004. Accessed on-line http://www.medscape.com/viewarticle/467074 (posted 01/20/2004).

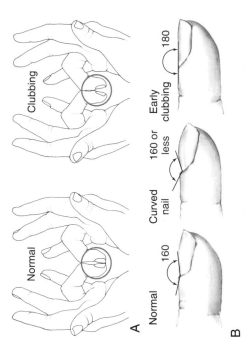

Normal | Clubbing

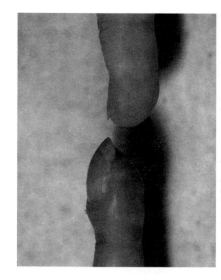

Fig. 4-34 • Rapid development of digital clubbing (fingers as shown on the left or toes, not shown) over the course of a 10-day to 2-week period requires immediate medical evaluation. Clubbing can be assessed using the Schamroth method shown in Fig. 4-35. (From Swartz MH: *Textbook of physical diagnosis*, ed 4, Philadelphia, 2001, WB Saunders.)

A

Normal | Curved nail | Early clubbing

160 | 160 or less | 180

B

Fig. 4-35 • Schamroth method. **A,** Assessment of clubbing by the Schamroth method. The client places the fingernails of opposite fingers together and holds them up to a light. If the examiner can see a diamond shape between the nails, there is no clubbing. Clubbing is identified by the absence of the diamond shape. It occurs first in the thumb and index finger. **B,** The index finger is viewed at its profile, and the angle of the nail base is noted (it should be about 160 degrees). The nail base is firm to palpation. Curved nails are a variation of normal with a convex profile. They may look like clubbed nails, but the angle between the nail base and the nail is normal (i.e., 160 degrees or less). Clubbing of nails occurs with congenital chronic cyanotic heart disease, emphysema, cystic fibrosis, and chronic bronchitis. In early clubbing the angle straightens out to 180 degrees, and the nail base feels spongy to palpation. (**A,** From Ignatavicius DD, Bayne MV: Assessment of the cardiovascular system. In Ignatavicius DD, Bayne MV, editors: *Medical-surgical nursing*, Philadelphia, 1993, WB Saunders. **B,** From Jarvis C: *Physical examination and health assessment*, Philadelphia, 2004, WB Saunders.)

can occur within 10 days in someone with an acute systemic condition such as a pulmonary abscess, malignancy, or polycythemia. Clubbing may be the first sign of a paraneoplastic syndrome associated with cancer. Clubbing can be assessed by the Schamroth method (Fig. 4-35).

Any positive findings in the nail beds should be viewed in light of the entire clinical presentation. For example, a positive Schamroth test without observable clinical changes in skin color, capillary refill time, or shape of the fingertips may not signify systemic disease but rather a normal anatomic variation of nail curvature.

Nail Patella Syndrome

Nail Patella Syndrome (NPS; also called Fong's Disease, Hereditary Onycho-Osteodysplasia ['HOOD'], or Turner-Kieser Syndrome) is a genetic disorder characterized by an absence or underdevelopment of nail bed changes as shown here (Fig. 4-36, *A*). Lack of skin creases is also a telltale sign (Fig. 4-37).

Nail abnormalities vary and range from a sliver on each corner of the nail bed to a full nail that is very thick with splits. Some people have brittle, underdeveloped, cracked, or ridged nails while others are absent entirely. They are often concave, causing them to split and flip up, catching on clothing and bedding. Often, the lunula (the light crescent "half-moons" of the nail near the cuticle) are pointed or triangular-shaped (Fig. 4-36, *B*).

The therapist may be the first to see this condition since skeletal and joint problems are a common feature with this condition. The elbows,

hips, and knees are affected most often. Absence or hypoplasia (underdevelopment) of the patella and deformities of the knee joint itself often give them a square shape. Knee instability with patellar dislocation is not uncommon due to malformations in the bones, muscles, and ligaments; there is often much instability in the knee joint.

The client may also develop scoliosis, glaucoma, and kidney disease. Medical referral to establish a diagnosis is important, as clients with NPS need annual screening for renal disease, biannual screening for glaucoma in adulthood, and magnetic resonance imaging (MRI) for orthopedic abnormalities before physical therapy is considered.[71]

When a client presents with skin or nail bed changes of any kind, taking a personal medical history and reviewing recent (last 6 weeks) and current medications can provide the therapist with important clues in knowing whether to make an

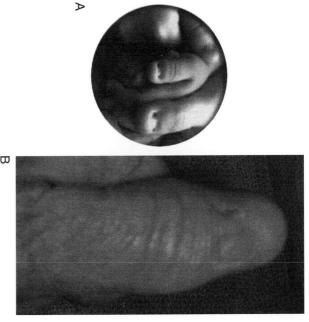

A

B

Fig. 4-36 • Nail-Patella Syndrome (NPS). Nail bed changes associated with NPS are presented here. Effects vary greatly between individuals but usually involve absence of part or all of the nail bed. For more photos of the skeletal changes associated with NPS, see http://members.aol.com/pacali/NPSpage.html (Accessed October 25, 2005). **A,** The thumbnails are affected the most with involvement decreasing towards the little finger. Nail changes occur more severely on the ulnar side of the affected nail. Toenails can be affected; it is often the little toenail that is involved.[71] **B,** Note the altered nail bed (more on the ulnar side) and especially the triangular-shaped lunula, a very distinctive sign of NPS. (Courtesy Nail Patella Syndrome Worldwide, 2005.)

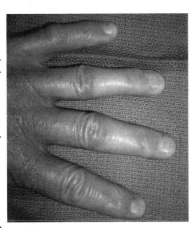

Fig. 4-37 • Nail changes are the most constant feature of NPS and may be absent, underdeveloped (hypoplastic), or abnormal in size or shape (dysplastic). Alternately, there may be longitudinal ridges, pitting, or discoloration. Note the lack of creases in the DIP joints of the fingers in this photo. The condition may be present at birth and usually presents symmetrically and bilaterally. (Courtesy Gary Ross, RN, BSN, Board Member, Nail Patella Syndrome Worldwide, 2005.)

immediate medical referral. Table 4-8 provides a summary of the most common skin changes encountered in a physical therapy practice and possible causes for each one.

▼ LYMPH NODE PALPATION

Part of the screening process for the therapist may involve visual inspection of the skin overlying lymph nodes and palpation of the lymph nodes. Look for any obvious areas of swelling or redness (erythema) along with any changes in skin color or pigmentation. Ask about the presence or recent history of sores or lesions anywhere on the body.

Keep in mind the therapist cannot know what the underlying pathology may be when lymph nodes are palpable and questionable. Performing a baseline assessment and reporting the findings is the important outcome of the assessment.

Whenever examining a lump or lesion, use the mnemonic in Box 4-10 to document and report findings on location, size, shape, consistency, mobility or fixation, and signs of tenderness. See also Box 4-17. Review *Special Questions to Ask: Lymph Nodes* at the end of this chapter for appropriate follow-up questions.

There are several sites where lymph nodes are potentially observable and palpable (Fig. 4-38). Palpation must be done lightly. Excessive pressure can press a node into a muscle or between two muscles. "Normal" lymph nodes usually are not visible or easily palpable. Not all visible or palpable lymph nodes are a sign of cancer. Infections, viruses, bacteria, allergies, thyroid conditions, and food intolerances can cause changes in the lymph nodes.

People with seasonal allergies or allergic rhinitis often have enlarged, tender, and easily palpable lymph nodes in the submandibular and supraclavicular areas. This is a sign that the immune system is working hard to stop as many perceived pathogens as possible.

Children often have easily palpable and tender lymph nodes because their developing immune system is continuously filtering out pathogens. Anyone with food intolerances or celiac sprue can have the same lymph node response in the inguinal area.

Studies show lymph node changes occur after total hip arthroplasty. The presence of polyethylene or metal debris in lymph nodes of the ipsilateral side have been demonstrated.[72]

The therapist is most likely to palpate enlarged lymph nodes in the neck, supraclavicular, and axillary areas during an upper quadrant examination

TABLE 4-8 ▼ Common Causes of Skin and Nail Bed Changes

Skin/nail bed changes	Possible cause
Dermatitis	Pulmonary malignancy, allergic reaction
Loss of turgor or elasticity	Dehydration
Rash (see Fig. 4-11)	Viruses (chicken pox, measles, Fifth disease)
	Systemic conditions: meningitis, lupus, hives, lupus, rosacea)
	Sexually transmitted diseases
	Lyme disease
	Parasites (e.g., lice, scabies)
	Reaction to chemicals, medications, food
	Malignancy, neoplastic syndromes
Hemorrhage (petechiae, ecchymosis, purpura) (see Fig. 4-13)	NSAIDs
	Anticoagulants (heparin, coumadin/warfarin, aspirin)
	Hemophilia
	Thrombocytopenia (low platelet level) and anything that can cause thrombocytopenia)
	Neoplasm; paraneoplastic syndrome
	Domestic violence
	Aging
Skin color	Jaundice (yellow, green, orange): hepatitis
	Chronic renal failure (yellow-brown)
	Cyanosis (pale, blue): anxiety, hypothermia, lung disease, congestive heart disease, venous obstruction
	Rubor (dusky red): arterial insufficiency
	Sunburn (red): radiation recall or radiation dermatitis
	Tan, black, blue: skin cancer
Hyperpigmentation	Addison's disease, ACTH-producing tumors
	Sarcoidosis
	Pregnancy
	Leukemia
	Hemochromatosis
	Celiac sprue (malabsorption)
	Scleroderma
	Chronic renal failure
	Hereditary (non-pathognomic)
	Low dose radiation
Café-au-lait (hyperpigmentation) (see Fig. 4-10)	Neurofibromatosis (more than 5 lesions)
	Albright's syndrome
	Urticaria pigmentosa (less than 5 lesions)
Hypopigmentation (vitiligo)	Albinism
	Sun exposure
	Steroid injections
	Hyperthyroidism
	Stomach cancer
	Pernicious anemia
	Diabetes mellitus
	Autoimmune diseases
	High dose radiation
Mongolian spots (see Fig. 4-23)	Blue-black discoloration: normal in certain people groups
Xanthomas (see Fig. 4-15)	Disorders of lipid metabolism
	Primary biliary cirrhosis
	Diabetes mellitus (uncontrolled)
Nail Bed Changes	
Onycholysis (see Fig. 4-29)	Graves' disease, psoriasis, reactive arthritis, nail picking

TABLE 4-8 ▼ Common Causes of Skin and Nail Bed Changes—cont'd

Skin/nail bed changes	Possible cause
Koilonychia (see Fig. 4-30)	Congenital or hereditary Hypochromic anemia Iron deficiency Diabetes mellitus (chronic, uncontrolled) Psoriasis Syphilis Rheumatic fever Thyroid dysfunction
Beau's lines (see Fig. 4-31)	Acute systemic illness Chemotherapy Peripheral vascular disease (PVD) Eating disorders Cirrhosis (chronic alcohol use) Recent heart attack Local trauma
Splinter hemorrhages (see Fig. 4-32)	Heart attack Bacterial endocarditis Vasculitis Renal failure Any systemic insult
Leukonychia (see Fig. 4-33)	Acquired or congenital Acquired: hypocalcemia, hypochromic anemia, Hodgkin's disease, renal failure, malnutrition, heart attack, hepatic cirrhosis, arsenic poisoning
Paronychia	Fungal infection Bacterial infection
Digital clubbing (see Fig. 4-34)	*Acute:* Pulmonary abscess, malignancy, polycythemia, paraneoplastic syndrome *Chronic:* COPD, cystic fibrosis, congenital heart defects, cor pulmonale
Absent or underdeveloped nail bed (s) (see Figs. 4-36 and 4-37)	Nail Patella Syndrome (NPS) Congenital
Pitting	Psoriasis

ACTH, Adrenocorticotropic hormone.

(Fig. 4-39), Virchow's node, a palpable enlargement of one of the supraclavicular lymph nodes may be palpated in the supraclavicular area in the presence of primary carcinoma of thoracic or abdominal organs. Virchow's node is more often found on the left side.

Posterior cervical lymph node enlargement can occur during the icteric stage of hepatitis (see Table 9-3). Swelling of the regional lymph nodes often accompanies the first stage of syphilis that is usually painless. These glands feel rubbery, freely movable, and are not tender on palpation. This may be followed by a general lymphadenopathy palpable in the posterior cervical or epitrochlear nodes (located in the inner condyle of the humerus).

The axillary lymph nodes are divided into three zones (Fig. 4-40). Only zones I and II are palpable.

Zone I nodes are superficial and palpable with the client sitting (preferred) or supine with the client's arm supported by the examiner's hand and forearm. Gently palpate the entire axilla for any lymph nodes.

Zone II lymph nodes are palpated with the client in sitting position. Zone II lymph nodes are below the clavicle in the area of the pectoralis muscle. The examiner must reach deep into the axilla to palpate for these lymph nodes.

To examine the right axilla, the examiner supports the client's right arm with his or her own right forearm and hand (reverse for palpation of the left axillary lymph nodes) (Fig. 4-41). This will help ensure relaxation of the chest wall musculature. Lift the client's upper arm up from under the elbow while reaching the fingertips of the left hand up as high as possible into the axilla.

and the potential for cancer recurrence. The most up-to-date recommendation is for physician evaluation of all suspicious lymph nodes.

▶ MUSCULOSKELETAL SCREENING EXAMINATION

Muscle pain, weakness, poor coordination, and joint pain can be caused by many systemic disorders such as hypokalemia, hypothyroidism, dehydration, alcohol or drug use, vascular disorders, GI disorders, liver impairment, malnutrition, vitamin deficiencies, and psychologic factors.

In a screening examination of the musculoskeletal system, the client is observed for any obvious deformities, abnormalities, disabilities, and asymmetries. Inspection and palpation of the skin, muscles, soft tissues, and joints often takes place simultaneously.

Assess each client from the front, back, and each side. Some general examination principles include[73]:

- Let the client know what to expect; offer simple but clear instructions and feedback.
- When comparing sides, test the "normal" side first.
- Examine the joint above and below the "involved" joint.
- Perform active, passive, and accessory or physiologic movements in that order unless circumstances direct otherwise.
- Resisted isometric movements (break test) follow accessory or physiologic motion.
- Resisted isometric motion is done in a physiologic neutral position (open pack position); the joint should not move.
- Painful joint motion or painful empty end feel of a joint should not be forced.
- Inspect and palpate the skin and surrounding tissue for erythema, swelling, masses, tenderness, temperature changes, and crepitus.
- The forward bend and full squat positions as well as walking on toes and heels and hopping on one leg are useful general screening tests.
- Perform specific special tests last based on client history, and results of the screening interview and clinical findings so far.

The *Guide* suggests key tests and measures to include in a comprehensive screening and specific testing process of the musculoskeletal system including:

- Patient/Client History (demographics, social and employment history, family and personal history, results of other clinical tests)

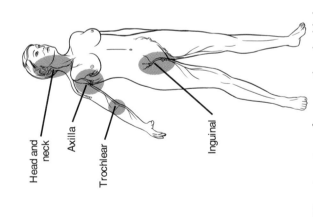

Fig. 4-38 • Locations of most easily palpable lymph nodes. Epitrochlear nodes are located on the medial side of the arm above the elbow in the depression above and posterior to the medial condyle of the humerus. Horizontal and vertical chains of inguinal nodes may be palpated in the same areas as the femoral pulse. Popliteal lymph nodes (not shown) are deep but may be palpated in some clients with the knee slightly flexed.

The examiner's fingertips will be against the chest wall and should be able to feel the rib cage (and any palpable lymph nodes). As the client's arm is lowered slowly, allow the fingertips to move down over the rib cage. Feel for the central nodes by compressing them against the chest wall and muscles of the axilla. The examiner may want to repeat this motion a second or third time until becoming more proficient with this examination technique.

Whenever the therapist encounters enlarged or palpable lymph nodes, ask about a past medical history of cancer (Case Example 4-3), implants, mononucleosis, chronic fatigue, allergic rhinitis, and food intolerances. Ask about a recent cut or infection in the hand or arm. Tender, moveable nodes may be present associated with these conditions, pharyngeal or dental infections, and other infectious diseases.

Lymph nodes that are hard, immovable, and nontender raise the suspicion of cancer, especially in the presence of a previous history of cancer. Previous editions of this textbook mentioned that any change in lymph nodes present for more than one month in more than one location was a red flag. This has changed with the increased understanding of cancer metastases via the lymphatic system

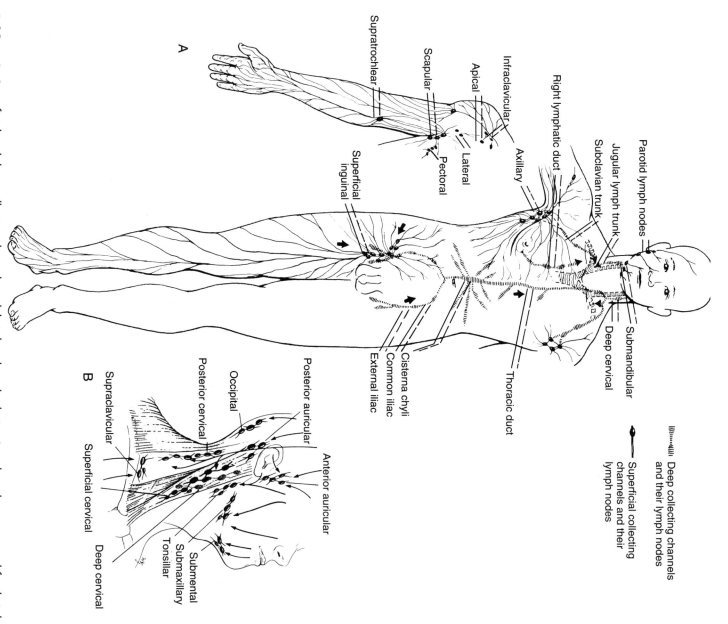

Fig. 4-39 • A, Superficial and deep collecting channels and their lymph node chains. Lymph nodes are named for their location. **B,** Lymph nodes of the neck and the direction of their drainage. The head and neck areas are divided into the anterior and posterior triangles divided by the sternocleidomastoid muscle. There are an estimated 75 lymph nodes on each side of the neck. The deep cervical chain is located in the anterior triangle, largely obstructed by the overlying sternocleidomastoid muscle. **(A,** From Jacob SW, Francone CA: *Elements of anatomy and physiology,* ed 2, Philadelphia, 1989, WB Saunders. **B,** From Swartz M: *Textbook of physical diagnosis,* Philadelphia, 1989, WB Saunders.)

Parotid lymph nodes
Jugular lymph trunk
Subclavian trunk
Right lymphatic duct
Infraclavicular
Apical
Scapular
Supratrochlear
Axillary
Lateral
Pectoral
Superficial inguinal

Submandibular
Deep cervical
Thoracic duct
Cisterna chyli
Common iliac
External iliac

A

B
Supraclavicular
Superficial cervical
Posterior cervical
Occipital
Posterior auricular
Anterior auricular
Tonsillar
Submaxillary
Submental
Deep cervical

Deep collecting channels and their lymph nodes
Superficial collecting channels and their lymph nodes

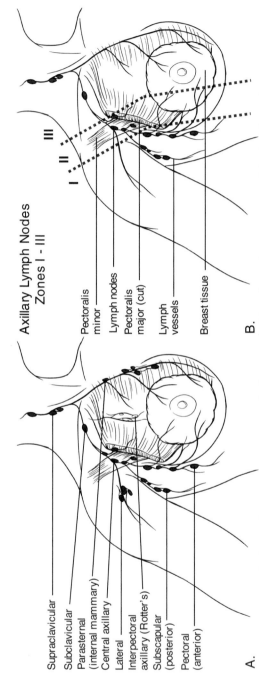

Supraclavicular
Subclavicular
Parasternal
(internal mammary)
Central axillary
Lateral
Interpectoral
axillary (Rotter's)
Subscapular
(posterior)
Pectoral
(anterior)

A.

Axillary Lymph Nodes
Zones I - III

Pectoralis
minor
Lymph nodes
Pectoralis
major (cut)
Lymph
vessels
Breast tissue

B.

Fig. 4-40 • A, The breast has an extensive network of venous and lymphatic drainage. Most of the lymphatic drainage empties into axillary nodes. The main lymph node chains and lymphatic drainage are labeled as shown here. **B,** Axillary lymph nodes are divided into three zones based on anatomical sites. Only Zones I and II are palpable.

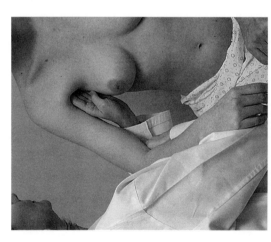

Fig. 4-41 • Palpation of Zone II lymph nodes in the sitting position. See description in text. (From Seidel HM, Ball JW, Dains JE: *Mosby's physical examination handbook*, ed 3, St. Louis, 2003, Mosby.)

- Aerobic Capacity and Endurance
- Anthropometric Characteristics
- Arousal, Attention, and Cognition
- Environmental, Home, and Work Barriers
- Ergonomics and Body Mechanics
- Gait, Locomotion, and Balance
- Motor Function (Motor Control and Motor Learning)

- Muscle Performance (Strength, Power, and Endurance)
- Posture
- Range of Motion
- Self-care and Home Management
- Work, Community, and Leisure Integration or Reintegration

These steps lead to a diagnostic classification or, when appropriate, to a referral to another practitioner.[12] Assessing joint or muscle pain is discussed in greater depth in Chapter 3 (see also Appendix B-16).

▶ NEUROLOGIC SCREENING EXAMINATION

Much of the neurologic examination is actually completed in conjunction with other parts of the physical assessment. Acute insult or injury to the neurologic system may cause changes in neurologic status requiring frequent reassessment. Systemic disease can produce nerve damage; careful assessment can help pinpoint the area of pathology.

There are six major areas to assess:

1. Mental and Emotional Status
2. Cranial Nerves
3. Motor Function (Gross motor and fine motor)
4. Sensory Function (Light touch, vibration, pain, and temperature)
5. Reflexes
6. Neural Tension

CASE EXAMPLE 4-3 Lymphadenopathy

A 73-year-old woman was referred to a physical therapy clinic by her oncologist with a diagnosis of cervical radiculopathy. She had a history of uterine cervical cancer 20 years ago and a history of breast cancer 10 years ago.

Treatment included a hysterectomy, left radical mastectomy, radiation therapy, and chemotherapy. She has been cancer free for almost 10 years. When seen by the physician, her family physician, oncologist, and neurologist actually all evaluated her before being referred to the physical therapist.

Examination by a physical therapist revealed obvious lymphadenopathy of the left cervical and axillary lymph nodes. When asked if the referring physician (or other physicians) saw the "swelling," she told the therapist that she had not disrobed during her medical evaluation and consultation.

The question for us as physical therapists in a situation like this one is how to proceed?

Several steps must be taken. First, the therapist must document all findings. If possible, photographs of the chest, neck, and axilla should be obtained.

Second, the therapist must ascertain whether or not the physician is already aware of the problem and has requested physical therapy as a palliative measure. Requesting the physician's dictation or notes from the examination is essential.

Contact with the physician will be important soon after obtaining the records, either to confirm the request as palliative therapy or to report your findings and confirm the need for medical reevaluation.

If it turns out that the physician is, indeed, unaware of these physical findings, it is best to make a problem list identified as "outside the scope of a physical therapist" when returning the client to the physician. Be careful to avoid making any statements that could be misconstrued as a medical diagnosis.

It is highly advised that the therapist offer to make the appointment for the client and do so immediately. We recommend writing a brief letter with the pertinent findings and ending with one of two one-liners:

What do you think?

Please advise.

Documentation of findings and recommendations must be complete even if the client declines. Every effort must be made to get the client to a physician. This may require follow-up phone calls and some persistence on the part of the therapist.

As always start with the client's history and note any previous trauma to the head or spine along with reports of headache, confusion (increased confusion), dizziness (see Appendix B-10), seizures, or other neurologic signs and symptoms. Note the presence of any incoordination, tremors, weakness, or abnormal speech patterns.

As mentioned previously, neurologic symptoms with no apparent cause such as paresthesias, dizziness, and weakness may actually be symptoms of depression. This is particularly true if the neurologic symptoms are symmetrical or not anatomic.[74]

Follow Up Questions

- Have you ever been in a car accident?
  If yes, did you lose consciousness, have a concussion, or a fractured skull?
- Have you ever been knocked out, unconscious, or have a concussion at any time?
- Have you ever had a seizure?
- Have you ever been paralyzed in your arms or legs?
- Have you ever broken your neck or back?

Clinical Signs and Symptoms of
Neurologic Impairment

- Confusion/increased confusion
- Depression
- Irritability
- Drowsiness/lethargy
- Dizziness/lightheadedness
- Loss of consciousness
- Blurred vision or other change in vision
- Slurred speech or change in speech pattern
- Headache
- Balance/coordination problems
- Weakness

Continued on p. 228

- Change in memory
- Change in muscle tone for individual with previously diagnosed neurologic condition
- Seizure activity
- Nerve palsy; transient paralysis

If there are no positive findings upon gross examination of the nervous system (e.g., reflexes, muscle tone assessment, gross manual muscle testing, sensation), further testing may not be required. For example, sensory function is not assessed if motor function is intact and there are no client reports of specific sensory problems or changes.

Keep in mind that fatigue and side effects of medications can affect the results of a neurologic exam. Give instructions clearly and take the time needed to map out an areas of deficit observed during the initial screening examination.

Mental Status

See the previous discussion on General Survey in this chapter.

Cranial Nerves

A neurologic screening exam may not involve a survey of the cranial nerves unless the therapist finds reason to perform a more focused neurologic exam. Most of these tests are performed as part of the musculoskeletal exam. See previous discussion (Musculoskeletal Screening Examination) in this chapter.

Specific tests such as tandem walking, Romberg's test, diadochokinesia (rapid, alternating movements of the hands or fingers such as repeatedly alternating forearm pronation to supination, the finger-to-nose/finger-to-finger, and thumb-to-finger opposition tests) can be added for more in-depth screening. Demonstrate all test maneuvers in order to prevent poor performance from a lack of understanding rather than from neurologic impairment.

Motor Function

Motor and cerebellar function can be screened most easily by observation of gait, posture, balance, strength, coordination, muscle tone, and motion.

Sensory Function

Screening for sensory function can begin with superficial pain (pinprick) and light touch (cotton ball) on the extremities. Show the client the items you will be using and how they will be used. For light touch, dab the skin lightly; do not stroke.

Tests are done with the client's eyes closed. Ask the client to tell you where the sensation is felt or to identify "sharp" or "dull." Apply the stimulus randomly and bilaterally over the face, neck, upper arms, hands, thighs, lower legs, and feet. Allow at least 2 seconds between the time the stimulus is applied and the next one is given. This avoids the summation effect.

Follow up with temperature using test tubes filled with hot and cold water and vibration using a low-pitch tuning fork over peripheral joints. Temperature can be omitted if pain sensation is normal. Apply the stem of the vibrating tuning fork to the distal interphalangeal joint of fingers and interphalangeal joint of the great toe, elbow, and wrist. Ask the client to tell you when vibration is first felt and when it stops. Remember aging adults often lose vibratory sense in the great toe and ankle on both sides.

Other tests include proprioception (joint position sense), kinesthesia (movement sense), stereognosis (identification of common object placed in the hand), graphesthesia (identifying number or letter when drawn on the palm of the hand), and two-point discrimination. Again, all tests should be performed on both sides.

Reflexes

Deep tendon reflexes (DTRs) are tested in a screening examination at the

- Jaw (Cranial nerve V)
- Biceps (C5-6),
- Brachioradialis (C5-6)
- Triceps (C7-8)
- Patella (L3-4)
- Achilles (S1-2)

These reflexes are assessed for symmetry and briskness using the following scale:

0 No response, absent

1 Low normal, diminished; slight muscle contraction

2 Normal, visible muscle twitch and movement of arm/leg

3 More brisk than normal, exaggerated; may not indicate disease

4 Hyperactive; very brisk, clonus; spinal cord disorder suspected

A change in 1 or more DTRs is a yellow (caution) flag. Some individuals have very brisk reflexes normally, while others are much more hyporeflexive. Whenever encountering increased (hyper-) or

TABLE 4-9 ▼ Cranial Nerve Function and Assessment

Cranial nerve	Type	Function	Assessment
I Olfactory	Sensory	Sense of smell	Able to identify common odors (e.g.; coffee, vanilla, orange or peppermint) with eyes closed Close one nostril and test one nostril at a time
II Optic	Sensory	Visual acuity	Visual acuity; test each eye separately with Snellen eye chart If literate, able to read printed material
III Oculomotor	Motor	Extraocular eye movement Pupil constriction and dilation	Assess cranial nerves III, IV, and VI together: Look for equal pupil size and shape; equal response to light and accommodation; inspect eyelids for drooping (ptosis) Follow finger with eyes without moving head (six points in an H pattern; gaze test) Convergence (move finger towards client's nose)
IV Trochlear	Motor	Upward and downward movement of eyeball	See Cranial nerve III; assess directions of gaze; visual tracking
V Trigeminal	Mixed	Sensory nerve to skin of face	Corneal reflex: client looks up and away, examiner lightly touches opposite cornea with wisp of cotton (look for blink in both eyes or report by client of blinking sensation) Facial sensation: apply sterile, sharp item to forehead, cheek, jaw; repeat with dull object; client reports "sharp" or "dull"; if abnormal, test for temperature, vibration, and light touch
		Motor nerve to muscles of jaw (mastication)	Ask client to clench teeth together as you palpate muscles over temples (temporal muscle) and jaw (masseter) on each side Look for symmetric tone (normal) or muscle atrophy, deviation of jaw to one side, or fasciculations (abnormal)
VI Abducens	Motor	Lateral movement of eyeballs	See Cranial nerve III; assess directions of gaze
VII Facial	Mixed	Facial expression	Look for symmetry with facial expressions (e.g., frown, smile, raise and lower eyebrows, puff cheeks out, close eyes tightly)
VIII Acoustic (auditory, vestibulocochlear)	Sensory	Hearing	Assess ability to hear spoken word and whisper Examiner stands behind client with hands on either side of client's head/ears; rub candy wrapper or fingers together to make noise on one side, ask client to identify which side noise is coming from Examiner stands 18 inches behind client and whispers 3 numbers
IX Glossopharyngeal	Mixed	Taste Gag, swallow	Client identifies sour or sweet taste on back of tongue Gag reflex (sensory IX and motor X) and ability to swallow
X Vagus	Mixed	Sensation of pharynx, voice, swallow	Client says, "Ah." Observe for normal palate and pharynx movement Listen for hoarseness or nasal quality in voice Observe for difficulty swallowing
XI Spinal Accessory	Motor	Movement of head and shoulders	Client is able to shrug shoulders and turn head against resistance Observe shoulders from behind for trapezius atrophy and/or asymmetry (abnormal finding)
XII Hypoglossal	Motor	Position and movement of tongue	Client can stick out tongue to midline and move it from side to side Client can move tongue toward nose and chin Clear articulation in speech pattern

decreased (hypo-) reflexes, the therapist routinely follows several guidelines:

Follow up Questions

- Test reflexes above and below and from side to side in order to gauge overall reflexive response. A "normal" hyperreflexive response will be present in most, if not all, reflexes. The same is true for generalized hyporeflexive responses.

- Offer the client distraction while testing through conversation or by asking such silly questions as, "What color is your tooth-brush?" "What day of the week were you born?" or "Count out loud backwards by three starting at 89."

- Retest unusual reflexes later in the day or on another day.

- Have another clinician test your client.

The isolated DTR that does not fit the client's physiologic pattern must be considered a red flag. As discussed in Chapter 2, one red flag by itself does not require immediate medical follow-up. But a hyporesponsive patellar tendon reflex that is reproducible and is accompanied by back, hip, or thigh pain in the presence of a past history of prostate cancer offers a different picture altogether.

A diminished reflex may be interpreted as the sign of a possible "space-occupying lesion"—most often, a disc protruding from the disc space and either pressing on a spinal nerve root or irritating the spinal nerve root (i.e., chemicals released by the herniation in contact with the nerve root can cause nerve root irritation).

Tumors (whether benign or malignant) can also press on the spinal nerve root, mimicking a disc problem. A small lesion can put just enough pressure to irritate the nerve root, resulting in a hyperreflexive DTR. A large tumor can obliterate the reflex arc resulting in diminished or absent reflexes. Either way, changes in DTRs must be considered a yellow or red flag sign to be documented, reported, and further investigated.

Superficial (cutaneous) reflexes (e.g., abdominal, cremasteric, plantar) can also be tested using the handle of the reflex hammer. The abdominal reflex is elicited by applying a stroking motion with a cotton-tipped applicator (or handle of the reflex hammer) toward the umbilicus. A positive sign of neurologic impairment is observed if the umbilicus moves toward the stroke. The test can be repeated in each abdominal quadrant (upper abdominal T7-T9; lower abdominal T11-T12).

The cremasteric reflex is elicited by stroking the thigh downward with a cotton-tipped applicator (or handle of the reflex hammer). A normal response in males is an upward movement of the testicle (scrotum) on the same side. The absence of a cremasteric reflex is indication of disruption at the T12-L1 level. Testing the cremasteric reflex may help the therapist identify neurologic impairment in any male with suspicious back, pelvic, groin (including testicular), and/or anterior thigh pain.

The plantar reflex occurs when the sole of the foot is stroked and the toes plantarflex downward.

Neural Tension

Excessive nerve tightness or adhesion can cause adverse neural tension in the peripheral nervous system. When the nerve cannot slide or glide in its protective sheath, neural extensibility and mobility are impaired. The clinical result can be numbness, tingling, and pain. This could be caused by disc protrusion, scar tissue, or spine changes including cancer metastases.[76,77]

A positive neural tension test does not tell the therapist what is the underlying etiology—only that the peripheral nerve is involved. History and physical examination is still very important in assessing the clinical presentation.

Someone with full range of motion accompanied by negative articular signs but with impaired neural extensibility and mobility raises a yellow flag. A second look at the history and a more thorough neurologic exam may be warranted.

Reducing symptoms with neural mobilization does not rule out the possibility of cancer. A red flag is raised with any client who responds well to neural mobilization but experiences recurrence of symptoms. This could be a sign that the tumor has grown larger, once again interfering with neural mobility.

REGIONAL SCREENING EXAMINATION

Head and Neck

Screening of the head and neck areas takes place when client history and report of symptoms or clinical presentation warrant this type of examination. The head and neck assessment provides information about the general health of multiple systems including integumentary, neurologic, respiratory, endocrine, hepatic, and gastrointestinal.

The head, hair and scalp, and face are observed for size, shape, symmetry, cleanliness, and presence of infection. Position of the head over the spine and in relation to midline and range-of-motion testing of the cervical spine and temporomandibular joints can be part of the screening and posture assessment.

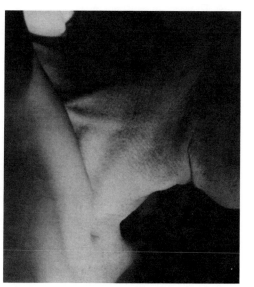

Fig. 4-42 ▲ Jugular venous distention is a sign of overhydration or heart disease, especially congestive heart failure and requires immediate medical attention if not previously reported. Inspect the jugular veins with the client sitting up at a 90-degree angle and again with the head at a 30- to 45-degree angle. The cervical spine should be in a neutral position. Correlate findings of this exam with results from palpation of carotid arteries for bruits (rate and rhythm) and auscultation of the carotid arteries for bruits. (From Daily EK, Schroeder JP: *Techniques in bedside hemodynamic monitoring,* ed 2, St. Louis, 1981, Mosby.)

The eyes can be examined for changes in shape, motor function, and color (conjunctiva and sclera). Conducting an assessment of cranial nerves II, III, and IV also will help screen for visual problems. The therapist should be aware that there are changes in the way older adults perceive color. This kind of change can affect function and safety; for example, some older adults are unable to tell when floor tiles end and the bathtub begins in a bathroom. Stumbling and loss of balance can occur at boundary changes.

Assessment of cranial nerves (see Table 4-9), regional lymph nodes (see discussion, this chapter), carotid artery pulses (see Fig. 4-1), and jugular vein patency (Fig. 4-42) are part of the head and neck screening examination. Therapists in a primary care setting may also examine the position of the trachea and thyroid for obvious deviations or palpable lesions.

Headaches are common and often the result of specific foods, stress, muscle tension, hormonal fluctuations, nerve compression, or cervical spine or temporomandibular joint dysfunction. Most headaches are acute and self limited. Headaches can be a symptom of a serious medical condition and should be assessed carefully (see Appendix B-15; see also the discussion of viscerogenic causes of head and neck pain in Chapter 14.)

Upper and Lower Extremities

The extremities are examined through a systematic assessment of various aspects of the musculoskeletal, neurologic, vascular, and integumentary systems. Inspection and palpation are two techniques used most often during the examination. A checklist can be very helpful (Box 4-15).

Peripheral Vascular Disease

Peripheral vascular disease (PVD; both arterial and venous conditions) is a common problem observed in the extremities of older adults, especially those with a history of heart disease. Knowing the risk factors for any condition, but especially problems like PVD helps the therapist know when to screen. These conditions, including risk factors, are discussed in greater depth in Chapter 6.

The first signs of vascular disease are often skin changes (see Box 4-12). The therapist must watch out for common risk factors including bedrest or prolonged immobility, use of intravenous catheters, obesity, myocardial infarction, heart

---

BOX 4-15 ▲ Extremity Examination Checklist

- Inspect skin for color, scratch marks, inflammation, track marks, bruises, heat, or other obvious changes (see Box 4-10)
- Observe for hair loss or hair growth
- Observe for asymmetry, contour changes, edema, obvious atrophy, fractures or deformities; measure circumference if indicated
- Assess palpable lesions (see Box 4-10)
- Palpate for temperature, moisture, and tenderness
- Palpate pulses
- Palpate lymph nodes
- Check nail bed refill (normal: capillary refill time under 2-3 seconds for fingers and 3-4 seconds for toes)
- Observe for clubbing, signs of cyanosis, other nail bed changes
- Observe for peripheral vascular disease (PVD; see Box 4-12); listen for femoral bruits if indicated; test for thrombophlebitis
- Assess joint ROM and muscle tone
- Perform gross MMT (gross strength test); grip and pinch strength
- Sensory testing: light touch, vibration, proprioception, temperature, pinprick
- Assess coordination (UEs: dysmetria, diadochokinesia; LEs: gait, heel-to-shin test)
- Test deep tendon reflexes

failure, pregnancy, post-operative patients, and any problems with coagulation.

Screening assessment of peripheral arterial disease (PAD) can be done using the ankle-brachial index (ABI). In fact, the American Diabetes Association recommends screening for anyone with diabetes who is 50 years old or older. Others who can benefit from screening include clients with risk factors for PAD such as smoking, advancing age, hypertension, hyperlipidemia, and symptoms of claudication.

Baseline ABI should be taken on both sides for anyone who has (or may have) PAD. Clients with diabetes who have normal ABI levels should be retested periodically.[75,76] The ABI is the ratio of the systolic blood pressure in the ankle divided by the systolic blood pressure at the arm:

$$SBP_{ankle}/SBP_{arm}$$

Assess ankle SBP using both the dorsalis pedis pulse and the posterior tibial pulse. Divide the higher SBP from each leg by the higher brachial systolic pressure (i.e., if the SBP is higher in the right arm use that figure for the calculations in both legs).

Normal ABI values lie in the range of 0.91 to 1.3. A general guideline is provided in Table 4-10. Recall what was said earlier in this chapter about normal blood pressures in the legs versus the arms: SBP in the legs is normally 10 to 20 percent higher than the brachial artery pressure in the arms resulting in an ABI greater than 1.0. PAD obstruction is indicated when the ABI values fall to less than or equal to 1.0.

Rubor on dependency is another test used to observe the adequacy of arterial circulation. Place the client in the supine position and observe the color of the soles of the feet. Normal feet should be pink or flesh colored in Caucasians and tan or brown in clients with dark skin tones. The feet of clients with impaired circulation are often chalky white (Caucasians) or gray or white in clients with darker skin.

Elevate the legs to 45 degrees (above the heart level). For clients with compromise of the arterial blood supply, any color present will quickly disappear in this position; in other words, the elevated foot develops increased pallor. No change (or little change) is observed in the normal individual. Bring the individual to a sitting position with the legs dangling. Venous filling is delayed following foot elevation. Color change in the lower leg and foot may take 30 seconds or more and will be a very bright red (dependent rubor).[16,77]

Venous Thromboembolism

Another condition affecting the extremities is venous thrombophlebitis or venous thromboembolism (VTE), a common complication seen in clients with cancer or following abdominal or pelvic surgery (especially orthopedic surgery such as total hip and total knee replacements), major trauma, or prolonged immobilization. Other risk factors are discussed in Chapter 6.

VTE is an inflammation of a vein associated with thrombus formation affecting superficial or deep veins of the extremities. Superficial vein thrombophlebitis typically involves the veins of the upper extremities and is more commonly associated with trauma (e.g., insertion of intravenous lines [IVs] and catheters in the subclavian vein). Deep vein thrombophlebitis usually involves the deep veins of the legs, primarily the calf.

Deep venous thrombosis (DVT) can become dislodged and travel as an embolus where it can become lodged in the pulmonary artery, leading to comorbidity or even death from acute coronary syndrome and stroke. DVTs are often asymptomatic, making screening a key component in the prevention of this potentially life-threatening problem.[78]

Many clinicians use Homan's sign as physical evidence of DVTs. The test uses slow dorsiflexion of the foot or gentle squeezing of the affected calf to elicit deep calf pain. Homan's sign is not specific for DVT because a positive Homan's sign is possible with Achilles tendinitis and muscle injury of the gastrocnemius and plantar muscle.

Autar DVT Risk Assessment Scale (Table 4-11) is a much more sensitive and specific test devel-

---

TABLE 4-10 ▼ Ankle Brachial Index Reading*

Indicators of Peripheral Arterial Disease

1.0-1.3	Normal (blood pressure at the ankle and arm are the same; no significant narrowing or obstruction of blood flow)
0.8-1.0	Mild peripheral arterial occlusive disease
0.5-0.8	Moderate peripheral arterial occlusive disease
Less than 0.5	Severe peripheral arterial occlusive disease
Less than 0.2	Ischemic or gangrenous extremity

* Different sources offer slightly different ABI values for normal to severe PAD. Some sources use values between 0.90 and 0.97 as the lower end of normal. Values greater than 1.3 are not considered reliable because calcified vessels show falsely elevated pressures. The therapist should follow guidelines provided by the physician or facility. Data from Sacks D, et al.: Position statement on the use of the ankle brachial index in the evaluation of patients with peripheral vascular disease. A consensus statement developed by the Standards Division of the Society of Interventional Radiology, J Vasc Interv Radiol 13:353, 2002.

TABLE 4-11 ▼ Autar DVT Scale

Category	Possible score (points)	Score (points)
Age (years)	10-30	0
	31-40	1
	41-50	2
	51-60	3
	61+	4
BMI (Wt kg)/(Hgt m)²	16-19	0
	20-25	1
	26-30	2
	31-40	3
	41+	4
Mobility	Ambulant	0
	Limited (walks with aids)	1
	Very limited (needs help)	2
	Chair bound	3
	Bed rest	4
Special DVT Risk	Birth control pills (less than 35 years old)	1
	Birth control pills (35 years old/older)	2
	Pregnant/up to 6 wks postpartum	3
Trauma Risk Factors (Score only preoperatively; score only one item)	Head or chest	1
	Head and chest	2
	Pelvic, abdominal, or thoracic	2
	Orthopedic (below waist)	3
	Spinal	4
Surgical Risk Factors (Score only one item)	Minor surgery (<30 minutes)	1
	Major surgery	2
	Emergency major	3
	Pelvic	3
	Spinal	3
	Lower limb	4
High Risk Diseases	Ulcerative colitis	1
	Anemia (sickle cell, polycythemis, hemolytic)	2
	Chronic heart disease	3
	Myocardial infarction	4
	Malignancy	5
	Varicose veins	6
	Previous DVT or CVA	7
Results based on total score	Less than or equal to: 6	TOTAL SCORE: No risk
	7-10	Low risk (less than 10%)
	11-14	Moderate risk (11-40%)
	15 Equal to or more than:	High risk (more than 40%)

BMI, Body mass index; see text for web links for easy calculation; *DVT*, deep venous thrombosis; *CVA*, cerebrovascular accident.
From Autar R. Nursing assessment of clients at risk of deep vein thrombosis (DVT): the Autar DVT scale, *J Advanced Nursing* 23(4): 763-770, 1996. Reprinted with permission of Blackwell Scientific.

oped as a predictive index of DVT. Seven risk categories are included: increasing age, build and body mass index (BMI), immobility, special DVT risk, trauma, surgery, and high-risk disease.[79,80]

A similar (less comprehensive) tool, the Clinical Decision Rule (CDR) developed by Wells and col-

leagues,[81-83] frequently discussed in the general medical literature, can also be used by therapists (Table 4-12).[84] The CDR incorporates signs, symptoms, and risk factors for DVT and should be used in all cases of suspected DVT.

The CDR is used more widely in the clinic, but the Autar scale is more comprehensive and incor-

TABLE 4-12 ▼ Wells' Clinical Decision Rule for DVT

Clinical presentation	Score
Previously diagnosed DVT	1
Active cancer (within 6 months of diagnosis or receiving palliative care)	1
Paralysis, paresis, or recent immobilization of lower extremity	1
Bedridden for more than 3 days or major surgery in the last 4 weeks	1
Localized tenderness in the center of the posterior calf, the popliteal space, or along the femoral vein in the anterior thigh/groin	1
Entire lower extremity swelling	1
Unilateral calf swelling (more than 3 mm larger than uninvolved side)	1
Unilateral pitting edema	1
Collateral superficial veins (nonvaricose)	1
An alternative diagnosis is as likely (or more likely) than DVT (e.g., cellulitis, postoperative swelling, calf strain)	−2
Total Points	

Key

−2 to 0	Low probability of DVT	(3%)
1 to 2	Moderate probability of DVT	(17%)
3 or more	High probability of DVT	(75%)

Medical consultation is advised in the presence of low probability; medical referral is required with moderate or high score.
From Wells PS, Anderson DR, Bormanis J, et al: Value of assessment of pretest probability of deep-vein thrombosis in clinical management, *Lancet* 350:1795-1798, 1997. Used with permission.

porates BMI, postpartum status, and the use of oral contraceptives as potential risk factors.

Research shows some physical therapists may not be referring clients to a physician for additional workup when the individual's risk for developing DVT warrants referral.[85] Medical consultation is advised for anyone with a low probability of DVT; medical referral is required for any individual suspected of having DVT.

The Chest and Back (Thorax)

A screening examination of the thorax requires the same basic techniques of inspection, palpation, and auscultation. Once again, keep in mind this is a screening examination. Being familiar with normal findings of the chest and thorax will help the therapist identify abnormal results requiring further evaluation or referral. Only basic screening tools are included. Specialized training may be required for some acute care or primary care settings.

Chest and Back: Inspection[23]

Inspect the client while he or she is sitting upright without support if possible. Observe the client's

thorax from the front, back, side, and over the shoulder (looking down over the anterior chest). Note any skin changes, signs of skin breakdown, and signs of cyanosis or pallor, scars, wounds, bruises, lesions, nodules, or superficial venous patterns.

Note the shape and symmetry of the thorax from the front and back. Observe posture and spinal alignment. Record the presence of any deformities. Estimate the anterior-posterior diameter compared to the transverse diameter. Look at the angle of the costal margins at the xiphoid process. Observe the client for muscular development and nutritional status by noting the presence of underlying adipose tissue and the visibility of the ribs.

Assess respiratory rate, depth, and rhythm or pattern of breathing while the client is breathing normally. Watch for symmetry of chest wall movement, costal versus abdominal breathing, the use of accessory muscles, and bulging or retraction of the intercostal spaces.

Chest and Back: Palpation

Palpation of the thorax is usually combined with inspection to save time. Breast examination and lymph node assessment may be part of the screening exam of the chest in males and females (see discussion later in this section).

Palpation can reveal skin changes and alert the therapist to conditions that relate to the client's respiratory status. Look for crepitus, a crackly, crinkly sensation in the subcutaneous tissue. Feel for vibrations during inspiration as described next.

Palpate the entire thorax (anterior and posterior) for tactile fremitus by placing the palms of both hands (examiner's) over the client's upper anterior chest at the second intercostal space (Fig. 4-43). The normal response is a feeling of vibrations of equal intensity during vocalizations on either side of the midline, front to back.

Tactile fremitus is found most commonly in the upper chest near the bronchi around the second intercostal space. Stronger vibrations are felt whenever air is present; the absence of air such as occurs with atelectasis is marked by an absence of vibrations. Fluid outside the lung pressing on the lung increases the force of vibration.

Increased tactile fremitus often accompanies inflammation, infection, congestion, or consolidation of a lung or part of a lung. Diminished tactile fremitus may indicate the presence of pleural effusion or pneumothorax.[23] Record the location, beginning and ending points, and note whether the tactile fremitus is increased or decreased. Confirm all findings with auscultation; a medical evaluation with chest X-ray provides the differential diagnosis.

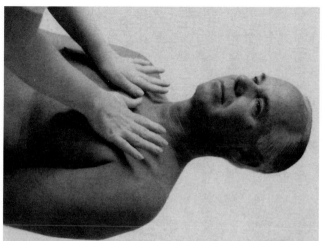

Fig. 4-43 • Palpating for tactile fremitus. Place the palmar surfaces of both hands on the client's chest at the second intercostal space. Ask the client to say "99" repeatedly as you gradually move your hands over the chest, systematically comparing the lung fields. Start at the center and move out toward the arms. Drop the hands down one level and move back toward the center. Continue until the complete lung fields have been assessed. Repeat the exam on the client's back. The normal response is a feeling of vibrations of equal intensity during vocalizations on either side of the midline, front to back. (From *Expert 10-minute physical examinations.* St. Louis, 1997, Mosby.)

Assess respiratory excursion and symmetry with the client in the supine position. Stand in front of your client and place your thumbs along the client's costal margins wrapping your fingers around the rib cage. Observe how far the thumbs move apart (range and symmetry) during chest expansion (normal breathing and deep breathing). Normal respiratory excursion will separate the thumbs by 1¼ to 2 inches. Assess respiratory excursion at more than one level, front to back.

The presence of costovertebral tenderness should be followed up with Murphy's percussion test (see Fig. 4-51). Bone tenderness over the lumbar spinous processes is a red flag symptom for osseous disorders such as fracture, infection, or neoplasm and requires a more complete evaluation.

Chest and Back: Percussion

Chest and back percussion is an advanced skill beyond the screening examination. The skilled clinician can use percussion of the chest and back to identify the left ventricular border of the heart and

the depth of diaphragmatic excursion in the upper abdomen during breathing. Percussion can also help identify disorders that impair lung ventilation, such as stomach distention, hemothorax, lung consolidation, and pneumothorax.[23]

Dullness over the lungs during percussion may indicate a mass or consolidation (e.g., pneumonia). Hyperresonance over the lungs may indicate hyperinflated or emphysemic lungs. Decreased diaphragmatic excursion on one side occurs with pleural effusion, diaphragmatic excursion (phrenic nerve) paralysis, tension pneumothorax, stomach distention (left side), hepatomegaly (right side), or atelectasis. Clients with chronic obstructive pulmonary disease (COPD) often have decreased excursion bilaterally as a result of a hyperinflated chest depressing the diaphragm.

Chest and Back: Lung Auscultation

In a screening exam the therapist should listen for normal breath sounds and air movement through the lungs during inspiration and expiration. Taking a deep breath or coughing clears some sounds. At times the examiner instructs the client to take a deep breath or cough and listens again for any changes in sound. With practice and training, the therapist can identify 1 of 4 abnormal sounds heard most often in clients with pulmonary involvement: crackles, wheezing, gurgles, and pleural friction rub.

Crackles (formerly called rales) is the sound of air moving through an airway filled with fluid. It is heard most often on inspiration and sounds like strands of hair being rubbed together under a stethoscope. Crackles are normal sounds in the morning as the alveolar spaces open up. Have the client take a deep breath to complete this process first before listening.

Abnormal crackles can be heard during exhalation in clients with pneumonia or congestive heart failure and during inhalation with the re-expansion of atelectatic areas. Crackles are described as fine (soft and high pitched), medium (louder and low pitched), or coarse (moist and more explosive).

Wheezing is the sound of air passing through a narrowed airway blocked by mucus secretions and usually occurs during expiration (wheezing on inspiration is a sign of a more serious problem). It is frequently described as a high-pitched, musical whistling sound. Wheezing is most often associated with asthma or emphysema. Take careful note when the wheezing goes away in any client who presents with wheezing. Disappearance of wheezing occurs when the person is not breathing.

Gurgles (formerly called rhonchi) is defined as air moving through thick secretions partially

obstructing airflow and is almost always associated with bronchitis. These loud, low-pitched rumbling sounds can be heard on inspiration or expiration and may be cleared by coughing.

Pleural friction rub makes a high pitched scratchy sound heard when a hand is cupped over the ear and scratched along the outside of the hand. It is caused by inflamed pleural surfaces and can be heard on inspiration and/or expiration. The pleural linings should move over each other smoothly and easily. In the presence of inflammation (pleuritis, pleurisy, pneumonia, tumors), the inflamed tissue (parietal pleura) is rubbing against other inflamed, irritated tissue (visceral pleura) causing friction.

Assess for *egophony* by asking the client to say and repeat the "ee" sound during auscultation of the lung fields. The "aa" sound heard as the client says the "ee" sound indicates pleural effusion or lung consolidation. *Bronchophony*, a clear and audible "99" sound suggests the sound is traveling through fluid or a mass; the sound should be muffled in the healthy adult. Finally, assess for consolidation using *whispered pectoriloquy*. Ask the client to whisper "1-2-3" as you listen to the chest and back. The examiner should hear a muffled noise (normal) instead of a clear and audible "1-2-3" (consolidation).

Describe sounds heard, the location of the sounds on the thorax, and when the sounds are heard during the respiratory cycle (inspiration vs. expiration). Have the client gently cough (bronchial secretions causing a "gurgle" will often clear with a cough) and listen again. Compare results with the first exam (and with the baseline if available). The decision to refer a client for further evaluation is based on history, clinical findings, client distress, vital signs, and any associated signs and symptoms observed or reported.

Chest and Back: Heart Auscultation

The same general principles for auscultation of lung sounds apply to auscultation of heart sounds. The therapist's primary responsibility in a screening examination is to know what "normal" heart sounds are like and report any changes (absence of normal sounds or presence of additional sounds).

The normal cardiac cycle correlates with the direction of blood flow and consists of two phases: systole (ventricles contract and eject blood) and diastole (ventricles relax and atria contract to move blood into the ventricles and fill the coronary arteries).

Normal heart sounds (S1 and S2) occur in relation to the cardiac cycle. Just before S1, the mitral and tricuspid valves are open, and blood from the atria is filling the relaxed ventricles (see Fig. 6-1). The ventricles contract and raise pressure, beginning the period called systole.

Pressure in the ventricles increases rapidly, forcing the mitral and tricuspid valves to close causing the first heart sound (S1). The S1 sound produced by the closing of the AV valves is *lubb*; it can be heard at the same time the radial or carotid pulse is felt.

As the pressure inside the ventricles increases, the aortic and pulmonic valves open and blood is pumped out of the heart into the lungs and aorta. The ventricle ejects most of its blood and pressure begins to fall causing the aortic and pulmonic valves to snap shut. The closing of these valves produces the *dubb* (S2) sound. This marks the beginning of the diastole phase.

S3 (third heart sound), S4 (fourth heart sound), heart murmurs, and pericardial friction rub are the most common extra sounds heard. S3, also known as a ventricular gallop, is a faint, low-pitched *lubb-dup-ah* sound heard directly after S2. It occurs at the beginning of diastole and may be heard in healthy children and young adults as a result of a large volume of blood pumping through a small heart. This sound is also considered normal in the last trimester of pregnancy. It is not normal when it occurs as a result of volume overload associated with congestive heart failure.

S4, also known as an atrial gallop, occurs in late diastole (just before S1) if there is a vibration of the valves or ventricular walls from resistance to filling. It is usually considered an abnormal sound (*ta-lup-dubb*), but may be heard in athletes with well-developed heart muscles.

Heart murmurs are swishing sounds made as blood flows across a stiff or incompetent valve, or through an abnormal opening in the heart wall. Most murmurs are associated with valve disease (stenosis, insufficiency) but they can occur with a wide variety of other cardiac conditions. They may be normal in children and during the third trimester of pregnancy.

A pericardial friction rub associated with pericarditis is a scratchy, scraping sound that is heard louder during exhalation and forward bending. The sound occurs when inflamed layers of the heart viscera (see Fig. 6-5) rub against each other causing friction.

Auscultate the heart over each of the six anatomical landmarks (Fig. 4-44), first with the diaphragm (firm pressure) and then with the bell (light pressure) of the stethoscope. Use a Z-path to include all landmarks while covering the entire surface area of the heart. Practice at each site until

1. Aortic area (right 2nd intercostal space, ICS)
2. Pulmonic area (left 2nd ICS)
3. Erb's point (left 3rd ICS); murmurs are best heard at this point using the stethoscope bell
4. Tricuspid (left 5th ICS at sternum)
5. Mitral or apical point of maximal impulse (PMI), (left 5th ICS medial to the midclavicular line)
6. Epigastric area (just below the tip of the sternum)

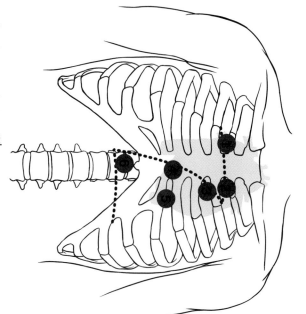

Fig. 4-44 • Cardiac anatomical landmarks. Inspect and palpate the anterior chest, auscultate all six anatomical landmarks shown.

you can hear the rate and rhythm, S1 and S2, extra heart sounds, including murmurs.

Practice at each site until you can hear the rate and rhythm, S1 and S2, extra heart sounds, including murmurs. Murmurs are not heard with a bell (listen for murmurs with the diaphragm); S3 and S4 are heard with the bell.

As with lung sounds, describe heart sounds heard, rate and rhythm of the sounds, the location of the sounds on the thorax, and when the sounds are heard during the cardiac cycle. The decision to refer a client for further evaluation is based on history, age, risk factors, presence of pregnancy, clinical findings, client distress, vital signs, and any associated signs and symptoms observed or reported.

Chest: Clinical Breast Examination (CBE)

Although the third edition of this text specifically said, "breast examination is not within the scope of a physical therapist's practice," this practice is changing.

As the number of cancer survivors increases in the United States, therapists treating post-mastectomy women and clients of both genders with lymphedema are on the rise. Cancer recurrence after mastectomy with or without reconstruction is possible. Recurrences after reconstructive surgery have been detected first on physical examination.[86-88]

With direct and unrestricted access of consumers to physical therapists in many states and with the expanded role of physical therapists in primary care, advanced skills have become necessary. For some clients, clinical breast exam (CBE) is an appropriate assessment tool in the screening process.[89]

CBE AND THE GUIDE

The *Guide* includes a concise description of the physical therapist in primary care and our respective roles in primary and secondary prevention.[12] Currently the *Guide* does not specifically include, nor exclude examination of breast tissue, but does include examination of the integument.

The *Guide* does not discriminate what parts of the body may, or may not, be examined as a part of professional practice. The section on examination of the integumentary system identifies the need to perform visual and palpatory inspection of the skin for abnormalities.

It is recognized that the *Guide* is a guide to practice that is intended to be revised periodically to reflect current physical therapy practice. Determining whether CBE should be included or excluded from the scope of a physical therapist's practice is the responsibility of each individual state.

If the therapist receives proper training to perform CBEs,* he or she must make sure this examination is allowed according to the state practice act for the state(s) in which the therapist is conducting CBEs. In some states it is allowed by exclu-

---

* The American Cancer Society and National Cancer Institute support the provision of cancer screening procedures by qualified health specialists. With additional training, physical therapists can qualify.

An introductory course to breast cancer and clinical breast examination for the physical therapist is available. Charlie McGarvey, PT, MS and Catherine Goodman, MBA, PT present the course in various sites around the U.S. and upon request.

A certified training program is also available through *MammaCare Specialist*. The program is offered to health care professionals at training centers in the United States. The course teaches proficient breast examination skills. For more information, contact: http://www.mammacare.com/professional_training.htm.

sion, meaning it is not mentioned and therefore included. When moving to a new state, the therapist is advised to take the time to review and understand that state's practice act.

SCREENING FOR EARLY DETECTION OF BREAST CANCER

The goal of screening examinations is early detection of breast cancer. Breast cancers that are detected because they are causing symptoms tend to be relatively larger and are more likely to have spread beyond the breast. In contrast, breast cancers found during screening examinations are more likely to be small and still confined to the breast.

The size of a breast neoplasm and how far it has spread are the most important factors in predicting the prognosis for anyone with this disease. According to the American Cancer Society (ACS) early detection tests for breast cancer saves many thousands of lives each year; many more lives could be saved if health care providers took advantage of these tests. Following the American Cancer Society's guidelines for the early detection of breast cancer improves the chances that breast cancer can be diagnosed at an early stage and treated successfully.[90,91]

CBE detects a small portion of cancers (4.6% to 5.9%) not found by mammography.[92] It may be important for women who do not receive regular mammograms, either because mammography is not recommended (e.g., women aged 40 and younger) or because some women do not receive screening mammography as recommended.[93]

ACS guidelines for CBE recommend CBE every 3 years for women ages 20 to 39 (more often if there are risk factors; see Table 173). An annual CBE is advised every year for asymptomatic women ages 40 and older. Men can develop breast cancer, but this disease is about 100 times more common among women than men.[91]

Self-breast examination (SBE) is an option for women starting at age 20. Women should be educated about the benefits and limitations of the SBE. Regular BSE is one way for women to know how their breasts normally feel and to notice any changes. Advise all women during the client education portion of the physical therapy intervention to report any breast changes right away. The primary care provider should also review each client's method of performing a SBE (see Appendix D-6).

It is generally accepted that mammography screening reduces the risk of death from breast cancer (except, perhaps, among younger women, for whom the benefit of mammography is controversial), and that this risk reduction is achieved through the detection of malignancy at an earlier stage, when treatment is more efficacious.[94]

The ideal interval between screening mammography remains under investigation. In the United States, the U.S. Preventive Services Task Force recommends screening every 1 to 2 years while the American Cancer Society recommends annual screening from age 40 years. In Europe, most countries focus on women aged 50 years and older and recommend screening every two years.[95]

Mammograms do not identify all breast cancers; for this reason, a *thorough* CBE remains an essential part of breast screening to complement mammograms and reduce false-negative results.[96,97]

"Thorough" is defined as palpation of the area from the collarbone to the bottom of the rib cage, one dime-size area at a time, at three levels of pressure from just below the skin, down to the midbreast, and up against the chest wall. A thorough CBE by a specially trained practitioner should take at least five minutes per breast.[90]

It has been shown both in the laboratory and in the clinic that properly trained fingers can detect breast lesions as small as 3 mm in diameter.[98,99] As experts in the assessment and palpation of the integumentary and musculoskeletal systems, physical therapists are highly qualified professionals to receive this type of training.

PHYSICAL THERAPIST'S ROLE IN SCREENING FOR BREAST CANCER

Historically the upper quadrant screening examination conducted by physical therapists has not included CBE. Procedures have been confined to questions posed to clients during the interview regarding past medical history (e.g., cancer, lactation, abscess, mastitis) and questions to identify the possibility of breast pathology as the underlying cause for back or shoulder pain and/or other symptoms.[89]

As health care specialists with advanced observational and palpatory skills, physical therapists can play an important role in the identification of aberrant soft tissue lesions requiring further medical evaluation. Physical therapists are professionally trained experts in tissue integrity and possess highly developed skills in the detection of various types of abnormalities. Properly trained, physical therapists should be considered "qualified, health care specialists" as defined by the ACS in the provision of cancer screening when the history, clinical presentation, and associated signs and symptoms point to the need for CBE.[89]

A physical therapist conducting a CBE could miss a lump (false negative finding) and not send

the client for medical evaluation. However, this will most certainly occur if the therapist is not conducting a CBE to assess the integrity of the skin and soft tissues of the breast or axilla. Conversely, a physical therapist finding a lump or abnormality on CBE would refer the client to a physician for examination.[89]

A blueprint for the screening assessment is provided in Box 4-16 and Fig. 4-45. Standardized CBE and reporting of results has not been established. Best practice for CBE using inspection and palpation based on current recommendations[93,100] is presented in Appendix D-7. For a discussion of benign breast diseases and breast conditions that

---

BOX 4-16 ▼ Screening For Breast Disease

Upper Quadrant Examination

Many conditions can cause breast pain or refer pain to the breast (see Table 17-2). For anyone with neck, upper back, chest, scapular, or shoulder symptoms, a screening examination of the upper quadrant may be necessary. The physical therapy differential diagnosis requires determination of the underlying soft tissue involvement and assesses the need for medical referral. The screening examination includes past and current medical history, clinical examination, review of systems, and review of any associated signs and symptoms.

Client Interview

Past Medical History

Look for a history of trauma, recent birth, overuse, increased abdominal breathing (e.g., prolonged running, lifting), cardiovascular disease, cancer, GI involvement, or other systemic conditions that can refer pain/symptoms to the upper quadrant.

Ask about a previous history of breast disease of any kind (e.g., chronic mastitis, cancer, Paget's disease).

Assess Risk Factors

See Table 17-3.

Special Questions to Ask: Breast

- Have you ever had any breast surgery (implants, lumpectomy, mastectomy, reconstructive surgery, or augmentation)?
- Have you ever been treated for cancer of any kind? If yes, when? What?
- Do you have any discharge from your breasts or nipples? If yes, do you know what is causing this discharge? Have you received medical treatment for this problem?
- Have you noticed any other changes in your breast(s)? For example, are there any noticeable, bulging, or distended veins, puckering, swelling, or any other skin changes?
- Are you nursing an infant (lactating)?
- Have you examined yourself for any lumps or nodules and found any thickening or lump? If yes, has your physician examined/treated this? If no, do you examine your own breasts? (Follow-up

questions, e.g., last breast examination by self or health care professional)

- Have you been involved in any activities of a repetitive nature that could cause sore muscles (e.g., painting, washing walls, push-ups or other calisthenics, heavy lifting or pushing, overhead movements, prolonged running, or fast walking)?
- Have you recently been coughing excessively?
- Have you ever had angina (chest pain) or a heart attack (residual trigger points)?
- Have you been in a fight or hit, punched, or pushed against any object that injured your chest or breast (assault)?
- See also Special Questions to Ask: Lymph Nodes (this chapter and Appendix B-19)

Clinical Presentation

Visual Inspection (Posture, Skin, Breast)

Look for asymmetry, nipple retraction, ulceration, erythema, peau d'orange, or other skin changes. Have the client raise arms overhead. Assess the lower half of the breast and the inframammary folds. Have the client place hands on hips and press down to contract the pectoralis major muscles. Observe for any undetected asymmetries or changes. Have the client bend forward with arms relaxed at his/her sides. Again, look for any undetected asymmetries or changes.

Screening Assessment/Evaluation

- Manual muscle testing (MMT), neurologic screen (reflexes, sensation, proprioception), trigger point assessment
- Neck, shoulder, clavicle, sternum ROM (AROM, PROM, accessory motions)

Palpation

Palpate appropriate soft tissue structures according to history and evaluation results. This may include breast, axilla, and lymph nodes, especially the supraclavicular nodes since these are the typical nodes assessed during CBE procedures in order to stage the disease. Palpation of the breast is performed with the client in the supine position. The shoulder/scapular area may be supported with a small pillow or foam wedge.

BOX 4-16 ▼ Screening For Breast Disease—cont'd

Palpate from the mid-axillary line to the sternum and from the clavicle to inframammary fold. Assess the entire thickness of the breast parenchyma. Patterns of palpation include: horizontal strip, radial, circular, and vertical strip. There is some evidence to suggest that the vertical pattern (up and down pattern) is the most effective pattern for covering the entire breast, without missing any breast tissue (Barton et al., 1999).*

Other Clues

- Resisted movements reproduce pain/symptoms [look for musculoskeletal cause]
- Response to stretch (reduces or eliminates pain/symptoms) [look for musculoskeletal cause]
- Eliminated by treatment (stretching, trigger point therapy) [look for musculoskeletal cause]

- Assess effect of lower extremity exertion only [screen for cardiovascular disease]
- Assess for 3 P's: pain on *p*alpation (myalgia), change in symptoms with change in *p*osition, symptoms increase with respiratory movements (*p*leuritic pain)

Associated Signs and Symptoms of Breast Disease

Palpable breast nodules or lumps
Skin surface red, warm, edematous, firm, painful
Firm, painful site under the skin surface
Skin dimpling over the lesion with attachment of mass to surrounding tissues
Unusual nipple discharge
Pain aggravated by jarring or movement of the breasts
Pain that is not aggravated by resistance to isometric movements of the upper extremities

*From Barton M, Harris R, Fletcher S: Does this patient have breast cancer? The Screening Clinical Breast Examination. *JAMA* 282(13):1270-1280, 1999.

---

can refer pain to the shoulder, neck, or chest, see Chapter 17.)

When a suspicious mass is found during examination, it must be medically evaluated, even if the client reports a recent mammography was "normal."[93] Clinical signs and symptoms of breast disease are listed in Chapter 17. More in-depth discussion of the role of the physical therapist in primary care and cancer screening as it relates to integrating CBE into an upper quarter examination is available.[89]

Abdomen

Anyone presenting with primary pain patterns from pathology of the abdominal organs will likely see a physician rather than a physical therapist. For this reason, abdominal and visceral assessment is not generally part of the physical therapy evaluation. When the therapist suspects referred pain from the viscera to the musculoskeletal system, this type of assessment can be helpful in the screening examination.

Abdomen: Inspection

From a screening or assessment point of view, the abdomen is divided into 4 quadrants centered on the umbilicus (as shown in Figs. 4-46 and 4-47). During the inspection, any abdominal scars (and associated history) should be identified (see Fig. 4-7).

Note the color of the skin and the presence and location of any striae from pregnancy or weight

gain/loss, petechiae, or spider angiomas (see Fig. 9-3). A bluish discoloration around the umbilicus (Cullen's sign) or along the lower abdomen and flanks (Grey Turner's sign) may be the sign of a retroperitoneal bleed (e.g., pancreatitis, ruptured ectopic pregnancy, posterior perforated ulcer). The color may be a shade of blue-red, blue-purple, or green-brown, depending on the stage of hemoglobin breakdown.[23]

From a seated position next to the client, the therapist looks for any asymmetry. Repeat the same visual inspection while standing behind the client's head. Make note if the umbilicus is displaced in any direction or if there are any masses, pulsations, or movements of the abdomen. Visible peristaltic waves are not normal and may signal a GI problem. Document the presence of ascites (see Fig. 9-8).

Clients with an organic cause for abdominal pain usually are not hungry. Ask the client to point to the location of the pain. Pain corresponding to the epigastric, periumbilical, and lower midabdominal regions is shown in Fig. 8-2. If the finger points to the navel but the client seems well, there may be a psychogenic source of symptoms.[101]

Abdomen: Auscultation

In a screening examination, the therapist may auscultate the four abdominal quadrants for the presence of abdominal sounds. Expect to hear rumblings and gurgling sounds every few seconds throughout the abdomen.

Breast and Lymph Node Examination – Palpable Findings

Please refer to Appendix: Clinical Breast Examination (CBE) Recommended Procedures when conducting the assessment and completing this form.

Date: _____   First day (date) of last (menstrual) period: _____   Client's name: _____

Description of lump:
None (circle if exam results are normal); skip to lymph node assessment below

Location	Size (cm x cm)	Contour	Shape
Side: Right		Irregular	Describe:
		Smooth	
Record o'clock position			
Side: Left		Irregular	Describe:
		Smooth	
Record o'clock position			

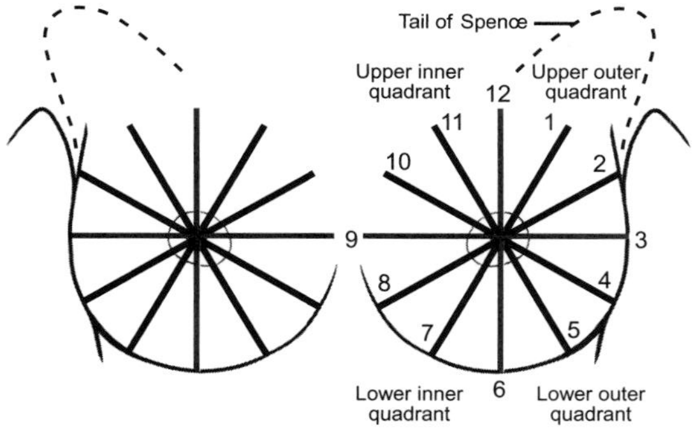

Note location of mass by quadrant, place on the clock and distance from the nipple

Tail of Spence

Upper inner quadrant / Upper outer quadrant
Lower inner quadrant / Lower outer quadrant

Density of lump/lesion	Tenderness	Mobility
Soft	Yes	Mobile
Rubbery	No	Fixed
Hard		

Description of lymph nodes:
None (exam results are normal)

Location	Zone (see Fig. 4-40)	Density	Mobility	Tenderness
Side: Right	I II III	Soft	Mobile	Yes
		Rubbery	Fixed	No
		Hard		
Side: Left	I II III	Soft	Mobile	Yes
		Rubbery	Fixed	No
		Hard		

Notes:

Note: Keep in mind the following general guidelines for breast lumps.
Refer all suspicious lesions or aberrant tissue for medical evaluation and diagnosis.

Benign	Malignant
Soft	Firm
Smooth	Irregular
Moveable	Fixed

Fig. 4-45 • Breast and lymph node examination.

The absence of sounds or very few sounds in any or all of the quadrants is a red flag and is most common in the older adult with multiple risk factors such as recent abdominal, back, or pelvic surgery and the use of narcotics or other medications.

As previously mentioned the therapist may auscultate the abdomen for vascular sounds (e.g., bruits) when the history (e.g., age over 65, history of coronary artery disease), clinical presentation (e.g., neck, back, abdominal, or flank pain), and associated signs and symptoms (e.g., syncopal episodes, signs and symptoms of peripheral vascular disease) warrant this type of assessment.

Listen for pulsations/bruits first before palpation as palpation may stir up the bowel contents and increase peristalsis, making auscultation more difficult.

Abdomen: Percussion and Palpation

Percussion over normal, healthy abdominal organs is an advanced skill even among doctors and nurses and is not a part of the physical therapy screening examination.

Palpation (light and deep) of all four abdominal quadrants is a separate skill used to assess for temperature changes, tenderness, and large masses. Keep in mind that even a skilled clinician will not be able to palpate abdominal organs in an obese person.

Most viscera in the normal adult are not palpable unless enlarged. Anatomical structures can be mistaken for an abdominal mass. Palpation is contraindicated in anyone with a suspected abdominal aortic aneurysm, appendicitis, known kidney disease, or who has had an abdominal organ transplantation.

When palpation is carried out, always explain to your client what test you are going to perform and why. Use proper draping and warm your hands. Have the client bend the knees with the feet flat on the exam table to put the abdominal muscles in a relaxed position. During palpation, if the person is ticklish, place his or her hand on top of your palpating hand. Ask him or her to breathe in and out slowly and regularly. The tickle response disappears in the presence of a truly acute abdomen.[102]

Start with a light touch, moving the fingers in a circular motion, slowly and gently. If the abdominal muscles are contracted, observe the client as he or she breathes in and out. The contraction is voluntary if the muscles are more strongly contracted during inspiration and less strong during expiration. Muscles firmly contracted throughout the

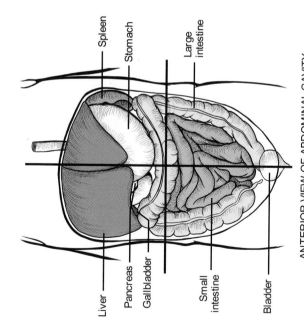

ANTERIOR VIEW OF ABDOMINAL CAVITY

Fig. 4-46 • Four abdominal (anterior) quadrants formed by two imaginary perpendicular lines running through the umbilicus. As a general rule, viscera in the RUQ can refer pain to the right shoulder; viscera in the LUQ can refer pain to the left shoulder; viscera in the lower quadrants are less specific and can refer pain to the pelvis, pelvic floor, groin, low back, hip, and sacroiliac/sacral areas. See also Figs. 3-4 and 3-5.

Labels: Spleen, Stomach, Large intestine, Liver, Pancreas, Gallbladder, Small intestine, Bladder

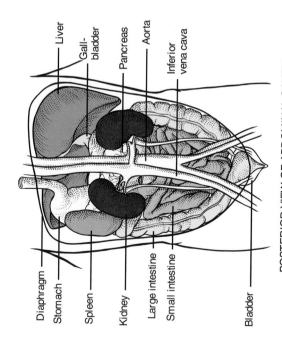

POSTERIOR VIEW OF ABDOMINAL CAVITY

Fig. 4-47 • Posterior view of the abdomen. The abdominal aorta passes from the diaphragm through the abdominal cavity, just to the left of the midline. It branches into the left and right common iliac arteries at the level of the umbilicus. Retroperitoneal bleeding from any of the posterior elements (e.g., stomach, spleen, aorta, kidneys) can cause back and/or shoulder pain.

Labels: Liver, Gallbladder, Pancreas, Aorta, Inferior vena cava, Diaphragm, Stomach, Spleen, Kidney, Large intestine, Small intestine, Bladder

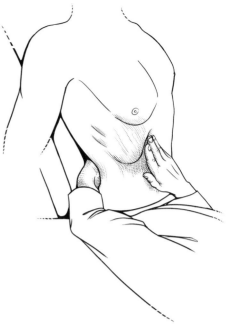

Fig. 4-48 • Palpating the liver. Place your left hand under the client's right posterior thorax (as shown) parallel to and at the level of the last two ribs. Place your right hand on the client's RUQ over the midclavicular line. The fingers should be pointing toward the client's head and positioned below the lower edge of liver dullness (previously mapped out by percussion). Ask the client to take a deep breath while pressing inward and upward with the fingers of the right hand. Attempt to feel the inferior edge of the liver with your right hand as it descends below the last rib anteriorly.

respiratory cycle (inspiration and expiration) are more likely to be involuntary, possibly indicating an underlying abdominal problem. To check for rebound tenderness, see Fig. 8-10.

LIVER

Liver percussion to determine its size and identify its edges is a skill beyond the scope of a physical therapist for a screening examination. Therapists involved in visceral manipulation will be most likely to develop this advanced skill.

To palpate the liver (Fig. 4-48), have the client take a deep breath as you feel deeply beneath the costal margin. During inspiration, the liver will move down with the diaphragm so that the lower edge may be felt below the right costal margin.

A normal adult liver is not usually palpable and palpation is not painful. Cirrhosis, metastatic cancer, infiltrative leukemia, right-sided congestive heart failure, and third-stage (tertiary) syphilis can cause an enlarged liver. The liver in clients with chronic obstructive pulmonary disease (COPD) is more readily palpable as the diaphragm moves down and pushes the liver below the ribs. The liver is often palpable 2 to 3cm below the costal margin in infants and young children. A palpable

If you come in contact with the bottom edge tucked up under the rib cage, the normal liver will feel firm, smooth, even, and rubbery. A palpable

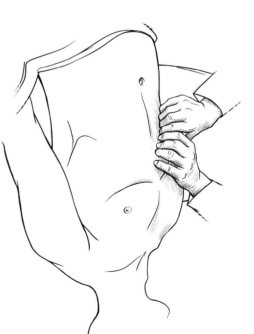

Fig. 4-49 • An alternate way to palpate the liver. Hook the fingers of one or both hands (depending on hand size) up and under the right costal border. As the client breathes in, the liver descends and the therapist may come in contact with the lower border of the liver. If this procedure elicits exquisite tenderness, it may be a positive *Murphy's sign* for acute cholecystitis (not the same as Murphy's percussion test [costovertebral tenderness] of the kidney depicted in Fig. 4-51).

hard or lumpy edge warrants further investigation. Some clinicians prefer to stand next to the client near his head, facing his feet. As the client breathes in, curl the fingers over the costal margin and up under the ribs to feel the liver (Fig. 4-49).

SPLEEN

As with other organs, the spleen is difficult to percuss, even more so than the liver, and is not part of a screening examination.

Palpation of the spleen is not possible unless it is distended and bulging below the left costal margin (Fig. 4-50). The spleen enlarges with mononucleosis and trauma. Do not continue to palpate an enlarged spleen because it can rupture easily. Report to the physician immediately how far it extends below the left costal margin and request medical evaluation.

GALLBLADDER AND PANCREAS

Likewise, the gallbladder tucked up under the liver (see Figs. 9-1 and 9-2) is not palpable unless grossly distended. To palpate the gallbladder, ask the person to take a deep breath as you palpate deep below the liver margin. Only an abnormally enlarged gallbladder can be palpated this way.

The pancreas is also inaccessible; it lies behind and beneath the stomach with its head along the

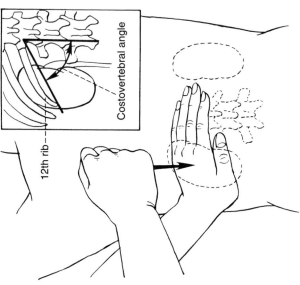

12th rib

Costovertebral angle

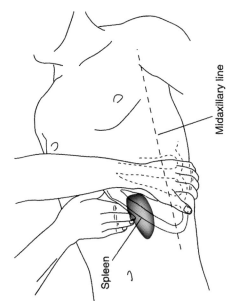

Spleen

Midaxillary line

Fig. 4-50 • Palpation of the spleen. The spleen is not usually palpable unless it is distended and bulging below the left costal margin. Left shoulder pain can occur with referred pain from the spleen. Stand on the person's right side and reach across the client with the left hand, placing it beneath the client over the left costovertebral angle. Lift the spleen anteriorly toward the abdominal wall. Place right hand on abdomen below left costal margin. Using findings from percussion gently press fingertips inward toward the spleen while asking client to take a deep breath. Feel for spleen as it moves downward towards fingers. (From Leasia MS, Monahan FD: *A practical guide to health assessment,* ed 2, Philadelphia, 2002, WB Saunders.)

Fig. 4-51 • Murphy's percussion also known as the test for *costovertebral tenderness.* Murphy's percussion is used to rule out involvement of the kidney and assess for pseudorenal pain (see discussion, Chapter 10). Indirect fist percussion causes the kidney to vibrate. To assess the kidney, position the client prone or sitting, and place one hand over the rib at the costovertebral angle on the back. Give the hand a percussive thump with the ulnar edge of your other fist. The person normally feels a thud but no pain. Reproduction of back and/or flank pain with this test is a red flag sign for renal involvement (e.g., kidney infection or inflammation). (From Black JM, Matassarin-Jacobs E, editors: *Luckmann and Sorensen's medical-surgical nursing,* ed 4, Philadelphia, 1993, WB Saunders.)

curve of the duodenum and its tip almost touching the spleen (see Fig. 9-1). A round, fixed swelling above the umbilicus that does not move with inspiration may be a sign of acute pancreatitis or cancer in a thin person.

KIDNEYS

The kidneys are located deep in the retroperitoneal space in both upper quadrants of the abdomen. Each kidney extends from approximately T12 to L3. The right kidney is usually slightly lower than the left.

Percussion of the kidney is accomplished using Murphy's percussion test (Fig. 4-51). To palpate the kidney, stand on the right side of the supine client. Place your left hand beneath the client's right flank. Flex the left metacarpophalangeal joints (MCPs) in the renal angle while pressing downward with the right hand against the right outer edge of the abdomen. This method compresses the kidney between your hands. The left kidney is usually not palpable because of its position beneath the bowel.

Kidney transplants are often located in the abdomen. The therapist should not percuss or palpate the kidneys of anyone with chronic renal disease or organ transplantation.

BLADDER

The bladder lies below the symphysis pubis and is not palpable unless it becomes distended and rises above the pubic bone. Primary pain patterns for the bladder are shown in Fig. 10-9. Sharp pain over the bladder or just above the symphysis pubis can also be caused by abdominal gas. The presence of associated gastrointestinal signs and symptoms and lack of urinary tract signs and symptoms may be helpful in identifying this pain pattern.

AORTIC BIFURCATION

It may be necessary to assess for an abdominal aneurysm, especially in the older client with back pain and/or who reports a pulsing or pounding sensation in the abdomen during increased activity or while in the supine position.

The ease with which the aortic pulsations can be felt varies greatly with the thickness of the abdominal wall and the anteroposterior diameter of the abdomen. To palpate the aortic pulse, the therapist should press firmly deep in the upper abdomen

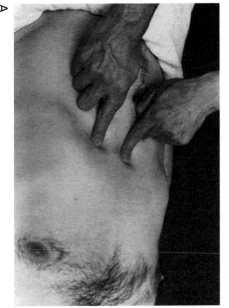

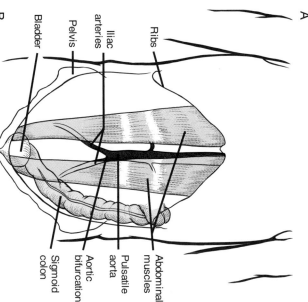

Fig. 4-52 • A, Place one hand or one finger on either side of the aorta as shown here. Press firmly deep in the upper abdomen just to the left of the midline. You may feel aortic pulsations. These pulsations are easier to appreciate in a thin person and more difficult to feel in someone with a thick abdominal wall or large anteroposterior diameter of the abdomen. Obesity and abdominal ascites or distension makes this more difficult. Use the stethoscope (bell) to listen for bruits. Bruits are abnormal blowing or swishing sounds heard on auscultation of the arteries. Bruits with both systolic and diastolic components suggest the turbulent blood flow of partial arterial occlusion. If the renal artery is occluded as well, the client will be hypertensive. **B,** Visualize the location of the aorta slightly to the left of midline and its bifurcation just below the umbilicus. The normal aortic pulse width is between 2.5 and 4.0 cm [some sources say the width must be no more than 3.0 cm; others list 4.0]. The pulse width expands at the aortic bifurcation (again, usually just below the umbilicus). An aneurysm can occur anywhere along the aorta; ninety-five percent (95%) of all abdominal aortic aneurysms occur just below the renal arteries. **(A,** From Boissonnault WG, editor: *Examination in physical therapy practice,* ed 2, New York, 1995, Churchill Livingstone.)

Labels on Fig. B: Ribs; Iliac arteries; Pelvis; Bladder; Sigmoid colon; Aortic bifurcation; Pulsatile aorta; Abdominal muscles

---

(slightly to the left of the midline) to find the aortic pulsations (Fig. 4-52, A).

The therapist can assess the width of the aorta by using both hands (one on each side of the aorta) and pressing deeply. The examiner's fingers along the outer margins of the aorta should remain the same distance apart until the aortic bifurcation. Where the aorta bifurcates (usually near the umbilicus), the width of the pulse should expand (Fig. 4-52, B). Throbbing pain that increases with exertion and is accompanied by a sensation of a heartbeat when lying down and of a palpable pulsating abdominal mass requires immediate medical attention.

SYSTEMS REVIEW . . . OR . . . REVIEW OF SYSTEMS?

When a physician conducts a systems review, the examination is a routine physical assessment of each system, starting with a general assessment of (ENT), followed by chest auscultation for pulmonary and cardiac function, palpation of lymph nodes, and so on.

The therapist does not conduct a systems review such as the medical doctor performs. The *Guide* uses the terminology "Systems Review" to describe a brief or limited exam of the anatomical and physiological status of the cardiovascular/pulmonary, integumentary, musculoskeletal, and neuromuscular systems.

As part of this Systems Review, the client's ability to communicate and process information are identified as well as any learning barriers such as hearing or vision impairment, illiteracy, or English as a second language (see *The Guide,* page 713/s705).

A more appropriate term for what the therapist does in the screening process may be a "Review of Systems." In the screening examination as presented in this text, after conducting an interview and assessment of pain type/pain patterns, the therapist may conduct a review of systems (ROS) first by looking for any characteristics of systemic disease in the history or clinical presentation.

Then the identified cluster(s) of associated signs and symptoms are reviewed to search for a potential pattern that will identify the underlying system involved (Box 4-17). The therapist may find cause to examine just the upper quadrant or just the lower quadrant more closely. A guide to physical assessment in a screening examination is provided (Table 4-13).

Therapists perform a ROS by categorizing all of the complaints and reported or observed associated

BOX 4-17 ▼ Review of Systems*

When conducting a general review of systems, ask the client about the presence of any other problems anywhere else in the body. Depending on the client's answer you may want to prompt him or her about any of the following common signs and symptoms associated with each system:

General Questions

___ Fever, chills, sweating (constitutional symptoms)
___ Appetite loss, nausea, vomiting (constitutional symptoms)
___ Fatigue, malaise, weakness (constitutional symptoms)
___ Excessive, unexplained weight gain or loss
___ Vital signs: blood pressure, temperature, pulse, respirations
___ Insomnia
___ Irritability
___ Hoarseness or change in voice, frequent or prolonged sore throat
___ Dizziness, falls

Integumentary (Include Skin, Hair, and Nails)

___ Recent rashes, nodules, or other skin changes
___ Unusual hair loss or breakage
___ Increased hair growth (hirsutism)
___ Nail bed changes
___ Itching (pruritus)

Musculoskeletal/Neurologic

___ Joint pain, redness, warmth, swelling, stiffness, deformity
___ Frequent or severe headaches
___ Vision or hearing changes
___ Vertigo
___ Paresthesias (numbness, tingling, "pins and needles" sensation)
___ Change in muscle tone
___ Weakness; atrophy
___ Abnormal deep tendon (or other) reflexes
___ Problems with coordination or balance; falling
___ Involuntary movements; tremors
___ Radicular pain
___ Seizures or loss of consciousness
___ Memory loss
___ Paralysis
___ Mood swings; hallucinations

Rheumatologic

___ Presence/location of joint swelling
___ Muscle pain, weakness
___ Skin rashes
___ Reaction to sunlight
___ Raynaud's phenomenon
___ Nail bed changes

Cardiovascular

___ Chest pain or sense of heaviness or discomfort
___ Palpitations
___ Limb pain during activity (claudication; cramps, limping)
___ Discolored or painful feet; swelling of hands and feet
___ Pulsating or throbbing pain anywhere, but especially in the back or abdomen
___ Peripheral edema; nocturia
___ Sudden weight gain; unable to fasten waist band or belt, unable to wear regular shoes
___ Persistent cough
___ Fatigue, dyspnea, orthopnea, syncope
___ High or low blood pressure, unusual pulses
___ Differences in blood pressure from side to side with position change (10 mm Hg or more; increase or decrease/diastolic or systolic; associated symptoms: dizziness, headache, nausea, vomiting, diaphoresis, heart palpitations, increased primary pain or symptoms)
___ Positive findings on auscultation

Pulmonary

___ Cough, hoarseness
___ Sputum, hemoptysis
___ Shortness of breath (dyspnea, orthopnea); altered breathing (e.g., wheezing, pursed-lip breathing)
___ Night sweats; sweats anytime
___ Pleural pain
___ Cyanosis, clubbing
___ Positive findings on auscultation (e.g., friction rub, unexpected breath sounds)

Psychologic

___ Sleep disturbance
___ Stress levels
___ Fatigue, psychomotor agitation
___ Changes in personal habits, appetite
___ Depression, confusion, anxiety
___ Irritability, mood changes

Gastrointestinal

___ Abdominal pain
___ Indigestion; heartburn
___ Difficulty in swallowing
___ Nausea/vomiting; loss of appetite
___ Diarrhea or constipation
___ Change in stools; change in bowel habits
___ Fecal incontinence
___ Rectal bleeding; blood in stool; blood in vomit
___ Skin rash followed by joint pain (Crohn's disease)

* Cluster of three to four or more lasting longer than 1 month.

BOX 4-17 ▲ Review of Systems*—cont'd

Hepatic/Biliary

___ Change in taste/smell
___ Anorexia
___ Feeling of abdominal fullness, ascites
___ Asterixis (muscle tremors)
___ Change in urine color (dark, cola-colored)
___ Light-colored stools
___ Change in stool color (yellow, green)
___ Skin changes (rash, itching, purpura, spider angiomas, palmar erythema)

Hematologic

___ Skin color or nail bed changes
___ Bleeding: nose, gums, easy bruising, melena
___ Hemarthrosis, muscle hemorrhage, hematoma
___ Fatigue, dyspnea, weakness
___ Rapid pulse, palpitations
___ Confusion, irritability
___ Headache

Genitourinary

___ Reduced stream, decreased output
___ Burning or bleeding during urination; change in urine color
___ Urinary incontinence, dribbling
___ Impotence, pain with intercourse
___ Hesitation, urgency
___ Nocturia, frequency
___ Dysuria (painful or difficult urination)
___ Testicular pain or swelling
___ Genital lesions
___ Penile or vaginal discharge
___ Impotence (males) or other sexual difficulty (males or females)
___ Infertility (males or females)
___ Flank pain

Gynecologic

___ Irregular menses, amenorrhea, menopause
___ Pain with menses or intercourse
___ Vaginal discharge, vaginal itching
___ Surgical procedures
___ Pregnancy, birth, miscarriage, and abortion histories
___ Spotting, bleeding-especially for the postmenopausal woman 12 months after last period (without hormone replacement therapy)

Endocrine

___ Hair and nail changes
___ Change in appetite, unexplained weight change
___ Fruity breath odor
___ Temperature intolerance, hot flashes, diaphoresis (unexplained perspiration)
___ Heart palpitations, tachycardia
___ Headaches
___ Low urine output, absence of perspiration
___ Cramps
___ Edema, polyuria, polydipsia, polyphagia
___ Unexplained weakness, fatigue, paresthesia
___ Carpal/tarsal tunnel syndrome
___ Periarthritis, adhesive capsulitis
___ Joint or muscle pain (arthralgia, myalgia), trigger points
___ Prolonged deep tendon reflexes
___ Sleep disturbance

Cancer

___ Constant, intense pain, especially bone pain at night
___ Unexplained weight loss (10% of body weight in 10-14 days); most clients in pain are inactive and gain weight
___ Loss of appetite
___ Excessive fatigue
___ Unusual lump(s), thickening, change in a lump or mole, sore that does not heal; other unusual skin lesions or rash
___ Unusual or prolonged bleeding or discharge anywhere
___ Change in bowel or bladder habits
___ Chronic cough or hoarseness, change in voice
___ Rapid onset of digital clubbing (10 to 14 days)
___ (Proximal) muscle weakness, especially when accompanied by change in one or more deep tendon reflexes

Immunologic

___ Skin or nail bed changes
___ Fever or other constitutional symptoms (especially recurrent or cyclical symptoms)
___ Lymph node changes (tenderness, enlargement)
___ Anaphylactic reaction
___ Symptoms of muscle or joint involvement (pain, swelling, stiffness, weakness)
___ Sleep disturbance

TABLE 4-13 ▼ Guide to Physical Assessment in a Screening Examination

General survey	Upper quadrant exam	Lower quadrant exam
Level of consciousness	Lymph node palpation	Lymph node palpation
Mental and emotional status	Head and neck	Lower limbs
Vision and hearing	Cranial nerves	• Muscle tone and strength
Speech	Upper limbs	• Trigger points
General appearance	• Muscle tone and strength	• Joint range of motion
Nutritional status	• Trigger points	• Reflexes
Level of self-care	• Joint range of motion	• Coordination
Body size and type (BMI)	• Reflexes	• Motor and sensory function
Obvious deformities	• Coordination	• Vascular assessment
Muscle atrophy	• Motor and sensory function	Abdomen
Body and breath odors	• Vascular assessment	• Inspection
Posture	Chest and back (heart and lungs)	• Auscultation
Movement patterns and gait	• Inspection	• Palpation
Use of assistive devices or mobility aids	• Palpation	
Balance and coordination	• Auscultation	
Inspect skin, hair, and nails	Clinical breast examination (CBE)	
Vital signs		

signs and symptoms. This type of review helps bring to the therapist's attention any signs or symptoms the client has not recognized, has forgotten, or thought unimportant. After compiling a list of the client's signs and symptoms, compare those to the list in Box 4-17. Are there any identifying clusters to direct the decision-making process? (Case Example 4-4)

For example, cutaneous (skin) manifestations and joint pain may occur secondary to systemic diseases such as Crohn's disease (regional enteritis), psoriatic arthritis, or as a delayed reaction to medications. Likewise, hair and nail changes, temperature intolerance, and unexplained excessive fatigue are cluster signs and symptoms associated with the endocrine system.

Changes in urinary frequency, flow of urine, or color of urine point to urologic involvement. Other groupings of signs and symptoms associated with each system are listed as mentioned in Box 4-17. If, for example, the client's signs and symptoms fall primarily within the genitourinary group, then turn to Chapter 10 for additional, pertinent screening questions listed at the end of the chapter. The client's answers to these questions will guide the therapist in making a final decision regarding physician referral (See the Case Study at the end of the chapter).

The therapist is not responsible for identifying the specific pathologic disease underlying the clinical signs and symptoms present. However, the alert therapist who recognizes clusters of signs and symptoms of a systemic nature will be more likely

to identify a problem outside the scope of physical therapy practice and make the appropriate referral. Early identification and intervention for many medical conditions can result in improved outcomes, including decreased morbidity and mortality.

▶ **PHYSICIAN REFERRAL**

All skin and nail bed lesions must be examined and evaluated carefully because any tissue irregularity may be a clue to malignancy. It is better to err on the side of being too quick to refer for medical evaluation than to delay and risk progression of underlying disease.

Medical evaluation is advised when the therapist is able to palpate a distended liver, gallbladder, or spleen. This is especially true in the presence of any cluster of signs and symptoms observed during the Review of Systems that are characteristic of that particular organ system.

Headaches that cannot be linked to a musculoskeletal cause (e.g., dysfunction of the cervical spine, thoracic spine, or temporomandibular joints; muscle tension, poor posture) may need further medical referral and evaluation. Conducting an upper quadrant physical screening assessment, including a neurologic screening may help in making this decision.

Vital Signs

Vital sign assessment is a very important and valuable screening tool. If the therapist does not

CASE EXAMPLE 4-4   Steps in the Screening Process

A 47-year-old man with low back pain of unknown cause has come to you for exercises. After gathering information from the client's history and conducting the interview, you ask him:

- Are there any other symptoms of any kind anywhere else in your body?

The client tells you he does break out into an unexpected sweat from time to time, but does not think he has a temperature when this happens. He has increased back pain when he passes gas or has a bowel movement, but then the pain goes back to the "regular" pain level (reported as 5 on a scale from 0 to 10).

Other reported symptoms include

- Heartburn and indigestion
- Abdominal bloating after meals
- Chronic bronchitis from smoking (3 packs/day)
- Alternating diarrhea and constipation

Do these symptoms fall into any one category? See Box 4-17.

What is the next step?

It appears that many of the symptoms are gastrointestinal in nature. Since the client has mentioned unexplained sweating, but no known fevers, take the time to measure all vital signs, especially body temperature.

Turn to the Special Questions to Ask at the end of Chapter 8 and scan the list of questions for any that might be appropriate with this client.

For example, find out about the use of nonsteroidal antiinflammatories (prescription and over-the-counter; be sure to include aspirin).

Follow up with

- Have you ever been treated for an ulcer or internal bleeding while taking any of these pain relievers?
- Have you experienced any unexpected weight loss in the last few weeks?
- Have you traveled outside the United States in the last year?
- What is the effect of eating or drinking on your abdominal pain? Back pain?
- Have the client pay attention to his symptoms over the next 24 to 48 hours:
  Immediately after eating
  Within 30 minutes of eating
  One to two hours later
- Do you have a sense of urgency so that you have to find a bathroom for a bowel movement or diarrhea right away without waiting?

Your decision to refer this client to a physician depends on your findings from the clinical examination and the client's responses to these questions. This does not appear to be an emergency since the client is not in acute distress. An elevated temperature or other unusual vital signs might speed along the referral process. Documentation of the screening process is important and the physician notified appropriately (by phone, fax, and/or report).

conduct any other screening physical assessment, vital signs should be assessed for a baseline value and then monitored. The following findings should always be documented and reported.

- Any of the yellow warning signs presented in Box 4-6.
- Individuals who report consistent ambulatory hypertension using out-of-office or at-home readings, adults who do not show a drop in BP at night (15 mm Hg lower than daytime measures), and older adults with diagnosed hypertension who have an excessive surge in morning BP measurements.
- African Americans with elevated blood pressure should be evaluated by a medical doctor.
- Pulse amplitude that fades with inspiration and strengthens with expiration

- Pulse increase over 20 BPM lasting more than 3 minutes after rest or changing position.
- Persistent low-grade (or higher) fever, especially associated with constitutional symptoms, most commonly sweats but also unintended weight loss, malaise, nausea, vomiting.
- Any unexplained fever without other systemic symptoms, especially in the person taking corticosteroids or otherwise immunosuppressed.
- Weak and rapid pulse accompanied by fall in blood pressure (pneumothorax).
- Clients who are neurologically unstable as a result of a recent CVA, head trauma, spinal cord injury, or other central nervous system insult

- Irregular pulse and/or irregular pulse combined with symptoms of dizziness or shortness of breath; tachycardia or bradycardia.

often exhibit new arrhythmias during the period of instability; when the client's pulse is monitored, any new arrhythmias noted should be reported to the nursing staff or physician.

- Always take BP in any client with neck pain, upper quadrant symptoms, or thoracic outlet syndrome (TOS).

Precautions/Contraindications to Therapy

The following parameters are listed as precautions/contraindications rather than one or the other because these signs and symptoms may have different significance depending on the client's overall health, age, medications taken, and other factors. What may be a precaution for one client may be a clear contraindication for another and vice versa.

- Resting heart rate 120 to 130 BPM*
- Resting systolic pressure 180 to 200 mm Hg*
- Resting diastolic pressure 105 to 110 mm Hg*
- Marked dyspnea
- Loss of palpable pulse or irregular pulse with symptoms of dizziness, nausea, or shortness of breath

Anemic individuals may demonstrate an increased normal resting pulse rate that should be monitored during exercise. Anyone with unstable blood pressure may require initial standing with a tilt table or monitoring of the blood pressure before, during, and after treatment. Check the nursing record for pulse rate at rest and blood pressure to use as a guide when taking vital signs in the clinic or at the patient's bedside.

Guidelines for Immediate Physician Referral

- Anyone with diabetes mellitus, who is immunocompromised, or who has a history of steroid and retroviral use now presenting with red, inflamed, swollen nail bed(s) or any skin lesion involving the feet must be referred for medical evaluation immediately.

- Any suspicious breast changes (e.g., unexplained nipple discharge, erythema, contour changes) must be reported to the physician immediately. Nipple discharge can occur during and after normal lactation or the use of oral contraceptives. Bloody discharge can occur during the last trimester of pregnancy or first 3 months of lactation.[93] The physician must decide when this finding is considered "normal" physiologically. Unilateral discharge is highly suspicious. Some medications can also produce nipple discharge (e.g., digitalis, tricyclic antidepressants, benzodiazepines, antipsychotics, isoniazid) as well as some drugs (e.g., marijuana, heroin).[103]
- Detection of palpable, fixed, irregular mass in the breast, axilla, or elsewhere requires medical referral or a recommendation to the client to contact a physician for evaluation of the mass. Suspicious lymph node enlargement or lymph node changes; generalized lymphadenopathy.[89]
- Unusual or suspicious findings during inspection, palpation, or auscultation of the chest or abdomen including positive Murphy's percussion test, Murphy's sign, the presence of rebound tenderness, or palpable distention of the spleen, liver, or gallbladder.
- Recurrent cancer can appear as a single lump, a pale or red nodule just below the skin surface, a swelling, a dimpling of the skin, or a red rash. Report any of these changes to a physician immediately.
- Immediate medical referral is advised for any client reporting new-onset of SOB who is tachypneic, diaphoretic, or cyanotic; any suspicion of anaphylaxis is also an emergency situation.
- Abrupt change in mental status, confusion or increasing confusion, and new onset of delirium requires medical attention.
- Outbreak of vesicular rash associated with herpes zoster. Medical referral within 72 hours of the initial appearance of skin lesions is needed; client will begin a course of antiretroviral medication to manage symptoms and help prevent postherpetic neuropathy.

---

* Unexplained or poorly tolerated by client.

⟳ KEY POINTS TO REMEMBER

✓ A head-to-toe complete physical assessment is an advanced clinical skill and a challenge even to the most skilled physician, physician assistant, or nurse practitioner. The therapist conducts a screening assessment using appropriate portions of the physical assessment.

✓ The therapist carries out certain portions of the physical assessment with every client by observing general health and nutrition, mental status, mood or affect, skin and body contours, mobility, and function.

✓ The therapist conducts a formal screening examination using the subjective and objective portions of the evaluation whenever the client history, age, gender, or other risk factors, or clinical presentation raise yellow or red warning flags.

✓ Measuring vital signs is a key component of the screening assessment. Vital signs, observations, and reported associated signs and symptoms are among the best screening tools available to the therapist. These same parameters can be used to plan and progress safe and effective exercise programs for clients who have true neuromuscular or musculoskeletal problems, but who also have other health concerns or comorbidities.

✓ Documentation of physical findings is important. From a legal point of view, if it is not documented, it was not assessed. Record important normal and abnormal findings.

✓ The therapist must be able to recognize normal and abnormal results when conducting inspection, palpation, percussion, and auscultation of the chest, thorax, and abdomen. The order of these tests is important and differs from chest and thorax to abdomen.

✓ Auscultation usually follows inspection and palpation of the chest and thorax. Examination of the abdomen should be performed in this order: inspection, auscultation, and then palpation, because palpation can affect findings on auscultation.

✓ The therapist should try to follow the same pattern every time to decrease the chances of missing an assessment parameter and to increase accuracy and thoroughness.

✓ Skin and nail bed assessment should be a part of every patient/client assessment.

✓ Changes in the skin and nail beds may be the first sign of inflammatory, infectious, and immunologic disorders and can occur with involvement of a variety of organs.

✓ Consider all integumentary and nail bed findings in relation to the client's age, ethnicity, occupation, and general health. When analyzing any signs and symptoms present, assess if this is a problem with the integumentary system versus an integumentary response to a systemic problem.

✓ The therapist may encounter enlarged or palpable lymph nodes. Keep in mind the therapist cannot know what the underlying pathology may be when lymph nodes are palpable and questionable. Performing a baseline assessment and reporting the findings is the important outcome of the assessment.

✓ With direct and unrestricted access of consumers to physical therapists in many states and the role of physical therapists in primary care, advanced skills have become necessary. For some clients, clinical breast exam (CBE) is an appropriate assessment tool in the screening process.

✓ Properly trained, physical therapists should be considered "qualified," health care specialists" as defined by the ACS in the provision of cancer screening when the history, clinical presentation, and associated signs and symptoms point to the need for CBE.

✓ When a suspicious mass is found during examination, it must be medically evaluated, even if the client reports a recent mammography was "normal."

✓ For therapists without adequate training in conducting a CBE, the screening process is confined to asking questions during the interview regarding past medical history (e.g., cancer, lactation, abscess, mastitis) and questions to identify the possibility of breast pathology as the underlying cause for back or shoulder pain and/or other symptoms.

✓ Medical referral is advised for any individual suspected of having DVT; medical consultation is advised for those with a low probability.

SUBJECTIVE EXAMINATION

Special Questions To Ask

Breath and Body Odors

[Introductory remarks]: Mrs. Smith, as part of a physical therapy exam we always look at our client's overall health and general physical condition. Do you have any other health concerns besides your shoulder/back (name the involved body part)?

Are you being treated by anyone for any other problems? [Wait for a response but add prompts as needed: chiropractor? acupuncturist? naturopath?]

[If you suspect urinary incontinence]: Are you having any trouble with leaking urine or making it to the bathroom on time?

(Ask appropriate follow-up questions about cause, frequency, severity, triggers, and so on; see Appendix B-5).

[If you suspect fecal incontinence]: Do you have trouble getting to the toilet on time for a bowel movement? Do you have trouble wiping yourself clean after a bowel movement?

(Ask appropriate follow-up questions about cause, frequency, severity, triggers, and so on).

[If you detect breath odor]: I notice an unusual smell on your breath. Do you know what might be causing this? (Ask appropriate follow-up questions depending on the type of smell you perceive; you may have to conduct an alcohol screening survey—see Chapter 2 or Appendices B-1 and B-2.

Skin

- Does the skin itch?
- Yellow skin (jaundice). Look for associated risk factors for hepatitis (see Box 9-2).
- Have you recently had a serious blood loss (possibly requiring transfusion)? (**Anemia;** also consider **jaundice/hepatitis posttransfusion**)
- Soft tissue lumps or skin lesions:
  How long have you had this?
  Has it changed in the last 6 weeks to 6 months?
  Has your doctor seen it?
  Does it itch, hurt, feel sore, or burn?
- Does anyone else in your household have anything like this?
- Have you taken any new medications (prescribed or over-the-counter) in the last 6 weeks?
- Have you traveled somewhere new in the last month?
- Have you been exposed to anything in the last month that could cause this?
  (Consider exposure due to occupational, environmental, and hobby interests.)

Do you have any other skin changes anywhere else on your body?

- Have you had a fever or sweats in the last 2 weeks? Are you having any trouble breathing or swallowing?
- Have you had any other symptoms of any kind anywhere else in your body?
- Surgical scars: Would you have any objections if I looked at (or examined) the scar tissue?

Lymph Nodes

Use the lymph node assessment form (see Fig. 4-45) to record and report baseline findings.

- [General screening question:] Have you examined yourself for any lumps or nodules and found any thickening or lump? *If yes*, has your physician examined/treated this?
- Do you have (now or recently) any sores, rashes, or lesions anywhere on your body? If any suspicious or aberrant lymph nodes are observed during palpation, ask the following question.

Have you (ever) had

- Cancer of any kind?
  If no, have you ever been treated with radiation or chemotherapy for any reason?
- Breast implants
- Mastectomy or prostatectomy
- Mononucleosis
- Chronic fatigue syndrome
- Allergic rhinitis
- Food intolerances, food allergies, or celiac sprue
- Recent dental work
- Infection of any kind
- Recent cut, insect bite, or infection in the hand or arm
- A sexually transmitted disease of any kind
- Sores or lesions of any kind anywhere on the body (including genitals)
  Breast: See Chapter 17 and Appendix B-7
  Headache: See Appendix B-15

Neurologic

- Have you ever been in a car accident?
  If yes, did you lose consciousness, have a concussion, or a fractured skull?
- Have you ever been knocked out, unconscious, or have a concussion at any time?
- Have you ever had a seizure?
- Have you ever been paralyzed in your arms or legs?
- Have you ever broken your neck or back?

CASE STUDY 4-1

REVIEW OF SYSTEMS

A 48-year-old male was seen at the hospital emergency department following a multiple car motor vehicle accident (MVA). X-rays were negative and the patient was diagnosed with an uncomplicated sprain/strain of the left hip. He was referred to the rehab clinic associated with the hospital for therapy within one week of the MVA.

Carry out a review of systems and group the following findings in appropriate clusters. Look for any patterns suggesting the need for further screening and/or impairment or dysfunction in any one particular organ system.

- Unable to palpate lymph nodes; obesity may have prevented an accurate assessment
- Symptoms worse after one month of soft tissue therapy
- Unable to ambulate more than five feet without assistance due to severe pain (self-rated as 8.5/10)
- Lumbar range of motion and left hip ROM limited due to pain
- Client reports night pain from time to time that wakes him up at night; sometimes he can get back to sleep easily; at other times, not so well
- Valsalva's maneuver: negative
- Initial complaint of low back and left hip pain described as "burning"
- Client was sweating profusely throughout initial exam; described intermittent "sweats" over the course of month long therapy
- Initial complaint of pain radiates down the left leg into the left foot occasionally; never present during sessions with the therapist
- Patellar deep tendon reflexes 2/3 (right:average/left:slightly brisk)
- Achilles deep tendon reflexes 0 (absent) due to edema
- 8 cm mass on client's left buttock developed one month after MVA; firm and cool to the touch; no bruising or skin color changes; gluteal musculature atrophied around the mass
- Alert but agitated from time to time
- Blood pressure 120/80 bilateral upper extremities
- Heart rate 72 beats per minute, steady
- Height: 6'3" Weight: 300 pounds
- No saddle anesthesia reported; no bowel or bladder dysfunction reported; no sexual dysfunction reported
- Any movement of the left hip increases low back and left hip pain

- Bilateral straight leg raise to 80 degrees without reproducing symptoms
- Signs of venous stasis in the feet and lower legs; client reports these have been present since before the accident
- Marked pitting edema of both ankles
- Gross Manual Muscle Test (MMT):
  Right hip flexion 5/5
  Left hip flexion 2/5
  Ankle (right or left) 5/5
- Lower extremity sensation: within normal limits (WNL)
- Lab Values from Emergency Department intake exam:
  Hemoglobin   116 g/dl (mildly decreased)
  Serum lactate dehydrogenase levels   (Normal)

There is no "right" or "wrong" way to approach this; just different methods. Using the client history, clinical presentation, and associated signs and symptoms presented throughout this text, we suggest:

HISTORY
- Significant history of trauma

CLINICAL PRESENTATION
- Pain pattern: Progressive, unremitting, radiating pain; night pain; pain described as "burning"; aggravated by any movement of the left hip
- Left hip flexor weakness
- Alert, but agitated
- Mass on left buttock with gluteal muscle atrophy at that site
- Signs of chronic venous stasis in lower extremities; bilateral pitting edema

ASSOCIATED SIGNS AND SYMPTOMS
- Constitutional symptoms: unexplained perspiration

REVIEW OF SYSTEMS
- The most significant cluster of findings seems to be neurologic: "burning" pain that radiates, muscle weakness, agitation, and progressive presentation of pain pattern. The new onset of a soft tissue mass is of great concern.
- There is no mention in the client's chart of changes (worsening/improving) of muscle strength over the course of treatment.
- Chronic pitting edema with signs of venous stasis suggests a peripheral vascular disorder.

CASE STUDY 4-1—cont'd

ADDITIONAL CLUES

- Client is not better after physical therapy intervention; in fact, client is worse.

There are enough red flags here to suggest further screening is needed if not immediate referral.

Age (over 40)

Left buttock mass with muscle atrophy

Chronic venous stasis present before the accident

Screening may be nothing more than asking some of the same questions as presented in the intake interview as well as conducting some of the same tests again. For example:

Past Medical History:

Previous health history (especially including previous/current history of cancer, vascular or cardiac disease)

Review information collected using the Documentation Template for Physical Therapist Client Management, *Guide*, Appendix. Ask yourself:

Have I left anything out that is important?

Any history of drug or alcohol use/abuse?

Recent history of medications, over-the-counter drugs, nutraceuticals?

Recent history of infections?

Previous history of any surgeries? Remember back and/or hip pain can occur even years later after orthopedic surgery, for example from infection, implant loosening, fracture, hemorrhage or other complication.

CLINICAL PRESENTATION:

Any signs of liver impairment (liver flap, nail bed changes, symptoms of carpal tunnel syndrome, angiomas, palmar erythema)?

Changes in muscle strength or deep tendon reflexes?

Left hip pain: conduct tests for psoas abscess (iliopsoas and obturator tests) or other infectious/inflammatory processes such as appendicitis (McBurney's Point), peritonitis (Blumberg rebound test).

ASSOCIATED SIGNS AND SYMPTOMS:

Effect of food on symptoms (especially pain at night)

Any significant weight loss?

Take the client's temperature

Changes in vital signs

From Busse JW: Delayed Diagnosis of Non-Hodgkin's Lymphoma: A Case Report. *Journal of the Neuromusculoskeletal System* 9(2):60-64, Summer 2001.

PRACTICE QUESTIONS

1. When assessing the abdomen, what sequence of physical assessment is best?
   a. Auscultation, inspection, palpation, percussion
   b. Inspection, percussion, auscultation, palpation
   c. Inspection, auscultation, percussion, palpation
   d. Auscultation, inspection, percussion, palpation

2. A line drawn down the middle of a lesion with two different halves suggest:
   a. A malignant lesion
   b. A benign lesion
   c. A normal presentation
   d. A skin reaction to medications

3. Pulse strength graded as 1+ means:
   a. Easily palpable, normal
   b. Present occasionally
   c. Pulse diminished, barely palpable
   d. Within normal limits

4. During auscultation of an adult client with rheumatoid arthritis, the heart rate gets stronger as she breathes in and decreases as she breathes out. This sign is:
   a. Characteristic of lung disease
   b. Typical in coronary artery disease
   c. A normal finding
   d. Common in anyone with pain

5. How do you plan or modify an exercise program for a client with cancer without the benefit of blood values?

6. Body temperature should be taken as part of vital sign assessment:
   a. Only for clients who have not been seen by a physician
   b. For any client who has musculoskeletal pain of unknown origin
   c. For any client reporting the presence of constitutional symptoms, especially fever or night sweats
   d. (b) and (c)
   e. All of the above

7. When would you consider listening for femoral bruits?

8. A 23-year old female presents with new onset of skin rash and joint pain followed two weeks later by GI symptoms of abdominal pain, nausea, and diarrhea. She has a previous history of Crohn's disease, but this condition has been stable for several years. She does not think her current symptoms are related to her Crohn's disease. What kind of screening assessment is needed in this case?
   a. Vital signs only
   b. Vital signs and abdominal auscultation
   c. Vital signs, neurologic screening examination, and abdominal auscultation
   d. No further assessment is needed; there are enough red flags to advise this client to seek medical attention.

9. A 76-year old man was referred to physical therapy after a total hip replacement (THR). The goal is to increase his functional mobility. Is a health assessment needed since he was examined just before the surgery two weeks ago? The physician conducted a systems review and summarized the medical record by saying the client was in excellent health and a good candidate for THR.

10. You notice a new client has an unusual (strong) breath odor. How do you assess this?

11. Why does postural orthostatic hypotension occur upon standing for the first time in a young adult who has been supine in skeletal traction for 3 weeks?

REFERENCES

1. Danielson K, Solheim K: *Essential physical assessment skills*, Eau Claire, Wisconsin, PESI HealthCare, 2003.
2. Holden U: Dementia in acute units: confusion, *Nurs Stand* 9(17):37-39, 1995.
3. Sarter M, Mahoney J, Craft T, et al: Microsphere embolism-induced cortical cholinergic deafferentation and impairments in attentional performance, *Eur J Neuroscience* 21(11):3117-3132, June 2005.
4. Jennett B, Bond M: Assessment of outcome after severe brain damage, *Lancet* 1(7905):480-484, 1975.
5. Rowlett R: *Glasgow coma scale*, University of Carolina at Chapel Hill. Available at: www.unc.edu/~rowlett/units/scales/glasgow.htm. Accessed November 14, 2004.
6. The Internet Stroke Center: Stroke scales and clinical assessment tools. Available at: http://www.strokecenter.org/trials/scales/index.htm. Accessed November 14, 2004.
7. National Institutes of Health: *Calculate your body mass index*. Available at: http://nhlbisupport.com/bmi/bmicalc.htm. Accessed November 11, 2004.
8. Dr. Steven B. Hall's Body Mass Index seeker. Available at: http://www.halls.md/body-mass-index/bmi.htm. Accessed November 11, 2004.
9. National Center for Chronic Disease Prevention and Health Promotion: *Body mass index for children and teens*. Available at: http://www.cdc.gov/nccdphp/dnpa/bmi/bmi-for-age.htm. Accessed November 11, 2004.

10. Frese EM, Richter RR, Burlis TV: Self-reported measurement of heart rate and blood pressure in patients by physical therapy clinical instructors, *Physical Therapy* 82(12):1192-1200, 2002.

11. Billek-Sawhney B, Sawhney R: Cardiovascular considerations in outpatient physical therapy, *J Orthop Sports Phys Ther* 27:57, 1998.

12. Guide to the Physical Therapist Practice, ed 2 (revised). *Physical Therapy* 81(1):2003, Alexandria Virginia. American Physical Therapy Association.

13. American College of Sports Medicine (ACSM): *Resource manual for guidelines for exercise testing and prescription*, ed 3, Philadelphia, 1998, Lippincott, Williams, and Wilkins.

14. Bates B, Bickley LS, Hoekelman RA: *A guide to physical examination and history taking*, ed 8, Philadelphia, 2002, J.B. Lippincott.

15. Phoenix Publishing Product No. 4009-01: Thermister. Available at: http://www.phoenixpub.com/store/ [no financial or other benefit is derived by the authors of this textbook from posting this weblink].

16. Pullen RL: Using an ear thermometer, *Nursing2003* 33(5):24, 2003.

17. Hardwick KD: Insightful options, *Rehab Magazine* 15(7):30-33, 2002.

18. Ostchega Y, Prineas RJ, Paulose-Ram R, et al: National health and nutrition examination survey 1999-2000: effect of observer training and protocol standardization on reducing blood pressure measurement error, *J Clin Epidemiol* 56:768-774, 2003.

19. Personal communication with oncology staff (nurses and physical therapists) across the United States, 2005.

20. Pfalzer C: Personal communication, 2005.

21. Levin DK: Measuring blood pressure in legs, *Medscape Internal Medicine* 6(1), 2004. Retrieved June 10, 2006 from http://www.medscape.com/viewarticle/471829

22. The Seventh Report of the Joint National Committee on Prevention, Detection, Evaluation, and Treatment of High Blood Pressure (JNC-7), NIH Publication No. 03-5233, May 2003. National Heart, Lung, and Blood Institute (NHLBI).

23. *Expert 10-Minute Physical Examinations*, St. Louis, 1997, Mosby.

24. Hemingway TJ, Guss DA, Abdelnur D: Arm position and blood pressure measurement, *Ann Intern Med* 140(1):74-75, 2004.

25. Franklin SS: Pulse pressure as a risk factor, *Clin Exp Hypertens* 26(7-8):645-652, 2004.

26. American College of Sports Medicine: *ACSM guidelines for exercise testing and prescription*, ed 6, Philadelphia, 2000, Lippincott, Williams, and Wilkins.

27. Hussain SF: Progestogen-only pills and high blood pressure: is there an association? A literature review, *Contraception* 69(2):89-97, 2004.

28. Burkman R, Schlesselman JJ, Zieman M: Safety concerns and health benefits associated with oral contraception, *Am J Obstet Gynecol* 190(4 Suppl):S5-S22, 2004.

29. Hillegass EA, Sadowsky HS: *Essentials of cardiopulmonary physical therapy*, ed 2, Philadelphia, 2001, W.B. Saunders.

30. American Heart Association: *Postural orthostatic hypotension*. Available at: http://www.phoenixpub.com/store/ [no financial or other benefit is derived by the authors of this textbook from posting this weblink].

31. American Heart Association Updates Recommendations for Blood Pressure Measurements, Available at: http://www.americanheart.org. Accessed March 2, 2005.

32. Kario K: Morning surge and variability in blood pressure. A new therapeutic target? *Hypertension* 45(4):485-486, Feb. 21, 2005

33. Saunders E: Managing hypertension in African-American patients, *J Clin Hypertens (Greenwich)* 6(4 Suppl 1):19-25, 2004.

34. International Society on Hypertension in Blacks (ISHIB). Available at: http://www.ishib.org/. Accessed November 02, 2004.

35. Douglas JG, Bakris GL, Epstein M, et al: Management of high blood pressure in African Americans: consensus statement of the Hypertension in African Americans Working Group of the International Society on Hypertension in Blacks, *Arch Intern Med* 163(5):521-522, 2003.

36. National Heart, Lung, and Blood Institute (NHLBI): Fourth report on the diagnosis, evaluation, and treatment of high blood pressure in children and adolescents, *Pediatrics* 114(2):555-576, 2004.

37. Rocchini AP: Coarctation of the aorta and interrupted aortic arch, In Moller JH, Hoffmann U, editors: *Pediatric cardiovascular medicine*, New York, NY, 2000, Churchill Livingstone; p. 570.

38. Mourad A, Carney S, Gillies A, et al: Arm position and blood pressure: a risk factor for hypertension? *J Hum Hypertens* 17:389-395, 2003.

39. Netea RT, Lenders JW, Smits P, et al: Both body and arm position significantly influence blood pressure measurement, *J Hum Hypertens* 17:459-462, 2003.

40. Kario K, Tobin JN, Wolfson LI, et al: Lower standing systolic blood pressure as a predictor of falls in the elderly: a community-based prospective study, *J Am Coll Cardiol* 38(1):246-252, 2001.

41. Qui C, von Strauss E, Winblad B, et al: Decline in blood pressure over time and risk of dementia: a longitudinal study from the Kungsholmen project, *Stroke* 35(8):1810-1815. Epub July 01, 2004.

42. Verghese J, Lipton RB, Hall CB, et al: Low blood pressure and the risk of dementia in very old individuals, *Neurology* 61(12):1667-1672, 2003.

43. Pullen RL: Caring for a patient on pulse oximetry, *Nursing2003* 33(9):30, 2003.

44. Rupp JF, Kaplan DL: Pruritus—causes—cures, part 1, *Consultant* 39(11):3157-3160, 1999.

45. Webster GF: Common skin disorders in the elderly, *Clinical Cornerstone* 4(1):39-44, 2001.

46. Candelli M, Carloni E, Nista EC, et al: *Helicobacter pylori* eradication and acne rosacea resolution: cause—effect or coincidence? *Dig Liver Dis* 36(2):163, 2004.

47. Diaz C, O'Callaghan CJ, Khan A, et al: Rosacea: a cutaneous marker of Helicobacter pylori infection? Results of a pilot study, *Acta Derm Venereol* 83(4):282-286, 2003.

48. Rebora A: The management of rosacea, *Am J Clin Dermatol* 3(7):489-496, 2002.

49. Yazici Y, Erkan D, Scott R, et al: The skin: a map to rheumatic diseases, *J Musculoskel Med* 18(1):43-53, 2001.

50. Lyme Disease Foundation: Community Education. Available at: http://www.lyme.org/communityed.html [click on brochure or picture gallery or www.lyme.org/gallery/rashes.html]. Accessed January 5, 2005.

51. Guillot B, Bessis D, Dereure O: Mucocutaneous side effects of antineoplastic chemotherapy, *Expert Opin Drug Saf* 3(6):579-587, 2004.

52. Borroni G, Vassallo C, Brazzelli V, et al: Radiation recall dermatitis, panniculitis, and myositis following cyclophosphamide therapy: histopathologic findings of a patient affected by multiple myeloma, *Am J Dermatopathol* 26(3):213-216, June 2004.

53. Friedlander PA, Bansal R, Schwartz L, et al: Gemcitabine-related radiation recall preferentially involves internal tissues and organs, *Cancer* 100(9):1793-1799, May 1, 2004.

54. Centers for Disease Control and Prevention: Tracking the hidden epidemics 2000: trends in STDs in the United States, 2000. Available at: http://www.cdc.gov/nchstp/od/news/RevBrochure1pdftoc.htm. Accessed October 30, 2004.

55. Centers for Disease Control and Prevention: Sexually transmitted Disease Surveillance, 2000. Atlanta, Georgia: U.S. Department of Health and Human Services, 2001.

56. Goodman CC, Boissonnault WG, Fuller K: *Pathology: implications for the physical therapist*, ed 2, 2003.

57. Primary and secondary syphilis—United States, 2002, *MMWR* 52(46):1117-1120, 2003. Available at: http://www.cdc.gov/mmwr/

58. Heffelfinger J: *Syphilis trends in the U.S*, Presented at the 2004 National STD Convention, Philadelphia, PA, March 8-11, 2004.

59. American Social Health Association: The truth about HSV-1 and HSV-2. Available at: http://www.herpes.com/hsv1-2.html Accessed on November 5, 2004.

60. Walker BW: Getting the lowdown on herpetic whitlow, *Nursing2004* 34(7):17, 2004.

61. Omori M: Herpetic whitlow, *eMedicine* 2004.

62. Mudd SS, Findlay JS: The cutaneous manifestations and common mimickers of physical child abuse, *J Pediatr Health Care* 18(3):123-129, 2004.

63. Stanley WJ: Nailing a key assessment. Learn the significance of certain nail anomalies, *Nursing2003* 33(8):50-51, August 2003.

64. Callen J, Jorizzo J, Bologna J, et al: *Dermatological signs of internal disease*, ed 3, Philadelphia, 2003, W.B. Saunders.

65. Epstein E: *Common skin disorders*, ed 5, Philadelphia, 2001, W.B. Saunders.

66. Hordinsky MK, Sawaya ME, Scher RK, et al: *Atlas of hair and nails*, Philadelphia, 2000, Churchill Livingstone.

67. Mir MA: *Atlas of clinical diagnosis*, ed 2, Philadelphia, 2003, W.B. Saunders.

68. Arndt KA, Wintroub BU, Robinson JK, et al: *Primary care dermatology*, Philadelphia, 1997, W.B. Saunders.

69. Rabar D, Combemale P, Peyron P: Doxycycline-induced photo-onycholysis, *J Travel Med* 116):386-387, 2004.

70. Maino Kimberly, Stashower ME: Traumatic transverse leukonychia, *SKINmed* 3(1):53-55, 2004. Accessed on-line: http://www.medscape.com/viewarticle/467074 (posted 01/20/2004).

71. Sweeney E, Fryer A, Mountford R, et al: Nail patella syndrome: a review of the phenotype aided by developmental biology, *J Med Genet* 40:153-162, 2003.

72. Hicks DL, Judkins AR, Sickel JZ, et al: Granular histiocytosis of pelvic lymph nodes following total hip arthroplasty, *J Bone Joint Surg* 78A:482-496, 1996.

73. Hosford D: On-Line University: *The Hosford's differential diagnosis tables*, Available at: http://www.ptcentral.com/university/diagnose_pdf/html. Accessed December 28, 2005.

74. Smith NL: *The effects of depression and anxiety on medical illness*, University of Utah, Stress Medicine Clinic, 2002.

75. Sheehan P: Diabetes and PAD: consensus statement urges screening, *Medscape Cardiology* 8(1), 2004. Available at: http://www.medscape.com/viewarticle/467520. Accessed December 31, 2004.

76. Mohler ER: Peripheral arterial disease, *Archives of Internal Medicine* 163(19):2306-2314, 2003.

77. Merli GJ, Weitz HH, Carabasi A: *Peripheral vascular disorders*, Philadelphia, 2004, Elsevier Science.

78. Tepper S, McKeough M: Deep venous thrombosis: risks, diagnosis, treatment interventions, and prevention, *Acute Care Perspectives* 9(1):1-7, 2000.

79. Autar R: Nursing assessment of clients at risk of deep vein thrombosis (DVT): the Autar DVT scale, *J Adv Nurs* 23(4):763-770, 1996.

80. Autar R: Calculating patients' risk of deep vein thrombosis, *Br J Nurs* 7(1):7-12, 1998.

81. Wells PS, Hirsch J, Anderson DR, et al: Accuracy of clinical assessment of deep-vein thrombosis, *Lancet* 345:1326-1330, 1995.

82. Wells PS, Anderson DR, Bormanis J, et al: Value of assessment of pretest probability of deep-vein thrombosis in clinical management, *Lancet* 350:1795-1798, 1997.

83. Wells PS, Hirsch J, Anderson DR, et al: A simple clinical model for the diagnosis of deep vein thrombosis combined with impedance plethysmography: potential for an improvement in the diagnostic process, *J Intern Med* 243:15-23, 1998.

84. Riddle DL, Wells PS: Diagnosis of lower-extremity deep vein thrombosis in outpatients, *Physical Therapy* 84(8):729-735, 2004.

85. Riddle DL, Hillner BE, Wells PS, et al: Diagnosis of lower-extremity deep vein thrombosis in outpatients with musculoskeletal disorders: a national survey study of physical therapists, *Physical Therapy* 84(8):717-728, 2004.

86. Shaikh N, LaTrenta G, Swistel A, et al: Detection of recurrent breast cancer after TRAM flap reconstruction, *Annals of Plastic Surgery* 47(6):602-607, 2001.

87. Devon RK, Rosen MA, Mies C, et al: Breast reconstruction with a transverse rectus abdominis myocutaneous flap: spectrum of normal abnormal MR imaging findings, *Radiographics* 24(5):1287-1299.

88. Mustonen P, Lepisto J, Papp A, et al: The surgical and oncological safety of immediate breast reconstruction, *Eur J Surg Oncol* 30(8):817-823, 2004.

89. Goodman CC, McGarvey CL: The role of the physical therapist in primary care and cancer screening: integrating clinical breast examination (CBE) in the upper quarter examination, *Rehabilitation Oncology* 21(2):4-11, 2003.

90. American Cancer Society (ACS): *Cancer reference information*. Available at: http://www.cancer.org/docroot/CRI/content/CRI_2_4_3X_Can_breast_cancer_be_found_early_5.asp? Accessed December 13, 2004.

91. Smith RA, Saslow D, Sawyer KA, et al: American cancer society guidelines for breast cancer screening: update 2003, *Cancer J Clin* 53(3):141-169, 2003.

92. Bancej C, Decker K, Chiarelli A, et al: Contribution of clinical breast examination to mammography screening in the early detection of breast cancer, *J Med Screen* 10:16-21, 2003.

93. Saslow D, Hannan J, Osuch J, et al: Clinical breast examination: practical recommendations for optimizing performance and reporting, *Cancer J Clin* 54:327-344, 2004.

94. White E, Miglioretti DL, Yankaskas BC, et al: Biennial versus annual mammography and the risk of late-stage breast cancer, *J Natl Cancer Inst* 96(24):1832-1839, December 2004.

95. Barclay L, Lie D: Biennial screening as good as annual mammography for women older than 49 years, *Medscape medical news*. Available at www.medscape.com/viewarticle/496129. Accessed December 23, 2004.

96. Park BW, Kim SI, Kim MH, et al: Clinical breast examination for screening of asymptomatic women: the importance of clinical breast examination for breast cancer detection, *Yonsei Medical Journal* 41(3):312-318, 2000.

97. Shen Y, Zelen M: Screening sensitivity and sojourn time from breast cancer early detection clinical trials: mammograms and physical examinations, *Journal of Clinical Oncology* 19(15):3490-3499, 2001.

98. Pennypacker HS, Naylor L, Sander AA, et al: Why can't we do better breast examinations? *Nurse Practitioner Forum* 10(3):122-128, 1999.

99. Bloom H, Criswell E, Pennypacker H, et al: Major stimulus dimensions determining detection of simulated breast lesions, *Percep Psychophys* 20:163-167, 1982.

100. McDonald S, Saslow D, Aleiati MH: Performance and reporting of clinical breast examination: a review of the literature, *Cancer J Clin* 54:345-361, 2004.

101. Potter PA, Weilitz PB: *Pocket guide to health assessment*, ed 5, St. Louis, 2003, Mosby.

102. Schnur W: Tickle me not, *Postgrad Med* 96(6):35, 1994.

103. Dains JE, Baumann LC, Scheibel P: *Advanced health assessment and clinical diagnosis in primary care*, ed 2, St. Louis, 2003, Mosby.

Viscerogenic Causes of Neuromusculoskeletal Pain and Dysfunction

The blood consists of two major components: plasma, a pale yellow or gray-yellow fluid; and formed elements, erythrocytes (red blood cells, or RBCs), leukocytes (white blood cells, or WBCs), and platelets (thrombocytes). Blood is the circulating tissue of the body; the fluid and its formed elements circulate through the heart, arteries, capillaries, and veins.

The *erythrocytes* carry oxygen to tissues and remove carbon dioxide from them. *Leukocytes* act in inflammatory and immune responses. The *plasma* carries antibodies and nutrients to tissues and removes wastes from tissues. *Platelets*, together with *coagulation factors* in plasma, control the clotting of blood.

Primary hematologic diseases are uncommon, but hematologic manifestations secondary to other diseases are common. Cancers of the blood are discussed in Chapter 13.

In the physical therapist's practice, symptoms of blood disorders are most common in relation to the use of nonsteroidal antiinflammatory drugs (NSAIDs) for inflammatory conditions, neurologic complications associated with pernicious anemia, and complications of chemotherapy or radiation.

SIGNS AND SYMPTOMS OF HEMATOLOGIC DISORDERS

There are many signs and symptoms that can be associated with hematologic disorders. Some of the most important indicators of dysfunction in this system include problems associated with exertion (often minimal exertion) such as dyspnea, chest pain, palpitations, severe weakness, and fatigue. Neurological symptoms such as headache, drowsiness, dizziness, syncope, or polyneuropathy can also indicate a variety of possible problems in this system.

Significant skin and fingernail bed changes that can occur with hematologic problems might include pallor of the face, hands, nail beds, and lips; cyanosis or clubbing of the fingernail beds and wounds or easy bruising or bleeding in skin, gums, or mucous membranes, often with no reported trauma to the area. The presence of blood in the stool or emesis or severe pain and swelling in joints and muscles should also alert the physical therapist to the possibility of a hematologic-based systemic disorder and can sometimes be a critical indicator of bleeding disorders that can be life threatening.

Many hematologic-induced signs and symptoms seen in the physical therapy practice occur as a result of medications. For example, chronic or long-term use of steroids and nonsteroidal antiinflammatories can lead to gastritis and peptic ulcer with gastrointestinal bleeding and subsequent iron deficiency anemia. Leukopenia, a common problem occurring during

chemotherapy, or as a symptom of certain types of cancer, can produce symptoms of infections such as fever, chills, tissue inflammation, severe mouth, throat and esophageal pain, and mucous membrane ulcerations.

Thrombocytopenia (decreased platelets) associated with easy bruising and spontaneous bleeding is a result of the pharmacologic treatment of common conditions seen in a physical therapy practice such as rheumatoid arthritis and cancer. More about this condition will be included later in this chapter.

▶ CLASSIFICATION OF BLOOD DISORDERS

Erythrocyte Disorders

Erythrocytes (red blood cells) consist mainly of hemoglobin and a supporting framework. Erythrocytes transport oxygen and carbon dioxide; they are important in maintaining normal acid-base balance. There are many more erythrocytes than leukocytes (600 to 1). The total number is determined by gender (women have fewer erythrocytes than men), altitude (less oxygen in the air requires more erythrocytes to carry sufficient amounts of oxygen to the tissues), and physical activity (sedentary people have fewer erythrocytes, athletes have more).

Disorders of erythrocytes are classified as follows (not all of these conditions are discussed in this text):

• Anemia (too few erythrocytes)
• Polycythemia (too many erythrocytes)
• Poikilocytosis (abnormally shaped erythrocytes)
• Anisocytosis (abnormal variations in size of erythrocytes)
• Hypochromia (erythrocytes deficient in hemoglobin)

Anemia

Anemia is a reduction in the oxygen-carrying capacity of the blood as a result of an abnormality in the quantity or quality of erythrocytes. Anemia is not a disease but is a symptom of any number of different blood disorders. Excessive blood loss, increased destruction of erythrocytes, and decreased production of erythrocytes are the most common causes of anemia.[1]

In the physical therapy practice, anemia-related disorders usually occur in one of four broad categories:

1. Iron deficiency associated with chronic gastrointestinal (GI) blood loss secondary to NSAID use;

2. Chronic diseases or inflammatory diseases, such as rheumatoid arthritis or systemic lupus erythematosus;
3. Neurologic conditions (pernicious anemia); and
4. Infectious diseases, such as tuberculosis or AIDS, and neoplastic disease or cancer (bone marrow failure).

Anemia with neoplasia may be a common complication of chemotherapy or develop as a consequence of bone marrow metastasis.[2] Anemia can also occur as a symptom of leukemia.

CLINICAL SIGNS AND SYMPTOMS

Deficiency in the oxygen-carrying capacity of blood may result in disturbances in the function of many organs and tissues leading to various symptoms that differ from one person to another. Slowly developing anemia in young, otherwise healthy individuals is well tolerated, and there may be no symptoms until hemoglobin concentration and hematocrit fall below one half of normal (see values inside book cover).

However, rapid onset may result in symptoms of dyspnea, weakness and fatigue, and palpitations, reflecting the lack of oxygen transport to the lungs and muscles. Many people can have moderate-to-severe anemia without these symptoms. Although there is no difference in normal blood volume associated with severe anemia, there is a redistribution of blood so that organs most sensitive to oxygen deprivation (e.g., brain, heart, muscles) receive more blood than, for example, the hands and kidneys.

Changes in the hands and fingernail beds (Table 5-1) may be observed during the inspection/observation portion of the physical therapy evaluation (see Table 4-8 and Box 4-15). The physical therapist should look for pale palms with normal-colored creases (severe anemia causes pale creases as well). Observation of the hands should be done at the level of the client's heart. In addition, the anemic client's hands should be warm; if they are cold, the paleness is due to vasoconstriction.

Pallor in dark-skinned people may be observed by the absence of the underlying red tones that normally give brown or black skin its luster. The brown-skinned individual demonstrates pallor with a more yellowish-brown color, and the black-skinned person will appear ashen or gray.

Systolic blood pressure may not be affected, but diastolic pressure may be lower than normal, with an associated increase in the resting pulse rate. Resting cardiac output is usually normal in people with anemia, but cardiac output increases with exercise more than it does in people without

TABLE 5-1 ▼ Changes Associated with Hematologic Disorders

Changes	Causes
Skin	
Light, lemon-yellow tint	Untreated pernicious anemia
White, waxy appearance	Severe anemia resulting from acute hemorrhage
Gray-green yellow	Chronic blood loss
Gray tint	Leukemia
Pale hands or palmar creases	Anemia
Nail Bed	
Brittle	Long-standing iron deficiency anemia
Concave (rather than convex)	Long-standing iron deficiency anemia
Oral Mucosa/Conjunctiva	
Pale or yellow color	Anemia

CASE EXAMPLE 5-1 Anemia

A 72-year-old woman, status post-hip fracture, was treated surgically with nails (used for the fixation of the ends of fractured bones) and was referred to physical therapy for follow-up treatment before hospital discharge. The physician's preoperative examination and surgical report were unremarkable for physical therapy precautions or contraindications.

When the therapist met with the client for the first time, she had already been ambulating alone in her room from the bed to the bathroom and back using a hospital wheeled walker. She was wearing thigh length support hose, hospital gown, and open heeled slippers from home. Although the nursing report indicated she was oriented to time and place, she seemed confused and required multiple verbal cues to follow the physical therapist's directions.

After ambulating a distance of approximately 50 feet using her wheeled walker and standby assistance from the therapist, the client reported that she could not "catch her breath" and asked to sit down. She placed her hand over her heart and commented that her heart was "fluttering." Blood pressure and pulse measurements were taken and recorded as

145/72 mm Hg (blood pressure) and 90 bpm (pulse rate).

The physical therapist consulted with nursing staff immediately regarding this episode and was given the "go ahead" to complete the therapy session. The physical therapist documented the episode in the medical record and left a note for the physician, briefly describing the incident and ending with the question: Are there any medical contraindications to continuing progressive therapy?

Result: A significant fall in hemoglobin (Hb) often occurs after hip fracture and surgical intervention secondary to the blood loss caused by the fracture and surgery. Other contributing factors may include blood transfusion and alcoholic liver cirrhosis.[4,5]

In this case, although the physician did not offer a direct reply to the physical therapist, the physician's notes indicated a suspected diagnosis of anemia. Follow-up blood work was ordered and the diagnosis was confirmed. Nursing staff conferred with the physician, and the therapist was advised to work within the patient's tolerance using perceived exertion as a guide while monitoring pulse and blood pressure.

anemia. As the anemia becomes more severe, resting cardiac output increases and exercise tolerance progressively decreases until dyspnea, tachycardia, and palpitations occur at rest.

Diminished exercise tolerance is expected in the client with anemia. Exercise testing and prescribed exercise(s) in clients with anemia must be instituted with extreme caution and should proceed very gradually to tolerance and/or perceived exertion levels.[3] In addition, exercise for any anemic client should be first approved by his or her physician (Case Example 5-1).

Clinical Signs and Symptoms of Anemia

- Skin pallor (palms, nail beds) or yellow-tinged skin (mucosa, conjunctiva)
- Fatigue and listlessness
- Dyspnea on exertion accompanied by heart palpitations and rapid pulse (more severe anemia)

Continued on p. 264

- Chest pain with minimal exertion
- Decreased diastolic blood pressure
- CNS manifestations (pernicious anemia):
  - Headache
  - Drowsiness
  - Dizziness, syncope
  - Slow thought processes
  - Apathy, depression
  - Polyneuropathy

Polycythemia

Polycythemia (also known as erythrocytosis) is characterized by increases in both the number of red blood cells and the concentration of hemoglobin. People with polycythemia have increased whole blood viscosity and increased blood volume.

The increased erythrocyte production results in this thickening of the blood and an increased tendency toward clotting. The viscosity of the blood limits its ability to flow easily, diminishing the supply of blood to the brain and to other vital tissues. Increased platelets in combination with the increased blood viscosity may contribute to the formation of intravascular thrombi.

There are two distinct forms of polycythemia: primary polycythemia (also known as polycythemia vera) and secondary polycythemia. *Primary polycythemia* is a relatively uncommon neoplastic disease of the bone marrow of unknown etiology. *Secondary polycythemia* is a physiologic condition resulting from a decreased oxygen supply to the tissues. It is associated with high altitudes, heavy tobacco smoking, radiation exposure, and chronic heart and lung disorders, especially congenital heart defects.

CLINICAL SIGNS AND SYMPTOMS

The symptoms of this disease are often insidious in onset with vague complaints. The most common first symptoms are shortness of breath and fatigue. The affected individual may be diagnosed only secondary to a sudden complication (e.g., stroke or thrombosis). Increased skin coloration and elevated blood pressure may develop as a result of the increased concentration of erythrocytes and increased blood viscosity.

Gout is sometimes a complication of primary polycythemia, and a typical attack of acute gout may be the first symptom of polycythemia. Gout is a metabolic disease marked by increased serum urate levels (hyperuricemia), which cause painfully arthritic joints. Uric acid level is an end product of purine metabolism. Purine metabolism is altered by excessive cellular proliferation and breakdown associated with increased red cells,

granulocytes, and platelets. Hyperuricemia is uncommon in secondary polycythemia because the cellular proliferation is not as extensive as in primary polycythemia.

Blockage of the capillaries supplying the digits of either the hands or the feet may cause a peripheral vascular neuropathy with decreased sensation, burning, numbness, or tingling. This small blood vessel occlusion can also contribute to the development of cyanosis and clubbing. If the underlying disorder is not recognized and treated, the person may develop gangrene and have subsequent loss of tissue.

Watch for increase in blood pressure and elevated hematocrit levels.

Clinical Signs and Symptoms of

Polycythemia

Clinical signs and symptoms of polycythemia (whether primary or secondary) are directly related to the increase in blood viscosity described earlier and may include

- General malaise and fatigue
- Shortness of breath
- Intolerable pruritus (skin itching) **(poly-cythemia vera)***
- Headache
- Dizziness
- Irritability
- Blurred vision
- Fainting
- Decreased mental acuity
- Feeling of fullness in the head
- Disturbances of sensation in the hands and feet
- Weight loss
- Easy bruising
- Cyanosis (blue hue to the skin)
- Clubbing of the fingers
- Splenomegaly (enlargement of spleen)
- Gout
- Hypertension

* This condition of skin itching is particularly related to warm conditions, such as being in bed at night or in a bath and is called the "hot bath sign."

Sickle Cell Anemia

Sickle cell disease is a generic term for a group of inherited, autosomal recessive disorders characterized by the presence of an abnormal form of hemoglobin, the oxygen-carrying constituent of erythrocytes. A genetic mutation resulting in a single amino acid substitution in hemoglobin causes the hemoglobin to aggregate into long

CASE EXAMPLE 5-2 Sickle Cell Anemia

A 20-year-old African-American woman came to physical therapy with severe right knee joint pain. She could recall no traumatic injury but reported hiking 2 days previously in the Rocky Mountains with her brother, whom she was visiting (she was from New York City).

A general screen for systemic illness revealed frequent urination over the past 2 days. She also complained of stomach pain, but she thought this was related to the stress of visiting her family. Past medical history included one other similar episode when she had acute pneumonia at the age of 11 years. She stated that she usually felt fatigued but thought it was because of her active social life and busy professional career. She is a nonsmoker and a social drinker (1 to 3 drinks per week).

On examination, the right knee was enlarged and inflamed, with joint range of motion limited by the local swelling. In fact, pain, swelling, and guarded motion in the joint prevented a complete evaluation. Given that restraint, there were no other physical findings, but not all special tests were completed. The neurologic screen was negative.

This woman was treated for local joint inflammation, but the combination of change in altitude, fatigue, increased urination, and stomach pains alerted the therapist to the possibility of a systemic process despite the client's explanation for the fatigue and stomach upset. Because the client was from out of town and did not have a local physician, the therapist telephoned the hospital emergency department for a telephone consultation. It was suggested that a blood sample be obtained for preliminary screening while the client continued to receive physical therapy. Laboratory results included the following:

- Hct 30%   (normal 35% to 47%)
- Hb 10g/dl   (normal 12 to 15g/dl)
- WBC 20,000/mm³ (normal 4500 to 11,000/mm³)

Based on these findings, the client was admitted to the hospital and diagnosed as having sickle cell anemia. It is likely that the change in altitude, the emotional stress of visiting family, and the physical exertion precipitated a "crisis." She received continued physical therapy treatment during her hospital stay and was discharged with further follow-up planned in her home city.

Adapted from Jennings B: Nursing role in management: hematological problems. In Lewis S, Collier I, editors: *Medical-surgical nursing: assessment and management of clinical problems*, St Louis, 1992, Mosby, pp 664-714. Used with permission.

---

chains, altering the shape of the cell. This sickled or curved shape causes the cell to lose its ability to deform and squeeze through tiny blood vessels, thereby depriving tissue of an adequate blood supply.

The two features of sickle cell disorders, chronic hemolytic anemia and vaso-occlusion, occur as a result of obstruction of blood flow to the tissues and early destruction of the abnormal cells. Anemia associated with this condition is merely a symptom of the disease and not the disease itself, despite the term *sickle cell anemia*.

CLINICAL SIGNS AND SYMPTOMS

A series of "crises," or acute manifestations of symptoms, characterize sickle cell disease. Some people with this disease have only a few symptoms, whereas others are affected severely and have a short life span. Cerebrovascular accidents (CVAs) are a frequent and severe manifestation.

Stress from viral or bacterial infection, hypoxia, dehydration, emotional disturbance, extreme temperatures, fever, strenuous physical exertion, or fatigue may precipitate a crisis. Pain caused by the blockage of sickled red blood cells (RBCs) forming sickle cell clots is the most common symptom; it may be in any organ, bone, or joint of the body. Painful episodes of ischemic tissue damage may last 5 or 6 days and manifest in many different ways, depending on the location of the blood clot (Case Example 5-2).

Clinical Signs and Symptoms of Sickle Cell Anemia

- Pain
  - Abdominal
  - Chest
  - Headaches

Continued on p. 266

Lymphocytes produce antibodies and react with antigens, thus initiating the immune response to fight infection. *Monocytes* are the largest circulating blood cells and represent an immature cell until they leave the blood and travel to the tissues where they form macrophages in response to foreign substances such as bacteria. *Granulocytes* contain lysing agents capable of digesting various foreign materials and defend the body against infectious agents by phagocytosing bacteria and other infectious substances.

Disorders of leukocytes are recognized as the body's reaction to disease processes and noxious agents. The therapist will encounter many clients who demonstrate alterations in the blood leukocyte (WBC) concentration as a result of acute infections or chronic systemic conditions. The leukocyte count also may be elevated (leukocytosis) in women who are pregnant, in clients with bacterial infections, appendicitis, leukemia, uremia, or ulcers, in newborns with hemolytic disease and normally at birth. The leukocyte count may drop below normal values (*leukopenia*) in clients with viral diseases (e.g., measles), infectious hepatitis, rheumatoid arthritis, cirrhosis of the liver, and lupus erythematosus, and also after treatment with radiation or chemotherapy.

Leukocytosis

Leukocytosis characterizes many infectious diseases and is recognized by a count of more than 10,000 leukocytes/mm^3. It can be associated with an increase in circulating neutrophils (neutrophilia), which are recruited in large numbers early in the course of most bacterial infections.

Leukocytosis is a common finding and is helpful in aiding the body's response to any of the following:

- Bacterial infections
- Inflammation or tissue necrosis (e.g., infarction, myositis, vasculitis)
- Metabolic intoxications (e.g., uremia, eclampsia, acidosis, gout)
- Neoplasms (especially bronchogenic carcinoma, lymphoma, melanoma)
- Acute hemorrhage
- Splenectomy
- Acute appendicitis
- Pneumonia
- Intoxication by chemicals
- Acute rheumatic fever

- Bone and joint crises from the ischemic tissue, lasting for hours to days and subsiding gradually
  - Low-grade fever
  - Extremity pain
  - Back pain
  - Periosteal pain
  - Joint pain, especially in the shoulder and hip
- Vascular complications
  - Cerebrovascular accidents (affects children and young adults most often)
  - Chronic leg ulcers
  - Avascular necrosis of the femoral head
  - Bone infarcts
- Pulmonary crises
  - Bacterial pneumonia
  - Pulmonary infarction (less common)
- Neurologic manifestations
  - Convulsions
  - Drowsiness
  - Coma
  - Stiff neck
  - Paresthesias
  - Cranial nerve palsies
  - Blindness
  - Nystagmus
- Hand-foot syndrome
  - Fever
  - Pain
  - Dactylitis (painful swelling of the dorsum of hands and feet)
- Splenic sequestration crisis (occurs before adolescence)
  - Liver and spleen enlargement due to trapped erythrocytes
  - Subsequent spleen atrophy due to repeated blood vessel obstruction
- Renal complications
  - Enuresis (bed-wetting)
  - Nocturia (excessive urination at night)
  - Hematuria (blood in the urine)
  - Pyelonephritis
  - Renal papillary necrosis
  - End-stage renal failure (elderly population)

Leukocyte Disorders

The blood contains three major groups of leukocytes including:

1. Lymphoid cells (lymphocytes, plasma cells);
2. Monocytes; and
3. Granulocytes (neutrophils, eosinophils, and basophils).

Clinical Signs and Symptoms of
Leukocytosis

These clinical signs and symptoms are usually associated with symptoms of the conditions listed earlier and may include

- Fever
- Symptoms of localized or systemic infection
- Symptoms of inflammation or trauma to tissue

Leukopenia

Leukopenia, or reduction of the number of leukocytes in the blood below 5000 per microliter, can be caused by a variety of factors. Unlike leukocytosis, leukopenia is never beneficial.

Leukopenia can occur in many forms of bone marrow failure such as that following antineoplastic chemotherapy or radiation therapy, in overwhelming infections, in dietary deficiencies, and in autoimmune diseases.

It is important for the physical therapist to be aware of the client's most recent white blood cell count prior to and during the course of physical therapy. If the client is immunosuppressed, infection is a major problem. Constitutional symptoms such as fever, chills, or sweats warrant immediate medical referral.

Nadir, or the lowest point the white blood count reaches, usually occurs 7 to 14 days after chemotherapy or radiation therapy. At this time, the client is extremely susceptible to opportunistic infections and severe complications. The importance of good handwashing and hygiene practices cannot be overemphasized when treating any of these people.

Clinical Signs and Symptoms of
Leukopenia

- Sore throat, cough
- High fever, chills, sweating
- Ulcerations of mucous membranes (mouth, rectum, vagina)
- Frequent or painful urination
- Persistent infections

Leukemia

Leukemia is a disease arising from the bone marrow and involves the uncontrolled growth of immature or dysfunctional white blood cells; a complete discussion of this cancer is found in Chapter 13.

Platelet Disorders

Platelets (thrombocytes) function primarily in hemostasis (stopping bleeding) and in maintaining capillary integrity (see normal values listed inside book cover). They function in the coagulation (blood clotting) mechanism by forming hemostatic plugs in small ruptured blood vessels or by adhering to any injured lining of larger blood vessels.

A number of substances derived from the platelets that function in blood coagulation have been labeled "platelet factors." Platelets survive approximately 8 to 10 days in circulation and are then removed by the reticuloendothelial cells. *Thrombocytosis* refers to a condition in which the number of platelets is abnormally high, whereas *thrombocytopenia* refers to a condition in which the number of platelets is abnormally low.

Platelets are affected most often by anticoagulant drugs, including aspirin, heparin, warfarin (Coumadin), and other newer antithrombotic drugs now appearing on the market (e.g., Arixtra). Platelet levels can also be affected by diet (presence of lecithin preventing coagulation or vitamin K from promoting coagulation), by exercise that boosts the production of chemical activators that destroy unwanted clots, and by liver disease that affects the supply of vitamin K. Platelets are also easily suppressed by radiation and chemotherapy.

Thrombocytosis

Thrombocytosis is an increase in platelet count that is usually temporary. It may occur as a compensatory mechanism after severe hemorrhage, surgery, and splenectomy; in iron deficiency and polycythemia vera; and as a manifestation of an occult (hidden) neoplasm (e.g., lung cancer).

It is associated with a tendency to clot because blood viscosity is increased by the very high platelet count, resulting in intravascular clumping (or thrombosis) of the sludged platelets. Peripheral blood vessels, particularly in the fingers and toes are affected.

Thrombocytosis remains asymptomatic until the platelet count exceeds 1 million/mm³. Other symptoms may include splenomegaly and easy bruising.

Clinical Signs and Symptoms of
Thrombocytosis

- Thrombosis
- Splenomegaly
- Easy bruising

Thrombocytopenia

Thrombocytopenia, a decrease in the number of platelets (less than 150,000/mm^3) in circulating blood, can result from decreased or defective platelet production or from accelerated platelet destruction.

There are many causes of thrombocytopenia (Box 5-1). In a physical therapy practice the most common causes seen are bone marrow failure from radiation treatment, leukemia, or metastatic cancer; cytotoxic agents used in chemotherapy; and drug-induced platelet reduction, especially among adults with rheumatoid arthritis treated with gold or inflammatory conditions treated with aspirin or other NSAIDs.

Primary bleeding sites include bone marrow or spleen; secondary bleeding occurs from small blood vessels in the skin, mucosa (e.g., nose, uterus, gastrointestinal tract, urinary tract, and respiratory tract), and brain (intracranial hemorrhage).

CLINICAL SIGNS AND SYMPTOMS

Severe thrombocytopenia results in the appearance of multiple petechiae (small, purple, pinpoint hemorrhages into the skin), most often observed on the lower legs. Gastrointestinal bleeding and bleeding into the central nervous system associated with severe thrombocytopenia may be life-threatening manifestations of thrombocytopenic bleeding.

The physical therapist must be alert for obvious skin, joint, or mucous membrane symptoms of thrombocytopenia, which include severe bruising, external hematomas, joint swelling, and the presence of multiple petechiae observed on the skin or gums. These symptoms usually indicate a platelet count well below 100,000/mm^3. Strenuous exercise or any exercise that involves straining or bearing down could precipitate a hemorrhage, particularly

of the eyes or brain. Blood pressure cuffs must be used with caution and any mechanical compression, visceral manipulation, or soft tissue mobilization is contraindicated without a physician's approval.

People with undiagnosed thrombocytopenia need immediate physician referral. Exercise guidelines for thrombocytopenia can be found in Goodman et al, *Pathology: Implications for the Physical Therapist*, 2nd ed (Table 39-7).

Clinical Signs and Symptoms of Thrombocytopenia

- Bleeding after minor trauma
- Spontaneous bleeding
  - Petechiae (small red dots)
  - Ecchymoses (bruises)
  - Purpura spots (bleeding under the skin)
  - Epistaxis (nosebleed)
- Menorrhagia (excessive menstruation)
- Gingival bleeding
- Melena (black, tarry stools)

Coagulation Disorders

Hemophilia

Hemophilia is a hereditary blood-clotting disorder caused by an abnormality of functional plasma-clotting proteins known as factors VIII and IX. In most cases, the person with hemophilia has normal amounts of the deficient factor circulating, but it is in a functionally inadequate state. Persons with hemophilia bleed longer than those with normal levels of functioning factors VIII or IX, but the bleeding is not any faster than would occur in a normal person with the same injury.

CLINICAL SIGNS AND SYMPTOMS

Bleeding into the joint spaces (hemarthrosis) is one of the most common clinical manifestations of hemophilia. It may result from an identifiable trauma or stress or may be spontaneous, most often affecting the knee, elbow, ankle, hip, and shoulder (in order of most common appearance).

Recurrent hemarthrosis results in hemophiliac arthropathy (joint disease) with progressive loss of motion, muscle atrophy, and flexion contractures. Bleeding episodes must be treated early with factor replacement and joint immobilization during the period of pain. This type of affected joint is particularly susceptible to being injured again, setting up a cycle of vulnerability to trauma and repeated hemorrhages.

BOX 5-1 ▼ Causes of Thrombocytopenia

- Bone marrow failure
- Radiation
- Aplastic anemia
- Leukemia
- Metastatic carcinoma
- Cytotoxic agents (chemotherapy)
- Medications
  - Nonsteroidal antiinflammatory drugs (including aspirin)
  - Methotrexate
  - Gold
  - Coumadin/warfarin

Hemarthroses are not common in the first year of life but increase in frequency as the child begins to walk. The severity of the hemarthrosis may vary (depending on the degree of injury) from mild pain and swelling, which resolves without treatment within 1 to 3 days, to severe pain with an excruciatingly painful, swollen joint that persists for several weeks and resolves slowly with treatment.

Bleeding into the muscles is the second most common site of bleeding in persons with hemophilia. Muscle hemorrhages can be more insidious and massive than joint hemorrhages. They may occur anywhere but are common in the flexor muscle groups, predominantly the iliopsoas, gastrocnemius, and flexor surface of the forearm, and they result in deformities such as hip flexion contractures, equinus position of the foot, or Volkmann's deformity of the forearm. For a more in-depth discussion of hemophilia and the clinical signs and symptoms associated with it, see Goodman et al, *Pathology: Implications for the Physical Therapist*, ed 2 (Table 13-11).

When bleeding into the psoas or iliacus muscle puts pressure on the branch of the femoral nerve supplying the skin over the anterior thigh, loss of sensation occurs. Distention of the muscles with blood causes pain that can be felt in the lower abdomen, possibly even mimicking appendicitis when bleeding occurs on the right side. In an attempt to relieve the distention and reduce the pain, a position with hip flexion is preferred.

Clinical Signs and Symptoms of Acute Hemarthrosis

- Aura, tingling, or prickling sensation
- Stiffening into the position of comfort
- Decreased range of motion
- Pain
- Swelling
- Tenderness
- Heat

Clinical Signs and Symptoms of Muscle Hemorrhage

- Gradually intensifying pain
- Protective spasm of the muscle
- Limitation of movement at the surrounding joints
- Muscle assumes the position of comfort (usually shortened)
- Loss of sensation

Clinical Signs and Symptoms of Gastrointestinal Involvement

- Abdominal pain and distention
- Melena (blood in stool)
- Hematemesis (vomiting blood)
- Fever
- Low abdominal/groin pain due to bleeding into wall of large intestine or iliopsoas muscle
- Flexion contracture of the hip due to spasm of the iliopsoas muscle secondary to retroperitoneal hemorrhage

Two tests are used to distinguish an iliopsoas bleed from a hip bleed:

1. When the client flexes the trunk, severe pain is produced in the presence of *iliopsoas bleeding*, whereas only mild pain is found with a hip hemorrhage.
2. When the hip is gently rotated in either direction, severe pain is experienced with a *hip hemorrhage*, but is absent or mild with iliopsoas bleeding.

Over time, the following complications may occur:

- Vascular compression causing localized ischemia and necrosis
- Replacement of muscle fibers by nonelastic fibrotic tissue causing shortened muscles and thus producing joint contractures
- Peripheral nerve lesions from compression of a nerve that travels in the same compartment as the hematoma, most commonly affecting the femoral, ulnar, and median nerves
- Pseudotumor formation with bone erosion

PHYSICIAN REFERRAL

Understanding the components of a client's past medical history that can affect hematopoiesis (production of blood cells) can provide the physical therapist with valuable insight into the client's present symptoms, which are usually already well known to the attending physician.

For example, the effects of certain drugs, exposure to radiation, or recent cytotoxic cancer chemotherapy can affect bone marrow. Whenever uncertain, the physical therapist is encouraged to contact the physician by telephone for discussion and clarification of the client's medical symptoms.

A history of excessive menses, a folate-poor diet, alcohol abuse, drug ingestion, family history of anemia, and family roots in geographic areas where red blood cell enzyme or hemoglobin abnormalities are prevalent represent some important

findings. The presence of any one or more of these factors should alert the physical therapist to the need for medical referral when the client is not already under the care of a physician or when new signs or symptoms develop.

In addition, exercise for *anemic* clients must be instituted with extreme caution and should first be approved by the client's physician. Clients with undiagnosed thrombocytopenia need immediate medical referral. The physical therapist must be alert for obvious skin or mucous membrane symptoms of *thrombocytopenia*. The presence of severe bruising, hematomas, and multiple petechiae usually indicates a platelet count well below normal. With clients who have been diagnosed with *hemophilia*, medical referral should be made when any painful episode develops in the muscle(s) or joint(s). Pain usually occurs before any other evidence of bleeding. Any unexplained symptom may be a signal of bleeding.

Guidelines for Immediate Medical Attention

- Signs and symptoms of thrombocytopenia (decreased platelets) (e.g., excessive or spontaneous bleeding, petechiae, severe bruising) previously unseen or unreported to the physician

Guidelines for Physician Referral

- Consultation with the physician may be necessary when establishing or progressing

an exercise program for a client with known anemia
- New episodes of muscle or joint pain in a client with hemophilia; pain usually occurs before any other evidence of bleeding. Any unexplained symptom(s) may be a signal of bleeding; coughing up blood in this population group must be reported to the physician

Clues to Screening for Hematologic Disease

These clues will help the therapist in the decision making process:

- Previous history (delayed effects) or current administration of chemotherapy or radiation therapy
- Chronic or long-term use of aspirin or other NSAIDs (drug-induced platelet reduction)
- Spontaneous bleeding of any kind (e.g., nosebleed, vaginal/menstrual bleeding, blood in the urine or stool, bleeding gums, easy bruising, hemarthrosis), especially with a previous history of hemophilia
- Recent major surgery or previous transplantation
- Rapid onset of dyspnea, chest pain, weakness, and fatigue with palpitations associated with recent significant change in altitude
- Observed changes in the hands and fingernail beds (see Table 5-1 and Fig. 4-30)

✓ KEY POINTS TO REMEMBER

- ✓ Anemia may have no symptoms until hemoglobin concentration and hematocrit fall below one half of normal.
- ✓ Weakness, fatigue, and dyspnea are early signs of anemia.
- ✓ Exercise for anyone who is anemic must be instituted gradually per tolerance and/or perceived exertion levels with physician approval.
- ✓ Platelet level below 10,000 (thrombocytopenia) can be life threatening. Platelet transfusions are usually given for platelet counts below this level in adults and children who have chemotherapy-induced thrombocytopenia. Multiple bruises and petechiae may be the only sign.
- ✓ For clients with known thrombocytopenia, exercise programs must avoid the Valsalva (or bearing down) movement, and caution must be used to avoid further injury by bumping against objects.

- ✓ During the inspection/observation portion of the objective examination, screen both hands for skin or nail bed changes indicative of hematologic involvement.
- ✓ For the client with hemophilia, bleeding episodes must be treated early with factor replacement and joint immobilization during the period of pain. Never apply heat to a bleeding or suspected bleeding area.
- ✓ Pain may be the only symptom of a joint or muscle bleed for the client with hemophilia. Any painful or unexplained symptom in this population must be screened medically. Coughing up blood is not a normal finding with hemophilia and should be reported to the physician immediately.
- ✓ The National Hemophilia Foundation (NHF) publishes additional materials for physical therapists. These can be ordered by calling the NHF at (212) 328-3700.

SUBJECTIVE EXAMINATION

Special Questions to Ask

Past Medical History

- Have you recently been told you are anemic?

- Have you recently had a serious blood loss (possibly requiring transfusion)? (**Anemia;** also consider **jaundice/hepatitis posttransfusion**)

- Have you ever been told that you have a congenital heart defect (also chronic lung/heart disorders)? (**Polycythemia:** also chronic lung/heart **history of heavy tobacco use**)

- Do you have a history of bruising easily, nose bleeds, or excessive blood loss?* (**Polycythemia, hemophilia, thrombocytopenia**)

  For example, do you bleed or bruise easily after minor trauma, surgery, or dental procedures? Has any previous bleeding been severe enough to require a blood transfusion?

- Have you been exposed to occupational or industrial gases, such as chlorine gas, mustard gas, Agent Orange, napalm?

Associated Signs and Symptoms

- Do you experience shortness of breath, heart palpitations, or chest pain with slight exertion (e.g., climbing stairs) or even just at rest? (**Anemia**)

- Alternate or additional questions: Do you ever have trouble catching your breath?

  Are there any activities you have had to stop doing because you don't have enough energy or breath? [Therapist: Be aware of the clients who stop doing certain activities because they become

  short of breath. For example, they no longer go up and down stairs in their homes and choose to avoid this activity . . . or the client who can't complete all of his or her shopping at one time. They may not report being short of breath because they have decreased their activity level to accommodate for the change in their pulmonary capacity.]

- **For persons at elevations above 3500 feet:** Have you recently moved from one geographic location to another? (**Polycythemia**)

- Do you ever have episodes of dizziness, blurred vision, headaches, fainting, or a feeling of fullness in your head? (**Polycythemia**)

- Do you have recurrent infections and low-grade fever such as colds, influenza-like symptoms, or other upper respiratory infections? (**Abnormal leukocytes**)

- Do you have black, tarry stools (**bleeding into the gastrointestinal tract**) or blood in urine (**genitourinary tract**)?

- **For women (anemia, thrombocytopenia):** Do you frequently have prolonged or excessive bleeding in association with your menstrual flow? (Excessive may be considered to be measured by the use of more than four tampons each day; prolonged menstruation usually refers to more than 5 days—both of these measures are subjective and must be considered along with other factors, such as the presence of other symptoms, personal menstrual history, placement in the life cycle [i.e., in relation to menopause].)

---

* Symptoms beginning in infancy or childhood suggest a congenital hemostatic defect, whereas symptoms beginning later in life indicate an acquired disorder, such as secondary to drug-induced defect of platelet function, a common cause of easy bruising and excessive bleeding. This bruising or bleeding occurs usually in association with trauma, menstruation, dental work, or surgical procedures. Drug-induced bruising or bleeding may also occur with use of aspirin and aspirin-containing compounds; nonsteroidal antiinflammatory agents such as ibuprofen (Motrin) and naproxen (Naprosyn) (see Table 8-3) and penicillins, because these drugs inhibit platelet function to some extent.

CASE STUDY

REFERRAL

You are working in a hospital setting and you have received a physician's referral to ambulate and exercise a patient who was involved in a serious automobile accident 10 days ago. The patient had internal injuries that required immediate abdominal surgery and 600 ml of blood transfused within 24 hours postoperatively. His condition is considered to be medically "stable."

CHART REVIEW

What specific medical information should you look for in the medical record before beginning your evaluation?

Name, age, and occupation:

Past medical history: Previous myocardial infarcts, history of heart disease, diabetes (type)

Surgical report: Type of surgery, locations of scar, any current contraindications

Were there any other injuries? If yes, what were these and what is the current status of each injury?

Body weight:

Pulmonary status: Is the patient a cigarette or pipe smoker (or other tobacco user)? Is the patient currently receiving oxygen or respiratory therapy? Is there a recommendation for how many litres (L) of oxygen per minute can be used during exercise? What was the patient's pulmonary status after the accident and postoperatively?

Laboratory report: Hematocrit/hemoglobin levels. Anemia?

Current status: Nursing reports of the patient's complaints of any kind (e.g., symptoms of dyspnea or heart palpitations from rapid loss of blood). Has the patient been out of bed at all yet? If yes, when? How far did he walk? How much assistance was required? Did he have symptoms of orthostatic hypotension? Does the patient have any gastrointestinal symptoms? Is patient oriented to time, place, and person? Are there any dietary or fluid restrictions to be observed while the patient is in the physical therapy department? Is he on an intravenous line?

Vital signs: Blood pressure
Presence of fever
Resting pulse rate
Pulse oximetry (if available)

Current medications: Be aware of the purpose for each medication and its potential side effects.

Are there any known discharge plans at this time?

PRACTICE QUESTIONS

1. If rapid onset of anemia occurs after major surgery, which of the following symptom patterns might develop?
   a. Continuous oozing of blood from the surgical site
   b. Exertional dyspnea and fatigue with increased heart rate
   c. Decreased heart rate
   d. No obvious symptoms would be seen

2. Chronic GI blood loss sometimes associated with use of nonsteroidal antiinflammatory drugs (NSAIDs) can result in which of the following problems?
   a. Increased incidence of joint inflammation
   b. Iron deficiency
   c. Decreased heart rate and bleeding
   d. Weight loss, fever, and loss of appetite

3. Under what circumstances would you consider asking a client about a recent change in altitude or elevation?

4. Preoperatively, clients cannot take aspirin or antiinflammatory medications because these:
   a. Decrease leukocytes
   b. Increase leukocytes
   c. Decrease platelets
   d. Increase platelets
   e. None of the above

5. Skin color and nail bed changes may be observed in the client with:
   a. Thrombocytopenia resulting from chemotherapy
   b. Pernicious anemia resulting from Vitamin B₁₂ deficiency
   c. Leukocytosis resulting from AIDS
   d. All of the above

6. In the case of a client with hemarthrosis associated with hemophilia, what physical therapy intervention would be contraindicated?

7. Bleeding under the skin, nosebleeds, bleeding gums, and black stools require medical evaluation as these may be indications of:
   a. Leukopenia
   b. Thrombocytopenia
   c. Polycythemia
   d. Sickle cell anemia

8. Describe the two tests used to distinguish an iliopsoas bleed from a joint bleed.

9. What is the significance of *nadir?*

10. When exercising a client with known anemia, what two measures can be used as guidelines for frequency, intensity, and duration of the program?

REFERENCES

1. Holcomb S: Anemia, Pointing the way to a deeper problem, *Nursing 2001* 31(7):36-42, 2001.
2. Goodman CC, Boissonault WG, Fuller K: *Pathology: implications for the physical therapist.* Philadelphia, 2003, WB Saunders.
3. Callahan L, Woods K et al: Cardiopulmonary responses to exercise in women with sickle cell anemia, *American Journal Respiratory Critical Care Medicine* 165(9):1309-1316, 2002.
4. Lombardi G, Rizzi E et al: Epidemiology of anemia in older patients with hip fracture, *J Am Geriatr Soc* 44(6):740-741, 1996.
5. Mackenzie C: Hip fracture in the elderly, *Best Practice of Medicine,* Merck Medicus, Thomson Micromedex, March 2002.

Screening for Cardiovascular Disease

The cardiovascular system consists of the heart, capillaries, veins, and lymphatics and functions in coordination with the pulmonary system to circulate oxygenated blood through the arterial system to all cells. This system then collects deoxygenated blood from the venous system and delivers it to the lungs for reoxygenation (Fig. 6-1).

Heart disease remains the leading cause of death in industrialized nations. In the United States alone, cardiovascular disease (CVD) is responsible for approximately one million deaths each year. More than one in four Americans has some form of cardiovascular disease. The American Heart Association reports that about half of all deaths from heart disease are sudden and unexpected.

Fortunately, during the last two decades cardiovascular research has greatly increased our understanding of the structure and function of the cardiovascular system in health and disease. Despite the formidable statistics regarding the prevalence of CVD, during the last 15 years a steady decline in mortality from cardiovascular disorders has been witnessed. Effective application of the increased knowledge regarding CVD and its risk factors will assist health care professionals to educate clients in achieving and maintaining cardiovascular health.

Information about heart disease is changing rapidly. Part of the therapist's intervention includes patient/client education. The therapist can access up-to-date information at many useful web sites (Box 6-1).

SIGNS AND SYMPTOMS OF CARDIOVASCULAR DISEASE

Cardinal symptoms of cardiac disease usually include chest, neck and/or arm pain or discomfort, palpitation, dyspnea, syncope (fainting), fatigue, cough, diaphoresis, and cyanosis. Edema and leg pain (claudication) are the most common symptoms of the vascular component of a cardiovascular pathologic condition. Symptoms of cardiovascular involvement should also be reviewed by system (Table 6-1).

Chest Pain or Discomfort

Chest pain or discomfort is a common presenting symptom of cardiovascular disease and must be evaluated carefully. Chest pain may be cardiac or noncardiac in origin and may radiate to the neck, jaw, upper trapezius muscle, upper back, shoulder, or arms (most commonly the left arm).

Radiating pain down the arm follows the pattern of ulnar nerve distribution. Pain of cardiac origin can be experienced in the somatic areas because the heart is supplied by the C3-T4 spinal segments, referring visceral pain to the corresponding somatic area (see Fig. 3-3). For example, the heart and the diaphragm, supplied by the C5-6 spinal segment, can refer pain to the shoulder (see Figs. 3-4 and 3-5).

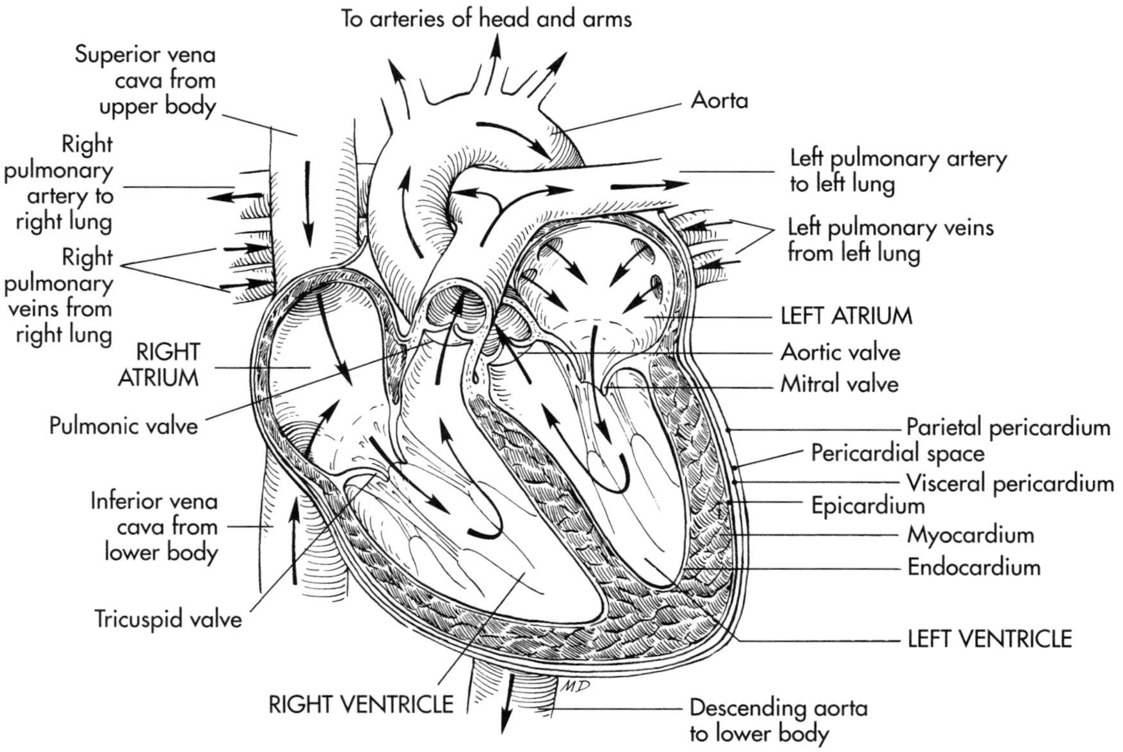

Fig. 6-1 • Structure and circulation of the heart. Blood entering the left atrium from the right and left pulmonary veins flows into the left ventricle. The left ventricle pumps blood into the aorta. From the systemic circulation, blood returns to the heart through the superior and inferior venae cavae. From there the right ventricle pumps blood into the lungs through the right and left pulmonary arteries. A thick layer of connective tissue called the *septum* separates the left and right chambers of the heart. The top of the heart (*atria*) is also separated from the bottom of the heart (*ventricles*) by connective tissue, which does not conduct electrical activity and serves as an electrical barrier or insulator. (From Black JM, Matassarin-Jacobs E, editors: *Luckmann and Sorenson's medical-surgical nursing*, ed 4, Philadelphia, 1993, WB Saunders, p. 1093.)

Labels on figure:

- Superior vena cava from upper body
- Right pulmonary artery to right lung
- Right pulmonary veins from right lung
- Pulmonic valve
- RIGHT ATRIUM
- Inferior vena cava from lower body
- Tricuspid valve
- RIGHT VENTRICLE
- To arteries of head and arms
- Descending aorta to lower body
- Aorta
- Left pulmonary artery to left lung
- Left pulmonary veins from left lung
- LEFT ATRIUM
- Aortic valve
- Mitral valve
- Parietal pericardium
- Pericardial space
- Epicardium
- Visceral pericardium
- Myocardium
- Endocardium
- LEFT VENTRICLE

BOX 6-1 ▼ Informational Websites

American Heart Association

http://www.americanheart.org

The American Heart Association has also developed a validated health-risk appraisal instrument called the RISKO scale. Anyone can use this tool to assess individual risk (www.americanheart.org/risk/quiz.html).

The American Heart Association also has a web site just for health care professionals. They offer comprehensive information on cardiovascular and cerebrovascular medicine. You can access clinical summaries of new papers and journal articles from well-known publications.

http://www.my.americanheart.org/portal/professional

American Stroke Association

The American Stroke Association is a division of the American Heart Association with updated information for consumers on strokes as well as a special link just for health care professionals.

http://www.strokeassociation.org

National Cholesterol Education Program

This web site offers a risk assessment tool for estimating the 10-year risk of developing coronary vascular disease (heart attack and coronary death) based on recent data from the Framingham Heart Study.

http://hin.nhlbi.nih.gov/atpiii/calculator.asp?usertype = prof

American College of Cardiology

http://www.acc.org

The American College of Cardiology offers the latest professional information on heart disease, research, and treatment. A special feature is the availability of clinical statements and guidelines that can be printed or downloaded.

Elsevier Science

http://www.cardiosource.com

This site is offered by collaboration between the American College of Cardiology Foundation and Elsevier Science. It includes a drug database, case studies for self-study, and a library with access to journal abstracts and reference texts.

National Heart, Lung, and Blood Institute

http://www.nhlbi.nih.gov/index.htm

The National Heart, Lung, and Blood Institute (NHLBI) at the National Institutes of Health (NIH) offers information for health care professionals and consumers. Research results, clinical guidelines, and information for women and heart disease are available.

Heart Center Online

http://www.heartcenteronline.com

Physicians provide patient education on cardiac conditions, medical devices, procedures, and tests. There is also a prevention center with a focus on lifestyle issues and nutrition, video library, and an entire section on transtelephonic monitoring.

TABLE 6-1 ▼ Cardiovascular Signs and Symptoms by System

System	Symptoms
General	Weakness
	Fatigue
	Weight change
	Poor exercise tolerance
	Peripheral edema
Integumentary	Pressure ulcers
	Loss of body hair
	Cyanosis (lips and nail beds)
Central nervous system	Headaches
	Impaired vision
	Dizziness of syncope
Pulmonary	Labored breathing, dyspnea
	Productive cough
Genitourinary	Urinary frequency
	Nocturia
	Concentrated urine
	Decreased urinary output
Musculoskeletal	Chest, shoulder, back, neck, jaw, or arm pain
	Myalgias
	Muscular fatigue
	Muscle atrophy
	Edema
	Claudication
Gastrointestinal	Nausea and vomiting
	Ascites (abdominal distention)

Modified from Goodman CC, Boissonnault WG: *Pathology: implications for the physical therapist*, Philadelphia, 1998, WB Saunders.

Cardiac-related chest pain may arise secondary to angina, myocardial infarction, pericarditis, endocarditis, mitral valve prolapse, or dissecting aortic aneurysm. Location and description (frequency, intensity, and duration) vary according to the underlying pathologic condition (see each individual condition).

Cardiac chest pain is often accompanied by associated signs and symptoms, such as nausea, vomiting, diaphoresis, dyspnea, fatigue, pallor, or syncope. These associated signs and symptoms provide the therapist with red flags to identify musculoskeletal symptoms of a systemic origin.

Noncardiac chest pain can be caused by an extensive list of disorders requiring screening for

medical disease. For example, cervical disk disease and arthritic changes can mimic atypical chest pain. Chest pain that is attributed to anxiety, trigger points, cocaine use, and other noncardiac causes is discussed in Chapter 17.

Palpitation

Palpitation, the presence of an irregular heartbeat, may also be referred to as arrhythmia or dysrhythmia, which may be caused by a relatively benign condition (e.g., mitral valve prolapse, "athlete's heart," caffeine, anxiety, exercise) or a severe condition (e.g., coronary artery disease, cardiomyopathy, complete heart block, ventricular aneurysm, atrioventricular valve disease, mitral or aortic stenosis).

The sensation of palpitations has been described as a bump, pound, jump, flop, flutter, or racing sensation of the heart. Associated symptoms may include lightheadedness or syncope. Palpated pulse may feel rapid or irregular, as if the heart "skipped" a beat.

Occasionally, a client will report "fluttering" sensations in the neck. Generally, unless accompanied by other symptoms, these sensations in the neck are caused by anxiety, random muscle fasciculation, or minor muscle strain or overuse.

Palpitations can be considered physiologic (i.e., when less than six occur per minute, this may be considered within normal function of the heart). However, palpitation lasting for hours or occurring in association with pain, shortness of breath, fainting, or severe lightheadedness requires medical evaluation. Palpitation in any person with a history of unexplained sudden death in the family requires medical referral.

Clients describing "palpitations" or similar phenomena may not be experiencing symptoms of heart disease. Palpitations may occur as a result of an overactive thyroid, secondary to caffeine sensitivity, as a side effect of some medications, and with the use of drugs such as cocaine. Encourage the client to report any such symptoms to the physician if this information has not already been brought to the physician's attention.

Dyspnea

Dyspnea, also referred to as breathlessness or shortness of breath, can be cardiovascular in origin, but it may also occur secondary to a pulmonary pathologic condition (see also Chapter 7, fever, certain medications, allergies, poor physical conditioning, or obesity). Early onset of dyspnea may be described as having to breathe too much or

as an uncomfortable feeling during breathing after exercise or exertion.

Shortness of breath with mild exertion (dyspnea on exertion [DOE]), when caused by an impaired left ventricle that is unable to contract completely, results in the lung's inability to empty itself of blood. Pulmonary congestion and shortness of breath then occur. With severe compromise of the cardiovascular or pulmonary systems, dyspnea may occur at rest.

The severity of dyspnea is determined by the extent of disease. Thus the more severe the heart disease is, the easier it is to bring on dyspnea. Extreme dyspnea includes paroxysmal nocturnal dyspnea (PND) and orthopnea (breathlessness that is relieved by sitting upright with pillows used to prop the trunk and head).

PND and sudden, unexplained episodes of shortness of breath frequently accompany congestive heart failure (CHF). During the day the effects of gravity in the upright position and the shunting of excessive fluid to the lower extremities permit more effective ventilation and perfusion of the lungs, keeping the lungs relatively fluid free, depending on the degree of CHF. PND awakens the person sleeping in the recumbent position because the amount of blood returning to the heart and lungs from the lower extremities increases in this position.

Anyone who cannot climb a single flight of stairs without feeling moderately to severely winded or who awakens at night or experiences shortness of breath when lying down should be evaluated by a physician. Anyone with known cardiac involvement who develops progressively worse dyspnea must also notify the physician of these changes.

Dyspnea relieved by specific breathing patterns (e.g., pursed-lip breathing) or by specific body position (e.g., leaning forward on the arms to lock the shoulder girdle) is more likely to be pulmonary than cardiac in origin. Because breathlessness can be a terrifying experience for many persons, any activity that provokes the sensation is avoided, thus quickly reducing functional activities.

Cardiac Syncope

Cardiac syncope (fainting) or more mild lightheadedness can be caused by reduced oxygen delivery to the brain. Cardiac conditions resulting in syncope include arrhythmias, orthostatic hypotension, poor ventricular function, coronary artery disease, and vertebral artery insufficiency.

Lightheadedness that results from orthostatic hypotension (sudden drop in blood pressure) may occur with any quick change in a prolonged position (e.g., going from a supine position to an upright posture or standing up from a sitting position) or physical exertion involving increased abdominal pressure (e.g., straining with a bowel movement, lifting). Any client with aortic stenosis is likely to experience lightheadedness as a result of these activities.

Noncardiac conditions such as anxiety and emotional stress can cause hyperventilation and subsequent lightheadedness (vasovagal syncope). Side effects such as orthostatic hypotension may also occur during the period of initiation and regulation of cardiac medications (e.g., vasodilators).

Syncope that occurs without any warning period of lightheadedness, dizziness, or nausea may be a sign of heart valve or arrhythmia problems. Since sudden death can thus occur, medical referral is recommended for any unexplained syncope, especially in the presence of heart or circulatory problems or if the client has any risk factors for heart attack or stroke.

Examination of the cervical spine may include vertebral artery tests for compression of the vertebral arteries.[1-4] If signs of eye nystagmus, changes in pupil size, or visual disturbances and symptoms of dizziness or lightheadedness occur, care must be taken concerning any treatment that follows. It has been suggested, however, that other factors, such as individual sensitivity to extreme head positions, age, and vestibular responsiveness, could affect the results of these tests.[5]

Fatigue

Fatigue provoked by minimal exertion indicates a lack of energy, which may be cardiac in origin (e.g., coronary artery disease, aortic valve dysfunction, cardiomyopathy, or myocarditis) or may occur secondary to a neurologic, muscular, metabolic, or pulmonary pathologic condition. Often fatigue of a cardiac nature is accompanied by associated symptoms, such as dyspnea, chest pain, palpitations, or headache.

Fatigue that goes beyond expectations during or after exercise, especially in a client with a known cardiac condition, must be closely monitored. It should be remembered that beta-blockers prescribed for cardiac problems can also cause unusual fatigue symptoms.

For the client experiencing fatigue without a prior diagnosis of heart disease, monitoring vital signs may indicate a failure of the blood pressure to rise with increasing workloads. Such a situation may indicate cardiac output that is inadequate in meeting the demands of exercise. However, poor exercise tolerance is often the result of deconditioning, especially in the older

adult population. Further testing (e.g., exercise treadmill test) may be helpful in determining whether fatigue is cardiac-induced.

Cough

Cough (see also Chapter 7) is usually associated with pulmonary conditions, but it may occur as a pulmonary complication of a cardiovascular pathologic complex. Left ventricular dysfunction, including mitral valve dysfunction resulting from pulmonary edema or left ventricular CHF, may result in a cough when aggravated by exercise, metabolic stress, supine position, or PND. The cough is often hacking and may produce large amounts of frothy, blood-tinged sputum. In the case of CHF, cough develops because a large amount of fluid is trapped in the pulmonary tree, irritating the lung mucosa.

Cyanosis

Cyanosis is a bluish discoloration of the lips, and nail beds of the fingers and toes that accompanies inadequate blood oxygen levels (reduced amounts of hemoglobin). Although cyanosis can accompany hematologic or central nervous system disorders, most often visible cyanosis accompanies cardiac and pulmonary problems.

Edema

Edema in the form of a 3-pound or greater weight gain or a gradual, continuous gain over several days that results in swelling of the ankles, abdomen, and hands combined with shortness of breath, fatigue, and dizziness may be red-flag symptoms of CHF.

Other accompanying symptoms may include jugular vein distention (JVD) and cyanosis (of lips and appendages). Right upper quadrant pain described as a constant aching or sharp pain may occur secondary to an enlarged liver in this condition.

Right heart failure and subsequent edema can also occur secondary to cardiac surgery, venous valve incompetence or obstruction, cardiac valve stenosis, coronary artery disease, or mitral valve dysfunction.

Noncardiac causes of edema may include pulmonary hypertension, kidney dysfunction, cirrhosis, burns, infection, lymphatic obstruction, use of nonsteroidal antiinflammatory drugs (NSAIDs), or allergic reaction.

When edema and other accompanying symptoms persist despite rest, medical referral is required. Edema of a cardiac origin may require

electrocardiogram (ECG) monitoring during exercise or activity (the physician may not want the client stressed when extensive ECG changes are present), whereas edema of peripheral origin requires treatment of the underlying etiologic complex.

Claudication

Claudication or leg pain occurs with peripheral vascular disease (PVD) (arterial or venous), often occurring simultaneously with coronary artery disease. Claudication can be more functionally debilitating than other associated symptoms, such as angina or dyspnea, and may occur in addition to these other symptoms. The presence of pitting edema along with leg pain is usually associated with vascular disease.

Other noncardiac causes of leg pain (e.g., sciatica, pseudoclaudication, anterior compartment syndrome, gout, peripheral neuropathy) must be differentiated from pain associated with peripheral vascular disease. Low back pain associated with pseudoclaudication often indicates spinal stenosis. The discomfort associated with pseudoclaudication is frequently bilateral and improves with rest or flexion of the lumbar spine (see also Chapter 14).

Vascular claudication may occur in the absence of physical findings, but is usually accompanied by skin discoloration and trophic changes (e.g., thin, dry, hairless skin) in the presence of vascular disease. Core temperature, peripheral pulses, and skin temperature should be assessed. Cool skin is more indicative of vascular obstruction; warm to hot skin may indicate inflammation or infection. Abrupt onset of ischemic rest pain or sudden worsening of intermittent claudication may be due to thromboembolism and must be reported to the physician immediately.

If people with intermittent claudication have normal-appearing skin at rest, exercising the extremity to the point of claudication usually produces marked pallor in the skin over the distal third of the extremity. This postexercise cutaneous ischemia occurs in both upper and lower extremities and is due to selective shunting of the available blood to the exercised muscle and away from the more distal parts of the extremity.

Vital Signs

The therapist may see signs of cardiac dysfunction as abnormal responses of heart rate and blood pressure during exercise. The therapist must

remain alert to a heart rate that is either too high or too low during exercise, an irregular pulse rate, a systolic blood pressure that falls during exercise, a change in diastolic pressure greater than 15 to 20 mm Hg (Case Example 6-1).

Monitor vital signs in anyone with known heart disease. Some blood pressure lowering medications can keep a client's heart rate from exceeding 90 bpm. For these individuals the therapist can monitor heart rate, but use perceived rate of exertion (PRE) as a gauge of exercise intensity. See Chapter 4 for more specific information about vital sign assessment.

▶ CARDIAC PATHOPHYSIOLOGY

Three components of cardiac disease are discussed, including diseases affecting the heart muscle, diseases affecting heart valves, and defects of the cardiac nervous system (Table 6-2).

Conditions Affecting the Heart Muscle

In most cases a cardiopulmonary pathologic condition can be traced to at least one of three processes:

CASE EXAMPLE 6-1 Cardiac Impairment Affecting Balance

Chief Complaint: The 84-year-old woman was referred to outpatient physical therapy for gait training with a diagnosis of ataxia and "at risk" status for falls. The client's goal is to walk without staggering.

Social History: Retired, lives alone in a two-story house.

Past Medical History: Atrial fibrillation, hypertension, arthritis in both hands, visual impairment (right eye), allergies to Novocain and antibiotics, transient ischemic attacks (TIAs), recurrent pneumonia.

Current Medications: Diltiazem (calcium channel blocker), Toprol (antihypertensive, beta blocker), aspirin (nonsteroidal antiinflammatory), Oscal (antacid, calcium supplement)

Clinical Presentation: Client is independent with activities of daily living but slow to complete tasks. She goes up and down one flight of steep stairs 3 to 4 times a day, using a handrail. She is an independent community ambulator but admits to frequently "staggering" (ataxia) with several falls. Baseline testing:

1. Get-up-and-go test: 17 seconds (within normal limits)

2. Functional reach test: 8 inches (within normal limits)

Presence of other symptoms includes numbness along both feet that does not change with position. Shortness of breath with activity (short distance walking, ascending and descending 6 steps); recovers after a short rest. Thoracic kyphosis. Mild strength losses in hips, knees, and ankles. Reports of being "dizzy"

and "lightheaded," feeling like she is going to "fall out."

Vital signs:

Blood pressure (before activity)	136/79 mm Hg (arm and position not recorded)
Blood pressure (after activity)	132/69
10 minutes of activity)	
Pulse (before activity)	82 beats per minute
Pulse (after activity)	73 beats per minute

Assessment: This 84-year old client with a diagnosis of ataxia and risk of falls presented with fairly good bilateral lower extremity strength but had deficits in sensation and vision, increasing her risk for falling. She was quite resistant to using a cane for increased safety.

The client experienced an abnormal response to exercise in which the pulse rate and blood pressure decreased. She required several rest breaks during the exercise session due to "fading."

The therapist referred the client to her cardiologist for evaluation to determine medical stability before further intervention.

Result: Nuclear stress testing revealed blockage of two major coronary arteries requiring cardiac catheterization with balloon angioplasty and placement of a stent. The cardiologist confirmed the therapist's suspicions that the client's balance deficits from neuropathy and decreased vision were made worse by shortness of breath and lightheadedness from cardiac impairment.

Monitoring vital signs before and during exercise was a simple way to screen for underlying cardiovascular impairment.

From Goff T: Case report presented in partial fulfillment of DPT 910, *Principles of differential diagnosis*, Institute for Physical Therapy Education, Chester, Pennsylvania, 2005, Widener University. Used with permission.

TABLE 6-2 ▼ Cardiac Diseases

Heart muscle	Heart valves	Cardiac nervous system
Coronary artery disease	Rheumatic fever	Arrhythmias
Myocardial infarct	Endocarditis	Tachycardia
Pericarditis	Mitral valve	Bradycardia
Congestive heart failure	prolapse	
Aneurysms	Congenital	
	deformities	

1. Obstruction or restriction
2. Inflammation
3. Dilation or distention.

Any combination of these can cause chest, neck, back, and/or shoulder pain. Frequently, these conditions occur sequentially. For example, an underlying *obstruction*, such as pulmonary embolus, leads to *congestion*, and subsequent *dilation* of the vessels blocked by the embolus.

The most common cardiovascular conditions to mimic musculoskeletal dysfunction are angina, myocardial infarction, pericarditis, and dissecting aortic aneurysm. Other cardiovascular diseases are not included in this text because they are rare or because they do not mimic musculoskeletal symptoms.

Degenerative heart disease refers to the changes in the heart and blood supply to the heart and major blood vessels that occur with aging. As the population ages, degenerative heart disease becomes the most prevalent form of cardiovascular disease. Degenerative heart disease is also called atherosclerotic cardiovascular disease, arteriosclerotic cardiovascular disease, coronary heart disease (CHD), and coronary artery disease (CAD).

Hyperlipidemia

Hyperlipidemia refers to a group of metabolic abnormalities resulting in combinations of elevated serum total cholesterol (hypercholesterolemia), elevated low-density lipoproteins, elevated triglycerides (hypertriglyceridemia) and decreased high-density lipoproteins. These abnormalities are the primary risk factors for atherosclerosis and coronary artery disease.[6-8]

Statin medications (e.g., Zocor, Lipitor, Crestor, Lescol, Mevacor, Pravachol) are used to reduce LDL-cholesterol. While statins are generally well tolerated, there is a wide body of medical literature that associates the adverse reaction of myalgia and the more serious reaction of rhabdomyolysis with statin medications.[8,9] If detected early, statin-

related symptoms can be reversible with reduction of dose, selection of another statin, or cessation of statin use.[10,11]

SCREENING FOR SIDE EFFECTS OF STATINS

Myalgia is the most common myotoxic event associated with statins; joint pain is also reported. The incidence of myotoxic events appears to be dose-dependent. Rates of adverse events from statins vary in the literature from 5% up to 14%.[11,12]

Monitoring for elevated serum liver enzymes and creatine kinase are significant laboratory indicators of muscle and liver impairment.[13] Symptoms of mild myalgia (muscle ache or weakness without increased creatine [CK] levels), myositis (muscle symptoms with increased CK levels), or frank rhabdomyolysis (muscle symptoms with marked CK elevation; more than 10 times the normal upper limit) range from 1% to 7%.[8]

Muscular symptoms are more common in older individuals (Case Example 6-2).[8,14] Other risk factors include[15]

- Age over 80 (women more than men)
- Small body frame or frail
- Kidney or liver disease
- Drinks excessive grapefruit juice daily (more than 1 quart/day)
- Use of other medications (e.g., cyclosporine, some antibiotics, Verapamil, HIV protease inhibitors, some antidepressants)[15]
- Alcohol abuse (independently predisposes to myopathy)

Muscle aches and pain, unexplained fever, nausea, vomiting and dark urine can potentially be signs of myositis and should be referred to a physician immediately. Risk for statin-induced myositis is highest in people with liver disease, acute infection, and hypothyroidism. Screening for liver impairment (see Chapter 9) in people taking statins is an important part of assessing for rhabdomyolysis.[16]

Clinical Signs and Symptoms of Statin-Induced Side Effects

- Myalgia
- Unexplained fever
- Nausea, vomiting
- Signs and symptoms of liver impairment:
  Dark urine
  Asterixis (liver flap)
  Bilateral carpal tunnel syndrome
  Palmar erythema (liver palms)
  Spider angiomas
  Nail bed changes, skin color changes
  Ascites

CASE EXAMPLE 6-2 Statins and Myalgia

Referral: The client was a 53-year-old woman who complained of right-sided knee pain and stiffness and constant, bilateral thigh pain. She was referred by her orthopedic surgeon for physical therapy with a musculoskeletal diagnosis of osteoarthritis of both knees.

Medications: Lipitor (antilipemic for high cholesterol), Lopressor (anti-hypertensive, beta blocker), Ambien (sedative for insomnia), Naprosyn (anti-inflammatory). Dosage of the Lipitor was increased from 20 mg to 40 mg at the last physician visit.

Past Medical History: Hypertension, hypercholesterolemia, insomnia

Clinical Presentation: Pain pattern—Client reported constant but variable pain in the right knee, ranging from 2/10 at rest and 5/10 during and after weight-bearing activities. Morning stiffness was prominent, and the client described difficulty transitioning from prolonged sitting to standing. The client reported increased pain in the right knee after weight bearing for approximately five minutes.

In addition to the right-sided knee pain, the client also complained of a constant anterior thigh pain. This pain was described as a "flushing" sensation and was unchanged by position or motion. The intensity of the bilateral constant thigh pain was rated 3-4/10.

Complete physical examination of integument and gait inspection, muscle strength, and joint range of motion (ROM) was conducted and results recorded (on file). Findings from the lower quarter screen (LQS) were unremarkable. Lumbar ROM was WNL.

Neurologic screening exam—within normal limits

Review of Systems: Unremarkable; no other associated signs or symptoms reported. What are the red flags in this scenario?

Red Flags:

Age

Constant, bilateral myalgic pain unchanged by position or motion

Recent dosage change in medication

Is it safe to treat this client?

Physical therapy intervention can be implemented despite complaints of pain from an unknown origin. In the past 10 weeks prior to

the initial physical therapy examination, this client had been evaluated by a physician four times. The most recent evaluation was by an orthopedic surgeon one week prior to her initial evaluation.

Additionally, the client appeared to be otherwise in good health, her ROS was unremarkable. The presence of three red flags warrants careful observation of response to intervention, progression of current symptoms, or onset of any new symptoms.

Symptoms related to OA were expected to improve, while symptoms from a non-musculoskeletal origin were not expected to improve. The plan of care was explained to the client, and it was mutually agreed that if the constant thigh pain did not significantly improve within 4 weeks, the client would be referred back to her physician.

Result: Four weeks after the initial physical therapy visit symptoms of constant thigh pain had not resolved. The client had a follow up appointment with her orthopedic surgeon at which time she presented documentation of the physical therapy intervention to date and the therapist's concerns about the thigh pain.

The orthopedic surgeon reiterated his belief that the origin of her symptoms were due to OA. The client was instructed to continue physical therapy and to take Naprosyn as prescribed.

The client was discharged after receiving eight weeks of physical therapy intervention. At this juncture, the therapist believed that the client's right-sided knee symptoms were sufficiently improved and that the client could maintain or improve upon her current status by following her discharge instructions.

Furthermore, the myalgic thigh symptoms had not improved in the last eight weeks and the therapist did not feel the bilateral thigh myalgia would be improved by further physical therapy interventions.

The client was instructed to contact her primary care physician regarding her myalgic symptoms. Three days later, the client called her primary care physician rather than the physical therapy clinic. She had called her orthopedic surgeon rather than the primary care physician. According to the client, the orthopedic surgeon dismissed the association between the

CASE EXAMPLE 6-2 Statins and Myalgia—cont'd

thigh myalgia and the increased dosage of atorvastatin calcium (Lipitor). The client was again instructed to contact her primary care physician regarding the possibility of an adverse myalgic reaction to atorvastatin calcium (Lipitor). The client was also asked to contact the physical therapy clinic after being evaluated by her primary care physician.

Two weeks later, the client called and indicated her primary care physician evaluated her two days following our telephone conversation. The primary care physician discontinued the atorvastatin calcium (Lipitor). The client reported approximately a 50% reduction in the constant bilateral thigh myalgia after discontinuing the atorvastatin calcium (Lipitor).

The client was asked to contact the therapist in two or three weeks to provide an update of her status. Three weeks passed without hearing from the client. The therapist contacted the client by telephone. The client indicated that approximately four weeks following the discontinuation of the atorvastatin calcium (Lipitor)

her myalgic thigh complaints were fully resolved.

She stated that she would remain off the atorvastatin calcium (Lipitor) for a total of twelve weeks and then would receive clinical laboratory testing to evaluate serum cholesterol levels. The primary care physician would consider prescribing a different statin to control her hypercholesterolemia based on future cholesterol levels.

Summary: Medication used in many situations may have a significant effect on the health of the client and may alter the clinical presentation or course of the individual's symptoms. It is important to ask if the client is taking any new medication (over the counter or by prescription), nutraceutical supplements, and if there have been any recent changes in the dosages of current medications.

There is a wide body of medical literature that associates the adverse reaction of myalgia and the more serious reaction of rhabdomyolysis with statin medications. Therapists must perform good pharmacovigilance.

From Trumbore DJ: Case report presented in partial fulfillment of DPT 910. *Principles of differential diagnosis*, Institute for Physical Therapy Education, Chester, Pennsylvania, 2005, Widener University. Used with permission.

Coronary Artery Disease

The heart muscle must have an adequate blood supply to contract properly. As mentioned, the coronary arteries carry oxygen and blood to the myocardium. When a coronary artery becomes narrowed or blocked, the area of the heart muscle supplied by that artery becomes ischemic and injured, and infarction may result.

The major disorders caused by insufficient blood supply to the myocardium are angina pectoris and myocardial infarction. These disorders are collectively known as coronary artery disease (CAD), also called coronary heart disease or ischemic heart disease. CAD includes atherosclerosis (fatty buildup), thrombus (blood clot), and spasm (intermittent constriction).

CAD results from a person's complex genetic makeup and interactions with the environment, including nutrition, activity levels, and history of smoking. Susceptibility to CVD may be explained by genetic factors, and it is likely that an "atherosclerosis gene" or "heart attack gene" will be iden-

tified.[17] The therapeutic use of drugs that act by modifying gene transcription is a well-established practice in the treatment of CAD and essential hypertension.[18,19]

ATHEROSCLEROSIS

Atherosclerosis is the disease process often called arteriosclerosis or hardening of the arteries. It is a progressive process that begins in childhood. It can occur in any artery in the body, but it is most common in medium-sized arteries, such as those of the heart, brain, kidneys, and legs. Starting in childhood, the arteries begin to fill with a fatty substance, or lipids such as triglycerides and cholesterol, which then calcify or harden (Fig. 6-2).

This filler, called plaque, is made up of fats, calcium, and fibrous scar tissue, and lines the usually supple arterial walls, progressively narrowing the arteries. These arteries carry blood rich in oxygen to the myocardium (middle layer of the heart consisting of the heart muscle), but the atherosclerotic process leads to ischemia and to

necrosis of the heart muscle. Necrotic tissue gradually forms a scar, but before scar formation, the weakened area is susceptible to aneurysm development.

When fully developed, plaque can cause bleeding, clot formation, and distortion or rupture of a blood vessel (Fig. 6-3). Heart attacks and strokes are the most sudden and often fatal signs of the disease.

THROMBUS

When plaque builds up on the artery walls, the blood flow is slowed and a clot (thrombus) may form on the plaque. When a vessel becomes blocked with a clot, it is called thrombosis. Coronary thrombosis refers to the formation of a clot in one of the coronary arteries, usually causing a heart attack.

SPASM

Sudden constriction of a coronary artery is called a spasm; blood flow to that part of the heart is cut off or decreased. A brief spasm may cause mild symptoms that never return. A prolonged spasm may cause heart damage, such as an infarct. This process can occur in healthy persons who have no cardiac history, as well as in those who have known atherosclerosis. Chemicals like nicotine and cocaine may lead to coronary artery spasm; other possible factors include anxiety and cold air.

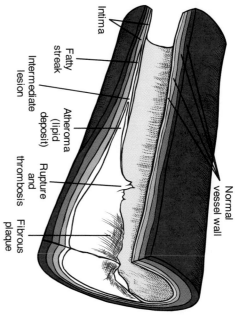

Fig. 6-2 • Hardening of the arteries. Atherosclerosis begins with an injury to the endothelial lining of the artery (intimal layer) that makes the vessel permeable to circulating lipoproteins. Penetration of lipoproteins into the smooth muscle cells of the intima produces "fatty streaks." A fibrous plaque large enough to decrease blood flow through the artery develops. Calcification with rupture or hemorrhage of the fibrous plaque is the final advanced stage. Thrombosis (stationary blood clot) may occur, further occluding the lumen of the blood vessel.

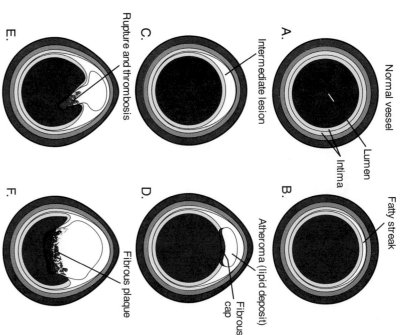

Fig. 6-3 • Updated model of atherosclerosis. New technology using intravascular ultrasound shows the whole atherosclerotic plaque and has changed the way we view things. The traditional model held that an atherosclerotic plaque in the blood vessel, particularly a coronary blood vessel, kept growing inward and obstructing flow until it closed off and caused a heart attack. This is not entirely correct. **A,** It is more accurate to say that in the normal vessel **B,** Penetration of lipoproteins into the smooth muscle cells of the intima produces fatty streaks and the start of a coronary lesion forms. **C** and **D,** The coronary lesion grows outward first in a compensatory manner to maintain the open lumen. This is called *positive remodeling*, as the blood vessel tries to maintain an open lumen until it can do so no more. **E,** Only then does the plaque (atheroma) begin to build up, gradually pressing inward into the lumen with obstruction of blood flow and possible rupture and thrombosis potentially leading to myocardial infarction or stroke. **F,** Vascular disease today is considered a disease of the wall. Some researchers like to say the disease is in the donut, not the hole of a donut, and that is a new concept.[20]

RISK FACTORS

In 1948 the United States government decided to investigate the etiology, incidence, and pathology of CAD by studying residents of a typical small town in the United States called Framingham, Massachusetts. Over the next multiple decades, various aspects of lifestyle, health, and disease were studied.

The research revealed important modifiable and nonmodifiable risk factors associated with death caused by CHD. Since that time, an additional category, contributing factors, has been added (Table 6-3). The American Heart Association has also developed a validated health-risk appraisal instrument called the RISKO scale. Anyone can use this tool to assess individual risk (www.americanheart.org/risk/quiz.html).

More recent research has identified other possible risk factors for and predictors of cardiac events, especially for those persons who have already had a heart attack. These additional risk factors include:

1. Exposure to bacteria such as *Chlamydia pneumoniae*, *Porphyromonas gingivalis*, and *Cytomegalovirus* organisms. [21-23]

2. Excess levels of homocysteine, an amino acid by-product of food rich in proteins

3. High levels of α-lipoprotein, a close cousin of low-density lipoprotein that transports fat throughout the body

4. High levels of fibrinogen, a protein that binds together platelet cells in blood clots [24]

5. Large amounts of C-reactive protein, a specialized protein necessary for repair of tissue injury. [25,26]

6. The presence of troponin T, a regulatory protein that helps heart muscle contract [27] and

7. The presence of diagonal earlobe creases [28,29]

Therapists can assist clients in assessing his or her 10-year risk for heart attack using a risk assessment tool from the National Cholesterol Education program available at http://hin.nhlbi.nih.gov/atpiii/calculator.asp?usertype=prof

WOMEN AND HEART DISEASE

Many women know about the risk of breast cancer, but in truth, they are 10 times more likely to die of cardiovascular disease. While 1 in 30 deaths is from breast cancer, 1 in 2.5 deaths are from heart disease. [30]

Women do not seem to do as well as men after taking medications to dissolve blood clots or after undergoing heart-related medical procedures. Of the women who survive a heart attack, 46% will be disabled by heart failure within 6 years. [31]

In general, the rate of coronary artery disease (CAD) is rising among women and falling among men. Men develop CAD at a younger age than women, but women make up for it after menopause. African-American women have a 70% higher death rate from CAD than white women. So whenever screening chest pain, keep in mind the demographics: older men and women, menopausal women, and black women are at greatest risk.

Diabetes alone poses a greater risk than any other factor in predicting cardiovascular problems in women. Women with diabetes are seven times more likely to have cardiovascular complications and about half of them will die of CAD. [32]

Studies have shown that women and men actually differ in the symptoms of CAD and in the manner in which acute MI can present. Women experience symptoms of CAD, which are more subtle and are "atypical" compared to the traditional symptoms such as angina and chest pain.

One of the most important primary signs of CAD in women is unexplained, severe episodic fatigue and weakness associated with decreased ability to carry out normal activities of daily living (ADLs). Because fatigue, weakness, and trouble sleeping are general types of symptoms, they are not as easily associated with cardiovascular events and are many times missed by health care providers in screening for heart disease. [33]

Symptoms of weakness, fatigue and sleeping difficulty and nausea have been reported as a common occurrence as much as a month prior to the development of acute MI in women (see Table 6-4). The classic pain of CAD is usually substernal chest pain characterized by a crushing, heavy, squeezing sensation commonly occurring during emotion or exertion. The pain of CAD in women, however may vary greatly from that in men (see further discussion, Myocardial Infarction, this chapter).

Risk reduction in women focuses on lifestyle changes such as smoking cessation, low fat, low cholesterol diet, increased intake of omega-3 fatty acids, increased fruit, vegetable, whole grain

TABLE 6-3 ▼ Risk Factors for Coronary Artery Disease

Modifiable risk factors	Nonmodifiable risk factors	Contributing factors
Physical inactivity	Age	Obesity
Cigarette smoking	Male gender	Response to stress
Elevated serum cholesterol	Family history	Personality
High blood pressure	Race	Peripheral vascular disease
	Postmenopausal (female)	Hormonal status
		Alcohol consumption

Modified from Reigle J, Ringel KA: Nursing care of clients with disorders of cardiac function. In Black JM, Matassarin-Jacobs E, editors: *Luckmann and Sorensen's medical-surgical nursing*, ed 4, Philadelphia, 1993, WB Saunders; p 1140.

intake, salt and alcohol limitation, and increased exercise and weight loss. If the woman has diabetes, strict glucose control is extremely important.[34]

CLINICAL SIGNS AND SYMPTOMS

Atherosclerosis, by itself, does not necessarily produce symptoms. For manifestations to develop there must be a critical deficit in blood supply to the heart in proportion to the demands of the myocardium for oxygen and nutrients (supply and demand imbalance). When atherosclerosis develops slowly, collateral circulation develops to meet the heart's demands. Often, symptoms of CAD do not appear until the lumen of the coronary artery narrows by 75% (see also Hypertension).

Although the arteries are rarely completely blocked, the deposits of plaque are often extensive enough to restrict blood flow to the heart, especially during exercise in a clinical practice when there is a need to deliver more oxygen-carrying blood to the heart. Like other muscles, the heart, when deprived of oxygen, may ache, causing chest pain or discomfort referred to as angina.

CAD is a progressive disorder, especially if left untreated. If the blood flow is entirely disrupted, usually by a clot that has formed in the obstructed region, some of the tissue that is supplied by the vessel can die, and a heart attack or even sudden cardiac death results.

When tissue loss is extensive enough to disrupt the electrical impulses that stimulate the heart's contractions, heart failure, chronic arrhythmias, and conduction disturbances may develop.

Angina

Acute pain in the chest, called angina pectoris, results from the imbalance between cardiac workload and oxygen supply to myocardial tissue. Angina is a symptom of obstructed or decreased blood supply to the heart muscle primarily from a condition called atherosclerosis.

Atherosclerosis is now recognized as an inflammatory condition affecting the coronary arteries as well as the peripheral vessels. It is often accompanied by hypertension and signs of peripheral vascular disease (PVD). Although the primary cause of angina is CAD, angina can occur in individuals with normal coronary arteries and with other conditions affecting the supply/demand balance.

As vessels become lined with atherosclerotic plaque, symptoms of inadequate blood supply develop in the tissues supplied by these vessels. A growing mass of plaque in the vessel collects platelets, fibrin, and cellular debris. Platelet aggregations are known to release prostaglandin capable of causing vessel spasm. This in turn promotes platelet aggregation, and a vicious spasm/pain cycle begins.

The present theory of heart pain suggests that pain occurs as a result of an accumulation of metabolites within an ischemic segment of the myocardium. The transient ischemia of angina or the prolonged, necrotic ischemia of a myocardial infarction sets off pain impulses secondary to rapid accumulation of these metabolites in the heart muscle.

The imbalance between cardiac workload and oxygen supply can develop as a result of disorders of the coronary vessels, disorders of circulation, increased demands on output of the heart, or damaged myocardium unable to utilize oxygen properly.

TYPES OF ANGINAL PAIN

There are a number of types of anginal pain, including chronic stable angina (also referred to as walk-through angina), resting angina (angina decubitus), unstable angina, nocturnal angina, atypical angina, new-onset angina, and Prinzmetal's or "variant" angina.

Chronic stable angina occurs at a predictable level of physical or emotional stress and responds promptly to rest or to nitroglycerin. No pain occurs at rest, and the location, duration, intensity, and frequency of chest pain are consistent over time.

Resting angina, or *angina decubitus*, is chest pain that occurs at rest in the supine position and frequently at the same time every day. The pain is neither brought on by exercise nor relieved by rest.

Unstable angina, also known as crescendo angina, preinfarction angina, or progressive angina, is an abrupt change in the intensity and frequency of symptoms or decreased threshold of stimulus, such as the onset of chest pain while at rest. The duration of these attacks is longer than the usual 1 to 5 minutes; they may last for up to 20 to 30 minutes. Pain or discomfort is unrelieved by rest or nitroglycerin signals a higher risk for myocardial infarction. Such changes in the pattern of angina require immediate medical follow up by the client's physician.

Nocturnal angina may awaken a person from sleep with the same sensation experienced during exertion. During sleep this exertion is usually caused by dreams. This type of angina may be associated with underlying CHF.

Atypical angina refers to unusual symptoms (e.g., toothache or earache) related to physical or emotional exertion. These symptoms subside with

rest or nitroglycerin. New-onset angina describes angina that has developed for the first time within the last 60 days.

Prinzmetal's angina produces symptoms similar to those of typical angina but is caused by coronary artery spasm. These spasms periodically squeeze arteries shut and keep the blood from reaching the heart. Coronary arteries are usually clear of plaque or physiologic changes causing obstruction of the blood vessels.

This form of angina occurs at rest, especially in the early hours of the morning, and can be difficult to induce by exercise. It is cyclic and frequently occurs at the same time each day. In postmenopausal women who are not undergoing hormone replacement therapy, the reduction in estrogen may cause coronary arteries to spasm, resulting in vasospastic (Prinzmetal's) angina.

CLINICAL SIGNS AND SYMPTOMS

The client may indicate the location of the symptoms by placing a clenched fist against the sternum. Angina radiates most commonly to the left shoulder and down the inside of the arm to the fingers; but it can also refer pain to the neck, jaw, teeth, upper back, possibly down the right arm, and occasionally to the abdomen (see Fig. 6-8).

Recognizing heart pain in women is more difficult because the symptoms are less reliable and often do not follow the classic pattern described earlier. Many women describe the pain in ways consistent with unstable angina, suggesting that they first become aware of their chest discomfort or have it diagnosed only after it reaches more advanced stages.

Some experience a sensation similar to inhaling cold air, rather than the more typical shortness of breath. Other women complain only of weakness and lethargy, and some have noted isolated pain in the midthoracic spine or throbbing and aching in the right biceps muscle (Fig. 6-4).

Pain associated with the angina and myocardial infarction occurring along the inner aspect of the arm and corresponding to the ulnar nerve distribution results from common connections between the cardiac and brachial plexuses.

Cardiac pain referred to the jaw occurs through internuncial (neurons connecting other neurons) fibers from cervical spinal cord posterior horns to the spinal nucleus of the trigeminal nerve. Abdominal pain produced by referred cardiac pain is more difficult to explain and may be due to the overflow of segmental levels to which visceral afferent nerve pathways flow (see Fig. 3-3). This overflow increases the chances that final common pain

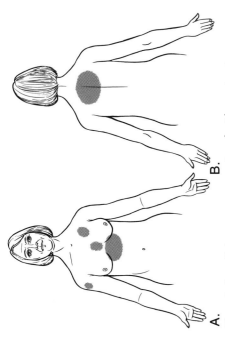

A.

B.

Fig. 6-4 • Pain patterns associated with angina in women may differ from patterns in men. Many presenting symptoms are subjective such as extreme fatigue, lethargy, breathlessness, or weakness. Isolated pain in the right mid-biceps may delay diagnosis. More classic pain patterns as shown in Fig. 6-8 are also possible.

pathways between the chest and the abdomen may occur.

The *sensation* of angina is described as squeezing, burning, pressing, choking, aching, or bursting. Chest pain can be brought on by a wide variety of noncardiac causes (see discussion of chest pain in Chapter 17).

In particular, angina is often confused with heartburn or indigestion, hiatal hernia, esophageal spasm, or gallbladder disease, but the pain of these other conditions is not described as sharp or knifelike.

The client often says the pain feels like "gas" or "heartburn" or "indigestion." Referred pain from a trigger point in the external oblique abdominal muscle can cause a sensation of heartburn in the anterior chest wall (see Fig. 17-7, *D*). A physician must make the differentiation between angina and heartburn, hiatal hernia, and gallbladder disease. The therapist can assess for trigger points; relief of symptoms with elimination of trigger points is an important diagnostic finding.

Clinical Signs and Symptoms of

Heartburn

- Frequent "heartburn" attacks
- Frequent use of antacids to relieve symptoms
- Heartburn wakes client up at night
- Acid or bitter taste in the mouth
- Burning sensation in the chest
- Discomfort after eating spicy foods
- Abdominal bloating and gas
- Difficulty in swallowing

Severity is usually mild or moderate. Rarely is the pain described as severe. The five-grade angina scale ranks angina as:

Grade 0 No angina
Grade 1 Light, barely noticeable
Grade 2 Moderately bothersome
Grade 3 Severe, very uncomfortable
Grade 4 Most pain ever experienced

As to *location*, 80% to 90% of clients experience the pain as retrosternal or slightly to the left of the sternum. The *duration* of angina as a direct result of myocardial ischemia is typically 1 to 3 minutes and no longer than 3 to 5 minutes. However, anger may last 15 to 20 minutes. Angina is relieved by rest or nitroglycerin (a coronary artery vasodilator).

People who have had coronary artery stents placed can experience angina if an occlusion occurs above, below or within the stent. Anyone with a stent who has chest pain should be immediately sent for referral to a physician.

Severity of pain is not a good prognostic indicator; some persons with severe discomfort live for many years, whereas others with mild symptoms may die suddenly. If the pain is not relieved by rest or up to 3 nitroglycerin tablets (taken one at a time at 5-minute intervals) in 10 to 15 minutes, the physician should be notified and the client taken to a cardiac care unit.

The client should take his or her own nitroglycerin. The therapist should not dispense medication but may assist the client in taking this medication. Nitroglycerin dilates the coronary arteries and improves collateral cardiac circulation, thus providing an increase in oxygen to the heart muscle and a decrease in symptoms of angina.

When screening for chest pain, a lack of objective musculoskeletal findings is always a red flag:

• Active range of motion (AROM) such as trunk rotation, side bending, shoulder motions does not reproduce symptoms
• Resisted motion (horizontal shoulder abduction/adduction) does not reproduce symptoms
• Heat and stretching do not reduce or eliminate symptoms

Clinical Signs and Symptoms of Angina Pectoris

• Gripping, viselike feeling of pain or pressure behind the breast bone
• Pain that may radiate to the neck, jaw, back, shoulder, or arms (most often the left arm in men)
• Toothache
• Burning indigestion
• Dyspnea (shortness of breath); exercise intolerance
• Nausea
• Belching

Myocardial Infarct

Myocardial infarct (MI), also known as a heart attack, coronary occlusion, or a "coronary," is the development of ischemia and necrosis of myocardial tissue. It results from a sudden decrease in coronary perfusion or an increase in myocardial oxygen demand without adequate blood supply. If the requirements for blood are not eased (e.g., by decreased activity), the heart attempts to continue meeting the increased demands for oxygen with an inadequate blood supply, which leads to an MI. Myocardial tissue death is usually preceded by a sudden occlusion of one or more of the major coronary arteries.

The myocardium receives its blood supply from the two large coronary arteries and their branches. Occlusion of one or more of these blood vessels (coronary occlusion) is one of the major causes of MI. The occlusion may result from the formation of a clot that develops suddenly when an atheromatous plaque ruptures through the sublayers of a blood vessel, or when the narrow, roughened inner lining of a sclerosed artery leads to complete thrombosis.

Although coronary thrombosis is the most common cause of infarction, many interrelated factors may be responsible, including coronary artery spasm, platelet aggregation and embolism, thrombus secondary to rheumatic heart disease, endocarditis, aortic stenosis, a thrombus on a prosthetic mitral or aortic valve, or a dislodged calcium plaque from a calcified aortic or mitral valve.

Coronary blood flow is affected by the tonus (tone) of the coronary arteries. Arteries "clogged" by plaque formation become rigid, and resultant spasm may be provoked by cold and by exercise, which explains the adverse effect of both factors on clients with angina.

CLINICAL SIGNS AND SYMPTOMS

There are some well-known pain patterns specific to the heart and cardiac system. Sudden death can be the first sign of heart disease In fact according to the American Heart Association, 63% of women who died suddenly of cardiovascular disease had no previous symptoms. Sudden death is the first symptom for half of all men who have a heart attack.

The onset of an infarct may be characterized by severe fatigue for several days before the infarct. The likelihood of having a heart attack in the morning hours is 40% higher than during the rest of the day.[35] The morning is when the body's clotting system is more active, blood pressure surges, heart rate increases, and there may be reduced blood flow to the heart.

Additionally, the levels and activity of stress hormones (e.g., catecholamines), which can induce vasoconstriction, increase in the morning. Combined with these factors are the increased mental and physical stresses that typically occur after waking. The shift worker would experience this same phenomenon in the evening or on arising.

Persons who have MIs may not experience any pain and may be unaware that damage is occurring to the heart muscle as a result of prolonged ischemia. The presence of silent infarction (SI) increases with advancing age, especially SI without a history of CAD.

Cardiac Arrest Researchers expect the number of Americans living with angina to grow as new treatments improve survival after heart attacks.[30] Failure to recognize prodromal symptoms in men or women may account for many cases of sudden cardiac death.[36]

Cardiac arrest strikes immediately and without warning. Signs of sudden cardiac arrest include[30]:
• Sudden loss of responsiveness. No response to gentle shaking.
• No normal breathing. The client does not take a normal breath when you check for several seconds.
• No signs of circulation. No movement or coughing.

If cardiac arrest occurs, call for emergency help and begin CPR immediately unless the client has a do not resuscitate (DNR) on file. Use an automated external defibrillator (AED) if available and appropriate.

Classic Warning Signs of Myocardial Infarction Those who do have warning signs of MI may have severe unrelenting chest pain described as "crushing pain" lasting 30 or more minutes that is not alleviated by rest or by nitroglycerin. This chest pain may radiate to the arms, throat, and back, persisting for hours (see Fig. 6-9).

Other symptoms include pallor, profuse perspiration, and possibly nausea and vomiting. The pain of an MI may be misinterpreted as indigestion because of the nausea and vomiting. A medical evaluation may be difficult because many clients have coexisting hiatal hernia, peptic ulcer, or gallbladder disease.

Cardiac pain patterns may differ for men and women. For many men, the most common report is a feeling of pressure or discomfort under the sternum (substernal), in the mid-chest region, or across the entire upper chest. It can feel like uncomfortable pressure, squeezing, fullness, or pain.

Pain may occur just in the jaw, upper neck, midback or down the arm without chest pain or discomfort. Pain may also radiate from the chest to the neck, jaw, mid back or down the arm(s). Pain down the arm(s) affects the left arm most often in the pattern of the ulnar nerve distribution. Radiating pain down both arms is also possible.

An MI may occur during exertion, exercise, or exposure to extremes of temperature, or it may occur while the person is at rest. A subtle variation on ischemia during exertion is an important one for the therapist.

The onset of an MI is known to be precipitated when working with the arms extended over the head. If the person becomes weak or short of breath while in this position, ischemia or infarction may be the cause of the pain and associated symptoms.

Because the infarction process may take up to 6 hours to complete, restoration of adequate myocardial perfusion is important if significant necrosis is to be limited. Deaths generally result from severe arrhythmias, cardiogenic shock, CHF, rupture of the heart, and recurrent MI.

Clinical Signs and Symptoms of
Myocardial Infarction

• May be silent (smokers, diabetics: reduced sensitivity to pain)
• Sudden cardiac death
• Prolonged or severe substernal chest pain or squeezing pressure
• Pain possibly radiating down one or both arms and/or up to the throat, neck, back, jaw, shoulders, or arms
• Feeling of indigestion
• Angina lasting for 30 minutes or more
• Angina unrelieved by rest, nitroglycerin, or antacids
• Pain of infarct unrelieved by rest or a change in position
• Nausea
• Sudden dimness or loss of vision or loss of speech
• Pallor
• Diaphoresis (heavy perspiration)
• Shortness of breath
• Weakness, numbness, and feelings of faintness

Warning Signs of Myocardial Infarction in Women

For women symptoms can be more subtle or "atypical." Chest pain or discomfort is less common in women, but still a key feature for some. Women describe heaviness, squeezing, or pain in the left side of the chest, abdomen, mid back (thoracic), shoulder, or arm with no mid chest symptoms.[37]

They often have prodromal symptoms up to one month before having a heart attack (Table 6-4).[36,38]

Fatigue, nausea, and lower abdominal pain may signal a heart attack. Many women pass these off as the flu or food poisoning. Other symptoms for women include a feeling of intense anxiety, isolated right biceps pain, or mid-thoracic pain, heartburn; sudden shortness of breath, or the inability to talk, move, or breathe; shoulder or arm pain; or ankle swelling or rapid weight gain.

In addition, she may describe palpitations or pain that is sharp and fleeting. Antacids may relieve it rather than rest or nitroglycerin. Women having an acute MI have also described a pain in the jaw, neck, shoulder, back, or ear and a feeling of intense anxiety, nausea, or shortness of breath. Many women do not associate these symptoms with having a heart attack and they may do nothing to seek help.[37]

Clinical Signs and Symptoms of Myocardial Ischemia in Women

- Heart pain in women does not always follow classic patterns
- Many women do experience classic chest discomfort
- Older female: mental status change or confusion may be common
- Dyspnea (at rest or with exertion)
- Weakness and lethargy (unusual fatigue; fatigue that interferes with ability to perform activities of daily living)
- Indigestion, heart burn, or stomach pain; mistakenly diagnosed or assumed to have gastroesophageal reflux disease (GERD)
- Anxiety or depression
- Sleep disturbance (woman awakens with any of the symptoms listed here)
- Sensation similar to inhaling cold air; unable to talk or breathe
- Isolated, continuous mid-thoracic or interscapular back pain
- Isolated right biceps aching
- Symptoms may be relieved by antacids (sometimes antacids work better than nitroglycerin)

TABLE 6-4 ▼ Heart Attack Symptoms in Women

One month before a heart attack		During a heart attack	
Unusual fatigue (71%)		Dyspnea (58%)	
Sleep disturbance (48%)		Weakness (55%)	
Dyspnea (42%)		Unusual fatigue (43%)	
Indigestion or GERD (39%)		Cold sweat (39%)	
Anxiety (36%)		Dizziness (39%)	
Heart racing (27%)		Nausea (36%)	
Arms weak/heavy (25%)		Arms weak/heavy (35%)	

McSweeney JC: Women's early warning symptoms of acute myocardial infarction, *Circulation* 108(21):2619-2623, 2003.

Pericarditis

Pericarditis is an inflammation of the pericardium, the sac-like covering of the heart. Specifically, it affects the parietal pericardium (fluid-like membrane between the fibrous pericardium and the epicardium) and the visceral (epicardium) pericardium (Fig. 6-5).

This inflammatory process may develop either as a primary condition or secondary to a number of diseases and conditions (e.g., influenza, HIV infection, tuberculosis, cancer, kidney failure, hypothyroidism, autoimmune disorders). Myocardial injury or trauma such as a heart attack, chest injury, chest radiation, or cardiac surgery can cause pericarditis. Very often the cause is unknown resulting in a diagnosis of idiopathic pericarditis.

Pericarditis may be acute or chronic (recurring); it is not known why pericarditis may be a single illness in some persons and recurrent in others. Chronic or recurring pericarditis is accompanied by a pericardium that is rigid, thickened, and scarred.

Previous infection may be mild or asymptomatic with postinfectious onset of pain occurring 1 to 3 weeks later. Because this condition can occur in any age group, a history of recent pericarditis in the presence of new onset of chest, neck, or left shoulder pain is important.

CLINICAL SIGNS AND SYMPTOMS

At first, pericarditis may have no external signs or symptoms. The symptoms of acute pericarditis vary with the cause but usually include chest pain and dyspnea, an increase in the pulse rate, and a rise in temperature. Malaise and myalgia may occur.

Over time, the inflammatory process may result in an accumulation of fluid in the pericardial sac,

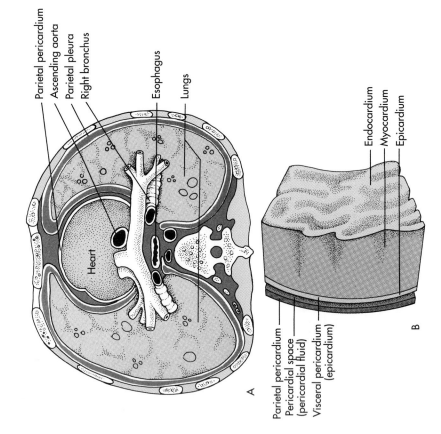

Parietal pericardium
Ascending aorta
Parietal pleura
Right bronchus

Esophagus

Lungs

Parietal pericardium
Pericardial space (pericardial fluid)
Visceral pericardium (epicardium)

Heart

A

Endocardium
Myocardium
Epicardium

B

Fig. 6-5 • The heart and associated layers of membranes. **A,** Cross section through the thorax just above the heart, emphasizing the lining of the cavity that contains the lungs (parietal pleura) and the lining of the cavity that contains the heart (parietal pericardium). **B,** Sagittal view of the layers of the heart.

TABLE 6-5 ▼ Characteristics of Cardiac Chest Pain

Angina	Myocardial infarct	Mitral valve prolapse	Pericarditis
Begins 3 to 5 minutes after exertion or activity ("lagtime"); 1-5 minutes	30 minutes-hour	Minutes to hours	Hours to days
Moderate intensity Tightness; chest discomfort	Severe (can be painless) Crushing pain; intolerable (can be painless)	Rarely severe May be asymptomatic; "sticking" sensation, not substernal	Varies; mild to severe Asymptomatic; sharp or cutting; can mimic MI
Can occur at rest or during sleep	Exertion	Often occurs at rest	Worse with breathing, swallowing, belching, neck or trunk movement
Usually occurs with exertion, emotion, cold, or large meal			
Subsides with rest or nitroglycerin; worse when lying down	Unrelieved by rest or nitroglycerin	Unrelieved by rest or nitroglycerin; may be relieved by lying down	Relieved by kneeling on all fours, leaning forward, sitting upright, or breatholding
Pain related to tone of arteries (spasm)	Pain related to heart ischemia	Mechanism of pain unknown	Pain related to inflammatory process

preventing the heart from expanding fully. The inflamed pericardium may cause pain when it rubs against the heart. Chest pain from pericarditis (see Fig. 6-10) closely mimics that of an MI since it is substernal, is associated with cough, and may

radiate to the left shoulder or supraclavicular area. It can be differentiated from MI by the pattern of relieving and aggravating factors (Table 6-5).

For example, the pain of an MI is unaffected by position, breathing, or movement, whereas the

pain associated with pericarditis may be relieved by kneeling on all fours, leaning forward, or sitting upright. Pericardial chest pain is often worse with breathing, swallowing, belching, or neck or trunk movements, especially side bending or rotation. The pain tends to be sharp or cutting and may recur in intermittent bursts that are usually precipitated by a change in body position. Pericarditis pain may diminish if the breath is held.

Clinical Signs and Symptoms of Pericarditis

- Substernal pain that may radiate to the neck, upper back, upper trapezius muscle, left supraclavicular area, down the left arm to the costal margins
- Difficulty in swallowing
- Pain relieved by leaning forward or sitting upright
- Pain aggravated by movement associated with deep breathing (laughing, coughing, deep inspiration)
- Pain relieved or reduced by holding the breath
- Pain aggravated by trunk movements (side bending or rotation) and by lying down
- History of fever, chills, weakness, or heart disease (a recent myocardial infarction accompanying the pattern of symptoms may alert the therapist to the need for medical referral to rule out cardiac involvement)
- Cough
- Lower extremity edema (feet, ankles, legs)

Congestive Heart Failure or Heart Failure

Heart failure, also called cardiac decompensation and cardiac insufficiency, can be defined as a physiologic state in which the heart is unable to pump enough blood to meet the metabolic needs of the body (determined as oxygen consumption) at rest or during exercise, even though filling pressures are adequate.

The heart fails when, because of intrinsic disease or structural defects, it cannot handle a normal blood volume, or in the absence of disease cannot tolerate a sudden expansion in blood volume (e.g., exercise). Heart failure is not a disease itself; instead, the term denotes a group of manifestations related to inadequate pump performance from either the cardiac valves or the myocardium.

Whatever the cause, when the heart fails to propel blood forward normally, congestion occurs in the pulmonary circulation as blood accumulates in the lungs. The right ventricle, which is not yet affected by congestive heart disease, continues to pump more blood into the lungs. The immediate result is shortness of breath and, if the process continues, actual flooding of the air spaces of the lungs with fluid seeping from the distended blood vessels. This last phenomenon is called pulmonary congestion or pulmonary edema.

Because a properly functioning heart depends on both ventricles, failure of one ventricle almost always leads to failure of the other ventricle. This is called ventricular interdependence. Right-sided ventricular failure (right-sided heart failure) causes congestion of the peripheral tissues and viscera. The liver may enlarge, the ankles may swell, and the client develops ascites (fluid accumulates in the abdomen).

Some clients have preexisting mild-to-moderate heart disease with no evidence of CHF. However, when the heart undergoes undue stress or deterioration from risk factors, compensatory mechanisms may be inadequate, and the heart fails.

Conditions that precipitate or exacerbate heart failure include hypertension, CAD, cardiomyopathy, heart valve abnormalities, arrhythmia, fever, infection, anemia, thyroid disorders, pregnancy, Paget's disease, nutritional deficiency (e.g., thiamine deficiency secondary to alcoholism), pulmonary disease, spinal cord injury, and hypervolemia from poor renal function.

Medications are frequently implicated in the development of CHF. Examples include cardiovascular drugs, antibiotics, central nervous system drugs (e.g., sedatives, hypnotics, antidepressants, narcotic analgesics), and antiinflammatory drugs (both nonsteroidal and steroidal).

CLINICAL SIGNS AND SYMPTOMS

The incidence of CHF increases with advancing age. Because of the increasing age of the U.S. population and newer medications and technologies that have increased survival at the expense of increased cardiovascular morbidity, the population affected by CHF is markedly increasing. In view of this increase, many individuals with a wide variety of heart and lung diseases will very likely develop CHF at some time during their lives, manifesting itself as pulmonary congestion or edema.[39]

Left Ventricular Failure Failure of the left ventricle causes either pulmonary congestion or a disturbance in the respiratory control mechanisms. These problems in turn precipitate respiratory distress. The degree of distress varies with the client's position, activity, and level of stress.

However, many persons with severely impaired ventricular performance may have few or no

symptoms, particularly if heart failure has developed gradually. Breathlessness, exhaustion, and lower extremity edema are the most common signs and symptoms of CHF.

Dyspnea is subjective and does not always correlate with the extent of heart failure. To some degree, exertional dyspnea occurs in all clients. The increased fluid in the tissue spaces causes dyspnea, at first on effort and then at rest, by stimulation of stretch receptors in the lung and chest wall and by the increased work of breathing with stiff lungs.

Paroxysmal nocturnal dyspnea (PND) resembles the frightening sensation of suffocation. The client suddenly awakens with the feeling of severe suffocation. Once the client is in the upright position, relief from the attack may not occur for 30 minutes or longer.

Orthopnea is a more advanced stage of dyspnea. The client often assumes a "three-point position," sitting up with both hands on the knees and leaning forward. Orthopnea develops because the supine position increases the amount of blood returning from the lower extremities to the heart and lungs. This gravitational redistribution of blood increases pulmonary congestion and dyspnea. The client learns to avoid respiratory distress at night by supporting the head and thorax on pillows. In severe heart failure the client may resort to sleeping upright in a chair.

Cough is a common symptom of left ventricular failure and is often hacking, producing large amounts of frothy, blood-tinged sputum. The client coughs because a large amount of fluid is trapped in the pulmonary tree, irritating the lung mucosa.

Pulmonary edema may develop when rapidly rising pulmonary capillary pressure causes fluid to move into the alveoli, resulting in extreme breathlessness, anxiety, frothy sputum, nasal flaring, use of accessory breathing muscles, tachypnea, noisy and wet breathing, and diaphoresis.

Cerebral hypoxia may occur as a result of a decrease in cardiac output, causing inadequate brain perfusion. Depressed cerebral function can cause anxiety, irritability, restlessness, confusion, impaired memory, bad dreams, and insomnia.

Fatigue and muscular cramping or weakness is often associated with left ventricular failure (Case Example 6-3). Inadequate cardiac output leads to hypoxic tissue and slowed removal of metabolic wastes, which in turn causes the client to tire easily. A common report is feeling tired after an activity or type of exertion that was easily accomplished previously. Disturbances in sleep and rest patterns may aggravate fatigue.

Nocturia (urination at night) develops as a result of renal changes that can occur in both right- and left-sided heart failure (but more evident in left-sided failure). During the day the affected individual is upright and blood flow is away from the

---

CASE EXAMPLE 6-3   Congestive Heart Failure—Muscle Cramping and Headache

A 74-year-old retired homemaker had a total hip replacement (THR) 2 days ago and remains as an inpatient with complications related to congestive heart failure. She has a previous medical history of gallbladder removal 20 years ago, total hysterectomy 30 years ago, and surgically induced menopause with subsequent onset of hypertension. Her medications include intravenous furosemide (Lasix), digoxin, and potassium replacement.

During the initial physical therapy session, the client complained of muscle cramping and headache but was able to complete the entire exercise protocol. Blood pressure was 100/76 mm Hg. Systolic measurement dropped to 90 mm Hg when the client moved from supine to standing. Pulse rate was 56 bpm with a pattern of irregular pulse beats. Pulse rate did not change with

postural change. Platelet count was 98,000 cells/mm^3.

Result: With congestive heart failure, the heart will try to compensate by increasing the heart rate. However, the digoxin is designed to increase cardiac output and lower heart rate. In normal circumstances postural changes result in an increase in heart rate, but when digoxin is used, this increase cannot occur so the person becomes symptomatic. Most of the clients like this one are also taking beta-blockers, which also prevent the heart rate from increasing when the blood pressure drops.

In a clinical situation such as this one, the response of vital signs to exercise must be monitored carefully and charted. Any unusual symptoms, such as the muscle cramping and headaches, and any irregular pulse patterns must also be reported and documented.

kidneys with reduced formation of urine. At night urine formation increases as blood flow to the kidneys improves.

Nocturia may interfere with effective sleep patterns, contributing to the fatigue associated with CHF. As cardiac output falls, decreased renal blood flow may result in oliguria (reduced urine output), a late sign of heart failure.

Clinical Signs and Symptoms of Left-Sided Heart Failure

- Fatigue and dyspnea after mild physical exertion or exercise
- Persistent spasmodic cough, especially when lying down, while fluid moves from the extremities to the lungs
- Paroxysmal nocturnal dyspnea (occurring suddenly at night)
- Orthopnea (person must be in the upright position to breathe)
- Tachycardia
- Fatigue and muscle weakness
- Edema (especially of the legs and ankles) and weight gain
- Irritability/restlessness
- Decreased renal function or frequent urination at night

Right Ventricular Failure Failure of the right ventricle may occur in response to left-sided CHF or as a result of pulmonary embolism (see cor pulmonale, Chapter 7). Right ventricular failure results in peripheral edema and venous congestion of the organs.

For example, as the liver becomes congested with venous blood, it becomes enlarged and abdominal pain occurs. If this occurs rapidly, stretching of the capsule surrounding the liver causes severe discomfort. The client may notice either a constant aching or a sharp pain in the right upper quadrant.

Dependent edema is one of the early signs of right ventricular failure. Edema is usually symmetric and occurs in the dependent parts of the body, where venous pressure is the highest. In ambulatory individuals, edema begins in the feet and ankles and ascends the lower legs. It is most noticeable at the end of a day and often decreases after a night's rest.

Many people experiencing this type of edema assume that it is a normal sign of aging and fail to report it to their physician. In the recumbent person, pitting edema may develop in the presacral area and, as it worsens, progress to the genital area and medial thighs (Case Example 6-4).

Cyanosis of the nail beds appears as venous congestion reduces peripheral blood flow. Clients with CHF often feel anxious, frightened, and depressed. Fears may be expressed as frightening nightmares, insomnia, acute anxiety states, depression, or withdrawal from reality.

CASE EXAMPLE 6-4 Congestive Heart Failure—Bilateral Pitting Edema

A 65-year-old man came to the clinic with a referral from his family doctor for "Hip pain—evaluate and treat." Past medical history included three total hip replacements of the right hip, open heart surgery 6 years ago, and persistent hypertension currently being treated with beta-blockers.

During the interview it was discovered that the client had experienced many bouts of hip pain, leg weakness, and loss of hip motion. He was not actually examined by his doctor, but had contacted the physician's office by phone, requesting a new P.T. referral.

On examination, large adhesed scars were noted along the anterior, lateral, and posterior aspects of the right hip, with significant bilateral hip flexion contractures. Pitting edema was noted in the right ankle, with mild swelling also observed around the left ankle. The client was unaware of this swelling. Further questions were negative for shortness of breath, difficulty in sleeping, cough, or other symptoms of cardiopulmonary involvement.

The bilateral edema could have been from compromise of the lymphatic drainage system following the multiple surgeries and adhesive scarring. However, with the positive history for cardiovascular involvement, bilateral edema, and telephone-derived referral, the physician was contacted by phone to notify him of the edema, and the client was directed by the physician to make an appointment.

The client was diagnosed in the early stages of congestive heart failure. Physical therapy to address the appropriate hip musculoskeletal problems was continued.

Clinical Signs and Symptoms of
Right-Sided Heart Failure

- Increased fatigue
- Dependent edema (usually beginning in the ankles)
- Pitting edema (after 5 to 10 pounds of edema accumulate)
- Edema in the sacral area or the back of the thighs
- Right upper quadrant pain
- Cyanosis of nail beds

Aneurysm

An aneurysm is an abnormal dilatation (commonly a saclike formation) in the wall of an artery, a vein, or the heart. Aneurysms occur when the vessel or heart wall becomes weakened from trauma, congenital vascular disease, infection, or atherosclerosis. This section could also be discussed under Peripheral Vascular Diseases because aneurysms of arterial blood vessels can result in some form of PVD.

Aneurysms are designated either venous or arterial and are also described according to the specific vessel in which they develop. *Thoracic aneurysms* usually involve the ascending, transverse, or descending portion of the aorta; *abdominal aneurysms* generally involve the aorta between the renal arteries and the iliac branches; *peripheral arterial aneurysms* affect the femoral and popliteal arteries.

THORACIC AND PERIPHERAL ARTERIAL ANEURYSMS

A dissecting aneurysm (most often a thoracic aneurysm) splits and penetrates the arterial wall, creating a false vessel. Thoracic aneurysms occur most frequently in hypertensive men between the ages of 40 and 70 years. Marked elevation of blood pressure may facilitate rapid disruption and final rupture of the aortic wall when a small tear in the intima has occurred.

The most common site for peripheral arterial aneurysms is the popliteal space in the lower extremities. Popliteal aneurysms cause ischemic symptoms in the lower limbs and an easily palpable pulse of larger amplitude. An enlarged area behind the knee may be present, seldom with discomfort.

ABDOMINAL AORTIC ANEURYSMS

An aneurysm is an abnormal dilation in a weak or diseased arterial wall causing a saclike protrusion. Aneurysms can occur anywhere in any blood

vessel, but the two most common places are the aorta and cerebral vascular system. The aneurysm may be dissecting, which means a tear has occurred between two layers of the intima and blood is flowing between these two layers rather than through the lumen.

Abdominal aortic aneurysms (AAAs) occur about four times more often than thoracic aneurysms. The natural course of an untreated AAA is expansion and rupture in one of several places, including the peritoneal cavity, the mesentery, behind the peritoneum, into the inferior vena cava, or into the duodenum or rectum.

The most common site for an AAA is just below the kidney (immediately below the takeoff of the renal arteries), with referred pain to the thoracolumbar junction (see Fig. 6-11). Aneurysms can be caused by:

- Trauma/weight lifting [aging athletes]
- Congenital vascular disease
- Infection
- Atherosclerosis

RISK FACTORS

The therapist should look for a history of known congenital heart disease, recent infection, or diagnosis of coronary artery disease (CAD; atherosclerosis). Many seniors are keeping active and fit by participating in activities at the gym, at home, or elsewhere that involve lifting weights. There is an increased risk of aneurysm for these clients. AAAs can be exacerbated by anticoagulant therapy (risk factor).

The therapist may be prescribing progressive resistive exercises that can have an adverse effect in an older adult with any of these etiologies (Case Example 6-5). Monitoring vital signs is important among exercising senior adults. Teaching proper breathing and abdominal support without using a Valsalva maneuver is important in any exercise program, but especially for those clients at increased risk for aortic aneurysm.

The U.S. Preventive Services Task Force now recommends one-time ultrasonographic screening for abdominal aortic aneurysm for men ages 65 to 75 who presently smoke or who have smoked in the past. No recommendation is made for or against men who have never smoked. Routine screening for women is not advised.[41]

Clients who have had orthopedic surgery involving anterior spinal procedures of any kind (e.g., spinal fusion, spinal fusion with cages, artificial disc replacement) are at risk for trauma to the aorta (rather than aortic aneurysm) from damage to blood vessels moved out of the way during

CASE EXAMPLE 6-5 Abdominal Aortic Aneurysm—Weight Lifting

A 72-year-old retired farmer has come to the physical therapist for recommendations about weight lifting. He had been following a regular program of weight lifting for almost 30 years, using a set of free weights purchased at a garage sale.

One year ago he experienced an abdominal aortic aneurysm that ruptured and required surgery. Symptoms at the time of the diagnosis were back pain at the thoracolumbar junction radiating outward toward the flanks bilaterally. The client is symptom-free and in apparent good health, taking no medications, and receiving no medical treatment at this time.

What are your recommendations for resuming his weight lifting program?

The hemodynamic stresses of weight lifting involve a rapid increase in systemic arterial blood pressure without a decrease in total peripheral vascular resistance. This principle combined with aortic degeneration may have contributed to the aortic dissection.[40]

Weight lifting in anyone with a history of aortic aneurysm is considered a contraindication. The therapist suggested a conditioning program, combining a walking/biking program with resistive exercises using a lightweight elastic band alternating with an aquatic program for cardiac clients. Given this client's history, a medical evaluation before initiating an exercise program is necessary.

CASE EXAMPLE 6-6 Abdominal Aortic Aneurysm—Hip Replacement

A therapist was ambulating with a 76-year-old woman post-hip arthroplasty in an acute care (hospital) setting. The patient complained of back pain with every step and asked to sit down. The pain went away when she sat down. Once she started walking again, the pain started again.

She asked the therapist to walk her to the bathroom. After helping her onto the toilet, the therapist waited as a standby assist outside the bathroom. When several minutes went by with no call or sound, the therapist knocked on the door. There was no response. The therapist repeated knocking and calling the patient's name.

Upon opening the bathroom door, the therapist found the patient slumped over on the toilet. Emergency help was summoned immediately. She was later diagnosed with an abdominal aortic aneurysm.

What are the red flags in this scenario?

Age

Pain with activity that is relieved with rest

Vital signs should be taken in a case of this type after the first complaint of pain with activity.

CLINICAL SIGNS AND SYMPTOMS

Most AAAs are asymptomatic; discovery occurs on physical or x-ray examination of the abdomen or lower spine for some other reason.

The most common symptom is awareness of a pulsating mass in the abdomen, with or without pain, followed by abdominal pain and back pain.

Internal bleeding can result in a distended abdomen, changes in blood pressure, changes in stool (e.g., melena, bloody diarrhea), and possible back and/or shoulder pain.

surgery. Internal bleeding can result in a distended abdomen, changes in blood pressure, changes in stool (e.g., melena, bloody diarrhea), and possible back and/or shoulder pain.

The therapist is most likely to observe rapid onset of severe neck or back pain (Case Example 6-6).

The client may report feeling a heartbeat in the abdomen or stomach when lying down. Back pain may be the only presenting feature. Groin pain and flank pain may be experienced because of increasing pressure on other structures.

The pain is usually described as sharp, intense, severe or knifelike in the abdomen, chest or anywhere in the back (including the sacrum). Pain may radiate to the chest, between the scapulae, or to the posterior thighs.

The location of the symptoms is determined by the location of the aneurysm. Most aortic aneurysms (95%) occur just below the renal arteries. Extreme pain described as "tearing" or "ripping" may be felt at the base of the neck along the back, particularly in the interscapular area, while dissection proceeds over the aortic arch and into the descending aorta. Symptoms are not relieved by a change in position.

The physical therapist can palpate the width of the arterial pulses; these pulses (e.g., aortic, femoral) should be uniform in width from the midline outward on either side (see Fig. 4-51). In adults older than 50, a normal aorta is not more than 3 cm (average 2.5 cm) wide.

The abdominal aorta passes posterior to the diaphragm (aortic hiatus) at the level of the T12 vertebral body and bifurcates at the level of the L4 vertebral body to form the right and left common iliac arteries. Watch for a widening of the pulse width before reaching the umbilicus. The pulse width expands normally at the aortic bifurcation, usually observed just below the umbilicus. Ninety-five percent of all AAAs occur just below the renal arteries.

Systolic blood pressure below 100 mm Hg and pulse rate over 100 beats per minute may indicate signs of shock. Other symptoms may include ecchymoses in the flank and perianal area; severe and sudden pain in the abdomen, paravertebral area, or flank; and lightheadedness and nausea with sudden hypotension.

The therapist may observe cold, pulseless lower extremities and/or blood pressure differences (more than 10 mm Hg) between the arms. Consistent with the model for a screening examination the therapist must look for screening clues in the history, pain patterns, and associated signs and symptoms. Knowledge of the clinical signs and symptoms of impending rupture or actual rupture of the aortic aneurysm is important.

If a client (usually a postoperative inpatient) has internal bleeding (rather than an aneurysm) from complications of anterior spinal surgery the therapist may note

- Distended abdomen
- Changes in blood pressure
- Changes in stool
- Possible back and/or shoulder pain

The client's recent history of anterior spinal surgery accompanied by any of these symptoms is enough to notify nursing or medical staff of these observations. Monitoring post-operative vital signs in these clients is essential.

Clinical Signs and Symptoms of

Aneurysm

- Chest pain with any of the following:
  - Palpable, pulsating mass (abdomen, popliteal space)
  - Abdominal "heartbeat" felt by the client when lying down
  - Dull ache in the midabdominal left flank or low back
  - Groin and/or leg pain
  - Weakness or transient paralysis of legs.

Ruptured Aneurysm

- Sudden, severe chest pain with a tearing sensation (see Fig. 6-10)
- Pain may extend to the neck, shoulders, between the scapulae, lower back, or abdomen; pain radiating to the posterior thighs helps distinguish it from a myocardial infarction
- Pain is not relieved by change in position
- Pain may be described as "tearing" or "ripping"
- Pulsating abdominal mass
- Other signs: cold, pulseless lower extremities, BP changes (more than 10 mm Hg difference in diastolic BP between arms; systolic BP less than 100 mm Hg)
- Pulse rate more than 100 beats/min
- Ecchymoses in the flank and perianal area
- Lightheadedness and nausea

Conditions Affecting the Heart Valves

The second category of heart problems includes those that occur secondary to impairment of the valves caused by disease (e.g., rheumatic fever or coronary thrombosis), congenital deformity, or infection such as endocarditis. Three types of valve deformities may affect aortic, mitral, tricuspid, or pulmonic valves: *stenosis*, *insufficiency*, or *prolapse*.

Stenosis is a narrowing or constriction that prevents the valve from opening fully, and may be caused by growths, scars, or abnormal deposits on the leaflets. *Insufficiency* (also referred to as regurgitation) occurs when the valve does not close properly and causes blood to flow back into the heart chamber. *Prolapse* affects only the mitral valve and occurs when enlarged valve leaflets bulge backward into the left atrium.

These valve conditions increase the workload of the heart and require the heart to pump harder to

force blood through a stenosed valve or to maintain adequate flow if blood is seeping back. Further complications for individuals with a malfunctioning valve may occur secondary to a bacterial infection of the valves (endocarditis).

Persons affected by diseases of the heart valves may be asymptomatic, and extensive auscultation with a stethoscope and diagnostic study may be required to differentiate one condition from another. In its early symptomatic stages cardiac valvular disease causes the person to become fatigued easily. As stenosis or insufficiency progresses, the main symptom of heart failure (breathlessness or dyspnea) appears.

Clinical Signs and Symptoms of Cardiac Valvular Disease

- Easy fatigue
- Dyspnea
- Palpitation (subjective sensation of throbbing, skipping, rapid or forcible pulsation of the heart)
- Chest pain
- Pitting edema
- Orthopnea or paroxysmal dyspnea
- Dizziness and syncope (episodes of fainting or loss of consciousness)

Rheumatic Fever

Rheumatic fever is an infection caused by streptococcal bacteria that can be fatal or may lead to rheumatic heart disease, a chronic condition caused by scarring and deformity of the heart valves. It is called rheumatic fever because two of the most common symptoms are fever and joint pain.

The infection generally starts with strep throat in children between the ages of 5 and 15 years and damages the heart in approximately 50% of cases. Rheumatic fever produces a diffuse, proliferative, and exudative inflammatory process.

The aggressive use of specific antibiotics in the United States had effectively removed rheumatic fever as the primary cause of valvular damage. However, in 1985 a series of epidemics of rheumatic fever occurred in several widely diverse geographic regions of the continental United States. Currently, the prevalence and incidence of cases have not approximated the 1985 record, but they have remained above baseline levels.[42]

CLINICAL SIGNS AND SYMPTOMS
The most typical clinical profile of a child or young adult with acute rheumatic fever is an initial cold or sore throat followed 2 or 3 weeks later by sudden or gradual onset of painful migratory joint symptoms in the knees, shoulders, feet, ankles, elbows, fingers, or neck. Fever of 37.2°C to 39.4°C (99°F to 103°F) and palpitations and fatigue are also present. Malaise, weakness, weight loss, and anorexia may accompany the fever.

The migratory arthralgias may last only 24 hours, or they may persist for several weeks. Joints that are sore and hot and contain fluid completely resolve, followed by acute synovitis, heat, synovial space tenderness, swelling, and effusion present in a different area the next day. The persistence of swelling, heat, and synovitis in a single joint or joints for more than 2 to 3 weeks is extremely unusual in acute rheumatic fever.

In the acute full-blown sequelae, shortness of breath and increasing nocturnal cough will also occur. A rash on the skin of the limbs or trunk is present in fewer than 2% of clients with acute rheumatic fever. Subcutaneous nodules over the extensor surfaces of the arms, heels, knees, or back of the head may occur.

All layers of the heart (epicardium, endocardium, myocardium, and pericardium) may be involved, and the heart valves are affected by this inflammatory reaction. The most characteristic and potentially dangerous anatomic lesion of rheumatic inflammation is the gross effect on cardiac valves, most commonly the mitral and aortic valves. If untreated, as many as 25% of clients will have mitral valvular disease 25 to 30 years later.

Rheumatic chorea (also called chorea or St. Vitus' dance) may occur 1 to 3 months after the strep infection and always is noted after polyarthritis. Chorea in a child, teenager, or young adult is almost always a manifestation of acute rheumatic fever. Other uncommon causes of chorea are systemic lupus erythematosus, thyrotoxicosis, and cerebrovascular accident, but these are unlikely in a child.

The client develops rapid, purposeless, non-repetitive movements that may involve all muscles except the eyes. This chorea may last for 1 week or several months or may persist for several years without permanent impairment of the central nervous system.

Initial episodes of rheumatic fever last months in children and weeks in adults. Twenty percent of children have recurrences within 5 years. Recurrences are uncommon after 5 years of good health and are rare after age 21 years.

Clinical Signs and Symptoms of
Rheumatic Fever

- Migratory arthralgias
- Subcutaneous nodules on extensor surfaces
- Fever and sore throat
- Flat, painless skin rash (short duration)
- Carditis
- Chorea
- Weakness, malaise, weight loss, and anorexia
- Acquired valvular disease

Endocarditis

Bacterial endocarditis, another common heart infection, causes inflammation of the cardiac endothelium (layer of cells lining the cavities of the heart) and damages the tricuspid, aortic, or mitral valve.

This infection may be caused by bacteria entering the bloodstream from a remote part of the body (e.g., skin infection, oral cavity), or it may occur as a result of abnormal growths on the closure lines of previously damaged valves or artificial valves. These growths called vegetations consist of collagen fibers and may separate from the valve, embolize, and cause infarction in the myocardium, kidney, brain, spleen, abdomen, or extremities.

RISK FACTORS

In addition to clients with previous valvular damage, injection drug users and postcardiac surgical clients are at high risk for developing endocarditis. Congenital heart disease and degenerative heart disease, such as calcific aortic stenosis, may also cause bacterial endocarditis. The prosthetic cardiac valve (valve replacement) has become more important as a predisposing factor for endocarditis because cardiac surgery is performed on a much larger scale than in the past.

This infection is often the consequence of invasive diagnostic procedures, such as renal shunts and urinary catheters, long-term indwelling catheters, or dental treatment (because of the increased opportunities for normal oral microorganisms to gain entrance to the circulatory system by way of highly vascularized oral structures). Individuals who are susceptible may take antibiotics as a precaution before undergoing any of these procedures.

CLINICAL SIGNS AND SYMPTOMS

A significant number of clients (up to 45%) with bacterial endocarditis initially have musculoske-

tal symptoms, including arthralgia, arthritis, low back pain, and myalgias. Half these clients will have only musculoskeletal symptoms without other signs of endocarditis.

The early onset of joint pain and myalgia is more likely if the client is older and has had a previously diagnosed heart murmur. Musculoskeletal problems make up a significant part of the clinical picture of infective endocarditis diagnosed in an injection drug user.

The most common musculoskeletal symptom in clients with bacterial endocarditis is *arthralgia*, generally in the proximal joints. The shoulder is the most commonly affected site, followed (in declining incidence) by the knee, hip, wrist, ankle, metatarsophalangeal, and metacarpophalangeal joints, and acromioclavicular joints.

Most endocarditis clients with arthralgias have only one or two painful joints, although some may have pain in several joints. Painful symptoms begin suddenly in one or two joints, accompanied by warmth, tenderness, and redness. Symmetric arthralgia in the knees or ankles may lead to a diagnosis of rheumatoid arthritis. One helpful clue: as a rule, morning stiffness is not as prevalent in clients with endocarditis as in those with rheumatoid arthritis or polymyalgia rheumatica.

Osteoarticular infections are diagnosed infrequently and most commonly in association with injection drug use. Most commonly affected sites include the vertebrae, the wrist, the sternoclavicular joints, and the sacroiliac joints. Often multiple joint involvement occurs.[43,44]

Endocarditis may produce destructive changes in the *sacroiliac joint*, probably as a result of seeding the joint by septic emboli. The pain will be localized over the SI joint, and the physician will use roentgenograms and bone scans to verify this diagnosis.

Almost one third of clients with bacterial endocarditis have *low back pain*; in many clients it is the principal musculoskeletal symptom reported. Back pain is accompanied by decreased range of motion and spinal tenderness. Pain may affect only one side, and it may be limited to the paraspinal muscles.

Endocarditis-induced low back pain may be very similar to that associated with a herniated lumbar disk; it radiates to the leg and may be accentuated by raising the leg or by sneezing. The key difference is that neurologic deficits are usually absent in clients with bacterial endocarditis.

Widespread diffuse *myalgias* may occur during periods of fever, but these are not appreciably different from the general myalgia seen in clients

with other febrile illnesses. More commonly, myalgia will be restricted to the calf or thigh. Bilateral or unilateral leg myalgias occur in approximately 10% to 15% of all clients with bacterial endocarditis.

The cause of back pain and leg myalgia associated with bacterial endocarditis has not been determined. Some suggest that concurrent aseptic meningitis may contribute to both leg and back pain. Others suggest that leg pain is related to emboli that break off from the infected cardiac valves. The latter theory is supported by biopsy evidence of muscle necrosis or vasculitis in clients with bacterial endocarditis.

Rarely, other musculoskeletal symptoms, such as osteomyelitis, nail clubbing, tendinitis, hypertrophic osteoarthropathy, bone infarcts, and ischemic bone necrosis, may occur.

Clinical Signs and Symptoms of
Endocarditis

- Arthralgias
- Arthritis
- Musculoskeletal symptoms
- Low back/sacroiliac pain
- Myalgias
- Petechiae/splinter hemorrhages
- Constitutional symptoms
- Dyspnea, chest pain
- Cold and painful extremities

Lupus Carditis

Systemic lupus erythematosus (SLE) is a multisystem clinical illness associated with the release of a broad spectrum of autoantibodies into the circulation (see Chapter 12). The inflammatory process mediated by the immune response can target the heart and vasculature of the client with SLE.

Except for pericarditis, clinically significant cardiac disease directly associated with systemic lupus erythematosus (SLE) is relatively infrequent, but because of the musculoskeletal involvement, it may be of major importance for the therapist. Primary lupus cardiac involvement may include pericarditis, myocarditis, endocarditis, or a combination of the three.

Pericarditis is the most common cardiac lesion associated with SLE, appearing with the characteristic substernal chest pain that varies with posture, becoming worse in recumbency and improving with sitting or bending forward. *Myocarditis* may occur and is strongly associated with skeletal myositis in SLE.

Congenital Valvular Defects

Congenital malformations of the heart occur in approximately 1 of every 100 infants born in the United States. The most common defects include (Fig. 6-6):

- Ventricular or atrial septal defect (hole between the ventricles or atria)
- Tetralogy of Fallot (combination of four defects)
- Patent ductus arteriosus (shunt caused by an opening between the aorta and the pulmonary artery)
- Congenital stenosis of the pulmonary, aortic, and tricuspid valves

These congenital defects require surgical correction and may be part of the client's past medical history. They are not conditions that are likely to mimic musculoskeletal lesions and are therefore not covered in detail in this text.

Congenital cardiovascular abnormalities, which are usually asymptomatic and often undiagnosed during life, are the main cause of sudden death in athletes. Aortic stenosis, hypertrophic cardiomyopathy, Marfan's syndrome, congenital coronary artery anomalies, and ruptured aorta are the most commonly reported causes of sudden death during the practice of a sports activity.[45,46]

Family history of any of these conditions, premature sudden unexpected syncope, or family member death is an indication for a thorough cardiovascular evaluation of the athlete before participation in sports.[47]

MITRAL VALVE PROLAPSE

Echocardiographic studies have advanced our knowledge of mitral valve prolapse (MVP) in the last 2 decades. A more precise definition of MVP has resulted in a more accurate estimate of prevalence rate (2% to 3%). This is equally distributed between men and women,[48,49] although men seem to have a higher incidence of complications.

MVP is characterized by mitral leaflet thickness with increased extensibility, decreased stiffness, and decreased strength compared to normal valves. This structural variation has many other names, including floppy valve syndrome, Barlow's syndrome, and click-murmur syndrome.

MVP appears to be due to connective tissue abnormalities in the valve leaflets or in response to abnormalities in left ventricular cavity geometry.[50] Normally, when the lower part of the heart contracts, the mitral valve remains firm and allows no blood to leak back into the upper chambers. In MVP the structural changes in the mitral valve allows one part of the valve, the leaflet, to billow

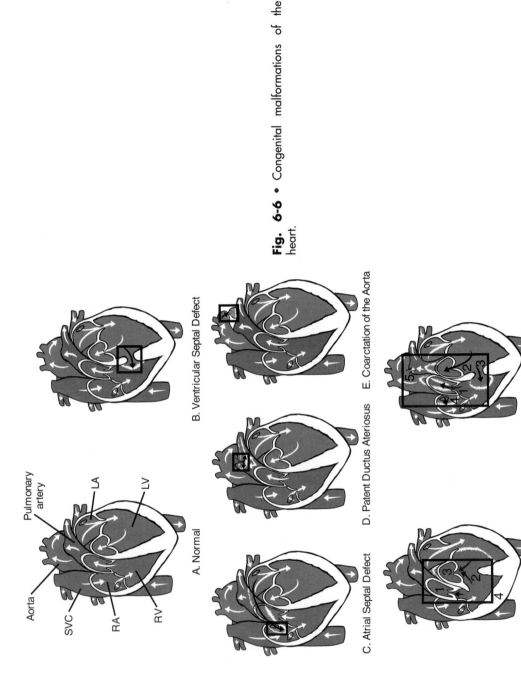

Fig. 6-6 • Congenital malformations of the heart.

A. Normal

B. Ventricular Septal Defect

C. Atrial Septal Defect

D. Patent Ductus Ateriosus

E. Coarctation of the Aorta

F. Tetrology of Fallot

G. Transposition of the Great Vessels

back into the upper chamber during contraction of the ventricle.

One or both of the valve leaflets may bulge into the left atrium during ventricular systole. This protrusion can often be heard through a stethoscope as a sound known as a "click." Leaking of blood backward through the mitral valve can also be heard and is referred to as a heart murmur.

Risk Factors MVP is a benign condition in isolation; however, it can be associated with a number of other conditions, especially the heritable connective tissue disorders such as Ehlers-Danlos syndrome, Marfan syndrome, and osteogenesis imperfecta. Other risk factors include endocarditis, myocarditis, atherosclerosis, systemic lupus erythematosus, muscular dystrophy, acromegaly, and cardiac sarcoidosis.

Clinical Signs and Symptoms Two thirds of the individuals with MVP experience no symp-

toms. Approximately one third experience occasional symptoms that are mildly to moderately uncomfortable—enough to interfere with the person's ability to enjoy an unrestricted life. Only about 1% suffer severe symptoms and lifestyle restrictions.

Almost all the symptoms of MVP syndrome are due to an imbalance in the autonomic nervous system, called dysautonomia. Frequently, when there is a slight variation in structure of the heart valve, there is also a slight variation in the function or balance of the autonomic nervous system (ANS).[50] This description in the autonomic innervation of the heart may account for the high incidence of MVP in fibromyalgia, a condition known to be associated with dysregulation or dysautonomia of the ANS.

Symptoms include profound fatigue that cannot be correlated with exercise or stress, cold hands

and feet, shortness of breath, chest pain, and heart palpitations. The most common triad of symptoms associated with MVP is fatigue, palpitations, and dyspnea (Fig. 6-7). Frequently occurring musculoskeletal findings in clients with MVP include joint hypermobility, temporomandibular joint (TMJ) syndrome, and myalgias.

Although the fatigue that accompanies MVP is not related to exertion, deconditioning from prolonged inactivity may develop, further complicating the picture. Chest pain associated with MVP can be severe but it differs from pain associated with MI (see Table 6-5). When there is an imbalance in the ANS, which controls contraction and relaxation of the chest wall muscles (the muscles of breathing), there may be inadequate relaxation between respirations. Over time these chest wall muscles go into spasm, resulting in chest pain.

It is important that the therapist evaluate the client with chest pain for trigger points. If palpation of the chest reproduces symptoms, especially radiating pain, deactivation of trigger points must be carried out followed by a reevaluation as part of the screening process for pain of a cardiac origin.

MVP is not life threatening but may be lifestyle threatening for the small number of persons (rare) who have more severe structural problems that may progress to the point at which surgical replacement of the valve is required. Sudden death is a recognized risk for cases of severe mitral regurgitation. To prevent infective endocarditis, the client may be given antibiotics prophylactically before any invasive procedures.

Mitral valve prolapse (MVP) is included in this section because of its increasing prevalence in the physical therapy client population. At presentation, usually the client with MVP has some other unrelated primary (musculoskeletal) diagnosis. During physical therapy intervention, the symptomatic MVP client may experience symptoms associated with MVP and require assurance or education regarding exercise and MVP.

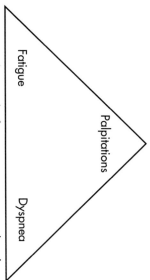

Fig. 6-7 • The triad of symptoms associated with mitral valve prolapse.

Palpitations

Fatigue

Dyspnea

Most individuals with MVP do not have to restrict their activity level or lifestyle; regular exercise is encouraged. Clients with mitral regurgitation (backward flow of blood into the left atrium) during exercise, but not at rest, have a higher rate of complications such as heart failure, syncope, and progressive mitral regurgitation requiring further medical treatment.[50]

Monitoring vital signs and observing or asking about additional signs and symptoms is important. Caution is advised in the use of weight training for the MVP client. Gradual buildup using light-weights and increased repetitions is recommended.

Clinical Signs and Symptoms of Mitral Valve Prolapse

- Profound fatigue; low exercise tolerance
- Chest pain; arm, back, or shoulder discomfort
- Palpitations or irregular heartbeat
- Tachycardia
- Migraine headache
- Anxiety, depression, panic attacks
- Dyspnea

Conditions Affecting the Cardiac Nervous System

The third component of cardiac disease is caused by failure of the heart's nervous system to conduct normal electrical impulses. The heart has its own intrinsic conduction system that allows the orderly depolarization of cardiac muscle tissue. Arrhythmias, also called dysrhythmias, are disorders of the heart rate and rhythm caused by disturbances in the conduction system.

Arrhythmias may cause the heart to beat too quickly (tachycardia), too slowly (bradycardia), or with extra beats and fibrillations. Arrhythmias can lead to dramatic changes in circulatory dynamics, such as hypotension, heart failure, and shock.

Clients who are neurologically unstable owing to recent cerebrovascular accident, head trauma, spinal cord injury, or other central nervous system insult often exhibit new arrhythmias during the period of instability (Case Example 6-7). These may be due to elevation of intracranial pressure, and once this has been controlled and returned to normal range, arrhythmias usually disappear.

Arrhythmias may also be triggered by environmental factors, abnormal thyroid function, and some medications. Clients who have preexisting arrhythmias, preexisting CAD, or CHF, may progress from "transient arrhythmias" to arrhythmias that do not disappear, with the potential for serious complications. Dizziness and loss of

CASE EXAMPLE 6-7   Cardiac Arrhythmia Cause of Transient Muscle Weakness

Referral: An 87-year-old man was admitted to a skilled nursing facility for short-term rehabilitation. Goal: Safely and independently navigate home environment on level surfaces and stairs with discharge to home within 2 to 3 months.

Medical Diagnosis: Mild left hemiparesis secondary to recent cerebrovascular accident (CVA)

Past Medical History: Urosepsis, seizure disorder, deep venous thrombosis (DVT), hypertension (HTN), congestive heart failure (CHF), myocardial infarction (MI), frequent falls, subdural hematoma with evacuation

Medications: Heparin (anticoagulant, antithrombotic), Lasix (diuretic for hypertension), Oscal (antacid, calcium supplement)

Systems Review:

Integument: Well-healed scar on head, postsurgical evacuation of subdural hematoma.

Musculoskeletal: Head position in sitting and standing is held in approximately 30° of lateral and forward flexion; full active head and neck range of motion present; overall flexed/stooped posture (left more than right); muscle strength-right trunk and right upper extremity: 4-/5; muscle strength-left trunk and left lower extremity: 3-/5.

Neuromuscular: Neurologic screening results consistent with upper motor neuron lesion; nonambulatory and requires moderate assistance for bed mobility and transfers; able to sit, stand, and walk with assistance of two and the use of a walker; patellar deep tendon reflexes (DTRs): right—within normal limits; left—+3; positive Babinski response on the left

Cardiovascular/Pulmonary: Vital Signs-blood pressure (142/80 mmHg, measured in right upper extremity, sitting); pulse rate-72 beats per minute; respiratory rate-18 breaths per minute; pulse oximeter (oxygen saturation)-97%

First Progress Report: Client made many functional gains during the first 4 weeks of rehab and was planning a trip home for 2 days but experienced multiple falls with several incidences of lacerations to the head requiring stitches.

Client also presented with multiple episodes of transient generalized weakness, increased postural instability, and increased bradykinesia. Episodes of weakness and falling were without warning and unrelated to activity but interfering with progress toward functional independence and discharge plans.

Vital signs: Radial and apical heart rate 72 beats per minute (BPM) with periodic and variable drops in heart rate to below 60 BPM with a low measurement of 37 BPM. Episodes of bradycardia lasted from 1 minute to 1 hour. Blood pressure fluctuated from 150/83 mmHg to 92/40 mmHg. Respiratory rate remained stable. Pulse oximetry levels varied from 91% to 97% with an occasional drop to 88% during transient episodes of weakness.

There was no complaint of, nor apparent shortness of breath, no complaint of dizziness, no syncope.

Referral: Client was referred to his primary physician with report of increasingly frequent periods of generalized muscle weakness with poor postural stability (cause unknown). Vital signs were reported.

Physician ruled out dehydration, renal insufficiency, anemia, and active bleeding as possible pathologies. EKG was obtained. He was eventually hospitalized and diagnosed with episodic bradycardia.

The client returned to the skilled nursing facility and continued to have multiple intermittent episodes of transient weakness and postural instability lasting from several minutes to several hours, affecting his progress towards independent functional mobility.

Second Progress Report: With each episode, vital signs were obtained. A significant drop in radial pulse was noted, along with decreased apical heart rate. This appeared to be the most significant finding. Blood pressure dropped during these incidents; however, it did not drop dangerously low except during several occurrences (82/40 mmHg); respiratory rate appeared stable with minimal alteration.

The nursing staff and physician were notified at the time of each occurrence. A 24-hour Holter monitor was ordered. The results were inconclusive because no sustained arrhythmias were noted.

A second cardiac evaluation identified a tachy-brady syndrome. The client received a pacemaker and appropriate medications. The

---

CASE EXAMPLE 6-7   Cardiac Arrhythmia Cause of Transient Muscle Weakness—cont'd

client was discharged to home 6 weeks later, independent in all functional mobility and ADLs.

Summary: Cardiac arrhythmia may be an underlying concern in patients with diagnosis of CVA. With the increasing population of over 65, and the increasing need for rehabilitative services in the aging adult population, understanding of the normal aging process versus disease states is imperative. Signs of pathology can be either overlooked or attributed to the age of the client or to the normal aging process.

Cardiac arrhythmia is an elusive state that may or may not produce overt symptoms. This case example suggests that although not documented in the literature yet, cardiac arrhythmia may cause transient weakness.

---

consciousness may occur when the arrhythmia results in a serious reduction in cardiac output, owing to loss of brain perfusion (not caused by transient ischemic attacks, as is often suspected).

The therapist should monitor pulse carefully before, during, and after exercise when working with any client who has had a stroke. Any pulse irregularities not already documented should be reported to the physician immediately and an EKG should be done to determine the nature of the irregularity.

The therapist may be the first health care professional to identify an arrhythmia that appears during exercise. In the early recovery period the therapist should monitor for these arrhythmias by taking the client's pulse. Arrhythmias should be reported to the physician (Case Example 6-8).

Fibrillation

The sinoatrial (SA) node (or cardiac pacemaker) initiates and paces the heartbeat. During an MI, damaged heart muscle cells, deprived of oxygen, can release small electrical impulses that may disrupt the heart's normal conduction pathway. These fibrillation impulses can occur in the atria or the ventricles.

If the heart attack develops suddenly into *ventricular* fibrillation, a potentially lethal arrhythmia, it can result in sudden death. Similarly, a heart damaged by CAD (with or without previous infarcts) can go into ventricular fibrillation. Ventricular fibrillation usually requires resuscitation and emergency electrical counter-shock (defibrillation) as life saving measures.

Atrial fibrillation, not an immediate lethal arrhythmia, is characterized by a total disorganization of atrial activity without effective atrial con-

traction. The upper chambers of the heart contract in an unsynchronized pattern, causing the atrium to quiver rather than to contract and often causing blood to pool, which allows for clots to form. These clots can break loose and travel to the brain, causing a stroke.

The therapist can easily and quickly screen individuals at risk and teach them to screen themselves by checking the pulse for the telltale signs of an irregular heartbeat. A regular heartbeat is characterized by a series of even and continuous pulsations, whereas an irregular heartbeat often feels like an extra or missed beat. To help determine the steadiness of the heartbeat, the therapist or individual keeps time by tapping the foot.

RISK FACTORS

Persons at risk for fibrillation who require screening include those who have had a previous heart attack or a history that includes high blood pressure, CHF, digitalis toxicity, pericarditis, or rheumatic mitral stenosis.

Other factors that can overstimulate the sinus node include excessive production of thyroid hormone (hyperthyroidism), alcohol and caffeine consumption, and high fevers. In many instances, particularly in younger persons, there is no apparent cause.

Recent studies have shown that presence of the organism *Helicobacter pylori* in the stomach is associated with persistent atrial fibrillation. In addition high concentrations of C-reactive proteins, which confirm the presence of systemic inflammation, are present in people with AF. A potential non-cardiovascular disease that predisposes to AF may be chronic gastritis caused by chronic *H. pylori* infection.[52]

CASE EXAMPLE 6-8   Unstable Cardiac Arrhythmia

Chief Complaint: A 62-year-old woman with a diagnosis of left lower extremity weakness was referred by her cardiologist to physical therapy. She also reported weakness and tingling in both legs from the knees down.

Past Medical History: Recent hospitalization for lung infection. Past history of hypertension, dizziness, and cardiac arrhythmia. Previous surgical history included thoracic outlet release 14 years ago.

Clinical Presentation: The client experienced worsening of symptoms with walking and climbing stairs; rest relieved her symptoms. Manual muscle test revealed weakness in the left hip flexor and external rotator muscles.

Client became diaphoretic with functional strength and exercise tolerance testing (repeated sit to stand and back to sitting). She reported the same response when doing housework.

Review of systems was significant for the cardiovascular system. Vital signs were as follows:

Blood pressure: 125/95 mm Hg (left arm, standing)/150/82 (supine)

Lower standing blood pressure is a risk factor for falls[51]

Apical pulse: 62 beats per minute; every third or fourth beat skipped; heart rate speeds up and then slows down after each skipped beat (cardiologist was aware of this pattern of irregularity; client was under medical treatment for cardiac arrhythmia)

What are the red flags here?
Age
History of cardiac arrhythmia

Diaphoresis is an abnormal response to exercise stress
Irregular heartbeat

Is it safe to proceed with physical therapy intervention since the client was referred by the cardiologist who is treating her for cardiac arrhythmia?

It is not always the case that the referring physician is aware of a client's current cardiovascular status. Referral may not always mean the client is appropriate for participation in an exercise program. Since the therapist noted the irregular heart rate, he was alert to the possibility of other signs of inappropriate exercise responses.

The main red flag here is the abnormal response to exercise stress in someone who is already being treated for a cardiac anomaly (arrhythmia). The variable blood pressure and irregular heartbeat suggest an unstable situation.

Result: In this case it just happened that the client was going from her appointment with the therapist to a visit with her family physician. A note summarizing the therapist's findings, including the vital signs and response to exercise was sent to the physician.

A copy of the letter was also faxed to the physician's office and to the cardiologist. The therapist followed up with a phone call to the client for an update on her status. The client was given an electrocardiogram (ECG), which was found to be abnormal and was admitted to the hospital for further testing.

The therapist was very instrumental in referring this client based on medical screening (i.e., systems review, exercise test). Information about the client's cardiovascular status gleaned by the therapist during the assessment was new and important for medical management.

Vernier DA: The meaning of screening. The application of vital signs should be used in physical therapy practice, *ADVANCE for Physical Therapists & PT Assistants* 15(18):47-49, 2004.

CLINICAL SIGNS AND SYMPTOMS

Symptoms of fibrillation vary depending on the functional state of the heart and the location of the fibrillation. Fibrillation may exist without symptoms. The affected individual is usually aware of the irregular heart action and reports feeling "palpitations." Careful questioning may be required

to pinpoint the exact description of sensations reported by the client.

Some individuals experience the symptoms of inadequate blood flow and low oxygen levels, such as dizziness, chest pain, and fainting. Chronic atrial fibrillation may cause CHF, which is often experienced as shortness of breath during

exercise and fluid accumulation in the feet and legs.

More than six palpitations occurring in a minute or prolonged, repeated palpitations, especially if accompanied by chest pain, dyspnea, fainting, or other associated signs and symptoms, should be reported to the physician.

Clinical Signs and Symptoms of
Fibrillation

- Subjective report of palpitations
- Sensations of fluttering, skipping, irregular beating or pounding, heaving action
- Dyspnea
- Chest pain
- Anxiety
- Pallor
- Nervousness
- Cyanosis

Sinus Tachycardia

Sinus tachycardia, defined as an abnormally rapid heart rate, usually taken to be more than 100 beats per minute, is the normal physiologic response to such stressors as fever, hypotension, thyrotoxicosis, anemia, anxiety, exertion, hypovolemia, pulmonary emboli, myocardial ischemia, CHF, and shock.

Sinus tachycardia is usually of no physiologic significance; however, in clients with organic myocardial disease, the result may be reduced cardiac output, CHF, or arrhythmias. Because heart rate is a major determinant of oxygen requirements, angina or perhaps an increase in the size of an infarction may accompany persistent tachycardia in clients with CAD.

CLINICAL SIGNS AND SYMPTOMS
The symptoms of tachycardia vary from one person to another and may range from an increased pulse to a group of symptoms that would restrict normal activity of the client. Anxiety and apprehension may occur, depending on the pain threshold and emotional reaction of the client.

Clinical Signs and Symptoms of
Sinus Tachycardia

- Palpitation (most common symptom)
- Restlessness
- Chest discomfort or pain
- Agitation
- Anxiety and apprehension

Sinus Bradycardia

In sinus bradycardia, impulses travel down the same pathway as in sinus rhythm, but the sinus node discharges at a rate less than 60 beats per minute. Bradycardia may be normal in athletes or young adults and is therefore asymptomatic.

In most cases sinus bradycardia is a benign arrhythmia and may actually be beneficial by producing a longer period of diastole and increased ventricular filling. In some clients who have acute MI, it reduces oxygen demands and may help minimize the size of the infarction.

Eye surgery, meningitis, intracranial tumors, cervical and mediastinal tumors, and certain disease states (e.g., MI, myxedema, obstructive jaundice, and cardiac fibrosis) may produce sinus bradycardia.

CLINICAL SIGNS AND SYMPTOMS
Syncope may be preceded by sudden onset of weakness, sweating, nausea, pallor, vomiting, and distortion or dimming of vision. Signs and symptoms remit promptly when the client is placed in the horizontal position.

Physician referral for sinus bradycardia is needed only when symptoms such as chest pain, dyspnea, lightheadedness, or hypotension occur.

Clinical Signs and Symptoms of
Sinus Bradycardia

- Reduced pulse rate
- Syncope

CARDIOVASCULAR DISORDERS

Hypertension (See also section on Blood Pressure in Chapter 4)

Blood pressure is the force against the walls of the arteries and arterioles as these vessels carry blood away from the heart. When these muscular walls constrict, reducing the diameter of the vessel, blood pressure rises; when they relax, increasing the vessel diameter, blood pressure falls.

A high blood pressure reading is usually a sign that the vessels cannot relax fully and remain somewhat constricted, requiring the heart to work harder to pump blood through the vessels. Over time the extra effort can cause the heart muscle to become enlarged and eventually weakened. The force of blood pumped at high pressure can also produce small tears in the lining of the arteries, weakening the arterial vessels. The evidence of this effect is most pronounced in the

vessels of the brain, the kidneys, and the small vessels of the eye.

Hypertension is a major cardiovascular risk factor, associated with elevated risks of cardiovascular diseases, especially MI, stroke, PVD, and cardiovascular death. Although diastolic changes were always evaluated closely, research now shows that the risks increase progressively as systolic pressure goes up and increased cardiovascular risk is consistent for men whose systolic blood pressure levels are near or slightly above normal.[53]

Hypertension is often considered in conjunction with peripheral vascular disorders for several reasons: both are disorders of the circulatory system, the course of both diseases are affected similar factors, and hypertension is a major risk factor in atherosclerosis, the largest single cause of PVD.

Hypertension is defined by an elevation of diastolic pressure, systolic pressure, or both measured on at least two separate occasions at least 2 weeks apart. This sequence of measurements indicates a sustained elevation of blood pressure. Medical researchers have developed classifications for blood pressure based on risk (see Table 4-5).

The guidelines were updated in 2003 by the Joint National Committee on Prevention, Detection, Evaluation, and Treatment of Hypertension (Case Example 6-9).[54] Preliminary recommendations for a "new definition" of hypertension were issued in 2005 by the American Society of Hypertension.[55]

The new proposed definition/classification is based on the idea that hypertension is a complex cardiovascular disorder, not a scale of blood pressure values. The new definition takes into account risk factors, early disease markers, and attempts to reflect the effects of hypertension on other organ systems. The goal of this risk-based approach is to identify individuals at any level of blood pressure who have a reasonable likelihood of future cardiovascular events.[55]

Simply stated the new guidelines emphasize the continuous relationship between blood pressure level and cardiovascular risk. The blood pressure classification scale used for diagnosis and treatment is based on total cardiovascular risk, not just blood pressure values. So for example, an individual with blood pressure values of 140/90 mm Hg (defined as Stage 1 or borderline hypertension) would not begin medical therapy in the absence of other risk factors. On the other hand, someone with much lower BP values (e.g., 120/75 mm Hg) might be treated immediately if other risk factors are present such as overweight or tobacco use.[55]

Pulse Pressure

The difference between the systolic and diastolic pressure readings (SBP minus DBP) is called pulse pressure. A widened pulse pressure often results from stiffening of the aorta secondary to atherosclerosis. Stroke volume or ventricular pressure (i.e., systolic BP) will increase. A BP of 150/80 would not be uncommon in a situation like this.

CASE EXAMPLE 6-9   Hypertension

Chief Complaint: A 70-year-old woman came to physical therapy with a diagnosis of left supraspinatus tendon strain.

Past Medical History: Cortisone injection to shoulder; recent normal ECG

Clinical Presentation: The client reported posterior left shoulder pain and lateral arm pain with occasional radiating pain down the arm to her hand. No other symptoms were reported. Vital signs were assessed:

Blood pressure: 170/95 (left arm, sitting)
Pulse: 82 beats per minute, regular
Should the client be referred for high blood pressure based on this information?

However, one high reading is not sufficient to render this diagnosis. Many other factors can influence blood pressure and should be evaluated (see Table 4-4).

The client was asked if she was ever diagnosed with high blood pressure or hypertension. She denied any personal history of known elevated blood pressure.

The client decided to have her blood pressure checked at the local health department once a week for the next two weeks. Each time the readings were above normal. She made a self-referral to her medical doctor. After a medical evaluation, she was placed on appropriate medication.

Data from Vernier DA: The meaning of screening. The application of vital signs should be used in physical therapy practice, *ADVANCE for Physical Therapists & PT Assistants* 15(18):47-49, 2004.

Widening of the pulse pressure is linked to a significantly higher risk of stroke and heart failure after the sixth decade. Some medications increase pulse pressure by lowering diastolic pressure more than systolic.[56]

Pulse pressure generally increases in direct proportion to the intensity of exercise as the SBP increases and DBP stays about the same.[57] A difference of more than 40 mm Hg is abnormal and should be reported.

Blood Pressure Classification

Hypertension can also be classified according to type (systolic or diastolic), cause, and degree of severity. *Primary (or essential) hypertension* is also known as *idiopathic hypertension* and accounts for 90% to 95% of all hypertensive clients.

Secondary hypertension results from an identifiable cause, including a variety of specific diseases or problems such as renal artery stenosis, oral contraceptive use, hyperthyroidism, adrenal tumors, and medication use.

Originally, birth control pills contained higher levels of estrogen, which was associated with hypertension, but today the estrogen and progestin contents of the pill are greatly reduced. The risk of high blood pressure with oral contraceptive use is now considered quite low but using oral contraceptives does still increase the risk of heart attack, stroke, and blood clots in certain women (e.g., age over 35, tobacco use, diabetes).

The risk may be increased for older women who smoke, but the risk for all women returns to normal after they discontinue the pill. The risk of venous thromboembolism associated with newer oral contraceptives remains under investigation.

Drugs that constrict blood vessels can contribute to hypertension. Among the most common are phenylpropanolamine in over-the-counter appetite suppressants, including herbal ephedra, pseudoephedrine in cold and allergy remedies, and prescription drugs such as monoamine oxidase (MAO) inhibitors (a class of antidepressant) and corticosteroids when used over a long period.

Intermittent elevation of blood pressure interspersed with normal readings is called *labile hypertension*, or *borderline hypertension*. Many older adults have a type of high blood pressure called *isolated systolic hypertension* (ISH) characterized by marked elevation of the systolic pressure (140 mm Hg or higher) but normal diastolic pressure (less than 90 mm Hg).[58]

ISH is a risk factor for stroke and death from cardiovascular causes. Elevated systolic pressure also raises the risk of heart attack, congestive heart failure, dementia, and end-stage kidney disease.[59]

Risk Factors

Modifiable risk factors for hypertension are primarily lifestyle factors such as stress, obesity, and poor diet or insufficient intake of nutrients (Table 6-6). Stress has been shown to cause increased peripheral vascular resistance and cardiac output and to stimulate sympathetic nervous system activity. Potassium deficiency can also contribute to hypertension.

JNC-7 (see Table 4-5) created a new blood pressure category called "prehypertension" to identify adults considered to be at risk for developing hypertension and to alert both individuals and health care providers of the importance of adopting lifestyle changes. Screening for prehypertension provides important opportunities to prevent hypertension and cardiovascular disease.[60]

Nonmodifiable risk factors include family history, age, gender, and race. The risk of hypertension increases with age as arteries lose elasticity and become less able to relax. There is a poorer prognosis associated with early onset of hypertension.

A sex-specific gene for hypertension may exist[61] because men experience hypertension at higher rates and at an earlier age than women do until after menopause. Hypertension is the most serious health problem for African-Americans (both men and women and at earlier ages than for whites) in the United States.

Clinical Signs and Symptoms

Clients with hypertension are usually asymptomatic in the early stages, but when symptoms do

TABLE 6-6 ▼ Risk Factors for Hypertension

Modifiable	Nonmodifiable
Smoking or tobacco use/abuse	African-American ethnicity
Type 2 diabetes	Age (60 or older)
High cholesterol	Postmenopausal status (including surgically-induced menopause)
Chronic alcohol use/abuse	Family history of cardiovascular disease (women younger than age 65; men younger than age 55)
Obesity	
Sedentary lifestyle	
Stress	
Diet, nutritional status; potassium deficiency	

occur, they include occipital headache (usually present in the early morning), vertigo, flushed face, nocturnal urinary frequency, spontaneous nosebleeds, and blurred vision.

Clinical Signs and Symptoms of
Hypertension

- Occipital headache
- Vertigo (dizziness)
- Flushed face
- Spontaneous epistaxis
- Vision changes
- Nocturnal urinary frequency

Transient Ischemic Attack

Hypertension is a major cause of heart failure, stroke, and kidney failure. Aneurysm formation and CHF are also associated with hypertension. Persistent elevated diastolic pressure damages the intimal layer of the small vessels, which causes an accumulation of fibrin, local edema, and, possibly, intravascular clotting.

Eventually, these damaging changes diminish blood flow to vital organs, such as the heart, kidneys, and brain, resulting in complications such as heart failure, renal failure, and cerebrovascular accidents or stroke.

Many persons have brief episodes of transient ischemic attacks (TIAs). The attacks occur when the blood supply to part of the brain has been temporarily disrupted. These ischemic episodes last from 5 to 20 minutes, although they may last for as long as 24 hours. TIAs are considered by some as a progression of cerebrovascular disease and may be referred to as "mini-strokes."

TIAs are important warning signals that an obstruction exists in an artery leading to the brain. Without treatment, 10% to 20% of people will go on to have a major stroke within 3 months, many within 48 hours.[62] Immediate medical referral is advised for anyone with signs and symptoms of TIAs, especially anyone with a history of heart disease, hypertension, or tobacco use. Other risk factors for TIAs include age (over 65), diabetes, and being overweight.

Clinical Signs and Symptoms of
Transient Ischemic Attack (TIA)

- Slurred speech, sudden difficulty with speech, or difficulty understanding others
- Sudden confusion, loss of memory, even loss of consciousness
- Temporary blindness or other dramatic visual changes

- Dizziness
- Sudden, severe headache
- Paralysis or extreme weakness, usually affecting one side of the body
- Difficulty walking, loss of balance or coordination
- Symptoms are usually brief, lasting only a few minutes but can persist up to 24 hours

Orthostatic Hypotension

(See also discussion on Hypotension in Chapter 4)

Orthostatic hypotension is an excessive fall in blood pressure of 20 mm Hg or more in systolic blood pressure or a drop of 10 mm Hg or more of both systolic and diastolic arterial blood pressure on assumption of the erect position with a 10% to 20% increase in pulse rate (Case Example 6-10). It is not a disease but a manifestation of abnormalities in normal blood pressure regulation.

This condition may occur as a normal part of aging or secondary to the effects of drugs such as hypertensives, diuretics, and antidepressants; as a result of venous pooling (e.g., pregnancy, prolonged bed rest, or standing); or in association with neurogenic origins. The last category includes diseases affecting the autonomic nervous system, such as Guillain-Barré syndrome, diabetes mellitus, or multiple sclerosis.

Orthostatic intolerance is the most common cause of lightheadedness in clients, especially those who have been on prolonged bed rest or those who have had prolonged anesthesia for surgery. When such a client is getting up out of bed for the first time, blood pressure, and heart rate should be monitored with the person in the supine position and repeated after the person is upright. If the legs are dangled off the bed, a significant drop in blood pressure may occur with or without compensatory tachycardia. This drop may provoke lightheadedness, and standing may even produce loss of consciousness.

These postural symptoms are often accentuated in the morning and are aggravated by heat, humidity, heavy meals, and exercise.

Clinical Signs and Symptoms of
Orthostatic Hypotension

- Change in blood pressure (decrease) and pulse (increase)
- Lightheadedness, dizziness
- Pallor, diaphoresis
- Syncope or fainting
- Mental or visual blurring
- Sense of weakness or "rubbery" legs

CASE EXAMPLE 6-10 Monitoring Vital Signs

Referral: An 83-year-old woman was referred to physical therapy for mobility training. Goal: Improve balance to prevent nursing home placement

Chief Complaints: Forgetfulness, two falls during the past three months, and inability to complete independent activities of daily living (ADLs)

Past/Current Medical History: Pernicious anemia, chronic venous insufficiency, noninsulin dependent diabetes, hypercholesterolemia, osteoporosis, progressive dementia, gastroesophageal reflux (GERD)

Medications/Supplements: Lasix for chronic edema in lower extremities secondary to venous insufficiency, Lipitor for elevated cholesterol, calcium for osteoporosis, Prilosec for GERD

Systems Review

Integument: Integument intact with good turgor.

Musculoskeletal: Strength 4/5 upper and lower extremities. ROM within functional limits. Thoracic kyphosis present.

Neuromuscular: Intact cranial nerves, independent transfers, impaired gait and balance.

Cardiovascular/pulmonary: Heart rate-65 beats per minute at rest; respiratory rate-16 breaths per minute; blood pressure-100/70 mm Hg (measured in sitting, right upper extremity).

Oral temperature: 100° with a regular pulse rate; finger pulse oximeter (oxygen saturation)-88% (rest) and 85% (walking with wheeled walker).

Further blood pressure assessment was conducted comparing measures in supine (110/70 mm Hg), sitting (100/70 mm Hg), and standing (90/65 mm Hg) with only slight increase in pulse rate (from 16 to 20 beats per minute) suggesting postural orthostatic hypotension (see discussion on postural orthostatic hypotension, Chapter 4). Client became diaphoretic during blood pressure testing.

Decreased breath sounds heard in right lower lobe during auscultation. Client reported productive cough and unusual fatigue.

What are the red flags in this case?

Age

Constitutional symptoms (low-grade fever, fatigue, unexplained diaphoresis)

Abnormal vital signs (blood pressure changes with change in position accompanied by increase in pulse rate, low oxygen saturation levels)

Productive cough, decreased breath sounds, right lower lobe

Result: The primary physician was contacted to discuss the therapist's concerns regarding the vital signs, constitutional symptoms, and signs and symptoms associated with the pulmonary system. The client was treated for unstable blood pressure and pneumonia.

Physical therapists can take a leadership role in the management of their clients. Every physical therapy examination should include, at a minimum, a baseline measurement of vital signs even without red flags or specific symptoms to suggest it.

Heins, P: Case report presented in partial fulfillment of DPT 910. *Principles of differential diagnosis*, Institute for Physical Therapy Education, Chester, Pennsylvania, 2005, Widener University. Used with permission.

Peripheral Vascular Disorders

Impaired circulation may be caused by a number of acute or chronic medical conditions known as peripheral vascular diseases (PVDs). PVDs can affect the arterial, venous, or lymphatic circulatory system.

Vascular disorders secondary to occlusive arterial disease usually have an underlying atherosclerotic process that causes disturbances of circulation to the extremities and can result in significant loss of function of either the upper or lower extremities.

Peripheral arterial occlusive diseases also can be caused by embolism, thrombosis, trauma, vasospasm, inflammation, or autoimmunity. The cause of some disorders is unknown.

Arterial (Occlusive) Disease

Arterial diseases include acute and chronic arterial occlusion (Table 6-7). Acute arterial occlusion may be caused by

1. Thrombus, embolism, or trauma to an artery.
2. Arteriosclerosis obliterans

TABLE 6-7 ▼ Comparison of Acute and Chronic Arterial Symptoms

Symptom analysis	Acute arterial symptoms	Chronic arterial symptoms
Location	Varies; distal to occlusion; may involve entire leg	Deep muscle pain, usually in calf, may be in lower leg or dorsum of foot.
Character	Throbbing	Intermittent claudication; feels like cramp, numbness, and tingling; feeling of cold
Onset and duration	Sudden onset (within 1 hour)	Chronic pain; onset gradual following exertion
Aggravating factors	Activity such as walking or stairs; elevation	Same as Acute Arterial
Relieving factors	Rest (usually within 2 minutes); dangling (severe involvement)	Same as Acute Arterial
Associated symptoms	6 P's: Pain, pallor, pulselessness, paresthesia, poikilothermia (coldness), paralysis (severe)	Cool, pale skin
At risk	History of vascular surgery, arterial invasive procedure, abdominal aneurysm, trauma (including injured arteries), chronic atrial fibrillation	Older adults; more males than females; inherited predisposition, history of hypertension, smoking, diabetes, hypercholesterolemia, obesity, vascular disease

Modified from Jarvis C: *Physical examination and health assessment,* Philadelphia, 1992, WB Saunders, p. 658.

3. Thromboangiitis obliterans or Buerger's disease
4. Raynaud's disease

Clinical manifestations of chronic arterial occlusion caused by peripheral vascular disease may not appear for 20 to 40 years. The lower limbs are far more susceptible to arterial occlusive disorders and atherosclerosis than are the upper limbs.

RISK FACTORS

Diabetes mellitus increases the susceptibility to coronary heart disease. People with diabetes have abnormalities that affect a number of steps in the development of atherosclerosis. Only the combination of factors, such as hypertension, abnormal platelet activation, and metabolic disturbances affecting fat and serum cholesterol, account for the increased risk.

Other risk factors include smoking, hypertension, hyperlipidemia (elevated levels of fats in the blood), and older age. Peripheral artery disease most often afflicts men older than 50, although women are at significant risk because of their increased smoking habits.

CLINICAL SIGNS AND SYMPTOMS

The first sign of vascular occlusive disease may be the loss of hair on the toes. The most important symptoms of chronic arterial occlusive disease are intermittent claudication (limping resulting from pain, ache, or cramp in the muscles of the lower extremities caused by ischemia or insufficient blood flow) and ischemic rest pain.

The pain associated with arterial disease is generally felt as a dull, aching tightness deep in the muscle, but it may be described as a boring, stabbing, squeezing, pulling, or even burning sensation. Although the pain is sometimes referred to as a cramp, there is no actual spasm in the painful muscles.

The location of the pain is determined by the site of the major arterial occlusion (see Table 14-7). Aortoiliac occlusive disease induces pain in the gluteal and quadriceps muscles. The most frequent lesion, which is present in about two thirds of clients, is occlusion of the superficial femoral artery between the groin and the knee, producing pain in the calf that sometimes radiates upward to the lower thigh. Occlusion of the popliteal or more distal arteries causes pain in the foot.

In the typical case of superficial femoral artery occlusion, there is a good femoral pulse at the groin but arterial pulses are absent at the knee and foot, although resting circulation appears to be good in the foot.

After exercise the client may have numbness in the foot as well as pain in the calf. The foot may be cold, pale, and chalky white, which is an indication that the circulation has been diverted to the arteriolar bed of the leg muscles. Blood in regions of sluggish flow becomes deoxygenated, inducing a red-purple mottling of the skin.

Painful cramping symptoms occur during walking and disappear quickly with rest. Ischemic rest pain is relieved by placing the limb in a dependent position, using gravity to enhance blood flow. In most clients the symptoms are constant and reproducible; that is, the client

who cannot walk the length of the house because of leg pain one day but is able to walk indefinitely the next does not have intermittent claudication.

Intermittent claudication is influenced by the speed, incline, and surface of the walk. Exercise tolerance decreases over time, so that episodes of claudication occur more frequently with less exertion. The differentiation between vascular claudication and neurogenic claudication is presented in Chapter 16 (see Table 16-5).

Ulceration and gangrene are common complications and may occur early in the course of some arterial diseases (e.g., Buerger's disease). Gangrene usually occurs in one extremity at a time. In advanced cases the extremities may be abnormally red or cyanotic, particularly when dependent. Edema of the legs is fairly common. Color or temperature changes and changes in nail bed and skin may also appear.

Clinical Signs and Symptoms of
Arterial Disease

- Intermittent claudication
- Burning, ischemic pain at rest
- Rest pain aggravated by elevating the extremity; relieved by hanging the foot over the side of the bed or chair
- Color, temperature, skin, nail bed changes
  Decreased skin temperature
  Dry, scaly, or shiny skin
  Poor nail and hair growth
- Possible ulcerations and gangrene on weight bearing surfaces (e.g., toes, heel)
- Vision changes (diabetic atherosclerosis)
- Fatigue on exertion (diabetic atherosclerosis)

Raynaud's Phenomenon and Disease

The term *Raynaud's phenomenon* refers to intermittent episodes during which small arteries or arterioles in extremities constrict, causing temporary pallor and cyanosis of the digits and changes in skin temperature.

These episodes occur in response to cold temperature or strong emotion (anxiety, excitement). As the episode passes, the changes in color are replaced by redness. If the disorder is secondary to another disease or underlying cause, the term *secondary Raynaud's phenomenon* is used.

Secondary Raynaud's phenomenon is often associated with connective tissue or collagen vascular disease, such as scleroderma, polymyositis/dermatomyositis, systemic lupus erythematosus, or rheumatoid arthritis. Raynaud's may occur as a long-term complication of cancer treatment. Unilateral Raynaud's phenomenon may be a sign of hidden neoplasm.

Raynaud's phenomenon may occur after trauma or use of vibrating equipment such as jackhammers, or it may be related to various neurogenic lesions (e.g., thoracic outlet syndrome) and occlusive arterial diseases.

Raynaud's disease is a primary vasospastic or vasomotor disorder, although it is included in this section under occlusive arterial because of the arterial involvement. It appears to be caused by

1. Hypersensitivity of digital arteries to cold
2. Release of serotonin
3. Congenital predisposition to vasospasm

Eighty percent of clients with Raynaud's disease are women between the ages of 20 and 49 years. Primary Raynaud's disease rarely leads to tissue necrosis.

Idiopathic Raynaud's disease is differentiated from secondary Raynaud's phenomenon by a history of symptoms for at least 2 years with no progression of the symptoms and no evidence of underlying cause.

CLINICAL SIGNS AND SYMPTOMS

The typical progression of Raynaud's phenomenon is pallor in the digits, followed by cyanosis accompanied by feelings of cold, numbness, and occasionally pain, and, finally, intense redness with tingling or throbbing.

The pallor is caused by vasoconstriction of the arterioles in the extremity, which leads to decreased capillary blood flow. Blood flow becomes sluggish and cyanosis appears; the digits turn blue. The intense redness (rubor) results from the end of vasospasm and a period of hyperemia as oxygenated blood rushes through the capillaries.

Clinical Signs and Symptoms of
Raynaud's Phenomenon and Disease

- Pallor in the digits
- Cyanotic, blue digits
- Cold, numbness, pain of digits
- Intense redness of digits

Venous Disorders

Venous disorders can be separated into acute and chronic conditions. Acute venous disorders include thromboembolism. Chronic venous disorders can be separated further into varicose vein formation and chronic venous insufficiency.

ACUTE VENOUS DISORDERS

Acute venous disorders are due to formation of thrombi (clots), which obstruct venous flow. Blockage may occur in both superficial and deep veins. Superficial thrombophlebitis is often iatrogenic, resulting from insertion of intravenous catheters or as a complication of intravenous sites.

Pulmonary emboli (see Chapter 7), most of which start as thrombi in the large deep veins of the legs, are an acute and potentially lethal complication of deep venous thrombosis.

Thrombus formation results from an intravascular collection of platelets, erythrocytes, leukocytes, and fibrin in the blood vessels, often the deep veins of the lower extremities. When thrombus formation occurs in the deep veins, the production of clots can cause significant morbidity and mortality resulting in a floating mass (embolus) that can occlude blood vessels of the lungs and other critical structures.[63]

Risk Factors Deep venous thrombosis (DVT) is a common disorder, affecting women more than men and adults more than children. Approximately one third of clients older than 40 who have had either major surgery or an acute MI develop DVT. The most significant clinical risk factors are age over 70 and previous thromboembolism[64,65] (Box 6-2).

Thrombus formation is usually attributed to (1) venous stasis, (2) hypercoagulability, or (3) injury to the venous wall. *Venous stasis* is caused by prolonged immobilization or absence of the calf muscle pump (e.g., because of illness, paralysis, or inactivity). Other risk factors include traumatic spinal cord injury; multiple trauma; CHF; obesity; pregnancy; and major orthopedic, gynecologic, abdominal, cardiac, renal or splenic surgery[66] (Case Example 6-11).

Hypercoagulability often accompanies malignant neoplasms, especially visceral and ovarian tumors. Oral contraceptives, selective estrogen receptor modulators (SERMs) (e.g., raloxifene) often used for osteoporosis related to menopause, and hematologic disorders also may increase the coagulability of the blood. In addition, previous spontaneous thromboembolism and increased levels of homocysteine are risk factors for venous as well as arterial thrombosis.[68]

The observed relationship of higher venous thrombosis risk with the use of third-generation oral contraceptives is an important consideration.[69,70] Third-generation contraceptives refer to the newest formulation of oral contraceptives with much lower levels of estrogen than those first administered.

The risk of having a blood clot depends on a number of factors. It increases with age and it also depends on what kind of oral contraceptive is being taken. Women using progestogen-only pills are at little or no increased risk of blood clots. The venous clots associated with the newest oral contraceptives typically develop in superficial leg veins and rarely result in pulmonary emboli.

Injury or trauma to the venous wall may occur as a result of intravenous injections, Buerger's disease, fractures and dislocations, sclerosing agents, and opaque mediator radiography.

Clinical Signs and Symptoms Superficial thrombophlebitis appears as a local, raised, red, slightly indurated (hard), warm, tender cord along the course of the involved vein.

In contrast, symptoms of deep venous thrombosis are less distinctive; about one half of clients are asymptomatic. The most common symptoms are pain in the region of the thrombus and unilateral swelling distal to the site (Case Example 6-12).

Other symptoms include redness or warmth of the leg, dilated veins, or low-grade fever possibly accompanied by chills and malaise. Unfortunately, the first clinical manifestation may be pulmonary embolism. Frequently, clients have thrombi in both legs even though the symptoms are unilateral.

Homans' sign (discomfort in the upper calf during gentle, forced dorsiflexion of the foot) is still

---

BOX 6-2 ▼	Risk Factors for Pulmonary Embolism (PE) and Deep Venous Thrombosis (DVT)

Previous personal/family history of thromboembolism
Congestive heart failure
Age (over 50 years)
Oral contraceptive use
Blood stasis
  Immobilization or inactivity
  Burns
  Obstetric/gynecologic conditions
  Obesity
  Spinal cord injured, stroke
Endothelial injury
  Neoplasm
  Recent surgical procedures
  Trauma or fracture of the legs or pelvis
Blood disorders (e.g., hypercoagulable state, clotting abnormalities)
History of infection, diabetes mellitus
Oral contraceptive use

CASE EXAMPLE 6-11 Deep Venous Thrombosis in a Spinal Cord-Injured Patient

Referral: An 18-year-old male with Down's syndrome fell and sustained a fracture at C2 with resultant spinal cord injury and flaccid quadriparesis. After medical treatment and stabilization, he was transferred to a rehabilitation facility.

Medications: Lovenox (anticoagulant, antithrombotic for DVT prevention)

Summary: This client had a long and extensive recovery and rehabilitation due to his diagnosis of Down's syndrome, English as a second language, high-level spinal cord injury, chronic pressure ulcers, and cardiovascular complications.

Eight months after the start of rehabilitation unilateral swelling, pain, and warmth developed in the left lower extremity. Elevating the leg did not relieve symptoms.

Circumference measurements around the left thigh, calf, and foot were 1 inch greater than around the right leg.

A DVT was highly suspected because the leg symptoms were unilateral. If the swelling were simply due to his legs being in the dependent position one would expect swelling in both of his legs. The client was in a high-risk category for developing a DVT.

He was also taken off Lovenox injections just 1 month prior to developing his symptoms. Weaning a client off percutaneous anti-coagulation therapy by six months is a generally accepted practice, continuing only with oral anti-coagulation therapy such as coumadin.[67] The client had been on Lovenox for 9 months.

Result: The client was diagnosed and treated for DVT and returned to the rehabilitation hospital. Repeat ultrasound the following month showed interval improvement without resolution of the DVT. Further medical treatment was instituted.

Although the risk of DVT is greater in the acute care phase, the therapist must remain alert to symptoms of DVT in at-risk clients with multiple comorbidities and complications. Use of the AUTAR Scale (see Table 4-11) or Wells' Clinical Decision Rule (see Table 4-12) is advised.

Even with medical treatment it should not be assumed that the condition has resolved until confirmed by medical testing. All precautions must remain in effect until released by the physician.

From Rosenzweig K: Case report presented in partial fulfillment of DPT 910. *Principles of differential diagnosis,* Institute for Physical Therapy Education, Chester, Pennsylvania, 2005, Widener University. Used with permission.

commonly assessed during physical examination. Unfortunately, it is insensitive and nonspecific. It is present in less than one third of clients with documented deep venous thrombosis. In addition, more than 50% of clients with a positive finding of Homans' sign do not have evidence of venous thrombosis.

Other more specific risk assessment and physical assessment tools are available for assessment of DVT and PVD (see ABI, AUTAR DVT Risk Assessment Scale, and Wells' Clinical Decision Rule [CDR] in Chapter 4).

The CDR may be used more widely in the clinic, but the AUTAR scale is more comprehensive and incorporates BMI, postpartum status, and the use of oral contraceptives as potential risk factors.

The Society of Interventional Radiology (SIR) now recommends that anyone being evaluated for

PVD should have ABI measurement done since this is a significantly more accurate screening measure for PVD.[71] Symptoms of superficial thrombophlebitis are relieved by bed rest with elevation of the legs and the application of heat for 7 to 15 days. When local signs of inflammation subside, the client is usually allowed to ambulate wearing elastic stockings.

Sometimes antiinflammatory medications are required. Anticoagulants such as heparin and warfarin are used to prevent clot extension.

Clinical Signs and Symptoms of
Superficial Venous Thrombosis

- Subcutaneous venous distinction
- Palpable cord
- Warmth, redness
- Indurated (hard)

CASE EXAMPLE 6-12 Deep Venous Thrombosis (DVT)

Referral: 96-year-old woman discharged from hospital to sub-acute center for rehabilitation.

Goal: Return to previous level of function if possible.

Chief Complaint: Fall with fracture of left pelvis; diffuse pain around left pelvic area rated 5/10 on the numeric rating scale; pain increases with weight bearing and movement. Conservative nonsurgical treatment was employed.

Past Medical History: Dementia, colon cancer

Current Medications: Acetaminophen 500 mg prn (for pain), warfarin daily (anticoagulant), Risperidone (for dementia), calcium carbonate/vitamin D (for osteoporosis)

Systems Review

Integument: Skin integrity within normal limits for client's age

Musculoskeletal: Muscle strength 3+/5 in both lower extremities; range of motion within functional limits for all but left hip; left hip flexion limited by pain at end of range; functional transfers, bed mobility, ambulation, and stairs with assistance; antalgic gait with decreased base of support, decreased stride/step length, minimal weight bearing on left leg

Neuromuscular: Standing balance fair, dynamic standing balance fair minus (F-) with a wheeled walker

Cardiovascular/pulmonary: Lower extremity pulses and circulation within normal limits for client's age (baseline). Two weeks later, affected foot and calf were edematous but reportedly pain free. Calf was tender to touch; leg was warm with discoloration of the affected limb.

Further Screening

Wells' Clinical Decision Rule for DVT

Clinical Presentation	Possible Score	Client's Score
Active cancer (within 6 months of diagnosis or receiving palliative care)	1	0
Paralysis, paresis, or recent immobilization of lower extremity	1	1
Bedridden for more than 3 days or major surgery in the last 4 weeks	1	0
Localized tenderness in the center of the posterior calf, the popliteal space, or along the femoral vein in the anterior thigh/groin	1	1
Entire lower extremity swelling	1	0
Unilateral calf swelling (more than 3 mm larger than uninvolved side)	1	1
Unilateral pitting edema	1	0
Collateral superficial veins (nonvaricose)	1	0
An alternative diagnosis is as likely (or more likely) than DVT (e.g., cellulitis, postoperative swelling, calf strain)	-2	0

Total Points 3

Key:

-2 to 0	Low probability of DVT (3%)
1 to 2	Moderate probability of DVT (17%)
3 or more	High probability of DVT (75%)

Medical consultation is advised in the presence of low probability; medical referral is required with moderate or high score.

From Wells PS, Anderson DR, Bormanis J, et al: Value of assessment of pretest probability of deep-vein thrombosis in clinical management, *Lancet* 350:1795-1798, 1997. Used with permission.

Result: Client was referred for medical evaluation of sudden change in the involved lower extremity. Recent pelvic fracture is a major risk factor for deep venous thrombosis, a potentially life-threatening condition. Duplex ultrasonography confirmed provisional medical diagnosis of DVT.

From Kehinde JA: Case report presented in partial fulfillment of DPT 910. *Principles of differential diagnosis*, Institute for Physical Therapy Education, Chester, Pennsylvania, 2005, Widener University. Used with permission.

Clinical Signs and Symptoms of

Deep Venous Thrombosis

- Unilateral tenderness or leg pain
- Unilateral swelling (difference in leg circumference)
- Warmth
- Discoloration
- Pain with placement of blood pressure cuff around calf inflated to 160 mm to 180 mm Hg

CHRONIC VENOUS DISORDERS

Chronic venous insufficiency, also known as postphlebitic syndrome, is identified by chronic swollen limbs; thick, coarse, brownish skin around the ankles; and venous stasis ulceration. Chronic venous insufficiency is the result of dysfunctional valves that reduce venous return, which thus increases venous pressure and causes venous stasis and skin ulcerations.

Chronic venous insufficiency follows most severe cases of deep venous thrombosis but may take as long as 5 to 10 years to develop. Education and prevention are essential, and clients with a history of deep venous thrombosis must be monitored periodically for life.

Lymphedema

The final type of peripheral vascular disorder, lymphedema, is defined as an excessive accumulation of fluid in tissue spaces. Lymphedema typically occurs secondary to an obstruction of the lymphatic system from trauma, infection, radiation, or surgery.

Postsurgical lymphedema is usually seen after surgical excision of axillary, inguinal, or iliac nodes, usually performed as a prophylactic or therapeutic measure for metastatic tumor. Lymphedema secondary to primary or metastatic neoplasms in the lymph nodes is common.

Clinical Signs and Symptoms of

Lymphedema

- Edema of the dorsum of the foot or hand
- Decreased range of motion, flexibility, and function
- Usually unilateral
- Worse after prolonged dependency
- No discomfort or a dull, heavy sensation; sense of fullness

▲ LABORATORY VALUES

The results of diagnostic tests can provide the therapist with information to assist in client education. The client often reports test results to the thera-

pist and asks for information regarding the significance of those results. The information presented in this text discusses potential reasons for abnormal laboratory values relevant to clients with cardiovascular problems.

A basic understanding of laboratory tests used specifically in the diagnosis and monitoring of cardiovascular problems can provide the therapist with additional information regarding the client's status.

Some of the tests commonly used in the management and diagnosis of cardiovascular problems include lipid screening (cholesterol levels, low-density lipoprotein/LDL levels, high-density lipoprotein/HDL levels, and triglyceride levels), serum electrolytes, and arterial blood gases (see Chapter 7).

Other laboratory measurements of importance in the overall evaluation of the client with cardiovascular disease include red blood cell values (e.g., red blood cell count, hemoglobin, and hematocrit). Those values (see Chapter 5) provide valuable information regarding the oxygen-carrying capability of the blood and the subsequent oxygenation of body tissues, such as the heart muscle.

Serum Electrolytes

Measurement of serum electrolyte values is particularly important in diagnosis, management, and monitoring of the client with cardiovascular disease, because electrolyte levels have a direct influence on the function of cardiac muscle (in a manner similar to that of skeletal muscle). Abnormalities in serum electrolytes, even in noncardiac clients, can result in significant cardiac arrhythmias and even cardiac arrest.

In addition, certain medications prescribed for cardiac clients can alter serum electrolytes in such a way that rhythm problems can occur as a result of the medication. The electrolyte levels most important to monitor include potassium, sodium, calcium, and magnesium (see inside back cover).

Potassium

Serum potassium levels can be lowered significantly as a result of diuretic therapy (particularly with loop diuretics such as Lasix [furosemide]), vomiting, diarrhea, sweating, and alkalosis. Low potassium levels cause increased electrical instability of the myocardium, life-threatening ventricular arrhythmias, and increased risk of digitalis toxicity.

Serum potassium levels must be measured frequently by the physician in any client taking a

digitalis preparation (e.g., Digoxin), because most of these clients are also undergoing diuretic therapy. Low potassium levels in clients taking digitalis can cause digitalis toxicity and precipitate life-threatening arrhythmias.

Increased potassium levels most commonly occur because of renal and endocrine problems or as a result of potassium replacement overdose. Cardiac effects of increased potassium levels include ventricular arrhythmias and asystole/flatline (complete cessation of electrical activity of the heart).

Sodium

Serum sodium levels indicate the client's state of water/fluid balance, which is particularly important in CHF and other pathologic states related to fluid imbalances. A low serum sodium level can indicate water overload or extensive loss of sodium through diuretic use, vomiting, diarrhea, or diaphoresis.

A high serum sodium level can indicate a water deficit state such as dehydration or water loss (e.g., lack of antidiuretic hormone [ADH]).

Calcium

Serum calcium levels can be decreased as a result of multiple transfusions of citrated blood, renal failure, alkalosis, laxative or antacid abuse, and parathyroid damage or removal. A decreased calcium level provokes serious and often life-threatening ventricular arrhythmias and cardiac arrest.

Increased calcium levels are less common but can be caused by a variety of situations, including thiazide diuretic use (e.g., Diuril [chlorothiazide]), acidosis, adrenal insufficiency, immobility, and vitamin D excess. Calcium excess causes atrioventricular conduction blocks or tachycardia and ultimately can result in cardiac arrest.

Magnesium

Serum magnesium levels are rarely changed in healthy individuals because magnesium is abundant in foods and water. However, magnesium deficits are often seen in alcoholic clients or clients with critical illnesses that involve shifting of a variety of electrolytes.

Magnesium deficits often accompany potassium and calcium deficits. A decrease in serum magnesium results in myocardial irritability and cardiac arrhythmias, such as atrial or ventricular fibrillation or premature ventricular beats (PVCs).

SCREENING FOR THE EFFECTS OF CARDIOVASCULAR MEDICATIONS

When a client is physically challenged, as often occurs in physical therapy, signs and symptoms develop from side effects of various classes of cardiovascular medications (Table 6-8).

For example, medications that cause peripheral vasodilation can produce hypotension, dizziness, and syncope when combined with physical therapy interventions that also produce peripheral vasodilation (e.g., hydrotherapy, aquatics, aerobic exercise).

On the other hand, cardiovascular responses to exercise can be limited in clients who are taking beta-blockers because these drugs limit the increase in heart rate that can occur as exercise increases the workload of the heart. The available pharmaceuticals used in the treatment of the conditions listed in Table 6-8 are extensive. Understanding of drug interactions and implications requires a more specific text.

The therapist must especially keep in mind that nonsteroidal antiinflammatory drugs (NSAIDs), often used in the treatment of inflammatory conditions, have the ability to negate the antihypertensive effects of angiotensin-converting enzyme (ACE) inhibitors. Anyone being treated with both NSAIDs and ACE inhibitors must be monitored closely during exercise for elevated blood pressure.

TABLE 6-8 ▼ Cardiovascular Medications

Condition	Drug class
Angina pectoris	Organic nitrates
	Beta-blockers
	Calcium channel (Ca^{2+}) blockers
Arrhythmias	Sodium channel blockers
	Beta-blockers
	Calcium channel (Ca^{2+})
	Agents prolonging depolarization
Congestive heart failure	Cardiac glycosides (digitalis)
	Diuretics
	ACE inhibitors
	Vasodilators
Hypertension	Diuretics
	Beta-blockers
	ACE inhibitors
	Vasodilators
	Calcium (Ca^{2+}) channel blockers
	Alpha (α_1)-blockers

Courtesy Susan Queen, Ph.D., P.T., University of New Mexico School of Medicine, Physical Therapy Program, Albuquerque, New Mexico.

Likewise, NSAIDs have the ability to decrease the excretion of digitalis glycosides (e.g., digoxin [Lanoxin] and digitoxin [Crystodigin]). Therefore levels of these glycosides can increase, thus producing digitalis toxicity (e.g., fatigue, confusion, gastrointestinal problems, arrhythmias).

Digitalis and diuretics in combination with NSAIDs exacerbate the side effects of NSAIDs. Anyone receiving any of these combinations must be monitored for lower-extremity (especially ankle) and abdominal swelling.

Diuretics

Diuretics, usually referred to by clients as "water pills," lower blood pressure by eliminating sodium and water and thus reducing the blood volume. Thiazide diuretics may also be used to prevent osteoporosis by increasing calcium reabsorption by the kidneys. Some diuretics remove potassium from the body, causing potentially life-threatening arrhythmias.

The primary adverse effects associated with diuretics are fluid and electrolyte imbalances, such as muscle weakness and spasms, dizziness, headache, incoordination, and nausea (Box 6-3).

Beta-Blockers

Beta-blockers relax the blood vessels and the heart muscle by blocking the beta receptors on the sinoatrial node and myocardial cells, producing a decline in the force of contraction and a reduction in heart rate. This effect eases the strain on the heart by reducing its workload and reducing oxygen consumption.

The therapist must monitor the client's perceived exertion and watch for excessive slowing of the heart rate (bradycardia) and contractility, resulting in depressed cardiac function. Other potential side effects include depression, worsening of asthma symptoms, sexual dysfunction, and fatigue. The generic names of beta-blockers end in "olol" (e.g., propranolol, metoprolol, atenolol, labetalol). Trade names include Inderal, Lopressor, and Tenormin.

Alpha-1 Blockers

Alpha-1 blockers lower the blood pressure by dilating blood vessels. The therapist must be observant for signs of hypotension and reflex tachycardia (i.e., the heart rate increases to compensate for the hypotension). Alpha-1 blockers all have the last name "zocin" (e.g., prazocin, terazocin, doxazocin; trade names include Minipress, Hytrin, Cardura).

ACE Inhibitors

Angiotensin-converting enzyme (ACE) inhibitors are highly selective drugs that interrupt a chain of molecular messengers that constrict blood vessels. They can improve cardiac function in individuals with heart failure and are used for persons with diabetes or early kidney damage. Rash and a persistent dry cough are common side effects. The generic names of ACE inhibitors end in "pril" (e.g., benazepril, captopril, enalapril, lisinopril). Trade names include Lotensin, Capoten, Vasotec, Prinivil, and Zestril. Newest on the market are ACE II inhibitors, such a Cozaar (losartan potassium) and Hyzaar (losartan potassium-hydrochlorothiazide).

Calcium Channel Blockers

Calcium channel blockers inhibit calcium from entering the blood vessel walls, where calcium

---

BOX 6-3 ▼ Potential Side Effects of Cardiovascular Medications

Abdominal pain*
Asthmatic attacks*
Bradycardia*
Cough
Dehydration
Difficulty swallowing*
Dizziness or fainting*
Drowsiness
Dyspnea* (shortness of breath or difficulty breathing)
Easy bruising
Fatigue
Headache
Insomnia†
Joint pain*
Loss of taste
Muscle cramps†
Nausea
Nightmares†
Orthostatic hypotension†
Palpitations†
Paralysis*
Sexual dysfunction†
Skin rash†
Stomach irritation†
Swelling of feet or abdomen†
Symptoms of congestive heart failure*
Shortness of breath
Swollen ankles
Coughing up blood
Tachycardia†
Unexplained swelling, unusual or uncontrolled bleeding†
Vomiting
Weakness

* Immediate physician referral.
† Notify physician.

works to constrict blood vessels. Side effects may include swelling in the feet and ankles, orthostatic hypotension, headache, and nausea.

There are several groups of calcium channel blockers. Those in the group that primarily interact with calcium channels on the smooth muscle of the peripheral arterioles all end with "pine" (e.g., amlodipine, felodipine, nisoldipine, nifedipine). Trade names include Norvasc, Plendil, Sular, and Adalat or Procardia.

A second group of calcium channel blockers works to dilate coronary arteries to lower blood pressure and suppress some arrhythmias. This group includes verapamil (Verelan, Calan, Isoptin) and diltiazem (Cardizem, Dilacor).

Nitrates

Nitrates such as nitroglycerin (e.g., nitroglycerin [Nitrostat, Nitro-Bid], isosorbide dinitrate [Iso-Bid, Isordil]) dilate the coronary arteries and are used to prevent or relieve the symptoms of angina. Headache, dizziness, tachycardia, and orthostatic hypotension may occur as a result of the vasodilating properties of these drugs.

There are other classes of drugs to treat various aspects of cardiovascular diseases separate from those listed in Table 6-8. Hyperlipidemia is often treated with medications to inhibit cholesterol synthesis. Platelet aggregation and clot formation are prevented with anticoagulant drugs such as heparin, warfarin (Coumadin), and aspirin, whereas thrombolytic drugs such as streptokinase, urokinase, and tissue-type plasminogen activator (t-PA) are used to break down and dissolve clots already formed in the coronary arteries.

Anyone receiving cardiovascular medications, especially in combination with other medications or over-the-counter drugs, must be monitored during physical therapy for red flag signs and symptoms and any unusual vital signs.

The therapist should be familiar with the signs or symptoms that require immediate physician referral and those that must be reported to the physician. Special Questions to Ask: Medications are available at the end of this chapter.

▶ PHYSICIAN REFERRAL

Referral by the therapist to the physician is recommended when the client has any combination of systemic signs or symptoms discussed throughout this chapter at presentation. These signs and symptoms should always be correlated with the client's history to rule out systemic involvement or to identify musculoskeletal or neurologic disorders

that would be appropriate for physical therapy intervention.

Clients often confide in their therapists and describe symptoms of a more serious nature. Cardiac symptoms unknown to the physician may be mentioned to the therapist during the opening interview or in subsequent visits.

The description and location of chest pain associated with pericarditis, MI, angina, breast pain, gastrointestinal disorders, and anxiety are often similar. The physician is able to distinguish among these conditions through a careful history, medical examination, and medical testing.

For example, compared with angina, the pain of true musculoskeletal disorders may last for seconds or for hours, is not relieved by nitroglycerin, and may be aggravated by local palpation or by exertion of just the upper body.

It is not the therapist's responsibility to differentiate diagnostically among the various causes of chest pain, but rather to recognize the systemic origin of signs and symptoms that may mimic musculoskeletal disorders.

The physical therapy interview presented in Chapter 2 is the primary mechanism used to begin exploring a client's reported symptoms; this is accomplished by carefully questioning the client to determine the location, duration, intensity, frequency, associated symptoms, and relieving or aggravating factors related to pain or symptoms.

Guidelines for Immediate Medical Attention

Sudden worsening of intermittent claudication may be due to thromboembolism and must be reported to the physician immediately. Symptoms of TIAs in any individual, especially those with a history of heart disease, hypertension, or tobacco use, warrant immediate medical attention.

In the clinic setting the onset of an anginal attack requires immediate cessation of exercise. Symptoms associated with angina may be reduced immediately, but should subside within 3 to 5 minutes of cessation of activity.

If the client is currently taking nitroglycerin, self-administration of medication is recommended. Relief from anginal pain should occur within 1 to 2 minutes of nitroglycerin administration; some women may obtain similar results with an antacid. The nitroglycerin may be repeated according to the prescribed directions. If anginal pain is not relieved in 20 minutes or if the client has nausea, vomiting, or profuse sweating, immediate medical intervention may be indicated.

Changes in the pattern of angina, such as increased intensity, decreased threshold of stimulus, or longer duration of pain, require immediate intervention by the physician. Pain associated with a myocardial infarction is not relieved by rest, change of position, or administration of nitroglycerin or antacids.

Clients in treatment under these circumstances should either be returned to the care of the nursing staff or, in the case of an outpatient, should be encouraged to contact their physicians by telephone for further instructions before leaving the physical therapy department. The client should be advised not to leave unaccompanied.

Guidelines for Physician Referral

- When a client has any combination of systemic signs or symptoms at presentation, refer him or her to a physician.
- Women with chest or breast pain who have a positive family history of breast cancer or heart disease should always be referred to a physician for a follow up examination.
- Palpitation in any person with a history of unexplained sudden death in the family requires medical evaluation. More than six episodes of palpitations in 1 minute or palpitations lasting for hours or occurring in association with pain, shortness of breath, fainting, or severe lightheadedness require medical evaluation.
- Anyone who cannot climb a single flight of stairs without feeling moderately to severely winded or who awakens at night or experiences shortness of breath when lying down should be evaluated by a physician.
- Fainting (syncope) without any warning period of lightheadedness, dizziness, or nausea may be a sign of heart valve or arrhythmia problems. Unexplained syncope in the presence of heart or circulatory problems (or risk factors for heart attack or stroke) should be evaluated by a physician.
- Clients who are neurologically unstable as a result of a recent cerebrovascular accident, head trauma, spinal cord injury, or other central nervous system insult often exhibit new arrhythmias during the period of instability. When the client's pulse is monitored, any new arrhythmias noted should be reported to the nursing staff or the physician.
- Cardiac clients should be sent back to their physician under the following conditions:
  • Nitroglycerin tablets do not relieve anginal pain.
  • Pattern of angina changes is noted.
  • Client has abnormally severe chest pain with nausea and vomiting.
  • Anginal pain radiates to the jaw or to the left arm.
  • Anginal pain is not relieved by rest.
  • Upper back feels abnormally cool, sweaty, or moist to touch.
  • Client develops progressively worse dyspnea.
  • Individual with coronary artery stent experiencing chest pain.
  • Client demonstrates a difference of more than 40 mm Hg in pulse pressure (SBP minus DBP = pulse pressure).
  • Client has any doubt about his or her present condition.

Clues to Screening for Cardiovascular Signs and Symptoms

Whenever assessing chest, breast, neck, jaw, back, or shoulder pain for cardiac origins, look for the following clues:

- Personal or family history of heart disease including hypertension
- Age (postmenopausal woman; anyone over 65)
- Ethnicity (Black women)
- Other signs and symptoms such as pallor, unexplained profuse perspiration, inability to talk, nausea, vomiting, sense of impending doom or extreme anxiety
- Watch for the three Ps.
  1. Pleuritic pain (exacerbated by respiratory movement involving the diaphragm, such as sighing, deep breathing, coughing, sneezing, laughing, or the hiccups; this may be cardiac if pericarditis or it may be pulmonary); have the client hold his or her breath and reassess symptoms—any reduction or elimination of symptoms with breath holding or the Valsalva maneuver suggests pulmonary or cardiac source of symptoms.
  2. Pain on palpation (musculoskeletal origin).
  3. Pain with changes in position (musculoskeletal or pulmonary origin; pain that is worse when lying down and improves when sitting up or leaning forward is often pleuritic in origin).
- If two of the three P's are present, a myocardial infarction or anginal pain occurs in approximately 5% to 7% of clients whose pain is reproducible by palpation. If the symptoms are altered by a change in positioning, this percentage drops to 2%, and if the chest pain is reproducible by respiratory movements, the likelihood of a coronary event is only 1%.[72]

- Chest pain may occur from intercostal muscle or periosteal trauma with protracted or vigorous coughing. Palpation of local chest wall will reproduce tenderness. However, a client can have both a pulmonary/cardiac condition with subsequent musculoskeletal trauma from coughing. Look for associated signs and symptoms (e.g., fever, sweats, blood in sputum).

- Angina is activated by physical exertion, emotional reactions, a large meal, or exposure to cold and has a lag time of 5 to 10 minutes. Angina does not occur immediately after physical activity. Immediate pain with activity is more likely musculoskeletal, thoracic outlet syndrome, or psychologic (e.g., "I do not want to shovel today").

- Chest pain, shoulder pain, neck pain, or temporomandibular pain occurring in the presence of coronary artery disease or previous history of myocardial infarction, especially if accompanied by associated signs and symptoms, may be cardiac.

- Upper quadrant pain that can be induced or reproduced by lower quadrant activity, such as biking, stair climbing, or walking without using the arms, is usually cardiac in origin.

- Recent history of pericarditis in the presence of new onset of chest, neck, or left shoulder pain; observe for additional symptoms of dyspnea, increased pulse rate, elevated body temperature, malaise, and myalgia(s).

- If an individual with known risk factors for congestive heart disease, especially a history of angina, becomes weak or short of breath while working with the arms extended over the head, ischemia or infarction is a likely cause of the pain and associated symptoms.

- Insidious onset of joint or muscle pain in the older client who has had a previously diagnosed heart murmur may be caused by bacterial endocarditis. Usually there is no morning stiffness to differentiate it from rheumatoid arthritis.

- Back pain similar to that associated with a herniated lumbar disk but without neurologic deficits especially in the presence of a diagnosed heart murmur, may be caused by bacterial endocarditis.

- Watch for arrhythmias in neurologically unstable clients (e.g., spinal cord, new cerebrovascular accidents [CVAs], or new traumatic brain injured [TBIs]); check pulse and ask about/observe for dizziness.

- Anyone with chest pain must be evaluated for trigger points. If palpation of the chest reproduces symptoms, especially symptoms of radiating pain, deactivation of the trigger points must be carried out and followed by a reevaluation as part of the screening process for pain of a cardiac origin (see Fig. 17-7 and Table 17-4).

- Symptoms of vascular occlusive disease include exertional calf pain that is relieved by rest (intermittent claudication), nocturnal aching of the foot and forefoot (rest pain), and classic skin changes, especially hair loss of the ankle and foot. Ischemic rest pain is relieved by placing the limb in a dependent position.

- Throbbing pain at the base of the neck and/or along the back into the interscapular areas that increases with exertion requires monitoring of vital signs and palpation of peripheral pulses to screen for aneurysm. Check for a palpable abdominal heartbeat that increases in the supine position.

- See also section on clues to differentiating chest pain in Chapter 17.

OVERVIEW   CARDIAC CHEST PAIN PATTERNS

▼ ANGINA (Fig. 6-8)

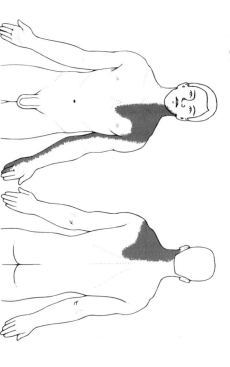

Fig. 6-8 • Pain patterns associated with angina. *Left,* Area of substernal discomfort projected to the left shoulder and arm over the distribution of the ulnar nerve. Referred pain may be present only in the left shoulder or in the shoulder and along the arm only to the elbow. *Right,* Occasionally, anginal pain may be referred to the back in the area of the left scapula or the interscapular region. Women can have the same patterns as shown for men in this figure or they may present as shown in Fig. 6-4. There may be no pain but rather a presenting symptom of extreme fatigue, weakness, or breathlessness.

Location:
Substernal/retrosternal (beneath the sternum)
Left chest pain in the absence of substernal chest pain (women)
Isolated midthoracic back pain (women)
Aching in the right biceps muscle (women)

Referral:
Neck, jaw, back, shoulder, or arms (most commonly the left arm)
May have only a toothache
Occasionally to the abdomen

Description:
Viselike pressure, squeezing, heaviness, burning indigestion

Intensity:*
Mild to moderate
Builds up gradually or may be sudden

Duration:
Usually less than 10 minutes
Never more than 30 minutes
Average: 3-5 minutes

Associated signs and
symptoms:
Extreme fatigue, lethargy, weakness (women)
Shortness of breath (dyspnea)
Nausea
Diaphoresis (heavy perspiration)
Anxiety or apprehension
Belching (eructation)
"Heartburn" (unrelieved by antacids) (women)
Sensation similar to inhaling cold air (women)
Prolonged and repeated palpitations without chest pain (women)

Relieving factors:
Rest or nitroglycerin
Antacids (women)

Aggravating factors:
Exercise or physical exertion
Cold weather or wind
Heavy meals
Emotional stress

* For each pattern reviewed, intensity is related directly to the degree of noxious stimuli.

OVERVIEW | **CARDIAC CHEST PAIN PATTERNS—cont'd**

▼ MYOCARDIAL INFARCTION (Fig. 6-9)

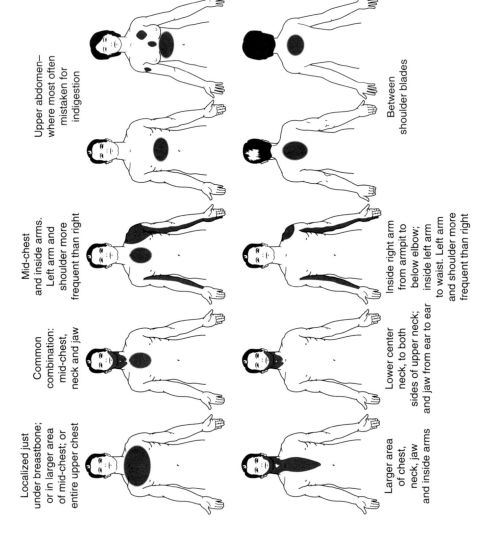

Localized just under breastbone; or in larger area of mid-chest; or entire upper chest

Common combination: mid-chest, neck and jaw

Mid-chest and inside arms. Left arm and shoulder more frequent than right

Upper abdomen—where most often mistaken for indigestion

Larger area of chest, neck, jaw and inside arms

Lower center neck, to both sides of upper neck; and jaw from ear to ear

Inside right arm from armpit to below elbow; inside left arm to waist. Left arm and shoulder more frequent than right

Between shoulder blades

Most common warning signs of heart attack

- Uncomfortable pressure, fullness, squeezing or pain in the center of the chest (prolonged)
- Pain that spreads to the throat, neck, back, jaw, shoulders, or arms
- Chest discomfort with lightheadedness, dizziness, sweating, pallor, nausea, or shortness of breath
- Prolonged symptoms unrelieved by antacids, nitroglycerin, or rest

Atypical, less common warning signs (especially women)

- Unusual chest pain (quality, location, e.g., burning, heaviness; left chest), stomach or abdominal pain
- Continuous midthoracic or interscapular pain
- Continuous neck or shoulder pain
- Isolated right biceps pain
- Pain relieved by antacids; pain unrelieved by rest or nitroglycerin
- Nausea and vomiting; flu-like manifestation without chest pain/discomfort
- Unexplained intense anxiety, weakness, or fatigue
- Breathlessness, dizziness

Fig. 6-9 • Early warning signs of a heart attack. Multiple segmental nerve innervations shown in Fig. 4-3 account for varied pain patterns possible. A woman can experience any of the various patterns described but is just as likely to develop atypical symptoms of pain as depicted here. (From Goodman CC, Boissonnault, WG, Fuller K: *Pathology: implications for the physical therapists,* ed 2, Philadelphia, 2003, WB Saunders. Fig 11-11, p. 408.)

OVERVIEW CARDIAC CHEST PAIN PATTERNS—cont'd

Location: Substernal, anterior chest
Referral: May radiate like angina, frequently down both arms
Description: Burning, stabbing, viselike pressure, squeezing, heaviness
Intensity: Severe
Duration: Usually at least 30 minutes; may last 1 to 2 hours
Residual soreness 1 to 3 days
Associated signs and
symptoms: None with a silent myocardial infarction
Dizziness, feeling faint
Nausea, vomiting
Pallor
Diaphoresis (heavy perspiration)
Apprehension, severe anxiety
Fatigue, sudden weakness
Dyspnea
May be followed by painful shoulder-hand syndrome (see text)
Relieving factors: None; unrelieved by rest or nitroglycerin taken every 5 minutes for 20 minutes
Aggravating factors: Not necessarily anything; may occur at rest or may follow emotional stress or
physical exertion

▼ PERICARDITIS (Fig. 6-10)

Location: Substernal or over the sternum, sometimes to the left toward the
cardiac apex
Referral: Neck, upper back, upper trapezius muscle, left supraclavicular area, down the
left arm, costal margins
Description: More localized than pain of myocardial infarction
Sharp, stabbing, knifelike
Intensity: Moderate-to-severe
Duration: Continuous; may last hours or days with residual soreness following
Associated signs and
symptoms: Usually medically determined associated symptoms (e.g., by chest auscultation
using a stethoscope); cough
Relieving factors: Sitting upright or leaning forward
Aggravating factors: Muscle movement associated with deep breathing (e.g., laughter, inspiration,
coughing)
Left lateral (side) bending of the upper trunk
Trunk rotation (either to the right or to the left)
Supine position

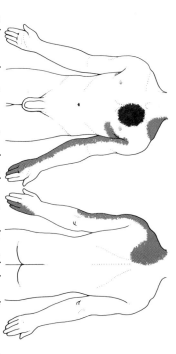

Fig. 6-10 • Substernal pain associated with pericarditis (*dark red*) may radiate anteriorly (*light red*) to the costal margins, neck, upper back, upper trapezius muscle, and left supraclavicular area or down the left arm.

O V E R V I E W   **CARDIAC CHEST PAIN PATTERNS—cont'd**

▼ **DISSECTING AORTIC ANEURYSM** (Fig. 6-11)

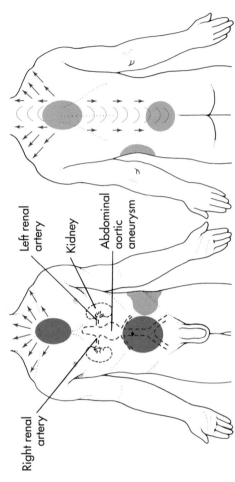

Fig. 6-11 • Most aortic aneurysms (more than 95%) are located just below the renal arteries and extend to the umbilicus, causing low back pain. Chest pain (*dark red*) associated with thoracic aneurysms may radiate (*see arrows*) to the neck, interscapular area, shoulders, lower back, or abdomen. Early warning signs of an impending rupture may include an abdominal heartbeat when lying down (not shown) or a dull ache in the midabdominal left flank or lower back (*light red*).

Location:	Anterior chest (thoracic aneurysm)
	Abdomen (abdominal aneurysm)
	Thoracic area of back
Referral:	Pain may move in the chest as dissection progresses
	Pain may extend to the neck, shoulders, interscapular area, or lower back
Description:	Knifelike, tearing (thoracic aneurysm)
	Dull ache in the lower back or midabdominal left flank (abdominal aneurysm)
Intensity:	Severe, excruciating
Duration:	Hours
Associated signs and symptoms:	Pulses absent
	Person senses "heartbeat" when lying down
	Palpable, pulsating abdominal mass
	Lower blood pressure in one arm
	Other medically determined symptoms
Relieving factors:	None
Aggravating factors:	Supine position accentuates symptoms

OVERVIEW NONCARDIAC CHEST PAIN PATTERNS

- Musculoskeletal disorders; see Chapters 14-18.
- Neurologic disorders; see Chapters 14-18.
- Pleuropulmonary disorders; see Chapter 7.
- Gastrointestinal disorders; see Chapter 8.
- Breast diseases; see Chapter 17.
- Anxiety states; see Chapter 3.

⚡ KEY POINTS TO REMEMBER

✓ Fatigue beyond expectations during or after exercise is a red-flag symptom.

✓ Be on the alert for cardiac risk factors in older adults, especially women, and begin a conditioning program before an exercise program.

✓ The client with stable angina typically has a normal blood pressure; it may be low, depending on medications. Blood pressure may be elevated when anxiety accompanies chest pain or during acute coronary insufficiency; systolic blood pressure may be low if there is heart failure.

✓ Cervical disk disease and arthritic changes can mimic atypical chest pain of angina pectoris, requiring screening through questions and musculoskeletal evaluation.

✓ If a client uses nitroglycerin, make sure that he or she has a fresh supply, and check that the physical therapy department has a fresh supply in a readily accessible location.

✓ Anyone being treated with both NSAIDs and ACE inhibitors must be monitored closely during exercise for elevated blood pressure.

✓ A person taking medications, such as beta-blockers or calcium channel blockers, may not be able to achieve a

target heart rate (THR) above 90 beats per minute. To determine a safe rate of exercise, the heart rate should return to the resting level 2 minutes after stopping exercise.

✓ Make sure that a client with cardiac compromise has not smoked a cigarette or eaten a large meal just before exercise.

✓ A 3-pound or greater weight gain or gradual, continuous gain over several days, resulting in swelling of the ankles, abdomen, and hands, combined with shortness of breath, fatigue, and dizziness that persist despite rest, may be red-flag symptoms of CHF.

✓ The pericardium (sac around the entire heart) is adjacent to the diaphragm. Pain of cardiac and diaphragmatic origin is often experienced in the shoulder because the heart and the diaphragm are supplied by the C5-6 spinal segment. The visceral pain is referred to the corresponding somatic area.

✓ Watch for muscle pain, cramps, stiffness, spasms, and weakness that cannot be explained by arthritis, recent strenuous exercise, a fever, a recent fall, or other common causes in clients taking statins to lower cholesterol.

SUBJECTIVE EXAMINATION

Special Questions to Ask

Past Medical History

- Has a doctor ever said that you have heart trouble? High blood pressure?
- Have you ever had a heart attack? *If yes, when?* Please describe.
- Do you associate your current symptoms with your heart problems?
- Have you ever had rheumatic fever, twitching of the limbs called St. Vitus' dance, or rheumatic heart disease?
- Have you ever had an abnormal electrocardiogram (ECG)?
- Have you ever had an ECG taken while you were exercising (e.g., climbing up and down steps or walking on a treadmill) that was not normal?
- Do you have a pacemaker, artificial heart, or any other device to assist your heart?
- For the therapist: Remember to review smoking, diet, lifestyle, exercise, and stress history (see family/personal history, Chapter 2).

Angina/Myocardial Infarct

- Do you have angina (pectoris) or chest pain or tightness?
  If yes, please describe the symptoms and tell me when it occurs.
  If no, have you ever had chest pain, dizziness, or shortness of breath during or after activity, exercise, or sport?
- Can you point to the area of pain with one finger? **(Anginal pain is characteristically demonstrated with the hand or fist on the chest.)**
- Is the pain close to the surface or deep inside? **(Pleuritic pain is close to the surface; anginal pain can be close to the surface but always also has a "deep inside" sensation.)**
  If yes, pursue further with the following questions:
- Do you ever have discomfort or tightness in your chest?
- Have you ever had a crushing sensation in your chest with or without pain down your left arm?
- Do you have pain in your jaw either alone or in combination with chest pain?
- If you climb a few flights of stairs fairly rapidly, do you have tightness or pressing pain in your chest?

- Do you get pressure or pain or tightness in the chest as if you were walking in the cold wind or facing a cold blast of air?
- Have you ever had pain or pressure or a squeezing feeling in the chest that occurred during exercise, walking, or any other physical or sexual activity?
- Have you been unusually tired lately **(possible new onset of angina in women)?**
- Do you get tired faster than others doing the same things?
- Has anyone in your family ever had or died from heart problems?
  If yes, did he/she die suddenly before age 50?

Associated Symptoms

- Do you ever have bouts of rapid heart action, irregular heartbeats, or palpitations of your heart?
- Have you ever felt a "heartbeat" in your abdomen when you lie down? *If yes,* is this associated with low back pain or left flank pain? **(Abdominal aneurysm)**
- Do you ever notice sweating, nausea, or chest pain when your current symptoms (e.g., back pain, shoulder pain) occur?
- Do you have frequent attacks of heartburn, or do you take antacids to relieve heartburn or acid indigestion? **(Noncardiac cause of chest pain [men], abdominal muscle trigger point, gastrointestinal disorder)**
- Do you get very short of breath during activities that do not make other people short of breath? **(Dyspnea)**
- Do you ever wake up at night gasping for air or have short breaths? **(Paroxysmal nocturnal dyspnea)**
- Do you ever need to sleep on more than one pillow to breathe comfortably? **(Orthopnea)**
- Do you ever get cramps in your legs if you walk for several blocks? **(Intermittent claudication)**
- Do you ever have swollen feet or ankles? *If yes,* are they swollen when you get up in the morning? **(Edema/congestive heart failure; NSAIDs)**
- Have you gained unexpected weight during a fairly short period of time (i.e., less than 1 week)? **(Edema, congestive heart failure)**
- Do you ever feel dizzy or have fainting spells? **(Valvular insufficiency, bradycardia,**

SUBJECTIVE EXAMINATION—cont'd

pulmonary hypertension, orthostatic hypotension)

- Have you had any significant changes in your urine (e.g., increased amount, concentrated urine, frequency at night, or decreased amount)? **(Congestive heart failure, diabetes, hypertension)**

- Do you ever have sudden difficulty with speech, temporary blindness, or other changes in your vision? **(Transient ischemic attacks)**

- Have you ever had sudden weakness or paralysis down one side of your body or just in an arm or a leg? **(Transient ischemic attacks)**

Medications

- Have you ever taken digitalis, nitroglycerin, or any other drug for your heart?

- Have you been on a diet or taken medications to lower your blood cholesterol?

- For the therapist: Any clients taking anticlotting drugs should be examined for hematoma, nosebleed, or other sites of bleeding. Protect client from trauma.

- Anyone taking cardiovascular medications (especially ACE inhibitors or digitalis glycosides) in combination with NSAIDs must be monitored closely (see text explanation).

- Any woman older than 35 and taking oral contraceptives who has a history of smoking

should be monitored for increases in blood pressure.

- Any woman taking third-generation oral contraceptives should be monitored for venous thrombosis.

For clients taking nitroglycerin

- Do you ever have headaches, dizziness, or a flushed sensation after taking nitroglycerin? (Most common side effects)

- How quickly does your nitroglycerin reduce or eliminate your chest pain? (Use as a guideline in the clinic when the client has angina during exercise; refer to a physician if angina is consistently unrelieved with nitroglycerin or rest after the usual period of time.)

For clients with breast pain (see questions, Chapter 17)

For clients with joint pain

- Have you had any recent skin rashes or dot-like hemorrhages under the skin? **(Rheumatic fever, endocarditis)** If yes, did this occur after a visit to the dentist?

- Do you notice any increase in your joint pain or symptoms 1 to 2 hours after you take your medication? **(Allergic response)**

- For new onset of left upper trapezius muscle/left shoulder pain: Have you been treated for any infection in the last 3 weeks?

CASE STUDY

REFERRAL

A 30-year-old woman with five children comes to you for an evaluation on the recommendation of her friend, who received physical therapy from you last year. She has not been to a physician since her last child was delivered by her obstetrician 4 years ago.

Her chief complaint is pain in the left shoulder and left upper trapezius muscle with pain radiating into the chest and referred pain down the medial aspect of the arm to the thumb and first two fingers.

When the medical history is being taken, the client mentions that she was told 5 years ago that she had a mitral valve prolapse secondary to rheumatic fever, which she had when she was 12 years old. She is not taking any medication, denies any palpitations, but complains of fatigue and has dyspnea after playing ball with her son for 10 or 15 minutes.

There is no reported injury or trauma to the neck or shoulder, and the symptoms subside with rest. Physical exertion, such as carrying groceries up the stairs or laundry outside, aggravates the symptoms, but she is uncertain whether just using her upper body has the same effect.

Despite the client's denial of injury or trauma, the neck and shoulder should be screened for any possible musculoskeletal or neurologic origin of symptoms. Your observation of the woman indicates that she is 30 to 40 pounds overweight. She confides that she is under physical and emotional stress by the daily demands made by seven people in her house.

She is not involved in any kind of exercise program outside of her play activities with the children. These two factors (obesity and stress) could account for her chronic fatigue and dyspnea, but that determination must be made by a physician. Even if you can identify a musculoskeletal basis for this woman's symptoms, the past medical history of rheumatic heart disease and absence of medical follow up would support your recommendation that the client should go to the physician for a medical checkup.

How do you rule out the possibility that this pain is not associated with a mitral valve prolapse and is caused instead by true cervical spine or shoulder pain?

It should be pointed out here that the therapist is not equipped with the skills, knowledge, or expertise to determine that the mitral valve prolapse is the cause of the client's symptoms.

However, a thorough subjective and objective evaluation can assist the therapist both in making a determination regarding the client's musculoskeletal condition and in providing clear and thorough feedback for the physician on referral.

SCREENING FOR MITRAL VALVE PROLAPSE

- Pain of a mitral valve must be diagnosed by a physician
- Mitral valve may be asymptomatic
- Positive history for rheumatic fever
- Carefully ask the client about a history of possible neck or shoulder pain, which the person may not mention otherwise
- Musculoskeletal pain associated with the neck or shoulder is more superficial than cardiac pain
- Total body exertion causing shoulder pain may be secondary to angina or myocardial ischemia and subsequent infarction, whereas movements of just the upper extremity causing shoulder pain are more indicative of a primary musculoskeletal lesion
- Does your shoulder pain occur during exercise, such as walking, climbing stairs, mowing the lawn, or during any other physical or sexual activity that does not require the use of your arm or shoulder?
- Presence of associated signs and symptoms, such as dyspnea, fatigue, or heart palpitations
- X-ray findings, if available, may confirm osteophyte formation with decreased intraforaminal spaces, which may contribute to cervical spine pain
- History of neck injury or overuse
- History of shoulder injury or overuse
- Results of objective tests to clear or rule out the cervical spine and shoulder as the cause of symptoms
- Presence of other neurologic signs to implicate the cervical spine or thoracic outlet type of symptoms (e.g., abnormal deep tendon reflexes, subjective report of numbness and tingling, objective sensory changes, muscle wasting or atrophy)
- Pattern of symptoms; a change in position may relieve symptoms associated with a cervical disorder.

PRACTICE QUESTIONS

1. Pursed-lip breathing in the sitting position while leaning forward on the arms relieves symptoms of dyspnea for the client with
   a. Orthopnea
   b. Emphysema
   c. Congestive heart failure
   d. (a) and (c)

2. Briefly describe the difference between myocardial ischemia, angina pectoris, and myocardial infarction.

3. What should you do if a client complains of throbbing pain at the base of the neck that radiates into the interscapular areas and increases with exertion?

4. What are the 3 Ps? What is the significance of each one?

5. When are palpitations clinically significant?

6. A 48-year-old woman with temporomandibular joint syndrome has been referred to you by her dentist. How do you screen for the possibility of medical (specifically cardiac) disease?

7. A 55-year-old male grocery store manager reports that he becomes extremely weak and breathless when he is stocking groceries on overhead shelves. What is the possible significance of this complaint?

8. You are seeing an 83-year-old woman for a home health evaluation after a motor vehicle accident (MVA) that required a long hospitalization followed by transition care in an intermediate care nursing facility and now home health care. She is ambulating short distances with a wheeled walker, but she becomes short of breath quickly and requires lengthy rest periods. At each visit the client is wearing her slippers and housecoat, so you suggest that she start dressing each day as if she intended to go out. She replies that she can no longer fit into her loosest slacks and she cannot tie her shoes.

Is there any significance to this client's comments, or is this consistent with her age and obvious deconditioning? Briefly explain your answer.

9. Peripheral vascular diseases include
   a. Arterial and occlusive diseases
   b. Arterial and venous disorders
   c. Acute and chronic arterial diseases
   d. All of the above
   e. None of the above

10. Which statement is the most accurate?
    a. Arterial disease is characterized by intermittent claudication, pain relieved by elevating the extremity, and history of smoking.
    b. Arterial disease is characterized by loss of hair on the lower extremities and throbbing pain in the calf muscles that goes away by using heat and elevation.
    c. Arterial disease is characterized by painful throbbing of the feet at night that goes away by dangling the feet over the bed.
    d. Arterial disease is characterized by loss of hair on the toes, intermittent claudication, and redness or warmth of the legs that is accompanied by a burning sensation.

11. What are the primary signs and symptoms of congestive heart failure?
    a. Fatigue, dyspnea, edema, nocturia
    b. Fatigue, dyspnea, varicose veins
    c. Fatigue, dyspnea, tinnitus, nocturia
    d. Fatigue, dyspnea, headache, night sweats

12. When would you advise a client in physical therapy to take his/her nitroglycerin?
    a. 45 minutes before exercise
    b. When symptoms of chest pain do not subside with 10 to 15 minutes of rest
    c. As soon as chest pain begins
    d. None of the above
    e. All of the above

REFERENCES

1. Aspinall W: Clinical testing for the cranioverterbral hypermobility syndrome. *J Orthop Sports Phys Ther* 12:180-181, 1989.
2. Magee DJ: *Orthopedic physical assessment*, ed 4, Philadelphia, 2002, WB Saunders.
3. Childs JD, Flynn TW, Fritz JM, et al: Screening for vertebrobasilar insufficiency in patients with neck pain: manual therapy decision-making in the presence of uncertainty, *JOSPT* 35(5):300-306, 2005.
4. Rivett DA: The premanipulative vertebral artery testing protocol: a brief review, *Physiotherapy* 23:9-12, 1995.
5. Thiel H, Wallace K, Donut J, et al: Effect of various head and neck positions on vertebral artery blood flow, *Clin Biomech* 9:105-110, 1994.
6. Trumbore DJ: Statins and myalgia: a case report of pharmacovigilance with implications for physical therapy case report presented in partial fulfillment of DPT 910, Principles of Differential Diagnosis, Institute for Physical

Therapy Education, Chester, Pennsylvania, 2005, Widener University. Used with permission.

7. Zhao H, Thomas G, Leung Y, et al: Statins in lipid-lowering therapy, *Acta Cardiol Sin* 19:1-11, 2003.

8. Rosenson RS: Current overview of statin-induced myopathy, *Am J Med* 116:408-416, 2004.

9. Roten L, Schoenenberger RA, Krahenbuhl S, et al: Rhabdomyolysis in association with simvastatin and amiodarone, *Ann Pharmacother* 38:978-81, 2004.

10. Tomlinson S, Mangione K: Potential adverse effects of statins on muscle: update, *Physical Therapy*, 85(5):459-465, 2005.

11. Pasternak RC, Smith SC, Bairey-Merz CN, et al: ACC/AHA/NHLBI clinical advisory on the use and safety of statins, *Circulation* 106:1024, 2002.

12. Ucar M, Mjorndal T, Dahlqvist R: HMG-CoA reductase inhibitors and myotoxicity, *Drug Saf* 22:441-57, 2000.

13. Baxter R, Moore J: Diagnosis and treatment of acute exertional rhabdomyolysis, *J Orthop Sports Phys Ther* 33(3):104-108, 2003.

14. Evans M, Rees A: Effects of HMG-CoA reductase inhibitors on skeletal muscle: are all statins the same? *Drug Saf* 25:649-63, 2002.

15. Using Crestor—and all statins—safely, *Harvard Heart Letter*, September 2005; p 3. More information available at www.health.harvard.edu/heartextra. Accessed: October 17, 2005.

16. Cholesterol drugs: very safe and highly beneficial, *Johns Hopkins Medical Letter: Health After 50* 13(12):3, 2002.

17. Prager GW, Binder BR: Genetic determinants: is there an "atherosclerosis gene"? *Acta Med Austriaca* 31(1):1-7, 2004.

18. Kurtz TW, Gardner DG: Transcription-modulating drugs: a new frontier in the treatment of essential hypertension, *Hypertension* 32(3):380-386, 1998.

19. Benson SC, Pershadsingh HA, Ho CI: Identification of telmisartan as a unique angiotensin II receptor antagonist with selective PPAR gamma-modulating activity, *Hypertension* 43(5):993-1002, 2004.

20. Horn HR: The impact of cardiovascular disease. On-line: http://www.medscape.com/viewarticle/466799_2, April 2004.

21. Davidson M: Confirmed previous infection with Chlamydia pneumoniae (TWAR) and its presence in early coronary atherosclerosis, *Circulation* 98(7):628-633, 1998.

22. Muhlestein, JB: Bacterial infections and atherosclerosis, *J Invest Med* 46(8):396-402, 1998.

23. Grayston JT, Kronmal RA, Jackson LA, et al: Azithromycin for the secondary prevention of coronary events, *NEJM* 352(16):1637-1645, 2005.

24. Toss H, Gnarpe J, Gnarpe H: Increased fibrinogen levels are associated with persistent *Chlamydia pneumoniae* infection in unstable coronary artery disease, *Eur Heart J* 19(4):570-577, 1998.

25. Anderson JL, Carlquist JF, Muhlestein JB, et al: Evaluation of C-reactive protein, an inflammatory marker, and infectious serology as risk factors of coronary artery disease and myocardial infarction, *J Am Coll Cardiol* 32(1):35-41, 1998.

26. Toth PP: C-reactive protein as a potential therapeutic target in patients with coronary heart disease, *Curr Atheroscler Rep* 7(5):333-334, 2005.

27. Morrow DA, Rifai N, Antman EM, et al: C-reactive protein is a potent predictor of mortality independently of and in combination with troponin T in acute coronary syndromes: a TIMI 11A substudy-thrombolysis in myocardial infarction, *J Am Coll Cardiol* 31(7):1460-1465, 1998.

28. Elliot WJ, Powel LH: Diagonal earlobe creases and prognosis in patients with suspected coronary artery disease, *Am J Med* 100(2):205-211, 1996.

29. Bahcelioglu M, Isik AF, Demirel D, et al: The diagonal ear lobe crease as sign of some diseases, *Saudi Med* 26(6):947-951, 2005.

30. American Heart Association (AHA): Heart and stroke encyclopedia. Available at: http://www.americanheart.org. Accessed August 17, 2005.

31. Gender matters: Heart disease risk in women, *Harvard Women's Health Watch* 11(9):1-3, 2004.

32. Cheek D: What's different about heart disease in women? *Nursing2003* 33(8):36-42, 2003.

33. LaGrossa J: Heart attack in women, *Advance Online Editions for Physical Therapists*, February 2, 2004. Available at: www.advanceforpt.com. Accessed October 17, 2005.

34. Barclay L, Vega C: AHA Updates Guidelines for cardiovascular disease prevention in women, CME 2004. Available at: www.medscape.com. Accessed October 17, 2005.

35. Cohen MC, Rohtla KM, Mittleman MA et al: Meta-analysis of the morning excess of acute myocardial infarction and sudden cardiac death, *Am J Cardiol* 79(11):1512-1516, 1997.

36. McSweeney JC: Women's early warning symptoms of acute myocardial infarction, *Circulation* 108(21):2619-2623, 2003.

37. Is it a heart attack? If you're a woman, will you know? *Berkeley Wellness Letter* 17(2):10, 2000.

38. Marrugat J: Mortality differences between men and women following first myocardial infarction, *JAMA* 280:1405-1409, 1998.

39. Cahalin LP: Heart failure, *Phys Ther* 76(5):517-533, 1996.

40. de Virgilio C: Ascending aortic dissection in weight lifters with cystic medial degeneration, *Ann Thorac Surg* 49(4):638-642, 1990.

41. U.S. Preventive Services Task Force (USPSTF): One-time screening in select subsets of men, *Annals Int Med* 142:198-202, 2005.

42. Hillman ND, Tani LY, Veasy LG, et al: Current status of surgery for rheumatic carditis in children, *Ann Thoracic Surg* 78(4):1403-1408, 2004.

43. Sapico FL, Liquette JA, Sarma RJ: Bone and joint infections in patients with infective endocarditis: review of a 4-year experience, *Clin Infect Dis* 22:783-787, 1996.

44. Vlahakis NE, Temesgen Z, Berbari EF, et al: Osteoarticular infection complicating enterococcal endocarditis, *Mayo Clin Proc* 78(5):623-628, 2003.

45. Cava JR, Danduran MJ, Fedderly RT, et al: Exercise recommendations and risk factors for sudden cardiac death, *Pediatr Clin North Am* 51(5):1401-1420, 2004.

46. Berger S, Kugler JD, Thomas JA, et al: Sudden cardiac death in children and adolescents: introduction and overview, *Pediatr Clin North Am* 51(5):1201-1209, 2004.

47. Bader RS, Goldberg L, Sahn DJ: Risk of sudden cardiac death in young athletes: which screening strategies are appropriate? *Pediatr Clin North Am* 51(5):1421-1441, 2004.

48. Freed LA, Benjamin EJ, Levy D, et al: Mitral valve prolapse in the general population the benign nature of echocardiographic features in the Framingham Heart Study, *J Am Coll Cardiol* 40(7):1298-1304, 2002.

49. Freed LA, Levy D, Levine RA, et al: Prevalence and clinical outcome of mitral valve prolapse, *NEJM* 341(1):1-7, 1999.

50. Hayek E, Gring CN, Griffin BP: Mitral valve prolapse, *Lancet* 365(9458):507-518, 2005.

51. Kario K, Tobin J, Wolfson L, et al: Lower standing systolic blood pressure as a predictor of falls in the elderly: a community-based prospective study, *J Am Coll Cardio* 38(1):246-252, 2001.

52. Montenero A, Mollichelli N, Zumbo F, et al: *Helicobacter pylori* and atrial fibrillation: a possible pathogenic link, *Heart* 91(7):960-961, 2005. Available at: http://www.heart.bmjjournals.com. Accessed October 17, 2005.

53. O'Donnell CJ, Ridker PM, Glynn RJ: Hypertension and borderline isolated systolic hypertension increase risks of cardiovascular disease and mortality in male physicians, *Circulation* 95(5):1132-1137, 1997.

54. National Heart, Lung, and Blood Institute (NHLBI): The Seventh Report of the Joint National Committee on Prevention, Detection, Evaluation, and Treatment of High Blood Pressure, NIH Publication No. 03-5233, May 2003. Available at www.nhlbi.nih.gov/. Accessed October 17, 2005.

55. Brookes L: The definition and consequences of hypertension are evolving. *Medscape Cardiology* 9(1):2005. Available at: http://www.medscape.com/viewarticle/506463. Accessed October 20, 2005.

56. Franklin SS: Pulse pressure as a risk factor, *Clin Exp Hypertens* 26(7-8), 645-652, 2004.

57. *ACSM's Guidelines for Exercise Testing and Prescription*, ed 6, Philadelphia, 2000, Lippincott, Williams, and Wilkins.

58. Chaudhry SI, Krumholz HM, Foody JM: Systolic hypertension in older persons, *JAMA* 292(9):1074-1080, 2004.

59. Your blood pressure: check that top number, *Johns Hopkins Medical Letter: Health After 50* 16(11):6-7, 2005.

60. Miller ER, Jehn ML: New high blood pressure guidelines create new at-risk classification: changes in blood pressure classification by JNC 7, *J Cardiovasc Nurs* 19(6):367-371, 2004.

61. O'Donnell CJ, Lindpaintner K, Larson MG, et al: Evidence for association and genetic linkage with hypertension and blood pressure in men but not women in the Framingham heart study, *Circulation* 97(18):1766-1772, 1998.

62. Treating a "mini stroke" to prevent a "major" stroke, *Johns Hopkins Medical Letter: Health After 50* 17(8):6-7, 2005.

63. Tepper S, McKeough M: Deep venous thrombosis: risks, diagnosis, treatment interventions, and prevention, *Acute Care Perspectives* 9(1):1-7, 2000.

64. Rosenzweig K: Differential diagnosis of deep vein thrombosis in a spinal cord injured client, Case report presented in partial fulfillment of DPT 910, Principles of Differential Diagnosis, Institute for Physical Therapy Education, Chester, Pennsylvania, 2005, Widener University.

65. Powell M: Duplex ultrasound screening for deep vein thrombosis in spinal cord injured patients at rehabilitation admission, *Arch Phys Med Rehab* 80:1044-1046, 1999.

66. Agnelli G, Sonaglia F: Prevention of venous thromboembolism, *Thromb Res* 97(1):V49-V62, 2000.

67. Ageno W: Treatment of venous thromboembolism, *Thromb Res* 97(1):V63-V72, 2000.

68. Bauer K: Hypercoagulable states, *Hematology* 10(Suppl 1):39, 2005.

69. Wu O, Robertson L, Langhorne P, et al: Oral contraceptives, hormone replacement therapy, thrombophilias, and risk of venous thromboembolism: a systematic review. The Thrombosis: Risk and Economic Assessment of Thrombophilia Screening (TREATS) Study, *Thromb Haemost* 94(1):17-25, 2005.

70. Gomes MP, Deitcher SR: Risk of venous thromboembolic disease associated with hormonal contraceptives and hormone replacement therapy: a clinical review, *Arch Intern Med* 164(18):1965-1976, 2004.

71. Sacks D, Bakal C, Beatty P, et al: Position statement on the use of the ankle brachial index in the evaluation of patients with peripheral vascular disease, *J Vasc Interv Radiol* 14(9 Pt 2):S389, 2003.

72. Bancroft B: Chest pain and the 3 P's, *Pathophysio Perspect*, March/April 1996.

Screening for Pulmonary Disease

For the client with neck, shoulder, or back pain at presentation, it may be necessary to consider the possibility of a pulmonary cause requiring medical referral. The most common pulmonary conditions to mimic those of the musculoskeletal system include pneumonia, pulmonary embolism, pleurisy, pneumothorax, and pulmonary artery hypertension.

As always, using the past medical history, risk-factor assessment, and clinical presentation, as well as asking about the presence of any associated signs and symptoms guides the screening process. In the case of pleuropulmonary disorders, the client's recent personal medical history may include a previous or recent upper respiratory infection or pneumonia.

Pneumothorax may be preceded by trauma, overexertion, or recent scuba diving. Each pulmonary condition will have its own unique risk factors that can predispose clients to a specific respiratory disease or illness.

A previous history of cancer, especially primary lung cancer or cancers that metastasize to the lungs (e.g., breast, bone) is a red flag and a risk factor for cancer recurrence. Risk-factor assessment also helps identify increased risk for other respiratory conditions or illnesses that can present as a primary musculoskeletal problem.

The material in this chapter will assist the therapist in treating both the client with a known pulmonary problem and the client having musculoskeletal signs and symptoms that may have an underlying systemic basis (Case Example 7-1).

▶ SIGNS AND SYMPTOMS OF PULMONARY DISORDERS

The most common sites for referred pain from the pulmonary system are the chest, ribs, upper trapezius, shoulder, and thoracic spine. The first symptoms may not appear until the client's respiratory system is stressed by the addition of exercise during physical therapy.

On the other hand, the client may present with what appears to be primary musculoskeletal pain in any one of those areas. Auscultation may reveal the first signs of pulmonary distress (see Chapter 4 for screening examination by auscultation).

The therapist must be careful when screening for dyspnea or shortness of breath, either with exertion or while at rest. If a client denies compromised breathing, look for functional changes as the client accommodates for difficulty breathing by reducing activity or exertion.

Exercise may induce pleural pain, coughing, hemoptysis, shortness of breath, and/or other abnormal changes in breathing patterns. When asked if the client is ever short of breath, the individual may say "no" because he or she has reduced activity levels to avoid dyspnea (see Appendix B-11).

CASE EXAMPLE 7-1 Bronchopulmonary Pain

A 67-year-old woman with a known diagnosis of rheumatoid arthritis has been treated as needed in a physical therapy clinic for the last 8 years. She has reported occasional chest pain described as "coming on suddenly, like a knife pushing from the inside out—it takes my breath away."

She missed 2 days of treatment because of illness, and when she returned to the clinic, the physical therapist noticed that she had a newly developed cough and that her rheumatoid arthritis was much worse. She says that she missed her appointments because she had the "flu."

Further questioning to elicit the potential development of chest pain on inspiration, the presence of ongoing fever and chills, and the changes in breathing pattern is recommended.

Positive findings beyond the reasonable duration of influenza (7 to 10 days) or an increase in pulmonary symptoms (shortness of breath, hacking cough, hemoptysis, wheezing or other changes in breathing pattern) raise a red flag indicating the need for medical referral.

This clinical case points out that clients currently undergoing physical therapy for a known musculoskeletal problem may be describing signs and symptoms of systemic disease.

Central nervous system (CNS) symptoms, such as muscle weakness, muscle atrophy, headache, loss of lower extremity sensation, and localized or radicular back pain may be associated with lung cancer and must be investigated by a physician to establish a medical diagnosis.

Pulmonary Pain Patterns

Pulmonary pain patterns are usually localized in the substernal or chest region over involved lung fields that may include the anterior chest, side, or back (Fig. 7-1). However, pulmonary pain can radiate to the neck, upper trapezius muscle, costal margins, thoracic back, scapulae, or shoulder. Shoulder pain may radiate along the medial aspect of the arm, mimicking other neuromuscular causes of neck or shoulder pain (see Fig. 7-10).

Pulmonary pain usually increases with inspiratory movements, such as laughing, coughing, sneezing, or deep breathing, and the client notes the presence of associated symptoms, such as dyspnea (exertional or at rest), persistent cough, fever, and chills. Palpation and resisted movements will not reproduce the symptoms, which may get worse with recumbency, especially at night or while sleeping.

The thoracic cavity is lined with pleura, or serous membrane. One surface of the pleura lines the inside of the rib cage (parietal) and the other surface covers the lungs (visceral). The parietal pleura is sensitive to painful stimulation, but the visceral pleura is insensitive to pain. This explains why pathology of the lungs may be painless until obstruction or inflammation is enough to press on the parietal pleura.

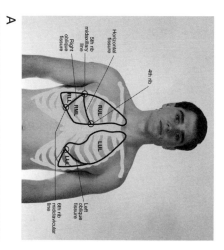
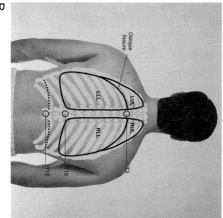

Fig. 7-1 • Pulmonary pain patterns are localized over involved lung fields affecting the anterior chest, side, or back. Radiating pain can also cause neck, shoulder, upper trapezius, rib, and/or scapular pain. **A,** Anterior chest. **B,** Posterior chest. The posterior chest is comprised primarily of lower lung lobes. The upper lobes occupy a small area from T1 to T3 or T4. (From Jarvis C: *Physical examination and assessment,* ed 3, Philadelphia, 2000, WB Saunders.)

Tracheobronchial Pain

Within the pulmonary system, the trachea and large bronchi are innervated by the vagus trunks, whereas the finer bronchi and lung parenchyma appear to be free of pain innervation. Tracheobronchial pain is referred to sites in the neck or anterior chest at the same levels as the points of irritation in the air passages (Fig. 7-2). This irritation may be caused by inflammatory lesions, irritating foreign materials, or cancerous tumors.

Pleural Pain

When the disease progresses enough to extend to the parietal pleura, pleural irritation occurs and results in sharp, localized pain that is aggravated by any respiratory movement. Clients usually note that the pain is alleviated by lying on the affected side, which diminishes the movement of that side of the chest called *autosplinting*.

Debate continues concerning the mechanism by which pain occurs in the parietal membrane. It has been long thought that friction between the two pleural surfaces (when the membranes are irritated and covered with fibrinous exudate) causes sharp pain. Other theories suggest that intercostal muscle spasm resulting from pleurisy or stretching of the parietal pleura causes this pain.

Pleural pain is present in pulmonary diseases such as pleurisy, pneumonia, pulmonary infarct (when it extends to the pleural surface, thus causing pleurisy), tumor (when it invades the parietal pleura), and pneumothorax. Tumor, especially bronchogenic carcinoma, may be accompanied by severe, continuous pain when the tumor tissue, extending to the parietal pleura through the lung, constantly irritates the pain nerve endings in the pleura.

Diaphragmatic Pleural Pain

The *diaphragmatic pleura* receives dual pain innervation through the phrenic and intercostal nerves. Damage to the phrenic nerve produces paralysis of the corresponding half of the diaphragm. The phrenic nerves are sensory and motor from both surfaces of the diaphragm.

Stimulation of the peripheral portions of the diaphragmatic pleura results in sharp pain felt along the costal margins, which can be referred to the lumbar region by the lower thoracic somatic nerves. Stimulation of the central portion of the diaphragmatic pleura results in sharp pain referred to the upper trapezius muscle and shoulder on the ipsilateral side of the stimulation (see Figs. 3-4 and 3-5).

Pain of cardiac and diaphragmatic origin is often experienced in the shoulder because the heart and diaphragm are supplied by the C5-C6 spinal segment, and the visceral pain is referred to the corresponding somatic area.

Diaphragmatic pleurisy secondary to pneumonia is common and refers sharp pain along the costal margins or upper trapezius, which is aggravated by any diaphragmatic motion, such as coughing, laughing, or deep breathing.

There may be tenderness to palpation along the costal margins, and sharp pain occurs when the client is asked to take a deep breath. A change in position (side bending or rotation of the trunk) does not reproduce the symptoms, which would be the case with a true intercostal lesion or tear.

Forceful, repeated coughing can result in an intercostal lesion in the presence of referred intercostal pain from diaphragmatic pleurisy, which can make differentiation between these two entities impossible without a medical referral and further diagnostic testing.

Pulmonary Physiology

The primary function of the respiratory system is to provide oxygen to and to remove carbon dioxide from cells in the body. The act of breathing, in which the oxygen and carbon dioxide exchange occurs, involves the two interrelated processes of ventilation and respiration.

Ventilation is the movement of air from outside the body to the alveoli of the lungs. Respiration is the process of oxygen uptake and carbon dioxide elimination between the body and the outside environment.

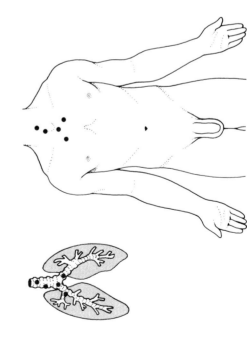

Fig. 7-2 ● Tracheobronchial pain is referred to sites in the neck or anterior chest at the same levels as the points of irritation in the air passages. The points of pain are on the same side as the areas of irritation.

Breathing is an automatic process by which sensors detect changes in the levels of carbon dioxide and continuously direct data to the medulla. The medulla then directs respiratory muscles that adjust ventilation. Breathing patterns can be altered voluntarily when this automatic response is overridden by conscious thought.

The major sensors mentioned here are the central chemoreceptors (located near the medulla) and the peripheral sensors (located in the carotid body and aortic arch). The central chemoreceptors respond to increases in carbon dioxide and decreases in pH in cerebrospinal fluid.

As carbon dioxide increases, the medulla signals a response to increase respiration. The peripheral chemoreceptor system responds to low arterial blood oxygen and is believed to function only in pathologic situations, such as when there are chronically elevated carbon dioxide levels (e.g., chronic obstructive pulmonary disease [COPD]).

Acid-Base Regulation

The proper balance of acids and bases in the body is essential to life. This balance is very complex and must be kept within the narrow parameters of a pH of 7.35 to 7.45 in the extracellular fluid. This number (or pH value) represents the hydrogen ion concentration in body fluid.

A reading of less than 7.35 is considered *acidosis* and a reading greater than 7.45 is called *alkalosis*. Life cannot be sustained if the pH values are less than 7 or greater than 7.8.

Living human cells are extremely sensitive to alterations in body fluid pH (hydrogen ion concentration); thus various mechanisms are in operation to keep the pH at a relatively constant level.

Acid-base regulatory mechanisms include chemical buffer systems, the respiratory system, and the renal system. These systems interact very closely to maintain a normal acid-base ratio of 20 parts of bicarbonate to 1 part of carbonic acid and thus to maintain normal body fluid pH.

The blood test used most often to measure the effectiveness of ventilation and oxygen transport is the arterial blood gas (ABG) test (Table 7-1). The measurement of arterial blood gases is important in the diagnosis and treatment of ventilation, oxygen transport, and acid-base problems.

The arterial blood gas test measures the amount of dissolved oxygen and carbon dioxide in arterial blood and indicates acid-base status by measurement of the arterial blood pH. In simple terms a low pH reflects increased acid build-up, and a high pH reflects an increased base build-up.

Pulmonary Pathophysiology
Respiratory Acidosis

Any condition that decreases pulmonary ventilation increases the retention and concentration of carbon dioxide from the lungs or when there is excess acid production from the tissues of the body. These problems are corrected by adjusting the ventilation or buffering the acid with bicarbonate.

Acid build-up occurs when there is an ineffective removal of carbon dioxide from the lungs or when there is excess acid production from the tissues of the body. These problems are corrected by adjusting the ventilation or buffering the acid with bicarbonate.

TABLE 7-1 ▼ Arterial Blood Gas Values*

pH	7.35-7.45
pCO_2 (partial pressure of carbon dioxide)	35-45 mm Hg
HCO_3 (bicarbonate ion)	22-26 mEq/L
pO_2 (partial pressure of oxygen)	75-100 mm Hg
O_2 saturation (oxygen saturation)	96%-100%
Panic Values	
pH	≤7.20 or >7.6
pCO_2	≤20 or >70 mm Hg
HCO_3	≤10 or >40 mEq/L
pO_2	≤40 mm Hg
O_2 saturation	≤60%

Normal pH level: The pH is inversely proportional to the hydrogen ion concentration in the blood. As the hydrogen ion concentration increases (acidosis), the pH decreases; as the hydrogen ion concentration decreases (alkalosis), the pH increases.

Normal pCO_2: The pCO_2 is a measure of the partial pressure of carbon dioxide in the blood. As the carbon dioxide level increases, the pH decreases (respiratory acidosis); as the carbon dioxide level decreases, the pH increases (respiratory alkalosis). pCO_2 measures the effectiveness of the body's ventilation system as CO_2 is removed.

Bicarbonate ion: HCO_3 is a measure of the metabolic portion of the acid-base function. As the bicarbonate value increases, the pH increases (metabolic alkalosis); as the bicarbonate value decreases, the pH decreases (metabolic acidosis).

Partial pressure of oxygen: The pO_2 is a measure of the partial pressure of oxygen in the blood and represents the status of alveolar gas exchange.

Oxygen saturation: O_2 saturation is an indication of the percentage of hemoglobin saturated with oxygen. When 95% to 100% of the hemoglobin binds and carries oxygen, the tissues are adequately perfused with oxygen. As the pO_2 decreases, the percentage of hemoglobin saturation also decreases. At oxygen saturation levels of less than 70%, the tissues are unable to carry out vital functions.

* Modified from Chernecky C, Berger B: *Laboratory tests and diagnostic procedures,* ed 4, Philadelphia, 2003, WB Saunders.

carbon dioxide (CO_2), hydrogen, and carbonic acid; this results in an increase in the amount of circulating hydrogen and is called respiratory acidosis.

If ventilation is severely compromised, CO_2 levels become extremely high and respiration is depressed even further, causing hypoxia as well.

During respiratory acidosis, potassium moves out of cells into the extracellular fluid to exchange with circulating hydrogen. This results in hyperkalemia (abnormally high potassium concentration in the blood) and cardiac changes that can cause cardiac arrest.

Respiratory acidosis can result from pathologic conditions that decrease the efficiency of the respiratory system. These pathologies can include damage to the medulla, which controls respiration, obstruction of airways (e.g., neoplasm, foreign bodies, pulmonary disease such as COPD, pneumonia), loss of lung surface ventilation (e.g., pneumothorax, pulmonary fibrosis), weakness of respiratory muscles (e.g., poliomyelitis, spinal cord injury, Guillain-Barré syndrome), or overdose of respiratory depressant drugs.

As hypoxia becomes more severe, diaphoresis, shallow rapid breathing, restlessness, and cyanosis may appear. Cardiac arrhythmias may also be present as the potassium level in the blood serum rises.

Treatment is directed at restoration of efficient ventilation. If the respiratory depression and acidosis are severe, injection of intravenous sodium bicarbonate and use of a mechanical ventilator may be necessary. Any client with symptoms of inadequate ventilation or CO_2 retention needs immediate medical referral.

Clinical Signs and Symptoms of

Respiratory Acidosis

- Decreased ventilation
- Confusion
- Sleepiness and unconsciousness
- Diaphoresis
- Shallow, rapid breathing
- Restlessness
- Cyanosis

Respiratory Alkalosis

Increased respiratory rate and depth decrease the amount of available CO_2 and hydrogen and create a condition of increased pH, or alkalosis. When pulmonary ventilation is increased, CO_2 and hydrogen are eliminated from the body too quickly and are not available to buffer the increasingly alkaline environment.

Respiratory alkalosis is usually due to *hyperventilation*. Rapid, deep respirations are often caused by neurogenic or psychogenic problems, including anxiety, pain, and cerebral trauma or lesions. Other causes can be related to conditions that greatly increase metabolism (e.g., hyperthyroidism) or overventilation of clients who are using a mechanical ventilator.

If the alkalosis becomes more severe, muscular tetany and convulsions can occur. Cardiac arrhythmias caused by serum potassium loss through the kidneys may also occur. The kidneys keep hydrogen in exchange for potassium.

Treatment of respiratory alkalosis includes reassurance, assistance in slowing breathing and facilitating relaxation, sedation, pain control, CO_2 administration, and use of a rebreathing device such as a rebreathing mask or paper bag. A rebreathing device allows the client to inhale and "rebreathe" the exhaled CO_2.

Respiratory alkalosis related to hyperventilation is a relatively common condition and might be present more often in the physical therapy setting than is respiratory acidosis. Pain and anxiety are common causes of hyperventilation, and treatment needs to be focused toward reduction of both of these interrelated elements. If hyperventilation continues in the absence of pain or anxiety, serious systemic problems may be the cause, and immediate physician referral is necessary.

If either respiratory acidosis or alkalosis persists for hours to days in a chronic and not life-threatening manner, the kidneys then begin to assist in the restoration of normal body fluid pH by selective excretion or retention of hydrogen ions or bicarbonate. This process is called *renal compensation*. When the kidneys compensate effectively, blood pH values are within normal limits (7.35 to 7.45) even though the underlying problem may still cause the respiratory imbalance.

Clinical Signs and Symptoms of

Respiratory Alkalosis

- Hyperventilation
- Lightheadedness
- Dizziness
- Numbness and tingling of the face, fingers, and toes
- Syncope (fainting)

Chronic Obstructive Pulmonary Disease

COPD, also called chronic obstructive lung disease (COLD), refers to a number of disorders that have in common abnormal airway structures resulting

in obstruction of air in and out of the lungs. The most important of these disorders are obstructive bronchitis, emphysema, and asthma.

Although bronchitis, emphysema, and asthma may occur in a "pure form," they most commonly coexist. For example, adult subjects with active asthma are as much as 12 times more likely to acquire COPD over time than subjects with no active asthma.[1]

COPD is a leading cause of morbidity and mortality among cigarette smokers. Other factors predisposing to COPD include air pollution, occupational exposure to irritating dusts or gases, hereditary factors, infection, allergies, aging, and potentially harmful drugs and chemicals.[2]

COPD rarely occurs in nonsmokers; however, only a minority of cigarette smokers develop symptomatic disease, suggesting that genetic factors may contribute to the development of COPD.[3]

In all forms of COPD narrowing of the airways obstructs airflow to and from the lungs (Table 7-2). This narrowing impairs ventilation by trapping air in the bronchioles and alveoli. The obstruction increases the resistance to airflow.

Trapped air hinders normal gas exchange and causes distention of the alveoli. Other mechanisms of COPD vary with each form of the disease. In the healthy adult the bottom margin of the respiratory diaphragm sits at T9 when the lungs are at rest. Taking a deep breath expands the diaphragm (and lungs) inferiorly to T11. For the client with COPD the lower lung lobes are already at T11 when the lungs are at rest from over expansion as a result of alveolar distention and hyperinflation.

COPD develops earlier in life than is usually recognized, making it the most underdiagnosed and undertreated pulmonary disease. Smoking cessation is the only intervention shown to slow decline in lung function. Identifying risk factors and recognizing early signs and symptoms of COPD increases the affected individual's chances of reduced morbidity through early intervention.[2]

BRONCHITIS

Acute Acute bronchitis is an inflammation of the trachea and bronchi (tracheobronchial tree) that is self-limiting and of short duration with few pulmonary signs. This condition may result from chemical irritation (e.g., smoke, fumes, gas) or may occur with viral infections such as influenza, measles, chickenpox, or whooping cough.

These predisposing conditions may become apparent during the subjective examination (i.e., Personal/Family History form or the Physical Therapy Interview). Although bronchitis is usually mild, it can become complicated in older clients and clients with chronic lung or heart disease. Pneumonia is a critical complication.

Clinical Signs and Symptoms of
Acute Bronchitis

- Mild fever from 1 to 3 days
- Malaise
- Back and muscle pain
- Sore throat
- Cough with sputum production, followed by wheezing
- Possibly laryngitis

Chronic Chronic bronchitis is a condition associated with prolonged exposure to nonspecific bronchial irritants and is accompanied by mucus hypersecretion and structural changes in the

---

TABLE 7-2 ▼ Respiratory Diseases: Summary of Differences

Disease	Primary area affected	Results
Bronchitis	Membrane lining bronchial tubes	Inflammation of lining
Bronchiectasis	Bronchial tubes (bronchi or air passages)	Bronchial dilation with inflammation
Pneumonia	Alveoli (air sacs)	Causative agent invades alveoli with resultant outpouring from lung capillaries into air spaces and continued healing process
Emphysema	Air spaces beyond terminal bronchioles (small airways)	Breakdown of alveolar walls; air spaces enlarged
Asthma	Bronchioles (small airways)	Bronchioles obstructed by muscle spasm, swelling of mucosa, thick secretions
Cystic fibrosis	Bronchioles	Bronchioles become obstructed and obliterated. Later, larger airways become involved. Plugs of mucus cling to airway walls, leading to bronchitis, bronchiectasis, atelectasis, pneumonia, or pulmonary abscess

bronchi (large air passages leading into the lungs). This irritation of the tissue usually results from exposure to cigarette smoke, long-term inhalation of dust or air pollution, and causes hypertrophy of mucus-producing cells in the bronchi.

In bronchitis, partial or complete blockage of the airways from mucus secretions causes insufficient oxygenation in the alveoli (Fig. 7-3). The swollen mucous membrane and thick sputum obstruct the airways, causing wheezing, and the client develops a cough to clear the airways. The clinical definition of a person with chronic bronchitis is anyone who coughs for at least 3 months per year for 2 consecutive years without having had a precipitating disease.

To confirm that the condition is chronic bronchitis, tests are performed to determine whether the airways are obstructed and to exclude other diseases that may cause similar symptoms, such as silicosis, tuberculosis, or a tumor in the upper airway. Sputum samples will be analyzed, and lung function tests may be performed.

Treatment is aimed at keeping the airways as clear as possible. Smokers are encouraged and helped to stop smoking. A combination of drugs may be prescribed to relieve the symptoms, including bronchodilators to open the obstructed airways and to thin the obstructive mucus so that it can be coughed up more easily.

Chronic bronchitis may develop slowly over a period of years, but it will not go away if untreated. Eventually, the bronchial walls thicken, and the number of mucous glands increases. The client is increasingly susceptible to respiratory infections,

during which the bronchial tissue becomes inflamed and the mucus becomes even thicker and more profuse.

Chronic bronchitis can be incapacitating and lead to more serious and potentially fatal lung disease. Influenza and pneumococcal vaccines are recommended for these clients.

Clinical Signs and Symptoms of Chronic Bronchitis

- Persistent cough with production of sputum (worse in the morning and evening than at midday)
- Reduced chest expansion
- Wheezing
- Fever
- Dyspnea (shortness of breath)
- Cyanosis (blue discoloration of skin and mucous membranes)
- Decreased exercise tolerance

BRONCHIECTASIS

Bronchiectasis is a form of obstructive lung disease that is actually a type of bronchitis. It is a progressive and chronic pulmonary condition that occurs after infections such as childhood pneumonia or cystic fibrosis.

Although bronchiectasis was once a common disease because of measles, pertussis, tuberculosis, and poorly treated bacterial pneumonias, the prevalence of bronchiectasis has diminished greatly since the introduction of antibiotics. It is characterized by abnormal and permanent dilatation of the large air passages leading into the lungs (bronchi) and by destruction of bronchial walls.

Bronchiectasis is caused by repeated damage to bronchial walls. The resultant destruction and bronchial dilatation reduce bronchial wall movement so that secretions cannot be removed effectively from the lungs, and the person is predisposed to frequent respiratory infections.

This vicious cycle of bacterial infection and inflammation of the bronchial wall leads to loss of ventilation and irreversible lung damage. Advanced bronchiectasis may cause pneumonia, cor pulmonale, or right-sided ventricular failure.

All pulmonary irritants, especially cigarette smoke, should be avoided. Postural drainage, adequate hydration, good nutrition, and bronchodilator therapy in bronchospasm are important components in treatment. Antibiotics are used during disease exacerbations (e.g., increased cough, purulent sputum, hemoptysis, malaise, and weight loss). The use of immunomodulatory

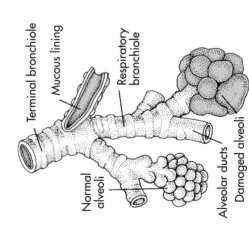

Terminal bronchiole

Mucous lining

Respiratory bronchiole

Normal alveoli

Alveolar ducts

Damaged alveoli

Fig. 7-3 • Chronic bronchitis may lead to the formation of misshapen or large alveolar sacs with reduced space for oxygen and carbon dioxide exchange. The client may develop cyanosis and pulmonary edema.

therapy to alter the host response directly and thereby reduce tissue damage is under investigation.[4,5]

Clinical Signs and Symptoms of Bronchiectasis

Clinical signs and symptoms of bronchiectasis vary widely, depending on the extent of the disease and on the presence of complicating infection, but may include:

- Chronic "wet" cough with copious foul-smelling secretions; generally worse in the morning after the individual has been recumbent for a length of time
- Hemoptysis (bloody sputum)
- Occasional wheezing sounds
- Dyspnea
- Sinusitis (inflammation of one or more paranasal sinuses)
- Weight loss
- Anemia
- Malaise
- Recurrent fever and chills
- Fatigue

EMPHYSEMA

Emphysema may develop in a person after a long history of chronic bronchitis in which the alveolar walls are destroyed, leading to permanent overdistention of the air spaces and loss of normal elastic tension in the lung tissue.

Air passages are obstructed as a result of these changes (rather than as a result of mucus production, as in chronic bronchitis). Difficult expiration in emphysema is due to the destruction of the walls (septa) between the alveoli, partial airway collapse, and loss of elastic recoil.

As the alveoli and septa collapse, pockets of air form between the alveolar spaces (called *blebs*) and within the lung parenchyma (called *bullae*). This process leads to increased ventilatory "dead space," or areas that do not participate in gas or blood exchange. The work of breathing is increased because there is less functional lung tissue to exchange oxygen and CO_2. Emphysema also causes destruction of the pulmonary capillaries, further decreasing oxygen perfusion and ventilation.

In advanced emphysema, oxygen therapy is usually necessary to treat the progressive hypoxemia that occurs as the disease worsens. Oxygen therapy is carefully titrated and monitored to maintain venous oxygen saturation levels at or slightly above 90%. Too much oxygen can depress the respiratory drive of a person with emphysema.

The drive to breathe in a normal person results from an increase in the arterial carbon dioxide level (pCO_2). Since the individual with emphysema chronically retains excessive amounts of carbon dioxide, an increased arterial pCO_2 is no longer an effective respiratory drive mechanism.

In the person with emphysema, low arterial oxygen levels are the respiratory drive triggers. Too much oxygen delivered as a treatment can then depress the respiratory drive, which is now reliant on lower levels of arterial oxygen.[6]

Types of Emphysema There are three types of emphysema. *Centrilobular emphysema* (Fig. 7-4), the most common type, destroys the bronchioles, usually in the upper lung regions. Inflammation develops in the bronchioles, but usually the alveolar sac remains intact. *Panlobular emphysema* destroys the more distal alveolar walls, most commonly involving the lower

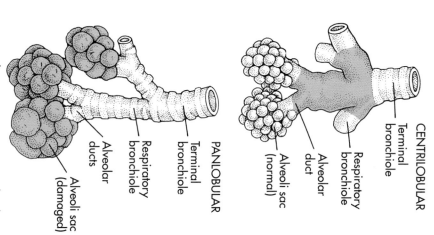

Fig. 7-4 • Emphysema traps air in the lungs so that expelling air becomes increasingly difficult. *Centrilobular* emphysema affects the upper airways and produces destructive changes in the bronchioles. *Panlobular* emphysema affects the lower airways and is more diffusely scattered throughout the alveoli.

CENTRILOBULAR
Terminal bronchiole
Respiratory bronchiole
Alveolar duct
Alveoli sac (normal)

PANLOBULAR
Terminal bronchiole
Respiratory bronchiole
Alveolar ducts
Alveoli sac (damaged)

lung. This destruction of alveolar walls may occur secondary to infection or to irritants (most commonly, cigarette smoke). These two forms of emphysema, collectively called centriacinar emphysema, occur most often in smokers.

Paraseptal (or *panacinar*) *emphysema* destroys the alveoli in the lower lobes of the lungs, resulting in isolated blebs along the lung periphery. Paraseptal emphysema is believed to be the likely cause of spontaneous pneumothorax.

Clinical Signs and Symptoms The irreversible destruction reduces elasticity of the lung and increases the effort to exhale trapped air, causing marked dyspnea on exertion later progressing to dyspnea at rest. Cough is uncommon.

The client is often thin, has tachypnea with prolonged expiration, and uses the accessory muscles for respiration. The client often leans forward with the arms braced on the knees to support the shoulders and chest for breathing. The combined effects of trapped air and alveolar distention change the size and shape of the client's chest, causing a barrel chest and increased expiratory effort.

As the disease progresses, there is a loss of surface area available for gas exchange. In the final stages of emphysema, cardiac complications, especially enlargement and dilatation of the right ventricle, may develop. The overloaded heart reaches its limit of muscular compensation and begins to fail (cor pulmonale).

The most important factor in the treatment of emphysema is smoking cessation. The main goals for the client with emphysema are to improve oxygenation and decrease CO₂ retention.

Pursed-lip breathing causes resistance to outflow at the lips, which in turn maintains intrabronchial pressure and improves the mixing of gases in the lungs. This type of breathing should be encouraged to help the client get rid of the stale air trapped in the lungs.

Exercise has not been shown to improve pulmonary function but is used to enhance cardiovascular fitness and train skeletal muscles to function more effectively. Routine progressive walking is the most common form of exercise.

Lung volume reduction surgery is available for some individuals and improves not only lung function and exercise performance, but also activities of daily function and quality of life.[7,8]

Clinical Signs and Symptoms of
Emphysema

- Shortness of breath
- Dyspnea on exertion
- Orthopnea (only able to breathe in the upright position) immediately after assuming the supine position
- Chronic cough
- Barrel chest
- Weight loss
- Malaise
- Use of accessory muscles of respiration
- Prolonged expiratory period (with grunting)
- Wheezing
- Pursed-lip breathing
- Increased respiratory rate
- Peripheral cyanosis

▶ INFLAMMATORY/INFECTIOUS DISEASE

Asthma

Asthma is a reversible obstructive lung disease caused by increased reaction of the airways to various stimuli. It is a chronic inflammatory condition with acute exacerbations that can be life-threatening if not properly managed. Our understanding of asthma has changed dramatically over the last decade.

Asthma was once viewed as a bronchoconstrictive disorder in which the airways narrowed, causing wheezing and breathing difficulties. Treatment with bronchodilators to open airways was the primary focus. Scientific evidence now supports the idea that asthma is primarily an inflammatory disorder in which the constriction of airways is a symptom of the underlying inflammation.

Asthma and other atopic disorders are the result of complex interactions between genetic predisposition and multiple environmental influences. The marked increase in asthma prevalence in the last 3 decades suggests environmental factors as a key contributor in the process of allergic sensitization.[9]

Fifteen million persons of all ages are affected by asthma in the United States. This represents a 61% increase over the last 15 years with a 45% increase in mortality during the last decade. Women are affected more than men, accounting for about 60% of the nearly 18 million cases of adult asthma. Hormones are thought to be a possible cause for this increase in incidence in women.[10]

Immune Sensitization and Inflammation

There are two major components to asthma. When the immune system becomes sensitized to an allergen, usually through heavy exposure in early life, an inflammatory cascade occurs, extending beyond the upper airways into the lungs.

The lungs become hyperreactive, responding to allergens and other irritants in an exaggerated way. This hyperresponsiveness causes the muscles working with known asthmatic clients should of the airways to constrict, making breathing more difficult (Fig. 7-5). The second component is inflammation, which causes the air passages to swell and the cells lining the passages to produce excess mucus, further impairing breathing.

Asthma may be categorized as conventional asthma, occupational asthma, or exercise-induced asthma (EIA), but the underlying pathophysiologic complex remains the same. Since the triggers or allergens vary, each person reacts differently.

Shortness of breath, wheezing, tightness in the chest, and cough are the most commonly reported symptoms, but other symptoms may also occur.

Clinical Signs and Symptoms

Anytime a client experiences shortness of breath, wheezing, and cough and comments, "I'm more out of shape that I thought," the therapist should ask

about a past medical history of asthma and review the list of symptoms with the client. Therapists working with known asthmatic clients should encourage them to maintain hydration by drinking fluids to prevent mucous plugs from hardening and to take prescribed medications.

Exercise- or hyperventilation-induced asthma potentially can be prevented by exercising in a moist, humid environment and by grading exercise according to client tolerance using diaphragmatic breathing. Any type of sustained running or cycling or activity in the cold is more likely to precipitate EIA (Box 7-1).

COMPLICATIONS

Status asthmaticus is a severe, life-threatening complication of asthma. With severe bronchospasm the workload of breathing increases five to ten times, which can lead to acute cor pulmonale. When air is trapped, a severe paradoxic pulse develops as venous return is obstructed. This condition is seen as a blood pressure drop of more than 10 mm Hg during inspiration.

Pneumothorax can develop. If status asthmaticus continues, hypoxemia worsens and acidosis begins. If the condition is untreated or not reversed, respiratory or cardiac arrest will occur. An acute asthma episode may constitute a medical emergency.

Medical treatment for the underlying inflammation and resulting airway obstruction is with antiinflammatory agents and bronchodilators to prevent, interrupt, or terminate ongoing inflammatory reactions in the airways. A new class of antiinflammatory agents known as leukotriene modifiers work by blocking the activity of chemicals called leukotrienes which are involved in airway inflammation. Reducing, eliminating, and avoiding allergens or triggers are important in self-care (see Box 7-1).

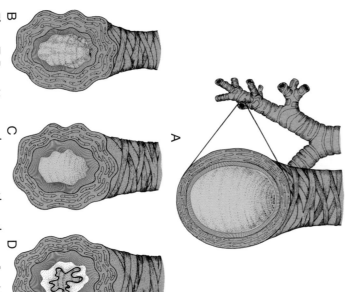

Fig. 7-5 • Airway changes with asthma. **A,** Normal bronchus: cross-section of a normal bronchus (mucous membrane in color). Healthy bronchioles accommodate a constant flow of air when open and relaxed. **B,** Asthma: airway inflammation begins. The smooth muscle surrounding the bronchus contracts and causes narrowing of the airway, called bronchospasm. **C,** The airway tissue swells; this edema of the mucous membrane further narrows airways. **D,** Mucus is produced, further compromising airflow.

BOX 7-1 ▼ Factors That May Trigger Asthma

- Respiratory infections, colds
- Cigarette smoke
- Allergic reactions to pollen, mold, animal dander, feather, dust, food, insects
- Indoor and outdoor air pollutants, including ozone
- Physical exertion or vigorous exercise
- Exposure to cold air or sudden temperature change
- Excitement or strong emotion, psychologic or emotional stress

Clinical Signs and Symptoms of

Asthma

Listen for

- Wheezing, however light
- Irregular breathing with prolonged expiration
- Noisy, difficult breathing
- Episodes of dyspnea
- Clearing the throat (tickle at the back of the throat or neck)
- Cough with or without sputum production, especially in the absence of a cold and/or occurring 5 to 10 minutes after exercise

Look for

- Skin retraction (clavicles, ribs, sternum)
- Hunched-over body posture; inability to stand, sit straight, or relax
- Pursed-lip breathing
- Nostrils flaring
- Unusual pallor or unexplained sweating

Ask about

- Restlessness during sleep
- Vomiting
- Fatigue unrelated to working or playing

Pneumonia

Pneumonia is an inflammation of the lungs and can be caused by (1) aspiration of food, fluids, or vomitus; (2) inhalation of toxic or caustic chemicals, smoke, dust, or gases; or (3) a bacterial, viral, or mycoplasmal infection. It may be primary or secondary (a complication of another disease); it often follows influenza.

The common feature of all types of pneumonia is an inflammatory pulmonary response to the offending organism or agent. This response may involve one or both lungs at the level of the lobe (lobar pneumonia) or more distally beginning in the terminal bronchioles and alveoli (bronchopneumonia). Bronchopneumonia is seen more frequently than lobar pneumonia and is common in clients with chronic bronchitis, particularly when these two situations coexist.

Infectious agents responsible for pneumonia are typically present in the upper respiratory tract and cause no harm unless resistance is lowered severely by some other factor, such as a severe cold, disease, alcoholism, or generally poor health (e.g., poorly controlled diabetes, chronic renal problems).

Older or bedridden clients are particularly at risk because of physical inactivity and immobility. Limited mobility causes normal secretions to pool in the airways and facilitates bacterial growth. Other risk factors predisposing a client to pneumonia are listed in Box 7-2.

Pneumocystis carinii is a protozoan organism that rarely causes pneumonia in healthy individuals. *Pneumocystis carinii* pneumonia (PCP) has been the most common life-threatening opportunistic infection in persons with acquired immune deficiency syndrome (AIDS). PCP also has been shown to be the first indicator of conversion from human immunodeficiency virus (HIV) infection to the designation of AIDS.

Clinical Signs and Symptoms

The onset of all pneumonias is generally marked by any of the following: fever, chills, sweats, pleuritic chest pain, cough, sputum production, hemoptysis, dyspnea, headache, or fatigue. Pneumocystis pneumonia causes a dry, hacking cough without sputum production.

The older client can have full-blown pneumonia and may appear with altered mental status

---

BOX 7-2 ▼ Risk Factors for Pneumonia

- Smoking
- Air pollution
- Upper respiratory infection (URI)
- Altered consciousness: alcoholism, head injury, seizure disorder, drug overdose, general anesthesia
- Endotracheal intubation
- Prolonged immobility
- Immunosuppressive therapy: corticosteroids, cancer chemotherapy
- Nonfunctional immune system: AIDS
- Severe periodontal disease
- Prolonged exposure to virulent organisms
- Malnutrition, dehydration
- Chronic diseases: diabetes mellitus, heart disease, chronic lung disease, renal disease, cancer
- Prolonged debilitating disease
- Inhalation of noxious substances
- Aspiration of oral/gastric material, foreign materials (e.g., Petroleum products)
- Chronically ill, older clients who have poor immune systems, often residing in group-living situations

(especially confusion) rather than fever or respiratory symptoms because of the changes in temperature regulation as we age. Anytime an older person has shoulder pain and confusion at presentation, consider the possibility of diaphragmatic impingement by an underlying lung pathologic condition. (Case Example 7-2)

The clinical manifestations of PCP are slow to develop; they include fever, tachypnea, tachycardia, dyspnea, nonproductive cough, and hypoxemia. A diffuse, bilateral pattern of alveolar infiltration is apparent on chest radiograph.

Hospitalization may be required for the immunocompromised client. Otherwise, if the client has an intact defense system and good general health, recuperation can take place at home with rest and supportive treatment. In the hospital rigorous handwashing by medical personnel is essential for reducing the transmission of infectious agents.

Clinical Signs and Symptoms of Pneumonia

- Sudden and sharp pleuritic chest pain that is aggravated by chest movement
- Shoulder pain
- Hacking, productive cough (rust-colored or green, purulent sputum)
- Dyspnea
- Tachypnea (rapid respirations associated with fever or pneumonia) accompanied by decreased chest excursion on the affected side
- Cyanosis
- Headache
- Fever and chills
- Generalized aches and myalgia that may extend to the thighs and calves
- Knees may be painful and swollen
- Fatigue
- Confusion in older adult or increased confusion in client with dementia or Alzheimer's

CASE EXAMPLE 7-2 Pneumonia

A 42-year-old man came to an outpatient physical therapy clinic with complaints of painful, swollen knees. Symptoms were first observed 10 days ago, and the left knee was reportedly worse than the right. Stiffness was reported in the morning on rising, with pain increasing as the day progressed. As a nonsmoker, the man reported his general health as "good" and noted that he had sprained his left ankle 2 months before the onset of knee pain.

The knee joints were not tender, warm, or red. Observable and palpable "boggy" fluid could be demonstrated in the popliteal spaces bilaterally. There was no sign of effusion when viewed anteriorly, and the test for a wave of fluid was negative.

All special tests for the hip and knee were negative, with full active and passive range of motion present. There was no known history of Baker's cysts (herniation of synovial tissue through a weakening in the posterior capsule wall) reported. There were no palpable myalgias of the lower leg musculature and no trigger points present.

The left ankle demonstrated some residual stiffness with a mild loss of plantar flexion. Joint accessory motions were consistent with a grade 1 lateral ankle sprain. Standing posture was unremarkable for possible contributing alignment problems.

The clinical presentation of this client was puzzling to the evaluating therapist. A brief screening for possible systemic origin of symptoms elicited no red-flag symptoms or history. Ongoing evaluation continued as treatment for both knees and the left ankle was initiated. After 3 weeks there were no changes in the clinical presentation of the knees. At that time the client developed a noticeable productive cough with greenish/yellow sputum but no other reported symptoms. Vital signs (including temperature) were unremarkable.

Given the unusual clinical presentation, lack of progress with treatment, and development of a productive cough, this client was referred to his family physician for a medical evaluation. A one-page letter outlining the therapist's findings and treatment protocol was sent with the client. A medical diagnosis of pneumonia was established. The physician noted that although the clinical presentation was unusual, knee involvement can occur with pneumonia. The pathophysiologic mechanism for this is unknown.

Tuberculosis

Tuberculosis (TB) is a bacterial infectious disease transmitted by the gram-positive, acid-fast bacillus *Mycobacterium tuberculosis*. Despite improved methods of detection and treatment, TB remains a worldwide health problem with increasing spread of a highly drug-resistant strain of TB present in almost every state in the United States.

Before the development of anti-TB drugs in the late 1940s, TB was the leading cause of death in the United States. Drug therapy, along with improvements in public health and general living standards, resulted in a marked decline in incidence. However, recent influxes of immigrants from developing Third World nations, rising homeless populations, and the emergence of HIV led to an increase in reported cases in the mid-1980s, reversing a 40-year period of decline.

Risk Factors

Although TB can affect anyone, certain segments of the population have an increased risk of contracting the disease (Box 7-3). The mycobacterium is usually spread by airborne droplet nuclei, which are produced when actively infected persons sneeze, sing, or cough.

Once released into the atmosphere, the organisms are dispersed and can be inhaled by a susceptible host. Brief exposure to a few bacilli rarely causes an infection. More commonly, it is spread with repeated close contact with an infected person.

Drug-resistant strains of TB have developed when the full course of treatment, lasting 6 to 9 months, is not completed. Once the infected person feels better and stops taking the prescribed medication, a new drug-resistant strain is passed along. Noncompletion of treatment among inner-city residents and the homeless presents a major factor in the failure to eradicate TB.

Drug resistant strains are also developing globally. Areas of the world with increased rates of drug-resistant disease include countries of the former Soviet Union (e.g., Estonia, Kazakhstan, Latvia, Lithuania, Usbekistan) and in Central Asia.

Families who adopt internationally should be aware of potential TB infection in children from some of the high-risk areas of the world. The vaccine BCG (bacille Calmette-Guerin) has been used in many foreign countries to attempt to prevent serious dissemination of TB infection in those countries.

The value of BCG is controversial since the protection it confers is short term. The CDC and the American Academy of Pediatrics strongly recom-

mend that history of BCG vaccination in a child from a high-risk part of the world should usually be ignored and all children adopted internationally should be skin tested for TB and treated if the disease is latent or active.[6]

TB most often involves the lungs, but extrapulmonary TB (XPTB) can also occur in the kidneys, bone growth plates, lymph nodes, and meninges and can be disseminated throughout the body.

Widespread dissemination throughout the body is termed *miliary tuberculosis* and is more common in people 50 years or older and very young children with unstable or underdeveloped immune systems.

On rare occasions TB will affect the hip joints and vertebrae, resulting in severe, arthritis-like damage, possibly even avascular necrosis of the

---

BOX 7-3 ▼ Risk Factors for TB

- Health care workers, especially those working in older hospitals (centralized ventilation), homeless shelters, or extended care facilities. Health care workers, including physical therapists must be alert to the need to use a special mask (particulate respirator) when cough-inducing procedures are being performed with any client with a risk for, or active TB
- Older adults, who constitute nearly half of the newly diagnosed cases of TB in the United States
- Overcrowded housing, most common among the economically disadvantaged; homeless, especially those people in crowded homeless shelters
- People who are incarcerated
- U.S. born non-Hispanic Blacks[11]
- Immigrants (including adopted children) from Southeast and Central Asia, Ethiopia, Mexico, Latin America, Eastern Europe
- Clients who are dependent on alcohol or other chemicals with resultant malnutrition, debilitation, and poor health
- Infants and children under the age of 5 years
- Clients with reduced immunity or malnutrition (e.g., anyone undergoing cancer therapy or steroid therapy) and those with HIV-positive lung cancer or head and neck cancer
- Persons with diagnosed rheumatoid arthritis. Data suggests increases in incidence could be due to new immunosuppressive treatments.[12]
- Persons with diabetes mellitus and/or end-stage renal disease
- People with a history of gastrointestinal disease (e.g., chronic malabsorption syndrome, upper gastrointestinal carcinomas, gastrectomy, intestinal bypass)

hip. Tuberculosis of the spine, referred to as Pott's disease is rare but can result in compression fracture of the vertebrae.

Pyogenic vertebral osteomyelitis can be caused by atypical organisms such as tuberculosis. As with other pyogenic infection, back pain is the most common symptom, but it is less severe as in other infections. Individuals from high-risk areas of the world, high-risk living conditions, and the immunocompromised and malnourished should be considered suspect for this condition.[14]

Clinical Signs and Symptoms

Clinical signs and symptoms are absent in the early stages of TB. Many cases are found incidentally when routine chest radiographs are made for other reasons. When systemic manifestations of active disease initially appear, the clinical signs and symptoms listed here may appear.

Tuberculin skin testing is done to determine whether the body's immune response has been activated by the presence of the bacillus. A positive reaction develops 3 to 10 weeks after the initial infection. A positive skin test reaction indicates the presence of a tuberculous infection but does not show whether the infection is dormant or is causing a clinical illness.

Chest x-ray films and sputum cultures are done as a follow-up to positive skin tests. All cases of active disease are treated, and certain cases of inactive disease are treated prophylactically.

Clinical Signs and Symptoms of Tuberculosis

• Fatigue
• Malaise
• Anorexia
• Weight loss
• Low-grade fevers (especially in late afternoon)
• Night sweats
• Frequent productive cough
• Dull chest pain, tightness, or discomfort
• Dyspnea

Systemic Sclerosis Lung Disease

Systemic sclerosis (SS) (scleroderma) is a restrictive lung disease of unknown etiologic origin characterized by inflammation and fibrosis of many organs (see Chapter 12). Fibrosis affecting the skin and the visceral organs is the hallmark of SS.

The lungs, highly vascularized and composed of abundant connective tissue, are a frequent target organ, ranking second only to the esophagus in visceral involvement.

The most common pulmonary manifestation of SS is interstitial fibrosis, which is clinically apparent in more than 50% of cases. Autopsy results suggest a prevalence of 75%, indicating the insensitivity of traditional tests such as pulmonary function tests and chest radiographs.

Clinical Signs and Symptoms

As discussed in Chapter 12, skin changes associated with SS generally preceded visceral alterations. Dyspnea on exertion and nonproductive cough are the most common clinical findings associated with SS. Rarely, these symptoms precede the occurrence of cutaneous changes of scleroderma.

Clubbing of the nails rarely occurs in SS because of the nearly universal presence of sclerodactyly (hardening and shrinking of connective tissues of fingers and toes). Peripheral edema may develop secondary to cor pulmonale, which occurs as the pulmonary fibrosis becomes advanced.

Pulmonary manifestations in systemic sclerosis include:

• *Common:* Interstitial pneumonitis and fibrosis and pulmonary vascular disease
• *Less common:* Pleural disease, aspiration pneumonia, pneumothorax, neoplasm, pneumoconiosis, pulmonary hemorrhage, and drug-induced pneumonitis

Pleural effusions may appear with orthopnea, edema, and paroxysmal nocturnal dyspnea if congestive heart failure occurs. Cystic changes in the parenchyma may progress to form pneumatoceles (thin-walled air-containing cysts) that may rupture spontaneously and produce a pneumothorax. Clients with SS have an increased incidence of lung cancer. Hemoptysis is often the first signal of pulmonary malignancy in individuals with SS.

The course of SS is unpredictable, from a mild, protracted course to rapid respiratory failure and death. Treatment of pulmonary complications, pulmonary hypertension, and interstitial lung disease remains difficult.

Clinical Signs and Symptoms of Systemic Sclerosis Lung Disease

• Dyspnea on exertion
• Nonproductive cough
• Peripheral edema (secondary to cor pulmonale)
• Orthopnea
• Paroxysmal nocturnal dyspnea (congestive heart failure)
• Hemoptysis

Neoplastic Disease

Lung Cancer (Bronchogenic Carcinoma)

Lung cancer is malignancy in the epithelium of the respiratory tract. At least a dozen different cell types of tumors are included under the classification of lung cancer.

Clinically, lung cancers are grouped into two divisions: small cell lung cancer and non–small cell lung cancer. The four major types of lung cancer include small cell carcinoma (oat cell carcinoma), and the types of non–small cell lung cancer, squamous cell carcinoma, adenocarcinoma, and large cell carcinoma.

Since the mid-1950s, lung cancer has been the most common cause of death from cancer in men. In 1987 lung cancer surpassed breast cancer to become the leading cause of cancer death in women in the United States.

The rate of lung cancer among women in the United States may be declining for some age groups. This decline is expected to continue through at least the year 2025. Sustaining that trend will require continued reductions in the number of female children who start to smoke and continued smoking cessation among addicted female smokers.[15]

RISK FACTORS

Smoking is the major risk factor for lung cancer, accounting for 82% of deaths caused by lung cancer.[16] Other risk factors are listed in Box 7-4. Compared with nonsmokers, heavy smokers (i.e., those who smoke more than 25 cigarettes a day) have a twentyfold greater risk of developing cancer.

States with strong anti-tobacco programs (e.g., Arizona, California) have the fewest current smokers, the most people who have quit smoking in some age groups, and the greatest drop in the death rate from lung cancer.[17] Quitting smoking

lowers the risk but the decrease is gradual and does not approach that of a nonsmoker.

The risk of lung cancer is increased in the smoker who is exposed to other carcinogenic agents, such as radon, asbestos, and chemical carcinogens. Internationally, the incidence of lung cancer is growing with industrialized nations having the highest rates.[18]

The increase of lung cancer mortality in the last decades can be entirely attributed to the trend of tobacco consumption. However, there is a lag time of many years between beginning smoking and the clinical manifestation of cancer. The therapist can have a key role in the prevention of lung cancer through risk-factor assessment and client education (see Chapter 2).

METASTASES

Metastatic spread of pulmonary tumors is usually to the long bones, vertebral column (especially the thoracic vertebrae), liver, and adrenal glands. Brain metastasis is also common, occurring in as many as 50% of cases.

Local metastases by direct extension may involve the chest wall, pleura, pulmonary parenchyma, or bronchi. Further local tumor growth may erode the first and second ribs and associated vertebrae, causing bone pain and paravertebral pain associated with involvement of sympathetic nerve ganglia.

The respiratory system is a common site for complications associated with cancer and cancer therapy. Several factors can lead to pulmonary complications. Immunosuppression caused by the underlying disease or the cancer therapy can lead to infectious disease.

In addition, the lungs contain an enormous capillary bed through which flows the entire venous circulation, making it a common site of metastasis from other primary cancers and pulmonary emboli. Carcinomas of the kidney, breast, pancreas, colon, and uterus are especially likely to metastasize to the lungs.

CLINICAL SIGNS AND SYMPTOMS

Clinical signs and symptoms of lung cancer often remain silent until the disease process is at an advanced stage. In many instances lung cancer may mimic other pulmonary conditions or may initially appear as chest, shoulder, or arm pain (Case Example 7-3).

Chest pain is a vague aching, and depending on the type of cancer, the client may have pleuritic pain on inspiration that limits lung expansion. Anorexia and weight loss occur in many clients

---

BOX 7-4 ▶ Risk Factors for Lung Cancer

- Age greater than 50 years
- Smoking or other tobacco use
- Previous tobacco-related cancer
- Passive (environmental) smoke
- Low consumption of fruit and vegetables
- Genetic predisposition
- Exposure to asbestos, uranium, radon
- Previous lung disease (e.g., COPD, pulmonary fibrosis, sarcoidosis)

CASE EXAMPLE 7-3 Neurologic Deficits in a Smoker

A 66-year-old man was referred by his primary care physician to physical therapy for weakness in the lower extremities. He also reported dysesthesia (pain with touch) in both legs from the knees down. The symptoms had been present for about 1 month before he saw his doctor. At the time of his physical therapy evaluation symptoms had been present for almost 2 months (client was delayed getting in to see a therapist due to his scheduling conflicts).

The client was a social worker who had never been married but had two children out of wedlock, had a history of chronic alcohol use, and reported a 60-pack-year history of tobacco use (pack years = number of packs/day × number of years; in this case the client had smoked two packs a day for the last 30 years).

Past medical history was negative for any previous significant injuries, illnesses, or hospitalizations. Both parents were killed in a car accident when the client was a child. Any other family history was unknown for the parents and unremarkable for the siblings.

Clinical examination revealed mild weakness in the distal muscle groups of the lower extremities (left weaker than right). Altered sensation was circumferential and included both lower legs equally. Tests for clonus and Babinski were negative. Deep tendon reflexes were equal bilaterally and within normal limits (WNL). Other neurologic screening tests were negative. There were no constitutional signs or symptoms reported or observed.

A program of strengthening and conditioning was started based on the physician's referral requesting strength training and clinical findings of muscular weakness. In the first 2 weeks of treatment, the client's weakness increased and he developed bilateral foot drop.

He started reporting episodes of dropping anything he lifted over 2 pounds. A quick screen-

ing examination showed bilateral weakness developing in the hands and wrists as well as the feet and ankles.

What are all the red flags in this case?

Age (over 50 years)

Significant smoking history

Alcohol use

Bilateral symptoms (hands and feet)

Progressive neurologic symptoms

Are there any other screening tests that can/should be done?

A screening physical examination should be conducted (see Chapter 4) and any significant findings noted and reported to the physician.

A general survey, vital signs, and chest auscultation would be a good place to start. It is possible that the client presentation (and certainly the new onset of symptoms) are unknown to the physician who saw him almost a month ago.

In fact the therapist observed signs of digital clubbing (hands only), oxygen saturation levels (SaO_2) consistently at 90%, and noted bilateral basilar crackles on lung auscultation.

The client was advised to make a follow-up appointment with the physician and the therapist faxed a letter of request for follow-up based on these new findings. The client also hand carried a copy of the therapist's letter to the medical appointment.

Result: The client was diagnosed with lung cancer with accompanying paraneoplastic syndrome (see discussion of paraneoplastic syndromes, Chapter 13). His condition worsened rapidly and he died 6 weeks later.

The family later came back to the therapist and expressed their appreciation for finding the problem early enough to make end-of-life decisions. Both children and three of the four siblings were able to visit with the gentleman before he died suddenly in his sleep.

with lung cancer, and can be a symptom of advanced disease.[19]

Hemoptysis (coughing or spitting up blood) may occur secondary to ulceration of blood vessels. Wheezing occurs when the tumor obstructs the bronchus. Dyspnea, either unexplained or out of proportion, is a red flag indicating the need for medical screening, as is unexplainable weight loss accompanied by dyspnea.

Centrally located tumors cause increased cough, dyspnea, and diffuse chest pain that can be referred to the shoulder, scapulae, and upper back.

This pain is the result of peribronchial or perivascular nerve involvement.

Other symptoms may include post-obstructive pneumonia with fever, chills, malaise, anorexia, hemoptysis, and fecal breath odor (secondary to infection within a necrotic tumor mass). If these tumors extend to the pericardium, the client may develop a sudden onset of arrhythmia (tachycardia or atrial fibrillation), weakness, anxiety, and dyspnea.

Peripheral tumors are most often asymptomatic until the tumor extends through visceral and parietal pleura to the chest wall. Irritation of the nerves causes localized sharp, pleuritic pain that is aggravated by inspiration.

Metastases to the mediastinum (tissue and organs between the sternum and the vertebrae, including the heart and its large vessels; trachea; esophagus; thymus; lymph nodes) may cause hoarseness or dysphagia secondary to vocal cord paralysis as a result of entrapment or local compression of the laryngeal nerve.

Apical (Pancoast's) tumors of the lung apex do not usually cause symptoms while confined to the pulmonary parenchyma. They can extend into surrounding structures and frequently involve the eighth cervical and first thoracic nerves within the brachial plexus.

A constellation of symptoms referred to as Pancoast's syndrome is produced in the distribution of the C8, T1, and T2 dermatomes. Extension of the tumor into the paravertebral sympathetic nerves results in Horner's syndrome, which consists of enophthalmos (backward displacement of the eye), ptosis (drooping eyelid), and miosis (pupil constriction).

The most common initial symptom is sharp (often posterior) shoulder pain produced by invasion of the brachial plexus and/or extension of the tumor into the parietal pleura, endothoracic fascia, first and second ribs, or vertebral bodies. There may be pain in the axilla and subscapular areas on the affected side (Case Example 7-4).

Pain may radiate up to the head and neck, across the chest, and/or down the medial aspect of the arm and hand (ulnar nerve distribution) (Fig. 7-6). There may be subsequent atrophy of the upper extremity muscles with weakness of the muscles of the hand.

Pulmonary symptoms such as cough, hemoptysis, and dyspnea are uncommon until late in the disease. Affected individuals are often treated for presumed cervical osteoarthritis or shoulder bursitis resulting in delay of diagnosis. The pain eventually progresses to become severe and constant,

eventually resulting in more thorough testing and accurate diagnosis.[20] The onset of pulmonary symptoms in any client with neck, shoulder, and/or arm pain should be a red flag symptom for the therapist.

Trigger points of the serratus anterior muscle (see Fig. 17-4) also mimic the distribution of pain caused by the eighth cervical nerve root compression. Trigger points can be ruled out by palpation and lack of neurologic deficits and may be confirmed by elimination with appropriate physical therapy intervention.

Paraneoplastic syndromes (remote effects of a malignancy; see explanation in Chapter 13) occur in 10% to 20% of lung cancer clients. These usually result from the secretion of hormones by the tumor acting on target organs, producing a variety of symptoms. Occasionally, symptoms of paraneoplastic syndrome occur before detection of the primary lung tumor.

As mentioned earlier, brain metastasis is common, occurring in as much as 50% of cases. About 10% of all individuals with lung cancer have CNS involvement at the time of diagnosis. Major clinical symptoms of brain metastasis result from increased intracranial pressure and may include headache, nausea, vomiting, malaise, anorexia, weakness, and alterations in mental processes. Localized motor or sensory deficits occur, depending on the location of lesions (see Chapter 13).

Metastasis to the spinal cord produces signs and symptoms of cord compression (see Table 13-6 and Appendix A-2) including back pain (localized or radicular), muscle weakness, loss of lower extremity sensation, bowel and bladder incontinence, and diminished or absent lower extremity reflexes (unilateral or bilateral).

Clinical Signs and Symptoms of

Lung Cancer

- Any change in respiratory patterns
- Recurrent pneumonia or bronchitis
- Hemoptysis
- Persistent cough
- Change in cough or development of hemoptysis in a chronic smoker
- Hoarseness or dysphagia
- Sputum streaked with blood
- Dyspnea (shortness of breath)
- Wheezing
- Sharp chest, upper back, shoulder, scapular, rib, or arm pain aggravated by inspiration or accompanied by respiratory signs and symptoms

Fig. 7-6 • Pancoast's tumors can present with changes in cutaneous dermatomal innervation. The shaded areas show the dermatomes affected when the superior (apical) sulcus tumors associated with Pancoast's syndrome invade the brachial plexus. Direct extension to the brachial plexus involving C8 and T1 result in symptoms affecting the C8, T1, and T2 dermatomes.

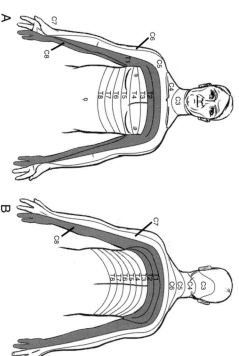

- Sudden, unexplained weight loss; anorexia
- Chest, shoulder, or arm pain
- Atrophy and weakness of the arm and hand muscles
- Fecal breath odor
- See also Clinical Signs and Symptoms of Paraneoplastic Syndrome, Brain Metastasis, and Metastasis to the Spinal Cord, Chapter 13; see Table 13-5 and Appendix A-2

GENETIC DISEASE OF THE LUNG

Cystic Fibrosis

Cystic fibrosis (CF) is an inherited disease of the exocrine ("outward-secreting") glands primarily affecting the digestive and respiratory systems.

This disease is the most common genetic disease in the United States, inherited as a recessive trait: both parents must be carriers, each having a defective copy of the CF gene. Each time two carriers conceive a child, there is a 25% chance that the child will have CF, a 50% chance that the child will be a carrier, and a 25% chance that the child will be a noncarrier. In the United States 5% of the population, or 12 million people, carry a single copy of the CF gene.

Because cysts and scar tissue on the pancreas were observed during autopsy when the disease was first being differentiated from other conditions, it was given the name *cystic fibrosis of the pancreas*. Although this term describes a secondary rather than primary characteristic, it has been retained.

In 1989 scientists isolated the cystic fibrosis gene located on chromosome 7. In healthy people a protein called cystic fibrosis transmembrane con-

ductance regulator (CFTR) provides a channel by which chloride (a component of salt) can pass in and out of cells.

Persons with CF have a defective copy of the gene that normally enables cells to construct that channel. As a result, salt accumulates in the cells lining the lungs and digestive tissues, making the surrounding mucus abnormally thick and sticky. These secretions, which obstruct ducts in the pancreas, liver, and lungs, and abnormal secretion of sweat and saliva are the two main features of CF.

Usually, CF manifests itself in early childhood, but there are some individuals who have a variant form the disease in which symptoms can appear during adolescence or adulthood. Symptoms tend to be milder and sweat chloride concentration may be normal.[21]

Obstruction of the bronchioles by mucous plugs and trapped air predisposes the client to infection, which starts a destructive cycle of increased mucus production with increased bronchial obstruction, infection, and inflammation with eventual destruction of lung tissue.

Clinical Signs and Symptoms

Pulmonary involvement is the most common and severe manifestation of CF. Obstruction of the airways leads to a state of hyperinflation and bronchiectasis. In time, fibrosis develops, and restrictive lung disease is superimposed on the obstructive disease.

Over time, pulmonary obstruction leads to chronic hypoxia, hypercapnia, and acidosis. Pneumothorax, pulmonary hypertension, and eventually cor pulmonale may develop. These are very poor prognostic indicators in adults. The course of

CASE EXAMPLE 7-4   Pancoast's Tumor

A 55-year-old man presented with shoulder pain radiating down the arm present for the last 3 months. His job as a mechanic required many hours with his arms raised overhead, which is what he thought was causing the problem.

He was diagnosed with cervical radiculopathy after cervical x-rays showed moderate osteoarthritic changes at the C678 levels. EMG studies confirmed the diagnosis and he was sent to physical therapy.

The client gave a history as a nonsmoker but mentioned his parents were chain-smokers and his wife of 35 years also smokes heavily. There was no other significant social or personal history. The client was adopted and did not know his family history.

The therapist conducted a physical screening examination and noted a slight drooping of the left eyelid, which the client attributed to fatigue and changes with middle age. Vital signs were unremarkable. Muscle atrophy and weakness were present in the left hand consistent with a C78 neurologic impairment. There were changes in the thumbs and index fingers on both sides with what looked like early signs of digital clubbing. The nail beds were spongy with a definite change in the shape of the distal phalanx.

When asked if there were any other symptoms of any kind anywhere else in the body the client mentioned a change in the way he perspires. He noticed his left face and armpit do not perspire like the right side. He could not remember when this change began but knew it was not something he had his whole life.

What are the red flag signs in this case?

Age

Exposure to passive tobacco smoke

Nailbed changes

Anhydrosis (lack of sweating)

Questionable changes in eyelid

What other screening tests might be appropriate?

A more careful neurologic examination is in order. Any findings to suggest impairment outside the parameters of the C678 nerve func-

tion might raise a yellow flag. Upper limb neurodynamic and neural tension tests are important; trigger point assessment is often helpful. A cranial nerve assessment also is advised due to the possible eye drooping observed.

Although the vital signs were unremarkable, the nailbed changes should prompt lung auscultation and a closer look at skin color, capillary refill time, and peripheral vascular assessment.

Result: No other neurologic findings were observed and the cranial nerve assessment was within normal limits with the exception of the eyelid drooping. The therapist also noticed the pupil in the left eye seemed smaller than the pupil on the right. Repeated attempts to use a penlight or darkness to change pupil size were unsuccessful.

Based on objective findings, the therapist started an intervention of neural mobilizations and gave the client a home program of postural exercises and self-neural mobilizations. A plan was outlined to integrate a strengthening program as soon as time would allow.

All findings were documented and sent to the physician. The client was not sent back to the physician but the physician, upon reading the therapist's notes, called the therapist and asked for further explanation of the therapist's findings. The physician was concerned and asked to have the client make a follow-up appointment.

Further medical testing brought about a diagnosis of Pancoast's tumor in the left upper lung lobe involving the brachial plexus and the first and second ribs. Horner's syndrome was also recognized as the cause of his drooping eye and anhydrosis.

Symptoms from the Horner syndrome resolved after radiotherapy; pain and weakness also improved after medical therapy. Physical therapy for rehabilitation was initiated after medical treatment, but the client developed progressive regional disease with distant metastases and died within 2 months.

CF varies from one client to another depending on the degree of pulmonary involvement.

Advances in treatment, including aerosolized antibiotics, mucus thinning agents, antiinflammatory agents, chest physical therapy, enzyme supplements, and nutrition programs, have extended the average life expectancy for CF sufferers into their early 20s, with maximal survival estimated at 30 to 40 years.

Because the genetic abnormality has been identified, considerable progress has been made in the development of gene therapy and preventive gene transfer for this disease.[22,23] Lung transplantation in older childhood and adolescence is a possible treatment option based on rapidly declining lung function.[24]

Clinical Signs and Symptoms of

Cystic Fibrosis

In Early or Undiagnosed Stages

- Persistent coughing and wheezing
- Recurrent pneumonia
- Excessive appetite but poor weight gain
- Salty skin/sweat
- Bulky, foul-smelling stools (undigested fats caused by a lack of amylase and tryptase enzymes)

In Older Child and Young Adult

- Infertility
- Nasal polyps
- Periostitis
- Glucose intolerance

Clinical Signs and Symptoms of

Pulmonary Involvement in Cystic Fibrosis

- Tachypnea (very rapid breathing)
- Sustained chronic cough with mucus production and vomiting
- Barrel chest (caused by trapped air)
- Use of accessory muscles for respiration and intercostal retraction
- Cyanosis and digital clubbing
- Exertional dyspnea with decreased exercise tolerance

Further complications include:
- Pneumothorax
- Hemoptysis
- Right-sided heart failure secondary to pulmonary hypertension

▲ OCCUPATIONAL LUNG DISEASES

Lung diseases are among the most common occupational health problems. They are caused by the inhalation of various chemicals, dusts, and other particulate matter present in certain work settings. Not everyone exposed to occupational inhalants will develop lung disease. Prolonged exposure combined with smoking increases the risk of developing occupational lung disease and increases the severity of these diseases.[25]

During the interview process, the therapist will ask questions about occupational and smoking history to identify the possibility of an underlying pulmonary pathologic condition (see Chapter 2 and Appendix B-13).

The most commonly encountered occupational lung diseases are occupational lung cancer, occupational asthma (also known as work-related asthma), asbestosis, mesothelioma, and byssinosis (brown lung disease). Other less common occupational lung diseases include hypersensitivity pneumonitis, acute respiratory irritation, and pneumoconiosis (black lung disease, silicosis).

The greatest number of occupational agents causing *asthma* are those with known or suspected allergic properties, such as plant and animal proteins (e.g., wheat, flour, cotton, flax, and grain mites). Exposures within the workplace can aggravate preexisting asthma.[26]

Asbestosis and *mesothelioma* occur as a result of asbestos exposure. Asbestos is the name of a group of naturally occurring minerals that separate into strong, very fine fibers. The fibers are heat-resistant and extremely durable, qualities that made asbestos useful in construction and industry.

Scarring of the lung tissue occurs in asbestosis as a result of exposure to the microscopic fibers of asbestos. Under certain circumstances fibers can be released and pose a health risk, such as lung cancer from inhaling the fibers. Mesothelioma is an otherwise rare cancer of the chest lining caused by asbestos exposure.

Byssinosis (brown lung disease) caused by dusts from hemp, flax, and cotton processing, results in chronic obstruction of the small airways impairing lung function. Textile workers are at greatest risk of disability from byssinosis.

Hypersensitivity pneumonitis, or allergic alveolitis, is most commonly due to the inhalation of organic antigens of fungal, bacterial, or animal origin. *Acute respiratory irritation* results from the inhalation of chemicals such as ammonia, chlorine, and nitrogen oxides in the form of gases, aerosols, or particulate matter. If such irritants reach the

lower airways, alveolar damage and pulmonary edema can result. Although the effects of these acute irritants are usually short-lived, some may cause chronic alveolar damage or airway obstruction.

Pneumoconioses, or "the dust diseases," result from inhalation of minerals, notably silica, coal dust, or asbestos. These diseases are most commonly seen in miners, construction workers, sandblasters, potters, and foundry and quarry workers. Occupational exposure to dust, fumes, or gases (including diesel) increases mortality due to COPD, even among workers who have never smoked.[27]

Pneumoconioses usually develop gradually over a period of years, eventually leading to diffuse pulmonary fibrosis, which diminishes lung capacity and produces restrictive lung disease.[27]

Home Remodeling

Home remodeling projects in the United States have increased dramatically in the last decade. Whether it is a do-it-yourself project or the occupants remain in the home during remodeling, problems can occur from dust inhalation and exposure to hazardous materials such as lead, asbestos, and creosote. Creosote is toxic (inhaled as fumes) and is a skin and eye irritant.

Lead poisoning is a serious problem in home remodeling projects throughout the United States. Special precautions to avoid lead poisoning must be followed if the home was built prior to 1978.

Lead poisoning can occur from inhaling paint dust (the result of sanding or scraping painted surfaces) and lead can be found in soil (children come into contact during play). Both sources of poisoning are common problems associated with remodeling projects.

Anyone presenting with a constellation of integumentary, musculoskeletal and/or neurologic symptoms accompanied by pulmonary involvement should be asked about the possibility of recent home remodeling projects and exposure to any of these materials.

Clinical Signs and Symptoms

Early symptoms of occupational-related lung disease depend on the specific exposure but may include noninflammatory joint pain, myalgia, cough, and dyspnea on exertion.

Chest pain, productive cough, and dyspnea at rest develop as the condition progresses. The therapist needs to be alert for the combination of significant arthralgias and myalgias with associated respiratory symptoms, accompanied by a past occupational and smoking history (see Appendix B-16).

Clinical Signs and Symptoms of

Occupational Lung Diseases

- Arthralgia
- Myalgia
- Chest pain
- Cough
- Dyspnea on exertion (progresses to dyspnea at rest)
- See also signs and symptoms of lung cancer in this chapter

▶ PLEUROPULMONARY DISORDERS

Pulmonary Embolism and Deep Venous Thrombosis

Pulmonary embolism (PE) involves pulmonary vascular obstruction by a displaced thrombus (blood clot), an air bubble, a fat globule, a clump of bacteria, amniotic fluid, vegetations on heart valves that develop with endocarditis, or other particulate matter. Once dislodged, the obstruction travels to the blood vessels supplying the lungs, causing shortness of breath, tachypnea (very rapid breathing), tachycardia, and chest pain.

The most common cause of PE is deep venous thrombosis (DVT) originating in the proximal deep venous system of the lower legs. The embolism causes an area of blockage, which then results in a localized area of ischemia known as a *pulmonary infarct*. The infarct may be caused by small emboli that extend to the lung surface (pleura) and result in acute pleuritic chest pain.

Risk Factors

Three major risk factors linked with DVT are blood stasis (e.g., immobilization because of bed rest, such as with burn clients, obstetric and gynecologic clients, and older or obese populations), endothelial injury (secondary to neoplasm, surgical procedures, trauma, or fractures of the legs or pelvis), and hypercoagulable states (see Box 6-2).

Other people at increased risk for DVT and PE include those with congestive heart failure, trauma, operation (especially hip, knee, and prostate surgery), age over 50 years, previous history of thromboembolism, malignant disease, infection, diabetes mellitus, inactivity or obesity, pregnancy, clotting abnormalities, and oral contraceptive use (see Chapter 6).

Prevention

Given the mortality of PE and the difficulties involved in its clinical diagnosis, prevention of DVT and PE is critical. A careful review of the Personal/Family History form (outpatient) or hospital medical chart (inpatient) may alert the therapist to the presence of factors that predispose a client to have a PE. Risk factor assessment is an important part of screening and prevention.

Although frequent changing of position, exercise, and early ambulation are necessary to prevent thrombosis and embolism, sudden and extreme movements should be avoided. Under no circumstances should the legs be massaged to relieve "muscle cramps," especially when the pain is located in the calf and the client has not been up and about.

Restrictive clothing and prolonged sitting or standing should be avoided. Elevating the legs should be accomplished with caution to avoid severe flexion of the hips, which will slow blood flow and increase the risk of new thrombi.

Deep Venous Thrombosis (see also Chapter 6)

Signs and symptoms include tenderness, leg pain, swelling (a difference in leg circumference of 1.4 cm in men and 1.2 cm in women is significant), and warmth. One may also see subcutaneous venous distention, discoloration, a palpable cord, and/or pain upon placement of a blood pressure cuff around the calf (considerable pain with the cuff inflated to 160 to 180 mm Hg).

A positive Homans' sign is still used clinically to diagnose DVT but has been shown to be an unreliable test for DVT.[29,30] Homans' sign is elicited by gentle squeezing of the affected calf or slow dorsiflexion of the foot on the affected side to elicit deep calf pain. In theory, the muscle are compressed or veins within the muscle are compressed or stretched causing deep calf pain. Only about half of all clients with DVT experience pain and Homan's sign.

Unfortunately, at least half the cases of DVT are asymptomatic, and in up to 30% of clients with clinical evidence of DVT, no DVT is demonstrable. A more sensitive and specific tool for predicting DVT is the Autar DVT Scale (see Table 4-11).

Clinical Signs and Symptoms of
Deep Venous Thrombosis (DVT)

- Unilateral tenderness or leg pain; dull ache or sensation of "tightness" in the area where the DVT is located

- Unilateral swelling (difference in leg circumference)
- Warmth
- Positive Homans' sign (unreliable test)
- Subcutaneous venous distention (superficial thrombus)
- Discoloration
- Palpable cord (superficial thrombus)
- Pain with placement around calf of blood pressure cuff inflated to 160 to 180 mm Hg

Pulmonary Embolism

Signs and symptoms of PE are nonspecific and vary greatly, depending on the extent to which the lung is involved, the size of the clot, and the general condition of the client.

Clinical presentation does not differ between younger and older persons. Dyspnea, pleuritic chest pain, and cough are the most common symptoms reported. Pleuritic pain is caused by an inflammatory reaction of the lung parenchyma or by pulmonary infarction or ischemia caused by obstruction of small pulmonary arterial branches.

Typical pleuritic chest pain is sudden in onset and aggravated by breathing. The client may also report hemoptysis, apprehension, tachypnea, and fever (temperature as high as 39.5° C, or 103.5° F). The presence of hemoptysis indicates that the infarction or areas of atelectasis have produced alveolar damage.

Clinical Signs and Symptoms of
Pulmonary Embolism (PE)

- Dyspnea
- Pleuritic (sharp, localized) chest pain
- Diffuse chest discomfort
- Persistent cough
- Hemoptysis (bloody sputum)
- Apprehension, anxiety, restlessness
- Tachypnea (increased respiratory rate)
- Tachycardia
- Fever

Cor Pulmonale

When a PE has been sufficiently massive to obstruct 60% to 75% of the pulmonary circulation, the client may have central chest pain, and acute cor pulmonale occurs. Cor pulmonale is a serious cardiac condition and an emergency situation arising from a sudden dilatation of the right ventricle as a result of PE.

As cor pulmonale progresses, edema, and other signs of right-sided heart failure develop. Symptoms are similar to those of congestive heart failure

from other causes: dyspnea, edema of the lower extremities, distention of the veins of the neck, and liver distention. The hematocrit is increased as the body attempts to compensate for impaired circulation by producing more erythrocytes.

Clinical Signs and Symptoms of

Cor Pulmonale

- Peripheral edema (bilateral legs)
- Chronic cough
- Central chest pain
- Exertional dyspnea or dyspnea at rest
- Distention of neck veins
- Fatigue
- Wheezing
- Weakness

Pulmonary Artery Hypertension (PAH)

Pulmonary artery hypertension (PAH) is a condition of vasoconstriction of the pulmonary arterial vascular bed. It can be either *primary* (rare) occurring mostly in young and middle aged women, or *secondary* occurring as a result of other clinical conditions such as pulmonary embolus, chronic lung disease, polycythemia, and heart abnormalities.

Normally, the pulmonary circulation has a low resistance and can accommodate large increases in blood flow during exertion. When pulmonary arterial vasoconstriction occurs and pulmonary arterial pressures rise above normal, the condition becomes self-perpetuating inducing further vasoconstriction in the pulmonary vasculature, structural abnormalities, and eventual right-sided heart failure (cor pulmonale).

The right ventricle must pump very hard against a narrowed, resistant pulmonary vascular bed thus resulting in pump failure.

Clinical Signs and Symptoms

Symptoms can be very subtle and difficult to recognize initially, especially in secondary PAH since underlying lung disease is usually present. PAH may present as dyspnea on exertion and later dyspnea at rest as well as dull, retrosternal chest pain, which often mimics angina pectoris. Fatigue and dizziness on exertion are also very common.[31]

Pleurisy

Pleurisy is an inflammation of the pleura (serous membrane enveloping the lungs) and is caused by infection, injury, or tumor. The membranous pleura that encases each lung consists of two close-fitting layers: the visceral layer encasing the lungs and

the parietal layer lining the inner chest wall. A lubricating fluid lies between these two layers.

If the fluid content remains unchanged by the disease, the pleurisy is said to be dry. If the fluid increases abnormally, it is a wet pleurisy or pleurisy with effusion (pleural effusion). If the wet pleurisy becomes infected with formation of pus, the condition is known as purulent pleurisy or empyema.

Pleurisy may occur as a result of many factors, including pneumonia, tuberculosis, lung abscess, influenza, systemic lupus erythematosus (SLE), rheumatoid arthritis, and pulmonary infarction. Any of these conditions is actually a risk factor for the development of pleurisy, especially in the aging adult population.

Pleurisy, with or without effusion associated with SLE, may be accompanied by acute pleuritic pain and dysfunction of the diaphragm.

Clinical Signs and Symptoms

The chest pain is sudden and may vary from vague discomfort to an intense stabbing or knifelike sensation in the chest. The pain is aggravated by breathing, coughing, laughing, or other similar movements associated with deep inspiration.

The visceral pleura is insensitive; pain results from inflammation of the parietal pleura. Because the latter is innervated by the intercostal nerves, chest pain is usually felt over the site of the pleuritis, but pain may be referred to the lower chest wall, abdomen, neck, upper trapezius muscle, and shoulder because of irritation of the central diaphragmatic pleura (Fig. 7-7).

Clinical Signs and Symptoms of

Pleurisy

- Chest pain
- Cough
- Dyspnea
- Fever, chills
- Tachypnea (rapid, shallow breathing)

Pneumothorax

Pneumothorax, or free air in the pleural cavity between the visceral and parietal pleurae, may occur secondary to pulmonary disease (e.g., when an emphysematous bulla or other weakened area on the lung ruptures) or as a result of trauma and subsequent perforation of the chest wall. Other risk factors include scuba diving and overexertion.

Pneumothorax is not uncommon after surgery or after an invasive medical procedure involving the chest or thorax. Air may enter the pleural space

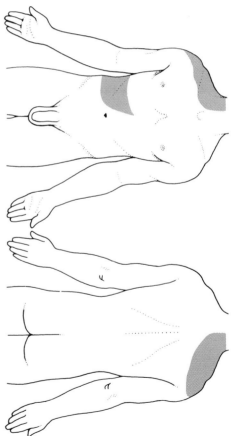

Fig. 7-7 • Chest pain over the site of pleuritis is usually perceived by the client. Referred pain (*light red*) associated with pleuritis may occur on the same side as the pleuritic lesion affecting the shoulder, upper trapezius muscle, neck, lower chest wall, or abdomen.

directly through a hole in the chest wall (open pneumothorax) or diaphragm. Pneumothorax associated with surgical management of patent ductus arteriosus (PDA) in neonates has been reported.[32]

Air may escape into the pleural space from a puncture or tear in an internal respiratory structure (e.g., bronchus, bronchioles, or alveoli). This form of pneumothorax is called closed or spontaneous pneumothorax.

Pneumothorax associated with scuba diving occurs as a result of arterial gas embolism (AGE). AGE is caused by pulmonary overinflation if the breathing gas cannot be exhaled adequately during the ascent. Inert gas bubbles cause impairment of pulmonary functions due to hypoxia.[33]

Extra-alveolar air (pulmonary barotrauma) from scuba diving can be overlooked resulting in serious neurologic sequelae. Scuba diving is contraindicated in anyone with asthma, hypertension, coronary heart disease, diabetes, or a history of pneumothorax.

Spontaneous pneumothorax occasionally affects the exercising individual and occurs without preceding trauma or infection. In a healthy individual, abrupt onset of dyspnea raises the suspicion of a spontaneous pneumothorax. Peak incidence for this type of pneumothorax is in adults between 20 and 40 years. Spontaneous pneumothorax in term newborn infants is significantly more likely in males with higher birth weights and with vacuum delivery.[34]

Idiopathic spontaneous pneumothorax (SP) is the result of leakage of air from the lung parenchyma through a ruptured visceral pleura into the pleural cavity. This rupture may be caused by an increased pressure difference between parenchymal airspace and pleural cavity. Another theory is that peripheral airway inflammation

leads to obstruction with airtrapping in the lung parenchyma, which precedes spontaneous pneumothorax.[35]

Clinical Signs and Symptoms

Symptoms of pneumothorax, whether occurring spontaneously or as a result of injury or trauma, vary depending on the size and location of the pneumothorax and on the extent of lung disease. When air enters the pleural cavity, the lung collapses, producing dyspnea and a shift of tissues and organs to the unaffected side.

The client may have severe pain in the upper and lateral thoracic wall, which is aggravated by any movement and by the cough and dyspnea that accompany it. The pain may be referred to the ipsilateral shoulder (corresponding shoulder on the same side as the pneumothorax), across the chest, or over the abdomen (Fig. 7-8). The client may be most comfortable when sitting in an upright position.

Other symptoms may include a fall in blood pressure, a weak and rapid pulse, and cessation of normal respiratory movements on the affected side of the chest (Case Example 7-5).

Clinical Signs and Symptoms of Pneumothorax

- Dyspnea
- Change in respiratory movements (affected side)
- Sudden, sharp chest pain
- Increased neck vein distention
- Weak and rapid pulse
- Fall in blood pressure
- Dry, hacking cough
- Shoulder pain
- Sitting upright is the most comfortable position

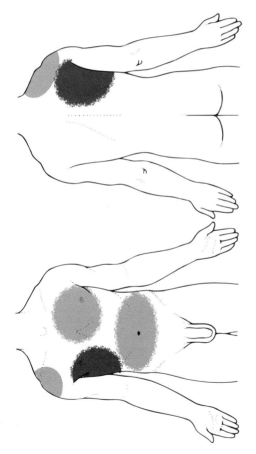

Fig. 7-8 • Possible pain patterns associated with pneumothorax: upper and lateral thoracic wall with referral to the ipsilateral shoulder, across the chest, or over the abdomen.

CASE EXAMPLE 7-5 Tension Pneumothorax

An 18-year-old male, who was injured in a motor vehicle accident (MVA), has come into the hospital physical therapy department with orders to begin ambulation. He had a long leg cast on his left leg and has brought a pair of crutches with him. This is the first time he has been out of bed in the upright position; he has not ambulated in his room yet.

Blood pressure measurement taken while the client was sitting in the wheelchair was 110/78 mm Hg. Pulse was easily palpated and measured at 72 BPM. The therapist gave the necessary instructions and assisted the client to the standing position in the parallel bars. Immediately on standing, this young man began to experience the onset of sharp midthoracic back pain and shortness of breath. He became pale and shaky, breaking out in a cold sweat.

The therapist assisted him to a seated position and asked the client if he was experiencing pain anywhere else (e.g., chest, shoulder, abdomen) while reassessing blood pressure. His blood pressure had fallen to 90/56 mm Hg, and he was unable to respond verbally to the questions asked. A clinic staff person was asked to telephone for immediate emergency help. While waiting for a medical team, the therapist noted a weak and rapid pulse, distention of the client's neck veins, and diminished respiratory movements.

This young man was diagnosed with tension pneumothorax caused by a displaced fractured rib. Untreated, tension pneumothorax can quickly produce life-threatening shock and bradycardia. Monitoring of the client's vital signs by the therapist resulted in fast action to save this young man's life.

▼ PHYSICIAN REFERRAL

It is more common for a therapist to be treating a client with a previously diagnosed musculoskeletal problem who now has chronic, recurrent pulmonary symptoms than to be the primary evaluator and health care provider of a client with pulmonary symptoms.

In either case the therapist needs to know what further questions to ask and which of the client's responses represent serious symptoms that require medical follow-up.

Shoulder or back pain can be referred from diseases of the diaphragmatic or parietal pleura or secondary to metastatic lung cancer. When clients have chest pain, they usually fall into two categories: those who demonstrate chest pain associated with pulmonary symptoms and those who have true musculoskeletal problems, such as intercostal strains and tears, myofascial trigger points, fractured ribs, or myalgias secondary to overuse.

Clients with chronic, persistent cough, whether that cough is productive or dry and hacking, may develop sharp, localized intercostal pain similar to

pleuritic pain. Both intercostal and pleuritic pain are aggravated by respiratory movements, such as laughing, coughing, deep breathing, or sneezing. Clients who have intercostal pain secondary to insidious trauma or repetitive movements, such as coughing, can benefit from physical therapy.

For the client with asthma, it is important to maintain contact with the physician if the client develops signs of asthma or any bronchial activity during exercise. The physician must be informed to help alter the dosage or the medications to maintain optimal physical performance.

The therapist will want to screen for medical disease through a series of questions to elicit the presence of associated systemic (pulmonary) signs and symptoms. Aggravating and relieving factors may provide further clues that can assist in making treatment or referral decision.

In all these situations, the referral of a client to a physician is based on the family/personal history of pulmonary disease, the presence of pulmonary symptoms of a systemic nature, or the absence of substantiating objective findings indicating a musculoskeletal lesion.

Guidelines for Immediate Medical Attention

- Abrupt onset of dyspnea accompanied by weak and rapid pulse and fall in blood pressure (pneumothorax), especially following motor vehicle accident, chest injury, or other traumatic event
- Chest, rib, or shoulder pain with neurologic symptoms following recent recreational or competitive scuba diving
- Client with symptoms of inadequate ventilation or carbon dioxide retention (see Respiratory Acidosis)
- Any red flag signs and symptoms in a client with a previous history of cancer, especially lung cancer

Guidelines for Physician Referral

- Shoulder pain aggravated by respiratory movements; have the client hold his or her breath and reassess symptoms; any reduction or elimination of symptoms with breath holding or the Valsalva maneuver suggests pulmonary or cardiac source of symptoms
- Shoulder pain that is aggravated by supine positioning; pain that is worse when lying down and improves when sitting up or leaning forward is often pleuritic in origin; abdominal contents push up against

diaphragm and, in turn, against the parietal pleura
- Shoulder or chest (thorax) pain that subsides with autosplinting (lying on the painful side) (For the client with asthma): Signs of asthma or bronchial activity during exercise
- Weak and rapid pulse accompanied by fall in blood pressure (pneumothorax)
- Presence of associated signs and symptoms, such as persistent cough, dyspnea (rest or exertional), or constitutional symptoms (see Boxes 1-3 and 4-18).

Clues to Screening for Pulmonary Disease

These clues will help the therapists in the decision making process:

- Age over 40 years
- History of cigarette smoking for many years
- Past medical history of breast, prostate, kidney, pancreas, colon, or uterine cancer
- Recent history of upper respiratory infection, especially when followed by noninflammatory joint pain of unknown cause
- Musculoskeletal pain exacerbated by respiratory movements (e.g., deep breathing, coughing, laughing)
- Respiratory movements are diminished or absent on one side (pneumothorax)
- Dyspnea (unexplained or out of proportion) especially when accompanied by unexplained weight loss
- Unable to localize pain by palpation
- Pain does not change with spinal motions (e.g., no change in symptoms with side bending, rotation, flexion, or extension)
- Pain does not change with alterations in position (possible exceptions: sitting upright is preferred with pneumothorax; symptoms may be worse at night with recumbency, sitting upright eases or relieves symptoms)
- Symptoms are increased with recumbency (lying supine shifts the contents of the abdominal cavity in an upward direction, thereby placing pressure on the diaphragm and, in turn, the lungs, referring pain from a lower lung pathologic condition)
- Presence of associated signs and symptoms, especially persistent cough, hemoptysis, dyspnea, and constitutional symptoms, most commonly sore throat, fever, and chills
- Autosplinting decreases pain
- Elimination of trigger points resolves symptoms confirms a musculoskeletal problem (or conversely, trigger point therapy does NOT

resolve symptoms raising a red flag for further examination and evaluation)

- Range of motion does not reproduce symptoms* (e.g., trunk rotation, trunk side bending, shoulder motions)

- Anytime an older person has shoulder pain and confusion at presentation, consider the possibility of diaphragmatic impingement by an underlying lung pathologic condition, especially pneumonia

* There are two possible exceptions to this guideline. Painful symptoms from an intercostal tear (secondary to forceful coughing caused by diaphragmatic pleurisy) will be reproduced by trunk side bending to the opposite side and trunk rotation to one or both sides. In such a case there is an underlying pulmonary pathologic condition, and a musculoskeletal component. Pleuritic pain can also be reproduced by trunk movements, but the therapist will be unable to localize the pain on palpation.

OVERVIEW PULMONARY PAIN PATTERNS

▼ **PLEUROPULMONARY DISORDERS** (Fig. 7-9)

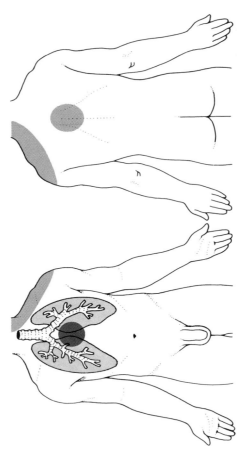

Fig. 7-9 • Primary pain patterns (dark red) associated with pleuropulmonary disorders, such as pulmonary embolus, cor pulmonale, pleurisy, or spontaneous pneumothorax, may vary, but they usually include substernal or chest pain. Pain over the involved lung fields (anterior, lateral, or posterior) may occur (not shown). Pain may radiate (light red) to the neck, upper trapezius muscle, ipsilateral shoulder, thoracic back, costal margins, or upper abdomen (the latter two areas are not shown).

Location:	Substernal or chest over involved lung fields—anterior, side, and back
Referral:	Often well localized (client can point right to the exact site of pain) without referral
	May radiate to neck, upper trapezius muscle, shoulder, costal margins, or upper abdomen
	Thoracic back pain occurs with irritation of the posterior parietal pleura
Description:	Sharp ache, stabbing, angina-like pressure, or crushing pain with pulmonary embolism
	Angina-like chest pain with severe pulmonary hypertension
Intensity:	Moderate
Duration:	Hours to days
Associated signs and symptoms:	Preceded by pneumonia or upper respiratory infection
	Wheezing
	Dyspnea (exertional or at rest)
	Hyperventilation

OVERVIEW   PULMONARY PAIN PATTERNS—cont'd

Tachypnea (increased respirations)
Fatigue, weakness
Tachycardia (increased heart rate)
Fever, chills
Edema
Apprehension or anxiety, restlessness
Persistent cough or cough with blood (hemoptysis)
Dry hacking cough (occurs with the onset of pneumothorax)
Medically determined signs and symptoms (e.g., by chest auscultation and chest radiograph)

Relieving factors:
Sitting
Some relief when at rest, but most comfortable position varies (pneumonia)
Pleuritic pain may be relieved by lying on the affected side
Breathing at rest

Aggravating factors:
Increased inspiratory movement (e.g., laughter, coughing, sneezing)
Symptoms accentuated with each breath

▼ LUNG CANCER

Location:
Anterior chest

Referral:
Scapulae, upper back, ipsilateral shoulder radiating along the medial aspect of the arm
First and second ribs and associated vertebrae and paravertebral muscles (apical or Pancoast's tumors)

Description:
Localized, sharp pleuritic pain (peripheral tumors)
Dull, vague aching in the chest
Neuritic pain of shoulders/arm (apical or Pancoast's tumors)
Bone pain caused by metastases to adjacent bone or to the vertebrae

Duration:
Constant

Intensity:
Moderate-to-severe

Associated signs and symptoms:
Dyspnea or wheezing
Hemoptysis (coughing up or spitting up blood)
Fever, chills, malaise, anorexia, and weight loss
Fecal breath odor
Tachycardia or atrial fibrillation (palpitations)
Muscle weakness or atrophy (e.g., Pancoast's tumor may involve the shoulder and the arm on the affected side)
Associated CNS symptoms:
Headache
Nausea
Vomiting
Malaise
Signs of cord compression:
Localized or radicular back pain
Weakness
Loss of lower extremity sensation
Bowel/bladder incontinence
Hoarseness, dysphagia (peripheral tumors)

Relieving factors:
None without medical intervention

Aggravating factors:
Inspiration: Deep breathing, laughing, coughing

⊘ KEY POINTS TO REMEMBER

✓ Pulmonary pain patterns are usually localized in the substernal or chest region over involved lung fields, which may include the anterior chest, side, or back (Figure 7-10; see also Fig. 7-9).

✓ Pulmonary pain can radiate to the neck, upper trapezius muscle, costal margins, thoracic back, scapulae, or shoulder.

✓ Shoulder pain caused by pulmonary involvement may radiate along the medial aspect of the arm, mimicking other neuromuscular causes of neck or shoulder pain.

✓ Pulmonary pain usually increases with inspiratory movements, such as laughing, coughing, sneezing, or deep breathing.

✓ Shoulder pain that is relieved by lying on the involved side may be "auto splinting," a sign of a pulmonary cause of symptoms.

✓ Shoulder pain that is aggravated when lying supine (arm/elbow supported) may be an indication of a pulmonary cause of symptoms.

✓ For anyone with pain patterns pictured here as presenting symptoms, especially in the absence of trauma or injury, check the client's personal medical history for previous or recurrent upper respiratory infection or pneumonia.

✓ Any client with symptoms of inadequate ventilation, pneumothorax, or CO_2 retention needs immediate medical referral.

✓ Clients with COPD who tend to retain CO_2 must be monitored carefully. Since clients with CO_2 retention have a decreased ventilatory drive unless oxygen levels are low, oxygen delivered by nasal cannula cannot get too high or the client will become apneic. There is a standard practice to increase oxygen levels administered by cannula during exercise with some clients who are compromised. Maintaining these levels around 1 to 2 liters/minute may be required with some clients who have COPD. Consult with respiratory therapy or nursing staff for optimal levels for this particular group of clients.

✓ CNS symptoms, such as muscle weakness, muscle atrophy, headache, loss of lower extremity sensation, and localized or radicular back pain, may be associated with lung cancer.

✓ Any CNS symptom may be the silent presentation of a lung tumor.

✓ Posterior leg or calf pain postoperatively may be caused by a thrombus and must be reported to the physician before physical therapy begins or continues.

✓ Hemoptysis or exertional/at rest dyspnea, either unexplained or out of proportion to the situation or person, is a red-flag symptom requiring medical referral.

✓ Any client with chest pain should be evaluated for trigger points and intercostal tears.

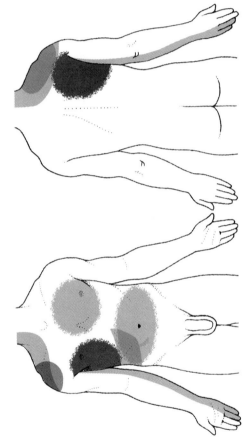

Fig. 7-10 • A composite picture of the pain patterns associated with many different impairments of the pulmonary parenchyma including pleuritis, pneumothorax, pulmonary embolism, cor pulmonale, and pleurisy. No single individual will present with all of these patterns at the same time. A composite illustration gives an idea of the wide range of referred pain patterns possible with pulmonary diseases or conditions. Remember that viscerogenic pain patterns do not usually present as discrete circles or ovals of pain as depicted here. This figure is an approximation of what the therapist might expect to hear the client describe associated with a pulmonary problem.

SUBJECTIVE EXAMINATION

Special Questions to Ask

Past Medical History

- Have you ever had trouble with breathing or lung disease such as bronchitis, emphysema, asthma, pneumonia, or blood clots?
- *If yes*: Describe what this problem was, when it occurred, and how it was treated.
- If the person indicated yes to asthma, either on the Personal/Family History form or to this question, ask:
- How can you tell when you are having an asthma episode?
- What triggers an asthma episode for you?
- Do you use medications during an episode? What is your current status?
- Do you have trouble with asthma during exercise?
- Do you time your medications with your exercise to prevent an asthma episode during exercise?
- Have you ever had tuberculosis?
- *If yes*: When did it occur, and how was it treated? What is your current status?
- When was your last test for tuberculosis? What was the test result?
- Have you had a chest x-ray film taken in the last 5 years?
- *If yes*: What were the results?
- Have you ever broken your nose, been told that you have a deviated septum (nasal passageway), nasal polyps, or sleep apnea? **(Hypoxia)**
- Have you ever had lung or heart surgery?
- *If yes*: What and when? **(Decreased vital capacity)**

Associated Signs and Symptoms

- Are you having difficulty breathing now?
- Do you ever have shortness of breath or breathlessness or cannot quite catch your breath?
- *If yes*: When does this happen? When you rest? When you lie flat, walk on level ground, or walk up stairs?
- How far can you walk before you feel breathless?
- What symptoms stop your walking (e.g., shortness of breath, heart pounding, chest tightness, or weak legs)?
- Are these episodes associated with night sweats, cough, chest pain, or bluish color around your lips or fingernails?
- Does your breathlessness seem to be related to food, pollen, dust, animals, season, stress, or strong emotion? **(Asthma)**
- Do you have any breathing aids (e.g., oxygen, nebulizer, inhaler, humidifier, air cleaner, or other aid)?

- Do you have a cough? (Note whether the client smokes, for how long, and how much.)
- *If yes* to cough, separate this cough from a smoker's cough by asking: When did it start? Is it related to smoking?
- Do you cough anything up? *If yes*: Describe the color, amount, and frequency.
- Are you taking anything to prevent this cough? *If yes*, does it seem to help?
- Are there occasions when you cannot seem to stop coughing?
- Do you ever cough up blood or anything that looks like coffee grounds? (Bright red fresh blood; brown or black older blood)
- Have you strained a muscle or your lower back from coughing?
- Does it hurt to touch your chest or take a deep breath, cough, sneeze, or laugh?
- Have you unexpectedly lost or gained 10 or more pounds recently?
  Gained: **Pulmonary edema, congestive heart failure, fat deposits under the diaphragm in the obese client reduces ventilation**
  Lost: **Emphysema, cancer**
- Do your ankles swell? **(Congestive heart failure)**
- Have you been unusually tired lately? **(Congestive heart failure, emphysema)**
- Have you noticed a change in your voice? **(Pathology of left hilum or trachea)**

Environmental and Work History Quick Survey (For full survey, see Appendix B-13):

- What kind of work do you do?
- Do you think your health problems are related to your work?
- Do you wear a mask at work?
- Are your symptoms better or worse when you're at home or at work?
  Follow-up if worse at work: Do others at work have similar problems?
  Follow-up if worse at home: Have you done any remodeling at home in the last 6 months?
- Have you been exposed to dusts, asbestos, fumes, chemicals, radiation, or loud noise?
- Have you ever served in any branch of the military?
  If yes, were you ever exposed to dusts, fumes, chemicals, radiation or other substances?
  Follow-up: It may be necessary to ask additional questions based on past history, symptoms, and risk factors present.

CASE STUDY

REFERRAL

A 65-year-old man has come to you for an evaluation of low back pain, which he attributes to lifting a heavy box 2 weeks ago. During the course of the medical history, you notice that the client has a persistent cough and that he sounds hoarse.

After reviewing the Personal/Family History form, you note that the client smokes two packs of cigarettes each day and that he has smoked at least this amount for at least 50 years. (One pack per day for 1 year is considered "one pack year.") This person has smoked an estimated 100 pack years; anyone who has smoked for 20 pack years or more is considered to be at risk for the development of serious lung disease.

What questions will you ask to decide for yourself whether this back pain is systemic?

PHYSICAL THERAPY INTERVIEW

Introduction to Client

It is important for me to make certain that your back pain is not caused by other health problems, such as prostate problems or respiratory infection, so I will ask a series of questions that may not seem to be related to your back pain, but I want to be very thorough and cover every possibility to obtain the best and most effective treatment for you.

Pain

From your history form I see that you associate your back pain with lifting a heavy box 2 weeks ago. When did you first notice your back pain (sudden or gradual onset)?

Have you ever hurt your back before or have you ever had pain similar to this episode in the past? **(Systemic disease: recurrent and gradually increases over time)**

Please describe your pain (supply descriptive terms if necessary)

How often do you have this pain?

FUPs: How long does it last when you have it? What aggravates your pain/symptoms? What relieves your pain/symptoms? How does rest affect your pain? Have you noticed any changes in your pain/symptoms since they first started to the present time?

Do you have any numbness in the groin or inside your legs? (Saddle anesthesia: **cauda equina**)

Pulmonary

I notice you have quite a cough and you sound hoarse to me. How long have you had this cough and hoarseness (when did it first begin)?

Do you have any back pain associated with this cough? Any other pain associated with your cough?

If yes: Have the person describe where, when, intensity, aggravating and relieving factors.

How does it feel when you take a deep breath? Does your lower back hurt when you laugh or take a deep breath?

When you cough, do you produce phlegm or mucus? If yes: Have you ever noticed any red streaks or blood in it?

Does your coughing or back pain keep you awake at night?

Have you been examined by a physician for either your cough or your back pain?

Have you had any recent chest or spine x-rays taken?

If yes: When and where? What were the results?

General Systemic

Have you had any night sweats, daytime fevers, or chills?

Do you have difficulty in swallowing **(Esophageal cancer, anxiety, cervical disc protrusion)**?

Have you had laryngitis over and over? **(Oral cancer)**

Urologic

Have you ever been told that you have a prostate problem or prostatitis?

If yes: Determine when this occurred, how it was treated, and whether the person had the same symptoms at that time that he is now describing to you.

Have you noticed any change in your bladder habits?

FUPS: Have you had any difficulty in starting or continuing to urinate?

Is there any burning or discomfort on urination?

Have you noticed any blood in your urine?

Have you recently had any difficulty with kidney stones or bladder or kidney infections?

Gastrointestinal

Have you noticed any change in your bowel pattern?

Have you had difficulty having a bowel movement?

CASE STUDY—cont'd

Do you find that you have soiled yourself without even realizing it? (**Cauda equina lesion**—this would require immediate referral to a physician)

Does your back pain begin or increase when you are having a bowel movement?

Is your back pain relieved after having a bowel movement?

Have you noticed any association between when you eat and when your pain/symptoms increase or decrease?

Final Question

Is there anything about your current back pain or your general health that we have not discussed that you think is important for me to know? (Refer to Special Questions to Ask in this chapter for other questions that may be pertinent to this client, depending on the answers to these questions.)

PHYSICIAN REFERRAL

As always, correlation of findings is important in making a decision regarding medical referral. If the client has a positive family history for respiratory problems (especially lung cancer) and if clinical findings indicate pulmonary involvement, the client should be strongly encouraged to see a physician for a medical check-up.

If there are positive systemic findings, such as difficulty in swallowing, persistent hoarseness, shortness of breath at rest, night sweats, fevers, bloody sputum, recurrent laryngitis, or upper respiratory infections *either in addition to or in association with* the low back pain, the client should be advised to see a physician, and the physician should receive a copy of your findings.

This guideline covers the client who has a true musculoskeletal problem but also has other health problems, as well as the client who may have back pain of systemic origin that is unrelated to the lifting injury 2 weeks ago.

PRACTICE QUESTIONS

1. If a client reports that the shoulder/upper trapezius muscle pain increases with deep breathing, how can you assess whether this results from a pulmonary or musculoskeletal cause?

2. Neurologic symptoms such as muscle weakness or muscle atrophy may be the first indication of:
   a. Cystic fibrosis
   b. Bronchiectasis
   c. Neoplasm
   d. Deep vein thrombosis

3. Back pain with radiating numbness and tingling down the leg past the knee does not occur as a result of:
   a. Postoperative thrombus
   b. Bronchogenic carcinoma
   c. Pott's disease
   d. Trigger points

4. Pain associated with pleuropulmonary disorders can radiate to the:
   a. Anterior neck
   b. Upper trapezius muscle
   c. Ipsilateral shoulder
   d. Thoracic spine
   e. (a) and (c)
   f. All of the above

PRACTICE QUESTIONS—cont'd

5. The presence of a persistent dry cough (no sputum or phlegm produced) has no clinical significance to the therapist. True or false?

6. Dyspnea associated with emphysema is the result of:
   a. Destruction of the alveoli
   b. Reduced elasticity of the lungs
   c. Increased effort to exhale trapped air
   d. (a) and (b)
   e. All of the above

7. What is the significance of autosplinting?

8. Which symptom has greater significance: dyspnea at rest or exertional dyspnea?

9. The presence of pain and anxiety in a client can often lead to hyperventilation. When a client hyperventilates, the arterial concentration of carbon dioxide will do which of the following?
   a. Increase
   b. Decrease
   c. Remain unchanged
   d. Vary depending on potassium concentration

10. Common symptoms of respiratory acidosis would be most closely represented by which of the following descriptions?
    a. Presence of numbness and tingling in face, hands, and feet
    b. Presence of dizziness and lightheadedness
    c. Hyperventilation with changes in level of consciousness
    d. Onset of sleepiness, confusion, and decreased ventilation

REFERENCES

1. Guerra S: Overlap of asthma and chronic obstructive pulmonary disease, *Curr Opin Pulm Med* 11(1):7-13, 2005.
2. Pauwels RA, Rabe KF: Burden and clinical features of chronic obstructive pulmonary disease (COPD), *Lancet* 364(9434):613-620, 2004.
3. Meyers DA, Larj MJ, Lange L: Genetics of asthma and COPD. Similar results for different phenotypes, *Chest* 126(2 Suppl):105S-110S, 2004.
4. Amsden GW: Anti-inflammatory effects of macrolides: an underappreciated benefit in the treatment of community-acquired respiratory tract infections and chronic inflammatory pulmonary conditions? *J Antimicrob Chemother* 55(1):10-21, 2005.
5. Rubin BK, Henke MO: Immunomodulatory activity and effectiveness of macrolides in chronic airway disease, *Chest* 125(2 Suppl):70S-78S, 2004.
6. Wisniewski A: Chronic bronchitis and emphysema: Clearing the air, *Nursing* 2003, 33(5): 44-49, 2003.
7. Goto Y, Kurosawa H, Mori N, et al: Improved activities of daily living, psychological state and health-related quality of life for 12 months following lung volume reduction surgery in patients with severe emphysema, *Respirology* 9(3):337-344, 2004.
8. Trow TK: Lung-volume reduction surgery for severe emphysema: appraisal of its current status, *Curr Opin Pulm Med* 10(2):128-132, 2004.
9. Upham JW, Holt PG: Environment and development of atopy, *Curr Opin Allergy Clin Immunol* 5(2):167-172, 2005.
10. Asthma in older women, *Harvard Women's Health Watch* 11(3):5-6, 2003.
11. Racial disparities in tuberculosis, selected Southeastern States, 1991-2002, *MMWR* 53(25):556-559, 2004.
12. Carmona L, Hernández-Garcia C, Vadillo C, et al: Increased risk of tuberculosis in patients with rheumatoid arthritis, *J Rheumatol*, 30:1436-1439, 2003.
13. Ogle J: Internationally adopted children need evaluation for tuberculosis, *Circle, Chinese Children Charities* 39:6-7, 2003.
14. Tay B, Deckey J, Hu S: Spinal infections, *J Amer Acad Orthop Surg* 10(3):188-197, 2002.
15. Jemal A, Ward E, Thun MJ: Contemporary lung cancer trends among U.S. women, *Cancer Epidemiol Biomarkers Prev* 14(3):582-585, 2005.
16. American Cancer Society: Anti-smoking efforts cut lung cancer deaths, *ACS News Center*. Available at: http://www.cancer.org/docroot/NWS/content/NWS_2_1x_Anti-Smoking_Efforts_Cut_Lung_Cancer_Deaths.asp. Accessed May 2, 2005.
17. Jemal A: Lung cancer trends in young adults: an early indicator of progress in tobacco control (United States), *Cancer Causes and Control* 14(6):579-585, 2003.
18. Porello P: Neoplasms, Lung. eMedicine. Available at www.emedicine.com/emerg/topic335.htm. Accessed May 2, 2005.
19. Kreamer K: Getting the lowdown on lung cancer, *Nursing* 2003, 33(11):36-42, 2003.
20. Arcasoy SM, Jett JR, Schild SE: Pancoast's syndrome and superior (pulmonary) sulcus tumors. UpToDate Patient Information. Sponsored by the American Society of General Internal Medicine and the American College of Rheumatology. Available at: http://patients.uptodate.com/topic.asp?file=lung_ca/12055 (version 13.2), June 2005.
21. Staton G: Chronic obstructive diseases of the lung, *ACP Medicine 2004*. Available at: www.medscape.com/viewarticle/494031. Posted 12-3-2004. Accessed April 28, 2005.
22. Griesenbach U, Geddes DM, Alton EW: Advances in cystic fibrosis gene therapy, *Curr Opin Pulm Med* 10(6):542-546, 2004.
23. Ostedgaard LS, Rokhlina T, Karp PH, et al: A shortened adeno-associated virus expression cassette for CFTR gene transfer to cystic fibrosis airway epithelia, *Proc Natl Acad Sci U S A* 102(8):2952-2957, 2005.
24. Rosenbluth DB, Wilson K, Ferkol T, et al: Lung function decline in cystic fibrosis patients and timing for lung transplantation referral, *Chest* 126(2):412-419, 2004.
25. American Lung Association: Occupational lung disease fact sheet, January 2004. Available at: http://www.lungusa.

org/site/pp.asp?c=dvLUK9OOE&b=35334. Accessed May 3, 2005.

26. National Institute for Occupational Safety and Health: Chapter 2: Respiratory Diseases. Worker Health Chartbook, 2004. Publication No. 2004-146.

27. Bergdahl IA, Toren K, Eriksson K, et al: Increased mortality in COPD among construction workers exposed to inorganic dust, *Eur Respir J* 23(3):402-406, 2004.

28. Pneumoconiosis prevalence among working coal miners examined in Federal Radiograph Surveillance programs, United States 1996-2002, *MMWR* 52(15):336-340, 2003.

29. O'Donnell T, Abbott W, Athanasoulis C, et al: Diagnosis of deep venous in the outpatient by venography, *Surg Gynecol Obstet* 150:69-74, 1980.

30. Molloy W, English J, O'Dwyer R, et al: Clinical findings in the diagnosis of proximal deep venous thrombosis, *Ir Med J* 75:119-120, 1982.

31. Holcomb S: Understanding pulmonary artery hypertension, *Nursing 2004* 34(9):50-54, 2004.

32. Jog SM, Patole SK: Diaphragmatic paralysis in extremely low birthweight neonates: is waiting for spontaneous recovery justified? *J Paediatr Child Health* 38(1):101-103, 2002.

33. Taylor DM, O'Toole KS, Ryan CM: Experienced, recreational scuba divers in Australia continue to dive despite medical contraindications, *Wilderness Environ Med* 13(3):187-193, 2002.

34. Al Tawil K, Abu-Ekteish FM, Tamimi O, et al: Symptomatic spontaneous pneumothorax in term newborn infants, *Pediatr Pulmonol* 37(5):443-446, 2004.

35. Smit HJ, Golding RP, Schramel FM, et al: Lung density measurements in spontaneous pneumothorax demonstrate airtrapping, *Chest* 125(6):2083-2090, 2004.

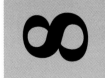

8

Screening for Gastrointestinal Disease

A great deal of new understanding of the enteric system and its relationship to other systems has been discovered over the last decade. For example, it is now known that the lining of the digestive tract from the esophagus through the large intestine (Fig. 8-1) is lined with cells that contain neuropeptides and their receptors. These substances, produced by nerve cells, are a key to the mind-body connection that contributes to the physical manifestation of emotions.[1,2]

In addition to the classic hormonal and neural negative feedback loops, there are direct actions of gut hormones on the dorsal vagal complex. The person experiencing a "gut reaction" or "gut feeling" may indeed be experiencing the direct effects of gut peptides on brain function.[3]

The association between the enteric system, the immune system, and the brain (now a part of the research referred to as psychoneuroimmunology or PNI) has been clearly established and forms an integral part of gastrointestinal (GI) symptoms associated with immune disorders such as fibromyalgia, systemic lupus erythematosus, rheumatoid arthritis, chronic fatigue syndrome, and others.

Researchers estimate that more than two thirds of all immune activity occurs in the gut. There are more T-cells in the intestinal epithelium than in all other body tissues combined. The gamma delta T cells form the forefront of the immune defense mechanism. They act as an early warning system in the cells lining the intestines, which are heavily exposed to microorganisms and toxins.[4,5] In some people, the wall of the gut seems to have been breached, either because the network of intestinal cells develops increased permeability (a syndrome referred to as "leaky gut") or perhaps because bacteria and yeast overwhelm it and migrate into the bloodstream.

Allowing undigested food or bacteria into the bloodstream sets in motion a chain of events as the immune system reacts. The body responds as if to an illness and expresses it in a number of ways such as a rash, diarrhea, GI upset, joint pain, migraines, and headache. The exact cause for these microscopic breaches remains unknown but food allergies, too much aspirin or ibuprofen, certain antibiotics, excessive alcohol consumption, smoking, or parasitic infections may be implicated.

All of these associations and new findings support the need for the therapist to assess carefully the possibility of GI symptoms present but unreported. This is especially important when considering the fact that GI tract symptoms can sometimes imitate musculoskeletal dysfunction.

GI disorders can refer pain to the sternal region, shoulder and neck, scapular region, mid-back, lower back, hip, pelvis, and sacrum. This pain can mimic primary musculoskeletal or neuromuscular lesions, causing confusion for the physical therapist or for the physician assessing the client's chief complaint.

Although these neuromusculoskeletal symptoms can occur alone and far from the actual site of the disorder, the client usually has other systemic

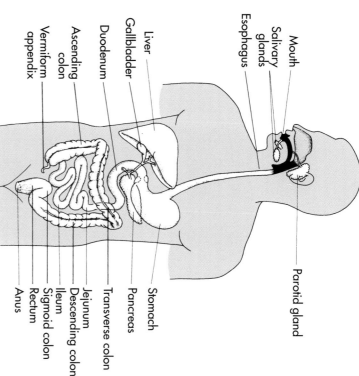

Fig. 8-1 • Organs of the digestive system; see also Fig. 9-1. (From Guyton AC: *Textbook of medical physiology,* ed 10, Philadelphia, 2000, WB Saunders.)

Mouth
Salivary glands
Esophagus
Parotid gland
Liver
Gallbladder
Duodenum
Ascending colon
Vermiform appendix
Stomach
Pancreas
Transverse colon
Jejunum
Descending colon
Ileum
Sigmoid colon
Rectum
Anus

signs and symptoms associated with GI disorders that should give the therapist who does a thorough investigation grounds for suspicion.

A careful interview to screen for systemic illness should include a few important questions concerning the client's history, prescribed medications, and the presence of any associated signs or symptoms that would immediately alert the therapist about the need for medical follow up. The most common intraabdominal diseases that refer pain to the musculoskeletal system are those that involve ulceration or infection of the mucosal lining. Drug-induced GI symptoms (e.g., antibiotic colitis, GI "blues" of nausea, vomiting, and anorexia from digitalis toxicity, NSAID-induced ulcers) can also occur with delayed reactions as much as 6 or 8 weeks after exposure to the medication.

SIGNS AND SYMPTOMS OF GASTROINTESTINAL DISORDERS

Any disruption of the digestive system can create symptoms such as pain, diarrhea, and constipation. The bowel is susceptible to altered patterns of normal motility caused by food, alcohol, tobacco, caffeine, drugs, physical and emotional stress, and lifestyle (e.g., lack of regular exercise). Gastrointestinal effects of chemotherapy include nausea

and vomiting, anorexia, taste alteration, weight loss, oral mucositis, diarrhea, and constipation.

Symptoms, including pain, can be related to various GI organ disturbances and differ in character depending on the affected organ. The most clinically meaningful GI symptoms reported in a physical therapy practice include

- Abdominal pain
- Dysphagia
- Odynophagia
- GI bleeding (emesis, melena, red blood)
- Epigastric pain with radiation to the back
- Symptoms affected by food
- Early satiety with weight loss
- Constipation
- Diarrhea
- Fecal incontinence
- Arthralgia
- Referred shoulder pain
- Psoas abscess
- Tenderness over McBurney's point (see Appendicitis this chapter)

Abdominal Pain

As we enter into this next discussion on primary and referred abdominal pain patterns, be aware that each pain pattern has listed with it both the sympathetic nerve distribution to the viscera (i.e.,

autonomic nervous system innervation of the structure) and the anatomic location of radiating or referred pain from the viscera or GI segment involved in the primary pain patterns.

Whenever possible, labels are used to differentiate between sympathetic nerve innervations of the viscera and anatomic locations of the pain. For example, the small intestine (viscera) is innervated by T9 to T11 but refers (somatic) pain to the L3 to L4 (anatomic) lumbar spine.

Primary GI Visceral Pain Patterns

Visceral pain (internal organs) occurs in the midline because the digestive organs arise embryologically in the midline and receive sensory afferents from both sides of the spinal cord. The site of pain corresponds to dermatomes from which the diseased organ receives its innervation (see Fig. 3-3). Pain is not well localized because innervation of the viscera is multisegmental over up to eight segments of the spinal cord but with few nerve endings.

The most common primary pain patterns associated with organs of the GI tract are depicted in Fig. 8-2. Pain in the *epigastric region* occurs anywhere from the midsternum to the xiphoid process from the heart, esophagus, stomach, duodenum, gallbladder, liver, and other mediastinal organs corresponding to the T3 to T5 sympathetic nerve distribution. The client may report the pain radiates around the ribs or straight through the chest

to the thoracic spine at the T3 to T6 or T7 anatomic levels.

Pain in the *periumbilical region* (T9 to T11 nerve distribution) occurs with impairment of the small intestine (see Fig. 8-13), pancreas, and appendix. Primary pain in the periumbilical region usually sends the client to a physician. However, pain around the umbilicus may be accompanied by low back pain. In the healthy adult who is not obese and does not have a protruding abdomen, the umbilicus is level with the disc located anatomically between the L3 and L4 vertebral bodies.

The physical therapist is more likely to see a client with anterior abdominal and low back pain at the same level but with alternating presentation. In other words, first the client experiences periumbilical pain with or without associated GI signs and symptoms, then the painful episode resolves. Later, the client develops low back pain with or without GI symptoms, but does not realize there is a link between these painful episodes. It is at this point the client presents in a physical therapy practice.

Pain in the *lower abdominal region* (hypogastrium) from the large intestine and/or colon may be mistaken for bladder or uterine pain by its suprapubic location. Referred pain at the same anatomic level posteriorly corresponds to the sacrum (see Fig. 8-14). The large intestine and colon are innervated by T10 to L2 depending on the location (e.g., ascending, transverse, descending colon).

The abdominal viscera are ordinarily insensitive to many stimuli, such as cutting, tearing, or crushing, that when applied to the skin evokes severe pain. Visceral pain fibers are sensitive only to stretching or tension in the wall of the gut from neoplasm, distention, or forceful muscular contractions secondary to bowel obstruction or spasm. The rate that tension develops must be rapid enough to produce pain; gradual distention, such as with malignant obstruction, may be painless unless ulceration occurs.

Inflammation may produce visceral pain and ischemia (deficiency of blood) that subsequently produces pain by increasing the concentration of tissue metabolites in the region of the sensory nerve. Pain associated with ischemia is steady pain, whether this ischemia is secondary to vascular disease or due to obstruction causing strangulation of tissue.

Additionally, although the viscera experience pain, the visceral peritoneum (membrane enveloping organs) is insensitive to pain. Except in the presence of widespread inflammation or ischemia, it is possible to have extensive disease without

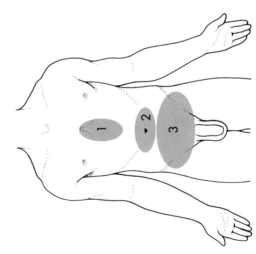

Fig. 8-2 • Visceral pain: (1) the epigastric region corresponding to T3-T5 sympathetic nerve distribution; (2) the periumbilical region (T10 sympathetic nerve distribution); the umbilicus is level with the disc located between the L3 and L4 vertebral bodies in the adult who is not overweight; and (3) the lower midabdominal or hypogastrium region (T10 to L2 sympathetic nerve distribution).

pain until the disease progresses enough to involve the parietal peritoneum.

Visceral pain is usually described as deep aching, boring, gnawing, vague burning, or deep grinding as opposed to the sharp, pricking, and knifelike qualities of cutaneous pain. When referred to the somatic regions of the low back, hip, or shoulder the sensation is vague and poorly localized because visceral afferents provide input over multiple segments of the spinal cord. As mentioned, afferents from different abdominal locations converge on the same dorsal nerve roots, which may be shared with the more precisely developed somatic sensory pathways.

Referred GI Pain Patterns

Sometimes visceral pain from a digestive organ is felt in a location remote from the usual anterior midline presentation. The referred pain site still lies within the dermatomes of the dorsal nerve roots serving the painful viscera. Such referred pain usually has the same qualities of visceral pain.

Afferent nerve impulses transmit pain from the esophagus to the spinal cord by sympathetic nerves from T5 to T10. Integration of the autonomic and somatic systems occurs through the vagus and the phrenic nerves. There can be referred pain from the esophagus to the mid-back and referred pain from the mid-back to the esophagus. For example, esophageal dysfunction can present as mid-thoracic spine pain and disc disease of the mid-thoracic spine can masquerade as esophageal pain.

Client history and the presence or absence of associated signs and symptoms will help guide the therapist. For example, a client with mid-back pain from esophageal dysfunction will not likely report numbness and tingling in the upper extremities or with discogenic disease. Likewise, disc involvement with referred pain to the esophagus will not cause melena or symptoms associated with meals.

Visceral afferent nerves from the liver, respiratory diaphragm, and pericardium are derived from C3 to C5 sympathetics and reach the central nervous system (CNS) via the phrenic nerve (see Fig. 3-3). The visceral pain associated with these structures is referred to the corresponding somatic area (i.e., the shoulder).

Afferent nerves from the gallbladder, stomach, pancreas, and small intestine travel through the celiac plexus (network of ganglia and nerves supplying the abdominal viscera) and the greater splanchnic nerves and enter the spinal cord from T6 to T9. Referred visceral pain from these visceral structures may be perceived in the mid-back and scapular regions.

Afferent stimuli from the colon, appendix, and pelvic viscera enter the 10th and 11th thoracic segments through the mesenteric plexus and lesser splanchnic nerves. Finally, the sigmoid colon, rectum, ureters, and testes are innervated by fibers that reach T11 to L1 segments through the lower splanchnic nerve and through the pelvic splanchnic nerves from S2 to S4. Referred pain may be perceived in the pelvis, flank, low back, or sacrum (Case Example 8-1).

Hyperesthesia (excessive sensibility to sensory stimuli) of skin and hyperalgesia (excessive sensibility to painful stimuli) of muscle may develop in the referred pain distribution. As mentioned in Chapter 3, in the early stage of visceral disease, sympathetic reflexes arising from afferent impulses of the internal viscera can be expressed first as sensory, motor, and/or trophic changes in the skin, subcutaneous tissues, and/or muscles. The client may present with itching, dysesthesia, skin temperature changes, perspiration, or dry skin.

The viscera do not perceive pain, but the sensory side is trying to get the message out that something is wrong by creating sympathetic sudomotor changes. When the afferent visceral pain stimuli are intense enough, discharges at synapses within the spinal cord cause this reflex phenomenon, usually transmitted by peripheral nerves of the same spinal segment(s). Thus the sudomotor changes occur as an automatic reflex along the distribution of the somatic nerve.

Remember from our discussion of viscerogenic pain patterns in Chapter 3 that any structure touching the respiratory diaphragm can refer pain to the shoulder, usually to the ipsilateral shoulder depending on where the direct pressure occurs. Anyone with upper back or shoulder pain and symptoms should be asked a few general screening questions about the presence of GI symptoms.

Referred pain to the musculoskeletal system can occur alone, without accompanying visceral pain, but usually visceral pain (or other symptoms) precedes the development of referred pain. The therapist will find that the client does not connect the two sets of symptoms or fails to report abdominal pain and GI symptoms when experiencing a painful shoulder or low back, thinking these are two separate problems. For a more complete discussion of the mechanisms behind viscerogenic referred pain patterns, see Chapter 3.

Most of what has been presented here has dealt with the sensory side of the clinical presentation.

CASE EXAMPLE 8-1   Colon Cancer

A 66-year-old university professor consulted with a physical therapist after twisting his back while taking the garbage out. He reported experiencing ongoing, painful low back symptoms 3 weeks after the incident. The objective assessment was consistent with a strain of the right paraspinal muscles with overall diminished lumbar spinal motion consistent with this gentleman's age. Given the reported mechanism of injury and the results of the examination consistent with a musculoskeletal problem, a medical screening examination was not included in the interview. A home exercise program was initiated including stretching and conditioning components.

When the client did not return for his follow up appointment, telephone contact was made with his family. The client had been hospitalized after collapsing at work. A medical diagnosis of colon cancer was determined. The family

reported he had been experiencing digestive difficulties "off and on" and low back pain for the past 3 years, always alternately and never simultaneously. The client died 6 weeks later.

In this case, the only red flag suggesting the need for medical screening was the client's age. However, the therapist did not ask about any associated signs and symptoms. We must always remember that even with a known and plausible reason for the injury, the client may wrongfully attribute symptoms to a logical event or occurrence. This man had been experiencing both abdominal symptoms and referred back pain, but since these episodes did not occur at the same time, he did not see a connection between them.

Always finish every interview with this question: "Are you having any other symptoms of any kind anywhere else in your body?"

There can be motor effects of GI dysfunction, too. For example contraction, guarding, and splinting of the rectus abdominis and muscles above the umbilicus can occur with dysfunction of the stomach, gallbladder, liver, pylorus, or respiratory diaphragm. Impairment of the ileum, jejunum, appendix, cecum, colon, and rectum are more likely to result in muscle spasm of the rectus abdominis below the umbilicus.[6]

At the same time, impairment of these GI structures can cause muscle dysfunction in the back (thoracic and lumbar spine) with loss of motion of the involved spinal segments. The clinical picture is one that is easily confused with primary pathology of the spinal segment.[6] Once again, the history and associated signs and symptoms help the therapist sort through the clinical presentation to reach a differential diagnosis. A thorough screening process is essential in such cases.

Dysphagia

Dysphagia is the sensation of food catching or sticking in the esophagus. This sensation may occur (initially) just with coarse, dry foods and may eventually progress to include anything swallowed, even thin liquids and saliva. Achalasia is a process by which the circular and longitudinal muscular fibers of the lower esophageal sphincter do not

relax. This disorder contributes to esophageal stricture. Closure (achalasia) of the esophageal sphincter may also create an obstruction of the esophagus.

Other possible GI causes of dysphagia include peptic esophagitis (inflammation of the esophagus) with stricture (narrowing), gastroesophageal reflux disease (GERD), and neoplasm (Case Example 8-2). Dysphagia may be a symptom of many other disorders unrelated to GI disease (e.g., stroke, Alzheimer's disease, Parkinson's disease). Certain types of drugs, including antidepressants, antihypertensives, and asthma drugs, can make swallowing difficult.

The presence of dysphagia requires prompt attention by the physician. Medical intervention is based on a subsequent endoscopic examination.

Odynophagia

Odynophagia, or pain during swallowing, can be caused by esophagitis or esophageal spasm. Esophagitis may occur secondary to GERD, the herpes simplex virus, or fungus caused by the prolonged use of strong antibiotics. Pain after eating may occur with esophagitis or may be associated with coronary ischemia.

To differentiate esophagitis from coronary ischemia: *upright positioning relieves esophagitis*

CASE EXAMPLE 8-2 Esophageal Cancer

An obese 88-year-old woman with a total knee replacement (TKR) was referred for rehabilitation because of loss of motion, joint swelling, and persistent knee pain. She was accompanied to the clinic for each session by one of her three daughters. Over a period of 2 or 3 weeks, each daughter commented on how much weight the mother had lost. When questioned, the client

complained of a loss of appetite and difficulty in swallowing, but she had been evaluated and treated only for her knee pain by the orthopedist. She was encouraged to contact her family doctor for evaluation of these red flag symptoms and was subsequently diagnosed with esophageal cancer.

BOX 8-1 ▼ Signs of Gastrointestinal Bleeding

Coffee ground emesis (vomit)
Bloody diarrhea
Bright red blood
Melena (dark, tarry stools)
Reddish or mahogany-colored stools

---

pain, whereas *cardiac pain* is relieved by nitroglycerin or by supine positioning. Both conditions require medical attention.

Gastrointestinal (GI) Bleeding

Gastrointestinal bleeding can appear as midthoracic back pain with radiation to the right upper quadrant. Bleeding may not be obvious; a hemoccult test may be required. A medical doctor should evaluate any type of bleeding. Ask about the presence of other signs such as blood in the vomit or stools (Box 8-1). *Coffee ground emesis* (vomit) may indicate a perforated peptic or duodenal ulcer.

Bloody diarrhea may accompany other signs of ulcerative colitis. Diarrhea and ulcerative colitis are discussed in greater depth separately in this chapter. *Bright red blood* usually represents pathology close to the rectum or anus and may be an indication of rectal fissures (e.g., history of anal intercourse) or hemorrhoids but can also occur as a result of colorectal cancer.

Melena, or black, tarry stool, occurs as a result of large quantities of blood in the stool. When asked about changes in bowel function, clients may describe black, tarry stools that have an unusual, noxious odor. The odor is caused by the presence of blood, and the black color arises as the digestive acids in the bowel oxidize red blood cells (e.g., bleeding esophageal varices, stomach, or duodenal ulceration). Melena is very sticky and does not clean well.

It may be necessary to ask about bowel smears on the under garments or difficulty getting wiped clean after a bowel movement. The following series may guide the therapist in this area:

Follow-Up Questions

• I would like to ask a few questions that may not seem related to your shoulder (back, hip, pelvic) pain, but these are very important in finding out what is causing your symptoms.
• Have you noticed any blood in your stools or change in the color or consistency of your bowel movements?
• Do you have any trouble wiping yourself clean after a bowel movement?
• Have you noticed any bowel smears on your underwear later after a bowel movement?

After going through the questions, it may be helpful to leave the back door open. Perhaps leave the client with this thought:

• If you do not know the answer right now or if you just have not noticed, please feel free to report back at a later time if you notice any changes.

Esophageal varices are dilated blood vessels, usually secondary to alcoholic cirrhosis of the liver. Blood that would normally be pumped back to the heart must bypass the damaged liver. The blood then "backs up" through the esophagus. Ruptured esophageal varices are an emergent, life-threatening condition. Vascular abnormalities of the stomach causing bleeding may include ulcers.

The client should be asked about the presence of any blood in the stool to determine whether it is melenic (from the upper GI tract) or bright red (from the distal colon or rectum). Ask about a history of NSAID use. Bleeding from internal or external hemorrhoids (enlarged veins inside or outside the rectum), rectal fissures, or colorectal carcinoma can cause bright red blood in the stools.

Rectal bleeding from anal lesions or fissures can occur in the homosexual population who are sexually active. Women engaging in anal intercourse can also be affected. A brief sexual history may be indicated in some cases.

Reddish or mahogany-colored stools can occur from eating certain foods such as beets or significant amounts of red food coloring but can also represent bleeding in the lower GI/colon. Medications that contain bismuth (e.g., Kaopectate, Pepto-Bismol, Bismatrol, Pink Bismuth) can cause darkened or black stools and the client's tongue may also appear black.

Clients who have received pelvic radiation for gynecologic, rectal, or prostate cancers have an increased risk for radiation proctitis, which can cause subsequent (delayed) rectal bleeding episodes. Be sure and ask about a past history of cancer and radiation treatment.

Epigastric Pain with Radiation

Epigastric pain perceived as intense or sharp pain behind the breastbone with radiation to the back may occur secondary to long-standing ulcers. For example, the client may be aware of an ulcer but does not relate the back pain to the ulcer. Close questioning related to GI symptoms can provide the therapist with knowledge of underlying systemic disease processes.

Anyone with epigastric pain accompanied by a burning sensation that begins at the xiphoid process and radiates up toward the neck and throat may be experiencing heartburn. Other common symptoms may include a bitter or sour taste in the back of the throat, abdominal bloating, gas, and general abdominal discomfort. Heartburn is often associated with gastroesophageal reflux disease (GERD). It can be confused with angina or heart attack when accompanied by chest pain, cough, and shortness of breath. A physician must evaluate and diagnose the cause of epigastric pain or heartburn.

A screening interview and evaluation is especially helpful when clients have neglected medical treatment for so long that epigastric back pain may in turn have created biomechanical changes in muscular contractions and spinal movement. These changes eventually create pain of a biomechanical nature.[7] The client then presents with enough true musculoskeletal findings such that a diagnosis of back dysfunction can be supported. However, the symptoms may be associated with a systemic problem. A good medical history can be a valuable tool in revealing the actual cause of the back pain.

Symptoms Affected by Food

Clients may or may not be able to relate pain to meals. Pain associated with gastric ulcers (located more proximally in the GI tract) may begin within 30 to 90 minutes after eating, whereas pain associated with duodenal or pyloric ulcers (located distally beyond the stomach) may occur 2 to 4 hours after meals (i.e., between meals). Alternatively stated, food is not likely to relieve the pain of a gastric ulcer, but it may relieve the symptoms of a duodenal ulcer.

The client with a duodenal ulcer may report pain during the night between midnight and 3:00 a.m. This pain should be differentiated from the nocturnal pain associated with cancer by its intensity and duration. More specifically, the gnawing pain of an ulcer may be relieved by eating, but the intense, boring pain associated with cancer is not relieved by any measures.

Ask the client with nighttime shoulder, neck, or back pain to eat something and assess the effect of food on these symptoms. Anyone whose musculoskeletal pain is altered (increased or decreased) or eliminated by food should be screened more thoroughly and referred for further medical evaluation when appropriate. Anyone with a previous history of cancer and nighttime pain must also be evaluated more closely. This is true even if eating has no effect on the client's symptoms.

Early Satiety

Early satiety occurs when the client feels hungry, takes one or two bites of food, and feels full. The sensation of being full is out of proportion with the time of the previous meal and the initial degree of hunger experienced. Vertebral compression fractures can occur from a variety of disorders including osteoporosis and can result in severe spinal deformity. This deformity, along with severe back pain can cause early satiety resulting in malnutrition.[8]

Constipation

Constipation is defined clinically as being a condition of prolonged retention of fecal content in the GI tract resulting from decreased motility of the colon or difficulty in expelling stool.

Common manifestations of this problem are hard stools, stools that are difficult to expel, infrequent stools, or a feeling of incomplete evacuation after defecation, and general discomfort. Constipated clients with tender psoas trigger points (TrPs) may report anterior hip, groin, or thigh pain when the fecal bolus presses against the TrPs.[9] Intractable constipation is called *obstipation* and

can result in a fecal impaction that must be removed. Back pain may be the overriding symptom of obstipation, especially in older adults who do not have regular bowel movements or who cannot remember the last bowel movement was several weeks ago (Case Example 8-3).

Changes in bowel habit may be a response to many other factors, such as diet (decreased fluid and bulk intake), smoking, side effects of medication, acute or chronic diseases of the digestive system, extra-abdominal diseases, personality, mood (depression), emotional stress, inactivity, prolonged bed rest, and lack of exercise (Table 8-1). Commonly implicated medications include narcotics, aluminum- or calcium-containing antacids (e.g., Alu-Tab, Basaljel, Tums, Rolaids), anticholinergics, tricyclic antidepressants, phenothiazines, calcium channel blockers, and iron salts.

Diets that are high in refined sugars and low in fiber discourage bowel activity. Transit time of the alimentary bolus from the mouth to the anus is influenced mainly by dietary fiber and is decreased with increased fiber intake. Additionally, motility can be decreased by emotional stress that has been correlated with personality. Constipation associated with severe depression can be improved by exercise.

People with low back pain may develop constipation as a result of muscle guarding and splinting that causes reduced bowel motility. Pressure on sacral nerves from stored fecal content may cause an *aching discomfort in the sacrum, buttocks, or thighs* (Case Example 8-4).

Because there are many specific organic causes of constipation, it is a symptom that may require further medical evaluation. It is considered a red flag symptom when clients with unexplained constipation have sudden and unaccountable changes in bowel habits or blood in the stools.

Diarrhea

Diarrhea, by definition, is an abnormal increase in stool liquidity and daily stool weight associated with increased stool frequency (i.e., more than three times per day). This may be accompanied by urgency, perianal discomfort, and fecal incontinence. The causes of diarrhea vary widely from one person to another, but food, alcohol, use of laxatives and other drugs, medication side effects, and travel may contribute to the development of diarrhea (Table 8-2).

Acute diarrhea, especially when associated with fever, cramps, and blood or pus in the stool, can accompany invasive enteric infection. Chronic diarrhea associated with weight loss is more likely to indicate neoplastic or inflammatory bowel disease. Extraintestinal manifestations such as arthritis or skin or eye lesions are often present in inflammatory bowel disease. Any of these combinations of symptoms must be reported to the physician.

Drug-induced diarrhea is associated most commonly with antibiotics. Diarrhea may occur as a direct result of antibiotic use and the GI symptom resolves when the drug is discontinued. Symptoms may also develop 6 to 8 weeks after first ingestion of an antibiotic. A more serious, less frequent, antibiotic-induced colitis with severe diarrhea is caused by *Clostridium difficile* (*C. difficile*).

This anaerobic bacterium colonizes the colon of 5% of healthy adults, but over 20% of hospitalized patients. Clients receiving enteral (tube) feedings are at higher risk for acquisition of *C. difficile* and associated severe diarrhea. *C. difficile* is the major cause of diarrhea in patients hospitalized for more than 3 days. It is spread in an oral-fecal manner and is readily transmitted from patient to patient by hospital personnel. Fastidious handwashing, use of gloves, and extremely careful cleaning of bathroom, bed linen, and associated items are helpful in decreasing transmission.[12]

Athletes using creatine supplements to enhance power and strength in performance may experience minor GI symptoms. Muscle cramps, diarrhea, loss of appetite, weight gain, and dizziness occur in about 8 percent of the individuals taking these supplements. Therapists working with athletes should keep this in mind when hearing reports of GI distress. Many sports players do not even know how much creatine they are taking or are taking more than the recommended dose. Players as young as 13 years old have reported using creatine supplements.[13,14]

For the client describing chronic diarrhea, it may be necessary to probe further about the use of laxatives as a possible contributor to this condition. Laxative abuse contributes to the production of diarrhea and begins a vicious cycle as chronic laxative users experience excessive secretion of aldosterone and resultant edema when they attempt to stop using laxatives. This edema and increased weight forces the person to continue to rely on laxatives. The abuse of laxatives is common in the eating disorder populations (e.g., anorexia, bulimia); affected persons may ingest up to 100 laxatives at a time.

Questions about laxative use can be asked tactfully during the Core Interview (see Chapter 2) when asking about medications, including over-the-counter drugs such as laxatives. Encourage the

CASE EXAMPLE 8-3 Obstipation

A 75-year-old Caucasian male was transported from his home to a hospital emergency department with acute onset of shortness of breath. He was intubated en route by ambulance personnel, secondary to hypoxemia and acute respiratory distress. Family members state that the patient has severe chronic obstructive pulmonary disorder (COPD) and uses continuous supplemental oxygen at home (usually 3 liters per minute). The client had no complaints of chest pain leading up to, or during, the episode.

While in the hospital, the client was hypotensive and started on dopamine. Chest x-ray revealed acute pulmonary edema consistent with congestive heart failure. He was treated with intravenous Lasix. Following removal of the NG tube, the client began to complain of severe low back pain and was started on Vicodin. MRI of the lumbar/sacral spine showed multiple levels of lumbar stenosis and facet sclerosis.

Four days post hospital admission, the client's oxygen saturation was 90% on 4 liters per minute of supplemental oxygen. The decision was made to transfer the client to a skilled nursing facility (SNF) with orders for activity as tolerated and physical therapy (evaluate and treat accordingly).

Medical Diagnoses

Acute respiratory
  failure
Hypoxemia
Congestive heart
  failure (CHF)
Pulmonary edema
COPD
Chronic low back pain
Degenerative joint
  disease (DJD)
Spinal stenosis

Past Medical History

Pulmonary asbestosis
Hypotension
Benign prostatic
  hypertrophy (BPH)
Non-Q myocardial
  infarction

Medications

Bactrim (antiinfective)
Ketoconazole (antifungal)
Plavix (Coronary Artery Disease prophylaxis;
  platelet aggregation inhibitor)
Aspirin (ASA); (Coronary Artery Disease pro-
  phylaxis)
Magnesium oxide (supplement)

K-dur (supplement)
Vasotec (antihypertensive; angiotensin-convert-
  ing enzyme [ACE] inhibitor)
Lasix (loop diuretic; CHF)
Percocet (opiate analgesic; back pain)
Colace (laxative)

Current Complaints

Client reports increased shortness of breath (SOB) with minor exertion and severe lumbar/sacral pain that has been constant over the last 3 days and appears to be getting worse.

Pain is described as "a dull ache" and is aggravated by movement. Minor relief is obtained through rest and use of pain medication. The client also reported recent lower abdominal discomfort, which he attributed to something he "ate for breakfast."

When asked about elimination patterns, he states that his bowel movements are not regular, but he "must have had one in the hospital." He "urinates frequently," has trouble starting a flow of urine, and does not void completely due to an enlarged prostate.

He reports a long history of progressive back pain without traumatic onset, starting in his 40s. His immediate goal is relief of back pain. His "normal" back pain is described as a 4 to 6 on a 0 to 10 scale. His current level of intensity is described as an 8/10 on pain medication.

Review of Systems

General

Oxygen saturation (pulse oximeter) while on
  4 liters of oxygen/minute: 92%
BP: 110/65 (seated, left arm)
RR: 16/minute HR: 86/minute (regular taken
  for one full minute)
Body temperature: 99.4 degrees

Neurologic

History of radicular pain symptoms in both
  lower extremities above the knee, but not
  present at this time
No observable atrophy of LE musculature
DTRs: +1 in bilateral patellar tendon; 0 for
  bilateral Achilles

CASE EXAMPLE 8-3 Obstipation—cont'd

MMT: Unable to perform due to back pain; decreased functional strength observed

Proprioception: Decreased in feet and ankles, bilaterally

Cardiovascular

Mild pitting edema (pedal: feet and ankles bilaterally) with 15-20 second rebound

2-3 pillow orthopnea

Digital clubbing, bilaterally

History of claudication with prolonged standing and ambulation

Pulmonary

Diminished breath sounds, especially at bases (auscultation)

Early exertional dyspnea

Gastrointestinal

Low abdominal pain/discomfort

Constipation

Genitourinary

Frequent urge to urinate

Difficulty starting flow

Decreased urine output

Musculoskeletal

Flexed postural stance (unable to straighten up due to pain)

Mild age-related ROM limitations noted

Muscle guarding and spasm in paravertebral musculature from T4 to L2

Balance, mobility, ambulation assessed and recorded

Evaluation: Although the client's back pain was made worse by movement, the presence of intense pain and constitutional symptom (low-grade fever) alerted the therapist to a possible systemic or viscerogenic cause of pain. The fact that the client could not remember his last bowel movement combined with abdominal pain was of concern. Change in bladder function was also of concern.

Prior to initiation of physical therapy services, the client was referred back to the attend-

ing physician. A brief summary of the client's neuromusculoskeletal impairments was presented, along with a description of the proposed intervention. A simple statement at the end was highlighted:

Intense back pain accompanied by low-grade fever

Abdominal pain and no recall of last bowel movement

Difficulty initiating and maintaining a flow of urine

Urinary frequency without a sense of void completion

Doctor

These symptoms are outside the scope of physical therapy intervention. Would you please evaluate before we begin rehab? Please advise if there are any recommended changes in the proposed program of intervention. Thank you.

Outcome

Physician ordered a urine culture, but attempts to obtain a sample were unsuccessful. The physician was unable to insert a straight catheter so the resident was sent to the hospital and a suprapubic catheter was inserted. He returned to the SNF 4 days later with the following diagnoses:

Bladder outlet obstruction

Urinary tract infection with E. coli

Prostate cancer, probably metastatic

Obstipation

When the resident returned to the SNF and was seen by P.T., there were no complaints of low back pain (beyond his lifetime baseline) and no lower abdominal discomfort. The neurologic deficits previously identified in both lower extremities were absent.

Summary: This is a good case to point out that medical personnel occasionally miss things that a physical therapist can find when conducting a screening exam and a review of systems. Recognizing red flags sent this client back to the physician sooner than later and ended needless painful suffering on his part.

From Joseph R. Clemente, DPT (submitted as part of a t-DPT requirement), New York, 2003.

TABLE 8-1 ▼ Causes of Constipation

Neurogenic	Muscular	Mechanical	Rectal lesions	Drugs/diet
Cortical, voluntary, or involuntary evacuation	Atony (loss of tone)	Bowel obstruction	Thrombosed hemorrhoids	Anesthetic agents (recent general surgery)
Central nervous system lesions	Severe malnutrition	Neoplasm	Perirectal abscess	Antacids (containing aluminum or calcium)
Multiple sclerosis	Metabolic defects	Volvulus (intestinal twisting)		Anticholinergics
Cord tumors	Hypothyroidism	Diverticulitis		Anticonvulsants
Tabes dorsalis	Hypercalcemia	Extraalimentary tumors		Antidepressants
Spinal cord lesions or tumors	Potassium depletion	Pregnancy		Antihistamines
Parkinson's	Hyperparathyroidism	Colostomy		Antipsychotics
Irritable bowel syndrome	Inactivity; chronic back pain			Barium sulfate
Dementia				Cancer chemotherapy (e.g., Oncovin)
				Iron compounds
				Diuretics
				Narcotics
				Lack of dietary bulk
				Renal failure (due to fluid restriction, phosphate binders)
				Myocardial infarction (narcotics for pain control)

CASE EXAMPLE 8-4 Constipated biker with leg pain

A 29-year-old male presented in the physical therapy clinic with inner thigh pain of the left leg of unknown cause over the last 3 weeks. The pain occurred most often when he had a bowel movement. He was training for an iron man competition (swimming, biking, running), but did not have any known injury or accident to attribute the symptom to.

When asked if there were any other symptoms anywhere else in his body, the client reported an inability to get an erection and a tendency toward constipation with hard stools. The therapist could find no clinical signs of muscle weakness, atrophy, or dysfunction. Postural alignment was symmetrical and without apparent problems. All provocation tests for hip, spine, sacrum, SI, and pelvis were negative. The client could complete a full squat without difficulty. Hop test and heel strike were both negative.

The client was screened for signs and symptoms associated with other possible causes of erectile dysfunction, such as diabetes, past history of testicular or prostate problems, past history of cancer, and possible sexual abuse. There was no red flag history or red flag signs and symptoms. Visual inspection of the lower half of the body revealed no signs of vascular compromise. The client denied any bladder problems or urinary incontinence.

Knowing that the pudendal nerve is responsible for penile erection, the therapist asked to see the client on his bicycle. Pressure on the nerve from a poorly constructed and minimally padded seat was a possible cause. The client was advised to change bike seats, change the seat height and tilt, and reassess symptoms in 2 weeks.

The client was also encouraged to stand up intermittently to relieve perineal pressure.

Result: The client reported complete cessation of all symptoms with the purchase of a bicycle seat with a cut-away middle. Since the obturator nerve passes below the symphysis pubis, it is likely bicycle seat compression on the nerve contributed to the inner thigh pain as well.

Bicycle seat neuropathy is not uncommon among long-distance bikers due to the cyclist supporting the body weight on a narrow seat. Vascular and/or neurologic compromise of the pudendal nerve is the most likely explanation for these symptoms.[10,11]

TABLE 8-2 ▼ Causes of Diarrhea

Malabsorption	Neuromuscular	Mechanical	Infectious	Nonspecific
Pancreatitis	Irritable bowel syndrome	Incomplete obstruction	Viral	Ulcerative colitis
Pancreatic carcinoma	Diabetic enteropathy	Neoplasm	Bacterial	Diverticulitis
Hyperthyroidism		Adhesions	Parasitic	Diet
Caffeine		Stenosis	Protozoal (Giardia)	Laxative abuse
		Fecal impaction		Food allergy
		Muscular incompetency		Antibiotics (Clostridium difficile)
		Postsurgical effect (ileal bypass)		Creatinine use
				Cancer chemotherapy (e.g., Fluorouracil)
				Lactose (milk) intolerance
				Psychogenic (nervous tension)

client to discuss bowel management without drugs at the next appointment with the physician.

Fecal Incontinence

Fecal incontinence may be described as an inability to control evacuation of stool and is associated with a sense of urgency, diarrhea, and abdominal cramping. Causes include partial obstruction of the rectum (cancer), colitis, and radiation therapy, especially in the case of women treated for cervical or uterine cancer. The radiation may cause trauma to the rectum that results in incontinence and diarrhea. Anal distortion secondary to traumatic childbirth, hemorrhoids, and hemorrhoidal surgery may also cause fecal incontinence.

Arthralgia

The relationship between "gut" inflammation and joint inflammation is well known, but not fully understood. Many inflammatory GI conditions have an arthritic component affecting the joints. For example, inflammatory bowel disease (ulcerative colitis and Crohn's disease) is often accompanied by rheumatic manifestations; peripheral joint arthritis and spondylitis with sacroiliitis are the most common of these manifestations.[15,16]

Researchers suggest a possible "interface" between the bowel and the articular surface of joints to explain this phenomenon.[17,18] It is hypothesized that an antigen crosses the gut mucosa and enters the joint setting up an immunologic response. Arthralgia with synovitis and immune-mediated joint disease may occur as a result of this immunologic response.[17] It is likely that an impaired antibacterial host defense and an uncontrolled pro-inflammatory response of the innate immune system are at fault.[19]

Joint arthralgia associated with gastrointestinal infection is usually asymmetric, migratory, and oligoarticular (affecting only one or two joints). This type of joint involvement is termed *reactive arthritis* when triggered by microbial infection such as *C. difficile* from the GI (and sometimes genitourinary or respiratory) tract. Other accompanying symptoms may include fever, malaise, skin rash or other skin lesions, nail bed changes (nails separate from the nail beds and become thin and discolored), iritis, or conjunctivitis.

The bowel and joint symptoms may or may not occur at the same time. Usually this type of arthralgia is preceded 1 to 3 weeks by diarrhea, urethritis, regional enteritis (Crohn's disease), or other bacterial infection. The knees, ankles, shoulders, wrists, elbows, and small joints of the hands and feet (listed in order of decreasing frequency) are the peripheral joints affected most often.[20]

A large knee effusion is a common presentation, but some clients have joint pain with minimal or no signs of inflammation. Muscle atrophy occurs when a chronic condition is present; in which case, there will be a history of previous GI and joint involvement. Stiffness, pain, tenderness, and reduced range of motion may be present, but with proper medical intervention, there is no permanent deformity.

Spondylitis with sacroiliitis may present as low back pain and morning stiffness that improves with activity and restriction of chest and spinal movement. Radiographic findings are consistent with those of classic ankylosing spondylitis with bilateral sacroiliac joint involvement and bony erosion and sclerosis of the symphysis pubis,

CASE EXAMPLE 8-5 Ruptured Spleen

A 23-year-old soccer player sustained a blow from the side as he was moving down the soccer field. He fell on his left side with the full force of his own body weight and the weight of the other player on top of him. He reported having "the wind knocked out of me" and sat out on the sidelines for 20 minutes. He resumed playing and completed the game. The next morning, he woke up with severe left shoulder pain and stopped by the office of a physical therapist located in the same building as his office. The objective examination was unremarkable for shoulder movement dysfunction, which was inconsistent with the client's complaint of "constant pain." The client was treated symptomati-

cally and instructed in pendulum exercises to maintain the joint motion.

He made a follow up appointment with the therapist for the next day, but before noon, he collapsed at work and was taken to a hospital emergency department. A diagnosis of ruptured spleen was made during emergency surgery. A ruptured spleen would have sent the typical adult for medical care much sooner, but this client was in excellent physical condition with a high tolerance for pain. Physical therapy intervention was not appropriate in this situation; an immediate medical referral was indicated given the history of trauma, sudden onset of symptoms, left shoulder pain (Kehr's sign), and constancy of pain.

ischial tuberosities, and iliac crests. Ultimately "bamboo spine" (see Fig. 12-3) will result.

Inflammation involving the sites of bony insertion of tendons and ligaments termed *enthesitis* is a classic sign of reactive arthritis. Tendon sheaths and bursae may also become inflamed. Ligaments along the spine and sacroiliac joints and around the ankle and midfoot may also show evidence of inflammation.

Heel pain is a frequent complaint, with swelling and tenderness located either posteriorly at the Achilles tendon insertion site, or inferiorly where the plantar fascia attaches to the calcaneus. Plantar fasciitis is common. Enthesopathy can also occur around the knee, ischial tuberosities, greater femoral trochanter, and costovertebral and manubriosternal joints.[21]

For a more complete discussion of joint pain and how to evaluate joint pain, see Chapter 3. A list of screening questions for joint pain is also reproduced in the Appendix as a quick reference in clinical practice.

Shoulder Pain

Pain in the left shoulder (Kehr's sign) can occur as a result of free air or blood in the abdominal cavity, such as a ruptured spleen causing distention. The Core Interview may help the client recall any precipitating trauma or injury, such as a sharp blow during an athletic event, a fall, or perhaps an automobile accident. The client may not connect these seemingly unrelated events with the present shoulder pain.

A ruptured ectopic pregnancy with retroperitoneal* bleeding into the abdominal cavity can also present as low abdominal and/or shoulder pain. Usually there is a history of sexual activity and missed menses in a woman of reproductive age.

Pancreatic disease can refer pain to the shoulder. When the head of the pancreas is involved, the client could have right shoulder pain, but more often it manifests as mid-back or mid-thoracic pain sometimes lateralized from the spine on either side. When the tail of the pancreas is diseased, pain can be referred to the left shoulder (see Fig. 3-4). Pain may also occur in the right shoulder when free air or blood is present in the abdominal cavity due to liver trauma (Case Example 8-5).

Obturator or Psoas Abscess

Abscess of the obturator or psoas muscle is a possible cause of lower abdominal pain, usually the consequence of spread of inflammation or infection from an adjacent structure. Since these muscles lie behind abdominal structures with no protective barrier, any infectious or inflammatory process affecting the abdominal or pelvic cavity can cause an obturator or psoas abscess (Fig. 8-3).

---

* Retroperitoneum refers to a position external or posterior to the peritoneum, the serous membrane lining the abdominopelvic walls. Retroperitoneal organs refer to viscera that lie against the posterior body wall and are covered by peritoneum on the anterior surface only (e.g., thoracic portion of the esophagus, pancreas, duodenal cap, ascending and descending colon, rectum).

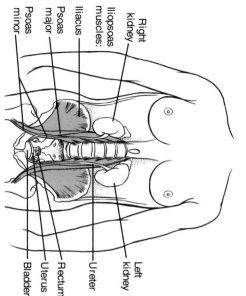

Right kidney
Iliopsoas muscles:
Iliacus
Psoas major
Psoas minor
Left kidney
Ureter
Rectum
Uterus
Bladder

Fig. 8-3 • The iliopsoas muscle is not separated from the abdominal or pelvic cavity. As this illustration shows, most of the viscera in the abdominal and pelvic cavities can come in contact with the iliopsoas muscle. Any infectious or inflammatory process present in either of these cavities can seed itself to the psoas muscle by direct extension.

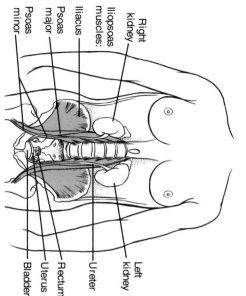

Psoas abscesses most commonly result from direct extension of intraabdominal infections such as diverticulitis, Crohn's disease, pelvic inflammatory disease (PID), and appendicitis (see also discussion on McBurney's point later in this chapter). Kidney infection or abscess can also cause psoas abscess. *Staphylococcus aureus* (staph infection) is the most common cause of psoas abscess secondary to vertebral osteomyelitis.

Peritonitis as a result of any infectious or inflammatory process can result in psoas abscess. Besides the diseases and conditions mentioned here, peritonitis can occur as a surgical complication. Look for a history of abdominal surgery of any kind, but especially the anterior approach to spinal surgery for disc removal, spinal fusion, and insertion of a cage or artificial disc implant.[22]

Regardless of the etiology, the abscess is usually confined to the psoas fascia, but can spread to the hip, upper thigh, or buttock. The iliacus muscle in the iliac fossa joins with the lower portion of the psoas muscle. Osteomyelitis of the ilium or septic arthritis of the sacroiliac joint can penetrate the muscle sheath of either muscle, producing an abscess of either the iliacus or psoas portion of the muscle.

In addition, abscesses of the pelvis, retroperitoneal area, and abdomen can spread bacteria or fungi to local vertebral areas causing spinal infections such as pyogenic vertebral osteomyelitis. From the lumbar spine, abscess formation may track along the psoas muscle and into the buttock muscle.

(piriformis fossa), the perianal region, the groin, and even the popliteal fossa.[23]

Clinical manifestations of a psoas or iliacus abscess include fever; night sweats; lower abdominal, pelvic, or back pain; or pain referred to the hip, medial thigh or groin (femoral triangle area), or knee. The right side is affected most often when associated with appendicitis. Both sides can be involved with generalized peritonitis, but usually that person has a clear systemic presentation and seeks medical evaluation. It is the unusual cases that a therapist will see, making it necessary to know both the typical pain patterns associated with systemic disease, as well as the atypical presentations.

Antalgic gait may develop with a psoas abscess secondary to a reflex spasm pulling the leg into internal rotation causing a functional hip flexion contracture. The affected individual may have pain with hip extension. Often a tender mass can be palpated in the groin. The therapist must assess for trigger points of the iliopsoas muscle. A psoas minor syndrome can be mistaken for appendicitis so be sure and assess for trigger points.[9]

Four tests can be performed to assess the possibility of systemic origin of painful hip or thigh symptoms (Box 8-2). Gently pick up the client's leg on the involved side and tap the heel. A painful expression and report of right lower quadrant pain may accompany peritoneal inflammation. If the client is willing and able, have him or her hop on one leg. The person with an inflamed peritoneum will clutch that side unable to complete the movement. The *iliopsoas muscle test* (Fig. 8-4) is performed when acute abdominal pain is a possible cause of hip or thigh pain. When an abscess forms on the iliopsoas muscle from an inflamed or perforated appendix or inflamed peritoneum, the iliopsoas muscle test causes pain felt in the right lower abdominal quadrant.* Alternately, the client lies on the pain-free side, and the therapist gently hyperextends the involved leg to stretch the psoas major muscle.

* Pain and tenderness in the lower left side of the abdomen may be caused by bowel perforation associated with diverticulitis.

BOX 8-2 ▼ Screening Tests for Psoas Abscess

Heel tap
Hop test
Iliopsoas muscle test
Palpate iliopsoas muscle

Additionally, palpate the iliopsoas muscle by placing the client in a supine position with hips and knees flexed and fully supported in a 90-degree position (Fig. 8-5). Palpate one third of the distance between the anterior superior iliac spine (ASIS) and the umbilicus. The client is asked to flex the hip gently to assist in isolating the iliopsoas muscle. Muscular tightness in the iliopsoas may result in radiating pain to the low back region during palpation, whereas inflammation or abscess will bring on painful symptoms in the right (or left depending on the underlying pathology) lower abdominal quadrant.

The *obturator muscle test* (Fig. 8-6) is also performed when the appendix could be the cause of referred pain to the hip. A perforated appendix or inflamed peritoneum can irritate the obturator muscle, producing right lower quadrant abdominal pain during the obturator test.

Although uncommon, psoas abscess still can be confused with a hernia. The therapist may perform evaluative tests to screen for a psoas abscess, but the physician must differentiate between an abscess and a hernia. Psoas abscess is often softer than a femoral hernia and has ill-defined borders,

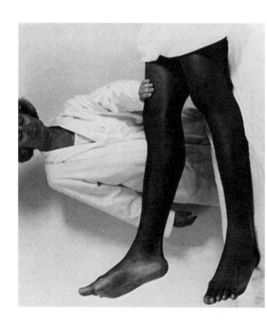

Fig. 8-4 • Iliopsoas muscle test. In the supine position, have the client actively perform a straight leg raise; apply resistance to the distal thigh as the client tries to hold the leg up. Alternately, ask the client to turn onto his or her side. Extend the person's uppermost leg at the hip. Increased abdominal, flank, or pelvic pain on either maneuver constitutes a positive sign, suggesting irritation of the psoas muscle by an inflamed appendix or peritoneum. (From Jarvis C: *Physical examination and health assessment,* Philadelphia, 2000, WB Saunders.)

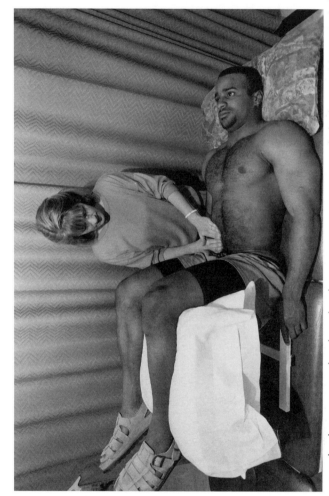

Fig. 8-5 • Palpating the iliopsoas muscle. Place the client in a supine position with the hips and knees both flexed and supported at a 90-degree angle. Slowly press fingers into abdomen approximately one third the distance from the anterior superior iliac spine (ASIS) toward the umbilicus. It may be necessary to ask the client to initiate slight hip flexion to help isolate the muscle and avoid palpating the bowel. Reproducing or causing lower quadrant, pelvic, or abdominal pain is considered a positive sign for iliopsoas abscess. Palpation may produce back pain or local muscular pain from shortened or contracted muscle. (From Goodman CC, Boissonnault WG: *Pathology: special implications for the physical therapist,* Philadelphia, 1998, WB Saunders.)

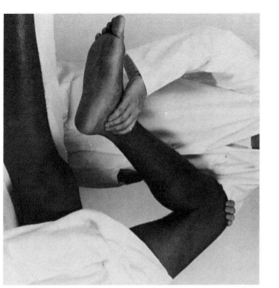

Fig. 8-6 • Obturator muscle test. In the supine position, perform active assisted motion, flexing at the hip and 90 degrees at the knee. Hold the ankle and rotate the leg internally and externally. A negative or normal response is no pain. A positive test for muscle affected by peritoneal infection or inflammation reproduces right lower quadrant abdominal or pelvic pain. (From Jarvis C: *Physical examination and health assessment,* Philadelphia, 2004, WB Saunders.)

Clinical Signs and Symptoms of
Psoas Abscess

- Fever ("hectic" fever pattern: up and down)
- Night sweats
- Abdominal pain
- Loss of appetite or other GI upset
- Back, pelvic, abdominal, hip, and/or knee pain
- Antalgic gait
- Palpable, tender mass

in contrast to the more sharply defined margins of the hernia. The major differentiating feature is the fact that a psoas abscess lies lateral to the femoral artery, whereas the femoral hernia is located medial to the femoral artery.[24]

▶ GASTROINTESTINAL DISORDERS

Gastroesophageal Reflux Disease (GERD)

GERD is an array of problems related to the backward movement of stomach acids and other stomach contents such as pepsin and bile into the esophagus, a phenomenon called acid reflux. Normally, some gastric contents move or reflux from the stomach into the esophagus, but in GERD, the process becomes pathologic producing symptoms that point to tissue injury in the esophagus and sometimes the respiratory tract.[25,26] In adults, GERD is usually caused by intermittent relaxation of the lower esophageal sphincter (LES).

Clinical Signs and Symptoms

Symptoms can include heartburn, chest pain, dysphagia, and a sense of a lump in the throat. Symptoms are sometimes mistaken for a heart attack. Less frequent symptoms can include wheezing, hoarseness, coughing, earache, sore throat, and difficulty swallowing. Sleep disturbance from nighttime coughing and heartburn can lead to fatigue and decreased daytime functioning. Complications of GERD may range from discomfort to severe strictures of the esophagus, esophagitis, aspiration pneumonia, and asthma.

Other serious consequences can be related to weight loss, GI blood loss, and Barrett's esophagitis, a precancerous condition. The relationship between GERD and asthma is poorly understood, but is thought to be a consequence of aspiration of gastric acid contents into the lung causing bronchospasm. Most adults with asthma also have GERD.[26,27]

GERD can occur in infants, but most "outgrow" it. Watch for frequent, forceful spitting up or vomiting, accompanied by irritability. Other alarm symptoms include respiratory distress, apnea, dysphagia, or failure to thrive. Watch for change in color, change in muscle tone, or choking and gagging.

Children may experience GERD in the same way adults do with abdominal or epigastric pain. Nighttime coughing, vomiting, and/or nausea are also possible. Neurologically impaired children and adults are at increased risk for reflux with aspiration. Fluid enters the upper airways from the esophagus, causing chronic respiratory problems, including recurrent pneumonia.

GERD should be treated in order to prevent a chronic condition from occurring with more serious consequences. Symptoms may be mild at first, but have a cumulative effect with increasing symptoms after the age of 40. Chronic GERD is a major risk factor for adenocarcinoma, an increasingly common cancer in white males in the United States.

Medical referral is advised for anyone who reports signs and symptoms of GERD. Some clients may need surgical treatment, now available with less invasive endoscopic techniques, but most can be treated with some simple changes in eating patterns, positioning, and medications. Drug

treatment includes antacids, H2 receptor blockers, and proton pump inhibitors (PPIs). Antacids such as Mylanta, Maalox, Tums, and Rolaids are available over the counter and do not reduce the acid, but merely neutralize it. H2 receptor blockers such as Tagamet (cimetidine), Zantac (ranitidine), and Pepcid (famotidine) reduce the amount of stomach acid produced by the stomach and are available over the counter.

PPIs such as Prilosec (omeprazole), Prevacid (lansoprazole), or Nexium (esomeprazole) are the most potent acid-suppressing agents available. These drugs actually inhibit acid formation rather than just neutralize it. The first PPI is now available over-the-counter; others are expected to become available as well. Caution is needed when using PPIs to self-treat without medical supervision. They can mask symptoms of serious GI disorders such as esophageal or stomach cancer. Diagnosis at an early, treatable stage may be delayed with serious implications.

Therapists must listen for client reports of headache, constipation or diarrhea, abdominal pain, or dizziness in anyone taking these medications. The client should be advised to notify his or her medical doctor with a report of these side effects.

Clinical Signs and Symptoms of

GERD

Typical Symptoms

- Heartburn
- Regurgitation with bitter taste in mouth
- Belching

Atypical Symptoms

- Chest pain unrelated to activity
- Sensation of a lump in the throat
- Difficulty swallowing (dysphagia)
- Painful swallowing (odynophagia)
- Wheezing, coughing, hoarseness
- Asthma
- Sore throat, laryngitis
- Weight loss
- Anemia

Peptic Ulcer

Peptic ulcer is a loss of tissue lining the lower esophagus, stomach, and duodenum. Gastric and duodenal ulcers are considered together in this section. Acute lesions that do not extend through the mucosa are called erosions. Chronic ulcers involve the muscular coat, destroying muscula-ture, and replacing it with permanent scar tissue at the site of healing.

Originally, all ulcers in the upper GI tract were believed to be caused by the aggressive action of hydrochloric acid and pepsin on the mucosa. They thus became known as "peptic ulcers," which is actually a misnomer.

It is now known that many of the gastric and duodenal ulcers are caused by infection with *H. pylori*, a corkscrew-shaped bacterium that bores through the layer of mucus that protects the stomach cavity from stomach acid. Ten percent of ulcers are induced by chronic use of nonsteroidal antiinflammatory drugs (NSAIDs), such as aspirin, ibuprofen, and naproxen, commonly taken by people with arthritis (Table 8-3).[28]

H. pylori ulcers are primarily located in the lining of the duodenum (upper portion of the small intestine that connects to the stomach) (Fig. 8-7). NSAID-induced ulcers occur primarily in the lining of the stomach, most frequently on the posterior wall, which accounts for back pain as an associated symptom.

Ulcers can be dangerous if left untreated, eroding into the stomach arteries and causing life-threatening bleeding or perforating the stomach and spreading infection. *H. pylori*-induced ulcers can recur after treatment. The recurrence rate is higher in clients with gastric ulcers and in people who smoke, consume alcohol, and use NSAIDs.[29] A past medical history of peptic ulcers in anyone with new onset of back or shoulder pain is a red flag requiring further screening and possible medical referral.

Clinical Signs and Symptoms

Clinical Signs and Symptoms

The cardinal symptom of peptic ulcer is epigastric pain that may be described as "heartburn" or as burning, gnawing, cramping, or aching located over a small area near the midline in the epigastrium near the xiphoid. Gastric ulcers are found along the distribution of the eighth thoracic nerve which causes pain in the upper epigastrium about one to two inches to the right of a spot halfway between the xiphoid and the umbilicus (see Fig. 8-12). Duodenal pain tends to present more in the right epigastrium, specifically a localized spot one to two inches above and to the right of the umbilicus because of its innervation by the tenth thoracic nerve.

The pain comes in waves that last several minutes (rather than hours) and may radiate below the costal margins into the back, or rarely, to the right shoulder. The daily pattern of pain is

TABLE 8-3 ▼ Nonsteroidal Antiinflammatory Drugs (NSAIDs)

Over-the-Counter		Prescription Non-selective (standard) COX-inhibitors		Prescription COX-2 Selective Inhibitors	
Generic	Common brand names	Generic	Common brand names	Generic	Common brand names
Aspirin	Anacin, Ascriptin*, Bayer*, Bufferin*, Ecotrin*, Excedrin*	Diclofenac sodium	Voltaren	Celecoxib	Celebrex
Ibuprofen	Advil, Motrin, Nuprin, Ibuprofen, various generic store brands	Diflunisal	Dolobid	Etoricoxib	Arcoxia
Ketoprofen	Orudis KT	Etodolac	Lodine	Rofecoxib	Vioxx†
Naproxen sodium	Aleve, various generic store brands	Fenoprofen calcium	Nalfon	Valdecoxib	Bextra†
		Flurbiprofen	Ansaid	Lumiracoxib	Prexige‡
		Ibuprofen	Motrin (prescription strength), others		
		Indomethacin	Indocin, others		
		Ketorolac	Toradol (short-term use only)		
		Ketoprofen	Orudis, Oruvail		
		Meclofenamate sodium	Meclomen		
		Mefenamic acid	Ponstel		
		Meloxicam	Mobic		
		Nabumetone	Relafen		
		Naproxen	Naprosyn, Naprelan		
		Naproxen sodium	Anaprox, Anaprox DS, EC-Naprosyn, others		
		Oxaprozin	Daypro		
		Phenylbutazone	Butazolidin, Cotylbutazone		
		Piroxicam	Feldene		
		Salsalate	Disalcid, Salaflex		
		Sulindac	Clinoril		
		Tolmetin sodium	Tolectin		

* These all have additives to minimize GI side effects but are known as aspirin products. Many non-selective (standard) NSAIDs are available over-the-counter at a lower dosage (e.g., 200 mg) and by prescription at a higher dosage (e.g., 500 mg). See discussion of peak effect for NSAIDs and time to impact underlying tissue impairment in chapter 2. Some prescription, non-selective COX inhibitors are available as extended release (Voltran XR, Indocin SR, Lodine XL, Oruvail), allowing once a day dosage.

† Removed from the market pending research results showing a link between drug use and risk of heart attack and stroke among individuals taking it 18 months or longer.

‡ As of 2006, the Food and Drug Administration has not yet granted approval for its sale in the United States; available in over 20 countries.

related to the secretion of acid and the presence of food in the stomach to act as a buffer.

Pain associated with duodenal ulcers is prominent when the stomach is empty, such as between meals and in the early morning. The pain may last from minutes to hours and may be relieved by antacids. Gastric ulcers are more likely to cause pain associated with the presence of food. Symptoms often appear for 3 or 4 days or weeks and then subside, reappearing weeks or months later.

Other symptoms of uncomplicated peptic ulcer include nausea, vomiting, loss of appetite, sometimes weight loss, and occasionally back pain. In duodenal ulcers, steady pain near the midline of the back (see Fig. 8-12) between T6 and T10 with radiation to the right upper quadrant may indicate perforation of the posterior duodenal wall.

Back pain may be the first and only symptom. Complications of hemorrhage, perforation, and obstruction may lead to additional symptoms that the client does not relate to the back pain. Bleeding may occur when the ulcer erodes through a blood vessel. It may present as vomited bright red blood or coffee-ground vomitus and by dark tarry stools (melena). The bleeding may vary from massive hemorrhage to occult (hidden) bleeding that occurs over a long period of time.

Symptoms associated with *H. pylori* include hal-itosis (bad breath) and a form of facial acne called

effects on the entire GI tract from the esophagus to the colon, although the most obvious clinical effect is on the gastroduodenal mucosa. GI impairment can be seen as subclinical erosions of the mucosa or more seriously, as ulceration with life-threatening bleeding and perforation.

The incidence of NSAID-related ulcer complications remains high despite the availability of newer gastroprotective NSAIDs such as cyclo-oxygenase-2 (COX-2) inhibitors (e.g., celecoxib, rofecoxib).[30] Cyclooxygenase (COX), a group of enzymes that facilitate chemical reactions exist in two forms: COX-1 and COX-2. COX 1 promotes proper GI function and blood clotting. COX-2 has a role in the preventing or reducing the inflammatory response.

Standard NSAIDs inhibit the actions of both types of cyclooxygenase so the client gets the antiinflammatory effect but at the expense of the GI system. COX-2 inhibitors suppress only COX 2. They can provide the same level of pain relief as standard NSAIDs with a lower risk of serious GI problems, but they are much more expensive than standard NSAIDs. Standard NSAIDs discourage the formation of blood clots, which can decrease the risk of heart attack or stroke; COX-2 inhibitors offer no cardioprotective benefit and may increase the risk of cardiovascular problems. If the newer agents are combined with even low-dose aspirin,* the safety of the COX-2 agent is partially negated.[31]

Infection with *H. pylori* bacteria increases the risk of ulcer disease threefold or more in people taking standard NSAIDs or low dose aspirin.[32] Clients receiving celecoxib, a COX-2 inhibitor may not have the same increased risk of ulcer formation in the presence of *H. pylori.* Data on this topic is limited at this time.[33,34]

COX-2 inhibitors are widely promoted as easier on the stomach than older NSAIDS, but not all clients are taking this newer generation of NSAIDs. For those who are taking COX-2s, preliminary studies show clients with a history of bleeding ulcer are at increased risk of recurrence so these clients must be monitored closely as well.[30] GI ulceration occurs in 15% to 30% of adults using NSAIDs,[35] but we must remember that physical and occupational therapists are seeing 90% of these people.

People with NSAID-induced GI impairment can be asymptomatic until the condition is advanced.

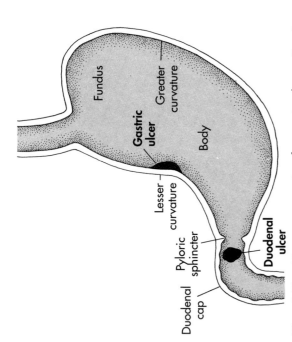

Fig. 8-7 • Most common sites for peptic ulcers. Gastric ulcers are found along the distribution on the eighth thoracic nerve with a corresponding pain pattern as described in Fig. 8-12. Pain patterns associated with duodenal ulcers correspond to the tenth thoracic nerve (Adapted from Ignatavicius DD, Bayne MV: *Medical-surgical nursing,* Philadelphia, 1991, WB Saunders.)

rosacea. Rosacea is characterized by a rosy appearance of the cheeks, nose, and chin. Facial flushing, red lines, and bumps over the nose may accompany rosacea.

Clinical Signs and Symptoms of

Peptic Ulcer

- "Heartburn" or epigastric pain aggravated by food (gastric ulcer); relieved by food, milk, antacids, or vomiting (duodenal ulcer)
- Night pain (12 midnight to 3:00 a.m.)–same relief as for epigastric pain (duodenal ulcer)
- Radiating back pain
- Stomach pain
- Right shoulder pain (rare)
- Lightheadedness or fainting
- Nausea
- Vomiting
- Anorexia
- Weight loss
- Bloody stools
- Black, tarry stools

Gastrointestinal Complications of NSAIDs

NSAIDs (see Table 8-3) have become increasingly popular by virtue of their analgesic, antiinflammatory, antipyretic, and antithrombotic (platelet-inhibitory) actions. NSAIDs have deleterious

*Low-dose aspirin is defined as 325 mg taken every other day or one "baby aspirin" containing 81 mg used for cardio-protection by people with or at risk for heart disease.

GI effects of NSAIDs are responsible for approximately 40% of hospital admissions among clients with arthritis. NSAID-induced GI bleeding is a major cause of morbidity and mortality among the aging adult population.[36]

For those who are symptomatic, the most common side effects of NSAIDs are stomach upset and pain, possibly leading to ulceration. Gastrointestinal complications of NSAID use include ulcerations, hemorrhage, perforation, stricture formation, and exacerbation of inflammatory bowel disease. Each NSAID has its own pharmacodynamic characteristics, and clients' responses to each drug may vary greatly.

Other possible adverse side effects of NSAIDs may include suppression of cartilage repair and synthesis, fluid retention and kidney damage, liver damage, skin reactions (e.g., itching, rashes, acne), and impairment of the nervous system such as headache, depression, confusion or memory loss, mood changes, and ringing in the ears.

Many people diagnosed with painful musculoskeletal conditions, especially arthritis, rely on NSAIDs to relieve pain and improve function. Anyone with a current history of NSAID use presenting with back or shoulder pain, especially when accompanied by any of the associated signs and symptoms listed for peptic ulcer, must be evaluated by a physician. The therapist should remain alert for the client taking multiple NSAIDs and simultaneously combining prescription and over-the-counter (OTC) NSAIDs or other drugs.

These drugs are potent renal vasoconstrictors, so look for increased blood pressure and ankle/foot edema. Take vital signs and visually inspect clients at risk for NSAID-induced impairments. Ask about muscle weakness, unusual fatigue, restless legs syndrome, polyuria, nocturia, or pruritus (signs of renal failure). In the aging adult, NSAID use may be associated with confusion and memory loss or increased confusion in the client with dementia or Alzheimer's disease. Report any associated signs and symptoms to the physician. Changing the dosage or switching to a different NSAID at the first sign of side effects can help clients avoid serious complications that can occur with prolonged use of an inappropriate dose or poorly tolerated NSAID.

Clinical Signs and Symptoms of
NSAID-Induced Impairment

- Asymptomatic
- Stomach upset (nausea) and stomach pain
- Indigestion, heartburn
- Skin reactions (itching, rash, acne)
- Tinnitus (ringing in the ears)
- CNS Changes
  - Headache
  - Depression
  - Confusion (older adult)
  - Memory loss (older adult)
  - Mood changes
- Renal Involvement
  - Muscle weakness
  - Unusual fatigue
  - Restless legs syndrome
  - Polyuria
  - Nocturia
  - Pruritus (skin itching)
  - Increased blood pressure
- New onset back (thoracic) or shoulder pain
- Pain relief after eating food
- Melena

Risk factor assessment is especially important in the primary care setting. Any identified risk factors should serve as red flags in any setting. The most predictive risk factors of serious GI events include: age, disability, NSAID dose, previous GI hospitalization, prior GI symptoms with NSAIDs, and use of prednisone (Box 8-3 and Case Example 8-6). See

---

BOX 8-3 ▲ Risk Factors for NSAID-Induced Gastropathy

- Age >65 years
- History of peptic ulcer disease or GI disease
- Smoking, alcohol use
- Oral corticosteroid use
- Anticoagulation or use of other anticoagulants (even when used for heart patients at a lower dose, e.g., 81 to 325 mg aspirin/day)
- Renal complications in clients with hypertension or congestive heart failure (CHF) or who use diuretics or ACE inhibitors
- Use of acid suppressants (e.g., H₂-receptor antagonists, antacids); these agents can mask the warning symptoms of more serious GI complications, leaving the client unaware of ongoing damage
- NSAIDs combined with selective serotonin reuptake inhibitors (SSRIs; antidepressants such as Prozac, Zoloft, Celexa, Paxil)

The newer COX-2 (cyclooxygenase) inhibitors such as Celebrex have reduced the incidence of GI disturbances, but this does not mean a client taking a COX-2 inhibitor cannot have NSAID-induced GI complaints. The risk of complications with COX-2 inhibitors is increased in the presence of any of the risk factors listed above.

CASE EXAMPLE 8-6   NSAIDs

Outpatient Orthopedic Client: A 72-year-old client with s/p left TKR×4 weeks. She did not attain 90-degrees knee flexion and continues to walk with a stiff leg. Her orthopedic surgeon has sent her to PT for rehab.

Past Medical History: Client reports generalized osteoarthritis. Previous left shoulder replacement 18 months ago. Very slow recovery and still does not have full shoulder ROM. Long-standing hearing impairment×60 years. Lost her left eye to macular degeneration 2 years ago.

Medications: Client reports the following drug use—Darvocet for pain 3x/day. Vioxx daily for arthritis. Also takes Feldene when her shoulder bothers her and daily ibuprofen.

Walks with a Trendelenburg gait and drags left leg using wheeled walker.

Current symptoms include left knee and shoulder pain, intermittent dizziness, sleep disturbance, finger/hand swelling in the afternoons, early morning nausea.

How do you assess for NSAID complications?

Review risk factors:
>65 years old
Shoulder pain
Ask about tobacco and alcohol use
Nausea . . . ask about other GI symptoms and previous history of peptic ulcer disease
Take blood pressure
Observe for peripheral edema (sacral and pedal)

How do you carry out a Review of Systems from a screening perspective and a Systems Review in accordance with the *Guide*?

After gathering all of the subjective and objective data, make a list of all the signs and symptoms. Are there any clusters or groups of signs and symptoms that fall into any particular category? These may or may not be associated with the primary neuromusculoskeletal problem as many clients have one or more other diseases, illnesses, or conditions (referred to as comorbidities) with additional clinical manifestations.

Start with general health. She reports:
Hearing and vision loss
Intermittent dizziness
Early morning nausea
Finger/hand swelling
Sleep disturbance

There is not much in the report about her general health. Make a note to consider asking a few more questions about her past and current general health. Ask how she would describe her overall health in one or two words.

Review her medications. She reports:
Darvocet 3/day for pain
Vioxx daily (COX-2 NSAID)
Feldene prn (standard or non-selective NSAID)
Ibuprofen daily (standard or non-selective NSAID)

Given how many forms of NSAIDs she is taking, ask yourself: Did I ask if there were any other symptoms or problems of any kind anywhere else in the body?

The remaining symptoms noted (positive Trendelenburg gait and antalgic gait, left shoulder and knee pain) fall into the musculoskeletal category. No other symptoms are noted.

Think now about the Systems Review as outlined by the *Guide*. Are there isolated groupings or clusters of signs and symptoms that fall into any of the other three diagnostic categories?

Neuromuscular
Cardiovascular/Pulmonary
Integumentary

Knowing what we do about the potential for GI and renal complications in some clients taking NSAIDs, make a mental note to do two things: 1) Assess risk factors for NSAID-induced gastropathy (see Box 8-3) and 2) Ask about the presence of previously unreported GI or renal signs and symptoms (see *Clinical Signs and Symptoms of NSAID-induced impairment*). If appropriate you can go through this list and ask Do you have any nausea? Stomach pain? Indigestion or heartburn?

Have you had any skin changes? You may want to prompt with: itching? Rash anywhere on your body?

Any ringing in the ears? Headaches? Depression or mood changes? Memory loss or confusion?

Have you had any trouble getting up out of a chair or bed? Difficulty with stairs? (muscle weakness) Shortness of breath? Unusual fatigue?

Are you urinating more often during the day? Getting up at night to empty your bladder? Do you have any trouble wiping yourself clean after a bowel movement? Any change in the color or smell of your stools?

Documentation, communication, and medical referral will be based on the results of your evaluation using a review mechanism like the one we just completed.

Chapter 2 for information on screening for the use of NSAIDs.

IS YOUR CLIENT AT RISK FOR NSAID-INDUCED GASTROPATHY?

Therapists also can estimate the risk of GI complications in clients with rheumatoid arthritis. The following tool can be used with clients who are taking NSAIDs of any kind for rheumatoid arthritis. This tool may prove valuable in assessing other patient populations as well.[37] This calculation can be used in one of several ways. First, clinical research is needed to substantiate the number of clients in a physical therapy practice who are at risk for serious NSAID-related gastropathy.

Second, charting a client's risk can help in the early identification of problems. Because prednisone use and NSAID dose are modifiable risk factors, early identification and referral to the physician can minimize the detrimental effects of NSAID-induced gastropathy. Clients with one or more risk factors for NSAID-associated GI ulcer should be prescribed preventive strategies such as acid-suppressive drugs and/or COX-2 inhibitors rather than standard NSAIDs.[38,39]

Third, from a fiscal point of view, every GI complication prevented lowers the cost of medical care in this country. Clients over 50 with comorbidities such as heart disease, renal disease, a history of ulcers, or taking prednisone or warfarin must be watched carefully.

The scoring system in Table 8-4 allows clinicians to estimate the risk of GI problems in clients with rheumatoid arthritis who are also taking NSAIDs.[40] The formula is based on age, history of NSAID symptoms, NSAID dose, and the American Rheumatism Association's (ARA) Functional Classes (Table 8-5).

NSAID dose used in this formulation is the fraction of the manufacturer's highest recommended dose. The manufacturer's highest recommended dose on the package insert is given a value of 1.00. The dose of each client is then normalized to this dose.

For example, the value 1.03 indicates the client is taking 103% of the manufacturer's highest recommended dose. Most often, clients are taking the highest dose recommended. They receive a 1.0. Anyone taking less will have a fraction percentage less than 1.0. Anyone taking more than the highest

TABLE 8-4 ▼ Calculating Your Client's Risk of NSAID-Induced Gastropathy

Risk is equal to the sum of:	Calculation	Points
Age in years	Multiply×2 =	
History of NSAID symptoms e.g., upper abdominal pain, bloating, nausea, heartburn, loss of appetite, vomiting	If yes, add 50 points	
ACR class (see Table 8-5)	Add 0, 10, 20 or 30 based on class 1-4	
NSAID dose (fraction of maximum recommended; see text explanation)	NSAID dose×15	
If currently using prednisone	Add 40 points	
TOTAL Score		
*Risk/year=[Total Score−100]÷40		

ACR, American College of Rheumatology.
* Higher total scores yield a greater predictive risk. The risk ranges from 0.0 (low risk) to 5.0 (high risk)
From Fries JF, et al: Nonsteroidal antiinflammatory drug-associated gastropathy: incidence and risk factor models, *Am J Med* 91(3):213-222, 1991.

TABLE 8-5 ▼ ACR Criteria for Classification of Functional Status in Rheumatoid Arthritis

Class 1	Completely able to perform usual ADLs (self-care, vocational, avocational)	Normal	0 points
Class 2	Able to perform usual self-care and vocational activities, but limited in avocational activities	Adequate	10 points
Class 3	Able to perform usual self-care activities, but limited in vocational and avocational activities	Limited	20 points
Class 4	Limited in ability to perform usual self-care, vocational, and avocational activities	Unable	30 points

ACR, American College of Rheumatology.

dose recommended will have a fraction percentage greater than 1.0. See formulation in Case Example 8-7.

To determine the risk (%) of hospitalization or death caused by GI complications over the next 12 months, subtract 100 from the total score obtained in Table 8-4, Calculating Your Client's Risk of NSAID-Induced Gastropathy, and divide the result by 40. Higher Total scores yield a greater predictive risk. The risk ranges from 0.0 (low risk) to 5.0 (high risk) (Case Example 8-7).

Diverticular Disease

The terms *diverticulosis* and *diverticulitis* are used interchangeably although they have distinct meanings. *Diverticulosis* is a benign condition in which the mucosa (lining) of the colon balloons out through weakened areas in the wall. Up to 60% of people over age 65 have these sac-like protrusions diagnosed typically when screening for colon cancer or other problems.

Diverticulitis describes the infection and inflammation that accompany a microperforation of one of the diverticula. Diverticulosis is very common, whereas complications resulting in diverticulitis occur in only 10% to 25% of people with diverticulosis. The most common cause of major lower intes-

tinal tract bleeding is diverticulosis. A significant number of cases of diverticular bleeding are associated with the use of NSAIDs in combination with diverticulosis. [41]

There is some controversy regarding whether diverticulosis is symptomatic, but perforation and subsequent infection causes symptoms of left lower abdominal or pelvic pain and tenderness in diverticulitis. For the therapist performing the iliopsoas and obturator tests, abdominal pain in the left lower quadrant may be caused by diverticular disease and should be reported to the physician. The diagnosis of diverticulitis is confirmed by accompanying fever, bloody stools, and elevated white blood cell count.

Clinical Signs and Symptoms of

Diverticulitis

- Left lower abdominal pain and tenderness
- Left pelvic pain
- Bloody stools

Appendicitis

Appendicitis is an inflammation of the vermiform appendix that occurs most commonly in adolescents and young adults. It is a serious disease

---

CASE EXAMPLE 8-7   Is Your Client At Risk for NSAID-Induced Gastropathy?

A 66-year-old woman with a history of rheumatoid arthritis (class 3) has been referred to physical therapy after three MCP-joint replacements.

Although her doctor has recommended maximum dosage of ibuprofen (800 mg tid; 2400 mg), she is really only taking 1600 mg/day. She says this is all she needs to control her symptoms.

She was taking prednisone before the surgery, but tapered herself off and has not resumed its use.

She has been hospitalized 3 times in the past 6 years for GI problems related to NSAID use, but does not have any apparent GI symptoms at this time.

Calculating her risk for serious problems with NSAID use, we have

Age in years	66 × 2 =	132
History of NSAID symptoms, e.g., abdominal pain, bloating, nausea	+50 points	50
ARA class (see Table 8-5)	add 0, 10, 20 or 30 based on class 1-4	20
Daily NSAID dose (fraction of maximum recommended)	1600 mg/2400 mg × 15 (0.67 × 15)	10
If currently using prednisone	add 40 points	0
TOTAL Score		212

Risk/year = [Total score − 100] + 40

Risk/year = [212 − 100] + 40

Risk/year = 112 + 40 = 2.80

The scores range from 0.0 (very low risk) to 5.0 (very high risk). A predictive risk of 2.8 is moderately high. This client should be reminded to report GI distress to her doctor immediately. Periodic screening for GI gastropathy is indicated with early referral if warranted.

usually requiring surgery. When the appendix becomes obstructed, inflamed, and infected, rupture may occur, leading to peritonitis.

Diseases that can be mistaken for appendicitis include Crohn's disease (regional enteritis), perforated duodenal ulcer, gallbladder attacks, and kidney infection on the right side, and for women, ruptured ectopic pregnancy, twisted ovarian cyst, or a hemorrhaging ovarian follicle at the middle of the menstrual cycle. Right lower lobe pneumonia sometimes is associated with prominent right lower quadrant pain.

Clinical Signs and Symptoms

The classic symptoms of appendicitis are pain preceding nausea and vomiting and low-grade fever in adults. Children tend to have higher fevers. Other symptoms may include coated tongue and bad breath.

The pain usually begins in the umbilical region and eventually localizes in the right lower quadrant of the abdomen over the site of the appendix. In retrocecal appendicitis, the pain may be referred to the thigh or right testicle (see Figure 8-9). Groin and/or testicular pain may be the only symptoms of appendicitis, especially in young, healthy, male athletes. The pain comes in waves, becomes steady, and is aggravated by movement, causing the client to bend over and tense the abdominal muscles or to lie down and draw the legs up to relieve abdominal muscle tension (Case Example 8-8).

Generalized peritonitis, whether caused by appendicitis or some other abdominal or pelvic inflammatory condition, can result in a "board-like" abdomen due to the spasm of the rectus abdominis muscles. Lean muscle mass deteriorates with aging, especially evident in the abdominal muscles of the aging population. The very old person may not present with this classic sign of generalized peritonitis because of the lack of toned abdominal muscles.

For this reason, the nursing home, skilled care facility, or home health therapist must evaluate the aging client who presents with hip or thigh pain for possible systemic origin (assess for Rebound Tenderness; see also McBurney's point, and specific tests for iliopsoas or obturator abscess).

Clinical Signs and Symptoms of Appendicitis

- Periumbilical and/or epigastric pain
- Right lower quadrant or flank pain
- Right thigh, groin, or testicular pain
- Abdominal muscular rigidity
- Positive McBurney's point
- Rebound tenderness (peritonitis)
- Positive hop test (hopping on one leg or jumping on both feet reproduces painful symptoms)
- Nausea and vomiting
- Anorexia
- Dysuria (painful/difficult urination)
- Low-grade fever
- Coated tongue and bad breath

CASE EXAMPLE 8-8   Appendicitis

Remember the 32-year-old female university student featured in Fig. 1-6? She had been referred to physical therapy with the provisional diagnosis: *Possible right oblique abdominis muscle tear/possible right iliopsoas muscle tear.* Her history included the sudden onset of "severe pain" in the right lower quadrant with accompanying nausea and abdominal distention. Aggravating factors included hip flexion, sit-ups, fast walking, and movements such as reaching, turning, and bending. Painful symptoms could be reproduced by resisted hip or trunk flexion, and tenderness/tightness was elicited on palpation of the right iliopsoas muscle compared with the left. A neurologic screen was negative.

Screening questions for general health revealed constitutional symptoms including fatigue, night sweats, nausea, and repeated episodes of severe, progressive pain in the right lower abdominal quadrant.

Although she presented with a musculoskeletal pattern of symptoms at the time of her initial evaluation with the physician, by the time she entered the physical therapy clinic her symptoms had taken on a definite systemic pattern. She was returned for further medical follow-up, and a diagnosis of appendicitis complicated by peritonitis was established. This client recovered fully from all her symptoms following emergency appendectomy surgery.

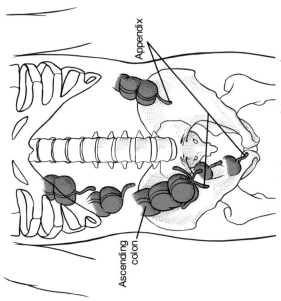

Appendix

Ascending colon

Fig. 8-9 • Variations in the location of the vermiform appendix. Negative tests for appendicitis using McBurney's point may occur when the appendix is located somewhere other than at the end of the cecum. In 50% of cases the appendix is retrocecal (behind the cecum) or retrocolic (behind the colon). See Fig. 8-10 for an alternate test.

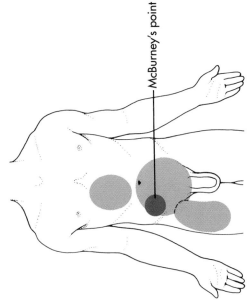

McBurney's point

Fig. 8-8 • The vermiform appendix and colon can refer pain to the area of sensory distribution for the eleventh thoracic nerve (T11). Primary (dark red) and referred (light red) pain patterns associated with the vermiform appendix are shown here with McBurney's point halfway between the ASIS and the umbilicus, usually on the right side. Gentle palpation of McBurney's point produces pain or exquisite tenderness. Rebound tenderness should also be assessed (see Fig. 8-10).

McBurney's Point

Parietal pain caused by inflammation of the peritoneum in acute appendicitis or peritonitis (from appendicitis or other inflammatory/infectious causes) may be located at McBurney's point (Fig. 8-8). The vermiform appendix receives its sympathetic supply from the 11th thoracic segment. In some people a branch of the 11th thoracic nerve pierces the rectus abdominis muscle and innervates the skin over McBurney's point. This may explain the hyperalgesia seen at this point in appendicitis.[6]

McBurney's point is located by palpation with the client in a fully supine position. Isolate the ASIS and the umbilicus; palpate for tenderness halfway between these two surface anatomic points. This method differs from palpation of the iliopsoas muscle, because the position used to locate the iliopsoas muscle is that of the client in a supine position, with hips and knees flexed in a 90-degree position, whereas McBurney's point is palpated with the client in the fully supine position.

The palpation point for the iliopsoas muscle is one third the distance between the ASIS and the umbilicus, whereas McBurney's point is halfway between these two points. Be aware that the location of the vermiform appendix can vary from individual to individual making the predictive value of this test less accurate (Fig. 8-9). Since the appen-

dix develops during the descent of the colon, its final position can be posterior to the cecum or colon. These positions of the appendix are called retrocecal or retrocolic, respectively. In about 50% of cases, the appendix is retrocecal or retrocolic.[42]

Both McBurney's point and the iliopsoas muscle are palpated for reproduction of symptoms to rule out appendicitis or iliopsoas abscess associated with appendicitis or peritonitis. One final test may be used to assess for the possibility of hip, pelvic, or flank pain from appendicitis, posterior penetrating ulcer, or peritonitis from any cause. After palpating for McBurney's point, if needed, perform the test for rebound tenderness (Fig. 8-10).

Pancreatitis

Pancreatitis* is an inflammation of the pancreas that may result in autodigestion of the pancreas by its own enzymes. Pancreatitis can be acute or chronic, but the therapist is most likely to see acute pancreatitis.

Acute pancreatitis can arise from a variety of etiologic factors, but in most instances, the specific

* The pancreas is both an exocrine gland and an endocrine gland. Its function in digestion is primarily an exocrine activity. This chapter focuses on digestive disorders associated with the pancreas. See Chapter 11 for pancreatic disorders associated with endocrine function.

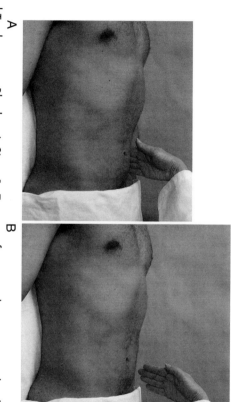

Fig. 8-10 • Rebound Tenderness or Blumberg's Sign. **A,** To assess for appendicitis or generalized peritonitis, place your hand on the abdomen in an area away from the suspected area of local inflammation. Palpate deeply and slowly. **B,** The palpating hand is then quickly removed. Pain induced or increased by quick withdrawal results from rapid movement of inflamed peritoneum and is called *rebound tenderness.* When rebound tenderness is present, the client will have pain or increased pain on the side of the inflammation when the palpatory pressure is released. Ask the client if it hurts as you are palpating or during the release. Since abdominal pain is increased uncomfortably with this test, save it for last when assessing abdominal pain during the physical examination. (From Jarvis C: *Physical examination and health assessment,* ed 4, Philadelphia, 2004, WB Saunders; Fig. 21-31, p 585.)

cause is unknown. Chronic alcoholism or toxicity from some other agent, such as glucocorticoids, thiazide diuretics, or acetaminophen, can bring on an acute attack of pancreatitis. A mechanical obstruction of the biliary tract may be present, usually because of gallstones in the bile ducts. Viral infections (e.g., mumps, herpesviruses, hepatitis) also may cause an acute inflammation of the pancreas.

Chronic pancreatitis is caused by long-standing alcohol abuse in more than 90% of adult cases. Chronic pancreatitis is characterized by the progressive destruction of the pancreas with accompanying irregular fibrosis and chronic inflammation.

Clinical Signs and Symptoms

The clinical course of most clients with *acute pancreatitis* follows a self-limited pattern. Symptoms can vary from mild, nonspecific abdominal pain to profound shock with coma and, ultimately, death. Abdominal pain begins abruptly in the midepigastrium, increases in intensity for several hours, and can last from days to more than a week.

The pain has a penetrating quality and radiates to the back. Pain is made worse by walking and lying supine and is relieved by sitting and leaning forward. The client may have a bluish discoloration of the periumbilical area as a physical manifestation of acute pancreatitis. This occurs in cases of severe hemorrhagic pancreatitis. Turner's sign is a

bluish discoloration of the flanks, also present in hemorrhagic pancreatitis.

Symptoms associated with *chronic pancreatitis* include persistent or recurrent episodes of epigastric and left upper quadrant pain with referral to the upper left lumbar region. Pathology of the head of the pancreas is more likely to cause epigastric and midthoracic pain from T5 to T9. Impairment of the tail of the pancreas (located to the left of midline; see Fig. 3-4) can refer pain to the left shoulder.

Anorexia, nausea, vomiting, constipation, flatulence, and weight loss are common. Attacks may last only a few hours or as long as 2 weeks; pain may be constant. In clients with alcohol-associated pancreatitis, the pain often begins 12 to 48 hours after an episode of inebriation. Clients with gallstone-associated pancreatitis typically experience pain after a large meal. Nausea and vomiting accompany the pain. Other symptoms include fever, tachycardia, jaundice, and malaise.

Clinical Signs and Symptoms of
Acute Pancreatitis

• Epigastric pain radiating to the back
• Nausea and vomiting
• Fever and sweating
• Tachycardia

Continued on p. 392

- Malaise
- Weakness
- Bluish discoloration of abdomen or flanks (severe hemorrhagic acute pancreatitis)
- Jaundice

Clinical Signs and Symptoms of
Chronic Pancreatitis

- Epigastric pain radiating to the back
- Upper left lumbar region pain
- Nausea and vomiting
- Constipation
- Flatulence
- Weight loss

Pancreatic Carcinoma

Pancreatic carcinoma is the fifth most common cause of death from cancer for women and fourth most common for men. The majority of pancreatic cancers (70%) arise in the head of the gland and only 20% to 30% occur in the body and tail (see Fig. 9-1). The latter usually have grown to a large size by the time the diagnosis is made, due to the absence of symptoms.

The most common symptoms of pancreatic cancer are anorexia and weight loss, epigastric/upper abdominal pain with radiation to the back, and jaundice secondary to obstruction of the bile duct. Jaundice is characterized by fatigue and yellowing of the skin and sclera of the eye. The urine may become dark like the color of a cola soft drink.

As with any pancreatic impairment, involvement of the head of the pancreas is more likely to cause epigastric and mid-thoracic pain (T5-T9), whereas, impairment of the tail of the pancreas (located to the left of midline; see Fig. 3-4) can refer pain to the left shoulder. Epigastric pain is often vague and diffuse. Radiation of pain into the lumbar region is common and sometimes is the only symptom.

The pain may become worse after the person eats or lies down. Sitting up and leaning forward may provide some relief, and this usually indicates that the lesion has spread beyond the pancreas and is inoperable. Other signs and symptoms include

Clinical Signs and Symptoms of
Pancreatic Carcinoma

- Epigastric/upper abdominal pain radiating to the back
- Low back pain may be the only symptom
- Jaundice
- Anorexia and weight loss
- Light-colored stools
- Constipation
- Nausea and vomiting
- Weakness

Inflammatory Bowel Disease

Inflammatory bowel disease (IBD) refers to two inflammatory conditions; it is *not* the same as irritable bowel syndrome (IBS) discussed separately:

- Ulcerative colitis (UC)
- Crohn's disease (CD) (also referred to as regional enteritis or ileitis)

Crohn's disease and ulcerative colitis are disorders of unknown etiology involving genetic and immunologic influences on the GI tract. Ulcerative colitis affects the large intestine (colon). Crohn's disease can affect any portion of the intestine from the mouth to the anus. Both diseases not only cause inflammation inside the intestine, but can also cause significant problems in other parts of the body.[43] These two diseases share many epidemiologic, clinical, and therapeutic features. Both are chronic, medically incurable conditions.

Extraintestinal manifestations occur frequently in clients with inflammatory bowel disease and complicate its management. The client may not know these signs and symptoms are associated with Crohn's disease. Manifestations involve the joints most commonly (see previous discussion of Arthralgia). The client with new onset of joint pain should be asked about a previous history of Crohn's disease.

Skin lesions may occur as either erythema nodosum (red bumps/purple knots over the ankles and shins) or pyoderma (deep ulcers or canker sores) of the shins, ankles, and calves. Ask about a recent history (last 6 weeks) of skin lesions anywhere on the body. Uveitis may cause red and painful eyes that are sensitive to light, but this condition does not affect the person's vision.

Nutritional deficiencies are the most common complications of IBD. Evidence to suggest increased intestinal permeability allowing increased exposure to foreign antigens has been

discovered.[44,45] Inflammation alone and the decrease in functioning surface area of the small intestine, increases food requirements, causing poor absorption.

Nutritional problems associated with the medical treatment of IBD may occur. The use of prednisone decreases vitamin D metabolism, impairs calcium absorption, decreases potassium supplies, and increases the nutritional requirement for protein and calories. Decreased vitamin D metabolism and impaired calcium absorption subsequently result in bone demineralization and osteoporosis.

Crohn's Disease

Crohn's disease (CD) is an inflammatory disease that most commonly attacks the terminal end (or distal portion) of the small intestine (ileum) and the colon. However, it can occur anywhere along the alimentary canal from the mouth to the anus. It occurs more commonly in young adults and adolescents but can appear at any age.

Clinical Signs and Symptoms

CD may have acute manifestations, but the condition is usually slow and nonaggressive. The client may present with mild intermittent symptoms months before the diagnosis is made. Fever may occur, with acute inflammation, abscesses, or rheumatoid manifestations.

Terminal ileum involvement produces pain in the periumbilical region with possible referred pain to the corresponding segment of the low back. Pain of the ileum is intermittent and felt in the lower right quadrant with possible associated iliopsoas abscess causing hip pain (see previous discussion of Psoas abscess). The client may experience relief of discomfort after passing stool or flatus. For this reason, it is important to ask whether low back pain is relieved after passing stool or gas.

Twenty-five percent of people with CD may present with arthritis or migratory arthralgias (joint pain). The person may present with monoarthritis (i.e, asymmetric pattern affecting one joint at a time), usually involving an ankle or knee, although elbows and wrists can be included.

Polyarthritis (involving more than one joint) or sacroiliitis (arthritis of the lower spine and pelvis) is common and may lead to ankylosing spondylitis in rare cases. Whether monoarthritic or polyarthritic, this condition comes and goes with the disease process and may precede repeat episodes of bowel symptoms by 1 to 2 weeks. With proper medical intervention, there is no permanent joint deformity.

Ulcerative Colitis

By definition, UC is an inflammation and ulceration of the inner lining of the large intestine (colon) and rectum. When inflammation is confined to the rectum only, the condition is known as ulcerative proctitis. UC is not the same as irritable bowel syndrome (IBS) or spastic colitis (another term for IBS).

Cancer of the colon is more common among clients with UC than among the general population. The incidence is greatly increased among those who develop UC before the age of 16 years and those who have had the condition for more than 30 years.

Clinical Signs and Symptoms

The predominant symptom of UC is rectal bleeding; mainly the left colon is involved; the small intestine is never involved. Clients often experience diarrhea, possibly 20 or more stools per day.

Nausea, vomiting, anorexia, weight loss, and decreased serum potassium may occur with severe disease. Fever is present during acute disease. Nocturnal diarrhea is usually present when daytime diarrhea is prominent.

The development of anemia depends on the degree of blood loss, severity of the illness, and dietary iron intake. Ankylosing spondylitis, anemia, and clubbing of the fingers are occasional findings. Clubbing (see Figs. 4-34 and 4-35) develops quickly within 7 to 10 days.

Medical testing and diagnosis are required to differentiate between these inflammatory conditions. Most often, the therapist is faced with clients presenting complaints of pain located in the shoulder, back, or groin that may have a GI origin and not be true musculoskeletal dysfunction at all.

Clinical Signs and Symptoms of Ulcerative Colitis and Crohn's Disease

- Diarrhea
- Constipation
- Fever
- Abdominal pain
- Rectal bleeding
- Night sweats
- Decreased appetite, nausea, weight loss
- Skin lesions
- Uveitis (inflammation of the eye)
- Arthritis
- Migratory arthralgias
- Hip pain (iliopsoas abscess)

Irritable Bowel Syndrome

Irritable bowel syndrome (IBS) has been called the "common cold of the stomach." It is a functional disorder of motility in the small and large intestines diagnosed according to specific bowel symptom clusters.

IBS is classified as a "functional" disorder because the abnormal muscle contraction identified in people with IBS cannot be attributed to any identifiable abnormality of the bowel. A lowered visceral pain threshold is commonly found with complaints of bloating and distention at lower volumes of colonic insufflation than normal controls.[46] In other words, affected individuals perceive unpleasant or inappropriate sensory experiences in the absence of any physiologic or pathophysiologic event. IBS rarely progresses and is never fatal.

Other descriptive names for this condition are spastic colon, irritable colon, nervous indigestion, functional dyspepsia, pylorospasm, spastic colitis, intestinal neuroses, and laxative or cathartic colitis.

IBS is the most common gastrointestinal disorder in Western society and accounts for 50% of subspecialty referrals. It is often linked with psychosocial factors. In cases where symptoms are severe and refractory to treatment, a history of mental, physical, or sexual abuse is suspected.[47-49] IBS is most common in women in early adulthood and there is a well-documented association between IBS and dysmenorrhea.[50,51] It is unclear whether this correlation represents diagnostic confusion or whether dysmenorrhea and IBS have a common physiologic basis.

As mentioned earlier in this chapter, emotional or psychologic responses to stress have a profound effect on brain chemistry, which in turn influences the enteric nervous system. Conversely, messages from the central nervous system are processed in the intestines by an elaborate neural network. Research is ongoing to find the biochemical links between psychosocial factors, physical disease, and somatic illness.

Clinical Signs and Symptoms

There is a highly variable complex of intermittent gastrointestinal symptoms, including nausea and vomiting, anorexia, foul breath, sour stomach, flatulence, cramps, abdominal bloating, and constipation and/or diarrhea. The client may report white mucus in the stools.

Pain may be steady or intermittent, and there may be a dull deep discomfort with sharp cramps in the morning or after eating. The typical pain pattern consists of lower left quadrant abdominal pain, constipation, and diarrhea. Symptoms seem to come and go with no apparent cause and effect that can be identified by the affected individual. Abdominal pain or discomfort is relieved by defecation.

These primary symptoms occur when the natural motility of the bowel (rhythmic peristalsis) is disrupted by stress, smoking, eating, and drinking alcohol. Rapid alterations in the speed of bowel movement create an obstruction to the natural flow of stool and gas. The resultant pressure build-up in the bowel produces pain and spasm.

The therapist should also be alert for the client with a known history of IBS now experiencing unexplained weight loss or persistent, severe diarrhea, possibly signaling disorders such as malignancy, inflammatory bowel disease (IBD), or celiac disease. Symptoms of IBS tend to disappear at night when the client is asleep. Nocturnal diarrhea, awakening the client from a sound sleep, is more often a result of organic disease of the bowel and is less likely to occur in IBS. Sudden return of symptoms after age 50 following prolonged remission must be evaluated medically, especially if there is blood in the stool.[52]

Clinical Signs and Symptoms of Irritable Bowel Syndrome

- Painful abdominal cramps
- Constipation
- Diarrhea
- Nausea and vomiting
- Anorexia
- Flatulence
- Foul breath

Colorectal Cancer

Colorectal cancer is the third most commonly diagnosed cancer and third most common cause of death from malignant disease for both men and women in the Western world.[53] Incidence increases with age, beginning around 40 years of age, and is higher in men than women. More African-American than Caucasian women are affected.[54]

Mortality can be significantly reduced by population screening by means of a simple fecal occult blood test (FOBT). Screening is particularly applicable to individuals belonging to high-risk groups, particularly those with a previous history of chronic inflammatory bowel disease (e.g., Crohn's disease, ulcerative colitis); adenomatous polyps; and hereditary nonpolyposis colon cancer.[55]

Clinical Signs and Symptoms

The presentation of colorectal carcinoma is related to the location of the neoplasm within the colon. Individuals are asymptomatic in the early stages, then develop minor changes in their bowel patterns (e.g., increased frequency of morning evacuation, sense of incomplete evacuation), and experience occasional rectal bleeding. When vague cramping pain or an aching pressure sensation occurs, it is usually associated with a palpable abdominal mass, although these symptoms are experienced before the identification of the mass. Acute pain is often indistinguishable from that of cholecystitis or acute appendicitis.

Fatigue and shortness of breath may occur secondary to the iron deficiency anemia that develops with chronic blood loss. Mahogany-colored stools may be present when there is blood mixed with the stool.* Bleeding with bright red blood is more common with a carcinoma of the left side of the colon. Pencil-thin stool may be described with cancer of the rectum.

When rectal tumors enlarge and invade the perirectal tissue, a sensation of rectal fullness develops and may progress to a dull, aching, perineal or sacral pain that can radiate down the legs when peripheral nerves are involved.

Clinical Signs and Symptoms of Colorectal Cancer

Early Stages

- Rectal bleeding, hemorrhoids
- Abdominal, pelvic, back, or sacral pain
- Back pain that radiates down the legs
- Changes in bowel patterns

Advanced Stages

- Constipation progressing to obstipation
- Diarrhea with copious amounts of mucus
- Nausea, vomiting
- Abdominal distention
- Weight loss
- Fatigue and dyspnea
- Fever (less common)

Acute Colonic Pseudo-obstruction

Acute colonic pseudo-obstruction (Ogilvie's syndrome) is a massive dilation of the cecum and proximal colon in the absence of actual mechanical

---

* The reddish-mahogany color associated with bleeding in the lower GI/colon differs from the melena or dark, tarry stools that occur when blood loss in the upper GI tract is oxidized before being excreted.

---

causes such as colonic obstruction.[56] This severe dilation of the colon may lead to spontaneous perforation of the colon, which is a life-threatening problem.

Ogilvie's syndrome is most commonly detected in surgical patients after trauma, burns, and GI tract surgery, or in medical patients who have severe metabolic, respiratory, and electrolyte disturbances. However, this complication has also been seen after hip arthroplasty. Possible explanations include acetabular trauma and heat generation from bone cement leading to damage to tissues close to the point of contact of the heated cement.

Other reported risks for development of this syndrome can be related to increased age, immobility, and use of client-controlled narcotic analgesia.[57] Symptoms include abdominal distention, nausea, vomiting, abdominal pain, and absent bowel movements. Bowel sounds may be absent or decreased and rebound tenderness is not usually present unless colon perforation has occurred and peritonitis is present.

▶ PHYSICIAN REFERRAL

A 67-year-old man is seeing you through home health care for a home program after discharge from the hospital 2 weeks ago for a total hip replacement. His recovery has been slowed by chronic diarrhea. A 25-year-old woman who is diagnosed as having a sacroiliac pain and joint dysfunction asks you what exercises she can do for constipation. A 44-year-old man with biceps tendinitis reports several episodes of fever and chills, diarrhea, and abdominal pain, which he contributes to "the stress of meeting deadlines on the job."

These are common examples of symptoms of a GI nature that are described by clients and are unrelated to current physical therapy treatment. These people may be seeking the therapist's advice as the only medical person with whom they have contact. Knowing the pain patterns associated with GI involvement and which follow-up questions to ask can assist the therapist in deciding when to suggest that the client return to a physician for a medical examination and treatment.

The client may not associate GI symptoms or already diagnosed GI disease with his or her musculoskeletal pain, which makes it necessary for the therapist to initiate questions to determine the presence of such GI involvement.

Taking the client's temperature and vital signs during the initial evaluation is recommended for

any person who has musculoskeletal pain of unknown origin. Fever, low-grade fever over a long period (even if cyclic), or sweats is indicative of systemic disease.

When appendicitis or peritonitis from any cause is suspected because of the client's symptoms, a physician should be notified immediately. The client should lie down and remain as quiet as possible. It is best to give her or him nothing by mouth because of the danger of aggravating the condition, possibly causing rupture of the appendix, or in case surgery is needed. Applications of heat are contraindicated for the same reason.

On the other hand, the therapist may be evaluating a client, who presents with shoulder, back, or groin pain and limitations that are not caused by true musculoskeletal lesions but rather the result of GI involvement. The presence of associated GI symptoms in the absence of conclusive musculoskeletal findings will alert the therapist to the possible need for medical referral. Correlate the *history with pain patterns* and any *unusual findings* that may indicate systemic disease.

Guidelines for Immediate Medical Attention

- Anytime appendicitis or iliopsoas/obturator abscess is suspected (positive McBurney's test, positive iliopsoas/obturator test, positive test for rebound tenderness)
- Anytime the therapist suspects retroperitoneal bleeding from an injured, damaged or ruptured spleen; ectopic pregnancy or (history of trauma; missed menses; positive Kehr's sign)

Guidelines for Physician Referral

- Clients who chronically rely on laxatives should be encouraged to discuss bowel management without drugs with their physician.
- Joint involvement accompanied by skin or eye lesions may be reflective of inflammatory bowel disease and should be reported to the physician if the physician is unaware of these extraintestinal manifestations.
- Anyone with a history of NSAID use presenting with back or shoulder pain, especially when accompanied by any of the associated signs and symptoms listed for peptic ulcer must be evaluated by a physician.
- Back pain associated with meals or relieved by a bowel movement (especially if accompanied by rectal bleeding) or with back pain and abdomi-

nal pain at the same level requires medical evaluation.
- Back pain of unknown cause that does not fit a musculoskeletal pattern, especially in a person with a previous history of cancer.

Clues to Screening for Gastrointestinal

These clues will help the therapist in the decision making process.

- Age over 45
- Previous history of NSAID-induced GI bleeding; NSAID use, especially chronic or multiple prescriptions and over-the-counter NSAIDs taken simultaneously
- Symptoms increase within 2 hours after taking NSAIDs or other medication
  - Symptoms are affected (increased or decreased) by food anywhere from immediately up to 2 to 4 hours later
- Presence of abdominal or GI symptoms occurring within 4 to 6 weeks of musculoskeletal symptoms, especially recurring or cyclical symptoms (systemic pattern)
- Back pain and abdominal pain at the same level, simultaneously or alternately, especially when accompanied by constitutional symptoms
- Shoulder, back, pelvic, or sacral pain:
  - Of unknown origin, especially with a past history of cancer
  - Affected by food, milk, antacids, or vomiting
  - Accompanied by constitutional symptoms
  - Back, pelvic, or sacral pain that is relieved or reduced by a bowel movement or accompanied by rectal bleeding
- Shoulder pain within 24 to 48 hours of laparoscopy, ruptured ectopic pregnancy, or traumatic blow or injury to the left side (Kehr's sign; see Chapter 18)
- Positive iliopsoas or obturator sign; positive McBurney's point; right (or left) lower quadrant abdominal or pelvic pain produced when palpating the iliopsoas muscle or tapping the heel of the involved side
- Joint pain or arthralgias preceded by skin rash, especially in the presence of a history of Crohn's disease
- When evaluated during early onset of referred pain, there is usually full and painless range of motion but, as time goes on, muscle splinting and guarding secondary to pain will produce altered movements as well

O V E R V I E W G A S T R O I N T E S T I N A L P A I N P A T T E R N S

▼ ESOPHAGEAL PAIN (Fig. 8-11)

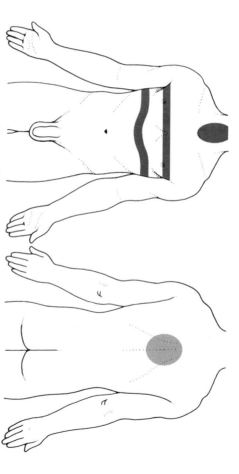

Fig. 8-11 • Nerve distribution of the esophagus is through T5 to T6 with primary pain around the xiphoid. Esophageal pain may be projected around the chest at any level corresponding to the esophageal lesion. Only two of the possible bands of pain around the chest are shown here. Similar symptoms can occur anywhere a lesion appears along the length of the esophagus.

Location:
Substernal discomfort at the level of the lesion
Lesion of upper esophagus: pain in the (anterior) neck
Lesion of lower esophagus: pain originating from the xiphoid process, radiating around the thorax

Referral:
Severe esophageal pain: pain referred to the middle of the back
Back pain may be the only symptom or may be the earliest symptom of esophageal cancer

Description:
Sharp, sticking, knifelike, stabbing
Strong burning pain (esophagitis)

Intensity:
Varies from mild discomfort to severe pain

Duration:
May be constant; associated with meals

Associated signs and symptoms:
Dysphagia, odynophagia, melena

Possible etiology:
Obstruction of the esophagus (neoplasm)
Esophageal stricture secondary to acid reflux (peptic esophagitis)
Esophageal stricture of unknown cause
Achalasia
Esophagitis or esophageal spasm
Esophageal varices (usually asymptomatic except bleeding)

O V E R V I E W **G A S T R O I N T E S T I N A L   P A I N   P A T T E R N S — cont'd**

▼ **STOMACH AND DUODENAL PAIN** (Fig. 8-12)

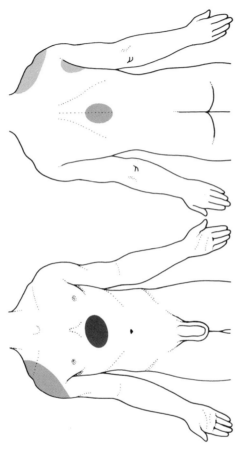

Fig. 8-12 • Stomach or duodenal pain *(dark red)* may occur anteriorly in the midline of the epigastrium or upper abdomen just below the xiphoid process. There is a tendency for the stomach and duodenum to refer pain posteriorly. Referred pain *(light red)* to the back occurs at the anatomic level of the abdominal lesion (T6 to T10). Other patterns of referred pain *(light red)* may include the right shoulder and upper trapezius or the lateral border of the right scapula.

Location:	Pain in the midline of the epigastrium
	Upper abdomen just below the xiphoid process
	One to two inches above and to the right of the umbilicus
Referral:	Common referral pattern to the back at the level of the lesion (T6 to T10)
	Right shoulder/upper trapezius
	Lateral border of the right scapula
Description:	Aching, burning ("heartburn"), gnawing, cramp-like pain (true visceral pain)
Intensity:	Can be mild or severe
Duration:	Comes in waves
Associated signs and symptoms:	Early satiety
	Melena
	Symptoms may be associated with meals
Possible etiology:	Peptic ulcers: gastric, pyloric, duodenal (history of NSAIDs)
	Stomach carcinoma
	Kaposi's sarcoma (most common malignancy associated with acquired immunodeficiency syndrome [AIDS]).

OVERVIEW GASTROINTESTINAL PAIN PATTERNS—cont'd

▼ SMALL INTESTINE PAIN (Fig. 8-13)

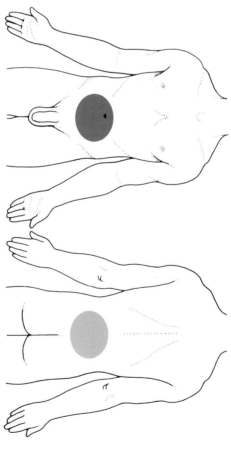

Fig. 8-13 ▪ Midabdominal pain (*dark red*) caused by disturbances of the small intestine is centered around the umbilicus (T9 to T11 nerve distribution) and may be referred (*light red*) to the low back area at the same anatomic level. Keep in mind the umbilicus is at the same level as the L3-L4 disc space in the average adult who is not obese or who has a protruding abdomen.

Location:	Midabdominal pain (about the umbilicus)
Referral:	Pain referred to the back if the stimulus is sufficiently intense or if the individual's pain threshold is low
Description:	Cramping pain
Intensity:	Moderate to severe
Duration:	Intermittent (pain comes and goes)
Associated signs and symptoms:	Nausea, fever, diarrhea Pain relief may not occur after passing stool or gas
Possible etiology:	Obstruction (neoplasm) Increased bowel motility Crohn's disease (regional enteritis)

OVERVIEW GASTROINTESTINAL PAIN PATTERNS—cont'd

▼ LARGE INTESTINE AND COLON PAIN (Fig. 8-14)

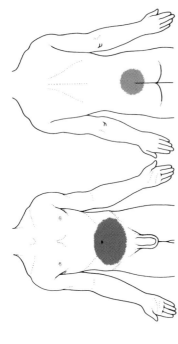

Fig. 8-14 • Pain associated with the large intestine and colon (*dark red*) may occur in the lower abdomen across either or both abdominal quadrants. Pain may be referred to the sacrum (*light red*) when the rectum is stimulated. The pattern of nerve supply varies depending on the segment: vermiform appendix, cecum, and ascending colon are supplied by the T10-T12 sympathetic fibers. Nerve distribution to the transverse colon is T12-L1 and the descending colon is supplied by L1-L2.

Location:	Lower midabdomen (across either or both quadrants)
	Poorly localized
Referral:	Pain may be referred to the sacrum when the rectum is stimulated
Description:	Cramping
Intensity:	Dull
Duration:	Steady
Associated signs and	Bloody diarrhea, urgency
symptoms:	Constipation
	Rectal pain; pain during defecation
	Pain relief may occur after defecation or passing gas
Possible etiology:	Ulcerative colitis
	Crohn's disease (regional enteritis)
	Carcinoma of the colon
	Long-term use of antibiotics
	Irritable bowel syndrome (IBS)

O V E R V I E W   GASTROINTESTINAL PAIN PATTERNS—cont'd

▼ PANCREATIC PAIN (Fig. 8-15)

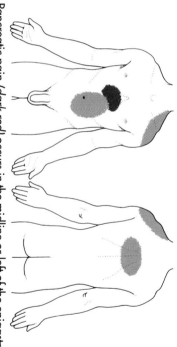

Fig. 8-15 • Pancreatic pain (*dark red*) occurs in the midline or left of the epigastrium, just below the xiphoid process, but may be referred (*light red*) to the left shoulder or to the mid-thoracic spine. Posterior pain may radiate or lateralize from the spine away from the midline. Sensory nerve distribution is from T5 to T9.

Location:	Midline or to the left of the epigastrium, just below the xiphoid process
Referral:	Referred pain in the middle or lower back is typical with pancreatic disease; more rarely, pain may be referred to the upper back, midscapular region. Somatic pain felt in the left shoulder may result from activation of pain fibers in the left diaphragm by an adjacent inflammatory process in the tail of the pancreas.
Description:	Burning, or gnawing abdominal pain
Intensity:	Severe
Duration:	Constant pain, sudden onset
Associated signs and symptoms:	Sudden weight loss
	Jaundice
	Nausea and vomiting
	Light-colored stools(carcinoma)
	Constipation
	Flatulence
	Tachycardia
	Symptoms may be unrelated to digestive activities (carcinoma)
	Weakness
	Symptoms may be related to digestive activities (carcinoma)
	Fever
	Malaise
Aggravating factors:	Walking and lying supine (pancreatitis)
Relieving factors:	Alcohol, large meals
	Sitting and leaning forward (pancreatitis, pancreatic carcinoma)
Possible etiology:	Pancreatitis
	Pancreatic carcinoma (primarily disease of men, occurs during the 6th and 7th decade)

O V E R V I E W | GASTROINTESTINAL PAIN PATTERNS—cont'd

▼ APPENDICEAL PAIN (See Fig. 8-8)

Location:	Right lower quadrant pain
Referral:	Well localized; first referred to epigastric or periumbilical area
	Referred pain pattern to the right hip and/or right testicle
Description:	Aching, comes in waves
Intensity:	Moderate to severe
Duration:	Steadily progresses over time (usually 12 hours with acute appendicitis)
Associated signs and symptoms:	Positive McBurney's point for tenderness
	Iliopsoas abscess may occur; positive iliopsoas muscle test or positive obturator test
	Anorexia, nausea, vomiting, low-grade fever
	Coated tongue and bad breath
	Dysuria (painful/difficult urination)

✔ KEY POINTS TO REMEMBER

✓ Gastrointestinal disorders can refer pain to the sternum, neck, shoulder, scapula, low back, sacrum, groin, and hip.

✓ When evaluated during early onset of referred pain, there is usually full and painless range of motion, but as time goes on, muscle splinting and guarding secondary to pain or as a component of motor nerve involvement will produce altered movements as well.

✓ The membrane that envelops organs (visceral peritoneum) is insensitive to pain so that, except in the presence of inflammation/ischemia, it is possible to have extensive disease without pain.

✓ Clients may not relate known GI disorders to current (or new) musculoskeletal symptoms.

✓ Sudden and unaccountable changes in bowel habits, blood in the stool, or vomiting red blood or coffee-ground vomitus are red flag symptoms requiring medical follow-up.

✓ Antibiotics and NSAIDs are the drugs that most commonly induce GI symptoms.

✓ Kehr's sign (left shoulder pain) occurs as a result of free air or blood in the abdominal cavity causing distention (e.g., trauma, ruptured spleen, laparoscopy, ectopic pregnancy).

✓ Epigastric pain radiating to the upper back or upper back pain alone can be the primary symptom of peptic ulcer, pancreatitis, or pancreatic carcinoma.

✓ Appendicitis and diseases of the intestines such as Crohn's disease and ulcerative colitis can cause abscess of the iliopsoas muscle, resulting in hip, thigh, or groin pain.

✓ Arthritis and migratory arthralgias occur in 25% of Crohn's disease cases.

Figs. 8-16 and 8-17 provide a summary of all the GI pain patterns described that can mimic the pain and dysfunction usually associated with musculoskeletal lesions.

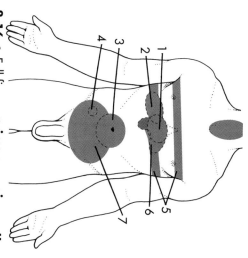

Fig. 8-16 • Full-figure **primary pain pattern:** (1) stomach/duodenum; (2) liver/gallbladder/common bile duct; (3) small intestine; (4) appendix; (5) esophagus; (6) pancreas; and (7) large intestine/colon.

SUBJECTIVE EXAMINATION

Special Questions to Ask

After completing the initial intake interview, if there is cause to suspect GI involvement, include any of the following additional questions that seem pertinent. It may be helpful to let the client know you will be asking some questions about overall health issues that may seem unrelated to their current symptoms but that are nevertheless important.

When asking questions about medications, look for long-term use of antibiotics, corticosteroids such as prednisone, or other hepatotoxic drugs. See Table 8-1 for a list of medications that can cause constipation.

Past Medical History

- (For the client with left shoulder pain): Have you sustained any injuries in the last week during a sports activity, fall, or automobile accident? Were you pushed down or pushed against something hard (assault)? Were you ever diagnosed with cancer of any kind? *If yes*, what, when, and has there been any follow-up?

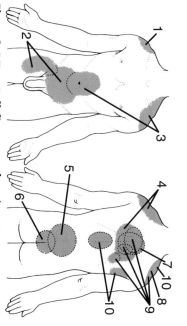

Fig. 8-17 • **Full-figure** referred pain patterns: (1) liver/gallbladder/common bile duct; (2) appendix; (3) pancreas; (4) pancreas; (5) small intestine; (6) colon; (7) esophagus; (8) stomach/duodenum; (9) liver/gallbladder/common bile duct; and (10) stomach/duodenum.

- Have you experienced any abdominal or intestinal problems, nausea, vomiting, episodes of night sweats or fever?
  - *If yes*, have you seen a physician about these problems or reported them to your physician?
  - For further follow-up questions related to this area, see Associated Signs and Symptoms below.
- Have you ever had an upset stomach or heartburn while taking your (NSAID) pain relievers like ibuprofen, naproxen (name the specific drug)?
- Have you ever been treated for an ulcer or internal bleeding while taking these (NSAID) pain relievers?
  - *If so, when?*
  - Do you still have any pain from your ulcer? Please describe.
- Have you ever had a colonoscopy, proctoscopy, or endoscopy? *If yes*, why and how long ago?
- Have you ever been diagnosed with cancer of any kind? *If yes*, what, when, and has there been any follow-up?
- (For the client with left shoulder pain): Have you sustained any injuries in the last week during a sports activity, fall, or automobile accident? Were you pushed down or pushed against something hard (assault)? **(Ruptured spleen: positive Kehr's sign)**

SUBJECTIVE EXAMINATION—cont'd

- Have you ever had radiation treatment? (**Rectal bleeding is a sign of radiation proctitis**)
- Have you ever had abdominal or spine (anterior retroperitoneal approach) surgery?
  - *If yes*, when and what type was it?
- Do you have hemorrhoids?
  - *If yes*, have you had surgery for your hemorrhoids? (**Most common cause of bright red blood coating stools**)

Associated Signs and Symptoms: Effects of eating/drinking

- Do you have any problems chewing or swallowing food? Do you have any pain when swallowing food or liquids? (**Dysphagia, odynophagia**)
- Have you been vomiting? (**Esophageal varices, ulcers**)
  - *If so*, how often?
  - Is your vomitus ever dark brown or black or look like it has coffee grounds in it? (**Blood**)
- Have you ever vomited, coughed up, or spit up blood?
- Have you experienced any loss of appetite or sudden weight loss in the last few weeks? (i.e., 10 to 15 pounds in 2 weeks without trying)
- Does eating relieve your symptoms? (**Duodenal or pyloric ulcer**)
  - *If yes*, how soon after eating?
- Does eating aggravate your symptoms? (**Gastric ulcer, gallbladder inflammation**)
- Does your pain occur 1 to 3 hours after eating or between meals? (**Duodenal or pyloric ulcers, gallstones, pancreatitis**)
- Have you ever had gallstones?
- Have you noticed any change in your symptoms after drinking alcohol? (**Alcohol-associated pancreatitis**)
- Have you ever awakened at night with pain? (**Duodenal ulcer, cancer**)
- Approximately what time does this occur? (**12 midnight to 3:00 a.m.: ulcer**)
- Can you relieve the pain in any way and get back to sleep. *If yes*, how? (**Ulcer: eating and antacids relieve/Cancer: nothing relieves**)
- Do you have a feeling of fullness after only one or two bites of food? (**Early satiety: esophagus, stomach and duodenum, or gallbladder**)

Associated Signs and Symptoms: Change in bowel habits

- Have you had any changes in your bowel movements (Normal frequency varies from three times a day to once every 3 or more days)? (**Constipation/bowel obstruction**)
  - *If yes* to constipation (see Table 8-1), do you use laxative or stool softeners? How often?
- Do you have diarrhea? (**Ulcerative colitis, Crohn's disease, long-term use of antibiotics, colonic obstruction, amebic colitis, angiodysplasia, creatine supplementation**)
  - Do you have more than two loose stools a day? *If so*, do you take medication for this problem? What kind of medication do you use?
  - Have you traveled outside of the United States within the last 6 months to 1 year? (**Amebic colitis associated with bloody diarrhea**)
- Do you have a sense of urgency so that you have to find a bathroom immediately without waiting?
- Do you ever have any blood in your stool, reddish Mahogany-colored stools, or dark, tarry stools that are hard to wipe clean? (**Bleeding ulcer, esophageal varices, colon or rectal cancer, hemorrhoids or rectal fissures; rectal lesions with bleeding can be caused by homosexual activity [men] or anal intercourse [women]**)
  - *If yes*, how often?
  - For the therapist: *If yes*, assess NSAID use and risk factors for NSAID-induced gastropathy.
  - Is the blood mixed in with the stool or does it coat the surface? (**Distal colon or rectum versus melena**)
- Do you ever have white mucus around or in your stools? (**Irritable bowel syndrome**)
- Do you ever have gray-colored stools? (**Lack of bile or caused by biliary obstruction such as hepatitis, gallstones, cirrhosis, pancreatic carcinoma, hepatotoxic drugs**)
- Are your stools ever pencil thin? (**Indicates bowel obstruction such as tumor or rectocele [prolapsed rectum] in women after childbirth**)
- Is your pain relieved after passing stool or gas? (**Yes: large intestine and colon; No: small intestine**)

CASE STUDY: CROHN'S

REFERRAL

A 21-year-old woman comes to you with complaints of pain on hip flexion when she lifts her right foot off the brake in the car. There are no other aggravating factors, and she is unaware of any way to relieve the pain when she is driving her car. Before the onset of symptoms, she jogged 5 to 6 miles/day, but could not recall any injury or trauma that might contribute to this pain. The Family/Personal History form indicates no personal illness but shows a complex, positive family history for heart disease, diabetes, ulcerative colitis, stomach ulcers, stomach cancer, and alcoholism.

PHYSICAL THERAPY INTERVIEW

It is suggested that the therapist use the physical therapy interview to assess the client's complaints today and follow up with appropriate additional questions, such as those noted here.

Introduction to Client

From your family history form, I notice that a number of your family members have reportedly been diagnosed with various diseases.

- Do you have any other medical or health-related problems?

- Have you sustained any injuries to the lower back, side, or abdomen in the last week—for example, during a sports activity, fall, or automobile accident? Were you pushed, kicked, or shoved against something?

Although the symptoms that you have described appear to be a musculoskeletal problem, I would like to check out the possibility of a urologic, abdominal, or gynecologic source of this irritation. I will ask you some additional questions that may seem to be unrelated to the problem with your hip, but which will help me put together the whole picture of the history, symptoms, and actual physical results from my examination today.

General Systemic

What other symptoms have you had with this problem? (After allowing the client to answer, you may prompt her by asking: For example, have you had any . . .)

- Numbness
- Fatigue
- Legs giving out from under you
- Burning, tingling sensation
- Weakness

Gastrointestinal

- Nausea
- Diarrhea
- Loss of appetite
- Feeling of fullness after only one or two bites of a meal
- Unexpected weight gain or loss (10 to 15 pounds without trying)
- Vomiting
- Constipation
- Blood in your stool
  (If yes to any of these, follow-up with *Special Questions to Ask* from this chapter.)

- Have you noticed any association between when you eat and your symptoms? (After allowing the client to respond, you may want to prompt her by asking whether eating relieves the pain or aggravates the pain.)

  Is your pain relieved or aggravated during or after you have a bowel movement?

Gynecologic

Since your hip/groin/thigh symptoms started, have you been examined by a gynecologist to rule out any gynecologic causes of this problem? *If no:*

- Have you ever been told that you have ovarian cysts, uterine fibroids, retroverted uterus, endometriosis, an ectopic pregnancy, or any other gynecologic problem?
- Are you pregnant or have you recently terminated a pregnancy either by miscarriage or abortion?
- Are you using an intrauterine contraceptive device (IUD)?
- Are you having any unusual vaginal discharge? (If yes to any of these questions, see the follow-up questions for women in Appendix B-32.)

Urologic

Have you had any problems with your kidneys or bladder? *If yes,* please describe.

Have you noticed any changes in your ability to urinate since your pain or symptoms started? (If no, it may be necessary to provide examples of what changes you are referring to; for example, difficulty in starting or continuing the flow of urine, numbness or tingling in the groin or pelvis, painful urination, urinary incontinence, blood in the urine.)

Have you had burning with urination during the last 1 to 3 weeks?

CASE STUDY: CROHN'S—cont'd

Objective Examination

Your objective examination reveals tenderness or palpation over the right anterior upper thigh muscles into the groin, with reproduction of the pain on resisted trunk flexion only. This woman attends daily ballet classes, stretches daily, and seems to be very active physically. All tests for flexibility were negative for tightness, including the Thomas' test for tight hip flexors.

Other special tests for hip and a neurologic screen had negative results. The client's temperature was normal when it was taken today during the intake screen of vital signs, but during the physical therapy interview, when specifically asked about fevers and night sweats, she indicated several recurrent episodes of night sweats during the last 3 months.

RESULTS

Although the client's complaints are primarily musculoskeletal, the absence of trauma, positive family history for systemic disease, limited musculoskeletal findings, and the client's remark concerning the presence of night sweats will alert the physical therapist to the need for a medical referral to rule out the possibility of a systemic origin of symptoms.

The client's condition gradually worsened during a 3-week period and reexamination by the physician led to an eventual diagnosis of Crohn's disease (regional gastroenteritis). The client was treated with medications that reduce abdominal inflammation and eliminated subjective reports of pain on active hip flexion. Performing the special tests for iliopsoas abscess may have provided valuable information and earlier medical referral if assessed during the initial evaluation.

PRACTICE QUESTIONS

1. Bleeding in the GI tract can be manifested as:
    a. Dysphagia
    b. Melena
    c. Psoas abscess
    d. Tenderness over McBurney's point
2. What is the significance of Kehr's sign?
    a. Gas, air, or blood in the abdominal cavity
    b. Infection of the peritoneum (peritonitis, appendicitis)
    c. Esophageal cancer
    d. Thoracic disc herniation masquerading as chest or anterior neck pain
3. What areas of the body can gastrointestinal (GI) disorders refer pain to?
    a. Sternum, shoulder, scapula
    b. Anterior neck, mid-back, lower back
    c. Hip, pelvis, sacrum
    d. All of the above
4. A 56-year old client was referred to PT for pelvic floor rehab. His primary symptoms are obstructed defecation and puborectalis muscle spasm. He wakes nightly with left flank pain. The pattern is low thoracic, laterally, but superior to iliac crest. Sometimes he has buttock pain on the same side. He doesn't have any daytime pain but is up for several hours at night. Advil and light activity do not help much. The pain is relieved or decreased with passing gas. He has very tight hamstrings and rectus femoris.

    Change in symptoms with gas or defecation is possible with:
    a. Thoracic disc disease
    b. Obturator nerve compression
    c. Small intestine disease
    d. Large intestine and colon dysfunction

PRACTICE QUESTIONS—cont'd

5. Name two of the most common medications taken by clients seen in a physical therapy practice likely to induce GI bleeding.
   a. Corticosteroids
   b. Antibiotics and antiinflammatories
   c. Statins
   d. None of the above

6. What is the significance of the psoas sign?

7. Which of the following are clues to the possible involvement of the GI system?
   a. Abdominal pain alternating with TMJ pain within a 2-week period
   b. Abdominal pain at the same level as back pain, occurring either simultaneously or alternately
   c. Shoulder pain alleviated by a bowel movement
   d. All of the above

8. A 65-year old client is taking OxyContin for a "sore shoulder." She also reports aching pain of the sacrum that radiates. The sacral pain can be caused by:
   a. Psoas abscess caused by vertebral osteomyelitis
   b. GI bleed causing hemorrhoids and rectal fissures
   c. Crohn's disease manifested as sacroiliitis
   d. Pressure on sacral nerves from stored fecal content in the constipated client taking narcotics

9. A 64-year old woman with chronic rheumatoid arthritis fell and broke her hip. Six months after her total hip replacement, she is still using a walker and complains of continued loss of strength and function. Her family practice physician has referred her to physical therapy for a home program to "improve gait and increase strength."

   The client reports frequent episodes of lightheadedness when her legs feel rubbery and weak. She is taking a prescription NSAID along with an OTC NSAID 3 times each day and has been taking NSAIDs 3 years continuously. There are no reported GI complaints or associated signs and symptoms, but after completing the intake interview and objective examination, you think there may be weakness associated with blood loss and anemia secondary to chronic NSAID use. How would you handle a case like this?

10. Body temperature should be taken as part of vital sign assessment:
    a. For every client evaluated
    b. For any client who has musculoskeletal pain of unknown origin
    c. For any client reporting the presence of constitutional symptoms, especially fever or night sweats
    d. (b) and (c)

REFERENCES

1. Pert CB, Dreher HE, Ruff MR: The psychosomatic network: foundations of mind-body medicine, *Altern Ther Health Med* 4(4):30-41, 1998.
2. Pert C: Paradigms from neuroscience: when shift happens, *Mol Interv* 3(7):361-366, 2003.
3. Mayer EA: Gut feelings: what turns them on? *Gastroenterology* 108(3):927-931, 1995.
4. Groh V and Spies T: Recognition of stress-induced MHC molecules by intestinal epithelial gamma delta T cells, *Science* 279:737-1740, 1998.
5. Wu J, et al: T-cell antigen receptor engagement and specificity in the recognition of stress-inducible MHC class I-related chains by human epithelial gamma delta T cells, *J Immunol* 169(3):1236-1240, 2002.
6. Rex L: evaluation and treatment of somatovisceral dysfunction of the gastrointestinal system, Edmonds, Washington, 2004, URSA Foundation.
7. Rose SJ, Rothstein JM: Muscle mutability: general concepts and adaptations to altered patterns of use, *Physical Therapy* 62:1773, 1982.
8. Ledlie J, Renfro M: Balloon kyphoplasty: one-year outcomes in vertebral body height restoration, chronic

9. Travell JG, Simons DG: *Myofascial pain and dysfunction: the trigger point manual*, Vol 2, Baltimore, 1992, Williams and Wilkins.
10. Oberpenning F, Roth S, Leusmann DB, et al: The Alcock syndrome: temporary penile insensitivity due to compression of the pudendal nerve within the Alcock canal, *J Urol* 151(2):423-425, 1994.
11. Weiss BD: Clinical syndromes associated with bicycle seats, *Clin Sports Med* 13(1):175-186, 1994
12. McQuaid K: Alimentary tract: antibiotic-associated colitis. In Tierney L, McPhee S, Papadakis M, editors: *Current medical diagnosis and treatment*, ed 43, New York, 2004, Lange; pp 596-597.
13. Smith J, Dahm DL: Creatine use among select population of high school athletes, *Mayo Clin Proc* 75(12):1257-1263, 2000.
14. Graham AS, Hatton RC: Creatine: a review of efficacy and safety, *J Am Pharm Assoc* 39(6):803-810, 1999.
15. Hellman D, Sone J: Arthritis and musculoskeletal disorders; reactive arthritis. In Tierney L, McPhee S, Papadakis M, editors: *Current medical diagnosis and treatment*, ed 43, New York, 2004, Lange; pp 821-822.

pain, and activity levels, *J Neurosurg (Spine I)* 98:36-42, 2003.

16. Palm O, et al: Prevalence of ankylosing spondylitis and other spondyloarthropathies among patients with inflammatory bowel disease: a population study (the IBSEN study), *Journal of Rheumatology* 29(3):511-515, 2002.

17. Inman RD: Arthritis and enteritis—an interface of protean manifestations, *Journal of Rheumatology* 14:406-410, 1987.

18. Gran JT, Husby G: Joint manifestations in gastrointestinal diseases, *Digestive Diseases* 10:295-312, 1992.

19. Baeten D, et al: Influence of the gut and cytokine patterns in spondyloarthropathy, *Clin Exp Rheumatol* 20(6 Suppl 28):S38-S42, 2002.

20. Sieper J et al: Diagnosing reactive arthritis: role of clinical setting in the value of serologic and microbiologic assays, *Arthritis Rheum* 46:319, 2002.

21. Mustafa K, Khan MA: Recognizing and managing reactive arthritis, *J Musculoskeletal Med* 13(6):28-41, 1996.

22. Burger EL: Lumbar disk replacement: restoring mobility, *Orthopedics* 27(4):386-288, 2004.

23. Tay B et al: Spinal infections, *J Amer Acad Orthop Surg* 10(3):188-197, 2002.

24. Goodman CC: The gastrointestinal system. In Goodman CC et al, editors: *Pathology: implications for the physical therapist*, ed 2, Philadelphia, 2003, WB Saunders; pp 628-666.

25. Rayhorn N, Argel N, Demchak K: Understanding gastroesophageal reflux disease, *Nursing2003* 33(10):37-41, 2003.

26. Sabesin SM, Fass R, Fisher R: Not all heartburn patients are equal: strategies for coping with gastroesophageal reflux disease (GERD), *Medscape Continuing Medical Education*.

27. Asthma in older women, *Harvard Women's Health Watch* 11(3):5, 2003.

28. Margolis S: Getting the right cure for ulcers, *Johns Hopkins Medical Letter* 10(1):1-2, 1998.

29. Miwa, H, Sakaki N, Sugano K, et al. Recurrent peptic ulcers in patients following successful *Helicobacter pylori* eradication: a multicenter study of 4940 patients, *Helicobacter* 9(1):9-16, 2004.

30. Chan FKL, Graham DY: Prevention of non-steroidal anti-inflammatory drug gastrointestinal complications—review and recommendations based on risk assessment, *Medscape Continuing Medical Education*.

31. Lanas A, Garcia-Rodriquez LA, Arroyo MT, et al: Risk of upper gastrointestinal ulcer bleeding associated with selective COX-2 inhibitors, traditional non-aspirin NSAIDs, aspirin, and combinations, *Gut* May 10, 2006 (Epub ahead of print).

32. McQuaid K: Alimentary tract: peptic ulcer disease. In Tierney L, McPhee S, Papadakis M, editors: *Current medical diagnosis and treatment*, ed 43, New York, 2004, Lange; pp 564-570.

33. Chan FK: Celecoxib versus diclofenac and omeprazole in reducing the risk of recurrent ulcer bleeding in patients with arthritis, *NEJM* 347(26):2104-2110, 2002.

34. Goldstein JL, et al: Incidence of outpatient physician claims for upper gastrointestinal symptoms among new users of celecoxib, ibuprofen, and naproxen in an insured population in the United States, *Am J Gastroenterol* 98(12):2627-2634, 1998.

35. Lefkowith JB: Cyclooxygenase-2 specificity and its clinical implications, *Am J Med* 106:43S-50S, 1999.

36. Chan F: Preventing recurrent upper gastrointestinal bleeding in patients with *Helicobacter pylori* infection who are taking low-dose aspirin or naproxen, *N Engl J Med* 344:967, 2001.

37. Peloso PM: NSAIDs: a Faustian bargain, *American Journal of Nursing* 100(6):34-43, 2000.

38. Sturkenboom MC, Burke TA, Dieleman JP, et al: Under-utilization of preventive strategies in patients receiving NSAIDs, *Rheumatology* (Oxford) 42(Suppl 3):iii23-31, 2003.

39. Goldstein JL: Challenges in managing NSAID-associated gastrointestinal tract injury, *Digestion* 69(Suppl 1):25-33, 2004.

40. Fries JF, et al: Nonsteroidal antiinflammatory drug-associated gastropathy: incidence and risk factor models, *Am J Med* 91(3):213-222, 1991.

41. Enns R: Acute lower gastrointestinal bleeding, Parts 1 and 2, *Can J Gastroenterology* 15:509-517, 2001.

42. Sadler TW: *Langman's medical embryology*, ed 9, Philadelphia, 2004, Lippincott, Williams & Wilkins.

43. Rayhorn N: Inflammatory bowel disease (IBD), *Nursing2003* 33(11):54-55, 2003.

44. Ma TY: Intestinal epithelial barrier dysfunction in Crohn's disease, *Proc Soc Exp Biol Med* 214(4):318-327, 1997.

45. Ma TY, Iwamoto GK, Hoa NT, et al: TNF-alpha-induced increase in intestinal epithelial tight junction permeability requires NF-kappa B activation, *Am J Physiol Gastrointest Liver Physiol* 286(3):G367-376, 2004.

46. Older K: Diagnosis of irritable bowel syndrome, *Gastroenterology* 122:1701, 2002.

47. McQuaid K: Alimentary tract: irritable bowel syndrome. In Tierney L, McPhee S, Papadakis M, editors: *Current medical diagnosis and treatment*, ed 43, New York, 2004, Lange; pp 592-596.

48. van Zanten SV: Diagnosing irritable bowel syndrome, *Rev Gastroenterol Disord* 3(Suppl 2):S12-17, 2003.

49. Salmon P, Skaife K, Rhodes J: Abuse, dissociation, and somatization in irritable bowel syndrome: towards an explanatory model, *J Behav Med* 26(1):1-18, 2003.

50. Crowell MD, Dubin NH, Robinson JC, et al: Functional bowel disorders in women with dysmenorrhea, *Am J Gastroenterol* 89:1973, 1994.

51. NIH: Irritable bowel syndrome, *NIH Publication* No. 03-693, April, 2003.

52. Lucak S: Diagnosing irritable bowel syndrome: what's too much, what's enough? *Medscape Medical Continuing Education*, on line, posted 3/12/04 on www.medscape.com/viewarticle 465760

53. Jemal A, Tiwari RC, Murray T, et al: Cancer statistics 2004, *CA Cancer J Clin* 54(1):8-29, 2004.

54. Sargent C, Murphy D: What you need to know about colorectal cancer, *Nursing2003* 33(2):37-41, 2003.

55. Smith R, et al: American Cancer Society guidelines for early detection of cancer, *CA Cancer J Clin* 52(1):8-22, 2002.

56. Schermer CR, et al: Ogilvie's syndrome in the surgical patient, a new therapeutic modality, *J Gastroenterol Surg* 3(2):173, 1999.

57. el Maraghy A, et al: Ogilvie's syndrome after lower extremity arthroplasty, *Can J Surg* 42(2):133, 1999.

As with many of the organ systems in the human body, the hepatic and biliary organs (liver, gallbladder, and common bile duct) (Fig. 9-1) can develop diseases that mimic primary musculoskeletal lesions. The musculoskeletal symptoms associated with hepatic and biliary pathologic conditions are generally confined to the mid-back, scapular, and right shoulder regions. These musculoskeletal symptoms can occur alone (as the only presenting symptom) or in combination with other systemic signs and symptoms discussed in this chapter.

▶ HEPATIC AND BILIARY SIGNS AND SYMPTOMS

The major causes of acute hepatocellular injury include hepatitis, drug-induced hepatitis, and ingestion of hepatotoxins. The physical therapist is most likely to encounter liver or gallbladder diseases manifested by a variety of signs and symptoms outlined in this section.

Taking a careful history and making close observations of the client's physical condition and appearance can detect telltale signs of hepatic disease. Most of the liver is contained underneath the rib cage and is largely inaccessible (Fig. 9-2). An enlarged liver that is palpable may be a red flag (see Fig. 4-48). Medical diagnosis of liver or gallbladder disease is made by x-ray examination or ultrasonic scanning of the gallbladder and computed tomography (CT) scanning of the abdomen, including the liver.

Other tests such as a cholescintigraphy may be used to track the flow of radioactivity into and out of the gallbladder to confirm gallstones. Blood tests may be used to look for signs of infection, obstruction, or jaundice. Laboratory tests useful in the diagnosis and treatment of liver and biliary tract disease are listed inside the back cover.

Skin and Nail Bed Changes

Skin changes associated with impairment of the hepatic system include *jaundice*, pallor, and orange or green skin. In some situations jaundice may be the first and only manifestation of disease. It is first noticeable in the sclera of the eye as a yellow hue when bilirubin reaches levels of 2 to 3 mg/dl. When the bilirubin level reaches 5 to 6 mg/dl, the skin becomes yellow.

Normally bilirubin, excreted in bile and carried to the small intestines, is reduced to a form that causes the stool to assume a brown color. Light-colored (almost white) stools and urine the color of tea or cola indicate an inability of the liver or biliary system to excrete bilirubin properly. Gall-bladder disease, hepatotoxic medications, or pancreatic cancer blocking the bile duct may cause light stools.

Other skin changes may include pruritus (itching), bruising, spider angiomas (Fig. 9-3), and palmar erythema (see Fig. 9-5). *Spider angiomas* (arterial spider, spider telangiectasis, vascular spider), branched dilations

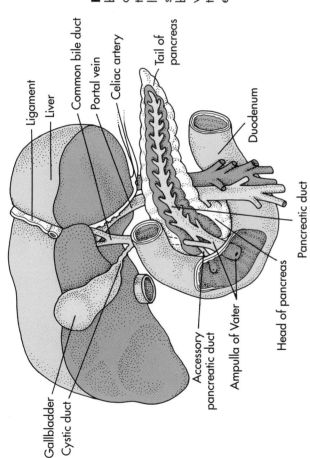

Ligament

Liver

Common bile duct

Portal vein

Celiac artery

Gallbladder

Cystic duct

Accessory pancreatic duct

Ampulla of Vater

Head of pancreas

Tail of pancreas

Duodenum

Pancreatic duct

Fig. 9-1 • Anatomy of the liver, gallbladder, common bile duct, and pancreas. The pear-shaped *gallbladder* is tucked up under the right side of the liver. The *pancreas* is located behind the stomach anterior to the L1 to L3 vertebral bodies. It is about 6 inches long, wide at one end (the head), then tapered through the body to the narrow end called the tail.

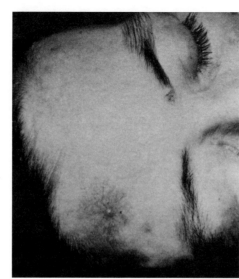

Fig. 9-3 • Spider Angioma. Permanently enlarged and dilated capillaries visible on the surface of the skin caused by vascular dilation are called *spider angiomas*. These capillary radiations can be flat (not shown) or raised in the center (as shown here). They present on the upper half of the body, primarily on the face, neck, chest, or abdomen and occur as a normal development or in association with pregnancy, chronic liver disease, or estrogen therapy. They do not go away when the underlying condition is treated; laser therapy is available to remove them for cosmetic reasons. (From Callen JP, Jorizzo JL, eds: *Dermatological signs of internal disease*, Philadelphia, 1988, WB Saunders.)

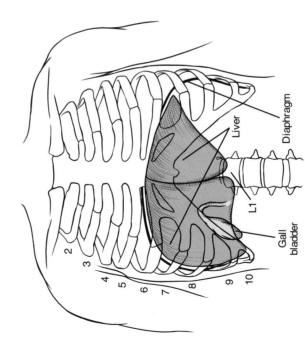

Liver

Diaphragm

L1

Gall bladder

2
3
4
5
6
7
8
9
10

Fig. 9-2 • Location of the liver and gallbladder. The *liver* is located just below the respiratory diaphragm, predominately on the right side, but with a portion crossing the midline to the left side. It is a large organ and spans many vertebral levels. The most superior part is the dome of the right lobe. The "peak" of the dome lies at about T8 or T9 during expiration. The inferior border of the left lobe is located just below the level of the left nipple and inclines downwards to the right at the tip of the 8th costal margin. The right lobe angles downward to the 9th and 10th costal margins. Posteriorly, the liver is located from approximately T9 to L1 at the midline. This varies from person to person and with inhalation (moves up a level or two) and exhalation (moves down). The fundus (base) of the *gallbladder* usually appears below the edge of the liver in contact with the anterior abdominal wall at the tip of the 9th right costal cartilage.

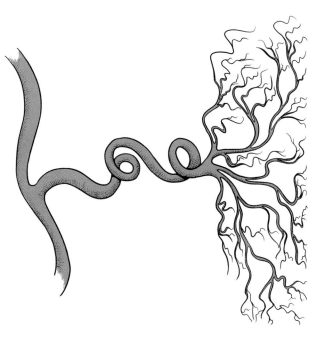

Fig. 9-4 • Arterial Spider. Schematic diagram of an arterial spider formed by a coiled arteriole that spirals up to a central point and then branches out into thin-walled vessels that merge with normal capillaries resembling a spider in appearance. Exposure to heat (e.g., hot tubs, warm shower) will cause temporary vasodilation. The skin lesion will appear larger until vasoconstriction occurs.

of the superficial capillaries resembling a spider in appearance (Fig. 9-4) may be vascular manifestations of increased estrogen levels (hyperestrogenism). Spider angiomas and palmar erythema both occur in the presence of liver impairment as a result of increased estrogen levels normally detoxified by the liver.

Palmar erythema (warm redness of the skin over the palms, also called *liver palms*) caused by an extensive collection of arteriovenous anastomoses especially affects the hypothenar and thenar eminences and pulps of the finger (Fig. 9-5). The soles of the feet may be similarly affected. The person may complain of throbbing, tingling palms.

Various forms of nail disease have been described in cases of liver impairment, such as the white nails of Terry (Fig. 9-6). Other nail bed changes such as white bands across the nail plate (leukonychia), clubbed nails (see Fig. 4-34), or koilonychia (see Fig. 4-30) can occur but these are not specific to liver impairment and can develop in the presence of other diseases as well.

Musculoskeletal Pain

Musculoskeletal pain associated with the hepatic and biliary systems includes thoracic pain between the scapulae, right shoulder, right upper trapezius,

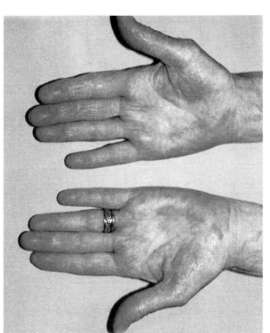

Fig. 9-5 • Palmer erythema caused by liver impairment presents as a warm redness of the skin over the palms and soles of the feet in the Caucasian population. Darker skin tones may change from a tan color to a gray appearance. Look for other signs of liver disease such as nail bed changes, spider angiomas, liver flap, and bilateral carpal or tarsal tunnel syndrome. Palmer erythema can occur in healthy individuals and in association with nonhepatic diseases. (From Barrison I, ed: *Gastroenterology in practice*, St. Louis, 1992, Mosby.)

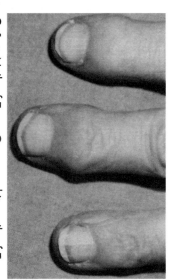

Fig. 9-6 • Nails of Terry. Opaque white nails of Terry in a patient with cirrhosis. Various forms of nail disease have been described in patients with cirrhosis. This is an example of the classic white nails of Terry characterized by an opaque nail plate with a narrow line of pink at the distal end instead of the more normal pink nail plate in the Caucasian. (From Callen JP, Jorizzo JL, eds: *Dermatological signs of internal disease*, Philadelphia, 1988, WB Saunders.)

right interscapular, or right subscapular areas (see Fig. 9-10 and Table 9-1).

Referred shoulder pain may be the only presenting symptom of hepatic or biliary disease. Pain from the superior ligaments of the liver and the superior portion of the liver capsule is transmitted by the phrenic nerves from the liver and the biliary system are connected through the celiac (abdominal) and splanchnic (visceral) plexuses to

TABLE 9-1 ▼ Referred Pain Patterns: Liver, Gallbladder, Common Bile Duct

Systemic causes	Location (see Figure 9-10)
Liver disease (abscess, cirrhosis, tumors, hepatitis)	Thoracic spine (T7-T10; midline to the right) Right upper trapezius and shoulder
Gallbladder	Right upper trapezius and shoulder Right interscapular area (T4 or T5-T8) Right subscapular area

the hepatic fibers in the region of the dorsal spine (see Fig. 3-3).

The celiac and splanchnic connections account for the intercostal and radiating interscapular pain that accompanies gallbladder disease. Although the innervation is bilateral, most of the biliary fibers reach the cord through the right splanchnic nerves, synapsing with adjacent phrenic nerve fibers innervating the diaphragm and producing pain in the right shoulder (see Fig. 3-4).

Hepatic osteodystrophy, abnormal development of bone, can occur in all forms of cholestasis (bile flow suppression) and hepatocellular disease, especially in the alcoholic person. Either osteomalacia or, more often, osteoporosis frequently accompanies bone pain from this condition. Vertebral wedging, vertebral crush fractures, and kyphosis can be severe; decalcification of the ribcage and pseudofractures[1] occur frequently.*

Osteoporosis associated with primary biliary cirrhosis and primary sclerosing cholangitis parallels the severity of liver disease rather than its duration. Painful osteoarthropathy may develop in the wrists and ankles as a nonspecific complication of chronic liver disease.

Rhabdomyolysis can occur as a result of acute trauma, overexertion, or in the case of liver impairment, from the use of cholesterol-lowering drugs called statins (e.g., Zocor, Lipitor, Crestor). Rhabdomyolysis, a potentially fatal condition involving the breakdown of muscle tissue, has been reported as a potential complication of all statin (choles-

---

* Pseudofractures, or Looser's zones, are narrow lines of radiolucency (areas of darkness on x-ray film) usually oriented perpendicular to the bone surface. This may represent a stress fracture that is repaired by laying down inadequately mineralized osteoid, or these sites may occur as a result of mechanical erosion caused by arterial pulsations since arteries frequently overlie sites of pseudofractures.

terol-lowering) drugs such as Zocor, Lipitor, or Crestor.[2]

Rhabdomyolysis is the most severe form of muscle disorder associated with statin use. Statin-associated myopathy is more likely characterized by muscle aches, cramps, soreness, and weakness. It may be accompanied by other symptoms of liver or renal involvement. Laboratory testing will show a creatine kinase (CK) level more than 10 times the upper limit of normal.

Although the literature reports the incidence of this severe myopathy with statin use as about 0.1% to 2.0% in clinical trials,[3] therapists report seeing cases more often than the low percentage would suggest.[4]

Statin-associated myopathy appears to occur more often in people with complex medical problems and/or taking other drugs, especially agents that share common metabolic pathways.[5] Other risk factors that increase the chances of this condition include excessive alcohol use, advancing age (over 80 years), recent history of surgery, and small physical stature.[2]

Neurologic Symptoms

Neurologic symptoms such as confusion, sleep disturbances, muscle tremors, hyperreactive reflexes, and asterixis may occur. When liver dysfunction results in increased serum ammonia and urea levels, peripheral nerve function can be impaired.

Ammonia from the intestine (produced by protein breakdown) is normally transformed by the liver to urea, glutamine, and asparagine, which are then excreted by the renal system. When the liver does not detoxify ammonia, ammonia is transported to the brain, where it reacts with glutamate (excitatory neurotransmitter), producing glutamine.

The reduction of brain glutamate impairs neurotransmission, leading to altered central nervous system metabolism and function. Asterixis and numbness/tingling (misinterpreted as carpal tunnel syndrome) can occur as a result of this ammonia abnormality, causing an intrinsic nerve pathologic condition (Case Example 9-1). There are many potential causes of carpal tunnel syndrome, both musculoskeletal and systemic (see Table 11-2). Careful evaluation is required (Box 9-1).

Pathophysiology

Asterixis (also called *flapping tremors* or *liver flap*) is a motor disturbance, specifically, the inability to maintain wrist extension with forward flexion of the upper extremities. Asterixis can be tested for by asking the client to dorsiflex the hand with the

CASE EXAMPLE 9-1   Carpal Tunnel Syndrome from Liver Impairment

A 45-year-old truck driver was diagnosed by a hand surgeon as having bilateral carpal tunnel syndrome (CTS) and referred to physical therapy. A screening examination was not performed during the evaluation. During the course of treatment, the client commented that he was seeing an acupuncturist, who told him that liver disease was the cause of his bilateral CTS.

The therapist suspected a history of alcohol abuse, which is a risk factor for liver disease.

Further questioning at that time indicated the lack of any other associated symptoms to suggest liver or hepatic involvement. However, because his symptoms were bilateral and there is a known correlation between liver disease and CTS, the referring physician was notified of these findings.

The client was referred for evaluation, and a diagnosis of liver cancer was confirmed. Physical therapy for CTS was appropriately discontinued.

BOX 9-1   ▼   Evaluating Carpal Tunnel Syndrome Associated with Liver Impairment

For any client presenting with bilateral carpal tunnel syndrome

- Ask about the presence of similar symptoms in the feet
- Ask about a personal history of liver or hepatic disease (e.g., cirrhosis, cancer, hepatitis)
- Look for a history of hepatotoxic drugs (see Box 9-3)
- Look for a history of alcoholism
- Ask about current or previous use of statins (cholesterol-lowering drugs such as Crestor, Lipitor, or Zocor)
- Look for other signs and symptoms associated with liver impairment (see Clinical Signs and Symptoms of Liver Disease)
- Test for signs of liver disease
  - Skin color changes
  - Spider angiomas
  - Palmer erythema (liver palms)
  - Nail bed changes (e.g., white nails of Terry, white bands, clubbing)
  - Asterixis (liver flap)

---

rest of the arm supported on a firm surface or with the arms held out in front of the body (Fig. 9-7).[6]

Observe for quick, irregular extensions and flexions of the wrist and fingers. Altered neurotransmission, specifically, impaired inflow of joint and other afferent information to the brainstem reticular formation, results in this movement dysfunction. Asterixis may be observed during blood pressure readings. Observe for flapping when the cuff is released. Watch for lack of concentration, fatigue, and other symptoms of encephalopathy (see Table 9-5).

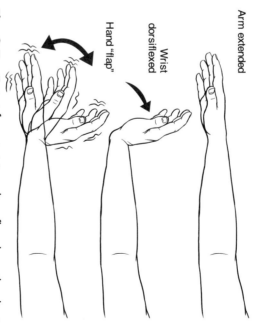

Arm extended

Wrist dorsiflexed

Hand "flap"

Fig. 9-7 • To test for asterixis or liver flap, have the client extend the arms, spread the fingers, extend the wrist, and observe for the abnormal "flapping" tremor at the wrist. If a tremor is not readily apparent, ask the client to keep the arms straight while gently hyperextending the client's wrist. There is an alternate method of testing for this phenomenon: have the client relax the legs in the supine position with the knees bent. The feet are flat on the table. As the legs fall to the sides, watch for a flapping or tremoring of the legs at the hip. The knees appear to come back towards the midline repeatedly.[6]

A careful history and close observation of the client are important in determining whether a person may need a medical referral for possible liver disease. Jaundice in the postoperative client is not uncommon, but it can be a potentially serious complication of surgery and anesthesia. Clues to screening for hepatic disease (see Clues to Screening for Hepatic Disease at the end of this chapter) should be taken into consideration when evaluating the clinical history and observations.

▶ HEPATIC AND BILIARY PATHOPHYSIOLOGY

Liver Diseases

Hepatitis

Hepatitis is an acute or chronic inflammation of the liver. It can be caused by a virus, a chemical, a drug reaction, or alcohol abuse. In addition, hepatitis can be secondary to disease conditions, such as an infection with other viruses (e.g., Epstein-Barr virus or cytomegalovirus).

VIRAL HEPATITIS

Viral hepatitis is an acute infectious inflammation of the liver caused by one of the following identified viruses: A, B, C, D, E, and G (Table 9-2).

Hepatitis is a major uncontrolled public health problem for several reasons: not all the causative agents have been identified, there are limited specific drugs for its treatment, its incidence has increased in relation to illicit drug use, and it can be communicated before the appearance of observable clinical symptoms.

Viral hepatitis is spread easily to others and usually results in an extended period of convalescence with loss of time from school or work. It is estimated that 60% to 90% of viral hepatitis cases are unreported because many cases are subclinical or involve mild symptoms.

Hepatitis A and E are transmitted primarily by the fecal-oral route. Common source outbreaks result from contaminated food or water. As people and foods, including produce, extend across the globe, the possibility of infection with these viruses increases.[7] Hepatitis A (HAV) must also be considered a potential problem in situations where fecal-oral communication along with food handling and/or unsanitary conditions occur. Some examples of potential sources of contact with HAV might include restaurants, day care centers, correctional institutions, sewage plants, and countries where these viruses are endemic.[8]

Hepatitis viruses B, C, D, and G are primarily blood borne pathogens that can be transmitted from percutaneous or mucosal exposures to blood or other body fluids from an infected person.

Hepatitis B virus (HBV) is usually transmitted by inoculation of infected blood or blood products or by sexual contact and is also found in body fluids (e.g., spinal, peritoneal, pleural) saliva, semen, and vaginal secretions. Hepatitis D virus must have Hepatitis B virus present to coinfect. Groups at risk include homosexuals and intravenous drug users; health care workers in any area where

---

Clinical Signs and Symptoms of
Liver Disease

- Sense of fullness of the abdomen
- Anorexia, nausea, and vomiting
- Skin changes and nail bed changes
  - Jaundice
  - Bruising
  - Spider angioma
  - Palmar erythema
  - White nails of Terry, other nail bed changes may be present
- Dark urine and light-colored or clay-colored feces
- Ascites (Fig. 9-8)
- Edema and oliguria (reduced urine secretion in relation to fluid intake)
- Right upper quadrant (RUQ) abdominal pain
- Musculoskeletal pain, especially right shoulder pain
- Myopathy (rhabdomyolysis in severe cases)
- Neurologic symptoms
  - Confusion
  - Sleep disturbances
  - Muscle tremors
  - Hyperactive reflexes
  - Asterixis (motor disturbance resembling body or extremity flapping)
  - Bilateral carpal/tarsal tunnel
- Pallor (often linked to cirrhosis or carcinoma)
- Gynecomastia (enlargement of breast tissue in men)

Clinical Signs and Symptoms of
Gallbladder Disease

- Right upper abdominal pain
- Jaundice (result of blockage of the common bile duct)
- Low-grade fever, chills
- Indigestion, nausea, feeling of fullness
- Excessive belching, flatulence (intestinal gas)
- Intolerance of fatty foods
- Persistent pruritus (skin itching)
- Sudden, excruciating pain in the mid-epigastrium with referral to the back and right shoulder (acute cholecystitis)
- Anterior rib pain (tip of 10th rib; can also affect ribs 11 and 12)

TABLE 9-2 ▼ Comparison of Major Types of Viral Hepatitis

Factor	Hepatitis A	Hepatitis B	Hepatitis C	Hepatitis D (delta agent)	Hepatitis E
Incidence	Endemic in areas of of poor sanitation; common in fall and early winter	Worldwide, especially in drug addicts, homosexuals, people exposed to blood products; occurs all year	Posttransfusion; those working around blood and blood products; occurs all year	Causes hepatitis only in association with hepatitis B and only presence of HbsAg; endemic in Mediterranean area	Parts of Asia, Africa, and Mexico, where sanitation is poor
Incubation period Risk factors	2-6 weeks Close personal contact or by handling feces-contaminated food or water	6 weeks-6 months Health care workers in contact with body secretions, blood, and blood products; hemodialysis and posttransfusion clients; homosexually active males and drug abusers; morticians; those receiving tattoos; workers, residents of correctional settings	6-7 weeks Similar to hepatitis B; healthcare workers in contact with blood and body fluids; blood transfusion recipients	Same as hepatitis B Same as hepatitis B	2-9 weeks Traveling or living in areas where incidence is high
Transmission	Infected feces, fecal-oral route*; may be airborne (if copious secretions); shellfish from contaminated water; also rarely parenteral; no carrier state	Parenteral, sexual contact, and fecal-oral route; carrier state	Contact with blood and body fluids; source of infection uncertain in many clients; carrier state	Coinfects with hepatitis B, close personal contact; carrier state	Fecal-oral route, food-borne or waterborne; no carrier state
Severity	Mortality low; rarely causes fulminating hepatic failure	More serious; may be fatal; mortality rate is up to 60%	Can lead to chronic hepatitis	Similar to hepatitis B; more severe if occurs with chronic active hepatitis B	Illness self-limiting; mortality rate in pregnant women is 10% to 20%
Prophylaxis and active or passive immunity	Hygiene; vaccine available; immune globulin	Hygiene; avoidance of risk factors; immune globulin (passive); hepatitis B vaccine (active); treatment with adefovir dipivoxil (Hepsera)	Hygiene; immune globulin (passive); treatment with Interferon alfacon-1 (Infergen) or pegylated interferons (peginterferon alpha-2a) and Ribavirin (viral inhibitor)	Hygiene; hepatitis B vaccine (active)	Hygiene; sanitation; no immunity

* The oral-fecal route of transmission is primarily from poor or improper handwashing and personal hygiene, particularly after using the bathroom and then handling food for public consumption. This route of transmission may also occur through shared use of razors and oral utensils such as straws, silverware, and toothbrushes.

contact with blood, blood products, or body fluids are likely; and residents and workers in correctional settings.[9]

Hepatitis C is transmitted similarly to HBV and HDV. Risk factors are also very similar with the addition of people who have received blood transfusions or organ transplants, including anterior cruciate ligament (ACL) reconstruction allograft.[10,11] There has been growing concern worldwide about the risk of occupational transmission of HCV. New findings, however, suggest that the transmission rate for health care workers is about 0.5% rather than the earlier reported 1.8%.[12]

Hepatitis G (HGV) designation has been applied to a virus that is percutaneously transmitted and associated with blood borne viral presence lasting approximately 10 years. HGV has been detected primarily in IV drug users, clients on hemodialysis, clients with hemophilia, and in a small percentage of blood donors. It does not appear to cause important liver disease or affect the response rate of those with chronic HBV or HCV to antiviral therapy.[13]

Hepatitis affects people in three stages: the initial or preicteric stage, the icteric or jaundiced stage, and the recovery period (Table 9-3). During the *initial* or *preicteric stage*, which lasts for 1 to 3 weeks, the person experiences vague gastrointestinal (GI) and general body symptoms. Fatigue, malaise, lassitude, weight loss, and anorexia are common.

Many people develop an aversion to food, alcohol, and cigarette smoke. Nausea, vomiting, diarrhea, arthralgias,* and influenza-like symptoms may occur. The liver becomes enlarged and tender (see Fig. 4-48), and intermittent itching (pruritus) may develop. From 1 to 14 days before the icteric stage, the urine darkens and the stool lightens as less bilirubin is conjugated and excreted.

The *icteric stage* is characterized by the appearance of jaundice, which peaks in 1 to 2 weeks and persists for 6 to 8 weeks. During this stage the acuteness of the inflammation subsides. The GI symptoms begin to disappear, and after 1 to 2 weeks of jaundice the liver decreases in size and becomes less tender. During the icteric stage the post-cervical lymph nodes and spleen are enlarged (see Fig. 4-50). Persons who have been treated with human immune serum globulin (ISG) may not develop jaundice.

The *recovery stage* lasts for 3 to 4 months, during which time the person generally feels well but fatigues easily.

People with mild-to-moderate acute hepatitis rarely require hospitalization. The emphasis is on preventing the spread of infectious agents and avoiding further liver damage when the underlying cause is drug-induced or toxic hepatitis. People with fulminant (severe, sudden intensity, sometimes fatal) hepatitis require special management because of the rapid progression of their disease and the potential need for urgent liver transplantation.

An entire spectrum of rheumatic diseases can occur concomitantly with hepatitis B and hepatitis C, including transient arthralgias, vasculitis, polyarteritis nodosa, rheumatoid arthritis (RA), fibromyalgia, lymphoma, Sjögren's syndrome, and persistent synovitis. Some conditions, such as RA and fibromyalgia, occur only in association with HCV, whereas others, such as polyarteritis nodosa, are observed in association with both forms of hepatitis.[14,15]

Rheumatic manifestations of hepatitis are varied early in the course of disease and can be

---

* There is a strong association between arthralgia and age with increasing incidence of joint involvement with increased age; arthralgia in children is much less common.

TABLE 9-3 ▼ Stages of Hepatitis

Initial/preicteric (1-3 weeks)	Icteric (2-4 weeks)	Recovery (3-4 months)
Dark urine	Jaundice	Easily fatigued
Light stools	GI symptoms subside	
Vague GI symptoms	Liver decreases in size and tenderness	
Constitutional symptoms	Enlarged spleen	
Fatigue	Enlarged post cervical lymph nodes	
Malaise		
Weight loss		
Anorexia		
Nausea/vomiting		
Diarrhea		
Aversion to food, alcohol, cigarette smoke		
Enlarged and tender liver		
Intermittent pruritus (itching)		
Arthralgias		

Modified from Goodman CC, Boissonnault WG: *Pathology: implication for the physical therapist*, Philadelphia, 2003, WB Saunders, p 676.

indistinguishable from mild RA. The therapist should be suspicious of anyone with risk factors for hepatitis, including injection drug use; previous blood transfusion, especially before 1991; hemodialysis; or other exposure to blood products/body fluids, such as a health care worker (Box 9-2) or a past history of hepatitis that currently appears with arthralgias. (Case Example 9-2)

Other red flag symptoms include joint or muscle pain that is disproportionate to the physical findings and the presence of palmar tendinitis in someone with RA and positive risk factors for hepatitis.

BOX 9-2 ▼ Risk Factors for Hepatitis

- Injection drug use
- Acupuncture
- Tattoo inscription or removal
- Ear or body piercing
- Recent operative procedure
- Liver transplant recipient
- Blood or plasma transfusion before 1991
- Hemodialysis
- Health care worker exposed to blood products or body fluids
- Exposure to certain chemicals or medications
- Unprotected homosexual/bisexual activity
- Severe alcoholism
- Travel to high risk areas
- Consumption of raw shellfish

Clinical Signs and Symptoms of Hepatitis A

Hepatitis A is often acquired in childhood as a mild infection with symptoms similar to the "flu" and may be misdiagnosed or ignored. It does not usually cause lasting damage to the liver, although the following symptoms may persist for weeks:

- Extreme fatigue
- Anorexia
- Fever
- Arthralgias and myalgias (generalized aching)
- Right upper abdominal pain
- Clay-colored stools
- Dark urine
- Icterus (jaundice)
- Headache
- Pharyngitis
- Alterations in the senses of taste and smell
- Loss of desire to smoke cigarettes or drink alcohol
- Low-grade fever
- Indigestion (varying degrees of nausea, heartburn, flatulence)

Clinical Signs and Symptoms of Hepatitis B

Hepatitis B may be asymptomatic but can include
- Jaundice (changes in skin and eye color)
- Arthralgias

Continued on p. 418

CASE EXAMPLE 9-2   Hepatitis C

A 43-year-old man, 1 year following traumatic injury to the right forearm, underwent surgery to transplant his great toe to function as a thumb. The surgery took place in another state, and the man, who had been a client in our facility before surgery, returned for postoperative rehabilitation.

Complaints of hives of the involved forearm, fatigue, depression, and increased perspiration were documented but attributed by his physician to recovery from the traumatic injury and the multiple operations. Medical records from the hospital consisted of therapy notes only.

Eventually, the client developed a yellowing of the sclerae (white outer coat of the eyeballs). Medical referral was requested, and the client was evaluated by an internal medicine specialist.

Hepatitis C was diagnosed, and full medical records then obtained revealed that although the man had donated his own blood in advance for the surgery, he was short by one unit of blood, which he received through a blood bank. The blood donation was attributed as the probable source of contamination.

Continued physical therapy intervention was modified to accommodate liver impairment with particular attention paid to activity level. The therapist also observed the client carefully for signs of fluid shift, such as weight gain and orthostasis; dehydration; pneumonia; and vascular problems.

- Rash (over entire body)
- Dark urine
- Anorexia, nausea
- Painful abdominal bloating
- Fever

CHRONIC HEPATITIS

Chronic hepatitis is the term used to describe an illness associated with prolonged inflammation of the liver after unresolved viral hepatitis or associated with *chronic active hepatitis* (CAH) of unknown cause. *Chronic* is defined as inflammation of the liver for 6 months or more. The symptoms and biochemical abnormalities may continue for months or years. It is divided into CAH and *chronic persistent hepatitis* (CPH) by findings on liver biopsy.

Chronic Active Hepatitis This type of hepatitis refers to seriously destructive liver disease that can result in cirrhosis. CAH is often a result of viral infection (HBV, HCV, and HDV), but it can also be secondary to drug sensitivity (e.g., methyldopa [Aldomet], an antihypertensive medication, and isoniazid [INH], an antitubercular drug).

Steroid therapy is sometimes recommended for clients with evidence of aggressive liver inflammation and necrosis (identified by liver biopsy) as a result of these drugs. If CAH is left untreated, its course is unpredictable and may range from progressive deterioration of liver function to spontaneous remissions and exacerbations.

Steroids may be used to treat CAH. They are usually prescribed for a period of 3 to 5 years. In addition, recombinant interferon-alpha-2b injections in low doses over a 6-month period have been shown to improve hepatic function in persons with CAH. Treatment of hepatitis C is relatively new and consists of the use of interferons (IFNs), a protein naturally occurring in the healthy body in response to infection such as the hepatitis virus.

Conventional interferon (IFNs) has been used for many years in the treatment of chronic hepatitis C in clients who persistently maintain HCV/RNA blood levels. Combining interferons with the drug ribavirin has resulted in better control of chronic HCV in some individuals but the treatment is not well tolerated because of side effects from the ribavirin.[16,17]

Pegylated interferons such as Pegasys (peginterferon alpha-2a) are new, improved forms of interferons that allow a decrease in dosage and offer improved efficacy. Peginterferons (PEGs) in combination with ribavirin are now considered the standard treatment for chronic HCV infection. These new PEG interferons do not eliminate the

known side effects associated with classical interferon treatment (e.g., fatigue, headache, myalgia, fever, anxiety, irritability, GI upset).[18]

Clinical Signs and Symptoms of
Chronic Active Hepatitis

The clinical signs and symptoms of chronic active hepatitis may range from asymptomatic to the person who is bedridden with cirrhosis and advanced hepatocellular failure. In the latter the prominent signs and symptoms may reflect multisystem involvement, including

- Fatigue
- Jaundice
- Abdominal pain
- Anorexia
- Arthralgia
- Fever
- Splenomegaly and hepatomegaly
- Weakness
- Ascites (see Fig. 9-8)
- Hepatic encephalopathy

Clinical Signs and Symptoms of
Chronic Persistent Hepatitis

- Right upper quadrant pain
- Anorexia
- Mild fatigue
- Malaise

Metabolic Disease The most common metabolic diseases that can cause chronic hepatitis and are of interest to a physical therapist are Wilson's disease and hematochromatosis, also termed *hemochromatosis*. Both these diseases are dealt with in greater detail as metabolic disorders in Chapter 11.

Wilson's disease is an autosomal recessive disorder in which biliary excretion of copper is impaired, and, as a consequence, total body copper is progressively increased. There may be mild-to-severe neurologic dysfunction, depending on the rate of hepatocyte injury.

Hemochromatosis is the most common genetic disorder (autosomal recessive defect in iron absorption) causing liver failure. Excessive iron is stored in various parenchymal organs with subsequent development of fibrosis. Arthralgias and arthropathy may develop and are often confused with RA or osteoarthritis. The second and third metacarpophalangeal joints are usually involved first.

Knees, hips, shoulders, and lower back may be affected. Acute synovitis with pseudogout of the knees has been observed.

NONVIRAL HEPATITIS

Nonviral hepatitis is considered to be a toxic or drug-induced form of liver inflammation. This type of hepatitis occurs secondary to exposure to alcohol, certain chemicals, or drugs such as anti-inflammatories, anticonvulsants, antibiotics, cytotoxic drugs for the treatment of cancer, antituberculars, radiographic contrast agents for diagnostic testing, antipsychotics, and antidepressants (Box 9-3).

Acetaminophen, the popular OTC pain reliever has been found to be the leading cause of sudden liver failure in adults in the United States. The drug is safe when taken properly, but even a small overdose in some people can trigger sudden liver failure. The use of this drug becomes even more dangerous with taken by individuals with an already impaired liver.[19]

The mechanism by which these agents induce overt injury may be dose-related and predictable or idiosyncratic and unpredictable, with the latter caused by an unusual susceptibility of the individual. Some drugs (e.g., oral contraceptives) may impair liver function and produce jaundice without causing necrosis, fatty infiltration of liver cells, or a hypersensitivity reaction.

Clinical Signs and Symptoms of
Toxic and Drug-Induced Hepatitis

These vary with the severity of liver damage and the causative agent. In most individuals symptoms resemble those of acute viral hepatitis:

- Anorexia, nausea, vomiting
- Fatigue and malaise
- Jaundice
- Dark urine
- Clay-colored stools
- Headache, dizziness, drowsiness (carbon tetrachloride poisoning)
- Fever, rash, arthralgias, epigastric or right upper quadrant pain (halothane anesthetic)

Cirrhosis

Cirrhosis is a chronic hepatic disease characterized by the destruction of liver cells and by the replacement of connective tissue by fibrous bands. As the liver becomes more and more scarred (fibrosed), blood and lymph flow become impaired, causing hepatic insufficiency and increased clinical manifestations. The causes of cirrhosis can be varied,

although alcohol abuse is the most common cause of liver disease in the United States.

In addition, about 25% of Americans have a problem called nonalcoholic fatty liver disease (NAFLD), defined as fatty infiltration of the liver

---

BOX 9-3 ▲ Common Hepatotoxic Agents

Analgesics
Acetaminophen
Aspirin
Diclofenac

Anesthetics
Halothane
Enflurane
Methoxyflurane
Chloroform

Anticonvulsants
Valproic acid
Phenytoin
Carbamazepine
Lamotrigine

Antidepressants/ antipsychotics
Monamine oxidase (MAO) inhibitors
Chlorpromazine and other phenothiazines

Antineoplastics
Methotrexate (related to cumulative dose)
Mercaptopurine
L-asparaginase
Carmustine, lomustine
Streptozocin

Antimicrobials
Chloramphenicol
Isoniazid (antitubercular)
Oxacillin
Erythromycin estolate
Novobiocin
Ketoconazole (antifungal)
Nitrofurantoin
Sulfonamides (class)
Minocycline
Tetracyclines (class)
Efavirenz (antiviral)
Nevirapine (antiviral)
Ritonavir (antiviral)

Cardiovascular
Quinidine sulfate
Amiodarone
Methyldopa

Hormonal
Oral contraceptives
Anabolic steroids
Oral hypoglycemics

Recreational Drugs
Alcohol
Cocaine
Ecstasy

Vitamins
Vitamin A (large doses)
Niacin (large doses)

Other
Carbon tetrachloride
Poisonous mushrooms
Heavy metals
Phosphorus
Tannic acid
Propylthiouracil
Diagnostic contrast agents

exceeding 5% to 10% by weight. NAFLD is an illness closely associated with diabetes and obesity and may make liver damage caused by other agents (e.g., alcohol, industrial toxins, hepatatrophic viruses) worse.[20]

Ten to 20% of people with NAFLD will develop liver inflammation leading to liver scarring and cirrhosis.[21] Prevention and treatment of both diabetes and obesity, and protection of the liver from toxins can help to limit the course of this disease.

The activity level of the client with damage from chronic liver impairment is determined by the symptoms. Because hepatic blood flow diminishes with moderate exercise, rest periods are advised and are adjusted according to the level of fatigue experienced by the client both during the exercise and afterward at home.

The person may return to work with medical approval but is advised to avoid straining, such as lifting heavy objects if portal hypertension and esophageal varices are a problem. Because stress decreases hepatic blood flow, any reduction of stress at home, at work, or during treatment is therapeutic.

Clinical Signs and Symptoms of
Cirrhosis

- Mild right upper quadrant pain (progressive)
- GI symptoms
  - Anorexia
  - Indigestion
  - Weight loss
  - Nausea and vomiting
  - Diarrhea or constipation
- Dull abdominal ache
- Ease of fatigue (with mild exertion)
- Weakness
- Fever

PROGRESSION OF CIRRHOSIS

As the cirrhosis progresses and hepatic insufficiency develops, a series of conditions emerges, including portal hypertension, ascites, and esophageal varices. Late symptoms affecting the entire body develop (Table 9-4).

Portal hypertension is elevated pressure in the portal vein (through which blood passes from the GI tract and spleen to the liver), occurring as portal blood meets increased resistance to flow in the fibrotic liver. The blood then backs up into esophageal, stomach, and splenic structures and bypasses the liver through collateral vessels.

Clinical Signs and Symptoms of
Portal Hypertension

- Ascites (see Fig. 9-8)
- Dilated collateral veins
  - Esophageal varices (upper GI)
  - Hemorrhoids (lower GI)
- Splenomegaly (enlargement of the spleen)
- Thrombocytopenia (decreased number of blood platelets for clotting)

Ascites is an abnormal accumulation of fluid containing large amounts of protein and electrolytes in the peritoneal cavity as a result of portal backup and loss of proteins (Fig. 9-8). For the physical therapist, abdominal hernias and lumbar lordosis observed in clients with ascites may present symptoms that mimic musculoskeletal involvement, such as groin or low-back pain (Case Example 9-3).

Esophageal varices are dilated veins of the lower esophagus that occur as a result of portal vein blood backup. These varices are thin-walled and can rupture, causing severe hemorrhage and sometimes death.

Clinical Signs and Symptoms of
Hemorrhage Associated with Esophageal Varices

- Restlessness
- Pallor
- Tachycardia
- Cooling of the skin
- Hypotension

Hepatic Encephalopathy (Hepatic Coma)

Hepatic coma is a neurologic disorder resulting from the inability of the liver to detoxify ammonia (produced from protein breakdown) in the intestine. Increased serum levels of ammonia are directly toxic to central and peripheral nervous system function, causing an array of neurologic symptoms. Flapping tremors (asterixis) and numbness/tingling (misinterpreted as carpal/tarsal tunnel syndrome) are common symptoms of this ammonia abnormality.

CLINICAL SIGNS AND SYMPTOMS

Clinical manifestations of hepatic encephalopathy vary, depending on the severity of neurologic involvement, and develop in four stages as the ammonia level increases in the serum. The accompanying clinical features are presented in Table 9-5.

TABLE 9-4 ▼ Clinical Manifestations of Cirrhosis

Body system	Clinical manifestations
Respiratory	Limited thoracic expansion (caused by ascites) Hypoxia Dyspnea Cyanosis Clubbing
Central nervous system (progressive to hepatic coma)	Subtle changes in mental acuity (progressive) Mild memory loss Poor reasoning ability Irritability Paranoia and hallucinations Slurred speech Asterixis (tremor of outstretched hands) Peripheral neuritis Peripheral muscle atrophy
Hematologic	Impaired coagulation/bleeding tendencies Nosebleeds Easy bruising Bleeding gums Anemia (usually caused by GI blood loss from esophageal varices)
Endocrine (caused by liver's inability to metabolize hormones)	Testicular atrophy Menstrual irregularities Gynecomastia (excessive development of breasts in men) Loss of chest and axillary hair
Integument (cutaneous and skin)	Severe pruritus (itching) Extreme dryness Poor tissue turgor Abnormal pigmentation Prominent spider angiomas Palmar erythema
Hepatic	Hepatomegaly (enlargement of the liver) Ascites Edema of the legs Hepatic encephalopathy (see Table 9-5)
Gastrointestinal (GI)	Anorexia Nausea Vomiting Diarrhea

For the physical therapist, the inpatient with impending hepatic coma has difficulty in ambulating and is unsteady. Protection from falling and seizure precautions must be taken. Skin breakdown in a client who is malnourished because of liver disease, immobile, jaundiced, and edematous can occur in less than 24 hours. Careful attention to skin care, passive exercise, and frequent changes in position are required.

Newborn Jaundice

Jaundice affects approximately 60% of newborn infants because liver function is somewhat slow to develop in the first few days of life. In a small percentage of infants, extreme jaundice can occur and if left untreated for too long can result in brain damage from toxic levels of bilirubin in the blood. It is critically important for all newborns to be screened for the development of this condition. Development of any color change in newborns needs immediate referral and testing for abnormal bilirubin levels.[23]

Liver Abscess

A liver abscess occurs when bacteria or protozoa destroy hepatic tissue and produce a cavity that

making it a primary metastatic site for tumors of the stomach, colorectum, and pancreas. It is also a common site for metastases from other primary cancers such as esophagus, lung, and breast.

Primary liver tumors (hepatocellular carcinoma [HCC]) are often associated with cirrhosis but can be linked to other predisposing factors, such as fungal infection (common in moldy foods of Africa), viral hepatitis, excessive use of anabolic steroids, trauma, nutritional deficiencies, and exposure to hepatotoxins.

Cholangiocarcinoma (CCC), a serious and often fatal form of liver cancer, is the second most common form of hepatic malignancy. CCC originates from the epithelium of the bile ducts and has many of the same risk factors as HCC, but pre-existing biliary disease is the primary risk factor.[24]

Several types of benign and malignant hepatic neoplasms can result from the administration of chemical agents. For example, adenoma (a benign tumor) can occur in recipients of oral contraceptives. Regression of the tumor occurs after withdrawal of the drug.

In most instances interference with liver function does not occur until approximately 80% to 90% of the liver is replaced by metastatic carcinoma or primary carcinoma. Signs of liver impairment are often late in the presentation making early detection and successful treatment less likely. The alert physical therapist may be the first to identify liver involvement when the neuromuscular or musculoskeletal systems are affected.

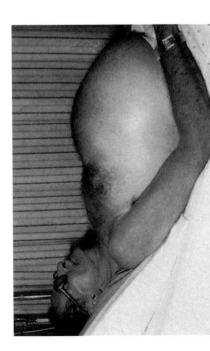

Fig. 9-8 • Ascites is an abnormal accumulation of serous (edematous) fluid in the peritoneal cavity associated with liver impairment, especially the portal and hepatic venous hypertension that accompanies cirrhosis of the liver. This condition also may be associated with other disorders such as advanced congestive heart failure, constrictive pericarditis, and hyperaldosteronism. Any condition affecting the peritoneum by producing increased permeability of the peritoneal capillaries and electrolyte disturbances can result in ascites. (From Swartz M: *Textbook of physical diagnosis: health and examination,* Philadelphia, 1989, WB Saunders.)

fills with infectious organisms, liquefied liver cells, and leukocytes. Necrotic tissue then isolates the cavity from the rest of the liver.

Even though liver abscess is relatively uncommon, it carries a mortality of 30% to 50%. This rate rises to more than 80% with multiple abscesses or other complications.

Clinical Signs and Symptoms of
Liver Abscess

Clinical signs and symptoms of liver abscess depend on the degree of involvement; some people are acutely ill, others are asymptomatic. Depending on the type of abscess, the onset may be sudden or insidious. The most common signs include

- Right abdominal pain
- Right shoulder pain
- Weight loss
- Fever, chills
- Diaphoresis
- Nausea and vomiting
- Anemia

Liver Cancer

Metastatic tumors to the liver occur 20 times more often than primary liver tumors. The liver filters blood coming from the gastrointestinal tract,

Clinical Signs and Symptoms of
Liver Neoplasm

If clinical signs and symptoms of liver neoplasm do occur (whether of primary or metastatic origin), these may include:

- Jaundice (icterus)
- Progressive failure of health
- Anorexia and weight loss
- Overall muscular weakness
- Epigastric fullness and pain or discomfort
- Constant ache in the epigastrium or mid-back
- Early satiety (cystic tumors)

GALLBLADDER AND DUCT DISEASES

Cholelithiasis

Gallstones are stonelike masses called calculi (singular: calculus) that form in the gallbladder possibly as a result of changes in the normal components of bile. Although there are two types

A 69-year-old man was seen at the Veteran's Administration (VA) Hospital outpatient physical therapy department following a left total hip replacement (THR) 2 weeks ago. The surgery was performed at a civilian hospital, but all his follow up care is through the VA. He had a long history of alcohol and tobacco use and medical intervention for heart disease, hypertension, and peripheral vascular disease.

The medical problem list (established by the physician) included

Liver cirrhosis secondary to alcoholism

Ascites secondary to portal hypertension

Coronary artery disease with hypertension

Peripheral vascular disease (arterial)

Mild vision loss secondary to macular degeneration

The client was referred to physical therapy for rehabilitation following his THR. During the examination the client reported various other musculoskeletal aches and pains including chronic low back pain present off and on for the last 6 months and new onset of groin pain on the left side (just since the THR).

Ascites can be a cause of low back and/or groin pain. How do you screen this client for a medical (vascular, liver) cause of the groin pain?

Past Medical History

Past history of cancer of any kind

Past history of abdominal or inguinal hernia

Clinical Presentation

Ask additional questions about pain pattern as discussed in Chapter 3

What do you think is causing your groin pain? Watch for red flag for possible vascular involvement; client describes pain as "throbbing"

Pain is worse 5 to 10 minutes after the start of activity involving the lower extremities and relieved by rest (intermittent claudication)

Visual inspection and palpation including observing for postural components (e.g., lumbar lordosis associated with ascites) as a contributing factor, abdominal or inguinal hernia, liver palpation, and lymph node palpation

Perform stretching and resistive movements to eliminate, reproduce, or aggravate symptoms; you may be limited in this assessment area because of THR precautions

Red flag: pain is not altered by stretching or resistive movement; pain cannot be reproduced with palpation

Past Medical History

Past history of cancer of any kind

Past history of abdominal or inguinal hernia

Assess for trigger points (e.g., adductor magnus) keeping in mind that common systemic perpetuating factors with myofascial pain include anemia and hypothyroidism as well as vitamin deficiency common with chronic alcohol use. Further screening may require assessing for risk factors and associated signs and symptoms for each of these conditions

Associated Signs and Symptoms

Ask the client about any other symptoms of any kind that may have developed just before or around the time of the onset of groin pain; offer some suggestions from the Overview section that appears later in this chapter.

As mentioned above, the therapist may have to ask about the presence of signs and symptoms associated with anemia and endocrine disease.

Should you send this client back to the doctor before continuing with physical therapy intervention?

It is very likely that this client will require referral to his physician. Your referral decision will be dependent on your findings, of course. For example, the presence of trigger points may warrant treatment first and reassessment for change in clinical presentation before making a final decision. Given the movement precautions this soon after a THR may prevent you from using positional release or stretch positions for trigger points. You may have to use alternate methods of trigger point release.

Remember true hip pain is often felt in the groin or deep buttock. There could be a problem with the hip implant (e.g., fracture, infection, loosening) causing the groin pain. There will be pain with active or passive motion of the hip joint. The pain increases with weight bearing.[22] If the physician does not know about this new groin pain, medical referral to reevaluate the implant is needed before continuing with a THR rehab protocol.

By continuing the screening process, the therapist can provide the physician with additional information to describe the problem. Communication is an important key element in the referral process. Provide the physician with a *brief* summary of your findings including a list of any unusual findings (see further discussion regarding physician in Chapter 1).

TABLE 9-5 ▼ Hepatic Encephalopathy

	Stages of Hepatic Encephalopathy		
Stage I (prodromal stage)	Stage II (impending stage)	Stage III (stuporous stage)	Stage IV (comatose stage)
Subtle symptoms may be overlooked	Tremor progresses to asterixis (liver flap)	Client can still be aroused	Client cannot be aroused; responds only to painful stimuli
Slight personality changes: Disorientation Confusion Euphoria or depression Forgetfulness Slurred speech	Resistance to passive movement (increased muscle tone) Lethargy Aberrant behavior Apraxia* Ataxia Facial grimacing and blinking	Hyperventilation Marked confusion Abusive and violent Noisy, incoherent speech Asterixis (liver flap) Muscle rigidity Positive Babinski† reflex Hyperactive deep tendon reflexes	No asterixis Positive Babinski reflex Hepatic fetor (musty, sweet odor to the breath caused by the liver's inability to metabolize the amino acid methionine)

* This type of motor apraxia can be best observed by keeping a record of the client's handwriting and drawings of simple shapes, such as a circle, square, triangle, rectangle. Check for progressive deterioration.
† A reflex action of the toes that is normal during infancy but abnormal after 12 to 18 months. It is elicited by a firm stimulus (usually scraping with the handle of a reflex hammer) on the sole of the foot from the heel along the lateral border of the sole to the little toe, across the ball of the foot to the big toe. Normally such a stimulus causes all the toes to flex downward. A positive Babinski reflex occurs when the great toe flexes upward and the smaller toes fan outward.

of stones, pigment and cholesterol stones, most types of gallstone disease in the United States, Europe, and Africa are associated with cholesterol stones.

Cholelithiasis, the presence or formation of gallstones, can be asymptomatic, detected incidentally during medical imaging. Problems arise if a stone leaves the gallbladder and causes obstruction somewhere else in the biliary system, presenting as biliary colic, cholecystitis, or cholangitis.

Cholelithiasis is the fifth leading cause of hospitalization among adults and accounts for 90% of all gallbladder and duct diseases. The incidence of gallstones increases with age, occurring in more than 40% of people older than 70. See Box 9-4 for risk factors to watch for in a client's history that correlate with the incidence of gallstones.

Clients with gallstones may be asymptomatic or may have symptoms of a gallbladder attack described in the next section. The prognosis is usually good with medical treatment, depending on the severity of disease, presence of infection, and response to antibiotics.

BOX 9-4 ▼ Risk Factors for Gallstones

- Age: Incidence increases with age
- Sex: Women are affected more than men before age 60
- Elevated estrogen levels
  Pregnancy
  Oral contraceptives
  Hormone therapy
  Multiparity (woman who has had two or more pregnancies resulting in viable offspring)
- Obesity
- Diet: High cholesterol, low fiber
- Diabetes mellitus
- Liver disease
- Rapid weight loss or fasting
- Taking cholesterol-lowering drugs (statins)
- Ethnicity (Stronger genetic predisposition in Native Americans, Mexican Americans)
- Genetics (family history of gallstones)

Biliary Colic

With biliary colic, the stone gets lodged in the neck of the gallbladder (cystic duct). Pain results as the gallbladder contracts and tries to push the stone through. The classic symptom of this problem is right upper abdominal pain that comes and goes in waves. The pain builds to a peak and then fades away.

Obstructions of the gallbladder can result in biliary stasis, delayed gallbladder emptying, and subsequent mixed stone formation. Stasis and delayed gallbladder emptying can occur with any pathologic conditions of the liver, hormonal influences, and pregnancy (usually third trimester when the developing fetus compresses the mother's gallbladder up against the liver).

Cholecystitis

Cholecystitis, blockage, or impaction of gallstones in the cystic duct (Fig. 9-9) leads to infection or inflammation of the gallbladder. This condition may be acute or chronic, causing painful distension of the gallbladder. The affected individual may feel

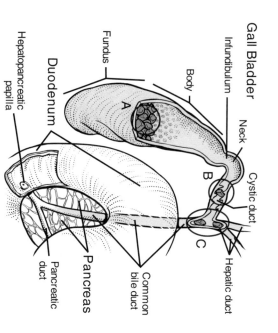

Gall Bladder

Infundibulum

Neck

Body

Fundus

Cystic duct

Hepatic duct

Duodenum

Common bile duct

Pancreas

Pancreatic duct

Hepatopancreatic papilla

Fig. 9-9 • The gallbladder and its divisions: fundus, body, infundibulum, and neck. **A,** Cholelithiasis, the presence or formation of gallstones, can be asymptomatic, detected incidentally during medical imaging. Problems arise if a stone leaves the gallbladder and causes obstruction somewhere else in the biliary system. **B,** If a gallstone enters the cystic duct and becomes lodged there, it can lead to cholecystitis (inflammation of the gallbladder). **C,** Obstruction of either the hepatic or common bile duct by stone or spasm blocks the exit of bile from the liver where it is formed. Jaundice is often the first symptom. If an infection develops and backs up into the liver, a condition called cholangitis can occur, a potentially life-threatening problem.

steady, severe pain that increases rapidly, lasting several minutes to several hours. Nausea, vomiting, and fever may be present.

Other causes of acute cholecystitis may be typhoid fever or a malignant tumor obstructing the biliary tract. Whatever the cause of the obstruction, the normal flow of bile is interrupted and the gallbladder becomes distended and ischemic.

Gallstones may also cause chronic cholecystitis (persistent gallbladder inflammation), in which the gallbladder atrophies and becomes fibrotic, adhering to adjacent organs. It is not unusual for affected clients to have repeated episodes before seeking medical attention.

Cholangitis

Gallstones lodged further down in the system in the common bile duct can cause cholangitis. Blocking the flow of bile at this point in the biliary tree can lead to jaundice. Infection can develop here and travel up to the liver, becoming a potentially life-threatening situation.

Clinical Signs and Symptoms

The typical pain of gallbladder disease has been described as colicky pain that occurs in the right upper quadrant of the abdomen after the person has eaten a meal that is high in fat (although food that provokes an attack of pain does not need to be "fatty"). However, the pain is not necessarily limited to the right upper quadrant, and more likely than not, it is constant, not colicky.

Like the stomach, pylorus, and duodenum, the liver and gallbladder can cause spasm of the rectus abdominis muscles above the umbilicus. This occurs when disturbances within the hepatic and biliary systems as part of the overall gastrointestinal system affect motor reflexes.

These disturbances can be reflected in muscular contractions of the spinal, abdominal, and other muscles supplied by the motor nerves from the anterior horn of the segment innervating the affected viscera.[25]

It looks just like a musculoskeletal problem, but the pain pattern is the result of viscero-somatic reflexes as discussed in Chapter 3 (Case Example 9-4). Ask about the timing of symptoms in relation to eating or drinking. Watch for symptoms that are worse immediately after eating (gallbladder inflammation) or pain and nausea 1 to 3 hours after eating (gallstones).

Muscle guarding and tenderness of the spinal musculature in the presence of constitutional symptoms (e.g., fever, sweats, chills, nausea) is another red flag. Ask about a previous history of

CASE EXAMPLE 9-4   Gallbladder Pain

A 48-year-old schoolteacher was admitted to the hospital following an episode of intense, sharp pain that started in the epigastric region and radiated around her thorax to the interscapular area. Her gallbladder had been removed 2 years ago, but she remarked that her current symptoms were "exactly like a gallbladder attack." The client was referred to physical therapy for "back care/education" on the day of discharge.

On examination, the client was in acute distress, unable to tolerate a full examination. She had not been able to transfer or ambulate independently. She was instructed in relaxation and breathing techniques to reduce her extreme level of anxiety associated with pain and given supportive reassurance. Instruction and assistance were provided in all transfers to minimize pain and maximize independent function. Given

her discharge status, outpatient physical therapy was recommended for follow up intervention.

She returned to physical therapy as planned and was provided with a back care program. She was also treated locally for scar tissue adhesion at the site of the gallbladder removal. Symptomatic relief was obtained in the first two sessions without recurrence of symptoms.

This case example is included to demonstrate how scar tissue associated with organ removal can reproduce visceral symptoms that are actually of musculoskeletal origin—the opposite concept of what is presented in this text. This may be more of an example of cellular memories sustaining a viscero-somatic reflex via the action of neuropeptides at the cellular level (see discussion of Psychoneuroimmunology in Chapter 3).

GI, liver, or gallbladder problems and review client's risk factors for hepatic involvement.

In the case of gallbladder disease, it is also possible to get tender points in the soma corresponding to visceral innervation. A gallbladder problem can result in a sore 10th rib tip (right side anteriorly) when messages from the viscera entering the spinal cord at the same level as the innervation of the rib are misinterpreted as a somatic problem. The gallbladder has most of its innervation from the right side of the cervical ganglia to the splanchnic nerves, which explains the predominance of right-sided somatic symptoms.

When visceral and cutaneous fibers enter the spinal cord at the same level, the nervous system may respond with sudomotor changes such as pruritus (itching of the skin) or a sore rib, instead of gallbladder symptoms. The clinical presentation appears as a biomechanical problem such as a rib dysfunction instead of nausea and food intolerances normally associated with gallbladder dysfunction.

Likewise, from our understanding of viscerogenic pain patterns based on embryologic development, we know that the visceral pericardium of the heart (see Fig. 6-5) is derived from the same embryologic tissue as the gallbladder. A gallbladder problem can also cause referred pain to the heart and must be ruled out by the physician as a possible cause of chest pain.

Clinical Signs and Symptoms of
Acute Cholecystitis

- Chills, low-grade fever
- Jaundice
- GI symptoms
- Nausea
- Anorexia
- Vomiting
- Tenderness over the gallbladder
- Tenderness on the tip of the 10th rib (right side anteriorly); called a "hot rib;" can also affect 11th and 12th ribs (right anterior)
- Severe pain in the right upper quadrant and epigastrium (increases on inspiration and movement)
- Pain radiating into the right shoulder and between the scapulae

Clinical Signs and Symptoms of
Chronic Cholecystitis

These may be vague or a sense of indigestion and abdominal discomfort after eating, unless a stone leaves the gallbladder and causes obstruction of the common duct (called choledocholithiasis), causing
- Biliary colic: severe, steady pain for 3 to 4 hours in the right upper quadrant

- Pain: may radiate to the mid-back between the scapulae (caused by splanchnic fibers synapsing with phrenic nerve fibers)
- Nausea (intolerance of fatty foods; decreased bile production results in decreased fat digestion)
- Abdominal fullness
- Heartburn
- Excessive belching
- Constipation and diarrhea

Primary Biliary Cirrhosis

Primary biliary cirrhosis (PBC) is a chronic, progressive, inflammatory disease of the liver that involves primarily the intrahepatic bile ducts and results in impairment of bile secretion. The disease, which often affects middle-aged women, begins with pruritus or biochemical evidence of cholestasis and progresses at a variable rate to jaundice, portal hypertension, and liver failure.

The cause of PBC is unknown, although various factors are being investigated. Many clients have associated autoimmune features, particularly Sjögren's syndrome, autoimmune thyroiditis, and renal tubular acidosis. In more rare cases, clients may exhibit sensory peripheral neuropathies of the hands and feet.

The most significant clinical problem for clients with PBC is bone disease characterized by impaired osteoblastic activity and accelerated osteoclastic activity. Calcium and vitamin D should be carefully monitored and appropriate replacement instituted. Physical activity following an osteoporosis protocol should be encouraged.

No specific treatment has been established yet for PBC other than liver transplantation or supportive measures for the clinical symptoms described.

Clinical Signs and Symptoms of
Primary Biliary Cirrhosis

- Pruritus
- Jaundice
- GI bleeding
- Ascites (see Fig. 9-8)
- Fatigue
- Right upper quadrant pain (posterior)
- Sensory neuropathy of hands/feet (rare)
- Osteoporosis (decreased bone mass)
- Osteomalacia (softening of the bones)
- Burning, pins and needles, prickling of the eyes
- Muscle cramping

Gallbladder Cancer

Gallbladder cancer is closely associated with gallstone disease, is usually late in diagnosis, and often has a very poor outcome. The primary associated risk factors include cholelithiasis (especially symptomatic, untreated), obesity, reproductive abnormalities, chronic gallbladder infections, and exposure to radon and certain industrial exposures including cellulose acetate fiber manufacturing. Testing and treatment of symptomatic gallstones is the only preventative measure identified at this time for gallbladder cancer.[26]

▲ PHYSICIAN REFERRAL

A careful history and close observation of the client are important in determining whether a person may need a medical referral for possible hepatic or biliary involvement. Any client with mid-back, scapular, or right shoulder pain (see Table 9-1) without a history of trauma (e.g., forceful movement of the spine, repetitive movements of the shoulder or back, or easy lifting) should be screened for possible systemic origin of symptoms.

For the physical therapist treating the inpatient population, jaundice in the postoperative individual is not uncommon, but can be a potentially serious complication of surgery and anesthesia.

Clinical management of jaundice is complicated by anything capable of damaging the liver, including physical stress associated with physical therapy intervention. Hypoxemia, blood loss, infection, and administration of multiple drugs can add additional physical stress.

When making the referral, it is important to report to the physician the results of your objective findings, especially when there is a lack of physical evidence to support a musculoskeletal lesion. The Special Questions to Ask may assist in assessing the client's overall health status.

Guidelines to Immediate
Physician Referral

- New onset of myopathy in any client, but especially the older adult, with a history of statin use (cholesterol-lowering drugs); look for other risk factors and other signs and symptoms of liver or renal impairment.

Guidelines to Physician Referral

- Obvious signs of hepatic disease, especially with a history of previous cancer or risk factors for hepatitis (see Box 9-2)

- Development of arthralgias of unknown cause in anyone with a previous history of hepatitis or risk factors for hepatitis
- Presence of bilateral carpal tunnel syndrome accompanied by bilateral tarsal tunnel syndrome unknown to the physician, asterixis, or other associated hepatic signs and symptoms
- Presence of sensory neuropathy of unknown cause accompanied by signs and symptoms associated with hepatic system impairment

Clues to Screening for Hepatic Disease

- Right shoulder/scapular and/or upper mid-back pain of unknown cause (see also Clues to Screening Shoulder Pain, Chapter 18)
- Shoulder motion is not limited by painful symptoms; client is unable to localize or pinpoint pain or tenderness
- Presence of GI symptoms, especially if there is any correlation between eating and painful symptoms
- Bilateral carpal/tarsal tunnel syndrome, especially of unknown origin; check for other signs of liver impairment such as liver flap, liver palms, and skin or nail bed changes (see Box 9-1)

- Personal history of cancer, liver, or gallbladder disease
- Personal history of hepatitis, especially with joint pain associated with rheumatoid arthritis or fibromyalgia accompanied by palmar tendinitis
- Recent history of statin use (cholesterol-lowering drugs such as Zocor, Lipitor, Crestor) or other hepatotoxic drugs
- Recent operative procedure (possible postoperative jaundice)
- Recent (within last 6 months) injection drug use, tattoo (receiving or removal), acupuncture, ear or body piercing, dialysis, blood or plasma transfusion, active homosexual activity, heterosexual sexual activity with homosexuals, consumption of raw shellfish (hepatitis)
- Changes in skin (yellow hue, spider angiomas, palmar erythema) or eye color (jaundice)
- Employment or lifestyle involving alcohol consumption (jaundice)
- Contact with jaundiced persons (health care worker handling blood or body fluids, dialysis clients, injection drug users, active homosexual sexual activity, heterosexual sexual activity with homosexuals)

▼ **LIVER PAIN** (Fig. 9-10)

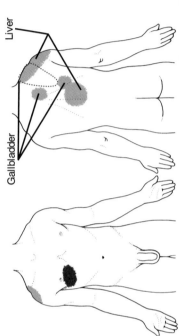

Fig. 9-10 ● The primary pain pattern from the liver, gallbladder, and common bile duct (*dark red*) presents typically in the midepigastrium or right upper quadrant of the abdomen. Innervation of the liver and biliary system is through the autonomic nervous system from T5 to T11 (see Fig. 3-3). Liver impairment is primarily reflected through the 9th thoracic distribution. Referred pain (*light red*) from the liver occurs in the thoracic spine from approximately T7 to T10 and/or to the right of midline, possibly affecting the right shoulder (right phrenic nerve). Referred pain from the gallbladder can affect the right shoulder by the same mechanism. The gallbladder can also refer pain to the right interscapular (T4 or T5 to T8) or right subscapular area.

OVERVIEW

LIVER/BILIARY PAIN PATTERNS—cont'd

Location:	Pain in the midepigastrium or right upper quadrant (RUQ) of abdomen
Referral:	Pain over the liver, especially after exercise (hepatitis) RUQ pain may be associated with right shoulder pain Both RUQ and epigastrium pain may be associated with back pain between the scapulae Pain may be referred to the right side of the midline in the interscapular or subscapular area (T7-T10)
Description:	Dull abdominal aching Sense of fullness of the abdomen or epigastrium
Intensity:	Mild at first, then increases steadily
Duration:	Constant

Associated signs and symptoms:	Nausea, anorexia (viral hepatitis)
	Early satiety (cystic tumors)
	Aversion to smoking for smokers (viral hepatitis)
	Aversion to alcohol (hepatitis)
	Arthralgias and myalgias (hepatitis A, B, or C)
	Headaches (hepatitis A, drug-induced hepatitis)
	Dizziness/drowsiness (drug-induced hepatitis)
	Low-grade fever (hepatitis A)
	Pharyngitis (hepatitis A)
	Extreme fatigue (hepatitis A, cirrhosis)
	Alterations in the sense of taste and smell (hepatitis A)
	Rash (hepatitis B)
	Dark urine, light- or clay-colored stools
	Ascites (see Fig. 9-8)
	Edema and oliguria
	Neurologic symptoms (hepatic encephalopathy)
	    Confusion, forgetfulness
	    Muscle tremors
	    Asterixis (Liver flap)
	    Slurred speech
	    Impaired handwriting
	Skin and nail bed changes
	Skin pallor (often linked with cirrhosis or carcinoma)
	Jaundice (skin and sclerae changes)
	Spider angiomas
	Palmar erythema (liver palms)
	Nail beds of Terry; leukonychia; digital clubbing; koilonychia
	Bleeding disorders
	    Purpura
	    Ecchymosis
	Diaphoresis (liver abscess)
	Overall muscular weakness (cirrhosis, liver carcinoma)
	Peripheral neuropathy (chronic liver disease)

Possible etiology:	Any liver disease
	    Hepatitis
	    Cirrhosis
	    Metastatic tumors
	Pancreatic carcinoma
	Liver abscess
	Medications: Use of hepatotoxic drugs

OVERVIEW LIVER/BILIARY PAIN PATTERNS—cont'd

▼ GALLBLADDER PAIN (see Fig. 9-10)

Location: Pain in the midepigastrium (may be perceived as heartburn)

Referral: RUQ of abdomen

RUQ pain may be associated with right shoulder pain

Both may be associated with back pain between the scapulae; back pain can occur alone as the primary symptom

Pain may be referred to the right side of the midline in the interscapular or subscapular area

Anterior rib pain (soreness or tender) at the tip of the 10th rib (less often, can also affect ribs 11 and 12)

Description: Dull aching

Deep visceral pain (gallbladder suddenly distends)

Biliary carcinoma is more persistent and boring

Intensity: Mild at first, then increases steadily to become severe

Duration: 2 to 3 hours

Aggravating factors: Respiratory inspiration

Eating

Upper body movement

Lying down

Associated signs and symptoms:
Dark urine, light stools

Jaundice

Skin: Green hue (prolonged biliary obstruction)

Persistent pruritus (cholestatic jaundice)

Pain and nausea occur 1 to 3 hours after eating (gallstones)

Pain immediately after eating (gallbladder inflammation)

Intolerance of fatty foods or heavy meals

Indigestion, nausea

Excessive belching

Flatulence (excessive intestinal gas)

Anorexia

Weight loss (gallbladder cancer)

Bleeding from skin and mucous membranes (late sign of gallbladder cancer)

Vomiting

Feeling of fullness

Low-grade fever, chills

Possible etiology: Gallstones (cholelithiasis)

Gallbladder inflammation (cholecystitis)

Neoplasm

Medications: Use of hepatotoxic drugs

▼ COMMON BILE DUCT PAIN (see Fig. 9-10)

Location: Pain in midepigastrium or RUQ of abdomen

Epigastrium: Heartburn (choledocholithiasis)

Referral: RUQ pain may be associated with right shoulder pain

Both may be associated with back pain between the scapulae

Pain may be referred to the right side of the midline in the interscapular or subscapular area

OVERVIEW

LIVER/BILIARY PAIN PATTERNS—cont'd

Description:	Dull aching
	Vague discomfort (pressure within common bile duct increasing)
	Severe, steady pain in RUQ (choledocholithiasis)
	Biliary carcinoma is more persistent and boring
Intensity:	Mild at first, increases steadily
Duration:	Constant
	3 to 4 hours (choledocholithiasis)
Associated signs and symptoms:	Dark urine, light stools
	Jaundice
	Nausea after eating
	Intolerance of fatty foods or heavy meals
	Feeling of abdominal fullness
	Skin: Green hue (prolonged biliary obstruction); pruritus (skin itching)
	Low-grade fever, chills
	Excessive belching (choledocholithiasis)
	Constipation and diarrhea (choledocholithiasis)
	Sensory neuropathy (primary biliary cirrhosis)
	Osteomalacia (primary biliary cirrhosis)
	Osteoporosis (primary biliary cirrhosis)
Possible etiology:	Common duct stones
	Common duct stricture (previous gallbladder surgery)
	Pancreatic carcinoma (blocking the bile duct)
	Medications: Use of hepatotoxic drugs
	Neoplasm
	Primary biliary cirrhosis
	Choledocholithiasis (obstruction of common duct)

🕐 KEY POINTS TO REMEMBER

✓ Primary signs and symptoms of liver diseases vary and can include GI symptoms, edema/ascites, dark urine, light-colored or clay-colored feces, and right upper abdominal pain.

✓ Neurologic symptoms, such as confusion, muscle tremors, and asterixis may occur.

✓ Skin changes associated with the hepatic system include pruritus, jaundice, pallor, orange or green skin, bruising, spider angiomas, and palmar erythema.

✓ Active, intense exercise should be avoided when the liver is compromised (jaundice or other active disease).

✓ Antiinflammatory and minor analgesic agents can cause drug-induced hepatitis. Nonviral hepatitis may occur postoperatively.

✓ When liver dysfunction results in increased serum ammonia and urea levels, peripheral nerve function is impaired. Flapping tremors (asterixis) and numbness/tingling (misinterpreted as carpal/tarsal tunnel syndrome) can occur.

✓ Musculoskeletal locations of pain associated with the hepatic and biliary systems include thoracic spine between scapulae, right shoulder, right upper trapezius, right interscapular, or right subscapular areas.

✓ Referred shoulder pain may be the only presenting symptom of hepatic or biliary disease.

✓ Gallbladder impairment can present as a rib dysfunction with tenderness anteriorly over the tip of the 10th rib (occasionally ribs 11 and 12 are also involved)

SUBJECTIVE EXAMINATION

Special Questions to Ask

Past Medical History

- Have you ever had an ulcer, gallbladder disease, your spleen removed, or hepatitis/jaundice?
  - *If yes* to hepatitis or jaundice: When was this diagnosed? How did you get this?
- Has anyone in your family ever been diagnosed with Wilson's disease (**excessive copper retention**) or hemochromatosis (**excessive iron absorption**)? (**Hereditary**)
- Do you work in a clinical laboratory, operating room, or with dialysis clients? (**Hepatitis**)
- Have you been out of the United States in the last 6 to 12 months? (**parasitic infection, country where hepatitis is endemic**)
- Have you worked in any setting that might be high risk for disease transmission such as a day care, correctional setting, or institutional setting? (**Hepatitis**)
- Have you had any recent contact with hepatitis or with a jaundiced person?
- Have you eaten any raw shellfish recently? (**Viral hepatitis**)
- Have you had any recent blood or plasma transfusion, blood tests, acupuncture, ear or body piercing, tattoos (including removal), or dental work done? (**Viral hepatitis**)
- Have you had a recent ACL reconstruction with an allograft? (**Hepatitis**)
- Have you had any kind of injury or trauma to your abdomen? (**Possible liver damage**)

For women: Are you currently using oral contraceptives? (**Hepatitis, adenoma**)

For the therapist:

- When asking about drug history, keep in mind that oral contraceptives may cause cholestasis (suppression of bile flow) or liver tumors. Some common over-the-counter drugs (e.g., acetaminophen) and some antibiotics, antitubercular drugs, anticonvulsants, cytotoxic drugs for cancer, antipsychotics, and antidepressants may have hepatotoxic effects. Ask about the use of cholesterol-lowering statins.

- Use questions from Chapter 2 to determine possible consumption of alcohol as a hepatotoxin.

Associated Signs and Symptoms

- Have you noticed a recent tendency to bruise or bleed easily? (**Liver disease**)
- Have you noticed any change in the color of your stools or urine? (**Dark urine, the color of cola and light- or clay-colored stools associated with jaundice**)
- Has your weight fluctuated 10 or 15 pounds or more recently without a change in diet? (**Cancer, cirrhosis, ascites, but also congestive heart failure**)
  - *If no,* have you noticed your clothes fitting tighter around the waist from abdominal swelling or bloating? (**Ascites**)
- Do you have a feeling of fullness after only one or two bites of food? (**Early satiety: stomach and duodenum, cystic tumors, or gallbladder**)
- Does your stomach feel swollen or bloated after eating? (**Abdominal fullness**)
- Do you have any abdominal pain? (Abdominal pain may be *visceral* from an internal organ [dull, general, poorly localized], *parietal* from inflammation of overlying peritoneum [sharp, precisely localized, aggravated by movement], or *referred* from a disorder in another site.)
- How does eating affect your pain? (**When eating aggravates symptoms: gastric ulcer, gallbladder inflammation**)
  - Are there any particular foods you have noticed that aggravate your symptoms?
  - *If yes,* which ones? (**Gallbladder: intolerance to fatty foods**)
- Have you noticed any unusual aversion to odors, food, alcohol, or (for people who smoke) smoking? (Jaundice)
- *For clients with only shoulder or back pain:* Have you noticed any association between when you eat and when your symptoms increase or decrease?

CASE STUDY HEPATITIS

REFERRAL

A 29-year-old male law student has come to you (self-referral) with headaches that developed after a motor vehicle accident 12 weeks ago. He was evaluated and treated in the emergency department of the local hospital and is not under the care of a primary care physician.

The headaches occur two to three times each week, starting at the base of the occiput and progressing up the back of his head to localize in the forehead bilaterally. The client has a sedentary lifestyle with no regular exercise, and he describes his stress level as being 6 on a scale from 0 to 10. The Family/Personal History form (see Fig. 2-2) indicates that he was diagnosed with hepatitis at the time of the accident.

PHYSICAL THERAPY INTERVIEW

What follow-up questions will you ask this client related to the hepatitis?

- I see from your History form that you have hepatitis.

- What type of hepatitis do you have? Give the client a chance to respond, but you may need to prompt with "type A," "type B," or "types C or D." Remember that hepatitis A is communicable before the appearance of any observable clinical symptoms. If he has been diagnosed, he is probably past this stage.

- Do you know how you initially came in contact with hepatitis? (Depending on the answer to the previous question, you may not need to ask this question).

Considerations requiring further questioning may include

- Illicit or recreational drug use

- Inadequate hygiene and poor handwashing in close quarters with travel companion

- Ingestion of contaminated food, water, milk, or seafood

- Recent blood transfusion or contact with blood/blood products

- *For type B:* Modes of sexual transmission

Remember the three stages when trying to determine whether this person may still be contagious. Hepatitis B can persist in body fluids indefinitely, requiring necessary precautions by you.

Hepatitis caused by medications or toxins is non-infectious hepatitis and is not communicable.

Transmissible hepatitis requires handwashing and hygiene precautions, including avoidance of any body fluids on your part through the use of protective gloves. This is especially true when treating a person with diabetes requiring fingerstick blood testing, when performing needle electromyograms, or providing open wound care, especially with debridement.

MEDICAL TREATMENT

- Did you receive any medical treatment? (immune globulin)

Immune serum globulin (ISG) is considered most effective in producing passive immunity for 3 to 4 months when administered as soon as possible after exposure to the hepatitis virus, but within 2 weeks after the onset of jaundice. Persons who have been treated with ISG may not develop jaundice, but those who have not received the gamma globulin usually develop jaundice.

- Are you currently receiving follow-up care for your hepatitis through a local physician?

This information will assist you in determining the appropriate medical source for further information if you need it and, in a case like this, assist you in choosing further follow up questions that may help you determine whether this person requires additional medical follow up.

Keep in mind that headaches can be persistent symptoms of hepatitis A. If the client is receiving no further medical follow up (especially if no serum globulin was administered initially), consider these follow up questions:

ASSOCIATED SYMPTOMS

- What symptoms did you have with hepatitis?

- Do you have any of those symptoms now?

- Are you experiencing any unusual fatigue or muscle or joint aches and pains?

- Have you noticed any unusual aversion to foods, alcohol, or cigarettes/smoke that you did not have before?

- Have you had any problems with diarrhea, vomiting, or nausea?

- Have you noticed any change in the color of your stools or urine? (1 to 4 days before the icteric stage, the urine darkens and the stool lightens)

- Have you noticed any unusual skin rash developing recently?

- When did you notice the headaches developing?

PRACTICE QUESTIONS

1. Referred pain patterns associated with hepatic and biliary pathologic conditions produce musculoskeletal symptoms in the
   a. Left shoulder
   b. Right shoulder
   c. Mid-back or upper back, scapular, and right shoulder areas
   d. Thorax, scapulae, right or left shoulder

2. What is the mechanism for referred right shoulder pain from hepatic or biliary disease?

3. Why does someone with liver dysfunction develop numbness and tingling that is sometimes labeled carpal tunnel syndrome?

4. When a client with bilateral carpal tunnel syndrome is being evaluated, how do you screen for the possibility of a pathologic condition of the liver?

5. What is the first most common sign associated with liver disease?

6. You are treating a 53-year-old woman who has had an extensive medical history that includes bilateral kidney disease with kidney removal on one side and transplantation on the other. The client is 10 years post-transplant and has now developed multiple problems as a result of the long-term use of immunosuppressants (cyclosporine to prevent organ rejection) and corticosteroids (prednisone). For example, she is extremely osteoporotic and has been diagnosed with cytomegalovirus and corticosteroid-induced myopathy. The client has fallen and broken her vertebra, ankle, and wrist on separate occasions. You are seeing her at home to implement a strengthening program and to instruct her in a falling prevention program, including home modifications. You notice the sclerae of her eyes are yellow-tinged. How do you tactfully ask her about this?

7. Clients with significant elevations in serum bilirubin levels caused by biliary obstruction will have which of the following associated signs?

   a. Dark urine, clay-colored stools, jaundice
   b. Yellow-tinged sclera
   c. Decreased serum ammonia levels
   d. *a* and *b* only

8. Preventing falls and trauma to soft tissues would be of utmost importance in the client with liver failure. Which of the following laboratory parameters would give you the most information about potential tissue injury?
   a. Decrease in serum albumin levels
   b. Elevated liver enzyme levels
   c. Prolonged coagulation times
   d. Elevated serum bilirubin levels

9. Decreased level of consciousness, impaired function of peripheral nerves, and asterixis (flapping tremor) would probably indicate an increase in the level of
   a. AST (aspartate aminotransferase)
   b. Alkaline phosphatase
   c. Serum bilirubin
   d. Serum ammonia

10. An inpatient who has had a total hip replacement with a significant history of alcohol use/abuse has a positive test for asterixis. This may signify
    a. Renal failure
    b. Hepatic encephalopathy
    c. Diabetes
    d. Gallstones obstructing the common bile duct

11. A decrease in serum albumin is common with a pathologic condition of the liver because albumin is produced in the liver. The reduction in serum albumin results in some easily identifiable signs. Which of the following signs might alert the therapist to the condition of decreased albumin?
    a. Increased blood pressure
    b. Peripheral edema and ascites
    c. Decreased level of consciousness
    d. Exertional dyspnea

REFERENCES

1. Key L, Bell NH: Osteomalacia and disorders of vitamin D metabolism. In Stein JH, editor: *Internal medicine*, ed 5, St Louis, 1998, Mosby.
2. Lenfant C: ACC/AHA/NHLBI Clinical advisory on the use and safety of statins, *Cardiology Review* 20(4Suppl):9-11, 2003.
3. Newman CB, Palmer G, Silbershatz H, et al: Safety of atorvastatin derived from analysis of 44 completed trials in 9,416 patients, *Am J Cardiol* 92(6):670-676, 2003.
4. Based on author's personal experience and communication with therapists in clinical practice across the country, 2004.
5. Ballantyne CM, Corsini A, Davidson MH, et al: Risk for myopathy with statin therapy in high-risk patients, *Arch Intern Med* 163(5):553-564, 2003.

6. Parnes A: Asterixis, *Trinity Student Medical Journal* 1:58, 2000. Available at: http://www.tcd.ie/tsmj.

7. Blumberg D, Low CM: Prevention of hepatitis A in a global community. *www.medscape.com/vicuprogram/2004*.

8. Grande P, Cronquist A: Public health dispatch, multistate outbreak of hepatitis A among young adult concert attendees, United States, 2003, *MMWR CDC* 52(35); 844-845, 2003. (*www.cdc.gov/mmwr/preview/mmwr/html/mm5235a5.htm*)

9. Weinbaum C, Lyerla C: Prevention and control of infections with hepatitis viruses in correctional settings. www.cdc.gov/mmwr/preview/mmwr/html/rr5201a1.htm; 1-33, Jan 24, 2003.

10. Parini S: Hepatitis C, *Nursing2003* 33(4):57, 2003.

11. Spencer KY, Chang MD: Anterior cruciate ligament reconstruction: allograft vs. autograft, *J of Arthroscopic and Related Surgery* 19(5):453, 2003.

12. Perry J, Jagger J: Statistically your risk of HCV infection has dropped, *Nursing2003* 33(6):82, 2003.

13. Friedman L: Liver, biliary tract and pancreas, diseases of the liver. In Tierney L, McPhee S, Papadakis M, editors: *Current medical diagnosis and treatment*, ed 43, New York, 2004, Lange; pp 629.

14. Lovy MR, Wener MH: Rheumatic disease: when is hepatitis C the culprit? *J Musculoskel Med* 13(4):27-35, 1996.

15. Rull M, Zonay L, Schumacher HR: Hepatitis C and rheumatic diseases, *J Musculoskel Med* 15(11):38-44, 1998.

16. Foster GR: Past, present, and future hepatitis C treatments, *Semin Liver Disease* Suppl 2:97-104, 2004.

17. Pearlman BL: Hepatitis C treatment update, *Am J Med* 117(5):344-352, 2004.

18. Pullen L: Hep-Hazard, *Hemaware* 9(2):54-56, 2004.

19. Liver function: two new threats, *The John Hopkins Medical Letter, Health After 50* 15(3):2-7, 2003. www.hopkinsafter50.com.

20. Salt WB: Nonalcoholic fatty liver disease (NAFLD): a comprehensive review, *J Insur Med* 36(1):27-41, 2004.

21. Younossi ZM, McCullough AJ, Ong JP, et al: Obesity and non-alcoholic fatty liver disease in chronic hepatitis C, *J Clin Gastroenterol* 38(8):705-709, 2004.

22. Kimbel DL: Hip pain in a 50-year-old woman with RA, *Journal of Musculoskeletal Medicine* 16(11):651-652, 1999.

23. Neonatal jaundice, unwelcome return for kernicterus, *Nursing2003* 33(11):35, 2003, www.aap.org.

24. Bisceglie A: Medscape gastroenterology conference coverage: hepatocellular carcinoma and cholangiocarcinoma, 12-8-2001. www.medscape.com/Medscape/CNO/2002/AASCD?pal-AASLD.html, 12-8-2001.

25. Rex L: *Evaluation and treatment of somatovisceral dysfunction of the gastrointestinal system*, Edmonds, Washington, 2004, URSA Foundation.

26. Lazeano-Ponce EC, Miquel JF: Epidemiology and molecular pathology of gallbladder cancer. *CA Cancer J Clin* 51(6):349, 2001.

Screening for Urogenital Disease

A 40-year-old athletic man comes to your clinic for an evaluation of back pain that he attributes to a very hard fall on his back while he was alpine skiing 3 days ago. His chief complaint is a dull, aching costovertebral pain on the left side, which is unrelieved by a change in position or by treatment with ice, heat, or aspirin. He stated that "even the skin on my back hurts." He has no previous history of any medical problems.

After further questioning, the client reveals that inspiratory movements do not aggravate the pain, and he has not noticed any change in color, odor, or volume of urine output. However, percussion of the costovertebral angle (see Fig. 4-51) results in the reproduction of the symptoms. This type of symptom complex may suggest renal involvement even without obvious changes in urine.

Whether secondary to trauma or of insidious onset, a client's complaints of flank pain, low back pain, or pelvic pain may be of renal or urologic origin and should be screened carefully through the subjective and objective examinations. Medical referral may be necessary.

SIGNS AND SYMPTOMS OF RENAL AND UROLOGICAL DISORDERS

This chapter is intended to guide the physical therapist in understanding the origins and relationships of renal, ureteral, bladder, and urethral symptoms. The urinary tract, consisting of kidneys, ureters, bladder, and urethra (Fig. 10-1), is an integral component of human functioning that disposes of the body's toxic waste products and unnecessary fluid and expertly regulates extremely complicated metabolic processes. The ureters, bladder, and urethra function primarily as transport vehicles for urine formed in the kidneys. The lower urinary tract is the last area through which urine is passed in its final form for excretion.

Formation and excretion of urine is the primary function of the renal nephron (the functional unit of the kidney) (Fig. 10-2). Through this process the kidney is able to maintain a homeostatic environment in the body. Besides the excretory function of the kidney, which includes the removal of wastes and excessive fluid, the kidney plays an integral role in the balance of various essential body functions, including the following:

- Acid base balance
- Electrolyte balance
- Control of blood pressure with renin
- Formation of red blood cells (RBCs)
- Activation of vitamin D and calcium balance

The failure of the kidney to perform any of these functions results in severe alteration and disruption in homeostasis and signs and symptoms resulting from these dysfunctions (Box 10-1).[1]

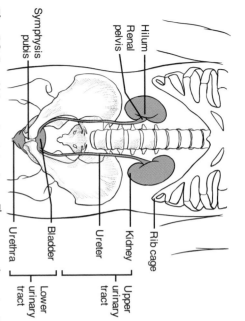

Fig. 10-1 • Urinary tract structures. The upper urinary tract is composed of the kidneys and ureters while the lower urinary tract is made up of the bladder and urethra. The upper portion of each kidney is protected by the rib cage, and the bladder is partially protected by the symphysis pubis.

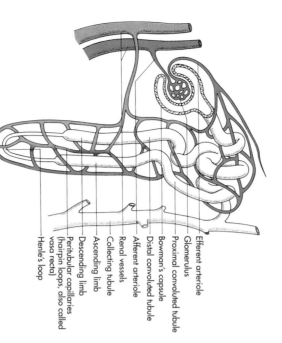

Fig. 10-2 • Components of the nephron. The afferent arteriole carries blood to the glomerulus for filtration through Bowman's capsule and the renal tubular system. (From Foster RL, Hunsberger MM, Anderson JJ: *Family-centered nursing care of children,* Philadelphia, 1989, WB Saunders.)

BOX 10-1 ▼ Signs and Symptoms of Genitourinary Disease

Constitutional Symptoms
- Fever, chills
- Fatigue, malaise
- Anorexia, weight loss

Musculoskeletal
- Unilateral costovertebral tenderness
- Low back, flank, inner thigh, or leg pain
- Ipsilateral shoulder pain

Urinary Problems
- Dysuria (painful burning or discomfort with urination)
- Nocturia (getting up more than once at night to urinate)
- Feeling that bladder has not emptied completely but unable to urinate more; straining to start a stream of urine or to empty bladder completely
- Hematuria (blood in urine; pink or red-tinged urine)
- Dribbling at the end of urination
- Frequency (need to urinate or empty bladder more than every 2 hours)
- Hesitancy (weak or interrupted urine stream)
- Proteinuria (protein in urine; urine is foamy)

Other
- Skin hypersensitivity (T10-L1)
- Infertility

Women
- Abnormal vaginal bleeding
- Painful menstruation (dysmenorrhea)
- Changes in menstrual pattern
- Pelvic masses or lesions
- Vaginal itching or discharge
- Pain during intercourse (dyspareunia)

Men
- Difficulty starting or continuing a stream of urine
- Discharge from penis
- Penile lesions
- Testicular or penis pain
- Enlargement of scrotal contents
- Swelling or mass in groin
- Sexual dysfunction

▼ THE URINARY TRACT

The upper urinary tract consists of the kidneys and ureters. The kidneys are located in the posterior upper abdominal cavity in a space behind the peritoneum (retroperitoneal space) (see Fig. 4-47). Their anatomic position is in front of and on both sides of the vertebral column at the level of T11 to L3. The right kidney is usually lower than the left.[2]

The upper portion of the kidney is in contact with the diaphragm and moves with respiration. The kidneys are protected anteriorly by the rib

cage and abdominal organs (see Fig. 4-46) and posteriorly by the large back muscles and ribs. The lower portions of the kidneys and the ureters extend below the ribs and are separated from the abdominal cavity by the peritoneal membrane.

The lower urinary tract consists of the bladder and urethra. From the renal pelvis, urine is moved by peristalsis to the ureters and into the bladder. The bladder, which is a muscular, membranous sac, is located directly behind the symphysis pubis and is used for storage and excretion of urine. The urethra is connected to the bladder and serves as a channel through which urine is passed from the bladder to the outside of the body.

Voluntary control of urinary excretion is based on learned inhibition of reflex pathways from the walls of the bladder. Release of urine from the bladder occurs under voluntary control of the urethral sphincter.

The male genital or reproductive system is made up of the testes, epididymis, vas deferens, seminal vesicles, prostate gland, and penis (Fig. 10-3).

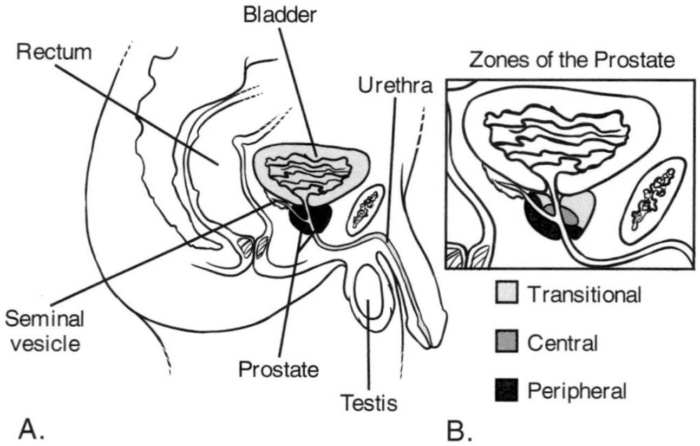

These structures are susceptible to inflammatory disorders, neoplasms, and structural defects.

In males the posterior portion of the urethra is surrounded by the prostate gland, a gland approximately 3.5 cm long by 3 cm wide (about the size of two almonds). Located just below the bladder, this gland can cause severe urethral obstruction when enlarged from a growth or inflammation resulting in difficulty starting a flow of urine, continuing a flow of urine, frequency, and/or nocturia.

The prostate gland is commonly divided into five lobes and three zones. Prostate carcinoma usually affects the posterior lobe of the gland; the middle and lateral lobes typically are associated with the nonmalignant process called benign prostatic hyperplasia (BPH).

▶ RENAL AND UROLOGICAL PAIN

Upper Urinary Tract (Renal/Ureteral)

The kidneys and ureters are innervated by both sympathetic and parasympathetic fibers. The kidneys receive sympathetic innervation from the lesser splanchnic nerves through the renal plexus, which is located next to the renal arteries. Renal vasoconstriction and increased renin release are associated with sympathetic stimulation. Parasympathetic innervation is derived from the vagus nerve, and the function of this innervation is not known.

Renal sensory innervation is not completely understood, even though the capsule (covering of the kidney) and the lower portions of the collecting system seem to cause pain with stretching (distention) or puncture. Information transmitted by renal and ureteral pain receptors is relayed by sympathetic nerves that enter the spinal cord at T10 to L1 (see Fig. 3-3).

Because visceral and cutaneous sensory fibers enter the spinal cord in close proximity and actually converge on some of the same neurons, when visceral pain fibers are stimulated, concurrent stimulation of cutaneous fibers also occurs. The visceral pain is then felt as though it is skin pain (hyperesthesia), similar to the condition of the alpine skier who stated that "even the skin on my back hurts." Renal and ureteral pain can be felt throughout the T10 to L1 dermatomes.

Renal pain (see Fig. 10-7) is typically felt in the posterior subcostal and costovertebral regions. To assess the kidney, the test for costovertebral angle tenderness can be included in the objective examination (see Fig. 4-51).

Ureteral pain is felt in the groin and genital area (see Fig. 10-8). With either renal pain or ureteral

Zones of the Prostate

Urethra

Bladder

Rectum

Seminal vesicle

Testis

Prostate

☐ Transitional
▨ Central
■ Peripheral

A.

B.

Fig. 10-3 • A, The prostate is located at the base of the bladder, surrounding a part of the urethra. It is innervated by T11-L1 and S2-S4 and can refer pain to the sacrum, low back, and testes (see Fig. 10-10). As the prostate enlarges, the urethra can become obstructed, interfering with the normal flow of urine. **B,** The prostate is composed of three zones. The transitional zone surrounds the urethra as it passes through the prostate. This is a common site for benign prostatic hyperplasia (BPH). The central zone is a cone-shaped section that sits behind the transitional zone. The peripheral zone is the largest portion of the gland and borders the other two zones. Most early tumors do not produce any symptoms because the urethra is not in the peripheral zone. It is not until the tumor grows large enough to obstruct the bladder outlet that symptoms develop. Tumors in the transitional zone, which houses the urethra, may cause symptoms sooner than tumors in other zones.

pain, radiation forward around the flank into the lower abdominal quadrant and abdominal muscle spasm with rebound tenderness can occur on the same side as the source of pain.

The pain can also be generalized throughout the abdomen. Nausea, vomiting, and impaired intestinal motility (progressing to intestinal paralysis) can occur with severe, acute pain. Nerve fibers from the renal plexus are also in direct communication with the spermatic plexus, and because of this close relationship, testicular pain may also accompany renal pain. Neither renal nor urethral pain is altered by a change in body position.

The typical renal pain sensation is aching and dull in nature but can occasionally be a severe, boring type of pain. The constant dull and aching pain usually accompanies distention or stretching of the renal capsule, pelvis, or collecting system. This stretching can result from intrarenal fluid accumulation, such as inflammatory edema, inflamed or bleeding cysts, and bleeding or neoplastic growths. Whenever the renal capsule is punctured, a dull pain can also be felt by the client. Ischemia of renal tissue caused by blockage of blood flow to the kidneys results in a *constant dull* or a *constant* sharp pain.

Ureteral obstruction (e.g., from a urinary calculus or "stone" consisting of mineral salts) results in distention of the ureter and causes spasm that produces intermittent or constant severe colicky pain until the stone is passed. Pain of this origin usually starts in the CVA and radiates to the ipsilateral lower abdomen, upper thigh, testis, or labium (see Fig. 10-8). Movement of a stone down a ureter can cause *renal colic*, an excruciating pain that radiates to the region just described and usually increases in intensity in waves of colic or spasm.

Chronic ureteral pain and renal pain tend to be vague, poorly localized, and easily confused with many other problems of abdominal or pelvic origin. There are also areas of *referred pain* related to renal or ureteral lesions. For example, if the diaphragm becomes irritated because of pressure from a renal lesion, shoulder pain may be felt (see Figs. 3-4 and 3-5). If a lesion of the ureter occurs *outside* the ureter, pain may occur on movement of the adjacent iliopsoas muscle (see Fig. 8-3).

Abdominal rebound tenderness results when the adjacent peritoneum becomes inflamed. Active trigger points along the upper rim of the pubis and the lateral half of the inguinal ligament may lie in the lower internal oblique muscle and possibly in the lower rectus abdominis. These trigger points can cause increased irritation and spasm of the detrusor and urinary sphincter muscles, producing urinary frequency, retention of urine, and groin pain.[3]

Pseudorenal Pain

Pseudorenal pain may occur secondary to radiculitis or irritation of the costal nerves caused by mechanical derangements of the costovertebral or costotransverse joints. Disorders of this sort are common in the cervical and thoracic areas, but the most common sites are T10 and T12.[4] Irritation of these nerves causes costovertebral pain that can radiate into the ipsilateral lower abdominal quadrant.

The onset is usually acute with some type of traumatic history, such as lifting a heavy object, sustaining a blow to the costovertebral area, or falling from a height onto the buttocks. The pain is affected by body position, and although the client may be awakened at night when assuming a certain position (e.g., sidelying on the affected side), the pain is usually absent on awakening and increases gradually during the day. It is also aggravated by prolonged periods of sitting, especially when driving on rough roads in the car. It may be relieved by changing to another position (Table 10-1).

Radiculitis may mimic ureteral colic or renal pain, but true renal pain is seldom affected by movements of the spine. Exerting pressure over the costovertebral angle (CVA) with the thumb may elicit local tenderness of the involved peripheral nerve at its point of emergence, whereas gentle percussion over the angle may be necessary

TABLE 10-1 ▼ Assessment for Pseudorenal Pain

History	Trauma (fall, assault, blow, lifting) • History of straining, lifting; accident or other mechanical injury to thoracic spine

Pain Pattern	• Back and/or flank pain occur at the same level as the kidney
	 • Affected by change in position
	   • Lying on the involved side increases pain
	   • Prolonged sitting increases pain
	   • Symptoms are reproduced with movements of the spine
	 • Costovertebral angle tenderness present on palpation

Associated Signs and Symptoms	None Murphy's percussion test is negative Report of bowel and bladder changes unlikely

to elicit renal pain, indicating a deeper, more visceral sensation. Fig. 4-51 illustrates percussion over the CVA (Murphy's percussion).

Lower Urinary Tract (Bladder/Urethra)

Bladder innervation occurs through sympathetic, parasympathetic, and sensory nerve pathways. Sympathetic bladder innervation assists in the closure of the bladder neck during seminal emission. Afferent sympathetic fibers also assist in providing awareness of bladder distention, pain, and abdominal distention caused by bladder distention. This input reaches the cord at T9 or higher. Parasympathetic bladder innervation is at S2, S3, and S4 and provides motor coordination for the act of voiding. Afferent parasympathetic fibers assist in sensation of the desire to void, proprioception (position sensation), and perception of pain.

Sensory receptors are present in the mucosa of the bladder and in the muscular bladder walls. These fibers are more plentiful near the bladder neck and the junctional area between the ureters and bladder.

Urethral innervation, also at the S2, S3, and S4 level, occurs through the pudendal nerve. This is a mixed innervation of both sensory and motor nerve fibers. This innervation controls the opening of the external urethral sphincter (motor) and an awareness of the imminence of voiding and heat (thermal) sensation in the urethra.

Bladder or urethral pain is felt above the pubis (suprapubic) or low in the abdomen (see Fig. 10-9). The sensation is usually characterized as one of urinary urgency, a sensation to void, and dysuria (painful urination). Irritation of the neck of the bladder or of the urethra can result in a burning sensation localized to these areas, probably caused by the urethral thermal receptors. See Box 10-2 for

causes of pain outside the urogenital system that present like upper or lower urinary tract pain of either an acute or chronic nature.

▶ RENAL AND URINARY TRACT PROBLEMS

Pathologic conditions of the upper and lower urinary tracts can be categorized according to primary causative factors. Inflammatory/infectious and obstructive disorders are presented in this section along with renal failure and cancers of the urinary tract.

When screening for any conditions affecting the kidney and urinary tract system, keep in mind factors that put people at increased risk for these problems (Case Example 10-1). Early screening and detection is recommended based on the presence of these risk factors.[5]

- Age over 60
- Personal or family history of diabetes or hypertension
- Personal or family history of kidney disease, heart attack, or stroke
- Personal history of kidney stones, urinary tract infections, lower urinary tract obstruction, or autoimmune disease
- African, Hispanic, Pacific Island, or Native American descent
- Exposure to chemicals (e.g., paint, glue, degreasing solvents, cleaning solvents), drugs, or environmental conditions
- Low birth weight

Inflammatory/Infectious Disorders

Inflammatory disorders of the kidney and urinary tract can be caused by bacterial infection, by changes in immune response, and by toxic agents such as drugs and radiation. Common infections of the urinary tract develop in either the upper or lower urinary tract (Table 10-2).

Upper urinary tract infections include kidney or ureteral infections. Lower urinary tract infections include cystitis (bladder infection) or urethritis (urethral infection). Symptoms of urinary tract infection (UTI) depend on the location of the infection in either the upper or lower urinary tract (although, rarely, infection could occur in both simultaneously).

Inflammatory/Infectious Disorders of the Upper Urinary Tract

Inflammations or infections of the upper urinary tract (kidney and ureters) are considered to be

---

BOX 10-2 ▼ Extraurologic Conditions Causing Urinary Tract Symptoms

Acute or chronic conditions affecting other viscera outside the urologic system can refer pain and symptoms to the upper or lower urinary tract. These can include:

- Perforated viscus (any large internal organ)
- Intestinal obstruction
- Cholecystitis (inflammation of the gallbladder)
- Pelvic inflammatory disease
- Tubo-ovarian abscess
- Ruptured ectopic pregnancy
- Twisted ovarian cyst
- Tumor (benign or malignant)

CASE EXAMPLE 10-1 ▪ Screening in the Presence of Risk Factors for Kidney Disease

A 66-year-old African American woman with a personal history of systemic lupus erythematosus (SLE) lost her balance and fell off the deck at her home. She sustained vertebral and rib fractures at T10 and T11. She is a retired paint factory worker. She reported daily exposure to paint and paint solvents during her 15 years of employment.

She was seen as a walk-in at the local medical clinic where she is a regular patient. She did not see the rheumatologist who was managing her SLE. The attending physician told her the injuries were "probably from the long-term use of prednisone for her lupus." She was referred to physical therapy by the attending physician for postural exercises.

During the interview, when asked, "Are you having any symptoms of any kind anywhere else in your body?" the client admitted to a pink color to her urine and some burning on urination. These symptoms have been present since the day after the fall 3 weeks ago.

There were no other signs or symptoms reported. Blood pressure measured 175/95 on three separate occasions. The client reported her blood pressure was elevated at the time of her visit to the doctor, but she thought it was caused by the stress of the fall.

Question: As you step back and conduct a Review of Systems, what are the red flags to suggest medical referral is needed? To whom do you refer this client?

Red flags:
- Age over 40 (age over 60 is a risk factor for kidney disease)
- African American descent (at risk for diabetes, kidney disease)
- Long-term use of NSAIDs (synergistic nephrotoxin in combination with certain chemicals such as paint and paint solvents)
- Elevated blood pressure
- Change in color and pattern of urination

The therapist may not recognize specific factors present that put the client at increased risk for kidney disease, but the obvious changes in urine color and pattern along with changes in blood pressure require medical referral.

Without the medical records, it is impossible to know what (if any) testing was done related to kidney function (e.g., urinalysis, blood test) at the time of the initial injury. A phone call to the referring physician is probably the best place to start. Documentation of the recent events and current red flag symptoms should be sent to the referring physician, the primary care physician, and the rheumatologist (if different from the primary care doctor).

Physical therapy intervention is still appropriate given her musculoskeletal injuries. Further medical assessment is warranted based on the development of symptoms unknown to the referring physician.

TABLE 10-2 ▾ Urinary Tract Infections

Upper urinary tract infection	Lower urinary tract infection
Renal infections, such as pyelonephritis (renal parenchyma, i.e., kidney tissue)	Cystitis (bladder infection) Urethritis (urethra infection)
Acute or chronic glomerulonephritis (glomeruli)	
Renal papillary necrosis	
Renal tuberculosis	

Renal infections, such as pyelonephritis (renal parenchyma) and acute and chronic glomerulonephritis (inflammation of the glomeruli of both kidneys). Less common conditions include renal papillary necrosis and renal tuberculosis.

Symptoms of upper urinary tract inflammations and infections are shown in Table 10-3. If the diaphragm is irritated, ipsilateral shoulder pain may occur. Signs and symptoms of renal impairment are also shown in Table 10-4 and, if present,

more serious because these lesions can be a direct threat to renal tissue itself.

The more common conditions include pyelonephritis (inflammation of the renal parenchyma) and acute and chronic glomerulonephritis (inflammation of the glomeruli of both kidneys). Less common conditions include renal papillary necrosis and renal tuberculosis.

TABLE 10-3 ▼ Clinical Symptoms of Infectious/Inflammatory Urinary Tract Problems

Upper urinary tract (kidney or ureteral infection)	Lower urinary tract (cystitis or urethritis)
Unilateral costovertebral tenderness	Urinary frequency
Flank pain	Urinary urgency
Ipsilateral shoulder pain	Low back pain
Fever and chills	Pelvic/lower abdominal pain
Skin hypersensitivity (hyperesthesia of dermatomes)	Dysuria (discomfort, such as pain or burning during urination)
Hematuria (blood [RBCs] in urine)	Hematuria
Pyuria (pus or white blood cells in urine)	Pyuria
Bacteriuria (bacteria in urine)	Bacteriuria
Nocturia (unusual or increased nighttime need to urinate)	Dyspareunia (painful intercourse)

are significant symptoms of impending kidney failure.

Inflammatory/Infectious Disorders of the Lower Urinary Tract

Both the bladder and urine have a number of defenses against bacterial invasion. These defenses are mechanisms such as voiding, urine acidity, osmolality, and the bladder mucosa itself, which is thought to have antibacterial properties.

Urine in the bladder and kidney is normally sterile, but urine itself is a good medium for bacterial growth. Interferences in the defense mechanisms of the bladder, such as the presence of residual or stagnant urine, changes in urinary pH or concentration, or obstruction of urinary excretion can promote bacterial growth.

Routes of entry of bacteria into the urinary tract can be *ascending* (most commonly up the urethra into the bladder and then into the ureters and kidney), *blood borne* (bacterial invasion through the bloodstream), or *lymphatic* (bacterial invasion through the lymph system, the least common route).[6]

A lower UTI occurs most commonly in women because of the short female urethra and the proximity of the urethra to the vagina and rectum. The rate of occurrence increases with age and sexual activity since intercourse can spread bacteria from the genital area to the urethra. Chronic health problems, such as diabetes mellitus, gout, hypertension, obstructive urinary tract problems, and medical procedures requiring urinary catheterization, are also predisposing risk factors for the development of these infections.[6]

Individuals with diabetes are prone to complications associated with urinary tract infections. Staphylococcus infection of the urinary tract may be a source of osteomyelitis, an infection of a vertebral body resulting from hematogenous spread or

local spread from an abscess into the vertebra. The infected vertebral body may gradually undergo degeneration and destruction, with collapse and formation of a segmental scoliosis.[7]

This condition is suspected from the onset of nonspecific low back pain, unrelated to any specific motion. Local tenderness can be elicited, but the initial x-ray finding is negative. Usually, a low-grade fever is present but undetected, or it develops as the infection progresses. This is why anyone with low back pain of unknown origin should have his or her temperature taken, even in a physical therapy setting.

Cystitis (inflammation with infection of the bladder), *interstitial cystitis* (inflammation without infection), and *urethritis* (inflammation and infection of the urethra) appear with a similar symptom progression (Case Example 10-2).

Interstitial cystitis (IC), chronic inflammation of the bladder, affects more than 700,000 individuals each year in the United States. As many as 90% of those affected are women. Several other disorders are associated with IC including allergies, inflammatory bowel syndrome, fibromyalgia, and vulvitis.[8]

Bladder pain associated with IC can vary from woman to woman and even within the same individual and may be dull, achy, or acute and stabbing. Discomfort while urinating also varies from mild stinging to intense burning. Sexual intercourse may ignite pain that lasts for days.[8]

Clients with any of the symptoms listed for the lower urinary tract in Table 10-3 at presentation should be referred promptly to a physician for further diagnostic work-up and possible treatment. Infections of the lower urinary tract are potentially very dangerous because of the possibility of upward spread and resultant damage to renal tissue. Some individuals, however, are asymptomatic, and routine urine culture and microscopic

---

CASE EXAMPLE 10-2 Bladder Infection

A 55-year-old woman came to the clinic with back pain associated with paraspinal muscle spasms. Pain was of unknown cause (insidious onset), and the client reported that she was "just getting out of bed" when the pain started. The pain was described as a dull aching that was aggravated by movement and relieved by rest (musculoskeletal pattern).

No numbness, tingling, or saddle anesthesia was reported, and the neurologic screening examination was negative. Sacroiliac (SI) testing was negative. Spinal movements were slow and guarded, with muscle spasms noted throughout movement and at rest. Because of her age and the insidious onset of symptoms, further questions were initiated to screen for medical disease.

This client was midmenopausal and was not taking any hormone replacement therapy (HRT). She had a bladder infection a month ago that was treated with antibiotics; tests for this were negative when she was evaluated and referred by her physician for back pain. Two weeks ago she had an upper respiratory infec-

tion (a "cold") and had been "coughing a lot." There was no previous history of cancer.

Local treatment to reduce paraspinal muscle spasms was initiated, but the client did not respond as expected over the course of five treatment sessions. Because of her recent history of upper respiratory and bladder infections, questions were repeated related to the presence of constitutional symptoms and changes in bladder function/urine color, force of stream, burning on urination, and so on. Occasional "sweats" (present sometimes during the day, sometimes at night) was the only red flag present. The combination of recent infection, failure to respond to treatment, and the presence of sweats suggested referral to the physician for early reevaluation.

The client did not return to the clinic for further treatment, and a follow-up telephone call indicated that she did indeed have a recurrent bladder infection that was treated successfully with a different antibiotic. Her back pain and muscle spasm were eliminated after only 24 hours of taking this new antibiotic.

---

examination are the most reliable methods of detection and diagnosis.

Older adults (both men and women) are at increased risk for UTI. They may present with non-specific symptoms, such as loss of appetite, nausea and vomiting abdominal pain, or change in mental status (e.g., onset of confusion, increased confusion). Watch for predisposing conditions that can put the older client at risk for UTI. These may include diabetes mellitus or other chronic diseases, immobility, reduced fluid intake, catheterization, and previous history of UTI or kidney stones.

Obstructive Disorders

Urinary tract obstruction can occur at any point in the urinary tract and can be the result of *primary* urinary tract obstructions (obstructions occurring within the urinary tract) or *secondary* urinary tract obstructions (obstructions resulting from disease processes outside the urinary tract).

A primary obstruction might include problems such as acquired or congenital malformations, strictures, renal or ureteral calculi (stones), poly-cystic kidney disease, or neoplasms of the urinary tract (e.g., bladder, kidney).

Secondary obstructions produce pressure on the urinary tract from outside and might be related to conditions such as prostatic enlargement (benign or malignant); abdominal aortic aneurysm; gyne-cologic conditions such as pregnancy, pelvic inflammatory disease, and endometriosis; or neoplasms of the pelvic or abdominal structures.

Obstruction of any portion of the urinary tract results in a backup or collection of urine behind the obstruction. The result is dilation or stretching of the urinary tract structures that are positioned behind the point of blockage.

Muscles near the affected area contract in an attempt to push urine around the obstruction. Pressure accumulates above the point of obstruction and can eventually result in severe dilation of the renal collecting system (hydronephrosis) and renal failure. The greater the intensity and duration of the pressure, the greater is the destruction of renal tissue.

Because urine flow is decreased with obstruction, urinary stagnation and infection or stone formation can result. Stones are formed because urine stasis permits clumping or precipitation of organic matter and minerals.

Lower urinary tract obstruction can also result in constant bladder distention, hypertrophy of bladder muscle fibers, and formation of herniated sacs of bladder mucosa. These herniated sacs result in a large, flaccid bladder that cannot empty completely. In addition, these sacs retain stagnant urine, which causes infection and stone formation.

Obstructive Disorders of the Upper Urinary Tract

Obstruction of the upper urinary tract may be sudden (acute) or slow in development. Tumors of the kidney or ureters may develop slowly enough that symptoms are totally absent or very mild initially, with eventual progression to pain and signs of impairment. *Acute* ureteral or renal blockage by a stone (calculus consisting of mineral salts), for example, may result in excruciating, spasmodic, and radiating pain accompanied by severe nausea and vomiting.

Calculi form primarily in the kidney. This process is called *nephrolithiasis*. The stones can remain in the kidney (renal pelvis) or travel down the urinary tract and lodge at any point in the tract. Strictly speaking, the term *kidney stone* refers to stones that are in the kidney. Once they move into the ureter, they become *ureteral stones*.

Ureteral stones are the ones that cause the most pain. If a stone becomes wedged in the ureter, urine backs up distending the ureter and causing severe pain. If a stone blocks the flow of urine, urine pressure may build up in the ureter and kidney causing the kidney to swell (hydronephrosis). Unrecognized hydronephrosis can sometimes cause permanent kidney damage.[9]

The most characteristic symptom of renal or ureteral stones is sudden, sharp, severe pain. If the pain originates deep in the lumbar area and radiates around the side and down toward the testicle in the male and the bladder in the female, it is termed *renal colic. Ureteral colic* occurs if the stone becomes trapped in the ureter. Ureteral colic is characterized by radiation of painful symptoms toward the genitalia and thighs (see Fig. 10-8).

Since the testicles and ovaries form in utero in the location of the kidneys and then migrate at full term following the pathways of the ureters, kidney stones moving down the pathway of the ureters cause pain in the flank. This pain radiates to the scrotum in males and the labia in females. For the same reason ovarian or testicular cancer can refer pain to the back at the level of the kidneys.

Renal tumors may also be detected as a flank mass combined with unexplained weight loss,

fever, pain, and hematuria. The presence of any amount of blood in the urine always requires referral to a physician for further diagnostic evaluation because this is a primary symptom of urinary tract neoplasm.

Clinical Signs and Symptoms of
Obstruction of the Upper Urinary Tract

- Pain (depends on the rapidity of onset and on the location)
  - Acute, spasmodic, radiating
  - Mild and dull flank pain
  - Lumbar discomfort with some renal diseases or renal back pain with ureteral obstruction
- Hyperesthesia of dermatomes (T10 through L1)
- Nausea and vomiting
- Palpable flank mass
- Hematuria
- Fever and chills
- Urge to urinate frequently
- Abdominal muscle spasms
- Renal impairment indicators (see inside front cover: Renal Blood Studies; see also Table 10-4)

Obstructive Disorders of the Lower Urinary Tract

Common conditions of (mechanical) obstruction of the lower urinary tract result in difficulty emptying urine from the bladder. Mechanical problems of the urinary tract result in difficulty emptying urine from the bladder. Improper emptying of the bladder results in urinary retention and impairment of voluntary bladder control (incontinence). Several possible causes of mechanical bladder dysfunction include pelvic floor dysfunction, UTIs, partial urethral obstruction, trauma, and removal of the prostate gland.

The nerves that carry pain sensation from the prostate do not localize the source of pain very precisely, and therefore it may be difficult for the man to describe exactly where the pain is coming from. Discomfort can be localized in the suprapubic region, in the penis and testicles, or it can be centered in the perineum or rectum (see Fig. 10-10).

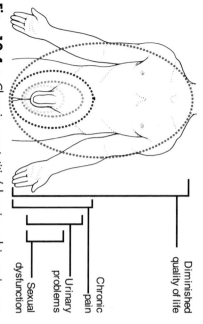

Fig. 10-4 • Chronic prostatitis/chronic pelvic pain syndrome (CP/CPPS) can have a serious impact on a man's quality of life as a result of voiding problems, chronic pelvic pain and discomfort, and sexual dysfunction with painful ejaculation, cramping or discomfort after ejaculation, and infertility.

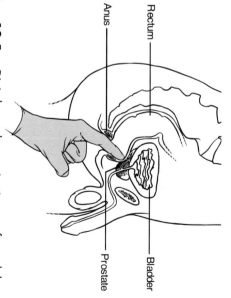

Fig. 10-5 • Digital rectal examination performed by a medical doctor or trained health care professional such as a nurse practitioner or physician's assistant puts pressure on the inflamed prostate reproducing painful symptoms associated with prostatitis.

PROSTATITIS

Prostatitis is a relatively common inflammation of the prostate causing prostate enlargement. This condition affects up to 10% of the adult male population accounting for the 2 million or more men who seek treatment annually in the United States.[10,11] It is often disabling, affecting men at any age, but typically found in men ages 40 to 70 years. Acute bacterial prostatitis occurs most often in men under age 35.

The NIH consensus classification of prostatitis includes four categories:

- Type I   Acute bacterial prostatitis
- Type II   Chronic bacterial prostatitis
- Type III Chronic prostatitis/Chronic Pelvic Pain Syndrome (CP/CPPS)
             A. Inflammatory
             B. Noninflammatory
- Type IV   Asymptomatic inflammatory prostatitis

Chronic (Type III, nonbacterial) prostatitis can be associated with pelvic pain syndrome, a chronic condition characterized primarily by pelvic pain. The symptoms of CP/CPPS appear to occur as a result of interplay between psychologic factors and dysfunction in the immune, neurologic, and endocrine systems.[12] Studies show a major impact on quality of life, urinary function, and sexual function along with chronic pain and discomfort (Fig. 10-4).[13,14]

The pain of prostatitis can be exacerbated by sexual activity, and some men describe pain upon ejaculation. A digital rectal examination by the physician will reproduce painful symptoms

when the prostate is inflamed or infected (Fig. 10-5).

In men with chronic prostatitis, voiding complaints similar to those caused by BPH are the predominant symptoms. These complaints include urgency, frequency, and nocturia (getting up at nighttime more than once); less frequently, men may complain of difficulty starting the urinary stream or a slow stream.

These symptoms typically differ from symptoms of BPH in that they are associated with some degree of discomfort before, during, or after voiding. Physical or emotional stress and/or irritative components of the diet (e.g., caffeine in coffee, soft drinks) commonly exacerbate chronic prostatitis symptoms.

The causes of prostatitis are unclear. Although it can be the result of a bacterial infection, many men have nonbacterial prostatitis of unknown cause. Risk factors for bacterial prostatitis include some sexually transmitted diseases (e.g., gonorrhea) from unprotected anal and vaginal intercourse, which can allow bacteria to enter the urethra and travel to the prostate.

Other risk factors include bladder outlet obstruction (e.g., stone, tumor, benign prostatic hyperplasia), diabetes mellitus, immunosuppression, and urethral catheterization. Neither prostatitis nor prostate enlargement is known to cause cancer, but men with prostatitis or BPH can develop prostate cancer as well.

The National Institutes of Health Prostatitis Symptom Index (NIH-CPSI) provides a valid

outcome measure for men with chronic prostatitis. The index may be useful in clinical practice as well as research protocols.[15] A less complete list of questions for screening purposes are most appropriate for men with low back pain and any of the risk factors or symptoms listed for **prostatitis** and may include the following.

Follow-Up Questions

- Do you ever have burning pain or discomfort during or right after urination?
- Does it feel like your bladder is not empty when you finish urinating?
- Do you have to go to the bathroom every 2 hours (or more often)?
- Do you ever have pain or discomfort in your testicles, penis, or the area between your rectum and your testicles (perineum)?
- Do you ever have pain in your pubic or bladder area?
- Do you have any discomfort during or after sexual climax (ejaculation)?

The therapist is reminded in asking these questions to offer clients a clear explanation for any questions asked concerning sexual activity, sexual function, or sexual history. There is no way to know when someone will be offended or claim sexual harassment. It is in your own interest to conduct the interview in the most professional manner possible.

There should be no hint of sexual innuendo or humor injected into any of your conversations with clients at any time. The line of sexual impropriety lies where the complainant draws it and includes appearances of misbehavior. This perception differs broadly from client to client.[16]

Prostatitis cannot always be cured but can be managed. Correct diagnosis is the key to the management of prostatitis. Screening men with red flag symptoms, history, and risk factors can result in early detection and medical referral.

Physical therapy has been shown to have some potential in helping men with chronic prostatitis. Physical therapy for this problem is more common in the European countries but is gaining support in the U.S. Intervention is directed toward reducing pelvic floor muscle tone and improving urinary function using electrostimulation, transrectal microwave hyperthermia, biofeedback, myofascial release, and transrectal mobilization of the pelvic ligaments.[17-20]

Clinical Signs and Symptoms of

Prostatitis

- Sudden moderate-to-high fever
- Chills
- Low back, inner thigh, and perineal pain
- Testicular or penis pain
- Urinary frequency and urgency
- Nocturia/(unusual voiding during the night)/sleep disturbance
- Dysuria (painful or difficult urination)
- Weak or interrupted urine stream (hesitancy)
- Unable to completely empty bladder
- Sexual dysfunction (e.g., painful ejaculation, cramping/discomfort after ejaculation, infertility)
- General malaise
- Arthralgia
- Myalgia

BENIGN PROSTATIC HYPERPLASIA

Benign prostatic hyperplasia (BPH; enlarged prostate) is a common occurrence in men older than 50. Like all cells in the body, cells in the prostate constantly die and are replaced by new cells. As men age, the ratio of new prostate cells to old prostate cells shifts in favor of lower cell death. With a lower cell turnover, there are more "old" cells than "new" ones and the prostate enlarges, squeezing the urethra and interfering with urination and sexual function. It is unclear why cell replacement is diminished, but it may be related to hormone changes associated with aging.

Prostate enlargement affects about half of all men between ages 60 and 69 and close to 80% of men between ages 70 and 90. Severity of signs and symptoms varies and only about half of men with prostate enlargement have problems noticeable enough to seek treatment.[21]

Because of the prostate's position around the urethra (see Fig. 10-3), enlargement of the prostate quickly interferes with the normal passage of urine from the bladder. Sexual function is not usually affected unless prostate surgery is required and sexual dysfunction occurs as a complication. If the prostate is greatly enlarged, chronic constipation may result.

Urination becomes increasingly difficult, and the bladder never feels completely empty. Straining to empty the bladder can stretch the bladder, making it less elastic. The detrusor becomes less efficient and urine collecting in the bladder can foster urinary tract infections.

If left untreated, loss of bladder tone and damage to the detrusor may not be reversible.

Continued enlargement of the prostate eventually obstructs the bladder completely, and emergency measures become necessary to empty the bladder. Like prostatitis, BPH cannot be cured but symptoms can be managed with medical treatment. Anyone with undiagnosed symptoms of BPH should seek medical evaluation as soon as possible. Screening questions for an **enlarged prostate** can include the following:

Follow-Up Questions

- Does it feel like your bladder is not empty when you finish urinating?
- Do you have to urinate again less than 2 hours after the last time you emptied your bladder?
- Do you have a weak stream of urine or find you have to start and stop urinating several times when you go to the bathroom?
- Do you have to push or strain to start urinating or to keep the urine flowing?
- Do you have any leaking or dribbling of urine from the penis?
- Do you get up more than once at night to urinate?

Clinical Signs and Symptoms of

Obstruction of the Lower Urinary Tract (Benign Prostatic Hyperplasia/Prostate Cancer)

Lower urinary tract symptoms of blockage are most commonly related to bladder or urethral pressure (e.g., prostate enlargement). This pressure results in bladder distention and subsequent pain. Common symptoms of lower urinary tract (LUT) obstruction include

- Bladder palpable above the symphysis pubis
- Urinary problems
  - Hesitancy: difficulty in initiating urination or an interrupted flow of urine
  - Small amounts of urine with voiding (weak urine stream)
  - Dribbling at the end of urination
  - Frequency: need to urinate often (more than every 2 hours)
  - Nocturia (unusual voiding during the night)/sleep disturbance
- Lower abdominal discomfort with a feeling of the need to void
- Low back and/or hip, upper thigh pain or stiffness
- Suprapubic or pelvic pain
- Difficulty having an erection
- Blood in urine or semen

PROSTATE CANCER

Prostate cancer is a slow growing form of cancer causing microscopic changes in the prostate in one third of all men by age 50. Carcinoma in situ is present in 50% to 75% of American men by age 75. Most of these changes are latent, meaning they produce no signs or symptoms or they are so slow growing (indolent) that they never cause a health threat.[22]

Even so, prostate cancer is the second most common type of cancer and second leading cause of death among men in this country. Of all the men who are diagnosed with cancer each year, about one third have prostate cancer.[23]

The number of new diagnosed cases of prostate cancer has dramatically increased over the last two decades (peaking in 1992), probably due to mass screening using a blood test to measure the prostate-specific antigen (PSA). PSA rises in men who have any changes in the prostate (e.g., tumor, infection, enlargement).[23] Despite the many controversies over "normal" levels of PSA, this test has shifted the detection of the majority of prostate cancer cases from late-stage to early-stage disease.[24]

Because more men are living longer and the incidence of prostate cancer increases with age, prostate cancer is becoming a significant health issue. Risk factors include advancing age, family history, ethnicity, and diet. Most men with prostate cancer are older than 65; the disease is rare in men younger than 45.

A man's risk of prostate cancer is higher than average if his brother or father had the disease. In fact, the more first-degree family members affected, the greater the person's risk of prostate cancer. It is more common in African American men compared to white or Hispanic men. It is less common in Asian and American Indian men.[22]

Some studies suggest a diet high in animal fat or meat may be a risk factor. Other risk factors may include low levels of vitamins or selenium, multiple sex partners, viruses, and occupational exposure to chemicals (including farmers exposed to herbicides and pesticides), cadmium, and other metals.[22]

Early prostate cancer often does not cause symptoms. But prostate cancer can cause any of the signs and symptoms listed in the box, Clinical Signs and Symptoms of Obstruction of the Lower Urinary Tract.

It is often diagnosed when the man seeks medical assistance because of symptoms of lower urinary tract obstruction or low back, hip, or leg

pain or stiffness (Case Example 10-3). There are four stages of prostate cancer[22]:

- Stage I or Stage A—The cancer cannot be felt during a rectal exam. It may be found when surgery is done for another reason, usually for BPH. There is no evidence that the cancer has spread outside the prostate.

- Stage II or Stage B—The tumor is large enough that it can be palpated during a rectal exam or found with a biopsy. There is no evidence that the cancer has spread outside the prostate.

- Stage III or Stage C—The cancer has spread outside the prostate to nearby tissues.

- Stage IV or Stage D—The cancer has spread to lymph nodes or to other parts of the body

Back pain and sciatica can be caused by cancer metastasis via the bloodstream of the lymphatic system to the bones of the pelvis, spine, or femur. Lumbar pain is predominant but the thoracolumbar pain can be painful as well depending on the location of the metastases. Prostate cancer is unique in that bone is often the only clinically detectable site of metastases. The resulting tumors tend to be osteoblastic (bone forming causing sclerosis), rather than osteolytic (bone lysing) (Fig. 10-6; see also Fig. 13-7).[25]

Symptoms of metastatic disease include bone pain, anemia, weight loss, lymphedema of the lower extremities and scrotum, and neurologic changes associated with spinal cord compression when spinal involvement occurs.

Incontinence

Urinary incontinence (UI) is the involuntary leakage of urine. According to the U.S. Department of Health and Human Services, incontinence is a vastly underdiagnosed and underreported problem affecting millions of Americans each year. The incidence of incontinence is expected to grow dramatically as the U.S. population continues to age.[26]

Urinary incontinence is not a disease, but rather a symptom of other underlying health conditions including trauma (e.g., childbirth, incest), diabetes, multiple sclerosis, Parkinson's disease, spinal injury, spina bifida, surgery, hormonal changes, medications, stroke dysfunction, urinary tract infections, neuromuscular conditions, constipation, or even dietary issues including caffeine intake.

Incontinent people may restrict their activities for fear of urine loss and concerns about odors in public. This reduction in social activity and impact on lifestyle can have profound effects on psychological well being and health including depression, skin breakdown, urinary tract infections, and urosepsis. The therapist can have an important role in the successful treatment of incontinence; therefore screening for this symptom is vital and should be a routine part of the health assessment for all adult clients, especially in a primary care setting.

There are four primary types of UI recognized in adults. These are based on the underlying anatomic or physiologic impairment and include: stress, urge, mixed (combination of urge and stress), and overflow.

Stress incontinence occurs when the support for the bladder or urethra is weak or damaged, but the bladder itself is normal. With stress incontinence, pressure applied to the bladder from coughing, sneezing, laughing, lifting, exercising, or other physical exertion increases abdominal pressure, and the pelvic floor musculature cannot counteract the urethral/bladder pressure. This type of

---

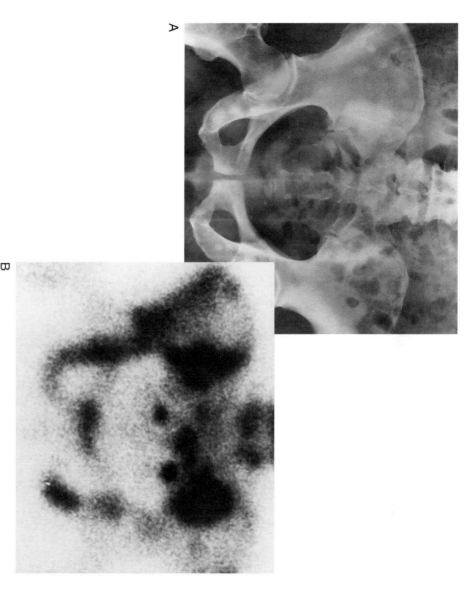

Fig. 10-6 • Widespread osteoblastic skeletal metastases in prostate adenocarcinoma. **A,** Anteroposterior radiograph of pelvis shows multiple sclerotic foci. **B,** Radioisotopic bone scan shows multiple foci of increased uptake in pelvis from the same patient. (From Dorfman HD, Czerniak B: *Bone tumors,* St. Louis, 1998, Mosby.)

incontinence causes 75% of all cases of urinary incontinence in women and is primarily related to urethral sphincter weakness, pelvic floor weakness, and ligamentous and fascial laxity.

Urge incontinence, now more commonly called overactive bladder, is the involuntary contraction of the detrusor muscle (smooth muscle of the bladder wall) with a strong desire to void (urgency) and loss of urine as soon as the urge is felt. The bladder involuntarily contracts or is unstable, or there may be involuntary sphincter relaxation. Urge incontinence is often idiopathic but can be caused by medications, alcohol, bladder infections, bladder tumor, neurogenic bladder, or bladder outlet obstruction.

Overflow incontinence is overdistention of the bladder and the bladder cannot empty completely. Urine leaks or dribbles out so the client does not have any sensation of fullness or emptying.

It may be caused by an acontractile or deficient detrusor muscle, a hypotonic or underactive detrusor muscle secondary to drugs, fecal impaction, diabetes, lower spinal cord injury, or disruption of the motor innervation of the detrusor muscle (e.g., multiple sclerosis).

In men, overflow incontinence is most often secondary to obstruction caused by prostatic hyperplasia, prostatic carcinoma, or urethral stricture. In women, this type of incontinence occurs as a result of obstruction caused by severe genital prolapse or surgical overcorrection of urethral detachment.

The client with incontinence from overflow will report a feeling that the bladder does not empty completely with an urge to void frequently including at night. Small amounts of urine are lost involuntarily throughout the day and night. There may be a weak stream or flow sometimes described as "dribbling."

The term *functional incontinence* describes another type of UI that occurs when the bladder is normal but the mind and body are not working together. Functional incontinence occurs from mobility and access deficits, such as being confined to a wheelchair or needing a walker to ambulate.[28]

Deficits in dexterity, such as weakness from a stroke or neuropathy and loss of motion from arthritis may keep the individual from getting pants unfastened or panties pulled down in time to avoid an accident. Altered mentation from dementia or Alzheimer's can also contribute to untimely urination without a urologic structural problem.

Causes of incontinence can range from urologic/gynecologic to neurologic, psychologic, pharmaceutical, or environmental. Anything that can interfere with neurologic function or produce obstruction can contribute to UI. There is a high prevalence of stress and urge incontinence in female elite athletes. The frequency of UI is significantly higher in eating disordered athletes.[29]

Risk factors for developing UI are listed in Box 10-3. Chronic constipation at any time, but especially during pregnancy, can lead to increased abdominal pressure, which can cause UI. Any condition leading to an enlarged abdomen (e.g., ascites, weight gain, pregnancy) with increased pressure on the bladder can contribute to incontinence.

Chemotherapy, radiation, surgery, and medications can cause disruptions in the cycle of micturition (urination) for many different physiologic reasons. For example, chemotherapy can increase fat deposits and decrease muscle mass, which increase the risk of bowel and bladder dysfunction.

Radiation alters tissue viability in the surrounding area, which can affect circulation to the organs and support from muscle, fascia, ligaments, and tendons.[31] Radiation can cause fibrotic contracted bladder tissue and damaged sphincter contributing to UI. Acute radiation prostatocystitis due to external beam radiation can cause frequency, nocturia, urgency, or urge incontinence as well as hematuria or transient urine retention.[32]

Surgery to remove tumors, lymph nodes, or the prostate can affect bladder control through alterations of blood and lymphatic circulation, innervation, and fascial support. Edema secondary to lymphatic system compromise can increase bladder (and bowel) dysfunction. Brain, spinal cord, or pelvic surgery can affect nervous control of the bowel and bladder.[31] Urge incontinence can occur as a result of bladder denervation from surgical injury.[32] Postprostatectomy UI (when incontinence is defined as any leak) occurs in up to 70%

Advancing age
Overweight/obese
Chronic cough
Chronic constipation
History of urinary tract infections
Enlarged abdomen (e.g., ascites, pregnancy, obesity, tumor)
Diabetes mellitus
Neurologic disorders
Medications
  Sedatives
  Diuretics
  Anticholinergics
  Alpha-adrenergic blockers
  Calcium channel blockers
  Antipsychotics
  Antidepressants
  Antiparkinsonian drugs
  Opioids
  Vincristine
  Angiotensin-converting enzyme (ACE) inhibitors
Caffeine, alcohol
Female gender (see below)

Specific to Women
Pregnancy (multiparity)
Vaginal or cesarean* birth
Previous bladder or pelvic surgery
Pelvic trauma or radiation
Bladder or bowel prolapse
Menopause (natural or surgically induced; estrogen deficiency)†
Tobacco use

Specific to Men
Enlarged prostate gland
Prostate or pelvic surgery
Radiation (acute and late complications) especially when combined with brachytherapy[32]

---

* Although the abdominal muscles are disrupted with a cesarean section and limit how much the woman can bear down on the bladder, abdominal tone and function are essential for pelvic muscle function.
† Urinary incontinence in middle-aged women may be more closely associated with mechanical factors such as childbearing, history of urinary tract infections, gynecologic surgery, chronic constipation, obesity, and exertion than with menopausal transition.[30]

---

of all cases but the rate of urine leak decreases as a result of time, medical treatment, and physical therapy intervention. UI is two times more common after prostatectomy than after radiation; surgical clients are three times more likely to use pads. Recovery occurs in most cases between 6 and 12 months after surgery.[32] Incontinence is not a

normal part of the aging process. When confronted with urinary incontinence in an older adult, consider some of the following causes of this disorder: infection, endocrine disorders, atrophic urethritis or vaginitis, restricted mobility, stool impaction (especially in smokers), alcohol or caffeine intake, and medications.

Smoking contributes to constipation and is often accompanied by chronic cough, which stresses the bladder. Some medications can lead to UI or aggravate already existing UI. Medications commonly involved with alterations in urinary continence include anticholinergic agents, calcium channel blockers, diuretics, sedatives, β-antagonists, and β-agonists.[33]

With any kind of incontinence, the onset of cervical spine pain at the same time that urinary incontinence develops is a red flag. These two findings would suggest there is a protrusion pressing on the spinal cord.

If a medical diagnosis for cervical disk protrusion has been established, referral would not be necessary. However, if incontinence is a new development from the time of the medical evaluation, the physician should be made aware of this information. Cervical spinal manipulation is considered contraindicated.

Many people are embarrassed about having an incontinence problem. It may help to introduce the subject by making a general statement such as "Many men and women have problems with bladder control. This is an area physical therapists can often help clients with so we routinely ask a few questions about bladder function."

Follow-Up Questions

Screening questions for incontinence can include

General:

Do you have any problems holding urine or emptying your bladder?

Do you ever leak urine or have accidents?

Do you wear pads to protect against urine leaking? Follow-up: How many do you use in a 24-hour period and how wet are they?

Are your activities limited because of urine leaking?

If the client answers "yes" to any of these questions, you may want to screen further with the following questions.

For stress incontinence:

Do you ever lose urine or wet your pants when you cough, sneeze, or laugh?

Do you lose urine or wet your pants when getting out of a chair, lifting, or exercising?

For overactive bladder (urge incontinence):

Do you have frequent, strong, or sudden urges to urinate and cannot get to the bathroom in time? For example:

When arriving home and getting out of the car?

When using a key to open the door?

When you hear water running?

Or when you run water over your hands?

When you go out into cold weather or put your hands in the freezer?

Do you get to the toilet and lose urine as you are pulling down your panties/shorts?

Do you urinate more than eight times a day?

Do you get up to go more than twice a night?

For overflow incontinence:

Do you dribble urine during the day and/or at night?

Can you urinate with a strong stream or does the urine dribble out slowly?

Does it feel like your bladder is empty when you are done urinating?

For functional incontinence:

Can you get to the toilet easily?

Do you have trouble getting to the bathroom on time?

Do you have trouble finding the bathroom or toilet?

Do you have accidents in the bathroom because you cannot get your pants unfastened or pulled down?

Renal Failure

A person is unlikely to seek treatment for renal problems from the physical therapist. However, patients/clients with renal failure may receive treatment for primary musculoskeletal lesions in both inpatient and outpatient clinics.

Renal failure exists when the kidneys can no longer maintain the homeostatic balances within the body that are necessary for life. Renal failure is classified as acute or chronic in origin and progression. *Acute renal failure* refers to the abrupt cessation of kidney activity, usually occurring over a period of hours to a few days. Acute renal failure is often reversible, with return of kidney function in 3 to 12 months.

Chronic renal failure, or irreversible renal failure (also known as end-stage renal disease or ESRD), is defined as a state of progressive decrease

in the ability of the kidney to filter fluids, metabolites, and electrolytes from the body, resulting in eventual permanent loss of kidney function. It can develop slowly over a period of years or can result from an episode of acute renal failure that does not resolve.

ESRD is a complex condition with multiple systemic complications. Diabetic nephropathy is the primary cause of ESRD, accounting for approximately 40% of newly diagnosed cases of ESRD. Individuals with diabetes and ESRD have higher morbidity and mortality rates than individuals with ESRD only.[34]

Risk factors for ESRD include age, diabetes mellitus, hypertension, chronic urinary tract obstruction and infection, and kidney transplantation. Hereditary defects of the kidneys, polycystic kidneys, and glomerular disorders such as glomerulonephritis can also lead to renal failure.

Chronic intake of certain medications and overthe-counter (OTC) drugs is also a factor in the development of renal disease. The increasing availability of OTC drugs has led to consumers treating themselves when they may lack the knowledge to do so safely. Age-related decline in renal function

combined with multiple medication use in the aging adult population increases the risk of hepatotoxicity.[35] Excessive consumption of acetaminophen and nonsteroidal antiinflammatory drugs, especially when combined with caffeine and/or codeine, are toxic to the kidneys.[36,37]

Clinical Signs and Symptoms

Failure of the filtering and regulating mechanisms of the kidney can be either acute (sudden in onset and potentially reversible) or chronic (called uremia, which develops gradually and is usually irreversible).

Individuals with either type of renal failure develop signs and symptoms characteristic of impaired fluid and waste excretion and altered renal regulation of other body metabolic processes, such as pH regulation, RBC production, and calcium-phosphorus balance.

Signs of renal impairment are shown in Table 10-4. The signs of actual renal failure are the same but more pronounced. In most cases of renal failure, urine volume is significantly decreased or absent. Edema becomes severe and can result in heart failure. Renal anemia is usually associated

---

TABLE 10-4 ▼ Systemic Manifestations of Renal Failure

System	Manifestation
General	Fatigue, malaise
Skin and nail beds	Pallor, ecchymosis, pruritus, dry skin and mucous membranes, thin/brittle nail beds, urine odor on skin, uremic frost (white urea crystals) on the face and upper trunk, poor wound healing
Skeletal	Osteomalacia, osteoporosis,* bone pain, myopathy, tendon rupture, fracture, joint pain, dependent edema
Neurologic	*CNS:* Recent memory loss, decreased alertness, difficulty concentrating, irritability, lethargy/sleep disturbance, coma, impaired judgment *PNS:* Muscle weakness, tremors, and cramping; restless leg syndrome, carpal tunnel syndrome, paresthesias
Eye, ear, nose, throat	Metallic taste in mouth, nosebleeds, uremic (urine-smelling) breath, pale conjunctiva, visual blurring
Cardiovascular	Hypertension, friction rub, congestive heart failure, pericarditis, cardiomyopathy, arrhythmia, Raynaud's phenomenon
Pulmonary	Dyspnea, pulmonary edema, crackles (rales), pleural effusion
Gastrointestinal	Anorexia, nausea, vomiting, hiccups, gastrointestinal bleeding
Genitourinary	Decreased urine output and other changes in pattern of urination (e.g., nocturia)
Metabolic/endocrine	Dehydration, hyperkalemia, metabolic acidosis, hypocalcemia, hyperphosphatemia, fertility and sexual dysfunction (e.g., impotence, loss of libido, amenorrhea), hyperparathyroidism
Hematologic	Anemia Thrombocytopenia

* Bone demineralization leads to a condition called renal osteodystrophy.
CNS, Central nervous system; *PNS,* peripheral nervous system.
From Goodman CC, Boissonnault WG, Fuller K: *Pathology: implications for the physical therapist,* ed. 2. Philadelphia, 2003, WB Saunders.

with extreme fatigue and intolerance to normal daily activities as well as a marked decrease in exercise capacity.[38]

In addition, the continuous presence of toxic waste products in the bloodstream (urea, creatinine, uric acid) results in damage to many other body systems, including the central nervous system, peripheral nervous system, eyes, gastrointestinal tract, integumentary system, endocrine system, and cardiopulmonary system.

Treatment of renal failure involves several elements designed to replace the lost excretory and metabolic functions of this organ. Treatment options include dialysis, dietary changes, and medications to regulate blood pressure and assist in replacement of lost metabolic functions, such as calcium balance and RBC production.

The choice of treatment options, such as dialysis, transplantation, or no treatment, depends on many factors, including the person's age, underlying physical problems, and availability of compatible organs for transplantation.[39] Untreated or chronic renal failure eventually results in death.

From a screening perspective, the therapist must be alert to the many complications associated with chronic renal failure and dialysis. Watch for signs and symptoms of fluid and electrolyte imbalances (see Chapter 11), dehydration (see Chapter 6), cardiac arrhythmias (see Chapter 11), and depression (see Chapter 3).

Clinical Signs and Symptoms of
Renal Impairment

Symptoms of upper urinary tract infection, particularly renal infection, can be categorized according to urinary tract manifestations or systemic manifestations caused by renal impairment (see Table 10-4). Clinical signs and symptoms of urinary tract involvement can include

- Unilateral costovertebral tenderness
- Flank pain
- Ipsilateral shoulder pain
- Fever and chills
- Skin hypersensitivity
- Hematuria (blood in urine)
- Pyuria (pus in urine)
- Bacteriuria (presence of bacteria in urine)
- Hypertension
- Decreased urinary output
- Dependent edema
- Weakness
- Anorexia (loss of appetite)
- Dyspnea
- Mild headache
- Proteinuria (protein in urine, urine may be foamy)
- Abnormal blood serum level, such as elevated blood urea nitrogen (BUN) and creatinine
- Anemia

Cancers of the Urinary Tract
Bladder Cancer

Bladder cancer is a common, major public health concern and it is strongly linked to cigarette smoking.[40] It is the fourth most common cancer in men and the tenth most common cancer in women. Bladder cancer is nearly three times more common in men than in women, thus it is typically diagnosed later in women and often at a more advanced stage.[41]

The exact cause of bladder cancer is not known, but certain risk factors have been identified which increase chances of developing this type of cancer.

- Age (over 40)
- Tobacco use (cigarette, pipe, and cigar smokers)
- Occupation (work place carcinogens such as rubber, chemical, leather industries; hairdressers, machinists, metal workers, printers, painters, textile workers, truck drivers)
- Infections (parasitic, usually in tropical areas of the world)
- Treatment with cyclophosphamide or arsenic (for other cancers)
- Race (whites highest; Asians lowest)
- Gender (men 2 to 3 times more likely than women)
- Previous personal history of bladder cancer
- Family history (some association but not clearly defined)[42,43]

Common symptoms of bladder cancer include blood in the urine, pain during urination, and urinary urgency or the feeling of urinary urgency without resulting urination. These symptoms are not sure signs of bladder cancer, but anyone with these symptoms should be referred to a physician for further follow up studies.

Measures that have been shown to reduce the risk of developing bladder cancer include cessation of smoking, adequate intake of fluids, intake of cruciferous vegetables, limiting exposure to workplace chemicals, and prompt treatment of bladder infections.

Renal Cancer

Cancer of the kidney (renal cancer) develops most often in people over the age of forty and has some associated risk factors. The following risk factors for renal cancer include

- Smoking (two times the risk as nonsmokers)
- Obesity
- Hypertension
- Long-term dialysis
- Van Hippel-Lindau (VHL) syndrome (genetic, familial syndrome)
- Occupation (coke oven workers in the iron and steel industry; asbestos and cadmium exposure)
- Gender (men twice more likely than women)

Common symptoms of renal cancer are very similar to those of bladder cancer and require immediate referral for follow up. These symptoms can include blood in the urine, pain in the side that does not go away, a lump or mass in the side or abdomen, weight loss, fever, and general fatigue or feeling of poor health.[44]

Clinical Signs and Symptoms of
Bladder and Renal Cancer

Bladder Cancer

- Blood in the urine
- Pain during urination
- Urinary urgency

Renal Cancer

- Blood in the urine
- Pain during urination
- Urinary urgency
- Flank or side pain
- Lump or mass in the side or abdomen
- Weight loss
- Fever
- General fatigue; feeling of poor health

Testicular Cancer[45]

The testicles (also called testes or gonads) are the male sex glands. They are located behind the penis in a pouch of skin called the scrotum (see Fig. 10-3). The testicles produce and store sperm and serve as the body's main source of male hormones. These hormones control the development of the reproductive organs and other male characteristics, such as body and facial hair, low voice, wide shoulders, and sexual function.

Testicular cancer is relatively rare and occurs most often in young men between the ages of 15 and 35 years old, although any male can be affected at any time (including infants). According to the National Cancer Institute's Surveillance, about 8000 men are diagnosed with testicular cancer each year (390 deaths annually).[23] The incidence of testicular cancer around the world has doubled in the past 30 to 40 years.

The cause of testicular cancer and even the risk factors remain unknown. Risk is higher than average for boys born with an undescended testicle (cryptorchidism). The cancer risk for boys with this condition is increased even if surgery is done to move the testicle into the scrotum. In the case of unilateral cryptorchidism, the risk of testicular cancer is increased in the normal testicle as well. This fact suggests testicular cancer is due to whatever caused the undescended testicle.

Having a brother or father with testicular cancer also increases an individual's risk. Other risk factors may include occupation (e.g., miners, oil and gas workers, leather workers, food and beverage processing workers, janitors, firefighters, utility workers) and HIV infection.

The risk of testicular cancer among white American men is about 5 to 10 times that of African American men and more than twice that of Asian American men. The risk for Hispanics is between that of Asians and non-Hispanic whites. The reason for this difference is unknown.

The testicular cancer rate has more than doubled among white Americans in the past 40 years but has not changed for African Americans. Worldwide, the risk of developing this disease is highest among men living in the United States and Europe and lowest among African and Asian men.

CLINICAL SIGNS AND SYMPTOMS

Testicular cancer can be completely asymptomatic. The most common sign is a hard, painless lump in the testicle about the size of a pea. There may be a dull ache in the scrotum and the man may be aware of tender, larger breasts. Other symptoms are listed in the box Clinical Signs and Symptoms of Testicular Cancer.

There are three stages of testicular cancer:

- Stage I—The cancer is confined to the testicle.
- Stage II—The cancer has spread to the retroperitoneal lymph nodes, located in the posterior abdominal cavity below the diaphragm and between the kidneys.
- Stage III—The cancer has spread beyond the lymph nodes to remote sites in the body, including the lungs, brain, liver, and bones.

If found early testicular cancer is almost always curable.[23] The American Cancer Society recommends monthly self-exam of the testicles for adolescents and men, starting at age 15. Testicular self-examination is an effective way of getting to know this area of the body and thus detecting testicular cancer at a very early, curable stage. The self-exam is best performed once each month during or after a warm bath or shower when

the heat has relaxed the scrotum (see Appendix D-8).

Men who have been treated for cancer in one testicle have about a 3% to 4% chance of developing cancer in the remaining testicle. If cancer does arise in the second testicle, it is nearly always a new disease rather than metastasis from the first tumor.

Metastases occur via the blood or lymph system. The most common place for the disease spread is to the lymph nodes in the posterior part of the abdomen. Therefore, lower back pain is a frequent symptom of later stage testicular cancer (Case Example 10-4). If the cancer has spread to the lungs, persistent cough, chest pain, and/or shortness of breath can occur. Hemoptysis (sputum with blood) may also develop.

Survivors of testicular cancer should be checked regularly by their doctors and should continue to perform monthly testicular self-examinations. Any unusual symptoms should be reported to the doctor immediately. Outcome even after a secondary testicular cancer is still excellent with early detection and treatment.

Clinical Signs and Symptoms
Testicular Cancer

- A lump in either testicle
- Any enlargement, swelling, or hardness of a testicle
- Significant loss of size in one of the testicles
- Feeling of heaviness in the scrotum and/or lower abdomen

Continued on p. 456

CASE EXAMPLE 10-4   Testicular Cancer

A 20-year-old track star and college football player developed back, buttock, and posterior thigh pain after a football injury. He was sent to physical therapy by the team physician with a diagnosis of "Sciatica; L4-5 radiculopathy. Please treat using McKenzie exercise program."

During the physical therapy interview, the client reported left low back pain and left buttock pain present for the last 2 weeks after being tackled from the right side in a football game. Symptoms developed approximately 12 hours after the injury. Pain was always present but was worse after sitting and better after standing.

On examination the client presented with major losses of lumbar spine range of motion in all planes. There was no observable lateral shift and lumbar lordosis was not excessive or reduced. Overall postural assessment was unremarkable.

He was able to lie flat in the prone position and perform a small prone press up without increasing any of his symptoms but he described feeling a "hard knot in my stomach" while in this position. When asked if he had any symptoms of any kind anywhere else in his body, the client replied that right after the injury, his left testicle swelled up but seemed better now. He denied any blood in the urine or difficulty urinating. Vital signs were within normal limits.

Even though the therapist thought the clinical findings supported a diagnosis of a derange-

ment syndrome according to the McKenzie classification, there were enough red flags to warrant further investigation.

The client was given an appropriate self-treatment program to perform throughout the day with instructions for self-assessment of his condition. In the meantime, the therapist contacted the physician with the following concerns:

- Palpable (non pulsatile) abdominal mass in the left upper abdominal quadrant (anterior)
- Reported left testicular swelling
- Age
- No imaging studies were done to confirm a discogenic lesion as the underlying cause of the symptoms

Result: Physician referral was made after a telephone discussion outlining the additional findings listed above. An abdominal CT scan showed a 20cm (5inch) abdominal mass pressing on the spinal nerves as the cause of the back pain. Further diagnostic testing revealed testicular cancer as the primary diagnosis with metastases to the abdomen causing the abdominal mass.

Surgery was performed to remove the testicle. The back pain was relieved within 3 days of starting chemotherapy. Physical therapy was discontinued for back pain but a new plan of care was established for exercise during cancer treatment.

- Dull ache in the lower abdomen or in the groin
- Sudden collection of fluid in the scrotum
- Pain or discomfort in a testicle or in the scrotum
- Enlargement or tenderness of the breasts
- Unexplained fatigue or malaise
- Infertility
- Low back pain (metastases to retroperitoneal lymph nodes)

▶ PHYSICIAN REFERRAL

The proximity of the kidneys, ureters, bladder, and urethra to the ribs, vertebrae, diaphragm, and accompanying muscles and tendinous insertions often can make it difficult to identify the client's problems accurately.

Pain related to a urinary tract problem can be similar to pain felt from an injury to the back, flank, abdomen, or upper thigh. The physical therapist is advised to question the client further whenever any of the signs and symptoms listed in Table 10-3 are reported or observed. Further diagnostic testing and medical examination must be performed by the physician to differentiate urinary tract conditions from musculoskeletal problems.

The physical therapist must be able to recognize the systemic origin of urinary tract symptoms that mimic musculoskeletal pain. Many conditions that produce urinary tract pain also include an elevation in temperature, abnormal urinary constituents, and changes in color, odor, or amount of urine.

These types of changes would not be observed or reported with a musculoskeletal condition, and the client may not mention them, thinking these symptoms do not have anything to do with the back, flank, or thigh pain present. The therapist must ask a few screening questions to bring this kind of information to the forefront.

When the physical therapist conducts a review of systems, any signs and symptoms associated with renal or urologic impairment should be correlated with the findings of the objective examination and combined with the medical history to provide a comprehensive report at the time of referral to the physician or other health care provider.

Diagnostic Testing

Screening of the composition of the urine is called *urinalysis* (UA), and UA is the commonly used method of determining various properties of urine. This analysis is actually a series of several tests of urinary components and is a valuable aid in the diagnosis of urinary tract or metabolic disorders.

Normal urinary constituents are shown (see inside front cover: Urine Analysis). Urine cultures are also very important studies in the diagnosis of UTIs. Anyone at risk for chronic kidney disease should be tested for markers of kidney damage. This is done by urinalysis for albumin (protein in the urine) and by blood serum for creatinine (waste product of muscle metabolism).

Various *blood studies* can be done to assess renal function (see inside front cover: Renal Blood Studies). These studies examine both the serum and cellular components of the blood for specific changes characteristic of renal performance. Substances that must be examined in the serum are those that are a *direct* reflection of renal function, such as creatinine, and others that are more *indirect* in renal evaluation, such as BUN, pH-related substances, uric acid, various ions, electrolytes, and cellular components (RBCs). (For a more in-depth discussion of laboratory values the reader is referred to a more specific source of information.)[46-48]

Guidelines for Immediate Medical Attention

- The presence of any amount of blood in the urine always requires a referral to a physician. However, the presence of abnormalities in the urine may not be obvious, and a thorough diagnostic analysis of the urine may be needed. Careful questioning of the client regarding urinary tract history, urinary patterns, urinary characteristics, and pain patterns may elicit valuable information relating to potential urinary tract symptoms.
- Presence of cervical spine pain at the same time that urinary incontinence develops. If a diagnosis of cervical disk prolapse has been made, the physician should be notified of these findings; referral may not be necessary, but communication with the physician to confirm this is necessary.
- Client with bowel/bladder incontinence and/or saddle anesthesia secondary to cauda equina lesion.

Guidelines for Physician Referral

Although immediate (emergency) medical attention is not required, medical referral is needed under the following circumstances:

- When the client has any combination of systemic signs and symptoms presented in this chapter. Damage to the urinary tract structures can occur with accident, injury, assault, or other trauma to the musculoskeletal structures

surrounding the kidney and urinary tract and may require medical evaluation if the clinical presentation or response to physical therapy treatment suggests it.

For example, the alpine skier discussed at the beginning of the chapter had a dull, aching costovertebral pain on the left side that was unrelieved by a change of position or by ice, heat, or aspirin. His pain is related directly to a traumatic episode, and musculoskeletal injury is a definite possibility in his case. He has no medical history of urinary tract problems and denies any changes in urine or pattern of urination. Because the pain is constant and unrelieved by usual measures and the location of the pain is approximate to renal structures, a medical follow up and urinalysis would be recommended.

OVERVIEW

RENAL AND UROLOGIC PAIN PATTERNS

▼ **KIDNEY** (Fig. 10-7)

- Men 45 years old or older
- In men, back pain accompanied by burning on urination, difficulty in urination, or fever may be

Clues Suggesting Pain of Renal/Urological Origin

- Positive Murphy's percussion test, especially with a recent history of renal or urologic infection.
- Back or shoulder pain accompanied by abnormal urinary constituents (e.g., change in color, odor, amount, flow of urine).

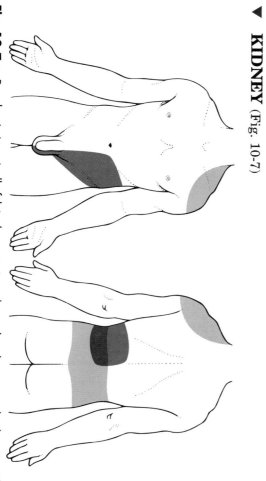

Fig. 10-7 • Renal pain is typically felt in the posterior subcostal and costovertebral region *(dark red)*. It can radiate across the low back *(light red)* and/or forward around the flank into the lower abdominal quadrant. Ipsilateral groin and testicular pain may also accompany renal pain. Pressure from the kidney on the diaphragm may cause ipsilateral shoulder pain.

associated with prostatitis; usually in such a case there is no limitation of back motion and no muscle spasm (until symptoms progress, causing muscle guarding and splinting)

- Blood in urine
- Change in urinary pattern such as increased or decreased frequency, change in flow of urine stream (weak or dribbling), and increased nocturia
- Presence of constitutional symptoms, especially fever and chills; pain is constant (may be dull or sharp, depending on the cause)
- Pain is unchanged by altering body position; side bending to the involved side and pressure at that level is "more comfortable" (may reduce pain but does not eliminate it)
- Neither renal nor urethral pain is altered by a change in body position; pseudorenal pain from a mechanical cause can be relieved by a change in position
- True renal pain is seldom affected by movements of the spine
- Straight leg–raising test is negative with renal colic appearing as back pain
- Back pain at the level of the kidneys in a woman with previous breast or uterine cancer (ovarian cancer)
- Assessment for pseudorenal pain is negative (see Table 10-1)

O V E R V I E W   RENAL AND UROLOGIC PAIN PATTERNS—cont'd

Location: Posterior subcostal and costovertebral region
            Usually unilateral

Referral: Radiates forward, around the flank or the side into the lower abdominal
            quadrant (T11 to T12), along the pelvic crest and into the groin
            Pressure from the kidney on the diaphragm may cause ipsilateral shoulder
            pain

Description: Dull, aching, boring

Intensity: Acute: Severe, intense
            Chronic: Vague and poorly localized

Duration: Constant

Associated signs and
symptoms: Fever, chills
            Increased urinary frequency
            Blood in urine
            Hyperesthesia of associated dermatomes (T9 and T10)
            Ipsilateral or generalized abdominal pain
            Spasm of abdominal muscles
            Nausea and vomiting when severely acute
            Testicular pain may occur in men
            Unrelieved by a change in position

▶ URETER (Fig. 10-8)

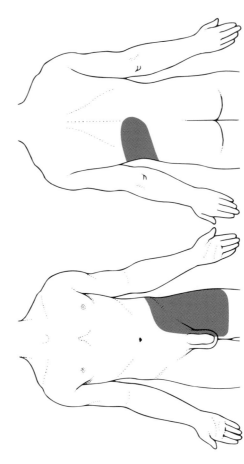

Fig. 10-8 • Ureteral pain may begin posteriorly in the costovertebral angle. It may then radiate anteriorly to the ipsilateral lower abdomen, upper thigh, testes, or labium.

Location: Costovertebral angle
            Unilateral or bilateral

Referral: Radiates to the lower abdomen, upper thigh, testis, or labium on the same
            side (groin and genital area)

Description: Described as crescendo waves of colic

Intensity: Excruciating, severe (Ureteral pain is commonly acute and caused by a
            kidney stone. Lesions outside the ureter are usually painless until advanced
            progression of the disease occurs.)

OVERVIEW RENAL AND UROLOGIC PAIN PATTERNS—cont'd

Duration: Ureteral pain caused by calculus is intermittent or constant without relief until treated or until the stone is passed
Rectal tenesmus (painful spasm of anal sphincter with urgent desire to evacuate the bowel/bladder; involuntary straining with little passage of urine or feces)

Associated signs and symptoms:
Nausea, abdominal distention, vomiting
Hyperesthesia of associated dermatomes (T10 to L1)
Tenderness over the kidney or ureter
Unrelieved by a change in position
Movement of iliopsoas may aggravate symptoms associated with a lesion outside the ureter (see Fig. 8-3)

▼ BLADDER/URETHRA (Fig. 10-9)

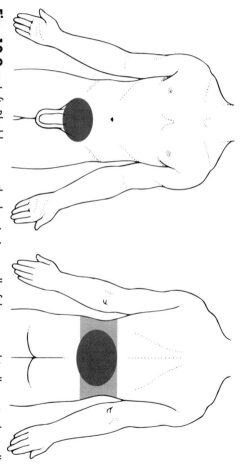

Fig. 10-9 • *Left,* Bladder or urethral pain is usually felt suprapubically or ipsilaterally in the lower abdomen. This is the same pattern for gas pain from the lower GI tract for some people. *Right,* Bladder or urethral pain may also be perceived in the low back area (*dark red:* primary pain center; *light red:* referred pain). Low back pain may occur as the first and only symptom associated with bladder/urethral pain, or it may occur along with suprapubic or abdominal pain or both.

Location: Suprapubic or low abdomen, low back
Referral: Pelvis

Description: Can be confused with gas
Sharp, localized

Intensity: Moderate-to-severe
Duration: Intermittent; may be relieved by emptying the bladder

Associated signs and symptoms:
Great urinary urgency
Tenesmus
Dysuria
Hot or burning sensation during urination

OVERVIEW   RENAL AND UROLOGIC PAIN PATTERNS—cont'd

▼ **PROSTATE** (Fig. 10-10)

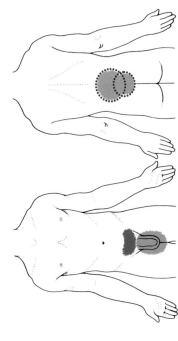

Fig. 10-10 • The prostate is segmentally innervated from T11-L1, S2-S4. Prostate problems can be painless. When pain occurs, the primary pain pattern is in the lower abdomen, suprapubic region (*dark red*), and perineum (between the rectum and testes; the latter is not pictured). Pain can be referred to the low back, sacrum, testes, and inner thighs (*light red*).

Symptoms of prostate involvement vary depending on the underlying cause (e.g., prostatitis vs. BPH vs. prostate cancer).

Location:	May be pain free; lower abdomen, suprapubic region
Referral:	Low back, pelvis, sacrum, perineum, inner thighs, testes; thoracolumbar spine with metastases (the latter is not pictured)
Description:	Persistent aching pain; pain is reproduced with digital rectal exam
Intensity:	Mild to severe; varies from person to person and can fluctuate for each individual on any given day
Duration:	Varies according to underlying cause
Associated signs and symptoms:	Chills and fever (prostatitis)
	Frequent and/or painful urination
	Urgency, hesitancy
	Nocturia
	Incomplete emptying of bladder
	Painful ejaculation
	Hematuria
	Arthralgia, myalgia

🕐 KEY POINTS TO REMEMBER

✓ Renal and urologic pain can be referred to the shoulder or low back.

✓ Lesions outside the ureter can cause pain on movement of the adjacent iliopsoas muscle.

✓ Radiculitis can mimic ureteral colic or renal pain, but true renal pain is seldom affected by movements of the spine.

✓ Inflammatory pain may be relieved by a change in position. Renal colic remains unchanged by a change in position.

✓ Low back, pelvic, or femur pain can be the first symptom of prostate cancer.

✓ Urinary incontinence is not a normal part of aging and should be evaluated carefully.

✓ With any kind of incontinence, the onset of cervical spine pain at the same time that urinary incontinence develops is a red flag and contraindicates the use of cervical spinal manipulation.

✓ Lower thoracic disc herniation can cause groin pain and/or leg pain, mimicking renal pain. The presence of neurologic changes such as bladder dysfunction can cause confusion when trying to differentiate a systemic from neuromusculoskeletal cause of symptoms. True renal pain is seldom affected by movements of the spine.

✓ Compare results of palpation and percussion tests.

✓ Testicular cancer with metastasis to the lymph system or bone can cause low back pain from pressure on the spinal nerves. Always watch for red flags even when an injury occurs; this is especially true in the young adult or athlete.

✓ Anyone with hypertension and/or diabetes (and/or other significant risk factors for renal disease) should be monitored carefully and consistently for any systemic signs and symptoms of renal impairment.

✓ People with diabetes are prone to complications associated with urinary tract infections.

✓ The sudden onset of nonspecific low back pain, unrelated to any specific motion may be an indication of osteomyelitis from spread of infection to the spine. Take the client's body temperature and ask him/her to monitor temperature for a few days to uncover the possibility of a low-grade fever associated with osteomyelitis. All the possible pain patterns discussed in this chapter are presented as follows:

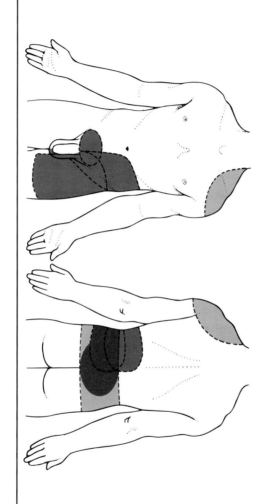

SUBJECTIVE EXAMINATION

Special Questions To Ask

Clients may be reluctant to answer the physical therapist's questions concerning bladder and urinary function. The physical therapist is advised to explain the need to rule out possible causes of pain related to the kidneys and bladder and to give the client time to respond if answers seem to be uncertain. For example, the physical therapist may ask the client to observe urinary function over the next 2 days. These questions should be reviewed again at the next appointment.

Past Medical History

- Have you had any problems with your prostate (for men), kidneys, or bladder? *If so,* describe.

SUBJECTIVE EXAMINATION—cont'd

- Have you ever had kidney or bladder stones? If so, when? How were these stones treated?
- Have you had an injury to your bladder or kidneys? *If so,* when? How was this treated? **(Be aware of unreported domestic abuse/ assault.)**
- Have you had any kidney or bladder infections in the past 6 months? How were these infections treated? Were they related to any specific circumstances **(e.g., pregnancy, intercourse, after strep throat or strep skin infections)?**
- Have you ever had surgery on your bladder or kidneys? *If so,* when and what?
- Have you had any hernias? *If yes,* when and how was this treated?
- Have you ever had cancer of any kind?
- Have you ever had testicular, kidney, bladder, or prostate cancer?
- Have you ever been treated with radiation or chemotherapy?

Special Questions To Ask: Bladder Control/Incontinence

Begin with a lead-in introduction to these questions such as:

Many people are embarrassed about having an incontinence problem. It may help to introduce the subject by making a general statement such as: "Many men and women have problems with bladder control. This is an area physical therapists can often help clients with so we routinely ask a few questions about bladder function."

General:

- Do you have any problems holding urine or emptying your bladder?
- Do you ever leak urine or have accidents?
- Do you wear pads to protect against urine leaking? Follow-up: How many do you use in a 24-hour period? How wet are they?
- Are your activities limited because of urine leaking?

If the male client answers "yes" to any of these questions, you may want to screen further with the following questions. See also Appendix B-27.

For Stress Incontinence:

- Do you ever lose urine or wet your pants when you cough, sneeze, or laugh?
- Do you lose urine or wet your pants when getting out of a chair, lifting, or exercising?

For Overactive Bladder (urge incontinence):

- Do you have frequent, strong, or sudden urges to urinate and cannot get to the bathroom in time? For example:
  - When arriving home and getting out of the car?
  - When using a key to open the door?
  - When you hear water running?
  - Or when you run water over your hands?
  - When you go out into cold weather or put your hands in the freezer?
- Do you get to the toilet and lose urine as you are pulling down your panties/shorts?
- Do you urinate more than every 2 hours in the daytime?
- Do you get up to go to the bathroom more than once a night?

  If yes, does this happen every night? Is it because you drink a large amount of fluids before bedtime?

For Overflow Incontinence:

- Do you dribble urine during the day and/or at night?
- Can you urinate with a strong stream or does the urine dribble out slowly?
- Does it feel like your bladder is empty when you are done urinating?

For Functional Incontinence:

- Can you get to the toilet easily?
- Do you have trouble getting to the bathroom on time?
- Do you have trouble finding the bathroom or toilet?
- Do you have accidents in the bathroom because you cannot get your pants unfastened or pulled down?

Special Questions to Ask: Urinary Tract Infection

- Have you had any side (flank) pain **(kidney or ureter)** or pain just above the pubic area **(suprapubic: bladder or urethra, prostate)?**
  - *If so,* what relieves this pain? Does a change in position affect it? **(Inflammatory pain** may be relieved by a change in position. **Renal colic** remains unchanged by a change in position.)
- During the last 2 to 3 weeks have you noticed a change in the amount or number of times that you urinate? **(Infection)**

SUBJECTIVE EXAMINATION—cont'd

- Do you ever have pain or a burning sensation when you urinate? (**Lower urinary tract irritation; prostatitis; venereal disease**)

- Does your urine look brown, red, or black? (Changes in urine color may be normal with some medications and foods such as beets or rhubarb.)

- Is your urine clear or cloudy? If not clear, describe. How often does this happen? (Could indicate **upper or lower urinary tract infection.**)

- Have you noticed an unusual or foul odor coming from your urine? (**Infection, secondary to medication**; may be normal after eating asparagus.)

For Women:

- When you urinate, do you have trouble starting or continuing the flow of urine? (**Urethral obstruction**)

- Have you noticed any unusual vaginal discharge during the time that you had pain (pubic, flank, thigh, back, labia)? (**Infection**)

- Have you noticed any changes in your sexual activity/function caused by your symptoms?

For Men:

- Have you noticed any unusual discharge from your penis during the time that you had pain (especially pain above the pubic area)? (**Infection**)

- Have you noticed any changes in your sexual activity/function caused by your symptoms?

Screening Questions to Ask: Prostatitis or Enlarged Prostate

- Have you ever had any problems with your prostate in the past?

Prostatitis

- Do you ever have burning pain or discomfort during urination?

- Does it feel like your bladder is not empty when you finish urinating?

- Do you have to go to the bathroom every 2 hours (or more often)?

- Do you ever have pain or discomfort in your testicles, penis, or the area between your rectum and your testicles (perineum)?

- Do you ever have pain in your pubic or bladder area?

- Do you have any discomfort during or after sexual climax (ejaculation)?

Enlarged prostate

- Does it feel like your bladder is not empty when you finish urinating?

- Do you have to urinate again less than 2 hours after you finished going to the bathroom last?

- Do you have a weak stream of urine or find you have to start and stop urinating several times when you go to the bathroom?

- Do you have an urge to go to the bathroom but very little urine comes out?

- Do you have to push or strain to start urinating or to keep the urine flowing?

- Do you have any leaking or dribbling of urine from the penis?

- How often do you get up to urinate at night?

The American Urologic Association recommends using the following scale when asking most of these screening questions. Some questions such as "How often do you get up at night?" requires a single number response. A total score of seven or more suggests the need for medical evaluation:

0	1	2	3	4	5
Not at all	Less than one time in five	Less than half the time	About half the time	More than half the time	Almost always

CASE STUDY

REFERRAL

The client is self-referred and states that he has been to your hospital-based outpatient clinic in the past. He has a very extensive chart containing his entire medical history for the last 20 years.

BACKGROUND INFORMATION

He is a 44-year-old man who describes his current occupation as "errand boy/gopher," which requires minimal lifting, bending, or strenuous physical activity. His chief complaint today is pain in the lower back, which comes and goes and seems to be aggravated by sitting. The pain is poorly described, and the client is unable to specify any kind of descriptive words for the type of pain, intensity, or duration.

SPECIAL QUESTIONS TO ASK

See Chapter 12 for Special Questions to Ask about the back. The client's answer to any questions related to bowel and bladder functions is either "I don't know" or "Well, you know," which makes a complete interview impossible.

SUBJECTIVE/OBJECTIVE FINDINGS

There are radiating symptoms of numbness down the left leg to the foot. The client denies any saddle anesthesia. Deep tendon reflexes are intact bilaterally, and the client stands with an obvious scoliotic list to one side. He is unable to tell you whether his symptoms are relieved or alleviated on performing a lateral shift to correct the curve. There are no other positive neuromuscular findings or associated systemic symptoms.

RESULT

After 3 days of treatment over the course of 1 week, the client has had no subjective improvement in symptoms. Objectively, the scoliotic shift has not changed. A second opinion is sought from two other staff members, and the consensus is to refer the client to his physician. The physician performs a rectal examination and confirms a positive diagnosis of prostatitis based on the results of laboratory tests. These test were consistent with the client's physical findings and previous history of prostate problems 1 year ago. The client was reluctant to discuss bowel or bladder function with the female therapist but readily suggested to his physician that his current symptoms mimicked an earlier episode of prostatitis.

It is not always possible to elicit thorough responses from clients concerning matters of genitourinary function. If the client hesitates or is unable to answer questions satisfactorily, it may be necessary to present the questions again at a later time (e.g., next treatment session), to ask a colleague of the client's sex to confer with the client, or to refer the client to his or her physician for further evaluation. Occasionally, the client will answer negatively to any questions regarding observed changes in urinary function and will then report back at the next session that there was some pathologic condition that was not noted earlier.

In this case a close review of the extensive medical records may have alerted the physical therapist to the client's previous treatment for the same problem, which he was reluctant to discuss.

PRACTICE QUESTIONS

1. Percussion of the costovertebral angle that results in the reproduction of symptoms:
   a. Signifies radiculitis
   b. Signifies pseudorenal pain
   c. Has no significance
   d. Requires medical referral

2. Renal pain is aggravated by:
   a. Spinal movement
   b. Palpatory pressure over the costovertebral angle
   c. Lying on the involved side
   d. All of the above
   e. None of the above

3. Important functions of the kidney include all the following *except:*
   a. Formation and excretion of urine
   b. Acid-base and electrolyte balance
   c. Stimulation of red blood cell production
   d. Production of glucose

4. Who should be screened for possible renal/urologic involvement?

5. What do the following terms mean?
   • Dyspareunia
   • Dysuria
   • Hematuria
   • Urgency

6. What is the difference between urge incontinence and stress incontinence?

7. What is the significance of "skin pain" over the T9/T10 dermatomes?

8. How do you screen for possible prostate involvement in a man with pelvic/low-back pain of unknown cause?

9. Explain why renal/urologic pain can be felt in such a wide range of dermatomes (i.e., from the T9 to L1 dermatomes).

10. What is the mechanism of referral for urologic pain to the shoulder?

REFERENCES

1. Cannon J: Recognizing chronic renal failure, the sooner, the better, *Nursing*2004 34(1):50-53, 2004.
2. Netter FH: *Atlas of human anatomy*, ed 2, Teterboro, New Jersey, 1997, Icon Learning Systems.
3. Simons DG, Travell JG, Simons LS: *Travell & Simons' myofascial pain and dysfunction: the trigger point manual*, ed 2, vol 1, Baltimore, 1999, Williams & Wilkins.
4. Smith DR, Raney FL, Jr: Radiculitis distress as a mimic of renal pain, *J Urol* 116:269, 1976.
5. National Kidney Foundation. K/DOQI clinical practice guidelines for chronic kidney disease: evaluation, classification, and stratification. Available at: http://www.kidney.org/professionals/doqi/kdoqi/p4_class_g3.htm. Accessed February 1, 2005.
6. Banishing urinary tract infections, *Harvard Women's Health Watch* 10(4):4-5, 2002.
7. Cailliet R: *Low back pain syndrome*, ed 5, Philadelphia, 1995, FA Davis.
8. Diagnosing and treating interstitial cystitis, *Harvard Women's Health Watch* 10(12):3, 2003.
9. Medical conditions, coping with kidney stones, *Harvard Women's Health Watch* 9(4):4-5, 2001.
10. Gurunadha Rao Tunuguntla HS, Evans CP: Management of prostatitis, *Prostate Cancer Prostatic Dis* 5(3):172-179, 2002.
11. Alexander RB: Treatment of chronic prostatitis, *Nat Clin Pract Urol* 1(1):2-3, 2004. Available on line: http://www.medscape.com/viewarticle/494378. Posted December 8, 2004.
12. Pontari MA, Ruggieri MR: Mechanisms in prostatitis/chronic pelvic pain syndrome, *J Urol* 172(3):839-845, 2004.
13. Tripp DA, Curtis NJ, Landis JR, et al: Predictors of quality of life and pain in chronic prostatitis/chronic pelvic pain syndrome: findings from the National Institutes of Health Chronic Prostatitis Cohort Study, *BJU* 94(9):1279-1282, 2004.

14. Schultz PL, Donnell RF: Prostatitis: the cost of disease and therapies to patients and society, *Curr Urol Rep* 5(4):317-319, 2004.
15. Litwin MS, McNaughton-Collins M, Fowler FL: Prostatitis: The National Institutes of Health Chronic Prostatitis Symptoms Index (NIH-CPSI), Smithshire, Illinois, 2002, Prostatitis Foundation. Retrieved July 25, 2006 from http://www.prostatitis.org/symptomindex.html.
16. Rex L: *Evaluation and treatment of somatovisceral dysfunction of the gastrointestinal system*, Edmonds, Washington, 2004, URSA Foundation.
17. Zvara P, Folsom JB, Plante MK: Minimally invasive therapies for prostatitis, *Curr Urol Rep* 5(4):320-326, 2004.
18. Sokolov AV: Transrectal microwave hyperthermia in the treatment of chronic prostatitis, *Urologiia* 5:20-26, 2003.
19. Cornel EB, van Haarst EP: *Chronic pelvic pain syndrome type 3 successfully treated with biofeedback physical therapy* (Abstract), Presented at the American Urological Association 2004 Annual Meeting, May 8-13, 2004, San Francisco, California. Available on line: http://www.prostatitis.org/AmericanUrologicalMeeting04.html.
20. Ruzaev ML, Levitskii EF, Kolmatsui IA: Rehabilitation of patients with chronic prostatitis in combination with reflex syndromes of lumbar osteochondrosis (Russian), *Vopr Kurortol Fizioter Lech Fiz Kult* 1:35-37, 2004.
21. Sheeler R: Enlarged prostate. Know when to seek treatment, *Mayo Clinic Health Letter* 22(8):1-3, 2004.
22. National Cancer Institute. Prostate cancer. Available at: http://www.nci.nih.gov/cancertopics/types/prostate. Posted June 21, 2004. Accessed February 2, 2005.
23. Jemal A, Murray T, Ward E, et al: Cancer statistics, CA *Cancer J Clin* 55(1):10-31, 2005.24. Carroll PR, Nelson WG: Report to the nation on prostate cancer: introduction, *Medscape Hematology-Oncology* 7(2), 2004. Available at: http://www.medscape.com/viewarticle/489635. Accessed February 3, 2005.
25. Logothetis CJ, Lin SH: Osteoblasts in prostate cancer metastasis to bone, *Nat Rev Cancer* 5(1):21-28, 2005.

26. U.S. Department of Health & Human Services. *Diseases and conditions*. Available at: www.hhs.gov/. Accessed February 7, 2005.

27. Shafik A, Shafik IA: Overactive bladder inhibition in response to pelvic floor muscle exercises, *World J Urol* 20(6):374-377, 2003.

28. Schultz JM: Urinary incontinence. Solving a secret problem, *Nursing2003* 33(11):5-10, 2003.

29. Bo K, Borgen JS: Prevalence of stress and urge urinary incontinence in elite athletes and controls, *Med Sci Sports Exerc* 33(11):1797-1802, 2001.

30. Sherburn M, Guthrie JR, Dudley EC, et al: Is incontinence associated with menopause? *Obstet Gynecol* 98(4):628-633, 2001.

31. Hulme J: *Regaining bowel and bladder control after cancer*, Missoula, Montana, 2003, Phoenix Publishers.

32. Grise P, Thurman S: Urinary incontinence following treatment of localized prostate cancer, *Cancer Control* 8(6):532-539, 2002. Available on-line at: http://www. medscape.com/viewarticle/423513.

33. Yim PS, Peterson AS: Urinary incontinence, *Postgrad Med* 99(5):137-150, 1996.

34. Evans N, Forsyth E: End-stage renal disease in people with type 2 diabetes: systemic manifestations and exercise implications, *Phys Ther* 84(5):454-463, 2004.

35. Peterson GM: Selecting nonprescription analgesics, *Am J Ther* 12(1):67-79, 2005.

36. Elseviers MM, De Broe ME: Analgesic abuse in the elderly. Renal sequelae and management, *Drugs Aging* 12(5):391-400, 1998.

37. National Kidney Foundation (NKF): *Can analgesics hurt kidneys?* Available at: http://www.kidney.org/atoz/atozPrint.cfm?id=23. Accessed February 5, 2005.

38. Holub C, Lamont M: The reliability of the six-minute walk test in patients with end stage renal disease, *Acute Care Perspectives*, 11(4):8-11, 2002.

39. Paton M: Continuous renal replacement therapy, *Nursing2003*, 33(6):40-50, 2003.

40. Best treatments for beating bladder cancer, *Johns Hopkins Medical Letter* 15(1):6-7, 2004.

41. Bladder cancer in women: no time to wait, *Harvard Women's Health Watch* 11(7):3-5, 2004.

42. National Cancer Institute: *What you need to know about bladder cancer*, www.cancer.gov/cancertopics/wyntk/bladder. Accessed September 2002.

43. Ongoing care of patients after primary treatment for their cancer: genitourinary cancers, bladder and kidney, *CA Cancer J Clin* 53(3):190-191, 2003.

44. National Cancer Institute: *What you need to know about kidney cancer*, www.cancer.gov/cancertopics/wyntk/kidneys. Accessed March 30, 2004.

45. American Cancer Society: *Detailed guide: testicular cancer. What are the risk factors for testicular cancer?* Available at: http://www.cancer.org. Accessed February 10, 2005.

46. Goodman CC, Boissonnault WG: *Pathology: implications for the physical therapist*, ed 2, Philadelphia, 2000, WB Saunders.

47. Polich S, Faynor S: Interpreting lab test values, *PT Magazine* 4(1):76-88, 1996.

48. Irion GL: Lab values update, *Acute Care Perspectives* 13(1):1, 3-5, 2004.

Endocrinology is the study of ductless (endocrine) glands that produce hormones. A hormone acts as a chemical agent that is transported by the bloodstream to target tissues, where it regulates or modifies the activity of the target cell.

The endocrine system cannot be understood fully without consideration of the effects of the nervous system on the endocrine system. The endocrine system works with the nervous system to regulate metabolism, water and salt balance, blood pressure, response to stress, and sexual reproduction.

The endocrine system is slower in response and takes longer to act than the nervous system in transferring biochemical information. The pituitary (hypophysis), thyroid, parathyroids, adrenals, and pineal are glands of the endocrine system whose functions are solely endocrine related and have no other metabolic functions (Fig. 11-1). The hypothalamus controls pituitary function and thus has an important indirect influence on the other glands of the endocrine system. Feedback mechanisms exist to keep hormones at normal levels.

The endocrine system meets the nervous system in a complex series of interactions that link behavioral-neural-endocrine-immunologic responses. The hypothalamus and the pituitary form an integrated axis that maintains control over much of the endocrine system. The discovery and study of this complex interface axis is called psychoneuroimmunology (PNI) and has provided a new understanding of interactive biologic signaling.

The hypothalamus exerts direct control over both the anterior and posterior portions of the pituitary gland and can synthesize and release hormones from its axon terminals directly into the blood circulation. These neurosecretory cells are so called because the neurons have a hormone-secreting function. Although neurons can have a hormone-secreting function, the opposite pathway is also present. Hormones that can stimulate the neural mechanism (e.g., acetylcholine) are called *neurohormones*. Acetylcholine is a neurotransmitter and a neurohormone. It is released at synapses to allow messages to pass along a nerve network, resulting in the release of both hormones and chemicals.

ASSOCIATED NEUROMUSCULAR AND MUSCULOSKELETAL SIGNS AND SYMPTOMS

The musculoskeletal system is composed of a variety of connective tissue structures in which normal growth and development are influenced strongly and sometimes controlled by various hormones and metabolic processes. Alterations in these control systems can result in structural changes and altered function of various connective tissues, producing systemic and musculoskeletal signs and symptoms (Table 11-1).

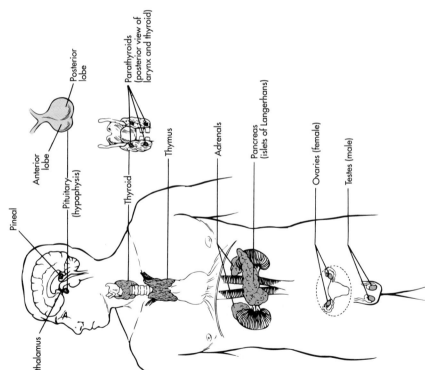

Fig. 11-1 • Location of the nine endocrine glands. (From Butts-Krakoff D: Structure and function: assessment of clients with metabolic disorders. In Black JM, Matassarin-Jacobs E, editors: *Luckmann and Sorensen's medical-surgical nursing*, ed 4, Philadelphia, 1993, Saunders, p. 1759.)

TABLE 11-1 ▼ Signs and Symptoms of Endocrine Dysfunction

Neuromusculoskeletal	Systemic
Signs and symptoms associated with rheumatoid arthritis	Excessive or delayed growth
Muscle weakness	Polydipsia
Muscle atrophy	Polyuria
Myalgia	Mental changes (nervousness, confusion, depression)
Fatigue	Changes in hair (quality and distribution)
Carpal tunnel syndrome	Changes in skin pigmentation
Synovial fluid changes	Changes in vital signs (elevated body temperature,
Periarthritis	pulse rate, increased blood pressure)
Adhesive capsulitis (diabetes)	Heart palpitations
Chondrocalcinosis	Increased perspiration
Spondyloarthropathy	Kussmaul's respirations (deep, rapid breathing)
Osteoarthritis	Dehydration or excessive retention of body water
Hand stiffness	
Arthralgia	

From Goodman CC, Boissonnault WG, Fuller KS: *Pathology: implications for the physical therapist*, Philadelphia, 2003, Saunders, p 323.

Muscle Weakness, Myalgia, and Fatigue

Muscle weakness, myalgia, and fatigue may be early manifestations of thyroid or parathyroid disease, acromegaly, diabetes, Cushing's syndrome, and osteomalacia. Proximal muscle weakness associated with endocrine disease is usually painless and unrelated to either the severity or the duration of the underlying disease. The muscular system is sometimes, but not

always, restored with effective treatment of the underlying condition.

Bilateral Carpal Tunnel Syndrome

Bilateral carpal tunnel syndrome (CTS), resulting from median nerve compression at the wrist, is a common finding in a variety of systemic and neuromusculoskeletal conditions but especially with certain endocrine and metabolic disorders (Table 11-2). The fact that the majority of persons with CTS are women at or near menopause suggests that the soft tissues about the wrist could be affected in some way by hormones. Thickening of the transverse carpal ligament in certain systemic disorders (e.g., acromegaly, myxedema) may be sufficient to compress the median nerve. Any condition that increases the volume of the contents of the carpal tunnel (e.g., neoplasm, calcium, and gouty tophi deposits) can compress the median nerve.

The signs and symptoms often associated with CTS include paresthesia, tingling, and numbness and/or pain with cutaneous distribution of the median nerve to the thumb, index, middle, and radial half of the ring finger. Nocturnal paresthesia is a common complaint, and this discomfort causes sleep disruption. It can be partially relieved by shaking of the hand. Pain may radiate into the palm and up the forearm and arm.[6]

It should be noted that bilateral tarsal syndrome affecting the feet also can occur either alone or in conjunction with CTS, although the incidence of myxedema.)[2-5]

TABLE 11-2 ▼ Causes of Carpal Tunnel Syndrome

Neuromusculoskeletal	Systemic
Amyloidosis	Alcohol
Anatomic sequelae of medical or surgical procedures	Arthritis (rheumatoid, gout, polymyalgia rheumatica)
Basal joint (thumb) arthritis	Benign tumors (lipoma, hemangioma, ganglia)
Cervical disc lesions	Leukemia (tissue infiltration)
Cervical spondylosis	Liver disease
Congenital anatomic differences	Medications
Cumulative trauma disorders (CTD)	NSAIDs
Peripheral neuropathy	Oral contraceptives
Poor posture (may also be associated with TOS)	Statins
Repetitive strain injuries (RSI)	Alendronate[1] (Fosamax)
Tendinitis	Multiple myeloma (amyloidosis deposits)
Trigger points	Obesity
Tenosynovitis	Pregnancy
Thoracic outlet syndrome (TOS)	Scleroderma
Wrist trauma (e.g., Colles' fracture)	Use of oral contraceptives
	Hemochromatosis
	Vitamin deficiency (especially vitamin B_6)
	Endocrine
	Acromegaly
	Diabetes mellitus
	Hormonal imbalance (menopause; posthysterectomy)
	Hyperparathyroidism
	Hyperthyroidism (Graves' disease)
	Hypocalcemia
	Hypothyroidism (myxedema)
	Gout (deposits of tophi and calcium)
	Infectious Disease
	Atypical mycobacterium
	Histoplasmosis
	Rubella
	Sporotrichosis

Modified from Goodman CC, Boissonnault WG: *Pathology: implications for the physical therapist*, Philadelphia, 2003, Saunders, Table 38-7, p 1149.

tarsal tunnel syndrome is not high. Bilateral median nerve neuritis can be characteristic of many systemic diseases, including rheumatoid arthritis, myxedema, localized amyloidosis, sarcoidosis, and infiltrative leukemia.[7,8]

Whenever a client presents with bilateral symptoms, it represents a red flag. With bilateral CTS the therapist can screen for medical disease by using the Special Questions to Ask: Bilateral Carpal Tunnel Syndrome section (see Appendix B-4).

Periarthritis and Calcific Tendinitis

Periarthritis (inflammation of periarticular structures, including the tendons, ligaments, and joint capsule) and calcific tendinitis occur most often in the shoulders of people who have endocrine disease. Treatment of the underlying endocrine impairment often improves the clinical picture; physical therapy intervention may have a temporary palliative effect.

Chondrocalcinosis

Chondrocalcinosis is the deposition of calcium salts in the cartilage of joints. When accompanied by attacks of goutlike symptoms, it is called *pseudogout*. Chondrocalcinosis is commonly seen on x-ray films as calcified hyaline or fibrous cartilage. There is an associated underlying endocrine or metabolic disease in approximately 5% to 10% of individuals with chondrocalcinosis (Table 11-3).

Spondyloarthropathy and Osteoarthritis

Spondyloarthropathy (disease of joints of the spine) and osteoarthritis occur in individuals with various metabolic or endocrine diseases, including hemochromatosis (disorder of iron metabolism with excess deposition of iron in the tissues; also known as *bronze diabetes and iron storage disease*),

ochronosis (metabolic disorder resulting in discoloration of body tissues caused by deposits of alkapton bodies), acromegaly, and diabetes mellitus.

Hand Stiffness and Hand Pain

Hand stiffness and hand pain, as well as arthralgias of the small joints of the hand, can occur with endocrine and metabolic diseases. Hypothyroidism is often accompanied by CTS; flexor tenosynovitis with stiffness is another common finding.

▶ ENDOCRINE PATHOPHYSIOLOGY

Disorders of the endocrine glands can be classified as primary (dysfunction of the gland itself) or secondary (dysfunction of an outside stimulus to the gland) and are a result of either an excess or an insufficiency of hormonal secretions.

Secondary dysfunction may also occur (iatrogenically) as a result of chemotherapy, surgical removal of the glands, therapy for a nonendocrine disorder (e.g., the use of large doses of corticosteroids resulting in Cushing's syndrome), or excessive therapy for an endocrine disorder.

Pituitary Gland
Diabetes Insipidus

Diabetes insipidus is caused by a lack of secretion of vasopressin (antidiuretic hormone [ADH]). This hormone normally stimulates the distal tubules of the kidneys to reabsorb water. Without ADH, water moving through the kidney is not reabsorbed but is lost in the urine, resulting in severe water loss and dehydration through diuresis.

Central or neurogenic diabetes insipidus, which is the most common type, can be idiopathic (primary) or related to other causes (secondary), such as pituitary trauma, head injury, infections such as meningitis or encephalitis, pituitary neoplasm, and vascular lesions such as aneurysms.

If the person with diabetes insipidus is unconscious or confused and is unable to take in necessary fluids to replace those fluids lost, rapid dehydration, shock, and death can occur. Because sleep is interrupted by the persistent need to void (nocturia), fatigue and irritability result.

Clinical Signs and Symptoms of Diabetes Insipidus

- Polyuria (increased urination)
- Polydipsia (increased thirst, which occurs subsequent to polyuria in response to the loss of fluid)

TABLE 11-3 ▼ Endocrine and Metabolic Disorders Associated with Chondrocalcinosis

Endocrine	Metabolic
Hypothyroidism	Hemochromatosis
Hyperparathyroidism	Hypomagnesemia
Acromegaly	Hypophosphatasia
	Ochronosis
	Oxalosis
	Wilson's disease

Modified from Louthrenoo W, Schumacher HR: Musculoskeletal clues to endocrine or metabolic disease, *J Musculoskel Med* 7(9):41, 1990.

- Dehydration
- Decreased urine specific gravity (1.001 to 1.005)
- Nocturia, fatigue, irritability
- Increased serum sodium (more than 145 mEq/dL; resulting from concentration of serum from water loss)

Syndrome of Inappropriate Secretion of Antidiuretic Hormone

Syndrome of inappropriate secretion of ADH (SIADH) is an excess or inappropriate secretion of vasopressin that results in marked retention of water in excess of sodium in the body. Urine output decreases dramatically as the body retains large amounts of water. Almost all the excess water is distributed within body cells, causing intracellular water gain and cellular swelling (water intoxication).

RISK FACTORS

Risk factors for the development of SIADH include pituitary damage caused by infection, trauma, or neoplasm; secretion of vasopressin-like substances from some types of malignant tumors (particularly pulmonary malignancies); and thoracic pressure changes from compression of pulmonary or cardiac pressure receptors, or both.

CLINICAL PRESENTATION

Symptoms of SIADH are the clinical opposite of symptoms of diabetes insipidus. They are the result of water retention and the subsequent dilution of sodium in the blood serum and body cells. Neurologic and neuromuscular signs and symptoms predominate and are directly related to the swelling of brain tissue and sodium changes within neuromuscular tissues.

Clinical Signs and Symptoms of Syndrome of Inappropriate Secretion of Antidiuretic Hormone

- Headache, confusion, lethargy (most significant early indicators)
- Decreased urine output
- Weight gain without visible edema
- Seizures
- Muscle cramps
- Vomiting, diarrhea
- Increased urine specific gravity (greater than 1.03)
- Decreased serum sodium (less than 135 mEq/dL; caused by dilution of serum from water)

Acromegaly

Acromegaly is an abnormal enlargement of the extremities of the skeleton resulting from hypersecretion of growth hormone (GH) from the pituitary gland. This condition is relatively rare and occurs in adults, most often owing to a tumor of the pituitary gland. In children, overproduction of GH stimulates growth of long bones and results in gigantism, in which the child grows to exaggerated heights. With adults, growth of the long bones has already stopped, so the bones most affected are those of the face, jaw, hands, and feet. Other signs and symptoms include amenorrhea (in women), diabetes mellitus, profuse sweating, and hypertension.

CLINICAL PRESENTATION

Degenerative arthropathy may be seen in the peripheral joints of a client with acromegaly, most frequently attacking the large joints. On x-ray studies, osteophyte formation may be seen, along with widening of the joint space because of increased cartilage thickness. In late-stage disease, joint spaces become narrowed, and occasionally chondrocalcinosis may be present.

Stiffness of the hand, typically of both hands, is associated with a broad enlargement of the fingers from bony overgrowth and with thickening of the soft tissue. Thickening and widening of the phalangeal tufts are typical x-ray findings, much of the pain and stiffness is believed to be due to premature osteoarthritis.

Carpal tunnel syndrome (CTS) is seen in up to 50% of people with acromegaly. The CTS that occurs with this growth disorder is thought to be caused by compression of the median nerve at the wrist from soft tissue hypertrophy or bony overgrowth or by hypertrophy of the median nerve itself.

Myopathy in people with acromegaly is commonly reported but poorly understood. Changes in muscle size and strength are associated with acromegaly and are probably multifactoral in origin. Screening individuals with acromegaly for muscle weakness and poor exercise tolerance is now recommended.[9]

About half the individuals with acromegaly have back pain. X-ray studies demonstrate increased intervertebral disc spaces and large osteophytes along the anterior longitudinal ligament (ALL), mimicking diffuse idiopathic skeletal hyperostosis (DISH).

DISH (also known as Forestier's disease) is characterized by abnormal ossification of the ALL,

resulting in an x-ray image of large osteophytes seemingly "flowing" along the anterior border of the spine. DISH is particularly common in the thoracic spine and has been reported to be more prevalent among persons with diabetes than among the nondiabetic population. DISH appears to be an age-related predisposition to ossification of tendon, joint capsule, and ligamentous attachments. Identification of the presence of DISH syndrome prior to surgery is important in the prevention of heterotropic bone formation.[10]

Clinical Signs and Symptoms of

Acromegaly

- Bony enlargement (face, jaw, hands, feet)
- Amenorrhea
- Diabetes mellitus
- Profuse sweating (diaphoresis)
- Hypertension
- Carpal tunnel syndrome
- Hand pain and stiffness
- Back pain (thoracic and/or lumbar)
- Myopathy and poor exercise tolerance

Adrenal Glands

The adrenals are two small glands located on the upper part of each kidney. Each adrenal gland consists of two relatively discrete parts: an outer cortex and an inner medulla. The outer cortex is responsible for the secretion of mineralocorticoids (steroid hormones that regulate fluid and mineral balance), glucocorticoids (steroid hormones responsible for controlling the metabolism of glucose), and androgens (sex hormones). The centrally located adrenal medulla is derived from neural tissue and secretes epinephrine and norepinephrine. Together, the adrenal cortex and medulla are major factors in the body's response to stress.

Adrenal Insufficiency

PRIMARY ADRENAL INSUFFICIENCY

Chronic adrenocortical insufficiency (hyposecretion by the adrenal glands) may be primary or secondary. Primary adrenal insufficiency is also referred to as *Addison's disease* (hypofunction), named after the physician who first studied and described the associated symptoms. It can be treated by the administration of exogenous cortisol (one of the adrenocortical hormones).

Primary adrenal insufficiency occurs when a disorder exists within the adrenal gland itself. This adrenal gland disorder results in decreased production of cortisol and aldosterone, two of the

primary adrenocortical hormones. The most common cause of primary adrenal insufficiency is an autoimmune process that causes destruction of the adrenal cortex.

The most striking physical finding in the person with primary adrenal insufficiency is the increased pigmentation of the skin and mucous membranes. This discoloration may vary in the white population from a slight tan or a few black freckles to an intense generalized pigmentation, which has resulted in persons being mistakenly considered to be of a darker-skinned race. Members of darker-skinned races may develop a slate-gray color that may be obvious only to family members.

Melanin, the major product of the melanocyte, is largely responsible for the coloring of skin. In primary adrenal insufficiency, the increase in pigmentation is initiated by the excessive secretion of melanocyte-stimulating hormone (MSH) that occurs in association with increased secretion of ACTH. ACTH is increased in an attempt to stimulate the diseased adrenal glands to produce and release more cortisol.

Most commonly, pigmentation is visible over extensor surfaces, such as the backs of the hands; elbows; knees; and creases of the hands, lips, and mouth. Increased pigmentation of scars formed after the onset of the disease is common. However, it is possible for a person with primary adrenal insufficiency to demonstrate no significant increase in pigmentation.

SECONDARY ADRENAL INSUFFICIENCY

Secondary adrenal insufficiency refers to a dysfunction of the gland because of insufficient stimulation of the cortex owing to a lack of pituitary ACTH. Causes of secondary disease include tumors of the hypothalamus or pituitary, removal of the pituitary, or rapid withdrawal of corticosteroid drugs. Clinical manifestations of secondary disease do not occur until the adrenals are almost completely nonfunctional and are primarily related to cortisol deficiency only.

Clinical Signs and Symptoms of

Adrenal Insufficiency

- Dark pigmentation of the skin, especially mouth and scars (occurs only with primary disease; Addison's)
- Hypotension (low blood pressure causing orthostatic symptoms)
- Progressive fatigue (improves with rest)
- Hyperkalemia (generalized weakness and muscle flaccidity)

- Gastrointestinal (GI) disturbances
- Anorexia and weight loss
- Nausea and vomiting
- Arthralgias, myalgias (secondary only)
- Tendon calcification
- Hypoglycemia

Cushing's Syndrome

Cushing's syndrome (hyperfunction of the adrenal gland) is a general term for increased secretion of cortisol by the adrenal cortex. When corticosteroids are administered externally, a condition of hypercortisolism called *iatrogenic Cushing's syndrome* occurs, producing a group of associated signs and symptoms. Hypercortisolism caused by excess secretion of ACTH (e.g., from pituitary stimulation) is called *ACTH-dependent Cushing's syndrome*.[11]

Therapists often treat people who have developed Cushing's syndrome after these clients have received large doses of cortisol (also known as hydrocortisone) or cortisol derivatives (e.g., dexamethasone) for a number of inflammatory disorders (Case Example 11-1).

It is important to remember that whenever corticosteroids are administered externally, the increase in serum cortisol levels triggers a nega-

tive feedback signal to the anterior pituitary gland to stop adrenal stimulation. Adrenal atrophy occurs during this time, and adrenal insufficiency will result if external corticosteroids are abruptly withdrawn. Corticosteroid medications must be reduced gradually so that normal adrenal function can return.

Because cortisol suppresses the inflammatory response of the body, it can mask early signs of infection. *Any unexplained fever without other symptoms should be a warning to the therapist of the need for medical follow-up.*

Clinical Signs and Symptoms of Cushing's Syndrome

- "Moonface" appearance (very round face; Fig. 11-2)
- Buffalo hump at the neck (fatty deposits)
- Protuberant abdomen with accumulation of fatty tissue and stretch marks
- Muscle wasting and weakness
- Decreased density of bones (especially spine)
- Hypertension
- Kyphosis and back pain (secondary to bone loss)
- Easy bruising

Continued on p. 474

CASE EXAMPLE 11-1 Cushing's Syndrome

A 53-year-old woman with Cushing's syndrome resulting from long-term use of cortisol for systemic lupus erythematosus reports the following problems:

- Hair and nail thinning and breaking easily
- Temperature intolerance (always cold)
- Muscle cramps
- Generalized weakness and fatigue

Her primary complaint and reason for referral to physical therapy is for sacroiliac (SI) joint pain as a result of stepping down off an uneven curb.

You realize the signs and symptoms are of an endocrine origin, but you do not know whether they are part of the Cushing's syndrome or a separate endocrine problem.

Should you send this client to a physician (or back to the referring physician)?

Not necessarily. This is more a case of need for additional information. Requesting a copy of the client's most recent physician's notes may

answer all of your questions. Reading the physician's systems review portion of the exam may reveal a record of these signs and symptoms with a corresponding medical problem list and plan.

If there is no mention of any of these associated signs and symptoms, a phone call to the physician's office may be the next step. If you speak with the physician directly, identify yourself and your connection with the client by name. Briefly mention why you are seeing this client and make the following observation:

"Mrs. Jones reports muscle cramps and generalized weakness that do not seem consistent with her SI problem. She complains of temperature intolerance and hair and nail bed changes. These symptoms are outside the scope of my practice.

Can you help me understand this? Are they part of her lupus, Cushing's syndrome, or something else?"

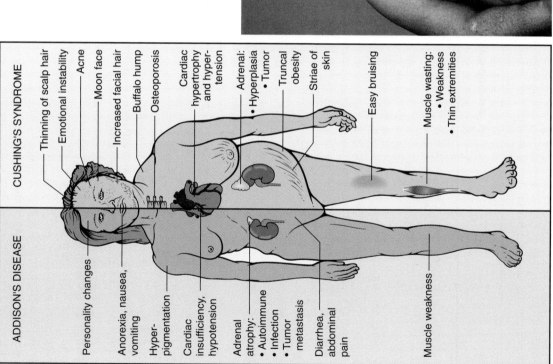

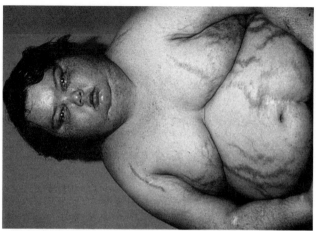

ADDISON'S DISEASE	CUSHING'S SYNDROME
	Thinning of scalp hair
	Emotional instability
	Acne
	Moon face
	Increased facial hair
	Buffalo hump
Personality changes	Osteoporosis
	Cardiac hypertrophy and hypertension
Anorexia, nausea, vomiting	
Hyper-pigmentation	Adrenal: • Hyperplasia • Tumor
Cardiac insufficiency, hypotension	Truncal obesity
Adrenal atrophy: • Autoimmune • Infection • Tumor metastasis	Striae of skin
Diarrhea, abdominal pain	Easy bruising
	Muscle wasting: • Weakness • Thin extremities
Muscle weakness	

Fig. 11-2 • A, Comparison of hyperfunction of the adrenal cortex (Addison's disease) and hypofunction (Cushing's syndrome). **B,** Individuals treated with corticosteroids can develop clinical features of Cushing's syndrome called *cushingoid features* including "moonface," obesity, and cutaneous striae as shown here. (From Damjanov I: *Pathology for the health-related profession,* ed 2, Philadephia, Saunders, 2000. Used with permission.)

- Psychiatric or emotional disturbances
- Impaired reproductive function (e.g., decreased libido and changes in menstrual cycle)
- Diabetes mellitus
- Slow wound healing
- *For women:* Masculinizing effects (e.g., hair growth, breast atrophy, voice changes)

EFFECTS OF CORTISOL ON CONNECTIVE TISSUE

Overproduction of cortisol or closely related glucocorticoids by abnormal adrenocortical tissue leads to a protein catabolic state. This overproduction causes liberation of amino acids from muscle tissue. The resultant weakened protein structures (muscle and elastic tissue) cause a protuberant abdomen, poor wound healing, generalized muscle weakness, and marked osteoporosis (demineralization of bone causing reduced bone mass), which is made worse by an excessive loss of calcium in the urine.

Excessive glucose resulting from this protein catabolic state is transformed mainly into fat and appears in characteristic sites, such as the

abdomen, supraclavicular fat pads, and facial cheeks. The change in facial appearance may not be readily apparent to the client or to the therapist, but pictures of the client taken over a period of years may provide a visual record of those changes.

The effect of increased circulating levels of cortisol on the muscles of clients varies from slight to very marked. There may be so much muscle wasting that the condition simulates muscular dystrophy. Marked weakness of the quadriceps muscle often prevents affected clients from rising out of a chair unassisted. Those with Cushing's syndrome of long duration almost always demonstrate demineralization of bone. In severe cases, this condition may lead to pathologic fractures, but it results more commonly in wedging of the vertebrae, kyphosis, bone pain, and back pain.

Obesity, diabetes, polycystic ovarian syndrome, and other metabolic/endocrine problems can resemble Cushing's syndrome. It is important to recognize critical indicators of this particular disorder such as excessive hair growth, moonface, mood disorders, and increased muscle weakness as indicators for further endocrine diagnostic testing.[12]

The poor wound healing that is characteristic of this syndrome becomes a problem when any surgical procedures are required. Inhibition of collagen formation with corticosteroid therapy is responsible for the frequency of wound breakdown in postsurgical clients.

Thyroid Gland

The thyroid gland is located in the anterior portion of the lower neck below the larynx, on both sides of and anterior to the trachea. The chief hormones produced by the thyroid are thyroxine (T_4), triiodothyronine (T_3), and calcitonin. Both T_3 and T_4 regulate the metabolic rate of the body and increase protein synthesis. Calcitonin has a weak physiologic effect on calcium and phosphorus balance in the body.

Genetics plays a role in thyroid disease. A family history of thyroid disease is a risk factor. Age and gender are also factors; most cases occur after age 50. Women are more likely than men to develop thyroid dysfunction.[12] Data gathered on the medical history of the orthopedic physical therapy outpatient population indicate a 7% incidence of thyroid disease in the female population.[13]

Thyroid function is regulated by the hypothalamus and pituitary feedback controls, as well as by an intrinsic regulator mechanism within the gland itself. Basic thyroid disorders of significance to physical therapy practice include goiter, hyperthyroidism, hypothyroidism, and cancer. Alterations in thyroid function produce changes in hair, nails, skin, eyes, GI tract, respiratory tract, heart and blood vessels, nervous tissue, bone, and muscle.

The risk of having thyroid diseases increases with age, but in people older than 60 years of age, it becomes more difficult to detect because it masquerades as other problems such as heart disease, depression, or dementia. Fatigue and weakness may be the first symptoms among older adults, often mistaken or attributed to normal aging. New-onset depression in the older adult population and anxiety syndromes are also symptoms that can indicate thyroid dysfunction.[14]

On the other hand, thyroid dysfunction can mimic signs and symptoms of aging such as hair loss, fatigue, and depression. The therapist may recognize problems early and make a medical referral, minimizing the client's symptoms. A simple and inexpensive blood test called a *thyroid-stimulating hormone (TSH) test* is usually recommended to show whether the thyroid gland is hyper or hypofunctioning.[15]

Goiter

Goiter, an enlargement of the thyroid gland, occurs in areas of the world where iodine (necessary for the production of thyroid hormone) is deficient in the diet. It is believed that when factors (e.g., a lack of iodine) inhibit normal thyroid hormone production, hypersecretion of TSH occurs because of a lack of a negative feedback loop. The TSH increase results in an increase in thyroid mass.

Pressure on the trachea and esophagus causes difficulty in breathing, dysphagia, and hoarseness. With the use of iodized salt, this problem has almost been eliminated in the United States. Although the younger population in the United States may be goiter free, older adults may have developed goiter during their childhood or adolescent years and may still have clinical manifestations of this disorder.

Clinical Signs and Symptoms of Goiter

- Increased neck size
- Pressure on adjacent tissue (e.g., trachea and esophagus)
- Difficulty in breathing
- Dysphagia
- Hoarseness

Thyroiditis

Thyroiditis is an inflammation of the thyroid gland. Causes can include infection and autoimmune processes. The most common form of this problem is a chronic thyroiditis called *Hashimoto's thyroiditis*. This condition affects women more frequently than men and is most often seen in the 30- to 50-year-old age group. Destruction of the thyroid gland from this condition can cause eventual hypothyroidism (Case Example 11-2).

Usually, both sides of the gland are enlarged, although one side may be larger than the other. Other symptoms are related to the functional state of the gland itself. Early involvement may cause mild symptoms of hyperthyroidism, whereas later symptoms cause hypothyroidism.

CASE EXAMPLE 11-2   Hashimoto's Thyroiditis

Referral: A 38-year-old woman with right-sided groin pain was referred to physical therapy by her physician. She says that the pain came on suddenly without injury. The pain is worse in the morning and hurts at night, waking her up when she changes position. The woman's symptoms are especially acute when she tries to stand up after sitting, with weight bearing impossible for the first 5 to 10 minutes.

The woman, who looks athletic, reports that before the onset of this problem, she was running 5 miles every other day without difficulty. The x-ray finding is reportedly within normal limits for structural abnormalities. Sed rate was 16 mm/hr.* The client has chronic sinusitis and has had two surgeries for that condition in the last 3 years. She is not a smoker and drinks only occasionally on a social basis.

This client was seen 6 weeks ago by another physical therapist, who tried ultrasound and stretching without improvement in symptoms or function.

Clinical Presentation: The physical therapy evaluation today revealed a positive Thomas test for right hip flexion contracture. However, it was difficult to assess whether there was a true muscle contracture or only loss of motion as a result of muscle splinting and guarding. Patrick's test (FABER's) for hip pathology and the iliopsoas test for intra-abdominal infection were both negative. Joint accessory motions appeared to be within normal limits, given that the movements were tested in the presence of some residual muscle tension

from protective splinting. A neurologic screen failed to demonstrate the presence of any neurologic involvement. Symptoms could be reproduced with deep palpation of the right groin area. There were no active or passive movements that could alter, provoke, change, or eliminate the pain. There were no trigger points in the abdomen or right lower quadrant that could account for the symptomatic presentation.

There was no apparent cause for her movement system impairment. Physical therapy intervention with soft tissue mobilization and proprioceptive neuromuscular facilitation techniques were initiated and used as a diagnostic tool. There was no change in the client's symptoms or clinical presentation as the therapist continued trying a series of physical therapy techniques.

Result: In a young and otherwise healthy adult, a lack of measurable, reportable, or observable progress becomes a red flag for further medical follow-up. The results of the physical therapy examination and lack of response to treatment constitute a valuable medical diagnostic tool.

Further laboratory results revealed a medical diagnosis of Hashimoto's thyroiditis. Treatment with thyroxine (T_4) resulted in resolution of the musculoskeletal symptoms. The correlation between groin pain and loss of hip extension with Hashimoto's remains unclear. Even so, response to the red flag (no change or improvement with intervention) resulted in a correct medical diagnosis.

---

* The sedimentation (SED) rate (an indication of possible infection or inflammation) was within normal limits for an adult woman.

Clinical Signs and Symptoms of

Thyroiditis

- Painless thyroid enlargement
- Dysphagia or choking
- Anterior neck, shoulder, or rib cage pain without biomechanical changes
- Gland sometimes easily palpable over anterior neck (warm, tender, swollen)

Hyperthyroidism

Hyperthyroidism (hyperfunction), or *thyrotoxicosis*, refers to those disorders in which the thyroid gland secretes excessive amounts of thyroid hormone. Graves' disease is a common type of excessive thyroid activity characterized by a generalized enlargement of the gland (or goiter leading to a swollen neck) and, often, protruding eyes caused by retraction of the eyelids and inflammation of the ocular muscles.

CLINICAL PRESENTATION

Excessive thyroid hormone creates a generalized elevation in body metabolism. The effects of thyrotoxicosis occur gradually and are manifested in almost every system (Fig. 11-3; Table 11-4).

In more than 50% of adults older than 70, three common signs are tachycardia, fatigue, and weight loss. In clients younger than 50, clinical signs and symptoms found most often include tachycardia, hyperactive reflexes, increased sweating, heat intolerance, fatigue, tremor, nervousness, polydipsia, weakness, increased appetite, dyspnea, and weight loss.[16]

Chronic periarthritis is also associated with hyperthyroidism. Inflammation that involves the periarticular structures, including the tendons, ligaments, and joint capsule, is termed *periarthritis*. The syndrome is associated with pain and reduced range of motion. Calcification, whether periarticular or tendinous, may be seen on x-ray studies. Both periarthritis and calcific tendinitis occur most often in the shoulder, and both are common findings in clients who have endocrine disease (Case Example 11-3).

Painful restriction of shoulder motion associated with periarthritis has been widely described among clients of all ages with hyperthyroidism. The involvement can be unilateral or bilateral and can worsen progressively to become adhesive capsulitis (frozen shoulder). Acute calcific tendinitis of the wrist also has been described in such clients. Although antiinflammatory agents may be needed for the acute symptoms, chronic periarthritis

usually responds to treatment of the underlying hyperthyroidism.

Proximal muscle weakness (most marked in the pelvic girdle and thigh muscles), accompanied by muscle atrophy known as *myopathy*, occurs in up to 70% of people with hyperthyroidism. Muscle strength returns to normal in about 2 months after medical treatment, whereas muscle wasting

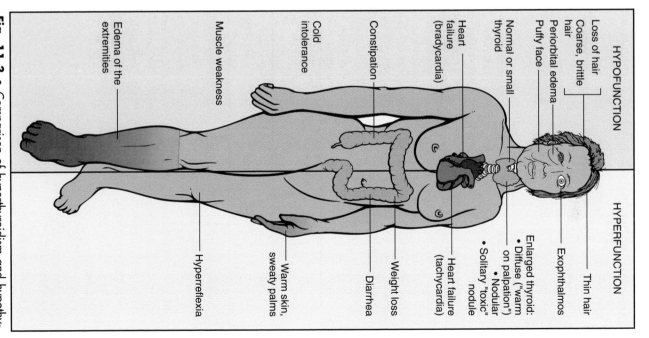

Fig. 11-3 • Comparison of hyperthyroidism and hypothyroidism. (From Damjanov I: *Pathology for the health-related profession*, ed 2, Philadephia, Saunders, 2000. Used with permission.)

HYPOFUNCTION

- Loss of hair
- Coarse, brittle hair
- Periorbital edema
- Puffy face
- Normal or small thyroid
- Constipation
- Heart failure (bradycardia)
- Cold intolerance
- Muscle weakness
- Edema of the extremities

HYPERFUNCTION

- Thin hair
- Exophthalmos
- Enlarged thyroid:
  - Diffuse ("warm on palpation")
  - Nodular
  - Solitary "toxic" nodule
- Weight loss
- Diarrhea
- Heart failure (tachycardia)
- Warm skin, sweaty palms
- Hyperreflexia

TABLE 11-4 ▼ Systemic Manifestations of Hyperthyroidism

CNS effects	Cardiovascular and pulmonary effects	Joint and integumentary effects	Ocular effects	GI effects	GU effects
Tremors	Increased pulse rate/tachycardia/palpitations	Chronic periarthritis	Weakness of the extraocular muscles (poor convergence, poor upward gaze)	Hypermetabolism (increased appetite with weight loss)	Polyuria (frequent urination)
Hyperkinesis (abnormally increased motor function or activity)	Arrhythmias (palpitations)	Capillary dilation (warm flushed, moist skin)			Amenorrhea (absence of menses)
	Weakness of respiratory muscles (breathlessness, hypoventilation)	Heat intolerance	Sensitivity to light	Increased peristalsis	Female infertility
Nervousness, irritability		Onycholysis (separation of the fingernail from the nail bed)	Visual loss	Diarrhea, nausea, and vomiting	First-trimester miscarriage
Emotional lability	Increased respiratory rate	Easily broken hair and increased hair loss	Spasm and retraction of the upper eyelids (bulging eyes), lid tremor	Dysphagia	and frequency of bowel movements
Weakness and muscle atrophy	Low blood pressure	Hyperpigmentation			
Increased deep tendon reflexes	Heart failure	Hard, purple area over the anterior surface of the tibia with itching erythema, and occasionally pain			
Fatigue					

CASE EXAMPLE 11-3 Graves' Disease (Hyperthyroidism)

A 73-year-old woman who has rheumatoid arthritis has just joined the Physical Therapy Aquatic Program. Despite the climate-controlled facility, she becomes flushed, demonstrates an increased respiratory rate that is inconsistent with her level of exercise, and begins to perspire profusely. She reports muscle cramping of the arms and legs and sudden onset of a headache.

Questions

- How would you handle this situation?
- Can this client resume the aquatic program when her symptoms have resolved?

Result: The client was quickly escorted from the pool. Her vital signs were taken and recorded for future reference. Later, the thera-

pist reviewed the client's health history and noted that the "thyroid medication" she reported taking was actually an antithyroid medication for Graves' disease.

The heat intolerance associated with the Graves' disease (hyperthermia secondary to accelerated metabolic rate) presents a potential contraindication for aquatic or pool therapy. Heat intolerance contributes to exercise intolerance, and the client was exhibiting signs and symptoms of heat stroke, even when exercising in a climate-controlled facility. The physician was notified of the symptoms and how quickly the onset occurred (after only 5 minutes of warm-up exercises). Strenuous exercise or a conditioning program should be delayed until symptoms of heat intolerance, tachycardia, or arrhythmias are under medical control.

THYROID STORM

Life-threatening complications with hyperthyroidism are rare but still important for the therapist to recognize. Unrecognized disease, untreated disease, or incorrect treatment can result in a condition called *thyroid storm.* In addition, precipitating factors such as trauma, infection, or surgery

resolves more slowly. In severe cases normal strength may not be restored for months.

The incidence of myasthenia gravis is increased in clients with hyperthyroidism, which in turn can aggravate muscle weakness. If the hyperthyroidism is corrected, improvement of myasthenia gravis follows in about two thirds of clients.

can turn well-controlled hyperthyroidism into a thyroid storm.

Thyroid storm includes severe tachycardia with heart failure, shock, and hyperthermia (up to 105.3 degrees F [40.7 degrees C]). Restlessness, agitation, abdominal pain, nausea and vomiting, and coma can occur. Medical referral is required to return the client to a normal thyroid state and prevent cardiovascular or hyperthermia collapse. Look for a recent history of the precipitating factors mentioned.

Hypothyroidism

Hypothyroidism (hypofunction) is more common than hyperthyroidism, results from insufficient thyroid hormone, and creates a generalized depression of body metabolism. Hypothyroidism in fetal development and infants is usually a result of absent thyroid tissue and hereditary defects in thyroid hormone synthesis. Untreated congenital hypothyroidism is referred to as *cretinism*.

The condition may be classified as either primary or secondary. *Primary hypothyroidism* results from reduced functional thyroid tissue mass or impaired hormonal synthesis or release (e.g., iodine deficiency, loss of thyroid tissue, autoimmune thyroiditis). *Secondary hypothyroidism* (which accounts for a small percentage of all cases of hypothyroidism) occurs as a result of inadequate stimulation of the gland because of pituitary disease.

RISK FACTORS

Women are 10 times more likely than men to have hypothyroidism. More than 10% of women over age 65 and 15% over age 70 are diagnosed with this disorder. Risk factors include surgical removal of the thyroid gland, external irradiation, and some medications (e.g., lithium, amiodarone).

CLINICAL PRESENTATION

As with all disorders affecting the thyroid and parathyroid glands, clinical signs and symptoms affect many systems of the body (Table 11-5). Because the thyroid hormones play such an important role in the body's metabolism, lack of these hormones seriously upsets the balance of body processes.

Among the primary symptoms associated with hypothyroidism are intolerance to cold, excessive fatigue and drowsiness, headaches, and weight gain. In women, menstrual bleeding may become irregular, and premenstrual syndrome (PMS) may worsen. Physical assessment often reveals dryness of the skin and increasing thinness and brittleness of the hair and nails. There may be nodules or other irregularities of the thyroid palpable during anterior neck examination.

Ichthyosis, or dry scaly skin (resembling fish scales; the word *ichthus*, which means "fish"), may be an inherited dermatologic condition (Fig. 11-4). It may also be the result of a thyroid condition. It must not be assumed that clients who present with this condition are merely in need of better hydration or regular use of skin lotion. A medical referral is needed to rule out underlying pathology.

Myxedema
A characteristic sign of hypothyroidism and more rarely associated with hyperthyroidism (Graves' disease) is *myxedema* (often used synonymously with *hypothyroidism*). Myxedema is a result of an alteration in the composition of the dermis and other tissues, causing connective tissues to be separated by increased amounts of mucopolysaccharides and proteins.

This mucopolysaccharide-protein complex binds with water, causing a nonpitting, boggy edema especially around the eyes, hands, and feet and in the supraclavicular fossae (Case Example 11-4). The binding of this protein-mucopolysaccharide complex causes thickening of the tongue and the laryngeal and pharyngeal mucous membranes. This results in hoarseness and thick, slurred speech, which are also characteristic of untreated hypothyroidism.

Clients who have myxedematous hypothyroidism may demonstrate synovial fluid that is highly distinctive. The fluid's high viscosity results in a slow fluid wave that creates a sluggish "bulge" sign visible at the knee joint. Often, the fluid contains calcium pyrophosphate dihydrate (CPPD) crystal deposits that may be associated with chondrocalcinosis (deposit of calcium salts in joint cartilage). Thus a finding of a highly viscous, "noninflammatory" joint effusion containing CPPD crystals may suggest to the physician possible underlying hypothyroidism.

When such clients with hypothyroidism have been treated with thyroid replacement, some have experienced attacks of acute pseudogout caused by CPPD crystals remaining in the synovial fluid.

Neuromuscular Symptoms
Neuromuscular symptoms are among the most common manifestations of hypothyroidism. Flexor tenosynovitis with stiffness often accompanies CTS in people with hypothyroidism. CTS can develop before other signs of hypothyroidism become evident. It is thought that this CTS arises from deposition of myxedematous tissue in the carpal tunnel area. Acroparesthesias may occur as a result of median

TABLE 11-5 ▼ Systemic Manifestations of Hypothyroidism

CNS effects	Musculoskeletal effects	Pulmonary effects	Cardiovascular effects	Hematologic effects	Integumentary effects	GI effects	GU effects
Slowed speech and hoarseness	Proximal muscle weakness	Dyspnea	Bradycardia	Anemia	Myxedema (periorbital and peripheral)	Anorexia	Infertility
Anxiety, depression	Myalgias	Respiratory muscle weakness	Congestive heart failure	Easy bruising	Thickened, cool, and dry skin	Constipation	Menstrual irregularity
Slow mental function (loss of interest in daily activities, poor short-term memory)	Trigger points	Pleural effusion	Poor peripheral circulation (pallor, cold skin, intolerance to cold, hypertension)		Scaly skin (especially elbows and knees)	Weight gain disproportionate to caloric intake	Heavy menstrual bleeding
	Stiffness, cramps						
	Carpal tunnel syndrome		Severe atherosclerosis		Carotenosis (yellowing of the skin)	Decreased absorption of nutrients	
Hearing impairment	Prolonged deep tendon reflexes (especially Achilles)		Angina		Coarse, thinning hair	Decreased protein metabolism (retarded skeletal and soft tissue growth)	
Fatigue and increased sleep	Subjective report of paresthesias without supportive objective findings		Elevated blood pressure		Intolerance to cold		
Headache	Muscular and joint edema		Increased cholesterol, triglycerides, LDL		Nonpitting edema of hands and feet	Delayed glucose uptake	
Cerebellar ataxia	Back pain		Cardiomyopathy		Poor wound healing	Decreased glucose absorption	
	Increased bone density				Thin, brittle nails		
	Decreased bone formation and resorption						

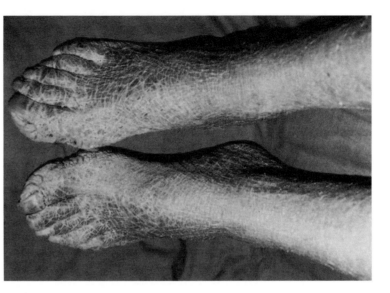

Fig. 11-4 • Ichthyosis of the legs in a woman with severe hypothyroidism. (From Callen JP, Jorizzo J, Greer KE, et al: *Dermatological signs of internal disease*, Philadelphia, Saunders, 1988. Used with permission.)

nerve compression at the wrist. The paresthesias are almost always located bilaterally in the hands. Most clients do not require surgical treatment because the symptoms respond to thyroid replacement.

Proximal muscle weakness sometimes accompanied by pain is common in clients who have hypothyroidism. As mentioned earlier, muscle weakness is not always related to either the severity or the duration of hypothyroidism and can be present several months before the diagnosis of hypothyroidism is made. Muscle bulk is usually normal; muscle hypertrophy is rare. Deep tendon reflexes are characterized by slowed muscle contraction and relaxation (prolonged reflex).

Characteristically, the muscular complaints of the client with hypothyroidism are aches and pains and cramps or stiffness. Involved muscles are particularly likely to develop persistent myofascial trigger points (TrPs). Of particular interest to the therapist is the concept that clinically any compromise of the energy metabolism of muscle aggravates and perpetuates TrPs. Treatment of the underlying hypothyroidism is essential in eliminating the TrPs,[17] but new research also supports the need for soft tissue treatment to achieve full recovery.[18]

There appears to be an association between hypothyroidism and fibromyalgia syndrome (FMS). Individuals with FMS and clients with undiagnosed myofascial symptoms may benefit from a medical referral for evaluation of thyroid function.[19-22]

Neoplasms

Cancer of the thyroid is a relatively uncommon, slow-growing neoplasm that rarely metastasizes. It is often the incidental finding in persons being treated for other disorders (e.g., musculoskeletal disorders involving the head and neck). Primary cancers of other endocrine organs are rare and are not encountered by the clinical therapist very often.

Risk factors for thyroid cancer include female gender, age over 40 years, Caucasian race, iodine deficiency, family history of thyroid cancer, and being exposed to radioactive iodine (I-131), especially as children. In addition, nuclear power plant fallout could expose large numbers of people to I-131 and subsequent thyroid cancer. The use of potassium iodide (KI) can protect the thyroid from the adverse effects of I-131 and is recommended to be made available in areas of the country near nuclear power plants in case of nuclear fallout. The initial manifestation in adults and especially in children is a palpable lymph node or nodule in the neck lateral to the sternocleidomastoid muscle in the lower portion of the posterior triangle overlying the scalene muscles[24] (Fig. 11-5).

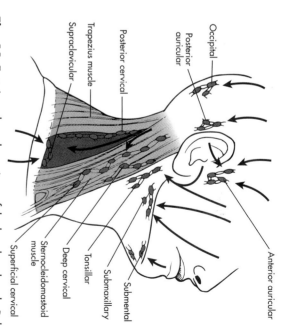

Fig. 11-5 • Lymph node regions of the head and neck. Palpable nodal disease associated with thyroid carcinoma is commonly located lateral to the sternocleidomastoid muscle in the lower portion of the posterior triangle overlying the scalene muscles (*dark red triangle*). (Modified from Swartz MH: *Textbook of physical diagnosis*, Philadelphia, 1989, Saunders.)

Occipital
Posterior auricular
Posterior cervical
Trapezius muscle
Supraclavicular
Anterior auricular
Superficial cervical
Submental
Submaxillary
Tonsillar
Deep cervical
Sternocleidomastoid muscle

CASE EXAMPLE 11-4 Myxedema

Referral: A 36-year-old African-American woman with a history of Graves' disease came to an outpatient hand clinic as a self-referral with painless swelling in both hands and feet. She had seen her doctor 6 weeks ago and was told that she did not have rheumatoid arthritis and should see a physical therapist.

Past Medical History: The woman had a 3-year history of Graves' disease, which was treated with thyroid supplementation. She had a family history of thyroid problems, maternal history of diabetes, and history of early death from heart attack (father). Aside from symptoms of hyperthyroidism, she did not have any health problems.

Clinical Presentation: There was a mild swelling apparent in the soft tissues of the fingers and toes. Presentation was painless and bilateral although asymmetric (second and third digits of the right hand were affected; third and fourth digits of the left hand were symptomatic).

The therapist was alerted to the unusual clinical presentation by the following signs:

- Thickening of the skin over the affected digits in the hands and feet
- Clubbing of all digits (fingers and toes)
- Nonpitting edema and thickening of the skin over the front of the lower legs down to the feet

The client did not think these additional symptoms were present at the time she saw her physician 6 weeks ago, but she could not remember exactly.

Result: The therapist was unsure if the symptoms present were normal manifestations of Graves' disease or an indication that the client's thyroid levels were abnormal. The physician was contacted with information about the additional signs and questions about this client's clinical presentation.

The physician requested a return visit from the client, at which time further testing was done. The skin changes and edema of the lower legs are called *pretibial myxedema*. Myxedema is more commonly associated with hypothyroidism. When accompanied by digital clubbing and new bone formation, the condition is called *thyroid acropachy*. This condition is seen most often in individuals who have been treated for hyperthyroidism.

Drug therapy for the thyroid function does not change the acropachy; treatment is palliative for relief of symptoms. Physical therapy intervention can be prescribed but has not been studied to prove effectiveness for this condition.

Parathyroid Glands

Two parathyroid glands are located on the posterior surface of each lobe of the thyroid gland. These glands secrete parathyroid hormone (PTH), which regulates calcium and phosphorus metabolism. Parathyroid disorders include hyperparathyroidism and hypoparathyroidism.

The therapist may see clients with parathyroid disorders in acute care settings and postoperatively because these disorders can result from diseases and surgical procedures. If damage or removal of these glands occurs, the resulting hypoparathyroidism (temporary or permanent) causes hypocalcemia, which can result in cardiac arrhythmias and neuromuscular irritability (tetany).

Disorders of the parathyroid glands may produce periarthritis and tendinitis. Both types of

A physician must evaluate any client with a palpable nodule because a palpable nodule is often clinically indistinguishable from a mass associated with a benign condition. The presence of new-onset hoarseness, hemoptysis, or elevated blood pressure is a red-flag symptom for systemic disease.

Clinical Signs and Symptoms of
Thyroid Carcinoma

- Presence of asymptomatic nodule or mass in thyroid tissue
- Nodule is firm, irregular, painless
- Hoarseness
- Hemoptysis
- Dyspnea
- Elevated blood pressure

inflammation may be crystal-induced and can be associated with periarticular or tendinous calcification.

Hyperparathyroidism

Hyperparathyroidism (hyperfunction), or the excessive secretion of PTH, disrupts calcium, phosphate, and bone metabolism. The primary function of PTH is to maintain a normal serum calcium level. Elevated PTH causes release of calcium by the bone and accumulation of calcium in the bloodstream.

Symptoms of hyperparathyroidism are related to this release of bone calcium into the bloodstream. This causes demineralization of bone and subsequent loss of bone strength and density. At the same time, the increase of calcium in the bloodstream can cause many other problems within the body, such as renal stones. The incidence of hyperparathyroidism is highest in postmenopausal women.[25]

The major cause of primary hyperparathyroidism is a tumor of a parathyroid gland, which results in the autonomous secretion of PTH. Renal failure, another common cause of hyperparathyroidism, causes hypocalcemia and stimulates PTH production. Hyperplasia of the gland occurs as it attempts to raise the blood serum calcium levels. Thiazide diuretics (used for hypertension) and lithium carbonate (used for some psychiatric problems) can exacerbate or even cause hyperparathyroid disorders.[26]

CLINICAL PRESENTATION

Many systems of the body are affected by hyperparathyroidism (Table 11-6). Proximal muscle weakness and fatigability are common findings and may be secondary to a peripheral neuropathic process. Myopathy of respiratory muscles with associated respiratory involvement often goes unnoticed. Striking reversal of muscle weakness and atrophy occur with successful treatment of the underlying hyperparathyroidism.

Other symptoms associated with hyperparathyroidism are muscle weakness, loss of appetite, weight loss, nausea and vomiting, depression, and increased thirst and urination (Case Example 11-5). Hyperparathyroidism can also cause GI problems, pancreatitis, bone decalcification, and psychotic paranoia (Fig. 11-6).

Bone erosion, bone resorption, and subsequent bone destruction from hypercalcemia associated with hyperparathyroidism occurs rarely today. In most cases, hypercalcemia is mild and detected before any significant skeletal disease develops. The classic bone disease *osteitis fibrosa cystica* affects persons with primary or renal hyperparathyroidism. Bone lesions called *Brown tumors* appear at the end stages of the cystic osteitis fibrosa. There are increasing reports of this condition in hyperparathyroidism secondary to renal failure because of the increasing survival rates of clients on hemodialysis.

Currently, skeletal manifestations of primary hyperparathyroidism are more likely to include bone pain secondary to osteopenia, especially diffuse osteopenia of the spine with possible vertebral fractures. In addition, a number of articular and periarticular disorders have been recognized in association with primary hyperparathyroidism. The therapist may encounter cases of ruptured tendons caused by bone resorption in clients with hyperparathyroidism.

Inflammatory polyarthritis may be associated with chondrocalcinosis and CPPD deposits in the synovial fluid. This erosion is called *osteogenic synovitis*. Concurrent illness and surgery (most often parathyroidectomy) are recognized inducers of acute arthritic episodes.

TABLE 11-6 ▼ Systemic Manifestations of Hyperparathyroidism

Early CNS symptoms	Musculoskeletal effects	GI effects	GU effects
Lethargy, drowsiness, paresthesia	Mild-to-severe proximal muscle weakness of the extremities	Peptic ulcers	Renal colic associated with kidney stones
Slow mentation, poor memory	Muscle atrophy	Pancreatitis	Hypercalcemia (polyuria, polydipsia, constipation)
Depression, personality changes	Bone decalcification (bone pain, especially spine; pathologic fractures; bone cysts)	Nausea, vomiting, anorexia	Kidney infections
Easily fatigued	Gout and pseudogout	Constipation	
Hyperactive deep tendon reflexes	Arthralgias involving the hands		
Occasionally glove-and-stocking distribution of sensory loss	Myalgia and sensation of heaviness in the lower extremities		
	Joint hypermobility		

CASE EXAMPLE 11-5   Rheumatoid Arthritis and Hyperparathyroidism

Referral: A 58-year-old man was referred to physical therapy by his primary care physician with a diagnosis of new-onset rheumatoid arthritis. Chief complaint was bilateral sacroiliac (SI) joint pain and pain on palpation of the hands and wrists.

When asked if he had any symptoms of any kind anywhere else in the body, he mentioned constipation, nausea, and loss of appetite. The family took the therapist aside and expressed concerns about personality changes, including apathy, depression, and episodes of paranoia. These additional symptoms were first observed shortly after the hand pain developed.

Past Medical History: The client had a motorcycle accident 2 years ago but reported no major injuries and no apparent residual problems. He had a family history of heart disease and hypertension but was not hypertensive at the time of the physical therapy interview. There was no other contributory personal or family past medical history.

Clinical Presentation: The therapist was unable to account for the sacroiliac joint pain. There were no particular movements that made it better or worse and no objective findings

to suggest an underlying movement system impairment.

Other red flags included age, bilateral hand and SI symptoms, gastrointestinal distress, and psychologic/behavioral changes observed by the family.

Result: The therapist contacted the referring physician with the results of her evaluation. During the telephone conversation, the therapist mentioned the family's concerns about the client's personality change and the fact that the client had bilateral symptoms that could not be provoked or relieved. Additional gastrointestinal symptoms were also discussed.

At the physician's request, the client completed a short course of physical therapy intervention with an emphasis on posture, core training, and soft tissue mobilization. The client returned to the physician for a follow-up examination 4 weeks later. His symptoms were unchanged.

After additional testing, the client was eventually diagnosed with hyperparathyroidism and treated accordingly. Both his hand and SI pain went away as well as most of the gastrointestinal problems.

Hypoparathyroidism

Hypoparathyroidism (hypofunction), or insufficient secretion of PTH, most commonly results from accidental removal or injury of the parathyroid gland during thyroid or anterior neck surgery. A less common form of the disease can occur from a genetic autoimmune destruction of the gland. Hypofunction of the parathyroid gland results in insufficient secretion of PTH and subsequent hypocalcemia, hyperphosphatemia, and pronounced neuromuscular and cardiac irritability.

CLINICAL PRESENTATION

Hypocalcemia occurs when the parathyroids become inactive. The resultant deficiency of calcium in the blood alters the function of many tissues in the body. These altered functions are described by the systemic manifestations of signs and symptoms associated with hypoparathyroidism (Table 11-7).

The most significant clinical consequence of hypocalcemia is neuromuscular irritability. This irritability results in muscle spasms, paresthesias, tetany, and life-threatening cardiac arrhythmias. Muscle weakness and pain have been reported along with hypocalcemia in clients with hypoparathyroidism.

Hypoparathyroidism is primarily treated through pharmacologic management with intravenous calcium gluconate, oral calcium salts, and vitamin D. Acute hypoparathyroidism is a life-threatening emergency and is treated rapidly with calcium replacement, anticonvulsants, and prevention of airway obstruction.

Pancreas

The pancreas is a fish-shaped organ that lies behind the stomach. Its head and neck are located in the curve of the duodenum, and its body extends horizontally across the posterior abdominal wall.

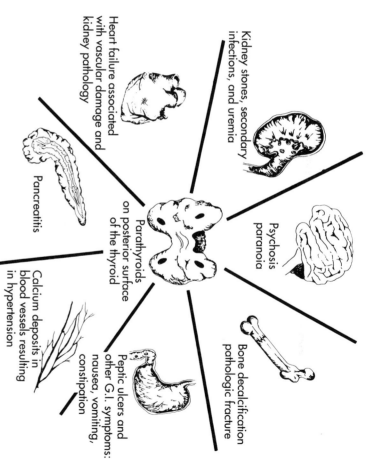

Fig. 11-6 • The pathologic processes of body structures as a result of excess parathyroid hormone. (From Muthe NC: *Endocrinology: a nursing approach,* Boston, 1981, Little, Brown, p 115.)

Kidney stones, secondary infections, and uremia

Heart failure associated with vascular damage and kidney pathology

Psychosis paranoia

Parathyroids on posterior surface of the thyroid

Pancreatitis

Calcium deposits in blood vessels resulting in hypertension

Bone decalcification pathologic fracture

Peptic ulcers and other G.I. symptoms: nausea, vomiting, constipation

TABLE 11-7 ▼ Systemic Manifestations of Hypoparathyroidism

CNS effects	Musculoskeletal effects*	Cardiovascular effects*	Integumentary effects	GI effects
Personality changes (irritability, agitation, anxiety, depression)	Hypocalcemia (neuromuscular excitability and muscular tetany, especially involving flexion of the upper extremity)	Cardiac arrhythmias	Dry, scaly, coarse, pigmented skin	Nausea and vomiting
	Spasm of intercostals muscles and diaphragm compromising breathing	Eventual heart failure	Tendency to have skin infections	Constipation or diarrhea
	Positive Chvostek's sign (twitching of facial muscles with tapping of the facial nerve in front of the ear)		Thinning of hair, including eyebrows and eyelashes	Neuromuscular stimulation of the intestine (abdominal pain)
			Fingernails and toenails become brittle and form ridges	

* The most common and important effects for the therapist to be aware of are the musculoskeletal and cardiovascular effects.

The pancreas has dual functions. It acts as both an *endocrine gland,* secreting the hormones insulin and glucagon, and an *exocrine gland,* producing digestive enzymes. Disorders of endocrine function are included in this chapter, whereas disorders of exocrine function affecting digestion are included in Chapter 8.

Diabetes Mellitus

Diabetes mellitus (DM) is a chronic disorder caused by deficient insulin or defective insulin action in the body. It is characterized by hyperglycemia (excess glucose in the blood) and disruption of the metabolism of carbohydrates, fats, and proteins. Over time, it results in serious small

vessel and large vessel vascular complications and neuropathies.

Type 1 DM is a condition in which little or no insulin is produced. It occurs in about 10% of all cases and usually occurs in children or young adults. Type 2 DM commonly occurs after age 40 and is a condition of defective insulin and/or impaired cell receptor binding of insulin. Table 11-8 depicts the major differences between type 1 and type 2 in presentation and treatment.

Native Americans, Latino Americans, Native Hawaiians, and some Asian Americans and Pacific Islanders have been identified at particularly high risk for type 2 diabetes mellitus and its complications.[27]

CLINICAL PRESENTATION

Specific physiologic changes occur when insulin is lacking or ineffective. Normally, the blood glucose level rises after a meal. A large amount of this glucose is taken up by the liver for storage or for use by other tissues, such as skeletal muscle and fat. When insulin function is impaired, the glucose in the general circulation is not taken up or removed by these tissues; thus it continues to accumulate in the blood. Because new glucose has not been "deposited" into the liver, the liver synthesizes more glucose and releases it into the general circulation, which increases the already elevated blood glucose level.

Protein synthesis is also impaired because amino acid transport into cells requires insulin.

The metabolism of fats and fatty acids is altered, and instead of fat formation, fat breakdown begins in an attempt to liberate more glucose. The oxidation of these fats causes the formation of ketone bodies. Because the formation of these ketones can be rapid, they can build quickly and reach very high levels in the bloodstream. When the renal threshold for ketones is exceeded, the ketones appear in the urine as acetone (ketonuria).

The accumulation of high levels of glucose in the blood creates a hyperosmotic condition in the blood serum. This highly concentrated blood serum then "pulls" fluid from the interstitial areas, and fluid is lost through the kidneys (osmotic diuresis). Because large quantities of urine are excreted (polyuria), serious fluid losses occur, and the conscious individual becomes extremely thirsty and drinks large amounts of water (polydipsia). In addition, the kidney is unable to resorb all the glucose, so glucose begins to be excreted in the urine (glycosuria).

Certain medications can cause or contribute to hyperglycemia. Corticosteroids taken orally have the greatest glucogenic effect. Any person with diabetes taking corticosteroid medications must be monitored for changes in blood glucose levels.

Other hormones produced by the body also affect blood glucose levels and can have a direct influence on the severity of diabetic symptoms. Epinephrine, glucocorticoids, and growth hormone can cause

TABLE 11-8 ▼ Primary Differences Between Type 1 and Type 2 Diabetes

Factors	Type 1	Type 2
Age of onset	Usually younger than 30	Usually older than 35 (Can be younger if history of childhood obesity)
Type of onset	Abrupt	Gradual
Endogenous (own) insulin production	Little or none	Below normal or above normal
Incidence	5%-10%	90%-95%
Ketoacidosis	May occur	Unlikely
Insulin injections	Required	Needed in 20% to 30% of clients
Body weight at onset	Normal or thin	80% are obese
Management	Diet, exercise, insulin	Diet, exercise, oral hypoglycemic agents or insulin
Etiology	Possible viral/autoimmune, resulting in destruction of islet cells	Obesity-associated insulin receptor resistance
Hereditary	Yes	Yes
Risk factors	May be autoimmune, environmental, genetic	Prediabetic Ethnicity • Native American • Hispanic/Latin • Native Hawaiian, Pacific Islanders

significant elevations in blood glucose levels by mobilizing stored glucose to blood glucose during times of physical or psychologic stress.

When persons with DM are under stress, such as during surgery, trauma, pregnancy, puberty, or infectious states, blood glucose levels can rise and result in the need for increased amounts of insulin. If these insulin needs cannot be met, a hyperglycemic emergency such as diabetic ketoacidosis can result.

It is essential to remember that clients with DM who are under stress will have increased insulin requirements and may become symptomatic even though their disease is usually well controlled in normal circumstances.

Clinical Signs and Symptoms of Untreated or Uncontrolled Diabetes Mellitus

The classic clinical signs and symptoms of untreated or uncontrolled diabetes mellitus usually include one or more of the following:

- Polyuria: increased urination caused by osmotic diuresis
- Polydipsia: increased thirst in response to polyuria
- Polyphagia: increased appetite and ingestion of food (usually only in type 1)
- Weight loss in the presence of polyphagia: weight loss caused by improper fat metabolism and breakdown of fat stores (usually only in type 1)
- Hyperglycemia: increased blood glucose level (fasting level greater than 126 mg/dL)
- Glycosuria: presence of glucose in the urine
- Ketonuria: presence of ketone bodies in the urine (by-product of fat catabolism)
- Fatigue and weakness
- Blurred vision
- Irritability
- Recurring skin, gum, bladder, or other infections
- Numbness/tingling in hands and feet
- Cuts/bruises that are difficult and slow to heal

DIAGNOSIS

To be diagnosed with diabetes, a person must have fasting plasma glucose (FPG) readings of 126 mg/dL or higher on two different days. The previous cutoff, set in 1979, was 140 mg/dL. This change occurred as a result of research showing that individuals with readings as low as the mid-120s have already started developing tissue damage from diabetes. A value greater than 100 mg/dL is considered "pre-diabetic" and is a risk factor for future diabetes and cardiovascular disease.

The American Diabetes Association offers consumers a risk test for diabetes (http://www.diabetes.org/risk-test.jsp). All adults should take this risk test; anyone 45 or older should be tested for diabetes every 3 years. Individuals with prediabetes should be tested every 1 to 2 years. The therapist can offer clients with pre-diabetes information on increased activity and exercise as a means of lowering their risk of developing diabetes.[28]

PHYSICAL COMPLICATIONS

At presentation, the client with DM may have a variety of serious physical problems. Infection and atherosclerosis are the two primary long-term complications of this disease and are the usual causes of severe illness and death in the person with diabetes.

Blood vessels and nerves sustain major pathologic changes in the person affected by DM. Atherosclerosis in both large vessels (macrovascular changes) and small vessels (microvascular changes) develops at a much earlier age and progresses much faster in the individual with DM. The blood vessel changes result in decreased blood vessel lumen size, compromised blood flow, and resultant tissue ischemia. The pathologic end-products are cerebrovascular disease (CVD), coronary artery disease (CAD), renal artery stenosis, and peripheral vascular disease.

Microvascular changes, characterized by the thickening of capillaries and damage to the basement membrane, result in diabetic nephropathy (kidney disease) and diabetic retinopathy (disease of the retina). Diabetes is the leading cause of kidney failure and new cases of blindness in the United States as of 2002.[27]

Poorly controlled DM can lead to various tissue changes that result in impaired wound healing. Decreased circulation to the skin can further delay or diminish healing. Skin eruptions called *xanthomas* (Fig. 11-7) may appear when high lipid levels (e.g., cholesterol and triglycerides) in the blood cause fat deposits in the skin over extensor surfaces such as the elbows, knees, back of the head and neck, and heels. Yellow patches on the eyelids are another sign of hyperlipidemia. Medical referral is required to normalize lipid levels.

PHYSICAL COMPLICATIONS OF DIABETES MELLITUS

- Atherosclerosis
  - Macrovascular disease

- Carpal tunnel syndrome (mononeuropathy; ischemia of median nerve)
  - Charcot's joint (diabetic arthropathy)
- Periarthritis
- Hand stiffness
  - Limited joint mobility (LJM) syndrome
  - Flexor tenosynovitis
  - Dupuytren's contracture
  - Complex Regional Pain Syndrome (CRPS)

Depression Depression is common in individuals with type 2 diabetes (see Box 3-10) and is linked with increased mortality in this population.[29] Adults with diabetes and depression are less likely to follow recommendations for nutrition and exercise. They are less likely to check their blood glucose levels routinely and more likely to take drug "holidays" from their other medications (e.g., for hyperlipidemia or hypertension). Clients with diabetes who are depressed are more likely to miss health care appointments for prevention and intervention.[30,31]

Diabetic Neuropathy Neuropathy is the most common chronic complication of long-term DM. Neuropathy in the client with DM is thought to be related to the accumulation in the nerve cells of sorbitol, a by-product of improper glucose metabolism. This accumulation then results in abnormal fluid and electrolyte shifts and nerve cell dysfunction. The combination of this metabolic derangement and the diminished vascular perfusion to nerve tissues contributes to the severe problem of diabetic neuropathy.

Risk Factors Other than glycemic control, there is no curative intervention for diabetic neuropathy. Identifying potentially modifiable risk factors for neuropathy is crucial; the therapist can have a key role in providing risk factor assessment for clients with diabetes.

Risk factors for the development of diabetic neuropathy include the duration and severity of diabetes, elevated triglycerides, higher body mass index, and a history of smoking or hypertension.[32,33]

Clinical Presentation Neuropathy may affect the central nervous system, peripheral nervous system, or autonomic nervous system. Peripheral neuropathy usually develops first as a sensory impairment of the extremities. Autonomic involvement is more common with long-standing disease.

Most common among the peripheral neuropathies are chronic sensorimotor distal symmetric polyneuropathy (DPN).[34] Polyneuropathy affects peripheral nerves in distal lower extremities, causing burning and numbness in the feet. It

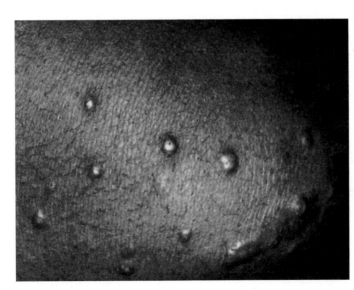

Fig. 11-7 • Multiple eruptive xanthomas over the extensor surface of the elbow in a client with poorly controlled diabetes. These lipid-filled nodules characterized by an intracellular accumulation of cholesterol develop in the skin, often around the extensor tendons. Medical referral is required; xanthomas in this population are a sign that the health-care team, including the therapist, must work with the client to provide further education about diabetes, gain better control of glucose levels, and prevent avoidable complications. These skin lesions will go away when the diabetes is under control. Xanthomas can occur in any condition with disturbances of lipoprotein metabolism (not just diabetes). (From Callen JP, Jorizzo J, Greer KE, et al: *Dermatological signs of internal disease*, Philadelphia, Saunders, 1988. Used with permission.)

Cerebrovascular disease (CVD)
Coronary artery disease (CAD)
Renal artery stenosis
Peripheral vascular disease (PVD)
- Microvascular disease
  Nephropathy
  Retinopathy
  Decreased microcirculation to skin/body organs
- Infection/impaired wound healing
- Neuropathy
- Autonomic (gastroparesis, diarrhea, incontinence, postural hypotension, decreased heart rate)
- Peripheral (polyneuropathy, diabetic foot)
- Diabetic amyotrophy

can result in muscle weakness, atrophy, and foot drop. Diabetic neuropathy can produce a syndrome of bilateral but asymmetric proximal muscle weakness called *diabetic amyotrophy.* Although the muscle enzyme levels are usually normal, muscle biopsy reveals atrophy of type II muscle fibers.

CTS (mononeuropathy) is also a common finding in persons with DM; it represents one form of diabetic neuropathy. As many as 5% to 16% of people with CTS have underlying diabetes. The mechanism is thought to be ischemia of the median nerve resulting from diabetes-related microvascular damage. This ischemia then causes increased sensitivity to even minor pressure exerted in the carpal tunnel area.

Autonomic involvement affects the pace of the heart beat, blood pressure, sweating, and bladder function and can cause symptoms such as erectile dysfunction and gastroparesis (delayed stomach emptying).[32]

Clinical Signs and Symptoms of
Diabetic Neuropathy (at least two or more are present)

Peripheral (Motor and Sensory)
- Sensory, vibratory impairment of the extremities
- Burning, stabbing, pain, or numbness distal lower extremities
- Extreme sensitivity to touch
- Muscle weakness and atrophy (diabetic amyotrophy)
- Absence of distal deep tendon reflexes (knee, ankle)
- Loss of balance
- Carpal tunnel syndrome

Autonomic
- Gastroparesis (delayed emptying of the stomach)
- Constipation or diarrhea
- Erectile dysfunction (sex drive unaffected; sexual function decreased)
- Urinary tract infections; urinary incontinence
- Profuse sweating
- Lack of oil production resulting in dry, cracked skin susceptible to bacteria and infection
- Pupillary adjustment restricted (difficulty seeing at night)
- Orthostatic hypotension
- Loss of heart rate variability

Charcot's joint, or neuropathic arthropathy, is a well-known complication of DM. This condition is due, at least in part, to the loss of proprioceptive

sensation that marks diabetic neuropathy. Severe degenerative arthritis similar to Charcot's joint has been noted in clients with CPPD crystal deposition disease. Shoulder, hand, and foot disorders are very common, and evaluation of clients with DM should include examination of these areas (Case Example 11-6).[35,36]

Clinical Signs and Symptoms of
Charcot's Joints

- Severe unilateral swelling (bilateral in 20% of cases but not bilateral at the same time)
- Increased skin warmth
- Redness
- Deep pressure sensation but significantly less pain than anticipated
- Normal x-rays initially but changes over time
- Joint deformity

The large- and small-vessel changes that occur with DM contribute to the changes in the feet of individuals with diabetes. Sensory neuropathy, which may lead to painless trauma and ulceration, can progress to infection. Neuropathy can result in drying and cracking of the skin, which creates more openings for bacteria to enter. The combination of all these factors can ultimately lead to gangrene and eventually require amputation. Prevention of these problems by meticulous care of the diabetic foot can reduce the need for amputation by 50% to 75%.

An annual foot screen by a health care provider is currently recommended for anyone with diabetes. This screen includes examination of toenails for length, thickness, and ingrown position. All calluses should be examined because ulceration can occur underneath them. General skin integrity, color, circulation, and structure should also be assessed.[37]

Whether a poorly controlled blood glucose level is a causative factor in the development of the long-term physical complications of diabetes is still controversial, but it does seem clear that these complications increase with the duration of the disease. Stable glycemic control, which prevents the fluctuation of blood glucose levels, has been shown to be helpful in decreasing neuropathic pain.[38]

Periarthritis Musculoskeletal disorders of the hand and shoulder, including periarthritis of the shoulder, is five times as common in this group as it is in individuals who do not have diabetes. The condition most often affects insulin-dependent people, and involvement is typically bilateral.

CASE EXAMPLE 11-6　Charcot Shoulder (Neuroarthropathy)

Referral: A 44-year-old wheelchair-dependent man with type 2 diabetes who was well-known to the physical therapy clinic came in with new symptoms of right shoulder pain. There was no known trauma or injury to account for the changes in his shoulder. He had previously been evaluated for an exercise program as part of his diabetes management.

Past Medical History: The client was involved in a rock-climbing accident 15 years ago. He has had multiple reconstructive surgeries for broken bones and frostbite of the lower extremities associated with the accident. He was diagnosed with type 2 diabetes 3 years ago and uses an insulin pump but does not have consistent control of his blood glucose levels over time.

The man remains active and has resumed rock climbing along with many other outdoor activities. This new onset of shoulder pain has limited his activities and impaired his ability to propel his wheelchair.

There is no other significant history to report. The client is a nonsmoker, drinks only occasionally and then only socially (one or two glasses of wine). He has not had any other symptoms; there have been no constitutional symptoms, loss of appetite, or other gastrointestinal problems.

Clinical Presentation: Cervical spine and elbow were cleared for any loss of motion, weakness, or other problems that might contribute to shoulder pain. Gross examination of motion and strength of the left shoulder revealed no problems. The skin was normal on both sides, no cervical or supraclavicular lymph node changes were observed or palpated, and no other observable changes in the upper quadrant were evident.

Range of motion of the right shoulder:
- Active and passive abduction were equal and limited to 60 degrees and painful.
- Active and passive flexion were equal and limited to 65 degrees and painful.
- Biceps and deltoid strength were both 4/5; upper trapezius and triceps strength was normal (5/5).
- Grip strength appeared normal.

Further neurologic screening exam revealed severely decreased proprioception of the entire right upper extremity; no other neurologic changes were observed or reported. Radial pulses intact and equal bilaterally.

Referral Decision: The therapist decided an x-ray might be helpful before initiating a program of physical therapy intervention. The client was very active and athletic and may have injured the joint or fractured the bone. Given the severity of his diabetic course over the last 3 years, an x-ray might be helpful in revealing any related arthritis that may be present.

The physician agreed with the therapist's assessment, and a radiographic examination was ordered.

Result: X-ray studies revealed destruction of two thirds of the right humeral head with microfractures and fragmentation throughout. The diagnosis of Charcot shoulder or neuroarthropathy was made. In this case, the therapist's knowledge of the client's past medical history and awareness of the physical complications possible with diabetes led to the referral decision before further damage was done to the bone and joint.

It is unusual for someone with this severe of a condition to present with only mild symptoms. His extreme athleticism and stoic attitude may have masked the intensity of his symptoms.

Hand Stiffness Diabetic stiff hand, limited joint mobility (LJM) syndrome, cheirarthritis (inflammation of the hand and finger joints), and diabetic contractures are common in both types of DM in direct relation to the presence and duration of microvascular complications.

Flexor tenosynovitis, caused by accumulation of excessive dermal collagen in the fingers, results in thickening and induration of the skin

The mechanism of this association is unclear, but it is believed to be related to fibroblast proliferation in the connective tissue structures around joints or to microangiopathy (disorder involving small blood vessels) involving the tendon sheaths. This periarthritic condition can behave unpredictably: It may regress spontaneously, remain stable, or progress to adhesive capsulitis or frozen shoulder.[39]

around the joints. This condition can lead to sclerodactyly (hardening and shrinking of fingers and toes), which in turn can mimic scleroderma.

Dupuytren's contracture has a strong association with DM. The syndrome is characterized by nodular thickening of the palmar fascia and flexion contracture of the digits. Clients usually have pain in the palm and digits, with decreased mobility and contracture of the fingers. In clients with diabetes, Dupuytren's contracture must be differentiated from LJM, which may involve the entire hand and is frequently bilateral, and from flexor tenosynovitis, which is marked by trigger finger.

Individuals with DM may develop complex regional pain syndrome (CRPS; formerly called *reflex sympathetic dystrophy (RSD) syndrome*), which is characterized by pain, hyperesthesia, vasomotor and dystrophic skin changes, and tenderness and swelling around the hands and feet.

INTERVENTION

Medical management of the client with diabetes is directed primarily toward maintenance of blood glucose values within the range of 80 to 120 mg/dL. The three primary treatment modalities used in the management of DM are diet, exercise, and medication (insulin and oral hypoglycemic agents; Table 11-9).

Recommended preventive care services such as yearly eye and foot examinations as well as measurements of glycosylated hemoglobin (A1C) two or more times per year are critical in the prevention of diabetic complications such as blindness, amputation, and cardiovascular disease.[40] A1C (also known as *glycosylated hemoglobin, glycated hemoglobin,* or *glycohemoglobin*) is an accurate, objective measurement of chronic glycemia in diabetes.

Most laboratories list the normal reference range as 4% to 6%. The goal is to maintain consistent A1C levels below 7%, which correlates to an average daily blood glucose below 170 mg/dL. The

---

TABLE 11-9 ▼ Types of Insulin and Insulin Action

Type	Name	Onset (hours)	Peak (hours)	Duration (hours)
Rapid-acting				
Insulin lispro	Humalog	Begins to work 5 min after injection	Peaks in about one hour	Continues to work for 2 to 4 hours
Insulin aspart	Novolog	5-10 min	1-3 hours	3-5 hours
Regular or short-acting	Humulin-R (human) Novolin-R (human) Iletin-pork	Reaches bloodstream in first 30 minutes after injection	2-3	Effective for about 3-6 hours
Intermediate-acting	NPH (Humulin N, Novolin N) Lente (Humulin L, Novolin L) NPH (Iletin-pork)	Reaches bloodstream in about 2-4 hours after injection	4-12	Effective for about 12 to 18 hours
Long-acting	Ultralente (Humulin U)	Reaches bloodstream 6-10 hours after injection	No peak (maintains consistent level)	Effective for 20 to 24 hours
	Glargine (lantus)	1hr		Effective for 10-16 hours
Premixed Insulins (combination of two types of insulin)	70/30 (%) NPH/regular 50/50 (%) NPH/regular 75/25 (%) (Humalog mix) 70/30 (%) (Novolog mix)	30 min to 1 hour	Depends on mixture	

Onset is how long it takes before the insulin reaches the bloodstream and starts to lower glucose levels.
Peak is the time when insulin reaches its maximum strength.
Duration defines how long the insulin continues to lower blood glucose.
Data from American Diabetes Association: The Basics of Insulin, 2005. Available on-line at http://www.diabetes.org. Accessed January 11, 2006.

A1C measurement gives the client and the therapist an indication of how successful diet, exercise, and medication are in controlling glucose levels over time. It can be used as a baseline from which to evaluate results of intervention.

The therapist can conduct a careful screening examination (Box 11-1). All individuals with type 2 diabetes should be screened at the time of diagnosis and annually thereafter for diabetic peripheral neuropathies. Individuals with type 1 diabetes should be screened 5 years after diagnosis and annually thereafter. Screening should include checking knee and ankle reflexes, examining sensory function in the feet, asking about neuropathic symptoms, and examining the distal extremities for ulcers, calluses, and deformities.[34]

EXERCISE-RELATED COMPLICATIONS

Any exercise can improve the body's ability to use insulin. Exercise causes a decrease in the amount of insulin the pancreas releases because muscle contractions are increasing blood glucose uptake.

For the person taking insulin, exercise adds to the effects of the insulin, dropping blood sugars to dangerously low levels. Exercise for the person with DM must be planned and instituted cautiously and monitored carefully because significant complications can result from exercise of higher intensity or longer duration.

Exercise-related complications can be prevented by careful monitoring of the client's blood glucose level before, during, and after strenuous exercise sessions (safe levels are individually determined but usually fall between 100 and 250 mg/dL). The following recommendations are general guidelines. Exceptions are common depending on the type of exercise, training level of the participant, expected glycemic pattern, and whether or not the individual is using an insulin pump.

If the blood glucose level is greater than 250 mg/dL at the start of the exercise, the client is experiencing a state of insulin deficiency. Exercise is likely to raise the blood sugars more; the exercise session should be postponed until the blood glucose level is under better control. If the blood glucose level is less than 100 mg/dL, a 10- to 15-g carbohydrate snack should be given and the glucose retested in 15 minutes to ensure an appropriate level.

Clients with active retinopathy and nephropathy should avoid high-intensity exercise that causes significant increases in blood pressure because such increases can cause further damage to the retinas and kidneys. Any exercise that places the head below the waist causing increased intrathoracic and intracranial pressures can also aggravate retinal problems. Screening for neuropathies by testing deep tendon reflexes and vibratory and position sense are also very important in the prevention of exercise-related complications such as ulcerations or fractures.

It is very important to have the client avoid insulin injection to active extremities within 1 hour of exercise because insulin is absorbed much more quickly in an active extremity. It is important to know the type, dose, and time of the client's insulin injections so that exercise is not planned for the peak activity times of the insulin.

Clients with type 1 diabetes may need to reduce the insulin dose or increase food intake when initiating an exercise program. During prolonged activities, a 10- to 15-g carbohydrate snack is recommended for each 30 minutes of activity. Activities should be promptly stopped with the development of any symptoms of hypoglycemia, and blood glucose should be tested. In addition, individuals with diabetes should not exercise

---

BOX 11-1 ▼ The Role of the Physical Therapist in Diabetes Screening

The therapist can provide education and prevention through the screening process including conducting periodic screening examinations for:

- Neuropathy
  - Assess for early signs of neuropathy (e.g., deep tendon reflexes, vibratory and position sense, touch)
  - Education in avoiding late complications of neuropathy (e.g., annual foot and hand screening, preventive foot care; periodic footwear evaluation)
- Assess for signs of neuropathic arthropathy (Charcot's joint)
- Monitor blood glucose levels in association with exercise
- Screen for neuromusculoskeletal disorders (e.g., adhesive capsulitis, Dupuytren disease, flexor tenosynovitis, carpal tunnel syndrome, complex regional pain syndrome)
- Monitor vital signs (especially blood pressure)
- Conduct periodic lower extremity vascular examination (see Box 4-15; Table 4-10)
- Screen for depression; monitor depression (see Appendix B-8; see Table 3-11)

The therapist can encourage the client to seek regular screening of:

- A1C levels
- Annual eye examination

alone. Partners, teammates, and coaches must be educated regarding the possibility of hypoglycemia and the way to manage it.

INSULIN PUMP DURING EXERCISE

People with type 1 diabetes (and some individuals with insulin-requiring type 2 diabetes) may be using an insulin pump. Continuous subcutaneous insulin infusion (CSII) therapy, known as *insulin pump therapy*, can bring the hormonal and metabolic responses to exercise close to normal for the individual with diabetes.

Although there are many benefits of pump use for active individuals with diabetes, there are a few drawbacks as well.[41] Exercise can speed the development of diabetic ketoacidosis (DKA) when there is an interruption of insulin delivery, which can quickly become a life-threatening condition.

Other considerations include the effect of excessive perspiration or water on the infusion set (needle into the skin at the infusion site gets displaced), ambient temperature (insulin degrades under extreme conditions of heat or cold), and the effect of movement or contact at the infusion site (this causes skin irritation).

Insulin pump users who have pre-exercise blood glucose levels less than 100mg/dL may not need a carbohydrate snack because they can reduce or suspend base insulin levels during an activity. The insulin reductions and required level of carbohydrate intake needed depends on the intensity and duration of the activity.[41]

The therapist should become familiar with the features of each pump in use by clients. Knowledge of basic guiding principles for exercise with diabetes and general recommendations for insulin regimen changes is also helpful.

Severe Hyperglycemic States

The two primary life-threatening metabolic conditions that can develop if uncontrolled or untreated DM progresses to a state of severe hyperglycemia (more than 400 mg/dL) are DKA and hyperglycemic, hyperosmolar, nonketotic coma (HHNC; Table 11-10).

DKA occurs with severe insulin deficiency caused by either undiagnosed DM or a situation in which the insulin needs of the person become greater than usual (e.g., infection, trauma, surgery, emotional stress). It is most often seen in the client with type 1 diabetes but can, in rare situations, occur in the client with type 2 diabetes. Medical treatment is necessary.

HHNC occurs most commonly in the older adult with type 2 diabetes. This complication is extremely serious and, in many cases, fatal. Factors that can precipitate this crisis are infections (e.g., pneumonia); medications that elevate the blood glucose level (e.g., corticosteroids); and procedures such as dialysis, surgery, or total parenteral nutrition (TPN).

There are specific clinical features that identify HHNC. Some of these are similar to those of DKA, such as severe hyperglycemia (1000 to 2000 mg/dL)

TABLE 11-10 ▼ Clinical Symptoms of Life-Threatening Glycemic States

Diabetic ketoacidosis (DKA)	Hyperosmolar, hyperglycemic state (HHS)	Hypoglycemia insulin shock
Gradual Onset	*Gradual Onset*	*Sudden Onset*
Thirst	Thirst	**Sympathetic activity**
Hyperventilation	Polyuria leading quickly to decreased urine output	Pallor
Fruity odor to breath		Perspiration
Lethargy/confusion	Volume loss from polyuria leading quickly to renal insufficiency	Irritability/nervousness
Coma		Weakness
Muscle and abdominal cramps	Severe dehydration	Hunger
	Lethargy/confusion	Shakiness
Polyuria, dehydration	Seizures	**CNS activity**
Flushed face, hot/dry skin	Coma	Headache
Elevated temperature	Abdominal pain and distention	Double/blurred vision
Blood glucose level >300 mg/dL	Blood glucose level >300 mg/dL	Slurred speech
Serum pH <7.3		Fatigue
		Numbness of lips/tongue
		Confusion
		Convulsion/coma
		Blood glucose level <70 mg/dL

and dehydration. The major differentiating feature between DKA and HHNC, however, is the absence of ketosis in HHNC.

Because it is likely that the therapist will work with clients who have diabetes, it is imperative that the clinical symptoms of DM and its potentially life-threatening metabolic states are understood. *If anyone with diabetes arrives for a clinical appointment in a confused or lethargic state or exhibiting changes in mental function, fingerstick glucose testing should be performed. Immediate physician referral is necessary.*

Hypoglycemia

Hypoglycemia (blood glucose of less than 70 mg/dL) is a major complication of the use of insulin or oral hypoglycemic agents. Hypoglycemia is usually the result of a decrease in food intake or an increase in physical activity in relation to insulin administration. It is a potentially lethal problem. The hypoglycemic state interrupts the oxygen consumption of nervous system tissue. Repeated or prolonged attacks can result in irreversible brain damage and death.

HYPOGLYCEMIA ASSOCIATED WITH DIABETES MELLITUS

Hypoglycemia during or after exercise can be a problem for anyone with diabetes. This condition results as glucose is used by the working muscles, if the circulating level of injected insulin is too high, or both. The degree of hypoglycemia depends on such factors as pre-exercise blood glucose levels, duration and intensity of exercise, and blood insulin concentration.

Clinical Presentation The severity and number of signs and symptoms depend on the individual client and the rapidity of the drop in blood glucose. It is important to note that clients can exhibit signs and symptoms of hypoglycemia when their elevated blood glucose level drops rapidly to a level that is still elevated (e.g., 400 to 200 mg/dL). The *rapidity* of the drop is the stimulus for sympathetic activity; even though a blood glucose level appears elevated, clients may still have hypoglycemia.

Clients receiving beta-adrenergic blockers (e.g., propranolol) can be at special risk for hypoglycemia by the actions of this medication. These beta-blockers inhibit the normal physiologic response of the body to the hypoglycemic state or block the appearance of the sympathetic manifestations of hypoglycemia. Clients may also have hypoglycemia during nighttime sleep (most often related to the use of intermediate- and long-acting

insulins given more than once a day), with the only symptoms being nightmares, sweating, or headache.

Intervention Hypoglycemia can be treated in the conscious client by immediate administration of sugar. It is always safer to give the sugar, even when there is doubt concerning the origin of symptoms (DKA and HHNC can also have similar central nervous system symptoms at presentation). Most often, 10 to 15 g of carbohydrate are sufficient to reverse the episode of hypoglycemia. Immediate-acting glucose sources should be kept in every physical therapy department (e.g., ½ cup of fruit juice or sugared cola, 8 oz of milk, two packets of sugar, 2-ounce tube of honey or cake-decorating gel).

Most people with diabetes carry a rapid-acting source of carbohydrate such as readily absorbable glucose tablets so that it is available for use if a hypoglycemic episode occurs. Some individuals use intramuscular glucagon. If the client loses consciousness, emergency personnel must be notified, and glucose will be administered intravenously.

Any episode or suspected episode of hypoglycemia must be treated promptly and must be reported to the client's physician. It is important to question each client who has diabetes regarding his or her individual response to hypoglycemia. Information regarding individual symptoms, frequency of episodes, and precipitating factors may be invaluable to the therapist in preventing or minimizing a hypoglycemic attack.

Other Hypoglycemic States

Other conditions that can cause hypoglycemic states are usually related to hormonal deficiencies (e.g., cortisol, glucagon, ACTH) or overproduction of insulin or insulin-like material from tumors.

Reactive hypoglycemia, also known as *functional hypoglycemia*, occurs after the intake of a meal and usually results from stomach or duodenal surgery. This condition involves rapid stomach emptying with rapid rises of glucose levels. Glucose then rapidly falls to below normal levels as an exaggerated response of insulin secretion develops. The cause of reactive hypoglycemia is unknown.

CLINICAL PRESENTATION

Clinical signs and symptoms of non-diabetes-related hypoglycemic states are the same as those described earlier for hypoglycemia related to DM. The client is warned to avoid fasting and simple sugars.

▲ INTRODUCTION TO METABOLISM

As noted earlier, the endocrine system works with the nervous system to regulate and integrate the body's metabolic activities. Although acid-base metabolism is not in itself a sign or a symptom, the consequences of an acid-base metabolism disorder can result in many clinical signs and symptoms.

The rate of metabolism can be increased by exercise, elevated body temperature (e.g., high fever), hormonal activity (e.g., thyroxine, insulin, epinephrine), and specific dynamic action that occurs after ingestion of a meal. All metabolic functions require proper fluid and acid-base balance.

Therapists are unlikely to evaluate someone with a primary musculoskeletal lesion that reflects an underlying metabolic disorder. However, many inpatients in hospitals and some outpatients may be affected by disturbances in acid-base metabolism and other specific metabolic disorders. Only those conditions that are likely to be encountered by a therapist are included in this text.

Fluid Imbalances

Fluid Deficit/Dehydration

Fluid deficit can occur as a result of two primary types of imbalance. There is either a loss of water without loss of solutes or a loss of both water and solutes.

The loss of body water without solutes results in the excess concentration of body solutes within the interstitial and intravascular compartments. To preserve equilibrium, water will then be forced to shift by osmosis from inside cells to these outside compartments.

If this state persists, large amounts of body water will be shifted and excreted (osmotic diuresis), and severe cellular dehydration will result. This type of imbalance can occur as a result of several conditions:

- Decreased water intake (e.g., unavailability, unconsciousness)
- Water loss without proportionate solute loss (e.g., prolonged hyperventilation, diabetes insipidus)
- Increased solute intake without proportionate water intake (tube feeding)
- Excess accumulation of solutes (e.g., high glucose levels such as in DM)

The second type of fluid imbalance results from a loss of *both* water and solutes. Causes of the loss of both water and solutes include hemorrhage, profuse perspiration (e.g., marathon runners), and loss of gastrointestinal tract secretions (e.g., vom-

iting, diarrhea, draining fistulas, ileostomy). Postsurgical patients who have had joint replacements, hip fractures, multiple trauma, or neurosurgery often lose blood and become hypovolemic despite efforts to maintain their homeostasis through blood transfusion and fluid replacement.

Severe losses of water or solutes (or both) can lead to dehydration and hypovolemic shock. It is important for the therapist to be aware of possible fluid losses or water shifts in any client who is already compromised by advanced age or by a situation, such as an ileostomy or tracheostomy, that results in a continuous loss of fluid. Because the response to fluid loss is highly individual, it is important to recognize the early clinical symptoms of fluid loss and to carefully monitor vital signs and clinical symptoms in clients who are at risk, especially the elderly, the very young, or the chronically ill.[42]

Athletes and normal adults may experience orthostatic hypotension when slightly dehydrated, especially when intense exercise increases the core body temperature. The normal vascular system can accommodate this effectively.

Clinical Signs and Symptoms of Dehydration or Fluid Loss

Early clinical signs and symptoms:

- Thirst
- Weight loss

As the condition worsens, other symptoms may include the following:

- Poor skin turgor
- Dryness of the mouth, throat, and face
- Absence of sweat
- Increased body temperature
- Low urine output
- Postural hypotension (increased heart rate by 10 beats/min and decreased systolic or diastolic blood pressure by 20 mm Hg when moving from a supine to a sitting position)
- Dizziness when standing
- Confusion
- Increased hematocrit

Fluid Excess

Fluid excess can occur in two major forms: water intoxication (excess of water without an excess of solutes) or edema (excess of both solutes and water).

Because the etiologic complex, symptoms, and outcomes related to these problems are substantially different, these fluid imbalances are discussed separately.

WATER INTOXICATION

Water intoxication (resulting in hyponatremia) is an excess of extracellular water in relationship to solutes. The extracellular fluid (ECF) becomes diluted, and water must then move into cells to equalize solute concentration on both sides of the cell membrane. High water consumption without solute replacement can result in hyponatremia, a potentially lethal situation.

Water excess can be caused by an accumulation of solute-free fluid. An increase in solute-free fluid usually occurs because of excess ADH (tumors, endocrine disorders) or intake of large amounts of only tap water without balanced solute ingestion. The latter situation occurs most often in older adults who drink additional water after having the flu, with its associated vomiting and diarrhea, or in athletes who have lost large amounts of body fluids during exercise that have been replaced with only water.

Symptoms of water intoxication are largely neurologic because of the shifting of water into brain tissues and resultant dilution of sodium in the vascular space.

Clinical Signs and Symptoms of

Water Intoxication

- Decreased mental alertness
  Other accompanying symptoms:
- Sleepiness
- Anorexia
- Poor motor coordination
- Confusion
  In a severe imbalance, other symptoms may include the following:
- Convulsions
- Sudden weight gain
- Hyperventilation
- Warm, moist skin
- Signs of increased intracerebral pressure
- Slow pulse
- Increased systolic blood pressure (more than 10 mm Hg)
- Decreased diastolic blood pressure (more than 10 mm Hg)
- Mild peripheral edema
- Low serum sodium
- Low hematocrit

EDEMA

An excess of solutes and water is called *isotonic volume excess.* The excess fluid is retained in the extracellular compartment and results in fluid accumulation in the interstitial spaces (*edema*).

Edema can be produced by many different situations, most commonly including vein obstruction, decreased cardiac output, endocrine imbalances, and loss of serum proteins (e.g., burns, liver disease, allergic reactions).

Clinical Signs and Symptoms of

Edema

- Weight gain (primary symptom)
- Excess fluid (several liters may accumulate before edema is evident)
- Dependent edema (collection of fluid in lower parts of the body)
- Pitting edema (finger pressed into edematous area leaves a persistent indentation in tissues)
- Increased blood pressure
- Neck vein engorgement (see Fig. 4-42)
- Effusions (pulmonary, pericardial, peritoneal)
- Congestive heart failure

Diuretic medications are used frequently to treat volume excess. Various diuretic medications may be used depending on the underlying cause of the problem and the desired effect of the drug. The most commonly used are the thiazide diuretics (e.g., chlorothiazide, hydrochlorothiazide). It is important to assess clients who take diuretic therapy for potential fluid loss and dehydration by observing for clinical symptoms of both.

These medications inhibit sodium and water resorption by the kidneys. Potassium is usually also lost with the sodium and water, so continuous replacement of potassium is a major concern for anyone receiving non–potassium-sparing diuretics. It is essential to monitor clients who take diuretics for signs and symptoms of potassium depletion.

It is also very important to check laboratory data for the potassium level in any client taking diuretics, particularly before exercise. Any value below the normal range (less than 3.5 mEq/L) is potentially dangerous and could result in a lethal cardiac arrhythmia even with moderate cardiovascular exercise.

For clients on diuretics, the therapist must observe for the appearance of symptoms consistent with dehydration or potassium depletion. Any concerns should be discussed with a physician before physical therapy intervention.

Clinical Signs and Symptoms of

Potassium Depletion

- Muscle weakness
- Fatigue

- Cardiac arrhythmias
- Abdominal distention
- Nausea and vomiting

Metabolic Disorders

Metabolic Syndrome

Metabolic syndrome is a group of signs and symptoms that are actually risk factors strongly linked to type 2 diabetes, cardiovascular disease, and stroke. This condition is characterized by insulin resistance and seems to be on the rise in Americans because of lifestyle and metabolic risk factors.

Insulin resistance is a generalized metabolic disorder in which the body cannot use insulin efficiently. Not only do the cells become resistant to insulin, but the cells themselves lose receptor sites (outside and inside the cell membrane). Insulin, which acts like a key to let glucose into the cells, cannot find a keyhole (receptor site) to open the door and let the glucose in.[43] This loss of receptor site and decreased receptor site receptivity is why the metabolic syndrome is also called the *insulin resistance syndrome*.

Some people are genetically predisposed to insulin resistance. Acquired factors, such as excess body fat and physical inactivity, can elicit insulin resistance and the metabolic syndrome in these people. Most people with insulin resistance have abdominal obesity. The biologic mechanisms at the molecular level between insulin resistance and metabolic risk factors are complex and not fully understood.[44]

RISK FACTORS

Serious health complications can be reduced by identifying risk factors early through screening. The dominant underlying risk factors for this syndrome appear to be abdominal obesity and insulin resistance. Other risk factors include family history of metabolic syndrome, type 2 diabetes, hypertension, elevated fasting glucose (100 mg/dL or more), elevated triglyceride levels (150 mg/dL or more), and low high-density lipoprotein (HDL) [men: less than 40 mg/dL; women: less than 50 mg/dL].

Clinical Signs and Symptoms of
Metabolic Syndrome

The metabolic syndrome is characterized by a group of metabolic risk factors in one person. They include the following[44]:

- Abdominal obesity (excessive fat tissue in and around the abdomen; increased waist size; men: equal or greater than 40 inches; women: equal or greater than 35 inches)
- Atherogenic dyslipidemia (blood fat disorders—high triglycerides, low HDL cholesterol, and high LDL cholesterol—that foster plaque buildups in artery walls)
- Elevated blood pressure (130/85 mm Hg or more)
- Insulin resistance or glucose intolerance (the body cannot properly use insulin or blood sugar)
- Prothrombotic state (e.g., high fibrinogen or plasminogen activator inhibitor–1 in the blood)
- Proinflammatory state (e.g., elevated C-reactive protein in the blood)

Metabolic Alkalosis

Metabolic alkalosis results from metabolic disturbances that cause either an increase in available bases or a loss of nonrespiratory body acids. Blood pH rises to a level greater than 7.45 (Table 11-11).

Common causes of metabolic alkalosis include excessive vomiting or upper gastrointestinal suctioning, diuretic therapy, or ingestion of large quantities of base substances such as antacids.

Decreased respirations may occur as the respiratory system attempts to compensate by buffering the basic environment. The lungs attempt to retain carbon dioxide (CO_2) and thus hydrogen ions (H).

It is important for the therapist to ask clients about the use of magnesium containing antacids because symptoms of alkalosis can affect muscular function by causing muscle fasciculation and cramping. Prevention of problems related to alkalosis may be accomplished by education of the client regarding antacid use.

Clinical Signs and Symptoms of
Metabolic Alkalosis

- Nausea
- Prolonged vomiting
- Diarrhea
- Confusion
- Irritability
- Agitation, restlessness
- Muscle twitching and muscle cramping
- Muscle weakness
- Paresthesias
- Convulsions
- Eventual coma
- Slow, shallow breathing

Metabolic Acidosis

Metabolic or nonrespiratory acidosis is an accumulation of fixed (nonvolatile) acids or a deficit of bases. Blood pH decreases to a level below 7.35 (see Table 11-11). Common causes of metabolic acidosis include DKA, lactic acidosis, renal failure, severe diarrhea, and drug or chemical toxicity.

Ketoacidosis occurs because insufficiency of insulin for the proper use of glucose results in increased breakdown of fat. This accelerated fat breakdown produces ketones and other acids. These acids accumulate to high levels. While the body attempts to neutralize these increased acids, the plasma bicarbonate (HCO_3) is used up.

Renal failure results in acidosis because the failing kidney not only is unable to rid the body of excess acids but also cannot produce necessary bicarbonate.

Lactic acidosis occurs as excess lactic acid is produced during strenuous exercise or when oxygen is insufficient for proper use of carbohydrate (CHO), glucose, and water (H_2O).

Intestinal and pancreatic secretions are highly alkaline so that *severe diarrhea* depletes the body

of these necessary bases. Metabolic acidosis can result from ingestion of large quantities of acetylsalicylic acid (salicylates); symptoms of possible metabolic acidosis should be carefully assessed in clients undergoing high-dose aspirin therapy.

Hyperventilation may occur as the respiratory system attempts to rid the body of excess acid by increasing the rate and depth of respiration. The result is an increase in the amount of carbon dioxide and hydrogen excreted through the respiratory system.

Clinical Signs and Symptoms of

Metabolic Acidosis

- Headache
- Fatigue
- Drowsiness, lethargy
- Nausea, vomiting
- Diarrhea
- Muscular twitching
- Convulsions
- Coma (severe)
- Rapid, deep breathing (hyperventilation)

TABLE 11-11 ▼ Laboratory Values: Uncompensated and Compensated Metabolic Alkalosis and Acidosis

	pH (7.35-7.45)	Arterial Blood Pco_2 (35-45 mm Hg)	HCO_3 (22-36 mEq/L)	Signs/Symptoms
Metabolic Alkalosis				
Uncompensated	>7.45	Normal	>26	Nausea Vomiting Diarrhea Confusion Irritability Agitation Muscle twitch Muscle cramp Muscle weakness Paresthesias Convulsions Slow breathing
Compensated	Normal	>45	>26	Decreased respiratory rate
Metabolic Acidosis				
Uncompensated	<7.35	Normal	<22	Headache Fatigue Nausea, vomiting Diarrhea Muscular twitching Convulsions Coma Hyperventilation
Compensated	Normal	<35	<22	Increased respiratory rate

Gout

Primary gout is the manifestation of an inherited inborn error of purine metabolism characterized by an elevated serum uric acid (hyperuricemia). Excess uric acid in the blood can result in tiny uric acid crystals forming that collect in the joints, triggering a painful inflammatory response.

Gout affects men predominantly, and the usual form of primary gout is uncommon before the third decade, with its peak incidence in the 40s and 50s. The frequency of gout in women approaches that in men after menopause when estrogen, which helps clear uric acid from the kidneys, declines dramatically.[45] Gout may occur as a result of another disorder or of its therapy. This is referred to as *secondary gout*. Secondary gout may be associated with neoplasm; renal disease; or other metabolic disorders, such as diabetes and hyperlipidemia (excess serum lipids).

RISK FACTORS

Increased serum uric acid levels are associated with middle age, obesity, white race, stress (including surgery and medical illness), and high dietary intake of purine-rich foods. A variety of medications (e.g., penicillin, insulin, or thiazide diuretics) may increase the serum uric acid level or decrease uric acid excretion, as may a number of acute or chronic disorders other than gout (Table 11-12).

High intake of meat (beef, pork, lamb) and seafood consumption has been associated with increased risk of gout, whereas high intake of low-

fat dairy products has been associated with a low risk. Purine-rich vegetables, protein intake, alcohol consumption, and body mass index are not associated with an increase in gout.[46]

Many diseases have a presentation similar to that of acute gouty arthritis. Gout and septic arthritis occasionally occur together. The diagnosis of gout must be based on the demonstration of monosodium urate crystals by synovial fluid analysis rather than on the clinical presentation alone.

CLINICAL PRESENTATION

Uric acid is usually dissolved in the blood until it is passed through the kidneys into the urine and then excreted. In individuals with gout, the uric acid changes into crystals (urate) that deposit in joints (causing gouty arthritis) and other tissues such as the kidneys, causing renal disease.

Most renal disease in clients with gout is the result of coexisting conditions such as hypertension or atherosclerosis. Renal dysfunction can occur as a result of urate-related parenchymal damage without the existence of other comorbidities. Urate nephropathy is relatively rare; the therapist is more likely to see a client receiving cyclosporine after a heart or kidney transplant who develops gout during the first year after the transplant.[47]

The most usual symptom of gout is acute monarticular arthritis. The individual may be awakened from sleep with exquisite pain in the affected joint; any pressure (even the touch of clothes or bed sheets) on the joint is intolerable. Redness and swelling occur within a few hours, sometimes accompanied by low-grade fever and chills. Untreated, the attack lasts from 10 days to 2 weeks. Later, episodes may develop more gradually, affecting more than one joint as the disease progresses.

The peripheral joints of the hands and feet are involved, with 90% of gouty clients having attacks in the metatarsophalangeal joint of the great toe. Other typical sites of initial involvement (in order of frequency) are the instep, ankle, heel, knee, and wrist, although any joint in the body may be involved.

In chronic gouty arthritis, periarticular and subcutaneous deposits of sodium urate (or urate salts) form; these are referred to as *tophus* (*tophi*). These deposits produce an acute inflammatory response that leads to acute arthritis and later to chronic arthritis. Enlarged tophi on the joints of the hands and feet may erupt and discharge chalky masses of urate crystals.

The formation of tophi is directly related to the elevation of serum urate; the higher the client's

---

TABLE 11-12 ▾ Causes of Secondary Hyperuricemia

Hematopoietic	Renal
Hemolytic anemia	Hemodialysis
Myeloproliferative disorders	Renal insufficiency
Polycythemia vera	Polycystic kidney disease
Myeloma	
	Drugs
Neoplastic	Low-dose aspirin
Leukemia	Diuretics
Lymphoma	Antineoplastic (cytotoxic) agents
Multiple myeloma	Alcohol
	Vitamin B$_{12}$
Endocrine	
Hypoparathyroidism	**Other**
Hyperparathyroidism	Chondrocalcinosis
Hypothyroidism	Psoriasis
Diabetes mellitus	Sarcoidosis
	Obesity
	Hyperlipidemia
	Starvation, dehydration
	Toxemia of pregnancy

From Wade JP, Liang MH: Avoiding common pitfalls in the diagnosis of gout, *J Musculoskel Med* 5(8):16-27, 1988.

serum urate concentration, the higher the rate of urate deposition in soft tissue. Before urate-lowering agents became available, 30% to 50% of people with acute gouty arthritis developed tophi. Today, chronic tophaceous gout is rarely seen.

The therapist should refer anyone taking urate-lowering drugs for gout who is having recurrent symptoms. It may be necessary to adjust medication levels. The therapist can reinforce the need for compliance with the management program and provide more education about controlling hypertension and obesity through diet and exercise. Avoidance of alcohol (especially beer), dehydration, and trauma to the extremities are other important components of effective management.[47]

Clinical Signs and Symptoms of

Gout

- Tophi: Lumps under the skin or actual eruptions through the skin of chalky urate crystals
- Joint pain and swelling (especially first metatarsal joint)
- Fever and chills
- Malaise
- Redness

PSEUDOGOUT

Pseudogout is an arthritic condition caused by calcium pyrophosphate dihydrate (CPPD) crystals. It occurs about one eighth as often as gout and may be hereditary or secondary to other disease processes (hyperparathyroidism is the most common one; Case Example 11-7).

Pseudogout is marked by attacks of goutlike symptoms, usually affecting a single joint (particularly the knee) and associated with chondrocalcinosis (deposition of calcium salts in joint cartilage). In anyone with pseudogout, routine x-ray studies of the knee and wrist frequently demonstrate cartilage calcification, or chondrocalcinosis. Because these changes are found in up to 10% of older adults, diagnosis must be made through aspiration of synovial fluid to identify the CPPD crystals.

Hemochromatosis

Hemochromatosis, also termed *hematochromatosis*, is an inborn error of iron metabolism. Mutations of the hemochromatosis (HFE) gene have been identified to help in better defining the type of disease present in an individual.[48]

The cardinal defect in hemochromatosis is the lack of regulation of iron absorption, but the exact

CASE EXAMPLE 11-7 Pseudogout

A 69-year-old man in previously good health complained of steadily increasing pain that had developed in his hands over the past several months. There was no history of occupational or accidental trauma.

Although the pain was present bilaterally, the pain in the left hand was more severe than in the right. The gentleman was right-hand dominant. There was a pattern of symptoms of increasing pain (described as deep aching) from morning to evening with a corresponding decrease in function.

Objective findings included reduced wrist range of motion in all directions bilaterally. There was no observed edema, warmth, or redness of the forearms, wrists, or hands. Although there were no reported symptoms at the elbow, left elbow extension and left forearm supination were also decreased by 25% as compared with the right side. Grip strength was reduced by 50% bilaterally for age and sex.

Neurologic screening was without significant findings. There were no trigger points corre-

sponding to the pain pattern present. No constitutional symptoms were reported, and vital signs were unremarkable.

Result: This man was treated by a hand therapist without significant changes in symptoms or function. In fact, he reported an increased inability to write with his right hand. The therapist suggested a medical evaluation with possible inclusion of x-ray examination. Physician assessment resulted in a diagnosis of calcium pyrophosphate dihydrate (CPPD) arthropathy (pseudogout) of unknown cause. Medical treatment included a prescription nonsteroidal antiinflammatory drug and return to physical therapy for continued symptomatic treatment addressing the loss of function.

Although a medical condition existed, physical therapy treatment was still warranted. In this case a medical differential diagnosis provided the client with necessary medical treatment and the physical therapist with information necessary to treat the client more specifically.

mechanism is unknown. The intestinal tract absorbs more iron than is required, thus producing an excess with progressive tissue damage in parenchymal organs from iron retention.

Hemochromatosis is found five to ten times more often in men than in women because women lose blood through menstruation and pregnancy. Men seldom have symptoms until after 50 years of age and are rarely symptomatic before 30 years of age. Because of menstrual blood loss, women display symptoms 10 years later than men (median age: 60 years).

Ascorbic acid (vitamin C) and alcohol seem to accelerate the absorption of dietary iron. The high incidence of alcoholism among clients with hemochromatosis (40%) supports this concept.

CLINICAL PRESENTATION

For many years, hemochromatosis was identified by a classic clinical triad of enlarged liver, skin hyperpigmentation, and diabetes. The term *bronze diabetes* was used to describe this presentation. Hyperpigmentation is caused by an increased number of melanocytes and a thinning of the epidermis. However, hemochromatosis may have many different signs and symptoms, confusing early diagnosis (Case Example 11-8).

In its early stages, hemochromatosis produces no symptoms because it takes many years of iron accumulation to produce warning signs or symptoms. Unfortunately, when the disease becomes evident, it is often too late because iron accumulation has caused irreversible tissue or end-organ

---

CASE EXAMPLE 11-8 Hemochromatosis

A 68-year-old man was admitted to the hospital after sustaining multiple fractures of unknown origin. He was referred to physical therapy for functional mobility, transfers, and active range of motion with prescribed limitations. The admitting physician was a third-year resident on an emergency department rotation.

When the client was seen by the physical therapist, there was obvious swelling and limited range of motion in the right shoulder. The skin was warm and tender over the shoulder joint.

The therapist also observed the following:

- Bony prominences involving the second and third metacarpophalangeal (MCP) joints
- Bony prominences over the wrists, elbows, knees, and ankles
- Palpable and audible crepitus of these same joints
- Gray discoloration to skin throughout the body and axial skeleton
- Very sparse axial hair and an unusual leathery texture to the skin

The client was a poor historian but mentioned a "liver problem" that he experienced years ago. When asked about any other problems anywhere else in the body, the client mentioned difficulty with sexual arousal, erection, and ejaculation over the last 6 months.

The therapist developed a plan of care based on the current medical problem list and physician's orders. She also made it a point to seek out the referring resident to review some of the more unusual findings and ask about the possible cause of these symptoms.

Result: Further testing revealed that this client had a hereditary disease called *hemochromatosis*. The condition is characterized by excessive iron absorption by the small intestine. Individuals with hemochromatosis lack an effective way to remove excess iron, and the iron begins to accumulate in the liver, pancreas, skin, heart, and other organs.

Excess iron accumulation in the body promotes oxidation and causes tissue injury, fatigue, arthralgia or arthritis, and skin changes. Complications can include hepatomegaly, diabetes, impotence (males), pulmonary involvement, and cardiac myopathy.

Medical treatment for this condition was required to prevent the condition from worsening. Treatment does not improve the associated arthritis in a case like this, but it does keep it from getting worse.

The therapist's careful observations and follow-up made a significant difference in this man's medical outcome.

Data from Sokolova Y: Acute shoulder pain and swelling in a 68-year-old man, *The Journal of Musculoskeletal Medicine* 17(11): 699-700, November 2000.

damage in the heart, liver, endocrine glands, skin, joints, bone, and pancreas. About half the clients with hemochromatosis will develop arthritis.

Hemochromatosis has a well-known association with chondrocalcinosis (deposition of calcium salts in the cartilage of joints). Acute attacks of synovitis can occur, which may resemble a rheumatoid flare. A biopsy of synovial tissue reveals iron deposition in the cells of the synovial lining that is noninflammatory.

Arthritis may be the presenting symptom of hemochromatosis, but it usually occurs after diagnosis and is more severe in adults older than 50. Arthritic manifestations are diverse, and joint damage occurs not from iron but from deposition of CPPD crystals.

The distribution of joint involvement may resemble rheumatoid arthritis, affecting the metacarpophalangeal (MCP) joints, in particular the second and third MCP joints. However, reduced MCP flexion is not accompanied by ulnar deviation. The arthritis can progress, and large joints may become involved, particularly the hips, knees, and shoulders.

Clinical Signs and Symptoms of

Hemochromatosis

- Arthropathy (joint disease)*
- Arthralgias
- Myalgias
- Progressive weakness
- Bilateral pitting edema (lower extremities)
- Vague abdominal pain
- Hypogonadism (lack of menstrual periods, impotence)*
- Congestive heart failure
- Hyperpigmentation of the skin (gray/blue to yellow)
- Loss of body hair
- Diabetes mellitus

---

* Unfortunately, even with treatment (removal of accumulated iron), arthritis, impotency, and sterility are not reversed.

Metabolic Bone Disease

Of the numerous metabolic disorders involving connective tissue, only the most commonly occurring diseases that would appear in a physical therapy setting are discussed in this text. These include osteoporosis, osteomalacia, and Paget's disease.

OSTEOPOROSIS

Osteoporosis, meaning "porous bone" and defined as a decreased mass per unit volume of normally

mineralized bone compared with age- and sex-matched controls, is the most prevalent bone disease in the world.

Osteoporosis is classified as *primary or secondary*. Primary osteoporosis is the deterioration of bone mass unassociated with other chronic illnesses or diseases. It is usually related to the aging process, including decreased gonadal function. Idiopathic, postmenopausal, and senile osteoporosis are included in the primary osteoporosis classification. *Postmenopausal osteoporosis* is associated with accelerated bone loss in the perimenopausal and postmenopausal period, accompanied by high fracture rates, particularly involving the vertebrae. *Senile osteoporosis*, or age-related osteoporosis, increases with advancing age; it is caused by the bone loss that normally accompanies aging.

Secondary osteoporosis may accompany various endocrine and metabolic disorders (e.g., hyperthyroidism, hyperparathyroidism, hypogonadism, Cushing's disease, and diabetes mellitus) that can produce associated osteopenia conditions (Table 11-13). *Endocrine-mediated bone loss* can produce osteoporosis because numerous endocrine hormones affect skeletal remodeling and hence skeletal mass.

Secondary osteoporosis is associated with other disorders that contribute to accelerated bone loss, such as chronic renal failure, rheumatoid arthritis, malabsorption syndromes related to gastrointestinal and hepatic disease, chronic respiratory disease, malignancies, and chronic chemical dependency (e.g., alcoholism).

Risk Factors The United States Preventive Services Task Force (USPSTF) now recommends that all women 65 years of age and older should be screened for osteoporosis. Despite the facts that approximately half of postmenopausal women will sustain an osteoporosis-related fracture and 15% will sustain a hip fracture in their lifetime, 75% of American women between the ages of 45 and 75 years have never discussed osteoporosis with their physician.[49,50]

Comparison of bone mineral density (BMD) to peak bone mass of women who are at peak bone mass is the designated T-score. T-scores are used as a method of describing severity of risk (Table 11-14). Therapists can be involved in primary prevention and education, encouraging and instructing consumers and clients in risk assessment and risk factor reduction (Fig. 11-8; Box 11-2).

Screening should begin at 60 years of age in women with key risk factors[53] (Box 11-3). Screening begins earlier for anyone who has a fracture

TABLE 11-13 ▼ Causes of Osteoporosis

Endocrine and metabolic	Other
Diabetes Mellitus (Type 1)	**Medications**
Glucocorticoid excess (Hyperadrenocorticism)	• Immunosuppressants (cyclosporine)
• Iatrogenic Cushing's syndrome	• Excess thyroid hormone
• Hyperadrenalism	• Glucocorticoids
Hyperthyroidism (thyrotoxicosis)	• Methotrexate
Hyperparathyroidism	• Anticonvulsants/seizure medications (e.g., dilantin, phenobarbital)
Hemochromatosis	
Acromegaly	**Nutritional**
Testicular insufficiency	• Anorexia nervosa; any eating disorder
	• Chronic alcohol use
	• Calcium/vitamin D deficiency
	• Chronic liver disease
	• Gastric bypass
	• Malabsorption syndromes (e.g., celiac sprue)
	Collagen/Genetic disorders
	• Ehlers-Danlos syndrome
	• Marfan syndrome
	• Osteogenesis imperfecta

TABLE 11-14 ▼ Bone Mineral Density T-Scores

Status	T-scores	Interpretation
Normal	–1.0 or above	T score (BMD) is within (or above) 1 SD of the young adult reference mean.
Osteopenia (low bone mass)	–1.0 to –2.5	T score is 1.0 to 2.5 SD below young adult mean for age.
Osteoporosis	–2.5 or less	T score is 2.5 or more SD below mean for age.
Severe osteoporosis	–2.5 or less with one or more fragility fractures	BMD is 2.5 or more SDs below mean for age.

The T score compares one person's bone mineral density (BMD) in standard deviations with the average peak BMD in healthy young persons. Sometimes, Z scores are used, which compare one individual's BMD with the mean BMD of persons in the same age group, rather than with the normal values listed for young adults.

The World Health Organization has proposed the clinical definition of osteoporosis in the table above based on epidemiologic data that link low bone mass with increased fracture risk.

In study populations of Caucasian postmenopausal women, a BMD that was lower than 2.5 standard deviation (SD) of normal peak bone mass was associated with a fracture prevalence; 50% of women with bone mass at this level had at least one bone fracture.[51] On the basis of these data, the WHO defined osteoporosis as BMD 2.5 or more SD below peak bone mass, osteopenia as bone mass between 1.0 and 2.5 SD below peak, and normal as 1.0 SD below normal peak bone mass or higher. The WHO criteria apply only to Caucasian, postmenopausal women, and not men, premenopausal women, or women of ethnicity other than Caucasian. T-scores for clinically significant low bone mass in other population groups are not yet available.

SD, Standard deviations; *BMD,* bone mineral density.

Data from World Health Organization, Criteria for Defining Bone Density, WHO, 1994.[51]

after age 50 or a maternal history of fracture after age 50.[58] Key risk factors include women who have body weight less than or equal to 125 pounds (57 kg),[58] and who do not currently use estrogen.

There is little known evidence to support the use of other individual risk factors such as smoking, caffeine or alcohol use, low calcium, or low vitamin D intake because those factors have not been shown to be independent predictors of low bone

density.[56] Medications used in high doses or for long-term use such as thyroid supplements, corticosteroids, anticoagulants, lithium, and anticonvulsants can contribute to the development of secondary osteoporosis.[59]

Primary prevention and education begins in childhood and adolescence, recognized as critical time periods for the development of normal peak bone mass. Diet and bone building exercise during

Osteoporosis Screening Evaluation

Name _____

Date _____

	YES	NO
1. Are you 65 years old or older?	☐	☐
2. Do you have a small, thin body?	☐	☐
3. Are you Caucasian or Asian?	☐	☐
4. Have any of your blood-related family members had osteoporosis?	☐	☐
5. Are you a postmenopausal woman?	☐	☐
6. Do you drink 2 or more ounces of alcohol each day? (1 beer, 1 glass of wine, or 1 cocktail = 1 ounce of alcohol)	☐	☐
7. Do you smoke more than 10 cigarettes each day?	☐	☐
8. Are you physically inactive? (Walking or similar exercise at least three times per week is average.)	☐	☐
9. Have you had both ovaries (with or without a hysterectomy) removed before age 40 years without treatment (hormone replacement)?	☐	☐
10. Have you ever been treated for or told you have rheumatoid arthritis? Have you been taking thyroid medication, antiinflammatories, or seizure medication for more than 6 months?	☐	☐
11. Have you ever broken your hip, spine, or wrist?	☐	☐
12. Do you drink or eat four or more servings of caffeine (carbonated beverages, tea, coffee, chocolate) per day?	☐	☐
13. Is your diet low in dairy products and other sources of calcium? (Three servings of dairy products or two doses of a calcium supplement per day are average.)	☐	☐

Fig. 11-8 • If you answer "yes" to three or more of these questions, you may be at greater risk for developing osteoporosis, or "brittle bone disease," and you should contact your physician for further information.

BOX 11-2 ▼ Osteoporosis Resources

National Osteoporosis Foundation

www.nof.org

Offers information for consumers and professionals about osteoporosis and its prevention. Includes information on bone density testing and risk factor assessment as well as a special web link, *Men and Osteoporosis*.

Harvard Center for Cancer Prevention

www.yourdiseaserisk.harvard.edu/

Offers consumers an opportunity to find out individual risk of developing five diseases, including cancer, diabetes, heart disease, osteoporosis, and stroke. Also includes tips on prevention for each of these diseases.

Medline Plus

http://www.nlm.nih.gov/medlineplus/ency/article/007197.htm

Information on bone mineral density testing, including normal values and how, when, and why the test is performed.

WebMD: Medical Tests

http://www.webmd.com/hw/osteoporosis/hw3738.asp

Offers the same information as provided by Medline Plus but also explains different techniques used to measure bone mineral density, how each one is done, and how to interpret the results.

Osteoporosis Education Project

http://www.betterbones.com/at_risk/questionnaire.htm

In addition to the osteoporosis screening evaluation presented in this chapter (see Fig. 11-8), consumers can take an osteoporosis fracture risk questionnaire offered by the Osteoporosis Education Project, a nonprofit organization dedicated to eduction and research on the topic of osteoporosis. The quiz is designed for both men and women of all ages.

Johns Hopkins SCORE Screening Quiz

http://www.hopkins-arthritis.som.jhmi.edu/other/osteo_update.html

The Simple Calculated Osteoporosis Risk Estimation (SCORE) is a 6-question screening questionnaire for osteoporosis with 89% sensitivity and 50% specificity in an ambulatory population of postmenopausal women. It is used to identify individuals who should be referred for bone densitometry testing.[52]

Fracture Index

An assessment tool for predicting fracture risk. This clinical assessment tool based on seven risk factors (age, T-score, personal or maternal fracture after age 50 years, weight, smoking status, use of arms to stand up from a chair) that can be used to assess a woman's risk of hip, vertebral, and nonvertebral fractures.

From Black DM, Steinbuch M, Palermo L, et al: An assessment tool for predicting fracture risk in postmenopausal women, *Osteoporosis International* 12(7):519-528, 2001.

this critical period are essential in the development of adequate bone mass.

Men can be affected, especially those who smoke, drink alcohol moderately, fail to maintain a calcium-rich diet, have a sedentary lifestyle, or have a family history of fractures or those undergoing dialysis or long-term steroid administration. Some data suggest that men do not receive treatment for osteoporosis or counseling for osteoporosis prevention as aggressively as women.[60]

Additionally, researchers are beginning to examine the environmental influences associated with industrialized countries such as the United States. For example, although menopause is universal, and the resulting estrogen deficiency is presumably similar for all women, differences in the occurrence of osteoporosis among countries cannot be explained only on the basis of estrogen deficiency.[61] Countries with the highest incidence of osteoporosis also have a high incidence of heart disease and the highest consumption of carbohydrates, fat, protein, salt, and caffeine.

Clinical Presentation

Osteoporosis is a silent disease with no visible signs or symptoms until bone loss is sufficient to result in fracture. Osteoporosis associated with aging involves fractures of the proximal femur and vertebrae as well as the hip, pelvis, proximal humerus, distal radius, and tibia.

Postmenopausal osteoporosis is associated with accelerated bone loss in the perimenopausal period accompanied by high fracture rates, particularly involving the vertebrae. Vertebral compression fracture will be likely in 25% of women older than 65 and 50% of women 80 years and older (Case Example 11-9).[70]

Mild-to-severe back pain and loss of height may be the only early signs observed. Changes in bone density do not show up on x-ray films until there is a 30% loss. The cardinal features of established osteoporosis are bone fracture, pain, and deformity.

More than half the women in the United States who are 50 years of age or older are likely to have radiologically detectable evidence of abnormally

---

BOX 11-3 ▲ Risk Factors for Osteoporosis

Residents in a nursing home, extended care, or skilled nursing facility have a fivefold to tenfold increase in fracture risk compared with community dwellers.[54] Therapists in these work settings have the potential to improve the recognition and management of osteoporosis in these populations, including reducing the number of fractures and falls.

Women
- Caucasian and Asian women are more likely to develop osteoporosis; African-American and Hispanic women have a significant risk for developing osteoporosis.[55]
- Gender: more common in women than men
- Age: postmenopausal (older than 65)
- Early or surgically induced menopause; menstrual dysfunction (amenorrhea)
- Family history of osteoporosis
- Family history and/or personal history of fractures
- Lifestyle*: cigarette smoking, excessive alcohol intake, inadequate calcium, little or no weight-bearing exercise
- Prolonged exposure to certain medications (more than 6 months):

  Thyroid medications, corticosteroids, antiinflammatories, anti seizure medication, aluminum-containing antacids, lithium, methotrexate, anticoagulants (heparin, warfarin), benzodiazepines (e.g., Lorazepam, diazepam), cyclosporine A (immuosuppressant), gonadotropic-releasing hormone agonists, Depo-Provera injections (contraceptives in adolescents)
- Some cancer treatments (oophorectomy, ovarian suppression, chemotherapy-induced ovarian failure, estrogen suppression, bone marrow transplantation)
- Thin, small-boned frame (weight less than or equal to 125 pounds or 57 kg)
- Chronic diseases that affect the kidneys, lungs, stomach, and intestines or alter hormones (especially if treated with corticosteroids); dialysis

Men
- Caucasian
- Gender: increasing incidence among men
- Advancing age
- Lifestyle: same as for women
- Prolonged exposure to medications (same as for women)
- Family history of osteoporosis
- History of prostate cancer with bilateral orchiectomy
- Undiagnosed low levels of testosterone
- Hypogonadism (long-term androgen deprivation therapy or ADT)
- Chronic diseases (as listed for women)

* Remains under investigation. There is little known evidence to support the use of other individual risk factors such as smoking, caffeine or alcohol use, low calcium, or low vitamin D intake because those factors have not been shown to be independent predictors of low bone density.[56] At least one study[57] reports that use of caffeine and antacids has no probable effect on bone mass in older women. The investigators also emphasized that it is weight, not body mass index, that is important. A 10 kg increase in weight reportedly implied a 6% increase in bone mineral density.

CASE EXAMPLE 11-9 Osteoporosis

Referral: A 77-year-old Caucasian woman was referred to outpatient physical therapy 1 month ago by her primary physician because of her complaint of gradual onset of low back pain (LBP) over the last 2 months. The physician's diagnosis was LBP secondary to osteoarthritis and osteoporosis. A recent radiology report indicated moderate osteoarthritis at L1-5 and radiolucency of the spine suggesting severe osteoporosis. No fractures or abnormal curvatures were noted.

Past Medical and Social History
- Osteoarthritis
- LBP secondary to L4/5 herniated disc; status postdiscectomy
- Osteoporosis (2-year history)

The client denied diabetes, high blood pressure, other heart diseases, or other health concerns.

She is a retired teacher who lives alone in an adult complex and still drives a car. She recently lost her second son in a motor vehicle accident 3 months ago and appears emotionally stressed from her loss. She has declined any counseling or medication suggested by her physician.

The client is highly motivated to improve so that she can go back to walking about 1 mile every other day; currently her pain level prevents her from this activity.

Medications
- Relafen 500 mg twice daily
- 5% Lidoderm patch applied dermally once a day for pain
- Norflex 100 mg twice daily to reduce muscle spasms

She has been on Fosamax 70 mg once a week for 2 years to improve her bone density loss caused by osteoporosis. The client reported little or no change in her pain level with the use of analgesics.

Clinical Presentation: During initial evaluation, LBP was graded as a 7/10 on the Visual Analogue Scale (VAS). Pain was localized to the low back without radiation; she described it as worse on getting up in the morning and after sitting or walking for a short period. Pain was progressively worse with walking, and the client stopped walking after 3 or 4 minutes. She denied any urinary or bowel incontinence.

On examination, the client presented with mild tenderness with palpation of L3-5 and mild paraspinal muscle spasms with slight loss of lumbar lordosis. There was no sensory loss noted with either upper/lower extremities or trunk and no pedal edema.

Range of motion (ROM): ROM was within normal limits (WNL) in both upper and lower extremities. Trunk flexion 0-76 degrees, trunk extension 0-13 degrees; all other motion: WNL. Manual muscle test (MMT): muscle strength for all extremities was grossly 5/5. Trunk extensors and abdominals were graded 4/5.

Straight leg raise (SLR): negative bilaterally; the client was unable to fully raise both legs because of hamstring tightness.

Normal deep tendon reflex (DTRs) for both quadriceps and Achilles tendons.

Intervention: Physical therapy intervention consisted of education on osteoporosis and its cause, prevention, treatment, and sequelae. Client was instructed in fall prevention and in making her apartment fall-proof.

Moist heat was applied to the low back for 15 minutes to reduce muscle spasm, increase muscle flexibility,[62] and reduce pain associated with osteoarthritis.[63]

Massage/soft tissue mobilization: This has been shown to be effective in reducing LBP when used in conjunction with other treatment modalities.[64]

Therapeutic exercise: Therapeutic exercise has been shown to be effective in the management of LBP.[65] In this case, single and double knee to chest exercises were done in the supine position, holding each one for 5 seconds. Single SLR supine and prone (double SLR was avoided because of its tendency to put great pressure on the spine, which may result in fracture in this client).

Walking on a treadmill: During the initial evaluation, the client was able to tolerate only 3½ minutes on the treadmill at 1.0 mph (zero grade) because of increasing pain. Treadmill walking was used to measure progress because one of the client's goals was to be able to walk up to 1 mile.

All exercises were progressed as client improved. A written handout was provided with

CASE EXAMPLE 11-9 Osteoporosis—cont'd

drawings and instructions for each exercise. Precautions were given to stop the exercise if experiencing shortness of breath, palpitation, or increased pain and to report these symptoms to the doctor. Any exercise that increased the pain was to be discontinued until the client checked with the therapist.

Outcome: The client showed remarkable improvement with her treatment. She was very diligent in performing her home exercise program (HEP) and following the therapist's instructions. She was highly motivated, attended all scheduled sessions, and was dedicated to achieving her goals.

By the third week of treatment, her pain had reportedly decreased, reduced from 7 to 4/10 on the VAS, trunk flexion was 0-94 degrees, and she was independent in her home exercise program as well as able to verbalize her fall prevention plan.

At 3 to 4 weeks, the client reported sudden increase in her LBP while getting out of bed. Pain was rated 6/10 and reported as constant but not getting worse. On examination, there was tenderness over L3-5, but it was not worse than previously reported.

There were mild low back muscle spasms, but no neurologic signs were noted and no abnormal curvature observed. This episode appeared to be an exacerbation episode. The primary care physician was notified, and the therapist was advised to continue intervention as planned. Treatment was continued as planned for 1 week without much improvement.

Result: The client returned to the physician for reevaluation. X-rays at that time diagnosed a compression fracture at L1. Further physical

therapy intervention was placed on hold pending orthopedic consult. She returned to physical therapy with a recommendation for lumbar corset, rest for 2 weeks, and continued physical therapy intervention.

Reflections: Compression fracture is a known complication of osteoporosis with or without neurologic deficit.[66] It is accepted that posterior midline tenderness is a red flag for spinal fracture; however, the absence of a posterior midline tenderness does not exclude significant spinal injury without trauma such as spinal compression fracture.[67] The therapist should remain alert to the possibility of a new vertebral fracture in anyone with osteoporosis who reports a substantial increase in low back pain.[68,69]

Signs and symptoms of compression fracture may be difficult to recognize, especially in a client who is already being treated for chronic LBP 2 years after discectomy for disc herniation.

It is not uncommon to see occasional flare-ups of pain in physical therapy clients who have been showing good improvement. A typical clinical scenario is the client who increases the frequency, intensity, or duration of activities, even adding activities he or she has been unable to enjoy previously because of back pain.

In some cases, clients overdo the home exercise program or add a new exercise suggested by a friend or seen on TV or at the gym. In some cases, there is no apparent reason for exacerbation of symptoms.

This case study demonstrates how any adverse change in pain level in an individual with osteoporosis undergoing physical therapy for back pain should not be dismissed as insignificant but should be thoroughly investigated, including medical referral when indicated.

Nubi, M: Case report presented in fulfillment of DPT 910, *Institute for Physical Therapy Education,* Widener University, Chester, Pennsylvania, 2005. Used with permission.

decreased bone mass (osteopenia) in the spine. More than a third of these women develop major orthopedic problems related to osteoporosis. Most fractures sustained by women older than 50 are secondary to osteoporosis.

Clinical Signs and Symptoms of

Osteoporosis

- Back pain: Episodic, acute low thoracic/high lumbar pain
- Compression fracture of the spine (postmenopausal osteoporosis)
- Bone fractures (age-related osteoporosis)
- Decrease in height (more than 1 inch shorter than maximum adult height)
- Kyphosis
- Dowager's hump
- Decreased activity tolerance
- Early satiety

OSTEOMALACIA

Osteomalacia is a softening of the bones caused by a vitamin D deficiency in adults and resulting from impaired mineralization in bone matrix. This failure in mineralization results in a reduced rate of bone formation. The deficiency may be due to lack of exposure to ultraviolet rays, inadequate intake of vitamin D in the diet, failure to absorb or use vitamin D, increased catabolism of vitamin D, a renal tubular defect, or a pathologically reduced number of vitamin D receptor sites in tissues.

The disease is characterized by decalcification of the bones, particularly those of the spine, pelvis, and lower extremities. X-ray examination reveals transverse, fracturelike lines in the affected bones and areas of demineralization in the matrix of the bone. These pseudofractures, known as *Looser's transformation zones*, are bilateral. The most common sites are the ribs, long bones, lateral scapular margin, upper femur, and pubic rami. As the bones soften, they become bent, flattened, or otherwise deformed. Looser's zones are believed to result from pressure on the softened bone by the nutrient arteries of its blood supply.

Severe bone pain, skeletal deformities, fractures, and severe muscle weakness and pain are common in people with osteomalacia. Clients typically complain of muscle weakness and pain that sometimes mimics polymyositis or muscular dystrophy.

A similar condition in children, occurring before epiphyseal plate closure, is called *rickets*. In children with rickets, x-ray findings include the well-known bowing of the long bones, in addition to widening, fraying, and clubbing of the areas of active bone growth. These areas especially include the metaphyseal ends of the long bones and the sternal ends of the ribs, the so-called rachitic rosary.

Clinical Signs and Symptoms of

Osteomalacia

- Bone pain
- Skeletal deformities
- Fractures
- Severe muscle weakness
- Myalgia

PAGET'S DISEASE

Paget's disease (osteitis deformans), named after Sir James Paget from the mid-1880s, is a focal inflammatory condition of the skeleton that produces disordered bone remodeling. Bone is resorbed and formed at an increased rate and in a haphazard fashion. As a result, the new bone is larger, less compact, more vascular, and more susceptible to fracture than normal bone.

Risk Factors Paget's disease is the most common skeletal disorder after osteoporosis, affecting men more often than women by a 3:2 ratio. Although Paget's disease affects 2% to 5% of the population older than 40, it is most commonly seen in people older than 70, most of whom are asymptomatic.[71] It is more prevalent in Europe and Australia and in people of Anglo-Saxon descent.

Genetic factors are important in the pathogenesis of Paget's disease; in many families, the disease is inherited in an autosomal-dominant manner. Specific genetic mutations are being identified.[72] Although the cause of this condition remains unknown, available evidence points to a slow viral infection in genetically predisposed individuals.[73] Evidence for a major genetic component is supported by 40% of affected individuals having affected first-degree relatives.

There are no known ways to prevent Paget's disease. Eating a healthy diet with sufficient calcium and vitamin D and getting exercise are critical in maintaining skeletal and joint function.[73]

Clinical Presentation The severity of involvement and associated clinical characteristics vary greatly. Although some people are asymptomatic, with very limited bone involvement, others manifest a disabling, painful form of Paget's disease that is characterized by skeletal pain and bones that are extremely deformed and easily fractured. Bones most commonly involved include (in decreas-

ing order) the pelvis, lumbar spine, sacrum, femur, tibia, skull, shoulders, thoracic spine, cervical spine, and ribs.

Bone pain associated with Paget's disease is described as aching, deep and boring, worse at night, and diminishing but not disappearing with physical activity. Muscular pain may be referred from involved bony structures or as a result of mechanical changes caused by joint deformities.

Other complications include a variety of nerve compression syndromes, secondary osteoarthritis, and vertebral compression and collapse. Rarely, Paget's disease converts to a malignant neoplasm (osteogenic sarcoma of the femur or humerus) in older adults with extensive Paget's disease. Metastases is common at the time of diagnosis; survival rates are very poor.[74]

Clinical Signs and Symptoms of
Paget's Disease

These depend on the location and severity of the bone lesions and may include the following:

- Pain and stiffness
- Fatigue
- Headaches and dizziness
- Bone fractures
- Vertebral compression and collapse
- Deformity
- Bowing of long bones
- Increased size and abnormal contour of clavicles
- Osteoarthritis of adjacent joints
- Acetabular protrusion
- Head enlargement
- Periosteal tenderness
- Increased skin temperature over long bones*
- Decreased auditory acuity (if skull is affected)
- Compression neuropathy
- Spinal stenosis
- Paresis
- Paraplegia
- Muscle weakness

* Increased skin temperature over affected long bones is a typical finding and is explained by soft tissue vascularity surrounding the bones.

▲ PHYSICIAN REFERRAL

Disorders of the endocrine and metabolic systems may appear with recognizable clinical signs and symptoms but almost always require a combination of clinical and laboratory findings for accurate identification.

The therapist is encouraged to complete a thorough Family/Personal History form, augmented by the screening interview, and careful clinical observations, to provide the physician with pertinent screening information when making a referral. When appropriate, the Osteoporosis Screening Evaluation (see Fig. 11-8; see also Appendix C-3) may be helpful. In most cases, the client who has suffered from an endocrine disorder has already been diagnosed and may have been referred for physical therapy for some other musculoskeletal complaint. Such clients may have musculoskeletal problems that can be affected by symptoms associated with hormone imbalances (see Tables 11-4 through 11-7).

Diseases of the endocrine-metabolic system such as diabetes, obesity, and thyroid abnormalities account for some of the most common disorders encountered in a physical therapy practice. In recent years, new laboratory techniques have greatly enhanced the physician's ability to diagnose these diseases.

Nevertheless, in many cases the disorder remains unrecognized until relatively late in its course; signs and symptoms may be attributed to some other disease process or musculoskeletal disorder (e.g., weakness may be the major complaint in Addison's disease). Thus any client who has any of the generalized signs and symptoms associated with the endocrine system (see Box 4-17) without an obvious or already known cause should be further evaluated by a physician.

Guidelines for Immediate
Medical Attention

- Any person with diabetes who is confused, lethargic, exhibiting changes in mental function, profuse sweating (without exercise), or demonstrating signs of DKA should receive medical attention. (Perform a fingerstick glucose test to help evaluate the situation.)

- Likewise, any episode or suspected episode of hypoglycemia must be treated promptly and reported to the client's physician.

- Signs of potassium depletion (e.g., muscle weakness or cramping, fatigue, cardiac arrhythmias, abdominal distention, nausea and vomiting) or fluid dehydration in a client who is taking non-potassium-sparing diuretics requires medical attention. Consultation with the physician is advised before exercising the individual.

- Signs of thyroid storm (tachycardia, elevated core body temperature, restlessness, agitation, abdominal pain, nausea, vomiting); observe clients with known history of hyperthyroidism

carefully postoperatively or following trauma or infection.

Guidelines for Physician Referral

- Any unexplained fever without other symptoms in a person taking corticosteroids may be an indication of infection and should be evaluated by a physician.

- Palpable nodules or a palpable mass in the supraclavicular area or the scalene triangle, or both (see Fig. 11-5), especially if accompanied by new-onset hoarseness, hemoptysis, or elevated blood pressure, must be evaluated by a physician.

- Any episode (especially a series of episodes) of hypoglycemia in the client with diabetes should be reported to the physician.

- The presence of multiple eruptive xanthomas on the extensor tendons of anyone with diabetes may signal uncontrolled glycemia and requires medical referral to normalize lipid levels; exercise remains a key to the management of this condition.

- Signs of fluid loss or dehydration in anyone taking diuretics should be reported to the physician.

- Recurrent arthritic symptoms in a client with gout who is already taking urate-lowering drugs require medical referral for review of medication.

Clues to Symptoms of Endocrine or Metabolic Origin

Past Medical History

- Endocrine or metabolic disease has been previously diagnosed. Bilateral CTS, proximal muscle weakness, and periarthritis of the shoulder(s) are common in persons with certain endocrine and metabolic diseases. Look for other associated signs and symptoms of endocrine or metabolic disease (see Box 4-17).

- Long-term use of corticosteroids can result in classic symptoms referred to as *Cushing's syndrome.*

Clinical Presentation

- Identified trigger points are not eliminated or relieved by trigger point therapy. Observe for signs and symptoms of hypothyroidism.

- Palpable lymph node(s) or nodule(s) in the scalene triangle (see Fig. 11-5), especially when accompanied by new-onset hoarseness, hemoptysis, or elevated blood pressure.

- Anyone with muscle weakness and fatigue who is taking diuretics may be experiencing symptoms of potassium depletion. Assess for cardiac arrhythmias, and ask about nausea and vomiting.

- Muscle fasciculation and cramping may be associated with antacid use (metabolic alkalosis).

Associated Signs and Symptoms

- Watch for anyone with arthralgias, hand pain and stiffness, or muscle weakness with an accompanying cluster of signs and symptoms of endocrine or metabolic disorders (see Box 4-17).

Clues to Recognizing Osteoporosis

- Pain is usually severe and localized to the site of fracture (usually midthoracic, lower thoracic, and lumbar spine vertebrae).

- Pain may radiate to the abdomen or flanks.

- Aggravating factors: prolonged sitting, standing, bending, or performing Valsalva's maneuver

- Alleviating factors: sidelying with hips and knees flexed

- Sitting up from supine requires rolling to the side first.

- Not usually accompanied by sciatica or chronic pain from nerve root impingement

- Tenderness to palpation over the fracture site

- Rib or spinal deformity, dowager's hump (cervical kyphosis)

- Loss of height

KEY POINTS TO REMEMBER

✓ Clients with a variety of endocrine and metabolic disorders commonly complain of fatigue, muscle weakness, and occasionally muscle or bone pain.

✓ Muscle weakness associated with endocrine and metabolic disorders usually involves proximal muscle groups.

✓ Periarthritis and calcific tendinitis of the shoulder is common in clients with endocrine issues. Symptoms usually respond to treatment of the underlying endocrine pathologic condition and are not likely to respond to physical therapy treatment.

✓ Carpal tunnel syndrome (CTS), hand stiffness, and hand pain can occur with endocrine and metabolic diseases.

✓ There is a correlation between hypothyroidism and fibromyalgia syndrome (FMS), which is being investigated. Any compromise of muscle energy metabolism aggravates and perpetuates trigger points (TrPs). Treatment of the underlying endocrine disorder is necessary to eliminate the TrPs, but myofascial treatment must be part of the recovery process to restore full function.

✓ Anyone with diabetes taking corticosteroid medications must be monitored for changes in blood glucose levels because these medications can cause or contribute to hyperglycemia.

✓ Exercise for the client with diabetes must be carefully planned because significant complications can result from strenuous exercise.

✓ Clients with DM who are under physical, emotional, or psychologic stress (e.g., hospitalization, pregnancy, personal problems) have increased insulin requirements; symptoms may develop in the person who usually has the disease under control.

✓ Exercise for the client with insulin-dependent diabetes should be coordinated to avoid peak insulin dosage whenever possible. Any client with known diabetes who appears confused or lethargic must be tested immediately by fingerstick for glucose level. Immediate medical attention may be necessary. Other precautions regarding diabetes mellitus for the therapist are covered in the text.

✓ When it is impossible to differentiate between ketoacidosis and hyperglycemia, administration of some source of sugar (glucose) is the immediate action to take.

✓ Early osteoporosis has no visible signs and symptoms. History and risk factors are important clues.

✓ Cortisol suppresses the body's inflammatory response, masking early signs of infection. Any unexplained fever without other symptoms should be a warning to the therapist of the need for medical follow-up.

✓ Excessive use of antacids can result in muscle fasciculation and cramping (see Alkalosis).

SUBJECTIVE EXAMINATION

Special Questions to Ask

Endocrine and metabolic disorders may produce subtle symptoms that progress so gradually that the person may be unaware of the significance of such findings. This requires careful interviewing to screen for potential physical and psychologic changes associated with hormone imbalances or other endocrine or metabolic disorders.

As always, it is important to be aware of client medications (whether over-the-counter or prescribed), the intended purpose of these drugs, and any potential side effects.

Past Medical History/Risk Factors

• Have you ever had head/neck radiation or cranial surgery? (**thyroid cancer, pituitary dysfunction**)

• Have you ever had a head injury? (**pituitary dysfunction**)

• Have you ever been told you have diabetes or that you have "sugar" in your blood?

• Have you ever been told that you have osteoporosis or brittle bones, fractures, or back problems? (**wasting of bone matrix in Cushing's syndrome, osteoporosis**)

SUBJECTIVE EXAMINATION—cont'd

- Have you ever been told that you have Cushing's syndrome?

Clinical Presentation

- Have you noticed any decrease in your muscle strength recently? (**growth hormone imbalance, ACTH imbalance, Addison's disease, hyperthyroidism, hypothyroidism**)
- Have you had any muscle cramping or twitching? (**metabolic alkalosis**)
  - *If yes,* do you take antacids with magnesium on a daily basis? How much and how often?
- Do you have any difficulty in going up stairs or getting out of chairs? (**muscle wasting secondary to large doses of cortisol**)

Associated Signs and Symptoms

- Have you noticed any changes in your vision, such as blurred vision, double vision, loss of peripheral vision, or sensitivity to light? (**thyrotoxicosis, hypoglycemia, diabetes mellitus**)
- Have you had an increase in your thirst or the number of times you need to urinate? (**adrenal insufficiency, diabetes mellitus, diabetes insipidus**)
- Have you had an increase in your appetite? (**diabetes mellitus, hyperthyroidism**)
- Do you bruise easily? (**Cushing's syndrome, excessive secretion of cortisol causes capillary fragility; small bumps/injuries produce bruising**)
- When you injure yourself, do your wounds heal slowly? (**growth hormone excess, ACTH excess, Cushing's syndrome**)
- Do you frequently have unexplained fatigue? (**hyperparathyroidism, hypothyroidism, growth hormone deficiency, ACTH imbalance, Addison's disease**)
  - *If yes,* what activities seem to be too difficult or tiring? (**muscle weakness caused by cortisol and aldosterone hypersecretion and adrenocortical insufficiency, hypothyroidism**)
- Have you noticed any increase in your collar size (goiter growth), difficulty in breathing or swallowing? (**goiter, Graves' disease, hyperthyroidism**)
  - *To the therapist:* Observe also for hoarseness.
- Have you noticed any changes in skin color? (**Addison's disease, hemochromatosis**) (e.g., overall skin color has become a darker shade of brown or bronze; occurrence of black freckles; darkening of palmar creases, tongue, mucous membranes)

For the Client with Diagnosed Diabetes Mellitus

- What type of insulin do you take? (see Table 11-9)
- What is your schedule for taking your insulin?
  - *To the therapist:* Coordinate exercise programs according to the time of peak insulin action. Do not schedule exercise during peak times.
- Do you ever have episodes of hypoglycemia or insulin reaction?
  - *If yes,* describe the symptoms that you experience.
- Do you carry a source of sugar with you in case of an emergency?
  - *If yes,* what is it, and where do you keep it in case I need to retrieve it?
- Have you ever had diabetic ketoacidosis (diabetic coma)?
  - *If yes,* describe any symptoms you may have had that I can recognize if this occurs during therapy.
- Do you use the fingerstick method for testing your own blood glucose levels?
  - *To the therapist:* You may want to ask the client to bring the test kit for use before or during exercise.
- Do you have difficulty in maintaining your blood glucose levels within acceptable ranges (70 to 100 mg/dL)?
  - *If yes, to the therapist:* You may want to take a baseline of blood glucose levels before initiating an exercise program.
- Do you ever have burning, numbness, or a loss of sensation in your hands or feet? (**diabetic neuropathy**)

CASE STUDY

REFERRAL

Paul Martin, a 45-year-old client with type 1 diabetes mellitus, has been receiving wound care for a foot ulcer during the last 2 weeks. Today, when he came to the clinic, he appeared slightly lethargic and confused. He indicated to you that he has had a "case of the flu" since early yesterday and that he had vomited once or twice the day before and once that morning before coming to the clinic. His wife, who had driven him to the clinic, said that he seemed to be "breathing fast" and urinating more frequently than usual. He has been thirsty, so he has been drinking "7-Up" and water, and those fluids "have stayed down okay."

PHYSICAL THERAPY INTERVIEW

- When did you last take your insulin? (Client may have forgotten because of his illness, forgetfulness, confusion, or just being afraid to take it while feeling sick with the "flu.")
- What type of insulin did you take?
- Do you have a source of sugar with you? If yes, where do you keep it? (This question should be asked during the initial physical therapy interview.)

- Have you contacted your physician about your condition?
- Have you done a recent blood glucose level (fingerstick)? If yes, when was the last time that this test was done?

WHAT WERE THE RESULTS?

To his wife: Your husband seems to be confused and is not himself. How long has he been like this? Have you observed any strong breath odor since this "flu" started? (Make your own observations regarding breath odor at this time.)

If possible, have the client perform a fingerstick blood glucose test on himself. This type of client should be sent immediately to his physician without physical therapy intervention. If he is hypoglycemic (unlikely under these circumstances), this condition should be treated immediately. It is more likely that this client is hyperglycemic and may have diabetic ketoacidosis. In either situation, he should not be driving, and arrangements should be made for transport to the physician's office.

PRACTICE QUESTIONS

1. What are the most common musculoskeletal symptoms associated with endocrine disorders?

2. What systemic conditions can cause carpal tunnel syndrome?

3. What are the mechanisms by which carpal tunnel syndrome occurs?

4. Disorders of the endocrine glands can be caused by:
   a. Dysfunction of the gland
   b. External stimulus
   c. Excess or insufficiency of hormonal secretions
   d. (a) and (b)
   e. (b) and (c)
   f. All the above

5. List three of the most common symptoms of diabetes mellitus.
   1. _____
   2. _____
   3. _____

PRACTICE QUESTIONS—cont'd

6. What is the primary difference between the two hyperglycemic states: diabetic ketoacidosis and hyperglycemic, hyperosmolar, nonketotic coma (HHNC)?

7. Is it safe to administer a source of sugar to a lethargic or unconscious person with diabetes?

8. Clients with diabetes insipidus would most likely come to the therapist with which of the following clinical symptoms?
   a. Severe dehydration, polydipsia
   b. Headache, confusion, lethargy
   c. Weight gain
   d. Decreased urine output

9. Clients who are taking corticosteroid medications should be monitored for the onset of Cushing's syndrome. You will need to monitor your client for which of the following problems?
   a. Low blood pressure, hypoglycemia
   b. Decreased bone density, muscle wasting
   c. Slow wound healing
   d. (b) and (c)

10. Signs and symptoms of Cushing's syndrome in an adult taking oral steroids may include:
    a. Increased thirst, decreased urination, and decreased appetite
    b. Low white blood cell count and reduced platelet count
    c. High blood pressure, tachycardia, and palpitations
    d. Hypertension, slow wound healing, easy bruising

11. Parathyroid hormone secretion is particularly important in the metabolism of bone. The client with an oversecreting parathyroid gland would most likely have:
    a. Increased blood pressure
    b. Pathologic fractures
    c. Decreased blood pressure
    d. Increased thirst and urination

12. Which A1C value is within the recommended range?
    a. 6%
    b. 8%
    c. 10%
    d. 12%

13. A 38-year old man comes to the clinic for low back pain. He has a new diagnosis of Graves' disease. When asked if there are any other symptoms of any kind, he replies, "increased appetite and excessive sweating." When you perform a neurologic screening examination, what might be present associated with the Graves' disease?
    a. Hyporeflexia but no change in strength
    b. Hyporeflexia with decreased muscle strength
    c. Hyperreflexia with no change in strength
    d. Hyperreflexia with decreased muscle strength

REFERENCES

1. Jones D, Savage R, Highton J: Synovitis induced by alendronic acid can present as acute carpal tunnel syndrome, *PubMed Central* 330(7482):74, 2005. Available on-line at: http://www.pubmedcentral.hin.gov. Accessed January 11, 2006.
2. Phalen GS: The carpal tunnel syndrome: seventeen years' experience in diagnosis and treatment of six hundred and fifty-four hands, *J Bone Joint Surg* 48A(2):211-228, 1966.
3. Grossman LA, Kaplan HJ, Ownby FD: Carpal tunnel syndrome: initial manifestation of systematic disease, *JAMA* 176:259-261, 1961.
4. Wluka AE, Cicuttini FM, Spector TD: Menopause, oestrogens, and arthritis, *Maturitas* 35(3):183-189, 2000.
5. Ferry S, Hannaford P, Warskyj M, et al: Carpal tunnel syndrome: a nested case-control study of risk factors in women, *Am J Epidemiol* 151(6):566-574, 2000.
6. Michlovitz S: Conservative interventions for carpal tunnel syndrome, *JOSPT* 34(10):591-598, 2004.
7. Grokoest AW, Demartini FE: Systemic disease and carpal tunnel syndrome, *JAMA* 155:635-637, 1954.
8. Katz JN: Clinical practice: carpal tunnel syndrome, *N Engl J Med* 346:1807, 2002.
9. McNab T, Khandwala H: Acromegaly as an endocrine form of myopathy: a case report and review of the literature, *Endocr Prac* 11(1):18-22, 2005. Available on-line at: www.medscape.com/viewarticle/501408. Accessed January 21, 2005.
10. Rothschild B: Hyperostosis associated with hip surgery? *J of Musculoskel Med* 21(5), 2004.
11. Holcomb S. Confronting Cushing's syndrome, *Nursing* 2005, 35(9):32-36, 2005.
12. Holcomb SS: Detecting thyroid disease, *Nursing* 2005 35(10):S4-S9, 2005.
13. Boissonnault WG, Koopmeiners MB: Medical history profile: orthopaedic physical therapy outpatients, *JOSPT* 20(1):2-10, July 1994.
14. President and Fellows of Harvard College, Harvard Medical School: Thyroid diseases—a special health report, Harvard Health Newsletter, 2004.
15. Ladenson P: What's new in ACP medicine: thyroid? *ACP Medicine* 2005. Available on-line at: http://www.medscape.com/viewarticle/506610. Accessed January 21, 2006.

16. Trivalle C, Doucet J, Chassagne P, et al: Differences in the signs and symptoms of hypothyroidism in older and younger patients, *JAGS* 1(44):50-53, 1996.

17. Lowe JC, Honeyman-Lowe G: *The metabolic treatment of fibromyalgia*, Lafayette, Colorado, McDowell Health Science Books, 2000.

18. Lowe JC, Lowe G: Facilitating the decrease in fibromyalgia pain during metabolic rehabilitation: an essential role for soft tissue therapies, *J Bodywork Movement Ther* 2(4):208-217, 1998.

19. Lowe JC, Reichman AJ, Honeyman GS, et al: Thyroid status of fibromyalgia patients, *Clin Bull Myofascial Ther* 3(1):47-53, 1998a.

20. Lowe JC, Reichman AJ, Yellin BA: A case-control study of metabolic therapy for fibromyalgia: long term follow-up comparison of treated and untreated patients, *Clin Bull Myofascial Ther* 3(1):65-79, 1998b.

21. Geenen R, Jacobs JW, Bijlsma JW: Evaluation and management of endocrine dysfunction in fibromyalgia, *Rheum Dis Clin North Am* 28(2):389-404, 2002.

22. Garrison RL, Breeding PC: A metabolic basis for fibromyalgia and its related disorders: the possible role of resistance to thyroid hormone, *Med Hypotheses* 61(2):182-189, 2003.

23. Johns Hopkins Medical Letter: An anti-nuclear shield for your thyroid 14(8):5-7, 2002.

24. Gagel RF, Goepfert H, Callender DL: Changing concepts in the pathogenesis and management of thyroid carcinoma, *CA Cancer J Clin* 46(5):261-283, 1996.

25. Strewler G: Primary hyperparathyroidism does not progress in most patients, *JAMA* (293):1772-1779, 2005.

26. Utiger R: The physician's perspective, *NEJM Health News*, 9(1):5, 2003.

27. Center for Disease Control and Prevention. Diabetes: National diabetes fact sheet for the United States, 2005. Available on-line at: http://www.cdc.gov/diabetes/pubs/factsheet05.htm. Accessed January 21, 2006.

28. Norris SL, Zhang X, Avenell A, et al: Long-term non-pharmacological weigh loss interventions for adults with prediabetes, *Cochrane Database Syst Rev* 2:CD005270, April 18, 2005.

29. Katon WJ, Rutter C, Simon G, et al: The association of comorbid depression with mortality in patients with type 2 diabetes, *Diabetes Care* 28(11):2668-2772, 2005.

30. Ciechanowski P, Russo J, Katon W, et al: Where is the patient? The association of psychosocial factors and missed primary care appointments in patients with diabetes, *Gen Hosp Psychiatry* 28(1):9-17, 2006.

31. Katon W, Cantrell CR, Sokol MC, et al: Impact of antidepressant drug adherence on comorbid medication use and resource utilization, *Arch Intern Med* 165(21):2497-2503, 2005.

32. Barclay L: Modifiable risk factors may be linked to risk of developing diabetic neuropathy, *Medscape Medical News*, March 31, 2005. Available on-line at: http://www.medscape.com/viewarticle/502295. Accessed on January 21, 2006.

33. Tesfaye S, Chaturvedi N, Eaton SE, et al: Vascular risk factors and diabetic neuropathy, *NEJM* 352(4):341-350, 2005.

34. Barclay L, Lie D: American Diabetes Association reviews diabetic neuropathies, *Medscape Medical News*, March 31, 2005. Available on-line at: http://www.medscape.com/viewarticle/498185. Accessed January 11, 2006.

35. Cagliero E, Apruzzese W, Perlmutter GS: Watch for hand, shoulder disorders in patients with diabetes, *Am J Med*, 112:487-490, 2002.

36. Cullen A, Ofuoglu O, Donthineni R: Neuropathic arthropathy of the shoulder, Charcot shoulder, *Medscape General Medicine* 7(1), 2005. Available on line at: www.medscape.com/viewarticle/496650). Accessed on January 21, 2006.

37. Scarborough P: Diabetes care; tests and measures for the foot and lower extremity, *Acute Care Perspectives* 11(4):1-6, 2002.

38. Boulton A: Treatment of symptomatic diabetic neuropathy, *Diabetes Metab Res Rev* 19 Suppl 1: S16-21, 2003.

39. Kelly J: Manipulation for frozen shoulder, *J of Musculoskel Med*, 2012):58, 2003.

40. Mukhtar Q, Pan L, Jack L et al: Prevalence of receiving multiple preventive care services among adults with diabetes—United States, 2002-2004, *MMWR*, 54(44):1130, 2005.

41. Colberg SR, Walsh J: Pumping insulin during exercise, *The Phys Sports Med* 30(4): on-line, April 2002. Available on-line at: http://www.physsportsmed.com/issues/2002/04_02/colberg.htm/ Accessed January 20, 2006.

42. Auber G: Taking the heat off: how to manage heat injuries, *Nursing* 2004, 34(7):50-52, 2004.

43. Appel SJ: Sizing up patients for metabolic syndrome, *Nursing 2005* 35(12):20-21, 2005.

44. American Heart Association: Metabolic syndrome, Posted 2005. Available on-line at: http://www.americanheart.org/presenter.jhtml?identifier = 475. Accessed January 18, 2006.

45. Chen L, Schumacher R: Gout and gout mimickers: 20 clinical pearls, *J Musculoskel Med*, 20(5):254-258, 2003.

46. Barclay L, Lie D: Dietary risk factors for gout clarified, *Medscape Medical News* March 10, 2004. Available on line at http://www.medscape.com/viewarticle/471444. Accessed January 21, 2006.

47. Wiese W, Sanders LS, Wortmann RL: Gout: effective strategies for acute and long-term control, *J Musculoskel Med* 21(10):510-519, 2004.

48. Stevens S, Edwards C: Recognizing and managing hemochromatosis and hemiarthropathy, *J Musculoskel Med* 21(4):212-225, 2004.

49. Edwards BJ, Brooks ER, Langman CB: Osteoporosis screening of postmenopausal women in the primary care setting; a case-based approach, *Gend Med* 1(2):70-85, 2004.

50. Feldstein AC, Nichols GA, Elmer JP, et al: Older women with fractures: patients falling through the cracks of guideline-recommended osteoporosis screening and treatment, *JBJS* 85-A(12):2294-2302, 2003.

51. The WHO Study Group: Assessment of fracture risk and its application to screening for postmenopausal osteoporosis, WHO Technical Report Series 843, Geneva, World Health Organization, 1994.

52. Lydick E, Cook K, Turpin J, et al: Development and validation of a simple questionnaire to facilitate identification of women likely to have low bone density, *Am J Man Care* 4:37-48, 1998.

53. Focus on Healthy Aging: Expert panel urges mass screening for osteoporosis, older women. *Mount Sinai School of Medicine* 6(1):2, 2003.

54. Elliott ME, Drinka PJ, Krause P, et al: Osteoporosis assessment strategies for male nursing home residents, *Maturitas* 48(3):225-233, July 2004.

55. National Osteoporosis Foundation (NOF): Standing tall for you. Prevention: who's at risk? Available at: http://www.nof.org. Accessed January 10, 2006.

56. Maricic M, Gluck O: Osteoporosis: 20 clinical pearls, *J of Musculoskel Med* 20(11):508-512, 2003.

57. Orwoll ES, Bauer DC, Vogt TM et al: Axial bone mass in older women, *Ann Intern Med* 124:187-196, 1996.

58. Black DM, Steinbuch M, Palermo L, et al: An assessment tool for predicting fracture risk in postmenopausal women, *Osteoporosis Int* 12(7):519-528, 2001.

59. Johns Hopkins Medical Letter: Bones are big news, *Health After 50* 17(1):4-5, 2005.

60. Kiebzak G, Beinart G, Perser K, et al: Under treatment of osteoporosis in men with hip fracture, *Arch Intern Med* 162(19):2217-2212, 2002.

61. Simmons G: *Far Eastern osteoporosis study*, Hong Kong, The Gordon Simmons Research Group Ltd., 1996.

62. Funk D, Swank Am, Adam KJ, Treolo D: Efficacy of moist heat pack application over static stretching on hamstring flexibility, *J Strength Cond Res* 15(1):123-126, 2001.

63. Daly MP, Berman BM: Rehabilitation of the elderly patient with osteoarthritis *Clin Geriatr Med* 9:783-801, 1993.

64. Cottingham JT, Maitland J: A three-paradigm treatment model using soft tissue mobilization and guided movement-awareness techniques for a patient with chronic low back pain: a case study, *JOSPT* 26(3):155-167, 1997.

65. Hayden JA, Van Tulder MW, Malmivaara AV, Koes BW. Meta-analysis: Exercise therapy for non-specific low back pain, *Ann Intern Med* 142(9):765-775, 2005.

66. Heggeness MH. Spinal fracture with neurological deficit in osteoporosis, *Osteoporos Int* 3(4):215-221, 1993.

67. D'Costa H, George G, Parry M, Pullinger R, Skinner D, Thomas S, Todd B, Wilson M: Pitfalls in the clinical diagnosis of vertebral fractures: a case series in which posterior midline tenderness was absent, *Emerg Med J* 22:330-332, 2005.

68. Nevitt MC, Ettinger B, Black DM, et al: The association of radiographically detected vertebral fractures with back pain and function: a prospective study, *Ann Intern Med* 128(10):793-800, 1998.

69. Fink HA, Milaetz DL, Palermo L, et al: What proportion of incident radiographic vertebral deformities is clinically diagnosed and vice versa? *J Bone Miner Res* 20(7):1216-1222, 2005.

70. DePalma M, Slipman C: Managing osteoporotic vertebral compression fractures, *J Musculoskel Med* 22(9):445-454, 2005.

71. Papapoulos SE: Paget's disease of bone: clinical, pathogenetic, and therapeutic aspects, *Baillieres Clin Endocrinol Metab* 11(1):117-143, 1997.

72. Daroszewska A, Ralston SH: Genetics of Paget's disease of bone, *Cli Sci* (London) 109(3):257-263, 2005.

73. Roodman GD, Windle JJ: Paget disease of bone, *J Clin Invest* 115(2):200-208, 2005.

74. American Academy of Orthopedic Surgeons: Paget's disease of bone, Oct. 2005. Available on-line at: http://www.orthoinfo.aaos.org, (See tumors). Accessed January 21, 2006.

75. Mankin HJ, Hornicek FJ: Paget's sarcoma: a historical and outcome review. *Clin Orthop Relat Res* 438:97-102, 2005.

Immunology, one of the few disciplines with a full range of involvement in all aspects of health and disease, is one of the most rapidly expanding fields in medicine today. Staying current is difficult at best, considering the volume of new immunologic information generated by clinical researchers each year. The information presented here is a simplistic representation of the immune system, with the main focus on screening for immune-induced signs and symptoms mimicking neuromuscular or musculoskeletal dysfunction.

Immunity denotes protection against infectious organisms. The immune system is a complex network of specialized organs and cells that has evolved to defend the body against attacks by "foreign" invaders. Immunity is provided by lymphoid cells residing in the immune system. This system consists of central and peripheral lymphoid organs (Fig. 12-1).

By circulating its component cells and substances, the immune system maintains an early warning system against both exogenous microorganisms (infections produced by bacteria, viruses, parasites, and fungi) and endogenous cells that have become neoplastic.

Immunologic responses in humans can be divided into two broad categories: humoral immunity, which takes place in the body fluids (extracellular) and is concerned with antibody and complement activities, and cell-mediated or cellular immunity, primarily intracellular, which involves a variety of activities designed to destroy or at least contain cells that are recognized by the body as being alien and harmful. Both types of responses are initiated by lymphocytes and are discussed in the context of lymphocytic function.

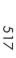

▼ USING THE SCREENING MODEL

As always in the screening evaluation of any client, the medical history is the most important variable, followed by any red flags in the clinical presentation and an assessment of associated signs and symptoms. Many immune system disorders have a unique chronology or sequence of events that define them. When the immune system may be involved, some important questions to ask include the following:

- How long have you had this problem? (acute vs. chronic)
- Has the problem gone away and then recurred?
- Have additional symptoms developed or have other areas become symptomatic over time?

Past Medical History

As mentioned, the family history is important when assessing the role of the immune system in presenting signs and symptoms. Persons with fibromyalgia or chronic pain often have a family history of alcoholism,

A recent history of surgery may be indicative of bacterial or reactive arthritis, which requires immediate medical evaluation.

Risk Factor Assessment

The cause and risk factors for many conditions related to immune system dysfunction remain unknown. Past medical history with a positive family history for systemic inflammatory or related disorders may be the only available red flag in this area.

Clinical Presentation

Symptoms of rheumatic disorders often include soft tissue and/or joint pain, stiffness, swelling, weakness, constitutional symptoms, Raynaud's phenomenon, and sleep disturbances. Inflammatory disorders such as RA and polymyalgia rheumatica are marked by prolonged *stiffness* in the morning lasting more than 1 hour. This stiffness is relieved with activity, but it recurs after the person sits down and subsequently attempts to resume activity. This is referred to as the gel phenomenon.

Specific arthropathies have a predilection for involving specific joint areas. For example, involvement of the wrists and proximal small joints of the hands and feet is a typical feature of RA. RA tends to involve joint groups symmetrically, whereas the seronegative spondyloarthropathies tend to be asymmetric. Psoriatic arthritis often involves the distal joints of the hands and feet.[1]

In anyone with *swelling*, especially single-joint swelling, it is necessary to distinguish whether this swelling is articular (as in arthritis), is periarticular (as in tenosynovitis), involves an entire limb (as with lymphedema), or occurs in another area (such as with lipoma or palpable tumors). The therapist will need to assess whether the swelling is intermittent, persistent, symmetric, or asymmetric and whether the swelling is minimal in the morning but worse during the day (as with dependent edema).

Generalized *weakness* is a common symptom of individuals with immune system disorders in the absence of muscle disease. If the weakness involves one limb without evidence of weakness elsewhere, a neurologic disorder may be present. Anyone having trouble performing tasks with the arms raised above the head, difficulty climbing stairs, or problems arising from a low chair may have muscle disease.

Nail bed changes are especially indicative of underlying inflammatory disease. For example, small infarctions or splinter hemorrhages (see Fig. 4-32) occur in endocarditis and systemic vasculitis.

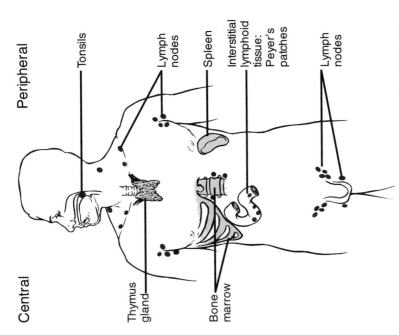

Fig. 12-1 • Organs of the immune system. Two thirds of the immune system resides in the intestines (intestinal lymphoid tissue), emphasizing the importance of diet and nutrition on immune system function.

depression, migraine headaches, gastrointestinal (GI) disorders, or panic attacks.

Clients with systemic inflammatory disorders may have a family history of an identical or related disorder such as rheumatoid arthritis (RA), systemic lupus erythematosus, autoimmune thyroid disease, multiple sclerosis, or myasthenia gravis. Other rheumatic diseases that are often genetically linked include seronegative spondyloarthropathy.

The seronegative spondyloarthropathies include a wide range of diseases linked by common characteristics such as inflammatory spine involvement (e.g., sacroiliitis, spondylitis), asymmetric peripheral arthritis, enthesopathy, inflammatory eye disease, and musculoskeletal and cutaneous features. All of these changes occur in the absence of serum rheumatoid factor (RF), which is present in about 85% of people with RA.[1]

This group of diseases includes ankylosing spondylitis (AS), reactive arthritis (ReA; such as Reiter's syndrome), psoriatic arthritis, and arthritis associated with inflammatory bowel disease (IBD; such as Crohn's disease or ulcerative colitis).

Characteristics of systemic sclerosis and limited scleroderma include atrophy of the fingertips, calcific nodules, digital cyanosis, and sclerodactyly (tightening of the skin). Dystrophic nail changes are characteristic of psoriasis. Spongy synovial thickening or bony hypertrophic changes (Bouchard's nodes) are present with RA and other hand deformities.

Associated Signs and Symptoms

With few risk factors and only the family history to rely upon, the clinical presentation is very important. Most of the immune system conditions and diseases are accompanied by a variety of associated signs and symptoms. Disease progression is common with different clinical signs and symptoms during the early phase of illness compared with the advanced phase.

Review of Systems

With many problems affecting the immune system, taking a step back and reviewing each part of the screening model (history, risk factors, clinical presentation, associated signs and symptoms) may be the only way to identify the source of the underlying problem. Remember to review Box 4-17 during this process.

For anyone with new onset of joint pain, a review of systems should include questions about symptoms or diagnoses involving other organ systems. In particular, the presence of dry, red, or irritated and itching eyes; chest pain with dyspnea; urethral or vaginal discharge; skin rash or photosensitivity; hair loss; diarrhea; or dysphagia should be assessed.

▶ IMMUNE SYSTEM PATHOPHYSIOLOGY

Immune disorders involve dysfunction of the immune response mechanism, causing overresponsiveness or blocked, misdirected, or limited responsiveness to antigens. These disorders may result from an unknown cause, developmental defect, infection, malignancy, trauma, metabolic disorder, or drug use. Immunologic disorders may be classified as one of the following:

- Immunodeficiency disorder
- Hypersensitivity disorder
- Autoimmune disorder
- Immunoproliferative disorder

Immunodeficiency Disorders

When the immune system is underactive, or hypoactive, it is referred to as being immunodeficient or immunocompromised, such as occurs in the case of anyone undergoing chemotherapy for cancer or taking immunosuppressive drugs after organ transplantation.

Acquired Immunodeficiency Syndrome

Human immunodeficiency virus (HIV) is a cytopathogenic virus that causes acquired immunodeficiency syndrome (AIDS). HIV has been identified as the causative agent, its genes have been mapped and analyzed, drugs that act against it have been found and tested, and vaccines against the HIV infection have been under development.

Acquired refers to the fact that the disease is not inherited or genetic but develops as a result of a virus. *Immuno* refers to the body's immunologic system, and *deficiency* indicates that the immune system is underfunctioning, resulting in a group of signs or symptoms that occur together called a *syndrome.*

People who are HIV-infected are vulnerable to serious illnesses called "opportunistic" infections or diseases, so named because they use the opportunity of lowered resistance to infect and destroy. These infections and diseases would not be a threat to most individuals whose immune systems functioned normally. *Pneumocystis carinii* pneumonia (PCP) continues to be a major cause of morbidity and mortality in the AIDS population.

HIV infection is the fifth leading cause of death for people who are between 25 and 44 years old in the United States. African-Americans represent about 12% of the total U.S. population but make up over half of all AIDS cases reported. AIDS is the leading cause of death for African-American men between the ages of 35 and 44. Overall estimates are that 850,000 to 950,000 U.S. residents are living with HIV infection, one quarter of whom are unaware of their infection. Approximately 40,000 new HIV infections occur each year in the United States, and approximately 5 million new HIV cases occur each year worldwide (Box 12-1).[2]

RISK FACTORS

Population groups at greatest risk include commercial sex workers (prostitutes) and their clients, homosexual men, injection drug users (IDUs), blood recipients, dialysis recipients, organ transplant recipients, fetuses of HIV-infected mothers, and people with sexually transmitted diseases (STDs). The latter group is estimated to have a 3 to 5 times higher risk for HIV infection compared with those having no STDs.

The rate of new cases of HIV among bisexual men of all races has started to rise again after a

- Male-to-male sexual contact
- Injection drug use (IDU)
- Both male-to-male sexual contact and IDU
- High-risk heterosexual contact (with someone of the opposite sex with HIV/AIDS or a risk factor for HIV)

Transmission occurs through *horizontal* transmission (from either sexual contact or parenteral exposure to blood and blood products) or through *vertical* transmission (from HIV-infected mother to infant). HIV is not transmitted through casual contact, such as the shared use of food, towels, cups, razors, or toothbrushes, or even by kissing. Despite substantial advances in the treatment of HIV, the number of new infections has not decreased in the past 10 years. Prevention of infection transmission by reduction of behaviors that might transmit HIV to others is critical.[7]

Transmission always involves exposure to some body fluid from an infected client. The greatest concentrations of virus have been found in blood, semen, cerebrospinal fluid, and cervical/vaginal secretions. HIV has been found in low concentrations in tears, saliva, and urine, but no cases have been transmitted by these routes. Breast-feeding is a route of HIV transmission from an HIV-infected mother to her infant. The reduction of HIV transmission through breast milk remains a challenge in many resource-poor settings.[8,9]

Any injectable drug, legal or illegal, can be associated with HIV transmission. It is not injection drug use that spreads HIV but the sharing of HIV-infected intravenous (IV) drug needles among individuals. Despite the perception that only IV injection is dangerous, HIV also can be transmitted through subcutaneous and intramuscular injection. Use of needles contaminated with blood for tattooing or body piercing are included in this category.

Public health organizations have changed their terminology, substituting the abbreviation *IDU* (injection drug user) for the earlier term *IVDU* (intravenous drug user). Injection drug users who sterilize their drug paraphernalia with a 1:10 solution of bleach to water before passing the needles are less likely to spread HIV. For further information regarding this or other HIV/AIDS-related questions, contact the CDC-INFO (formerly the CDC National AIDS Hotline) 24-hour/day, 7-days a week, at 1-800-342-2437 or 1-800-232-4636.

Blood and Blood Products Parenteral transmission occurs when there is direct blood-to-blood contact with a client infected with HIV. This can occur through sharing of contaminated needles and

---

BOX 12-1 ▼ Overview of AIDS in the United States

- **What it is:** AIDS, acquired immunodeficiency syndrome, is a contagious disease that destroys the T cells, a key component of the body's immune system.
- **What causes it:** AIDS is caused by the human immunodeficiency virus (HIV), spread through sexual contact, needles, or syringes shared by injection drug users (IDUs); transfusion of infected blood or blood products; or perinatal transmission (from infected birthing or breast-feeding mother to her infant).
- **Who gets it:** Primary persons infected with HIV have been homosexual men (men who have sex with men [MSM] and MSMs who have sex with women) and IDUs. The Centers for Disease Control and Prevention (CDC) estimate that heterosexual contact is responsible for 3% of male cases and 34% of female cases. Although 1 million Americans are infected, one fourth do not know they have it; as many as one third of adults tested never come back for the results.[3]
- **Diagnosis:** Screening for AIDs is conducted by testing a fingerstick sample of blood for the presence of antibodies to HIV-1. The test indicates only if a person has been exposed to the virus. A new "quick" test called OraQuick Rapid HIV Antibody Test is almost 100% accurate, and results are available within 20 minutes. A positive test requires additional confirmation testing.
- **Prognosis:** At present, there is no cure, but many people in the U.S. remain healthy and active with combination antiretroviral medications designed to attack HIV in various stages of its life cycle; when death occurs, it is usually as a result of "opportunistic" infections or cancers that the immunosuppressed body cannot resist. IDUs are four times more likely to die of AIDS than individuals infected through sexual contact.[4]

---

period of relative stability. Experts suggest the increase is due to erosion of safe sex practices. African-Americans (both men and women) are still 8 times as likely as whites to contract HIV, although the rate of newly diagnosed HIV infections among African-Americans is slowly declining.[5]

TRANSMISSION

Transmission of HIV occurs according to the following descending hierarchy:[6]

drug paraphernalia ("works"), through transfusion of blood or blood products, by accidental needle-stick injury to a health care worker, or from blood exposure to nonintact skin or mucous membranes. Health care workers who have contact with clients with AIDS and who follow routine instructions for self-protection are a very low risk group.

Almost all persons with hemophilia born before 1985 have been infected with HIV. Heat-treated factor concentrates, involving a method of chemical and physical processes that completely inactivate HIV, became available in 1985, eliminating the transmission of HIV to anyone with a clotting disorder who is receiving blood or blood products.

Additionally, HIV has been transmitted heterosexually from infected men with hemophilia to spouses or sexual partners in what is termed *the second wave* of infection and on to children born to infected couples. HIV infection in the United States is currently on the increase among women exposed via sexual intercourse with HIV-infected men. Minority women and women over the age of 50 are being affected more frequently than in prior years.[10]

CLINICAL SIGNS AND SYMPTOMS

Many individuals with HIV infection remain asymptomatic for years, with a mean time of approximately 10 years between exposure and development of AIDS. Systemic complaints such as weight loss, fevers, and night sweats are common. Cough or shortness of breath may occur with HIV-related pulmonary disease. GI complaints include changes in bowel function, especially diarrhea.

Cutaneous complaints are common and include dry skin, new rashes, and nail bed changes. Because virtually all these findings may be seen with other diseases, a combination of complaints is more suggestive of HIV infection than any one symptom.

Many persons with AIDS experience back pain, but the underlying causes may differ. Decrease in muscle mass with subsequent postural changes may occur as a result of the disease process or in response to medications. It is not uncommon for pain to develop in the back or another musculoskeletal location where there may have been a previous injury. This is more likely to occur when the T-cell count drops.

Bone disorders such as osteopenia, osteoporosis, and osteonecrosis have been reported in association with HIV, but the etiology and mechanism of these disorders are unknown. Prevalence reported varies from study to study; scientists are researching the influence of antiretroviral therapy and

lipodystrophy (absence or presence), severity of HIV disease, and overlapping risk factors for bone loss (e.g., smoking and alcohol intake). The therapist should conduct a risk factor assessment for bone loss in anyone with known HIV and educate clients about prevention strategies.[11]

Any woman at risk for AIDS should be aware of the possibility that recurrent or stubborn cases of vaginal candidiasis may be an early sign of infection with HIV. Pregnancy, diabetes, oral contraceptives, and antibiotics are more commonly linked to these fungal infections.

Side Effects of Medication The therapist should review the potential side effects from medication used in the treatment of AIDS. Delayed toxicity with long-term treatment for HIV-1 infection with antiretroviral therapy occurs in a substantial number of affected individuals.[12,13] The more commonly occurring symptoms include rash, nausea, headaches, dizziness, muscle pain, weakness, fatigue, and insomnia. Hepatotoxicity is a common complication; the therapist should be alert for carpal tunnel syndrome, liver palms, asterixis, and other signs of liver impairment (see Chapter 9).

Body fat redistribution to the abdomen, upper body, and breasts occurs as part of a condition called lipodystrophy associated with antiretroviral therapy. Other metabolic abnormalities, such as dysregulation of glucose metabolism (e.g., insulin resistance, diabetes), combined with lipodystrophy are labeled lipodystrophic syndrome (LDS). LDS contributes to problems with body image and increases the risk for cardiovascular complications.[14,15]

Clinical Signs and Symptoms of
Early Symptomatic HIV Infection

- Fever
- Night sweats
- Chronic diarrhea
- Fatigue
- Minor oral infections
- Headache
- (Women): Vaginal candidiasis
- Cough
- Shortness of breath
- Cutaneous changes (rash, nail bed changes, dry skin, telangiectasias, psoriasis, dermatitis)

Clinical Signs and Symptoms of
Advanced Symptomatic HIV Infection

- Kaposi's sarcoma
- Multiple purple blotches and bumps on skin

Continued on p. 522

- Hypertension (pulmonary and/or cardiac)
  - Dyspnea, syncope, fatigue, chest pain, nonproductive cough
- Opportunistic diseases (e.g., tuberculosis, *Pneumocystis carinii*, pneumonia, lymphoma, thrush; herpes I and II; toxoplasmosis; candidiasis)
  - Persistent dry cough
  - Fever, night sweats
  - Easy bruising
  - Thrush (thick, white coating on the tongue or throat accompanied by a sore throat)
  - Muscle atrophy and weakness
  - Back pain
  - Side effects of medication (see text)
  - HIV-related dementia (memory loss, confusion, behavioral change, impaired gait)
  - Distal symmetric polyneuropathy (pain, numbness, tingling, burning, weakness, atrophy)

AIDS and Other Diseases

AIDS is a unique disease—no other known infectious disease causes its damage through a direct attack on the human immune system. Because the immune system is the final mediator of human host–infectious agent interactions, it was anticipated early that HIV infection would complicate the course of other serious human diseases.

This has proved to be the case, particularly for tuberculosis and certain sexually transmitted infections such as syphilis and the genital herpes virus. Cancer has been linked with AIDS since 1981; this link was discovered with the increased appearance of a highly unusual malignancy, Kaposi's sarcoma. Since then, HIV infection has been associated with other malignancies, including non-Hodgkin's lymphoma (NHL), AIDS-related primary central nervous system lymphoma, and hepatocellular carcinoma.[16-18]

KAPOSI'S SARCOMA

Kaposi's sarcoma (KS) was first recognized as a malignant tumor of the inner walls of the heart, veins, and arteries in 1873 in Vienna, Austria. Before the AIDS epidemic, KS was a rare tumor that primarily affected older people of Mediterranean and Jewish origin.

Clinically, KS in HIV-infected, immunodeficient persons occurs more often as purplish-red lesions of the trunk and head. The lesion is not painful or contagious. It can be flat or raised and over time frequently progresses to a nodule. The mouth and many internal organs (especially those of the GI and respiratory tracts) may be involved either symptomatically or subclinically.

Prognosis depends on the status of the individual's immune system. People who die of AIDS usually succumb to opportunistic infections rather than to KS.

NON-HODGKIN'S LYMPHOMA

Approximately 3% of AIDS diagnoses in all risk groups and in all areas originate through discovery of NHL. The incidence of NHL increases with age and as the immune system weakens.

These malignancies are difficult to treat because clients often cannot tolerate the further immunosuppression that treatment causes. As with KS, prognosis depends largely on the initial level of immunity. Clients with adequate immune reserves may tolerate therapy and respond reasonably well. However, in people with severe immunodeficiency, survival is only 4 to 7 months on average. Clients diagnosed with HIV-related brain lymphomas have a very poor prognosis.

TUBERCULOSIS

Tuberculosis (TB) was considered a stable, endemic health problem, but now, in association with the HIV/AIDS pandemic, TB is resurgent. The recent emergence of multiple-drug–resistant TB, which has reached epidemic proportions in New York City, has created a serious and growing threat to the capacity of TB control programs (see Chapter 7).

In urban areas of the United States, the present upsurge in TB cases is occurring among young (aged 25 to 44 years) injection drug users, ethnic minorities, prisoners and prison staff (because of poorly ventilated and overcrowded prison systems), homeless people, and immigrants from countries with a high prevalence of TB.

The first major interaction between HIV and TB occurs as a result of the weakening of the immune system in association with progressive HIV infection. The great majority of individuals exposed to TB are infected but not clinically ill. Their subclinical TB infection is kept in check by an active, healthy immune system. However, when a TB-infected person becomes infected with HIV, the immune system begins to decline, and at a certain level of immune damage from HIV, the TB bacteria become active, causing clinical pulmonary TB.

TB is the only opportunistic infection associated with AIDS/HIV that is directly transmissible to household and other contacts. Therefore each individual case of active TB is a threat to community health.

Clinical Signs and Symptoms Pulmonary TB is the most common manifestation of TB disease in HIV-positive clients. When TB precedes the diagnosis of AIDS, disease is usually confined to the lung, whereas when TB is diagnosed after the onset of AIDS, the majority of clients also have extrapulmonary TB, most commonly involving the bone marrow or lymph nodes. Fever, night sweats, wasting, cough, and dyspnea occur in the majority of clients (see further discussion of tuberculosis in Chapter 7).

The standard tuberculin test is not reliable in persons with HIV infection or AIDS because the weakened immune system may simply be unable to respond to the test. As a result, the test is interpreted differently for a person who is HIV positive.

HIV NEUROLOGIC DISEASE

HIV neurologic disease may be the presenting symptom of HIV infection and can involve the central and peripheral nervous systems. HIV is a neurotropic virus and can affect neurologic tissues from the initial stages of infection. In the early course of the infection, the virus can cause demyelinization of central and peripheral nervous system tissues.[19] Signs and symptoms range from mild sensory polyneuropathy to seizures, hemiparesis, paraplegia, and dementia.

Central Nervous System Central nervous system (CNS) disease in HIV-infected clients can be divided into intracerebral space-occupying lesions, encephalopathy, meningitis, and spinal cord processes. Toxoplasmosis is the most common space-occupying lesion in HIV-infected clients. Presenting symptoms may include headache, focal neurologic deficits, seizures, or altered mental status.

AIDS dementia complex (HIV encephalopathy) is the most common neurologic complication and the most common cause of mental status changes in HIV-infected clients. It is characterized by cognitive, motor, and behavioral dysfunction. This disorder is similar to Alzheimer's dementia but has less impact on memory loss and a greater effect on time-related skills (i.e., psychomotor skills learned over time, such as playing piano or reading).

Early symptoms of AIDS dementia involve difficulty with concentration and memory, personality changes, irritability, and apathy. Depression and withdrawal occur as the dementia progresses. Motor dysfunction may accompany cognitive changes and may result in poor balance, poor coordination, and frequent falls.

Progressive multifocal leukoencephalopathy (PML), which produces localized lesions within the brain, causes demyelination in the brain and leads to death within a few months.

In addition to the brain, neurologic disorders related to AIDS and HIV may affect the spinal cord, appearing as myelopathies. A vacuolar myelopathy often appears in the thoracic spine and causes gradual weakness, painless gait disturbance characterized by spasticity, and ataxia in the lower extremities that progresses to include weakness of the upper extremities.

Structural and inflammatory abnormalities in the muscles of people with HIV have been reported to impair the muscle's ability to extract or utilize oxygen during exercise. Clinical manifestations of HIV-associated myopathies include proximal weakness, myalgia, abnormal electromyogram (EMG) activity, elevated creatine kinase, and decreased functioning of the muscle.[20]

Peripheral Nervous System Peripheral nerve disease is a common complication of the HIV infection. Peripheral nervous system syndromes include inflammatory polyneuropathies, sensory neuropathies, and mononeuropathies. An inflammatory demyelinating polyneuropathy similar to Guillain-Barré syndrome can occur in HIV-infected clients. Cytomegalovirus (CMV), a highly host-specific herpes virus that infects the nerve roots, may result in an ascending polyradiculopathy characterized by lower extremity weakness progressing to flaccid paralysis.

The most common neuropathy develops into painful sensory neuropathy with numbness and burning or tingling in the feet, legs, or hands. Immobility caused by painful neuropathies can result in deconditioning and eventual cardiopulmonary decline.

Clinical Signs and Symptoms of
HIV Neurologic Disease

- Difficulty with concentration and memory
- Personality changes (depressions, withdrawal, apathy)
- Headaches
- Seizures
- Paralysis (hemiparesis, paraplegia)
- Motor dysfunction (balance and coordination)
- Gradual weakness of extremities
- Numbness and tingling (peripheral neuropathy)
- Radiculopathy

Hypersensitivity Disorders

Although the immune system protects the body from harmful invaders, an overactive or overzealous

response is detrimental. When the immune system becomes overactive, or hyperactive, a state of hypersensitivity exists, leading to immunologic diseases such as allergies.

Although the word *allergy* is widely used, the term *hypersensitivity* is more appropriate. Hypersensitivity designates an increased immune response to the presence of an antigen (referred to as an *allergen*) that results in tissue destruction.

The two general categories of hypersensitivity reaction are immediate and delayed. These designations are based on the rapidity of the immune response. In addition to these two categories, hypersensitivity reactions are divided into four main types (I to IV).

Type I Anaphylactic Hypersensitivity ("Allergies")

ALLERGY AND ATOPY

Allergy refers to the abnormal hypersensitivity that takes place when a foreign substance (allergen) is introduced into the body of a person likely to have allergies. The body fights these invaders by producing the special antibody immunoglobulin E (IgE). This antibody (now a vital diagnostic sign of many allergies), when released into the blood, breaks down mast cells, which contain chemical mediators, such as histamine, that cause dilation of blood vessels and the characteristic symptoms of allergy.

Atopy differs from allergy because it refers to a genetic predisposition to produce large quantities of IgE, causing this state of clinical hypersensitivity. The reaction between the allergen and the susceptible person (i.e., allergy-prone host) results in the development of a number of typical signs and symptoms usually involving the GI tract, respiratory tract, or skin.

Clinical Signs and Symptoms Clinical signs and symptoms vary from one client to another according to the allergies present. With the Family/Personal History form used, each client should be asked what known allergies are present and what the specific reaction to the allergen would be for that particular person. The therapist can then be alert to any of these warning signs during treatment and can take necessary measures, whether that means grading exercise to the client's tolerance, controlling the room temperature, or appropriately using medications prescribed.

ANAPHYLAXIS

Anaphylaxis, the most dramatic and devastating form of type I hypersensitivity, is the systemic manifestation of immediate hypersensitivity. The implicated antigen is often introduced parenterally, such as by injection of penicillin or a bee sting. The activation and breakdown of mast cells systematically cause vasodilation and increased capillary permeability, which promote fluid loss into the interstitial space, resulting in the clinical picture of bronchospasms, urticaria (wheals or hives), and anaphylactic shock.

Initial manifestations of anaphylaxis may include local itching, edema, and sneezing. These seemingly innocuous problems are followed in minutes by wheezing, dyspnea, cyanosis, and circulatory shock. Clinical signs and symptoms of anaphylaxis are listed by system in Table 12-1.

TABLE 12-1 ▼ Clinical Aspects of Anaphylaxis by System

System	Signs and symptoms
General	Malaise, weakness
	Sense of illness
	Metallic taste
Dermal	Hives, erythema
	Edema of the lips, tongue
Mucosal	Periorbital edema
	Nasal congestion and pruritus
	Flushing or pallor, cyanosis
Respiratory	Sneezing
	Rhinorrhea
	Dyspnea
Upper airway	Hoarseness, stridor
	Tongue and pharyngeal edema
Lower airway	Dyspnea
	Acute emphysema
	Air trapping: asthma, bronchospasm
	Chest tightness; wheezing
Gastrointestinal	Increased peristalsis
	Vomiting
	Dysphagia
	Nausea
	Abdominal cramps
	Metallic taste in mouth
	Diarrhea (occasionally with blood)
Cardiovascular	Tachycardia
	Palpitations
	Hypotension
	Cardiac arrest
Central nervous system	Anxiety, seizures

Modified from Lawlor GJ, Rosenblatt HM: Anaphylaxis. In Lawlor GJ, Fischer TJ, Adelman DC, editors: *Manual of allergy and immunology: diagnosis and therapy*, ed 3, Boston, 1998, Lippincott Williams and Wilkins.

Clients with previous anaphylactic reactions (and the specific signs and symptoms of that individual's reaction) should be identified by using the Family/Personal History form. Identification information should be worn at all times by individuals who have had previous anaphylactic reactions. For identified and unidentified clients, immediate action is required when the person has a severe reaction. In such situations, the therapist is advised to call for emergency assistance.

Type II Hypersensitivity (Cytolytic or Cytotoxic)

A type II hypersensitivity reaction is caused by the production of autoantibodies against self cells or tissues that have some form of foreign protein attached to them. The autoantibody binds to the altered self cell, and the complex is destroyed by the immune system. Typical examples of this type of hypersensitivity are hemolytic anemias, idiopathic thrombocytopenia purpura (ITP), hemolytic disease of the newborn, and transfusion of incompatible blood. Blood group incompatibility causes cell lysis, which results in a hemolytic transfusion reaction. The antigen responsible for initiating the reaction is a part of the donor red blood cell (RBC) membrane.

Manifestations of a transfusion reaction result from intravascular hemolysis of RBCs.

Clinical Signs and Symptoms of
Type II Hypersensitivity

- Headache
- Back (flank) pain
- Chest pain similar to angina
- Nausea and vomiting
- Tachycardia and hypotension
- Hematuria
- Urticaria (skin reaction)

Type III Hypersensitivity (Immune Complex)

Immune complex disease results from formation or deposition of antigen-antibody complexes in tissues. For example, the antigen-antibody complexes may form in the joint space, with resultant synovitis, as in RA. Antigen-antibody complexes are formed in the bloodstream and become trapped in capillaries or are deposited in vessel walls, affecting the skin (urticaria), the kidneys (nephritis), the pleura (pleuritis), and the pericardium (pericarditis).

Serum sickness is another type III hypersensitivity response that develops 6 to 14 days after injection with foreign serum (e.g., penicillin, sulfonamides, streptomycin, thiouracils, hydantoin compounds). Deposition of complexes on vessel walls causes complement activation with resultant edema, fever, inflammation of blood vessels and joints, and urticaria.

Clinical Signs and Symptoms of
Type III Hypersensitivity

- Fever
- Arthralgias; synovitis
- Lymphadenopathy
- Urticaria
- Visceral inflammation (nephritis, pleuritis, pericarditis)

Type IV Hypersensitivity (Cell-Mediated or Delayed)

In cell-mediated hypersensitivity, a reaction occurs 24 to 72 hours after exposure to an allergen.

For example, type IV reactions occur after the intradermal injections of TB antigen. Graft-versus-host disease (GVHD) and transplant rejection are also type IV reactions. In GVHD, immunocompetent donor bone marrow cells (the graft) react against various antigens in the bone marrow recipient (the host), which results in a variety of clinical manifestations, including skin, GI, and hepatic lesions.

Contact dermatitis is another type IV reaction that occurs after sensitization to an allergen, commonly a cosmetic, adhesive, topical medication, drug additive (e.g., lanolin added to lotions, ultrasound gels, or other preparations used in massage or soft tissue mobilization), or plant toxin (e.g., poison ivy).

With the first exposure, no reaction occurs; however, antigens are formed. On subsequent exposures, hypersensitivity reactions are triggered, which leads to itching, erythema, and vesicular lesions. Anyone with known hypersensitivity (identified through the Family/Personal History form) should have a small area of skin tested before use of large amounts of topical agents in the physical therapy clinic. Careful observation throughout the episode of care is required.

Clinical Signs and Symptoms of
Type IV Hypersensitivity

- Itching
- Erythema
- Vesicular skin lesions
- Graft-versus-host disease (GVHD): skin, GI, hepatic dysfunction

Autoimmune Disorders

Autoimmune disorders occur when the immune system fails to distinguish self from nonself and misdirects the immune response against the body's own tissues. The body begins to manufacture antibodies called *autoantibodies* directed against the body's own cellular components or specific organs. The resultant abnormal tissue reaction and tissue damage may cause systemic manifestations varying from minimal localized symptoms to systemic multiorgan involvement with severe impairment of function and life-threatening organ failure.

The exact cause of autoimmune diseases is not understood, but factors implicated in the development of autoimmune immunologic abnormalities may include genetics (familial tendency), sex hormones (women are affected more often than men by autoimmune diseases), viruses, stress, cross-reactive antibodies, altered antigens, or environment.

Autoimmune disorders may be classified as organ-specific diseases or generalized (systemic) diseases. Organ-specific diseases involve autoimmune reactions limited to one organ. *Organ-specific autoimmune diseases* include thyroiditis, Addison's disease, Graves' disease, chronic active hepatitis, pernicious anemia, ulcerative colitis, and insulin-dependent diabetes. These diseases have been discussed in this text (see the chapter appropriate to the organ involved) and are not covered further in this chapter.

Generalized autoimmune diseases involve reactions in various body organs and tissues (e.g., fibromyalgia, rheumatoid arthritis, systemic lupus erythematosus, and scleroderma). Systemic autoimmune diseases lead to a sequence of abnormal tissue reaction and damage to tissue that may result in diffuse systemic manifestations.

Fibromyalgia Syndrome

Fibromyalgia syndrome (FMS) is a noninflammatory condition appearing with generalized musculoskeletal pain in conjunction with tenderness to touch in a large number of specific areas of the body and a wide array of associated symptoms. FMS is much more common in women than in men; it is 2 to 5 times more common than rheumatoid arthritis. It occurs in age groups from preadolescents to early postmenopausal women.[21] The condition is less common in older adults.

There is still much controversy over the exact nature of FMS and even debate over whether fibromyalgia is an organic disease with abnormal biochemical or immunologic pathologic aspects. Current theories suggest that it is a genetically predisposed condition with dysregulation of the neurohormonal and autonomic nervous systems. It may be triggered by viral infection, a traumatic event, or stress.

Controversy also exists regarding current use of the American College of Rheumatism (ACR) criteria for tender point count in clinical diagnosis of FMS. In fact, the original author of the used ACR criteria has suggested that counting the tender points was "perhaps a mistake" and advised against using it in clinical practice.[22]

Fibromyalgia has been differentiated from myofascial pain in that FMS is considered a systemic problem with multiple tender points as one of the key symptoms; there is usually a cluster of associated signs and symptoms. Myofascial pain is a localized condition specific to a muscle (trigger point, TrP) and may involve as few as one or several areas without associated signs and symptoms.

The hallmark of myofascial pain syndrome is the TrP, as opposed to tender points in FMS. Both disorders cause myalgia with aching pain and tenderness and exhibit similar local histologic changes in the muscle. Painful symptoms in both conditions are increased with activity, although fibromyalgia involves more generalized aching, whereas myofascial pain is more direct and localized (Table 12-2).

FMS has striking similarities to chronic fatigue syndrome (CFS), with a mix of overlapping symptoms (about 70%) that have some common biologic denominator. Diagnostic criteria for CFS focuses on fatigue, whereas the criteria for FMS focuses on

TABLE 12-2 ▼ Differentiating Myofascial Pain Syndrome from Fibromyalgia Syndrome

Myofascial pain syndrome	Fibromyalgia syndrome
Trigger points	Tender points
Localized musculoskeletal condition	Systemic condition
No associated signs and symptoms	Wide array of associated signs and symptoms
Etiology: overuse, repetitive motions; reduced muscle activity (e.g., casting or prolonged splinting)	Etiology: neurohormonal imbalance; autonomic nervous system dysfunction

pain, the two most prominent symptoms of these syndromes. Studies have shown that CFS and FMS are characterized by greater similarities than differences and involve both the central and peripheral nervous systems as well as the body tissues themselves (Box 12-2).[23]

CLINICAL SIGNS AND SYMPTOMS

The core features of FMS include widespread pain lasting more than 3 months and widespread local tenderness in all clients (Fig. 12-2). Primary musculoskeletal symptoms most frequently reported are (1) aches and pains, (2) stiffness, (3) swelling in soft tissue, (4) tender points, and (5) muscle spasms or nodules. Fatigue, morning stiffness, and sleep disturbance with nonrefreshed awakening may be present but are not necessary for the diagnosis.[24]

Nontender control points (such as midforehead and anterior thigh) have been included in the examination by some clinicians. These control points may be useful in distinguishing FMS from a conversion reaction, referred to as *psychogenic rheumatism*, in which tenderness may be present everywhere. However, evidence suggests that individuals with FMS may have a generalized lowered threshold for pain on palpation and the control points may also be tender on occasion. There is also an increased sensitivity to sensory stimulation such as pressure stimuli, heat, noise, odors and bright lights.[25]

Symptoms are aggravated by cold, stress, excessive or no exercise, and physical activity ("overdoing it"), including overstretching, and may be improved by warmth or heat, rest, and exercise, including gentle stretching.

Sleep disturbances in stage 4 of nonrapid eye movement sleep (needed for healing of muscle tissues), sleep apnea, difficulty getting to sleep or staying asleep, nocturnal myoclonus (involuntary arm and leg jerks), and bruxism (teeth grinding) cause clients with FMS to wake up feeling unrested and unrefreshed as if they had never gone to sleep (Box 12-3).

The ACR created the standard diagnostic tool currently used, although this is controversial, as mentioned. The presence of generalized body pain, prescribed number of tender points, and presence of associated symptoms are essential in the diagnostic process because numerous other diseases and conditions may appear with pain, tenderness, and some of the symptoms commonly associated with FMS. Several other treatable rheumatologic conditions can cause similar widespread pain and can be mistaken for FMS, such as systemic lupus erythematosus or polymyalgia rheumatica.

BOX 12-2 ▼ Fibromyalgia Web Links

• Fibromyalgia Network, providing educational materials on fibromyalgia syndrome (FMS) and chronic fatigue syndrome (CFS); very reliable source of information
http://www.fmnetnews.com

• American Fibromyalgia Syndrome Association, a non-profit organization dedicated to research, education and patient advocacy for fibromyalgia syndrome (FMS) and chronic fatigue syndrome (CFS)
http://www.afsafund.org

• National Fibromyalgia Association, a nonprofit organization to increase fibromyalgia awareness and improve treatment options
http://www.fmaware.org

• Fibromyalgia Research Foundation, with an emphasis on the metabolic basis of fibromyalgia and its treatment
http://www.drlowe.com

• Phoenix Publishing, website of physical therapist Janet A. Hulme, MA, PT, with personal care kits for the management of chronic pain/fibromyalgia. A self-care and treatment manual written by a physical therapist is available to help clients identify which one (or more) subtype they may be and offers specific treatment suggestions based on the subtypes, including modulating the autonomic nervous system through a process called Physiologic Quieting.
http:www.phoenixpub.com

Clinical Signs and Symptoms of Fibromyalgia Syndrome

• Myalgia (generalized aching)
• Fatigue (mental and physical)
• Sleep disturbances, nocturnal myoclonus, nocturnal bruxism
• Tender points of palpation
• Chest wall pain mimicking angina pectoris
• Tendinitis, bursitis
• Temperature dysregulation
   • Raynaud's phenomenon; cold-induced vasospasm (hypersensitivity to cold)
   • Hypothermia (mild decrease in core body temperature)
• Dyspnea, dizziness, syncope
• Headache (throbbing occipital pain)
• Morning stiffness (more than 15 minutes)
• Paresthesia (numbness and tingling)

Continued on p. 528

- Mechanical low back pain with sciatica-like radiation of pain
- Subjective swelling
- Irritable bowel symptoms
- Urinary urgency; irritable bladder syndrome
- Dry eyes/mouth (Sicca syndrome)
- Depression/anxiety
- Cognitive difficulties (e.g., short-term memory loss, decreased attention span)
- Premenstrual syndrome (PMS)
- Weight gain from physical inactivity because of pain and fatigue

Differential Diagnosis of Fibromyalgia

Frequently misdiagnosed, fibromyalgia syndrome is often confused with any of the following:

- Hypothyroidism
- Adult growth hormone deficiency (e.g., pituitary tumors, head trauma, AIDS)
- Polymyalgia rheumatica/giant cell arteritis
- Rheumatoid arthritis, seronegative
- Polymyositis/dermatomyositis
- Systemic lupus erythematosus
- Myofascial pain syndrome
- Metabolic myopathy (e.g., alcohol)
- Lyme disease
- Neurosis (depression/anxiety)
- Metastatic cancer
- Chronic fatigue syndrome
- Temporomandibular joint dysfunction
- Disc disease
- Myalgic side effect of medication (e.g., statins)
- Parasitic infection
- Depression, anxiety

Researchers are beginning to identify various subtypes of fibromyalgia and recognize the need for specific intervention based on the underlying subtype. These classifications are based on impairment of the autonomic nervous system. They include the following[26,27]:

- Hypoglycemia
- Hypothyroid
- Neurally mediated
- Immune system
- Reproductive hormone imbalance

A team approach to this condition requires medical evaluation and treatment as part of the intervention strategy for fibromyalgia. Therapists should refer clients suspected of having fibromyalgia for further medical follow-up.

Rheumatoid Arthritis

Rheumatoid arthritis (RA) is a chronic, systemic, inflammatory disorder of unknown cause that can affect various organs but predominantly involves the synovial tissues of the diarthrodial joints. There are more than 100 rheumatic diseases affecting joints, muscles, and extraarticular systems of the body.

Women are affected with RA 2 to 3 times more often than men; however, women who are taking or have taken oral contraceptives are less likely to develop RA. Although it may occur at any age, RA is most common in persons between the ages of 20 and 40 years.

RISK FACTORS

The etiologic factor or trigger for this process is as yet unknown. Support for a genetic predisposition comes from studies suggesting that RA clusters in families. One gene in particular (HLA-DRB1 on chromosome 6) has been identified in determining susceptibility. RA may be caused by a genetically susceptible person encountering an unidentified agent (e.g., virus, self-antigen), which then results in an immunopathologic response.[28] Researchers hypothesize that an infection could trigger an immune reaction that is mediated through multiple complex genetic mechanisms and continues clinically even if the organism is eradicated from the body.

Other nongenetic factors may also contribute to the development of RA. Because arthritis (and many related diseases) is more common in women, hormones have been implicated, but the relationship remains unclear. Environmental causes, such as chemicals (e.g., hair dyes, industrial pollutants), medications, food allergies, cigarette smoking, and stress remain under investigation as possible triggers for those individuals who are genetically susceptible to RA.

CLINICAL SIGNS AND SYMPTOMS

Clinical features of RA vary not only from person to person but also in an individual over the disease course. In most people, the symptoms begin gradually during a period of weeks or months. Frequently, malaise and fatigue prevail during this period, sometimes accompanied by diffuse musculoskeletal pain.

Symptoms of an inflammatory arthritis include the spontaneous onset of one or more swollen joints; morning stiffness lasting longer than 45 minutes; and diffuse joint pain and tenderness, particularly involving the metatarsophalangeal (MTP) or metacarpophalangeal (MCP) joints.

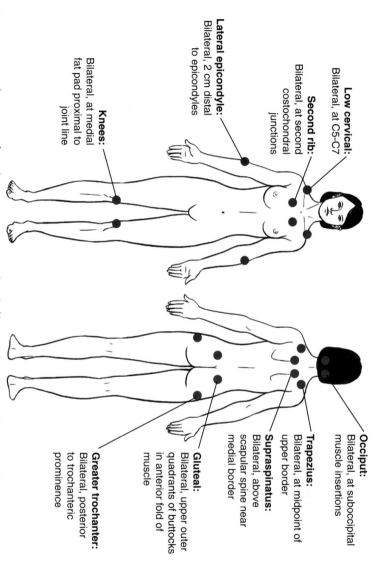

Occiput:
Bilateral, at suboccipital
muscle insertions

Trapezius:
Bilateral, at midpoint of
upper border

Supraspinatus:
Bilateral, above
scapular spine near
medial border

Gluteal:
Bilateral, upper outer
quadrants of buttocks
in anterior fold of
muscle

Greater trochanter:
Bilateral, posterior
to trochanteric
prominence

Low cervical:
Bilateral, at C5-C7
muscle insertions

Second rib:
Bilateral, at second
costochondral
junctions

Lateral epicondyle:
Bilateral, 2 cm distal
to epicondyles

Knees:
Bilateral, at medial
fat pad proximal to
joint line

Fig. 12-2 • Anatomic locations of tender points associated with fibromyalgia. According to the literature, digital palpation should be performed with an approximate force of 4 kg (enough pressure to indent a tennis ball), but clinical practice suggests much less pressure is required to elicit a painful response. For a tender point to be considered positive, the subject must state that the palpation was "painful." A reply of "tender" is not considered a positive response. As mentioned in the text, counting the number of points as part of the clinical diagnosis of FMS has been discounted; however, the presence of multiple tender points is still a key feature of FMS.

BOX 12-3 ▼ Fibromyalgia Syndrome (FMS) Screen

• Do you have trouble sleeping through the night?	YES NO
• Do you feel rested in the morning?	YES NO
• Are you stiff and sore in the morning?	YES NO
• Do you have daytime fatigue/exhaustion?	YES NO
• Can you do the grocery shopping on your own?	YES NO
• Can you do your regular daily activities?	YES NO
• Do your muscle pain and soreness travel (move around the body)?	YES NO
• Do you have tension/migraine headaches?	YES NO
• Do you have irritable bowel symptoms (e.g., nausea, diarrhea, stomach cramping)?	YES NO
• Do you have swelling, numbness, or tingling in your arms or legs?	YES NO
• Are you sensitive to temperature and humidity or changes in the weather?	YES NO
• Can you read a book or watch a movie and follow what is happening?	YES NO
• Does "brain fog" interfere with your activities or work?	YES NO

Key: Researchers have been unable to develop a reliable screening questionnaire for FMS because of the wide-ranging symptoms associated with this condition. This type of screening tool may help the therapist identify potential cases of FMS but should not be relied upon as the only evaluation instrument.

Inactivity, such as sleep or prolonged sitting, is commonly followed by stiffness. "Morning" stiffness occurs when the person arises in the morning or after prolonged inactivity. The duration of this stiffness is an accepted measure of the severity of the condition.

Clients should be asked: "After you get up in the morning, how long does it take until you are feeling the best you will feel for the day?" Pain and stiffness increase gradually as RA progresses and may limit a person's ability to walk, climb stairs, open doors, or perform other activities of daily living (ADLs). Weight loss, depression, and low-grade fever can accompany this process.

The inflammatory process may be under way for some time before swelling, tissue reaction, and joint destruction are seen. Structural damage usually begins between the first and second year of the disease. Early medical referral, followed by expedited diagnosis and intervention, results in a much more favorable outcome for persons with RA.

Studies have shown that 70% to 90% of persons with RA have significant joint erosions on x-ray by only 2 years after disease onset and that halting or slowing erosions should be initiated very early on in the course of the disease.[29] Having awareness of the group of symptoms that suggest inflammatory arthritis is critical. It is recommended that the criteria for referral of a person with early inflammatory symptoms include significant discomfort on the compression of the metacarpal and metatarsal joints, the presence of three or more swollen joints, and more than 1 hour of morning stiffness.[30]

Shoulder Chronic synovitis of the elbows, shoulders, hips, knees, and/or ankles creates special secondary disorders. When the shoulder is involved, limitation of shoulder mobility, dislocation, and spontaneous tears of the rotator cuff result in chronic pain and adhesive capsulitis.

Elbow Destruction of the elbow articulations can lead to flexion contracture, loss of supination and pronation, and subluxation. Compressive ulnar nerve neuropathies may develop related to elbow synovitis. Symptoms include paresthesias of the fourth and fifth fingers and weakness in the flexor muscle of the little finger.

Wrists The joints of the wrist are frequently affected in RA, with variable tenosynovitis of the dorsa of the wrists and, ultimately, interosseous muscle atrophy and diminished movement owing to articular destruction or bony ankylosis. Volar synovitis can lead to carpal tunnel syndrome.

Hands and Feet Forefoot pain may be the only small-joint complaint and is often the first one. Subluxation of the heads of the MTP joints and

shortening of the extensor tendons give rise to "hammer toe" or "cock up" deformities. A similar process in the hands results in volar subluxation of the MCP joints and ulnar deviation of the fingers. An exaggerated inflammatory response of an extensor tendon can result in a spontaneous, often asymptomatic rupture. Hyperextension of a proximal interphalangeal (PIP) joint and flexion of the distal interphalangeal (DIP) joint produce a swan neck deformity. The boutonnière deformity is a fixed flexion contracture of a PIP joint and extension of a DIP joint.

Cervical Spine Involvement of the cervical spine by RA tends to occur late in more advanced disease. Clinical manifestations of early disease consist primarily of neck stiffness that is perceived through the entire arc of motion. Inflammation of the supporting ligaments of C1-C2 eventually produces laxity, sometimes giving rise to atlantoaxial subluxation. Spinal cord compression can result from anterior dislocation of C1 or from vertical subluxation of the odontoid process of C2 into the foramen magnum.

Extra-Articular Extra-articular features, such as rheumatoid nodules, arteritis, neuropathy, scleritis, pericarditis, lymphadenopathy, and splenomegaly, occur with considerable frequency (Table 12-3). Once thought to be complications of RA, they are now recognized as being integral parts of the disease and serve to emphasize its systemic nature.

The subcutaneous nodules, present in approximately 25% to 35% of clients with RA, occur most commonly in subcutaneous or deeper connective tissues in areas subjected to repeated mechanical pressure, such as the olecranon bursae, the extensor surfaces of the forearms, the elbow, and the Achilles tendons.

Clinical Signs and Symptoms of

Rheumatoid Arthritis

- **S**welling in one or more joints
- **E**arly morning stiffness
- **R**ecurring pain or tenderness in any joint
- **I**nability to move a joint normally
- **O**bvious redness and warmth in a joint
- **U**nexplained weight loss, fever, or weakness combined with joint pain
- **S**ymptoms such as these that last for more than 2 weeks
- See also Table 12-3

Age-Related Differences One third of persons with RA acquire the disease after the age

TABLE 12-3 ▼ Extraarticular Manifestations of Rheumatoid Arthritis

Organ system	Extraarticular manifestations
Skin	Cutaneous vasculitis
	Rheumatoid nodules
	Ecchymoses/petechiae (drug-induced)
Eye	Episcleritis
	Scleritis
	Scleromalacia perforans
	Corneal ulcers/perforation
	Uveitis
	Retinitis
	Glaucoma
	Cataract
Lung	Pleuritis
	Diffuse interstitial fibrosis
	Vasculitis
	Rheumatoid nodules
	Caplan's syndrome
	Pulmonary hypertension
Heart and blood vessels	Pericarditis
	Myocarditis
	Coronary arteritis
	Valvular insufficiency
	Conduction defects
	Vasculitis
	Felty's syndrome
Nervous system	Mononeuritis multiplex
	Distal sensory neuropathy
	Cervical spine instability (spinal cord compression)

Modified from Andreoli TE et al: *Cecil essentials of medicine*, ed 3, Philadelphia, 1993, Saunders, p 566.

of 60 years. There are differences in presentation of the disease in older versus younger people. Onset in younger people is usually in 30- to 50-year-olds, with a 2:1 ratio of women to men; is polyarticular, involving small joints; and is gradual in onset with a positive RF. In the elderly population (age 60 years or older), joint involvement may be oligoarticular, involving large joints, and more abrupt in onset, with an equal ratio of women to men and a negative RF finding.[31]

Juvenile Idiopathic Arthritis Juvenile idiopathic arthritis (JIA, replaces the term JRA), a chronic inflammatory disorder that occurs during childhood, is made up of a heterogeneous group of diseases that share synovitis as a common feature. JIA has seven subcategories:

- Oligoarthritis JIA
- Polyarthritis JIA (positive RF)
- Polyarthritis JIA (negative RF)
- Systemic onset JIA
- Psoriatic JIA
- Enthesitis-related arthritis
- Other arthritis

Early recognition of JIA is key to timely initiation of treatment. For a diagnosis of JIA to be made, objective arthritis must be seen in one or more joints for at least 6 weeks in children younger than 16 years. Children should be screened for an array of symptoms, depending on the appropriate subcategory of disease. The number of joints involved, involvement of small joints, symmetry of joint involvement, uveitis risk, systemic features, and family history are important parts of this screening. It is important to educate parents regarding symptoms because parents are the first line of communication from their children to health care professionals.[32]

DIAGNOSIS

The clinical diagnosis of RA is based on careful consideration of three factors: the clinical presentation of the client, which is elucidated through history taking and physical examination; the corroborating evidence gathered through laboratory tests and radiography; and the exclusion of other possible diagnoses.

The physical presence of rheumatoid nodules and the presence of rheumatoid factor measured by laboratory studies are two indicators of RA, although some persons with actual rheumatoid factors are missed by commonly available methods.

Classification of RA (Table 12-4) is difficult in the early course of the disease, when articular symptoms are accompanied only by constitutional symptoms such as fatigue and loss of appetite, which are common to a number of chronic diseases. A full array of clinical signs and symptoms may not be manifest for 1 to 2 years. A diagnosis of RA is established on the presentation of four of the seven listed criteria with duration of joint signs and symptoms for at least 6 weeks.

Additional laboratory tests of significance in the diagnosis and management of RA include white blood cell (WBC) count, erythrocyte sedimentation rate, hemoglobin and hematocrit, urinalysis, and rheumatoid factor assay. The elevation of C-reactive protein (CRP) has been discovered in significant levels within 2 years preceding a confirmed diagnosis of RA. The increased levels of CRP may have clinical implications in the early prediction of later symptomatic inflammation.[33]

The number of WBCs will increase in the presence of joint inflammation, as will the erythrocyte

TABLE 12-4 ▼ American Rheumatism Association Criteria for Classification of Rheumatoid Arthritis*

Criteria	Definition
Morning stiffness	Morning stiffness in and around the joints lasting at least 1 hour
Arthritis of three or more joint areas	Simultaneous soft tissue swelling or fluid (not bony overgrowth alone) observed by a physician; the 14 possible joint areas are (right or left) PIP, MCP, wrist, elbow, knee, ankle, and MTP joints
Arthritis of hand joints	At least one joint area swollen as above in wrist, MCP, or PIP joint
Symmetric arthritis	Simultaneous bilateral involvement of the same joint areas as above (PIP, MCP, or MTP joints without absolute symmetry is acceptable)
Rheumatoid nodules	Subcutaneous nodules, over bony prominences or extensor surfaces
Serum rheumatoid factor	Abnormal amounts of serum rheumatoid factor
Radiographic changes	Radiographic changes typical of rheumatoid arthritis on posteroanterior hand and wrist radiographs, which must include erosions or bony decalcification localized to involved joints (osteoarthritis changes alone do not qualify)

Modified from Harris ED, Jr: Clinical features of rheumatoid arthritis. In Kelley WN et al: *Textbook of rheumatology*, ed 4, Philadelphia, 1993, Saunders, p 874.

* For classification purposes, a client is said to have rheumatoid arthritis if he or she has satisfied at least four of the above seven criteria. Criteria 1 through 4 must be present for at least 6 weeks. Clients with two clinical diagnoses are not excluded. Designation as classic, definite, or probable rheumatoid arthritis is no longer made.

MCP, Metacarpophalangeal; *MTP*, metatarsophalangeal; *PIP*, proximal interphalangeal.

sedimentation rate. Anemia may be present, and the rheumatoid factor will be elevated in clients with active RA. If the client's urinalysis reveals any protein, blood cells, or casts, systemic lupus erythematosus should be suspected. This type of abnormal urinalysis would necessitate further diagnostic evaluation and immediate physician referral (Case Example 12-1).

TREATMENT

Aggressive treatment of early arthritis with new medications has shown marked improvement in outcome. These medications have both immunosuppressive and biologic side effects that must be monitored. The emergence of therapeutic biologic agents such as antitumor necrosis factor (TNF) and biologic response modifiers called disease-modifying antirheumatic drugs (DMARDs) has led to suppression of symptoms of RA and slowed disease progression. Side effects and safety concerns are critical in the prevention of serious side effect–related problems, including the following:

- Congestive heart failure
- Serious infections due to immunosuppression (e.g., tuberculosis, listeria monocytogenes, coccidioidomycosis, histoplasmosis, viral hepatitis)
- Skin reactions (erythema, pruritis, rashes, urticaria, infection, eczema)[34]
- New onset symptoms of multiple sclerosis, optic neuritis, and transverse myelitis

- Hematologic abnormalities such as aplastic anemia, pancytopenia
- Increased risk of lymphomas

Screening should include a thorough epidemiologic history regarding previous exposure to tuberculosis.[35]

Polymyalgia Rheumatica

Polymyalgia rheumatica (PMR) is a systemic rheumatic inflammatory disorder with an unknown cause; there may be an autoimmune, viral, or stress-induced mechanism.

RISK FACTORS

PMR occurs almost exclusively in people over 55 years of age. The disease rarely occurs in persons under the age of 50, and it affects twice as many women as men. It is at least 10 times more prevalent in persons over 80 than in persons between the ages of 50 and 59, and it predominantly affects the Caucasian population.[36,37]

CLINICAL PRESENTATION

PMR is characterized by severe aching and stiffness primarily in the muscles, as opposed to the joints. Onset is usually very sudden and insidious. Areas commonly affected include the neck, shoulder girdle, and pelvic girdle. Joint pain is possible, and headache, weakness, and fatigue are commonly reported. The pain is usually more severe when the person gets up in the morning.

CASE EXAMPLE 12-1 Rheumatoid Arthritis

History: A 67-year-old woman with a 13-year history of rheumatoid arthritis requiring gold and methotrexate fell and fractured her right acetabulum, requiring a total hip replacement. She was referred to physical therapy through a home health agency for "aggressive rehabilitation." After 10 weeks she was walking unassisted after having progressed from a walker to a cane and participating in a swimming program sponsored by the local arthritis organization. She was discharged with a home program to continue working on strength and balance activities.

About 6 weeks later, the therapist received a telephone call from the client's husband, who reported that there had been a gradual decline in her walking and asked the therapist for a reevaluation. The woman came into the outpatient clinic and was examined with the following findings.

Clinical Presentation: The client had resumed the use of a cane, and her gait was characterized by wide-based stance, shortened steps, and trunk instability. She frequently took a few steps forward before tottering backward without falling. The client was unable to stand from a sitting position without assistance. When moving from a standing to a sitting position, she consistently fell backward.

When asked about the new onset of any other symptoms, the client noted urinary urge incontinence, and her husband commented that she had just started having difficulty remembering the dates of their children's birthdays and the names of their grandchildren.

The therapist performed both an orthopedic and a neurologic screening examination and measured vital signs. The client's blood pressure was 135/78 mmHg, resting pulse was 78 beats per minute, and body temperature was considered normal. The orthopedic examination was consistent with a total hip replacement 6 months ago, with mild hip flexor weakness and mild loss of hip motion on the left (compared with the right). However, the neurologic examination raised some red flags.

Muscle tone was increased in the lower extremities, with proprioception and deep tendon reflexes decreased in both feet (right more than left). Pinprick, light-touch, and two-point discrimination were normal. Romberg's sign was absent, but a test for dysmetria of the upper extremities revealed mild cogwheeling. There was an observable tremor when the client's arms were stretched out in front of her trunk.

Result: Given the history of a progressive gait disturbance, new onset of urge incontinence, and positive findings on a neurologic screening examination, this client was referred to her family physician for a medical evaluation.

The therapist explained to the client and her husband that these findings were not typical of someone who has had a total hip replacement or someone with rheumatoid arthritis (RA).

The client was examined by her family physician and referred to a neurologist. A magnetic resonance imaging (MRI) study was ordered, and a diagnosis of basilar impression was made. *Basilar impression* is the term used when the odontoid peg of C2 pushes up into the foramen magnum.

RA is a classic cause of this via atlantoaxial dislocation. The destructive inflammatory process of RA weakens ligaments that attach the odontoid to the atlas into the skull. The subsequent dislocation of the atlas on the axis can remain mobile, or it can become fixed, producing persistent symptoms.

Modified from Williams ME, Richman J, Scatliff J: A 67-year-old woman with a progressive gait disturbance, *JAGS* 44(7):843-846, 1996.

PMR is closely linked with giant cell or temporal arteritis. Giant cell arteritis (GCA) primarily affects the medium-sized muscular arteries, such as those that pass over the temples in the scalp. The temporal arteries become inflamed, subjecting them to damage. In GCA, the most common symptom is a severe headache on one or both sides of the head.

The ophthalmic arteries are affected in nearly half of all affected individuals, sometimes resulting in partial loss of vision or even sudden blindness. Early diagnosis of GCA is important to prevent blindness. The diagnosis of polymyalgia rheumatica is made on the basis of age, clinical presentation, and a very high sedimentation rate, or sed rate. The sed rate of the blood is a measure of the total inflammation in the body (Case Example 12-2).

Clinical Signs and Symptoms of
Polymyalgia Rheumatica

- Muscle pain or aching (proximal muscle groups: neck; shoulder and pelvic girdle)
- Stiffness upon arising in the morning or after rest
- Weakness, fatigue, malaise
- Low-grade fever, sweats
- Headache (temporal arteritis)
- Weight loss
- Depression
- Vision changes

PMR is self-limiting, typically lasting 2 to 3 years. In some cases, it goes away for reasons unknown. However, some persons may have a longer course of disease, requiring low-dose

---

CASE EXAMPLE 12-2 Polymyalgia Rheumatica

Current Complaint: The client was a 51-year-old female referred to physical therapy by her primary care physician for evaluation and treatment of persistent shoulder girdle pain and stiffness. The client reports that she had 1 or 2 days of fever and flulike symptoms associated with neck stiffness. The problem did not go away after the fever passed, and the symptoms gradually worsened.

A month later, both shoulders were particularly worse in the morning when she was waking up. It usually took her 3 to 4 hours before she was able to function properly. Her best moment in the day was late afternoon. Symptoms were persisting and also waking her up at night when she was trying to change positions. She tried to exercise and take nonsteroidal antiinflammatories (NSAIDs) in order to overcome the symptoms, but this did not help.

She saw her primary care physician for an annual physical but did not put much emphasis on these symptoms. She was given a prescription NSAID, which only minimally improved the symptoms. She again got in touch with her doctor, who referred her to physical therapy for evaluation of shoulder girdle pain.

Past Medical History: The client is postmenopausal and is no longer taking hormone replacement therapy (HRT). She has hyperten-

sion, which is controlled by medication. She had a C-section for delivery of twins in 1992 but no other surgeries. Family history reveals that her mother had Alzheimer's and passed away in December 2003. Her father had a stroke in 1991, which left him aphasic; he has hypertension, and a history of coronary artery disease with coronary artery bypass graft surgery in 1975. There was no family history of cancer.

The client is married, has three children, and works full-time in health care. Her desired outcome is to decrease the pain and stiffness in the shoulder area and get back to her full activities.

Current medications included Atenolol/Chlorthalidone 50/25 daily for blood pressure management; potassium 10 meq daily; aspirin 81 mg daily; calcium 1,000 mg daily. She was started on 10 mg prednisone by her primary care physician. There are no known allergies.

Evaluation

Examination: Tests and Measures

Cardiovascular/pulmonary: On initial evaluation at 3 PM, the patient's blood pressure was 120/80 mm/Hg and resting pulse was 68. The client routinely exercises using the treadmill and performs aerobic exercises three times per

CASE EXAMPLE 12-2 Polymyalgia Rheumatica—cont'd

week. Lungs were clear to auscultation. There was no history of angina, dyspnea, or chronic cough. In the mornings, there is some pain when coughing and on deep breathing.

Pain: Using a Visual Analog Scale, from 0 (no pain) to 10 (worst pain imaginable), pain was rated as 8/10 in the shoulder girdle area.

Posture: Mild kyphosis and a mild forward head (possible sign of osteoporosis), but otherwise unremarkable.

Gait: Gait examination revealed an antalgic gait due to pain. She was not using any assistive devices or orthotics.

Range of motion and strength: Full active and passive shoulder range of motion with moderate stiffness/pain on movement. There were no gross deformities or evidence of impingement. Hands, wrists, and elbows present painless full range of motion. Lower extremity evaluation revealed a prominent first left MTP (metatarsal phalangeal joint) but tibio-talar joints were fully mobile without pain. Knee and hip range of motion were normal on exam. There was no effusion or instability noted.

Neurologic exam: There was no focal or diffuse muscle strength deficit. Deep tendon reflexes were normal bilaterally. Cranial nerves and sensation were intact.

Work, community, and leisure: Client has reported she has had difficulty getting out of bed in the morning and difficulty with sleep because it's very painful when she changes positions at night. Lack of sleep has been affecting her work.

Red Flags

- Age: over 50
- Postmenopausal
- Persistent symptoms of shoulder girdle stiffness and pain for the last 3 months despite medication use
- The musculoskeletal examination of the upper quadrant is not consistent with

rheumatoid arthritis or other musculoskeletal problems.
- (No apparent red flags suggestive of cardiopulmonary involvement)

Result: The therapist contacted the physician by phone to discuss findings and concerns. A written report was faxed to the physician's office prior to the phone call. The physician ordered blood tests that showed the following results:

	Client's value	Reference range (female)
WBC	7.7	4.5–11.0/mm³
Hemoglobin	11.6	12–15g/dl
Hematocrit	33.6	35–47%
Platelets	410	150–400/mm³
Sedimentation rate	71*	1–25 mm/hr
Rheumatoid factor	36.3	less than 60 u/ml (units per milliliter)

* Outside normal range.

Client was diagnosed with polymyalgia rheumatica (PMR) with a recommendation for continued physical therapy intervention. Because of her prednisone use and the fact that she is postmenopausal, attention to management of the potential for osteoporosis must be included in the treatment plan. Client was advised to have a baseline DEXA scan to determine bone mineral density given her postmenopausal status and the fact that she is likely going to be on corticosteroids for some time.

Even though the client was seen by the physician before referral to physical therapy, there were enough red flags to warrant consultation before beginning physical therapy intervention. Early diagnosis can be important with PMR to prevent permanent disability, including visual loss when giant cell arteritis is present.

Anita Bemis-Dougherty, PT, MAS. Case report presented in fulfillment of DPT 910, Institute for Physical Therapy Education, Widener University, Chester, Pennsylvania, 2005. Used with permission.

steroids for much longer; a few have PMR for less than a year. Oral corticosteroids (especially prednisone) used to suppress the inflammation and treat the symptoms do not cure the illness.[39] These drugs usually afford prompt relief of symptoms, providing further diagnostic confirmation that PMR is the underlying problem.[36] The therapist must remain alert to the possibility of steroid-induced osteopenia and diabetes.

With medical intervention, most people with PMR (with or without GCA) do not have lasting disability. However, in GCA, if one or both eyes develop blindness before treatment becomes effective, the blindness may be permanent.

Systemic Lupus Erythematosus

Systemic lupus erythematosus (SLE) belongs to the family of autoimmune rheumatic diseases. It is known to be a chronic, systemic, inflammatory disease characterized by injury to the skin, joints, kidneys, heart and blood-forming organs, nervous system, and mucous membranes.

Lupus comes from the Latin word for wolf, referring to the belief in the 1800s that the rash of this disease was caused by a wolf bite. The characteristic rash of lupus (especially a butterfly rash across the cheeks and nose) is red, leading to the term *erythematosus.*

There are two primary forms of lupus: discoid and systemic. *Discoid lupus* is a limited form of disease confined to the skin presenting as coin-shaped lesions, which are raised and scaly (see Fig. 4-16). Discoid lupus rarely develops into systemic lupus. Individuals who develop the systemic form probably had systemic lupus at the outset, with the discoid lesions as the main symptom.

Systemic lupus is usually more severe than discoid lupus and can affect almost any organ or system of the body. For some people, only the skin and joints will be involved. In others, the joints, lungs, kidneys, blood, or other organs or tissues may be affected.

RISK FACTORS

The exact cause of SLE is unknown, although it appears to result from an immunoregulatory disturbance brought about by the interplay of genetic, hormonal, chemical, and environmental factors.

Some of the environmental factors that may trigger the disease are infections (e.g., Epstein-Barr virus), antibiotics (especially those in the sulfa and penicillin groups), exposure to ultraviolet (sun) light, and extreme physical and emotional stress, including pregnancy.

Although there is a known genetic predisposition, no known gene is associated with SLE. Lupus can occur at any age, but it is most common in persons between the ages of 15 and 40 years; it rarely occurs in older people. Women are affected 10 to 15 times more often than men, possibly because of hormones, but the exact relationship remains unknown.

SLE is more common in African-American, African-Caribbean, Hispanic-American, and Asian persons than in the Caucasian population. Other risk factors among African-American women include early tobacco use (before age 19) but not alcohol intake.[40]

CLINICAL SIGNS AND SYMPTOMS

There is no single characteristic clinical pattern of symptoms. Clients may differ dramatically in the relative severity and pattern of organ involvement. SLE can appear in one organ or many. Common organ involvement includes cutaneous lupus, polyarthritis, nephritis, and hematologic lupus.[41] Although these symptoms may not be present at disease onset, most persons develop manifestations of multisystem disease.

Musculoskeletal Changes Arthralgias and arthritis are the most common presenting manifestations of SLE. Acute migratory or persistent nonerosive arthritis may involve any joint, but typically the small joints of the hands, wrists, and knees are symmetrically involved. Lupus does not directly affect the spine, but syndromes such as costochondritis and cervical myofascial syndrome associated with SLE are commonly treated in a physical therapist practice.

One fourth of all persons with lupus develop progressive musculoskeletal damage with deforming arthritis, osteoporosis with fracture and vertebral collapse, and osteomyelitis. Often, these musculoskeletal complications occur as a result of the drugs necessary for treatment.

Approximately 30% of people with SLE have coexistent fibromyalgia, independent of race. Fibromyalgia is identified as a major contributor of pain and fatigue, but a medical differential diagnosis is required to rule out hypothyroidism, anemia, or pulmonary lupus (interstitial lung disease or pulmonary hypertension).

Peripheral Neuropathy Peripheral neuropathy may be motor, sensory (stocking-glove distribution), or mixed motor and sensory polyneuropathy. These may develop subacutely in the lower extremities and progress to the upper extremities. Numbness on the tip of the tongue and inside the mouth is also a frequent complaint.

Touch, vibration, and position sense are most prominently affected, and the distal limb reflexes are depressed (Case Example 12-3).

Clinical Signs and Symptoms of
Systemic Lupus Erythematosus

Although lupus can affect any part of the body, most people experience symptoms in only a few organs. The most common symptoms associated with lupus are listed here in order of declining prevalence.

- Constitutional symptoms (especially low-grade fever and fatigue)
- Achy joints (arthralgia)
- Arthritis (swollen joints)
- Arthralgia
- Skin rashes (malar)
- Pulmonary involvement (e.g., pleurisy, pleural effusion: chest pain, difficulty breathing, cough)
- Anemia
- Kidney involvement (e.g., lupus nephritis)
- Sun or light sensitivity (photosensitivity)

Continued on p. 538

CASE EXAMPLE 12-3   Systemic Lupus Erythematosus

Current Complaint: A 33-year-old woman with a known diagnosis of systemic lupus erythematosus came to the physical therapy clinic with the following report: "About 3 weeks ago, I was carrying a heavy briefcase with a strap around my shoulder. I put weight on my right leg and felt my hip joint slip in the back with immediate pain, and I was unable to put any weight on that leg. I moved my hip around in the socket and was able to get immediate relief from the pain, but it felt like it could catch at any time." The client also reported that "it feels like my left hip is 2 inches higher than my right."

Past Medical History: The client reported prolonged (over 7-year) use of prednisone and a past medical history of proteinuria and compromised kidney function. Muscle weakness 2 years ago resulted in a muscle biopsy and a diagnosis of "abnormal" muscle tissue of unknown cause. The client developed a staph infection from the biopsy, which resolved very slowly.

Other past medical history included a motor vehicle accident 2 years ago, at which time her knees went through the dashboard, which left both knees "numb" for a year after the accident.

Clinical Presentation: Aggravating and relieving factors from this visit fit a musculoskeletal pattern of symptoms, and objective examination was consistent with lumbar/sacroiliac mechanical dysfunction with a multitude of other compounding factors, including bilateral posterior cruciate ligament laxity, poor posture, obesity, and emotional lability.

Physical therapy treatment was initiated, but a week later, when the client woke up at night to go to the bathroom, she swung her legs over the edge of her bed and experienced immediate hip and diffuse low back pain and lower extremity weakness.

She went to the emergency department by ambulance and later was admitted to the hospital. She was evaluated by a neurologist (results unknown), recovered from her symptoms within 24 hours, and was released after a 3-day hospitalization. She was directed by her primary care physician to continue outpatient physical therapy services.

Result: After consulting with this client's physician, conservative symptomatic treatment was planned. Within 2 weeks, she experienced another middle-of-the-night acute exacerbation of symptoms. A subsequent magnetic resonance image resulted in a diagnosis of disc extrusion (annulus fibrosus perforated with discal material in the epidural space) at two levels (L4-L5 and L5-S1).

This case example is included to point out the complexity of treating a musculoskeletal condition in a client with a long-term chronic inflammatory disease process requiring years of steroidal antiinflammatory medications. Before including any resistive exercises, muscle energy techniques, or joint or self-mobilization techniques, the therapist must be aware of any clinically significant changes in bone density and the presence of developing osteoporosis.

- Hair loss
- Raynaud's phenomenon (fingers turning white or blue in the cold)
- CNS involvement:
  - Seizures
  - Headache
  - Peripheral neuropathy
  - Cranial neuropathy
  - Cerebral vascular accidents
  - Organic brain syndrome
  - Psychosis
  - Mouth, nose, or vaginal ulcers

Scleroderma (Progressive Systemic Sclerosis)

Scleroderma, one of the lesser-known chronic multisystem diseases in the family of rheumatic diseases, is characterized by inflammation and fibrosis of many parts of the body, including the skin, blood vessels, synovium, skeletal muscle, and certain internal organs such as kidneys, lungs, heart, and GI tract.

There are two major subsets: limited cutaneous (previously known as the CREST syndrome) and diffuse cutaneous scleroderma. The major differences between these two types are the degree of clinically involved skin and the pace of disease.

Limited scleroderma is often characterized by a long history of Raynaud's phenomenon before the development of other symptoms. Skin thickening is limited to the hands, frequently with digital ulcers. Esophageal dysmotility is common. Although limited scleroderma is generally a milder form than diffuse scleroderma, life-threatening complications can occur from small intestine involvement and pulmonary hypertension.

Children affected by juvenile localized scleroderma develop multiple extracutaneous manifestations in 25% of all cases. These extracutaneous features can include joint, neurologic (e.g., epilepsy, peripheral neuropathy, headache), vascular, and ocular changes. These manifestations are often unrelated to the site of the skin lesions and can be associated with multiple organ involvement. Even so, the risk of developing systemic sclerosis (SSc) is very low.[42]

Diffuse scleroderma has a much more acute onset, with many constitutional symptoms, arthritis, carpal tunnel syndrome, and marked swelling of the hands and legs. Widespread skin thickening occurs, progressing from the fingers to the trunk. Internal organ problems, including GI effects and pulmonary fibrosis (see the section on systemic sclerosing lung disease in Chapter 7), are common,

and severe life-threatening involvement of the heart and kidneys occurs.[43-45]

RISK FACTORS

Although the cause of scleroderma is unknown, researchers suspect a complex interaction of genetic and environmental factors. Scleroderma can occur in individuals of any age, race, or sex, but it occurs most commonly in young or middle-age women (ages 25 through 55).[46]

CLINICAL SIGNS AND SYMPTOMS

Skin Raynaud's phenomenon and tight skin are the hallmarks of SSc. Virtually all clients with SSc have Raynaud's phenomenon, which is defined as episodic pallor of the digits following exposure to cold or stress associated with cyanosis, followed by erythema, tingling, and pain. Raynaud's phenomenon primarily affects the hands and feet and less commonly the ears, nose, and tongue.

The appearance of the skin is the most distinctive feature of SSc. By definition, clients with diffuse SSc have taut skin in the more proximal parts of extremities, in addition to the thorax and abdomen. However, the skin tightening of SSc begins on the fingers and hands in nearly all cases. Therefore the distinction between limited and diffuse SSc may be difficult to make early in the illness.

Musculoskeletal Articular complaints are very common in progressive systemic sclerosis (PSS) and may begin at any time during the course of the disease. The arthralgias, stiffness, and arthritis seen may be difficult to distinguish from those of RA, particularly in the early stages of the disease. Involved joints include the MCPs, PIPs, wrists, elbows, knees, ankles, and small joints of the feet.

Muscle involvement is usually mild, with weakness, tenderness, and pain of proximal muscles of the upper and lower extremities. Late scleroderma is characterized by muscle atrophy, muscle weakness, deconditioning, and flexion contractures.

Viscera Skin changes, Raynaud's phenomenon, and involvement of the GI tract are the most common manifestation of SSc. Esophageal hypomotility occurs in more than 90% of clients with either diffuse or limited SSc. Similar changes occur in the small intestine, resulting in reduced motility and causing intermittent diarrhea, bloating, cramping, malabsorption, and weight loss. Inflammation and fibrosis can also affect the lungs, resulting in interstitial pulmonary fibrosis, a restrictive lung disease.[47]

The overall course of scleroderma is highly variable. Once remission occurs, relapse is uncommon. The diffuse form generally has a worse prognosis because of cardiac involvement, such as cardiomyopathy, pericarditis, pericardial effusions, or arrhythmias.

Clinical Signs and Symptoms of Scleroderma

Limited Cutaneous Sclerosis (lSSc)

- CREST syndrome
  Calcinosis (abnormal deposition of calcium salts in tissues; usually on the fingertips and over bony prominences)
  Raynaud's phenomenon persisting for years
  Esophageal dysmotility, dysphagia, heartburn
  Sclerodactyly (chronic hardening and shrinking of fingers and toes)
  Telangiectasia (spiderlike hemangiomas formed by dilation of a group of small blood vessels; occurs most commonly on the face and hands)

Diffuse Cutaneous Sclerosis (dSSc)

- Raynaud's phenomenon (acute onset)
- Trunk and extremity skin changes (swelling, thickening, hardening)
- Ulcerations of the fingers secondary to constriction of small blood vessels
- Polyarthralgia (joint pain affecting large and small joints with inflammation, stiffness, swelling, warmth, and tenderness)
- Tendon friction rubs
- Flexion contractures of large and small joints
- Visceral involvement
- Interstitial lung disease (dyspnea on exertion, chronic cough, pleurisy)
- Esophageal involvement
- Renal failure (headache, blurred vision, seizures, malaise)
- GI disease (bloating, cramps, diarrhea or constipation)
- Myocardial involvement (cardiomyopathy, pericarditis, pericardial effusions, arrhythmias)

Spondyloarthropathy

Spondyloarthropathy represents a group of noninfectious, inflammatory, erosive rheumatic diseases that target the sacroiliac joints, the bony insertions of the annulus fibrosi of the intervertebral discs, and the facet or apophyseal joints. This group of diseases includes ankylosing spondylitis (AS; also known as Marie-Strümpell disease), Reiter's syndrome, psoriatic arthritis, and arthritis associated with chronic inflammatory bowel disease (see discussion, Chapter 8).

Individuals with spondyloarthropathies are not seropositive for rheumatoid factor, and the progressive joint fibrosis present is associated with the genetic marker human leukocyte antigen (HLA-B27). Spondyloarthropathy is more common in men, who by gender have a familial tendency toward the development of this type of disease.

History Associated With Spondyloarthropathy

- Insidious onset of each episode of backache
- First episode of backache occurs before 30 years of age
- Each episode lasts for months
- Pain intensifies after rest
- Pain lessens with movement
- Family history of a spondyloarthropathy

ANKYLOSING SPONDYLITIS

Ankylosing spondylitis (AS) is a chronic, progressive inflammatory disorder of undetermined cause. It is actually more an inflammation of fibrous tissue affecting the entheses, or insertions of ligaments, tendons, and capsules into bone, than of synovium, as is common in other rheumatic disorders.

The sacroiliac joints, spine, and large peripheral joints are primarily affected, but this is a systemic disease with widespread effects. People with AS may experience arthritis in other joints, such as the hips, knees, and shoulders along with fever, fatigue, loss of appetite, and redness and pain of the eyes.

Although AS has always been more common in men, some studies now suggest that the disease has a more uniform sex distribution, but it may be milder in women with more peripheral joint manifestations than spinal disease.[48,49]

Diagnosis is delayed or inappropriate until disease progression can be identified radiographically.

Clinical Signs and Symptoms The classic presentation of AS is insidious onset of middle and low back pain and stiffness for more than 3 months in a person (usually male) under 40 years of age. It is usually worse in the morning, lasting more

than 1 hour, and is characterized as achy or sharp ("jolting"), typically localized to the pelvis, buttocks, and hips; this pain can be confused with sciatica. A neurologic examination will be within normal limits.

Paravertebral muscle spasm, aching, and stiffness are common, but some clients may have slow progressive limitation of motion with no pain at all. Most clients have sacroiliitis as the earliest feature seen on x-ray films before clinical involvement extends to the lumbar spine. A magnetic resonance imaging (MRI) examination can demonstrate acute and chronic changes of sacroiliitis, osteitis, discovertebral lesions, disc calcifications and ossification, arthropathic (joint) lesions, and complications such as fracture and cauda equina syndrome.[50]

On physical examination, decreased mobility in the anteroposterior and lateral planes will be symmetric. Reduction in lumbar flexion is an early sign of AS. The Schöber test is used to confirm reduction in spinal motion associated with AS.[51] The sacroiliac joint is rarely tender by direct palpation. As the disease progresses, the inflamed ligaments and tendons ossify (turn to bone), causing a rigid spine and the loss of lumbar lordosis. In the most severe cases, the spine becomes so completely fused that the person may be locked in a rigid upright position or in a stooped position, unable to move the neck or back in any direction.

Peripheral joint involvement usually (but not always) occurs after involvement of the spine. Typical extraspinal sites include the manubriosternal joint, symphysis pubis, shoulder, and hip joints. If the ligaments that attach the ribs to the spine become ossified, diminished chest expansion (<2 cm) occurs, making it difficult to take a deep breath. Chest wall stiffness seldom leads to respiratory disability as long as diaphragmatic movement is intact. This process of vertebral and costovertebral fusion results in the formation of syndesmophytes (Fig. 12-3). This reparative process also forms linear bone ossification along the outer fibers of the annulus fibrosus of the disc.

This bridging of the vertebrae is most prominent along the anterior longitudinal ligament and occurs earliest in the thoracolumbar region. Destructive changes of the upper and lower corners of the vertebrae (at the insertion of the annulus fibrosus of the disc) are responsible for the vertebral squaring. Late in the disease the vertebral column takes on an appearance that is referred to as "bamboo spine."

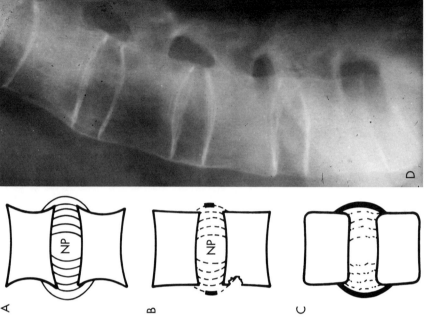

Fig. 12-3 • Pathogenesis of the syndesmophyte. The syndesmophyte, along with destruction of the sacroiliac joint, is the hallmark of the inflammatory spondyloarthropathies, such as ankylosing spondylitis. It should be distinguished from the osteophyte, which is characteristic of degenerative spondylosis. **A,** Normal intervertebral disc. The inner fibers of the annulus fibrosus are next to the nucleus pulposus (NP). The outer fibers insert into the periosteum of the vertebral body at least one third the distance toward the next end-plate. **B,** With early inflammation, the corners of the bodies are reabsorbed and appear to be square or even eroded. Fine deposits of amorphous apatite (calcium phosphate, a mineral constituent of bone) first appear on radiographs as thin, delicate calcification in the outer fibers of the midannulus. **C** and **D,** The process progresses to bridging calcification, with the syndesmophyte extending from one midbody to the next. Thus the spine takes on its bamboolike appearance on radiographs. (**A** to **C,** From Hadler NM: *Medical management of the regional musculoskeletal diseases,* Orlando, Fla, 1984, Grune & Stratton, p 5; **D,** From Bullough PG: *Bullough and Vigorita's orthopaedic pathology,* ed 3, London, Mosby-Wolfe, 1997, p 68.)

Extra-Articular Features Uveitis, conjunctivitis, or iritis occurs in nearly 25% of clients and follows a course that is unrelated to the severity of the joint disease. Ocular symptoms may precede

spinal symptoms by several weeks or even years. Pulmonary changes (chronic infiltrative or fibrotic bullous changes of the upper lobes) occur in 1% to 3% of persons with AS and may be confused with TB.

Cardiomegaly, conduction defects, and pericarditis are well-recognized cardiovascular complications of AS. Occasionally, renal manifestations precede other symptoms of AS.

Complications The very stiff osteoporotic spine of clients with AS is prone to *fracture* from even minor trauma. It has been estimated that the incidence of thoracolumbar fractures in ankylosing spondylitis is four times higher than that in the general population.[52] The most common site of fracture is the lower cervical spine. Risk of neurologic damage may be compounded by the development of epidural hematoma from lacerated vessels.

Severe neck or occipital pain possibly referring to the retroorbital or frontal area is the presenting symptom of *atlantoaxial subluxation*. This underappreciated entity may be either an early or a late manifestation, but it is frequently seen in clients with persistent peripheral arthritis.

Movement aggravates pain, and progressive myelopathy develops from cord compression, leading to motor/sensory disturbance in bladder and bowel control. The diagnosis of atlantoaxial subluxation is usually made from lateral x-ray views of the cervical spine in flexion and extension.

Spondylodiscitis (erosive and destructive lesions of vertebral bodies) is seen in clients with longstanding disease. Intervertebral disc lesions occur at multiple levels, especially in the thoracolumbar region.

Cauda equina syndrome is a late (rare) manifestation of the disease, with an average interval of 24 years between onset of AS and the syndrome.[53] The initial deficit is loss of sensation of the lower extremities, along with urinary and rectal sphincter disturbances and/or perineal pain and numbness or saddle anesthesia. Neurologic abnormalities in AS are usually related to nerve impingement or spinal cord trauma. Anyone with a known diagnosis of AS and a history of incontinence (bowel or bladder) or neurologic deficit should be evaluated for surgical intervention (e.g., laminectomy, lumboperitoneal shunting).[54]

Spinal stenosis occurs as a result of bony overgrowth of the spinal ligaments and facet joints. Symptoms of pain and numbness of the lower extremities are brought on by walking and relieved by rest.

Clinical Signs and Symptoms of Ankylosing Spondylitis

Early Stages

- Intermittent low back pain (nontraumatic, insidious onset; relieved by exercise or activity; persists beyond 3 months)
- Sacroiliitis (inflammation, pain, and tenderness in the sacroiliac joints)
- Spasm of the paravertebral muscles
- Loss of normal lumbar lordosis (positive Schöber's test)
- Intermittent, low-grade fever
- Fatigue
- Anorexia, weight loss
- Anemia
- Painful limitation of cervical joint motion

Advanced Stages

- Constant low back pain
- Loss of normal lumbar lordosis
- Ankylosis (immobility and consolidation or fusion) of the sacroiliac joints and spine
- Muscle wasting in shoulder and pelvic girdles
- Marked dorsocervical kyphosis
- Decreased chest expansion
- Arthritis involving the peripheral joints (hips and knees)
- Hip flexion in standing

Extraskeletal

- Cauda equina syndrome
  - Low back pain with or without sciatica
  - Loss of sensation in the lower extremities
  - Bowel and/or bladder changes (decreased anal sphincter tone, urinary retention, overflow incontinence)
  - Perineal pain or loss of sensation (saddle anesthesia)
  - Muscle weakness and atrophy
- Iritis or iridocyclitis (inflammation of the iris; occurs in 25% of all cases)
- Conjunctivitis
- Carditis (10% occurrence)
- Pericarditis and pulmonary fibrosis (rare)
- Prostatitis

REITER'S SYNDROME

Reiter's syndrome is characterized by a triad of arthritis, conjunctivitis, and nonspecific urethritis, although some clients develop only two of these three problems. Reiter's syndrome occurs mainly

in young adult men between the ages of 20 and 40 years, although women and children can be affected.

Risk Factors Reactive arthritis associated with Reiter's syndrome occurs in response to infection and typically begins acutely 2 to 4 weeks after venereal infections or bouts of gastroenteritis. Most cases occur in young men and are believed to result from venereal-acquired infections. Other infections, such as food-borne enteric infections, affect both men and women. The onset of Reiter's syndrome can be abrupt, occurring over several days or more gradually over several weeks.

HLA-B27, present in a high-frequency pattern, supports a genetic predisposition for the development of this syndrome after a person is exposed to certain bacterial infections or after sexual contact. Having HLA-B27 does not necessarily mean that the person will develop this syndrome but indicates that the person will have a greater chance of developing Reiter's syndrome than do persons without this marker.

Reiter's syndrome can be differentiated from AS by the presence of urethritis and conjunctivitis, the prominent involvement of distal joints, and the presence of asymmetric radiologic changes in the sacroiliac joints and spine.

Clinical Signs and Symptoms *Arthritis* associated with Reiter's syndrome often occurs precipitously and frequently affects the knees and ankles, lasting weeks to months. The distribution of the arthritis begins in the weight-bearing joints, especially of the lower extremities.

The arthritis may vary in severity from absence to extreme joint destruction. Involvement of the feet and spine is most common and is associated with HLA-B27 positivity. Affected joints are usually warm, tender, and edematous, with pain on active and passive movement. A dusky-blue discoloration or frank erythema accompanied by exquisite tenderness is a sign of a septic joint. Although the joints usually begin to improve after 2 or 3 weeks, many people continue to have pain, especially in the heels and back.

Low back and buttock pain are common in reactive arthritis; such pain is caused by sacroiliac or other spinal joint involvement. Sacroiliac changes seen on x-ray films are usually asymmetric and similar to those of AS. Small joint involvement, especially in the feet, is more common in Reiter's syndrome than in AS and is often asymmetric.

In addition to arthritis, inflammation typically occurs at bony sites where tendons, ligaments, or fascia have their attachments or insertions (enthe-ses). Enthesitis most commonly occurs at the inser-

tions of the plantar aponeurosis and Achilles tendon, on the calcaneus, leading to heel pain—one of the most frequent, distinctive, and disabling manifestations of the disease. Other common sites for enthesitis include ischial tuberosities, iliac crests, tibial tuberosities, and ribs, with associated musculoskeletal pain at sites other than joints (Case Example 12-4).

The *conjunctivitis* of Reiter's syndrome is mild and characterized by irritation with redness, tearing, and burning usually lasting a few days (or less commonly as long as several weeks). The process is ordinarily self-limiting.

Urethritis manifested by burning and urinary frequency is often the earliest symptom. A profuse and watery diarrhea can precede the onset of urethritis in Reiter's syndrome.

Clinical Signs and Symptoms of

Reiter's Syndrome

Articular Manifestations

- Polyarthritis (occurs several days or weeks after symptoms of infection appear)
- Sacroiliac joint changes
- Low back and buttock pain
- Small joint involvement, especially the feet (heel pain)
- Plantar fasciitis
- Low-grade fever
- Urethritis (when present, precedes other symptoms by 1 to 2 weeks)
- Conjunctivitis and iritis, bilaterally

Extraarticular Manifestations

- Skin involvement: inflammatory hyperkeratotic lesions of the toes, nails, and soles resembling psoriasis
- May be preceded by bowel infection: diarrhea, nausea, vomiting
- Anorexia and weight loss

PSORIATIC ARTHRITIS

Psoriatic arthritis (PsA) is a chronic, recurrent, erosive, inflammatory arthritis associated with the skin disease psoriasis. It is not just a variant of RA but is a distinct disease that combines features of both RA (e.g., joint pain, erythema, swelling, stiffness) and the spondyloarthropathies (e.g., enthesopathy; inflammation at insertion points of tendon, ligament, capsule; iritis). Psoriasis is quite common, affecting 1% to 3% of the general population. This arthritis occurs in one third of clients with psoriasis.

CASE EXAMPLE 12-4 Reiter's Syndrome

Past Medical History: At presentation, a 22-year-old man had left heel pain that had developed 3 weeks before his appointment in physical therapy. He could not attribute any trauma to the foot and was not involved in any sports or athletic activities. Previous medical history was minimal except for an appendectomy when he was 18 years old.

Clinical Presentation: The client reported that his pain was worst when he first got out of bed in the morning but improved with stretching and taking aspirin. He did not wear any orthotics or special shoes. The therapist did not ask about the presence of associated signs or symptoms.

No obvious gait abnormalities were observed. On palpation of the foot, there was no warmth, bruising, or redness in the area of the plantar fascia or calcaneus. Tenderness was reported along the plantar fascia, with a painful response to palpation of the tendinous attachment to the calcaneus. Ankle range of motion and muscle strength of the left lower leg were within normal limits. There was no tenderness of the surrounding bones, tendons, or muscles. A neurologic screen was also considered normal.

Intervention: The therapist treated this client by using a treatment protocol for plantar fasciitis, including ultrasound, deep friction massage, and stretching exercises. Symptoms subsided, and the client was discharged. He returned 6 weeks later with recurrence of the original symptoms and new onset of low back pain.

The therapist reevaluated the client, including an in-depth evaluation of postural components and performance of a back screening examination, but again did not ask any questions related to associated signs and symptoms. Before his next appointment, the client called and canceled further physical therapy treatment.

Result: A follow-up call determined that this young man had developed other symptoms, such as fever, red and itching eyes, and frequent urination. He went to a walk-in clinic, was referred to an internist, and received a diagnosis of Reiter's syndrome.

Whenever a client has musculoskeletal pain or symptoms of unknown cause, a series of questions must be posed to screen for medical disease. This is especially important when symptoms do not respond to treatment, when symptoms recur, or when new musculoskeletal symptoms develop.

Although joint pain, heel pain, or back pain usually occurs after the development of conjunctivitis, enteritis, or urethritis in Reiter's syndrome, this young man developed musculoskeletal symptoms first. At the time of the initial physical therapy evaluation, he was experiencing fatigue, low-grade fever, and malaise that he did not report. Asking the question "Are there any other symptoms of any kind anywhere in your body?" might have elicited the early red flag associated signs and symptoms for infection.

Past Medical History: Psoriatic arthritis (PsA) and reactive arthritis (formerly Reiter's syndrome) are two examples of spondyloarthropathy.

In contrast to RA, there is no gender predilection in PsA. Both sexes are affected equally, although women tend to develop symmetric polyarthritis, and spinal involvement is more common in men. PsA can occur at any age, although it usually occurs between the ages of 20 and 30 years. The onset of the arthritis may be acute or insidious and is usually preceded by the skin disease.

Risk Factors The cause of psoriasis and any risk factors for PsA are unknown. PsA is a complex, multifactorial disease; multiple genes are likely to

influence disease susceptibility and severity.[55] The presence of the histocompatibility complex marker HLA-B27 and other HLA antigens is not uncommon, and they occur in clients with peripheral arthritis and spondylitis.

The presence of these genetic markers may be associated with an increased susceptibility to unknown infectious or environmental agents or to primary abnormal autoimmune phenomena. There is some evidence to support dysregulated angiogenesis as a primary pathogenic mechanism in psoriatic arthritis.[56]

Clinical Signs and Symptoms *Skin lesions* that characterize psoriasis are readily recognized as piles of well-defined, dry, erythematous, often overlapping silver-scaled papules and plaques. These may appear in small, easily overlooked patches or may run together and cover wide areas. The scalp, extensor surfaces of the elbows and knees, back, and buttocks are common sites. The lesions, which do not usually itch, come and go and may be present for years (typically 5 to 10 years) before the onset of arthritis.

Nail lesions, including pitting, ridging (transverse grooves), cracking, onycholysis (loosening or separation of the nail; see Fig. 4-29), brown-yellow discoloration, and destruction of the nail, are the only clinical feature that may identify clients with psoriasis in whom arthritis is likely to develop. The nail changes may be mistaken for those produced by a fungal infection.

Arthritis appears as an early and severe sign in a symmetric distal distribution (DIP joints of fingers and toes before involvement of MCP and MTP joints) in half of all clients with PsA, which distinguishes it from RA. Severe erosive disease may lead to marked deformity of the hands and feet, called arthritis mutilans. Wrists, ankles, knees, and elbows can also be involved.

Clients report pain and stiffness in the inflamed joints, with morning stiffness that lasts more than 30 minutes. Other evidence of inflammation includes pain on stressing the joint, tenderness at the joint line, and the presence of effusion. Painful symptoms are aggravated by prolonged immobility and are reduced by physical activity.

Marked vertebral involvement can result in *ankylosis of the spine*. This differs from AS in a number of respects, most notably in the tendency for many of the syndesmophytes to arise not at the margins of the vertebral bodies but from the lateral and anterior surfaces of the bodies. *Sacroiliac changes*, including erosions, sclerosis, and ankylosis similar to that in Reiter's syndrome, occur in 10% to 30% of clients with PsA.

Soft-tissue involvement, similar to clinical manifestations of spondyloarthropathy, occurs often in PsA. Enthesitis, or inflammation at the site of tendon insertion or muscle attachment to bone, is frequently observed at the Achilles tendon, plantar fascia, and pelvic bones. Also common is tenosynovitis of the flexor tendons of the hands, extensor carpi ulnaris, and other sites.

Dactylitis, which occurs in more than one third of PsA clients, is marked by diffuse swelling of the whole finger. Inflammation in this typical "sausage

finger" extends to the tendon sheaths and adjacent joints.

Extra-articular features similar to those seen in clients with other seronegative spondyloarthropathies are frequently seen. These extraarticular lesions include iritis, mouth ulcers, urethritis, and, less commonly, colitis and aortic valve disease.

Clinical Signs and Symptoms of Psoriatic Arthritis (PsA)

- Fever
- Fatigue
- Dystrophic nail bed changes
- Polyarthritis
- Psoriasis
- Sore fingers (sometimes sausagelike swelling)

Unique Clinical Features of PsA

- DIP joint involvement
- Nail changes
- Dactylitis
- Spondylitis
- Iritis

Early recognition of this disorder is important because medical intervention with newer biologic agents can help prevent long-term complications such as permanent joint destruction and disability.[57]

Lyme Disease

In the early 1970s, a mysterious clustering of juvenile arthritis occurred among children in Lyme, Connecticut, and in surrounding towns. Medical researchers soon recognized the illness as a distinct disease, which they called Lyme disease. They were able to identify the deer tick infected with a spiral bacterium or spirochete (later named *Borrelia burgdorferi*) as the key to its spread.

The number of reported cases of Lyme disease, as well as the number of geographic areas in which it is found, has been increasing. Most cases are concentrated in the coastal northeast, the mid-Atlantic states, Wisconsin, Minnesota, Oregon, and northern California. Children may be more susceptible than are adults simply because they spend more time outdoors and are more likely to be exposed to ticks.

CLINICAL SIGNS AND SYMPTOMS

In most individuals, the first symptom of Lyme disease is a red rash, known as *erythema migrans*,

that starts as a small red spot that expands over a period of days or weeks, forming a circular, triangular, or oval rash. Sometimes the rash resembles a bull's-eye because it appears as a red ring surrounding a central clear area. The rash can range in size from that of a dime to the entire width of a person's back, appearing within a few weeks of a tick bite and usually at the site of the tick, which is often the axilla or groin. As infection spreads, several rashes can appear at different sites on the body.

Erythema migrans is often accompanied by flulike symptoms such as fever, headache, stiff neck, body aches, and fatigue. Although these symptoms resemble those of common viral infections, Lyme disease symptoms tend to persist or may occur intermittently over a period of several weeks to months.

Arthritis appears several months after infection with *Borrelia Burgdorferi*. Slightly more than half of the people who are not treated with antibiotics develop recurrent attacks of painful and swollen joints that last a few days to a few months. About 10% to 20% of untreated clients will go on to develop chronic arthritis.

In most clients, Lyme arthritis is monoarticular or oligoarticular (few joints), most commonly affecting the knee, but the arthritis can shift from one joint to another. Other large joints, such as the shoulder and elbow, are also commonly affected. Involvement of the hands and feet is uncommon, and it is these features that help differentiate Lyme arthritis from RA.[58]

Neurologic symptoms (including cognitive dysfunction referred to as neurocognitive symptoms) may appear because Lyme disease can affect the nervous system. Symptoms include stiff neck, severe headache associated with meningitis, Bell's palsy, numbness, pain or weakness in the limbs, or poor motor coordination. Memory loss, difficulty in concentrating, mood changes, and sleep disturbances have also been associated with Lyme disease. Nervous system involvement can develop several weeks, months, or even years following an untreated infection. These symptoms last for weeks or months and may recur.

Cardiac involvement occurs in less than 1% of the people affected by Lyme disease. Symptoms of irregular heartbeat, dizziness, and dyspnea occur several weeks after the infection and rarely last more than a few days or weeks. Recovery is usually complete.

Finally, although Lyme disease can be divided into early and later stages, each with a different set of complications, these stages may vary in duration, may overlap, or may even be absent. Clinical manifestations may first appear from 3 to 30 days after the tick bite but usually occur within 1 week.

Lyme disease is still mistaken for other ailments, including Guillain-Barré syndrome, multiple sclerosis, and fibromyalgia syndrome, and can be difficult to diagnose. The only distinctive hallmark unique to Lyme disease, the erythema migrans rash, is absent in at least one fourth of those who become infected. Many people are unaware that they have been bitten by a tick (Case Example 12-5).

In general, the sooner treatment is initiated, the quicker and more complete the recovery, with less chance for the development of subsequent symptoms of arthritis and neurologic problems. Following treatment for Lyme disease, some persons still have persistent fatigue and achiness, which can take months to subside.

Unfortunately, having had Lyme disease once is no guarantee that the illness will be prevented in the future. The disease can strike more than once in the same individual if she or he is reinfected with the Lyme disease bacterium.

Clinical Signs and Symptoms of
Lyme Disease

Early Infection (one or more may be present at different times during infection)

• Red rash (erythema migrans)
• Flulike symptoms (fever, headache, stiff neck, fatigue)
• Migratory musculoskeletal pain (joints, bursae, tendons, muscle, or bone)
• Neurologic symptoms:
  • Severe headache (meningitis)
  • Numbness, pain, weakness of extremities
  • Poor motor coordination
  • Cognitive dysfunction: Memory loss, difficulty in concentrating, mood changes, sleep disturbances

Less Common Symptoms

• Eye problems such as conjunctivitis
• Heart abnormalities and myocarditis

Late Infection (months to years after infection)

• Arthritis, intermittent or chronic
• Encephalopathy (mood and sleep disturbances)
• Neurocognitive dysfunction
• Peripheral neuropathy

CASE EXAMPLE 12-5 Lyme Disease

A 54-year-old business executive developed searing neck and back pain and was diagnosed as having a cervical disc protrusion. He was sent to physical therapy but had a very busy travel schedule and was unable to make even half of his scheduled appointments.

He chose to discontinue physical therapy, but his symptoms worsened and the pain became so intense that he was unable to go to work some mornings. He also started experiencing numbness in his right arm along the ulnar nerve distribution. He returned to physical therapy, but there was no discernible improvement subjectively, by client report, or objectively, as measured by functional improvement.

Anterior cervical discectomy was performed to remove the fifth cervical disc but with no change in symptoms postoperatively. There was

significant right extremity paresis, with maximal functional loss of the right hand and continued neck and back pain.

This client was eventually discharged from further physical therapy services and underwent a second surgical procedure, with no improvement in his condition. A year later, he telephoned the therapist to report that he had been diagnosed with Lyme disease. This man spent his vacations in the woods of Connecticut and Long Island, but this important piece of information was never gleaned from his past medical history.

Despite the lengthy time before diagnosis, the client was almost entirely recovered and ready to return to work after completing a course of antibiotics.

Autoimmune-Mediated Neurologic Disorders

Some neurologic disorders encountered by the therapist display features that suggest an immunologic basis for the disorder. Such diseases include multiple sclerosis (MS), Guillain-Barré syndrome, and myasthenia gravis. Other dysfunctions, such as amyotrophic lateral sclerosis (ALS) and acute disseminated encephalomyelitis, also associated with immunologic dysfunction but seen less often by the therapist, are not discussed.

Multiple Sclerosis

MS is the most common inflammatory demyelinating disease of the CNS, affecting areas of the brain and spinal cord but sparing the peripheral nerves. Symptoms appear usually between 20 and 40 years of age, with a peak onset of age 30 years. Onset is rare in children and in adults older than 50.

RISK FACTORS

Women are affected twice as often as men, and a family history of MS increases the risk tenfold. MS is not considered a hereditary disease, but a person who has a first-degree relative affected by the disease has an above-average risk for it.[59]

It would appear that MS susceptibility and age at onset are to some extent under genetic control. Environmental factors may affect onset; MS is five

times more prevalent in the temperate (colder) climates of North America and Europe than in tropical areas, even among people with similar genetic backgrounds. The reason may be lack of sunlight (less ultraviolet radiation needed for vitamin D).[60]

Evidence suggests that MS is an autoimmune disease, but the actual cause remains unknown. A virus or other infectious agent, toxins, vaccinations, stress,[61] and surgery are all thought to be possible triggers for the immune-mediated response, which is believed to destroy the CNS myelin.[62] According to the immune system hypothesis, T cells that have been called up against the virus, toxin, or stressor turn their focus to the myelin and continue to make intermittent attacks on it long after the initial infection or problem has resolved.

The disease is characterized by inflammatory demyelinating (destructive removal or loss) lesions that later form scars known as plaques, which are scattered throughout the CNS white matter, especially the optic nerves, cerebrum, and cervical spinal cord. When edema and inflammation subside, some remyelination occurs, but it is often incomplete. Axonal injury may cause permanent neurologic dysfunction.

The progression of MS is difficult to predict and depends on several factors, including the person's age and the intensity of onset, the neurologic status at 5 years after the onset, and the course of

exacerbations and remissions. The survival rate after the onset of symptoms is usually good, and death typically results from either respiratory or urinary infection.

CLINICAL SIGNS AND SYMPTOMS

Clinically, MS is characterized by multiple and varying signs and symptoms and by unpredictable and fluctuating periods of remissions and exacerbations. Symptoms may vary considerably in character, intensity, and duration. Symptoms can develop rapidly over a course of minutes or hours; less frequently, the onset may be insidious, occurring during a period of weeks or months.

Symptoms depend on the location of the lesions, and early symptoms demonstrate involvement of the sensory, pyramidal, cerebellar, and visual pathways or disruption of cranial nerves and their linkage to the brainstem.

Motor Symptoms Many persons with MS experience weakness in the extremities, leading to difficulty with ambulation, coordination, and balance, with ataxia or tremor present if lesions are in the cerebellum. Spasticity and hyperreflexia are common causes of disability with severe, uncontrollable spasms of the extremities. Profound fatigue or dysmetria (intention tremor) contribute to motor impairment.[63]

Difficulties with speech (slow, slurred) or chewing and swallowing can occur if the brainstem or cranial nerves are affected. Urinary frequency, urinary urgency, incontinence, urinary retention, or urinary hesitancy commonly characterizes motor and/or sensory bowel/bladder dysfunctions.

Sensory Symptoms Unilateral visual impairment (e.g., double vision, visual loss, red-green color blindness) that comes and goes as a result of optic neuritis is often the first indication of a problem. Optic neuritis occurs in about 20% of persons initially presenting with MS, while 40% may present with optic neuritis during the course of their disease.[64]

Extreme sensitivity to temperature changes is evident in more than 60% of the people diagnosed with MS. Elevated temperatures shorten the duration of the nerve impulse and worsen symptoms, whereas cooler temperatures actually restore conduction in blocked nerves and improve symptoms.

Paresthesias (numbness and tingling) accompanied by burning in the extremities can result in injury to the hands or feet. Lhermitte's sign (electric shock-like sensation down the spine and radiating to the extremities, initiated by neck flexion) is very suggestive of MS but can also occur with disc protrusion.

Clinical Signs and Symptoms of Multiple Sclerosis

(listed in declining order of frequency)

Symptoms

- Unilateral visual impairment
- Paresthesias
- Ataxia or unsteadiness
- Vertigo (sensation of rotation of self or surroundings)
- Fatigue
- Muscle weakness
- Bowel/bladder dysfunctions:
  - Frequency
  - Urgency
  - Incontinence
  - Retention
  - Hesitancy
- Speech impairment (slow, slurred speech)

Signs

- Optic neuritis
- Nystagmus
- Spasticity or hyperreflexia
- Babinski's sign
- Absent abdominal reflexes
- Dysmetria or intention tremor
- Labile or changed mood
- Lhermitte's sign

Guillain-Barré Syndrome (Acute Idiopathic Polyneuritis)

Guillain-Barré syndrome is a demyelination disease that affects the peripheral nervous system (especially spinal nerves) and is characterized by an abrupt onset of paralysis. The disease affects all age groups, and incidence is not related to race or sex.

RISK FACTORS

The exact cause of the disease is unknown, but it frequently occurs after an infectious illness. Upper respiratory infections, vaccinations, or viral infections such as measles, hepatitis, or mononucleosis commonly precede acute idiopathic polyneuritis by 1 to 3 weeks.

Like myasthenia gravis, acute idiopathic polyneuritis may be an autoimmune disease that occurs after surgery, a viral infection, or immunization. The immune system attacks its own myelin cells because they look similar to the molecules of the infecting virus. The immune system shifts into an accidental self-destructive overdrive.

CLINICAL SIGNS AND SYMPTOMS

The onset of acute idiopathic polyneuritis is generally characterized by a rapidly progressive weakness for a period of 3 to 7 days. It is usually symmetric, involving first the lower extremities, then the upper extremities, and then the respiratory musculature. Weakness and paralysis are frequently preceded by paresthesias and numbness of the limbs, but actual objective sensory loss is usually mild and transient.

Although muscular weakness is usually described as bilateral, progressing from the legs upward toward the arms, this syndrome may be missed when the client has unilateral symptoms that do not progress proximally.

Muscular weakness of the chest may appear early in this disease process as respiratory compromise. Respiratory involvement as such may be unnoticed until the person develops more severe symptoms associated with the Guillain-Barré syndrome.

The progression of paralysis varies from one client to another, often with full recovery from the paralysis. Usually symptoms develop over a period of 1 to 3 weeks, and the progression of paralysis may stop at any point. Once the weakness reaches a maximum (usually during the second week), the client's condition plateaus for days or even weeks before spontaneous improvement and eventual recovery begin, extending over a period of 6 to 9 months.

Cranial nerves, most commonly the facial nerve, can be involved. The tendon reflexes are decreased or lost early in the course of the illness. The incidence of residual neurologic deficits is higher than was previously recognized, and deficits may occur in as many as 50% of all cases.

TREATMENT

There is no immediate cure for this disease, but medical support is vital during the progression of symptoms, particularly in the acute phase when respiratory function may be compromised. Physical therapy is initiated at an early stage to maintain joint range of motion within the client's pain tolerance and to monitor muscle strength until active exercises can be initiated.

The usual precautions for clients immobilized in bed are required to prevent complications during the acute phase. A major precaution is to provide active exercise at a level consistent with the client's muscle strength. Overstretching and overuse of painful muscles may result in a prolonged recovery period or a lack of recovery (Case Example 12-6).

CASE EXAMPLE 12-6 Guillain Barré

A 67-year-old retired aeronautics engineer was referred to physical therapy by his physician for electrotherapy and therapeutic exercise. The physician's diagnosis was right-sided Bell's palsy. Past medical history was significant for an upper respiratory infection 2 weeks before the onset of his first symptoms.

The client reported difficulty in closing his eyes, chewing, and drinking, and he was unable to smile. There were no changes in sensation or hearing. During the neurologic examination, the client was unable to raise his eyebrows or close his eyes, and there was obvious facial drooping on both sides. A gross manual muscle test revealed full (5/5) muscle strength in all four extremities, but muscle stretch reflexes were absent in all four extremities.

Result: The therapist recognized three red-flag symptoms in this case: (1) recent upper respiratory infection followed by the development of neurologic symptoms; (2) progressive development of symptoms from right-sided to bilateral between the time the client was evaluated by the physician and went to the physical therapist; and (3) absent deep tendon reflexes, an inconsistent finding for Bell's palsy.

The therapist contacted the physician by telephone to relay this information and confirm the treatment plan given this new information. The physician requested that the client return for further medical testing, and a revised diagnosis of Guillain-Barré syndrome was made.

The client's clinical status stabilized, and he returned to the physical therapist. The treatment plan was modified accordingly. This case again demonstrates the importance of performing a careful examination, including screening for systemic disease and recognizing red-flag symptoms.

Clinical Signs and Symptoms of Guillain-Barré Syndrome (Acute Idiopathic Polyneuritis)

- Muscular weakness (bilateral, progressing from the legs to the arms to the chest and neck)
- Diminished deep tendon reflexes
- Paresthesias (without loss of sensation)
- Fever, malaise
- Nausea

Myasthenia Gravis

Myasthenia gravis (MG), an uncommon condition, develops when, for unknown reasons, antibodies produced by the immune system block receptors in muscles that receive signals of acetylcholine (a chemical messenger generated by nerve impulses), thus impairing muscle function.

MG may begin at any time in life, including in the newborn infant, but there are two major peaks of onset. In early-onset MG, at age 20 to 30 years, women are more often affected than men. In late-onset MG, after age 50 years, men are more often affected.

CLINICAL SIGNS AND SYMPTOMS

Clinically, the disease is characterized by muscle weakness and fatigability, most commonly in muscles controlling eye movement, chewing, swallowing, and facial expressions. Symptoms show fluctuations in intensity and are more severe late in the day or after prolonged activity. Speech may become unintelligible after prolonged periods of talking. Fluctuations also occur with superimposed illness, menses, and air temperature (worse with warming; improved with cold).

Fatigable and rapidly fluctuating asymmetric ptosis is a hallmark of the problem, since ocular muscle dysfunction is usually one of the first symptoms. The ice pack test, rest test, sleep tests, and peek sign are all useful in confirming the presence of MG (Box 12-4).[65]

Proximal muscles are affected more than distal muscles, and difficulty in climbing stairs, rising from chairs, combing the hair, or even holding up the head occurs. Cranial muscles, neck muscles, respiratory muscles, and muscles of the proximal limbs are the primary areas of muscular involvement. Neurologic findings are normal except for muscle weakness. There is no muscular atrophy or loss of sensation. Muscular weakness ranges from mild to life threatening (when involving respiratory muscles).

Clinical Signs and Symptoms of Myasthenia Gravis

- Muscle fatigability and proximal muscle weakness aggravated by exertion
- Respiratory failure from progressive involvement of respiratory muscles
- Ptosis (extraocular muscle weakness resulting in drooping of the upper eyelid)
- Diplopia (double vision)
- Dysarthria (slurred speech)
- Bulbar involvement
- Alteration in voice quality
- Dysphagia (difficulty swallowing)
- Nasal regurgitation
- Choking, difficulty in chewing

Immunoproliferative Disorders

Immunoproliferative disorders occur when abnormal reproduction or multiplication of the cells of the lymphoid system results in leukemia, lymphoma, and other related disorders. These have been covered in other parts of this text and are not discussed further in this chapter.

▶ PHYSICIAN REFERRAL

In most immunologic disorders, physicians must rely on the client's history and clinical findings in association with supportive information from diagnostic tests to make a differential diagnosis. Often, there are no definitive diagnostic tests, such as in the case of MS. The physician instead relies on objectively measured CNS abnormalities, a history of episodic exacerbations, and remissions of symptoms with progressive worsening of symptoms over time.

In the early stages of treating disorders such as MS, Guillain-Barré syndrome, and myositis, factors such as the effect of fatigue on the client's progress and fragile muscle fibers necessitate that the therapist keep close contact with the physician, who will use a physical examination and laboratory tests to determine the most opportune time for an exercise program. While the physician is monitoring serum enzyme levels and the overall medical status of the client, the therapist will continue to provide the physician with essential feedback regarding objective findings, such as muscle tenderness, muscle strength, and overall physical endurance.

A careful history and close clinical observations may elicit indications that the client is demonstrating signs and symptoms unrelated to a musculoskeletal disorder. Because the immune system can implicate many of the body systems, the therapist should not hesitate to relay to the physician any unusual findings reported or observed.

Guidelines for Immediate Medical Attention

- Anyone exhibiting signs and symptoms of anaphylactic shock, especially vocal hoarseness, difficulty breathing, and chest discomfort or tightness (see Table 12-1)
- New onset of joint pain with a recent history of surgery (**bacterial or reactive arthritis**)
- A dusky blue discoloration or erythema accompanied by exquisite tenderness is a sign of a septic (infected) joint; ask about a recent history of infection of any kind anywhere in the body; medical referral is advised

Guidelines for Physician Referral

- New onset of joint pain within 6 weeks of surgery, especially when accompanied by constitutional symptoms, rash, or skin lesions
- Symmetric swelling and pain in peripheral joints may be an early sign of rheumatoid arthritis; early medical intervention is critical to prevent erosive joint disease and disability.[29]
- Development of progressive neurologic symptoms within 1 to 3 weeks of a previous infection or recent vaccination
- Evidence of spinal cord compression in anyone with cervical rheumatoid arthritis who has progressed from generalized stiffness to new onset of cervical laxity (C1-C2 subluxation or dislocation)
- Presence of incontinence (bowel or bladder) in anyone with ankylosing spondylitis requires medical referral; surgical treatment of the underlying dural ectasia may be helpful.[54]
- Positive ptosis tests for myasthenia gravis (ice pack, rest, sleep tests)

Clues to Immune System Dysfunction

- Client with a history of rheumatoid arthritis taking disease-modifying antirheumatic drugs (DMARDs) who develops symptoms of drug toxicity (e.g., rash, petechiae/ecchymosis, photosensitivity, dyspnea, nausea/vomiting, lymph node swelling, edema, oral ulcers, diarrhea)
- Long-term use of NSAIDs or other antiinflammatory drugs, especially with new onset of GI symptoms; back or shoulder pain of unknown cause
- Long-term use of immunosuppressives or corticosteroids with onset of constitutional symptoms, especially fever
- Insidious onset of episodic back pain in a person younger than 40 who has a family history of spondyloarthropathy
- Joint pain preceded or accompanied by burning and urinary frequency (urethritis) and/or accompanied by eye irritation, crusting, redness, tearing, or burning usually lasting only a few days (**conjunctivitis; Reiter's syndrome**)
- Joint pain preceded or accompanied by skin rash or lesions (**psoriatic arthritis; Lyme disease; rheumatic fever**)
- New onset of inflammatory joint pain (especially monoarticular joint involvement) postoperatively, especially accompanied by extraarticular signs or symptoms such as rash, diarrhea, urethritis) (**reactive or bacterial arthritis**);

mouth ulcers (**Reiter's syndrome, systemic lupus erythematosus**); raised skin patches (**psoriatic arthritis**)

• Development of neurologic symptoms 1 to 3 weeks after an infection (**Guillain-Barré syndrome**)

⟲ KEY POINTS TO REMEMBER

✓ Pain in the knees, hands, wrists, or elbows may indicate an autoimmune disorder; aching in the bones can be caused by expanding bone marrow.

✓ True arthritis produces pain and limitation during both active and passive range of motion. Limitation from tendonitis is much worse during active range of motion.

✓ Any change in cough, pain, or fever and any change or new presentation of symptoms should be reported to the physician.

✓ Be alert to any warning signs of hypersensitivity response (allergic reaction) during therapy and be prepared to take necessary measures (e.g., graded exercise to client tolerance, control of room temperature, client use of medications).

✓ Immediate emergency procedures are required when a client has a severe allergic reaction (anaphylactic shock).

✓ For the client with Guillain-Barré syndrome, active exercise must be at a level consistent with the client's muscle strength. Overstretching and overuse of painful muscles may result in prolonged or lack of recovery.

✓ For the client with multiple sclerosis, treatment should take place in the coolest (temperature) setting possible.

✓ Increase in shoe size, marked fatigue, and onset of symptoms in the first year postpartum are important clues to the development of RA.

✓ For the client with rheumatoid arthritis or ankylosing spondylitis, the risk of fracture from the development of atlantoaxial subluxation necessitates the use of extreme caution in treatment procedures. The most common site of fracture is the lower cervical spine.

SUBJECTIVE EXAMINATION

Signs and symptoms of immune disorders can appear in any body system. A thorough review of the Family/Personal History form, subjective interview, and appropriate follow-up questions will help the therapist identify signs and symptoms that are not part of a musculoskeletal pattern. Special attention should be given to the question on the Family/Personal History form concerning general health. Clients with immune disorders or immunocompromised clients often have poor general health or recurrent infections.

Special Questions to Ask

When the immune system is involved, some important questions to ask include the following:

• How long have you had this problem? (acute vs. chronic)
• Has the problem gone away and then recurred?
• Have additional symptoms developed or have other areas become symptomatic over time?

Past Medical History

• Have you ever been told that you had/have an immune disorder, autoimmune disease,

SUBJECTIVE EXAMINATION—cont'd

or cancer? (Predisposes the person to other diseases)

- Have you ever had radiation treatment? (Diminishes blood cell production, predisposes to infection)
- Have you ever had an organ transplant (especially kidney) or removal of your thymus? **(Myasthenia gravis)**

Associated Signs and Symptoms

- Do you have difficulty with combing your hair; raising your arms; getting out of a bathtub, bed, or chair; or climbing stairs? **(Myasthenia gravis)**
- Do you have difficulty when raising your head from the pillow when you are lying down on your back? **(Myasthenia gravis)**
- Do you have difficulty with swallowing, or have you noticed any changes in your voice? **(Myasthenia gravis)**
- Have you noticed any changes in your skin texture or pigmentation? Do you have any skin rashes? **(Scleroderma, allergic reactions, systemic lupus erythematosus, rheumatoid arthritis, dermatomyositis, psoriatic arthritis, AIDS, Lyme disease)**
  - *If yes,* Have you noticed any association between the development of the skin rash and pain or swelling in any of your joints (or other symptoms)?
  - Do these other symptoms go away when the skin rash clears up?
  - Have you been exposed to ticks? For example, have you been out walking in the woods or in tall grass or in contact with pets? **(Lyme disease)**
- Have you had any recent vision problems? **(Multiple sclerosis, systemic lupus erythematosus)**
- Have you had any body tattooing or ear/body piercing done in the last 6 weeks to 6 months? **(AIDs, hepatitis)**
- Have you had any difficulties with urination—for example, a change in appearance of urine, accidents, increased frequency? **(Multiple sclerosis, myasthenia gravis, Reiter's syndrome)**

For the Person With Known Allergies (check the Family/Personal History form):

- What are the usual symptoms that you experience in association with your allergies?

- Describe a typical allergic reaction for you.
- Do the symptoms relate to physical changes (e.g., cold, heat, or dampness)?
- Do the symptoms occur in association with activities (e.g., exercise)?
- Do you take medication for your allergies?

For the Client Reporting Fatigue and Weakness:

- Do you feel tired all the time or only after exertion?
- Do you get short of breath after mild exercise or at rest?
- How much sleep do you get at night?
- Do you take naps during the day?
- Have you ever been told by a physician that you are anemic?
- How long have you had this weakness?
- Does it come and go, or is it persistent (there all the time)?
- Are you able to perform your usual daily activities without stopping to rest or nap?

For the Client With Sudden Onset of Joint Pain (Reiter's syndrome; see also Appendix: Special Questions to Ask: Joint Pain):

- Have you recently noticed any crusting, redness, or burning of your eyes?
- Have you noticed any burning when you urinate?
- Have you noticed an increase in the number of times you urinate?
- Have you had any bouts of diarrhea over the last 1 to 3 weeks (before the onset of joint pain)?
- *If yes* to any of these questions, have you ever been told you have a sexually transmitted infection such as herpes, genital warts, Reiter's disease, or other disease?

For the Client With Fever (fevers recurring every few days, fevers that rise and fall within 24 hours, and fevers that recur frequently should be documented and reported to the physician):

- When did you first notice this fever?
- Is it constant, or does it come and go?
- Does your temperature fluctuate?
- *If yes,* over what period of time does this occur?

CASE STUDY

REFERRAL

A 28-year-old Hispanic man has come to physical therapy for an evaluation without a medical referral. He has seen no medical practitioner for his current symptoms, consisting of an unusual gait pattern and weakness of the lower extremities, which he noticed during the last 2 days. He speaks English with a heavy accent, making it difficult to obtain a clear medical history, but the Personal/Family History form (see example in Fig. 2-2) indicates no previous or current health or medical problems of any kind. He does note that he has had influenza in the last 3 weeks but that he is fully recovered now.

PHYSICAL THERAPY INTERVIEW

Using the format outlined in the chapter on Interviewing as a Screening Tool (Chapter 2), begin with an open-ended question and follow up with additional appropriate questions incorporating the following:

Current Symptoms

- Tell me why you are here (open-ended question). Or you may prefer to say, "I notice from your intake form that you have had some weakness in your legs and a change in the way you walk. What can you tell me about this?"
- When did you first notice these changes?
- What did you notice that made you think that something was happening?
- Just before the development of these symptoms, did you injure yourself in any way that you can remember?
- Did you have a car accident, fall down, or twist your trunk or hips in any unusual way?
- Do you have any pain in your back, hips, or legs? If yes, use Figure 3-6 to elicit a further description.

Associated Symptoms

- Have you had any numbness or tingling in your back, buttocks, or hips or down your legs?
- Have you had any other changes in sensation in these areas, such as a burning or prickling feeling?
- Besides the flu have you had any other infection recently (e.g., head cold, upper respiratory infection, urinary tract infection)?
- Have you had a fever or elevated temperature in the last 48 hours?

- Do you think that you have a temperature right now?
- Have you noticed any other symptoms that I should know about?

Give the client time to answer the question. Prompt him or her if necessary with various suggestions (include any others that seem appropriate to the information and responses already given by the client; a similar checklist is provided in Fig. 3-6), such as the following:

- Nausea or dizziness
- Unusual fatigue
- Choking, difficulty with chewing
- Cold sweats during the day or night
- Skin rashes
- Shortness of breath with mild exertion (e.g., walking to the car or even at rest)
- Have you noticed any other respiratory, lung, or breathing problems?

- Diarrhea or constipation
- Recent headaches
- Vomiting
- Changes in vision or speech
- Joint pains

Final Question

Is there anything else you think that I should know about your current condition or general health that I have not asked yet?

Procedures to Carry Out During the First Session

Given the client's report of lower extremity weakness and antalgic gait of sudden onset without precipitating cause, the following possible problems should be assessed during the examination:

- Neurologic disease or disorder (immunologically based or otherwise), such as:
  - Discogenic lesion
  - Tumor
  - Myasthenia gravis (unlikely because of the man's age)
  - Guillain-Barré syndrome (recent history of the "flu")
  - Multiple sclerosis
  - AIDS dementia (unlikely given the way the history was presented)
  - Psychogenic disorder (e.g., hysteria, anxiety, alcoholism, or drug addiction)

Observation/Inspection

- Take the client's vital signs.
- Note any obvious changes, such as muscle atrophy, difficulty with breathing or swallowing, facial paralysis, intention tremor.

CASE STUDY—cont'd

- Describe the gait pattern: Observe for ataxia, incoordination, positive Trendelenburg position, balance, patterns of muscular weakness or imbalance, other gait deviations.

Neurologic Screening Examination

- All deep tendon reflexes
- Manual muscle testing of proximal-to-distal large muscle groups, looking for a pattern of weakness
- Babinski sign and clonus
- Gross sensory screen, looking for any differences in perceived sensation, proprioception, or vibration from one side to the other
- Test for dysmetria, balance, and coordination

Orthopedic Assessment

- Lower extremity range of motion (ROM): active and passive
- Back, lower quadrant evaluation protocol[67]

Testing Results

In the case of this client, the interview revealed very little additional information because he denied any other associated (systemic) signs or symptoms and denied bowel/bladder dysfunction, precipitating injury or trauma, and neurologic indications such as numbness, tingling, or paresthesias. Although he was difficult to understand, the therapist thought that the client had understood the questions and had answered them truthfully. Subjectively, he did not appear to be a malingerer or a hysterical/anxious individual.

The client's gait pattern could best be described as ataxic. His lower extremities would not support him fully, and he frequently lost his balance and fell down, although he denied any pain or warning that he was about to fall.

Objective findings revealed inconsistent results of muscle testing. The proximal muscles were more involved than the distal muscles (difference of one grade: proximal muscles = fair grade; distal muscles = good grade), but repeated tests elicited alternately strong, weak, or cogwheel responses, as if the muscles were moving in a ratcheting motion against resistance through the ROM.

The only other positive findings were slightly diminished deep tendon reflexes of the lower extremities compared with the upper extremities, but, again, these findings were inconsistent when tested over time.

Final Results

Because the subjective and objective examinations were so inconsistent and puzzling, the therapist asked another therapist to briefly examine this client. In turn, the second therapist decided to ask the client to return either at the end of the day or for the first appointment of the next day to reexamine him for any changes in the pattern of his symptoms. It was more convenient for him to return the next day, and he did.

At that time, it became clear that the therapist's difficulty in understanding the client had less to do with his use of English as a second language and more to do with an increasingly slurred speech pattern. His gait remained unchanged, but the muscle strength of the proximal pelvic muscles was consistently weak over several trials spread out during the therapy session, which lasted for 1 hour.

This time, the therapist checked the muscles of his upper extremities and found that the scapular muscles were also unable to move against any manual resistance. Deep tendon reflexes of the upper extremities were inconsistently diminished, and reflexes of the lower extremities were now consistently diminished.

The client was referred to a physician for further follow-up and was not treated at the physical therapy clinic that day. He was examined by his family physician, who referred him to a neurologist. A diagnosis of Guillain-Barré syndrome was confirmed when the client's symptoms progressed dramatically, requiring hospitalization.

PRACTICE QUESTIONS

1. Fibromyalgia syndrome is a
   a. Musculoskeletal disorder
   b. Psychosomatic disorder
   c. Neurosomatic disorder
   d. Noninflammatory rheumatic disorder

2. Which of the following best describes the pattern of rheumatic joint disease?
   a. Pain and stiffness in the morning gradually improves with gentle activity and movement during the day.
   b. Pain and stiffness accelerate during the day and are worse in the evening.
   c. Night pain is frequently associated with advanced structural damage seen on x-ray.
   d. Pain is brought on by activity and resolves predictably with rest.

3. Match the following skin lesions with the associated underlying disorder:
   a. Raised, scaly patches _____ Psoriatic arthritis
   b. Flat or slightly raised malar on the face _____ Systemic lupus erythematosus
   _____ HIV infection
   c. Petechiae _____ Scleroderma
   d. Tightening of the skin _____ Rheumatoid arthritis
   e. Kaposi's sarcoma _____ Allergic reaction
   f. Erythema migrans _____ Lyme disease
   g. Hives _____ Thrombocytopenia
   h. Subcutaneous nodules

4. A new client has come to you with a primary report of new onset of knee pain and swelling. Name three clues that this client might give from his medical history that should alert you to the possibility of immunologic disease.

5. A positive Schöber's test, is a sign of
   a. Reiter's syndrome
   b. Infectious arthritis
   c. Ankylosing spondylitis
   d. (a) or (b)
   e. (a) or (c)

6. What is Lhermitte's sign, and what does it signify?

7. Proximal muscle weakness may be a sign of
   a. Paraneoplastic syndrome
   b. Neurologic disorder
   c. Myasthenia gravis
   d. Scleroderma
   e. (b), (c), and (d)
   f. All of the above

8. Which of the following skin assessment findings in the HIV-infected client occurs with Kaposi's sarcoma?
   a. Darkening of the nail beds
   b. Purple-red blotches or bumps on the trunk and head
   c. Cyanosis of the lips and mucous membranes
   d. Painful blistered lesions of the face and neck

9. The most common cause of change in mental status of the HIV-infected client is related to:
   a. Meningitis
   b. Alzheimer's disease
   c. Space-occupying lesions
   d. AIDS dementia complex

10. Symptoms of anaphylaxis that would necessitate immediate medical treatment or referral are
    a. Hives and itching
    b. Vocal hoarseness, sneezing, and chest tightness
    c. Periorbital edema
    d. Nausea and abdominal cramping

REFERENCES

1. Klippel JH, editor: *Primer on the Rheumatic Diseases*, ed 12, Atlanta, Ga, Arthritis Foundation, 2001.
2. Centers for Disease Control and Prevention (CDC): HIV/AIDS Fact Sheet October 19, 2005. Available at: http://www.cdc.gov/omh/AMH/factsheets/hiv.htm. Accessed November 28, 2005.
3. Janssen RS, Onorato IM: Advancing HIV prevention: new strategies for a changing epidemic—United States, 2003, *MMWR* 52(15):329-332, 18, 2003.
4. Porter K, Babiker A, Bhaskaran K: Determinants of survival following HIV-1 seroconversion after the introduction of HAART, *Lancet* 362(9392):1267-1274, 2003.
5. Centers for Disease Control and Prevention National Prevention Information Network (NPIN): African-Americans. Available at: http://www.cdcnpin.org/scripts/population/afram.asp. Accessed November 28, 2005.
6. Espinoza L, Hall HI, Campsmith ML, et al: Trends in HIV/AIDS diagnoses—33 states, 2001-2004, *MMWR* 54(45):1149-1153, 2005.

7. Jaffe H, Janssen R: Incorporating HIV prevention into the medical care of persons living with HIV, *MMWR* 52 (RR 12):1-24, 2003.

8. McIntyre J: Preventing mother-to-child transmission of HIV: successes and challenges, *BJOG* 112(9):1196-1203, 2005.

9. Coutsoudis A: Infant feeding dilemmas created by HIV: South African experiences, *J Nutr* 135(4):956-959, 2005.

10. Kenny P: The changing face of AIDS, *Nursing 2004* 34(8):54-63, 2004.

11. Qaqish RB, Sims KA: Bone disorders associated with the human immunodeficiency virus: pathogenesis and management, *Pharmacotherapy* 24(10):1331-1346, 2004.

12. Abrescia N, D'Abbraccio M, Figoni M, et al: Hepatotoxicity of antiretroviral drugs, *Curr Pharm Des* 11(28):3697-3710, 2005.

13. Baba M: Advances in antiviral chemotherapy, *Uirusu* 55(1):69-75, 2005.

14. Malita FM, Karelis AD, Toma E, et al: Effects of different types of exercise on body composition and fat distribution in HIV-infected patients: a brief review, *Can J Appl Physiol* 30(2):233-245, 2005.

15. Sweet DE: Metabolic complications of antiretroviral therapy, *Top HIV Med* 13(2):70-74, 2005.

16. Carbone A, Gloghini A: AIDS-related lymphomas: from pathogenesis to pathology, *Br J Haematol* 130(5):662-670, 2005.

17. Kasamon YL, Ambinder RF: AIDS-related primary central nervous system lymphoma, *Hematol Oncol Clin North Am* 19(4):665-687, 2005.

18. Sherman M: Hepatocellular carcinoma: epidemiology, risk factors, and screening, *Semin Liver Dis* 25(2):143-154, 2005.

19. Deshpande A, Mrinal M, Patnaik M: Nonopportunistic neurologic manifestations of the human immunodeficiency virus: an Indian study, *eJIAS, Medscape General Medicine* 7(3):1-2, 2005. Available at: http://www.medscape.com/viewarticle/511865. Accessed on-line November 26, 2005.

20. Cade W, Peralta L, Keyser R: Aerobic exercise dysfunction in HIV: A potential link to physical disability, *Physical Therapy* 84(7): 655-664, 2004.

21. Hallegua DS, Wallace DJ: Managing fibromyalgia: a comprehensive approach, *J Musculoskel Med* 22(8):382-390, 2005.

22. Wolfe F: Stop using the American College of Rheumatology criteria in the clinic, *J Rheumatol* 30(8):1671-1672, 2003.

23. American Association for Chronic Fatigue Syndrome: CFS Conference Highlights: The merging of two syndromes, *Fibromyalgia Network* 61:4-70, 2003.

24. Leventhal L, Bouali H: Fibromyalgia: 20 clinical pearls, *J Musculoskeletal Med* 20(2):59-65, 2003.

25. Clauw D: Fibromyalgia: Correcting the misconceptions, *J Musculoskeletal Med* 20(10):467-472, 2003.

26. Hulme J: *Fibromyalgia: a handbook for self-care and treatment*, ed 3, Missoula, Mt, Phoenix, 2000. www.phoenix-pub.com; 1-800-549-8371.

27. Lowe JR: *The metabolic treatment of fibromyalgia*, McDowell Publishing Company, 1999. (Available from McDowell Publishing Company; phone: (303)-570-7231 or by email: McDPubCo@McDowellPublishing.com or on-line at http://www.McDowellPublishing.com).

28. Koch A: Targeting cytokines and growth factors in RA, *J Musculoskel Med* 22(3):130-136, 2005.

29. Freeston J, Keenan AM, Emery P: Spotting the early warning signs of aggressive RA, *J Musculoskel Med* 22(10):503-512, 2005.

30. Bykerk V, Keystone E: RA in primary care: 20 clinical pearls, *J Musculoskel Med* 21(3):133-146, 2004.

31. Yazici Y, Erkan D, Paget S: Inflammatory musculoskeletal diseases in the elderly, Part I, *J Musculoskel Med* 19(7):265-276, 2002.

32. Moorthy L, Onel K: Juvenile idiopathic arthritis: making the diagnosis, *J Musculoskel Med* 21(11):581-588, 2004.

33. Clinical Update: advances in rheumatology: new approaches to early diagnosis and treatment, *J Musculoskel Med* 21(10):509-560, 2004.

34. Flendrie M, Vissers WH, Creemers MC, et al: Dermatological conditions during TNR-alpha-blocking therapy in patients with rheumatoid arthritis: a prospective study, *Arthritis Res Ther* 7(3):R666-6676, 2005.

35. Taylor M, Furst D: Biologic response modifiers: Addressing the safety concerns, *J Musculoskel Med* 22(5):223-239, 2005.

36. Labbe P, Hardouin P: Epidemiology and optimal management of polymyalgia rheumatica, *Drugs Aging* 13(2):109-118, 1998.

37. Spiera R, Spiera H: Inflammatory diseases in older adults: polymyalgia rheumatica, *Geriatrics* 59(11):39-43, 2004.

38. Versluis RG, Papapoulous SE: Clinical risk factors as predictors of postmenopausal osteoporosis in general practice, *Brit J Gen Pract* 51(471):805-809, 2001.

39. Salvarani C, Cantini F, Bioardi L, et al: Polymyalgia rheumatica, *Best Pract Res Clin Rheumatol* 18(5):705-722, 2004.

40. Formica MK, Palmer JR, Rosenberg L, et al: Smoking, alcohol consumption, and risk of systemic lupus erythematosus in the Black Women's Health Study, *J Rheumatol* 30:1222-1226, 2003.

41. Petri M: Systemic lupus erythematosis: New management strategies, *J Musculoskel Med* 22(3):108-116, 2005.

42. Zulian F, Vallongo C, Woo P, et al: Localized scleroderma in childhood is not just a skin disease, *Arthritis Rheum* 52(9):2873-2881, 2005.

43. Steen VD: Clinical manifestations of systemic sclerosis, *Semin Cutan Med Surg* 17(1):48-54, 1998.

44. Steen VD: Autoantibodies in systemic sclerosis, *Semin Arthritis Rheum* 35(1):35-42, 2005.

45. Steen VD, Syzd A, Johnson JP, et al: Kidney disease other than renal crisis in patients with diffuse scleroderma, *J Rheumatol* 32(4):649-655, 2005.

46. Moxley G: Scleroderma and related diseases, WebMD Scientific American® Medicine. Posted 03/22/2004. Available at: www.medscape.com/viewarticle/472036. Accessed November 28, 2005.

47. Highland KB, Silver RM: New developments in scleroderma interstitial lung disease, *Curr Opin Rheumatol* 17(6):737-745, 2005.

48. Gomez KS, Raza K, Jones SD, et al: Juvenile onset ankylosing spondylitis: more girls than we thought? *J Rheumatol* 24(4):735-737, 1997.

49. Ostensen M, Ostensen H: Ankylosing spondylitis: the female aspect, *J Rheumatol* 25(1):120-124, 1998.

50. Levine DS, Forbat SM, Saifuddin A: MRI of the axial skeletal manifestations of ankylosing spondylitis, *Clin Radiol* 59(5):400-413, 2004.

51. Lewis R, Creamer P: Ankylosing spondylitis: early diagnosis and management, *J Musculoskel Med* 20(4):184-198, 2003.

52. Hitchon P, From A, Brenton M, et al: Fractures of the thoracolumbar spine complicating ankylosing spondylitis, *J Neurosurg (Spine 2)* 97:218-222, 2002.

53. Tullous MW, Skerhut HEI, Story JL, et al: Cauda equina syndrome of long-standing ankylosing spondylitis: case report and review of the literature, *J Neurosurg* 73:441-447, 1990.

54. Ahn NU, Ahn UM, Nallamshetty L, et al: Cauda equina syndrome in ankylosing spondylitis (the CES-AS syndrome): meta-analysis of outcomes after medical and surgical treatments, *J Spinal Disord* 14(5):427-233, 2001.

55. Korendowych E, McHugh N: Genetic factors in psoriatic arthritis, *Curr Rheumatol Rep* 7(4):306-312, 2005.

56. Leong TT, Faron U, Veale DJ: Angiogenesis in psoriasis and psoriatic arthritis: clues to disease pathogenesis, *Curr Rheumatol Rep* 7(4):325-329, 2005.

57. Qureshi AA, Husni ME, Mody E: Psoriatic arthritis and psoriasis: need for a multidisciplinary approach, *Semin Cutan Med Surg* 24(1):46-51, 2005.

58. Kalish R, Biggee B: Lyme disease: 20 clinical pearls, *J Musculoskel Med* 20(6):271-285, 2003.

59. Making sense of multiple sclerosis, *Harvard Women's Health Watch* 12(11):4-6, 2005.

60. Munger KL, Zhang SM, O'Reilly E, et al: Vitamin D intake and incidence of multiple sclerosis, *Neurology* 62(1):60-65, 2004.

61. Galea I, Newman TA, Gidron Y: Stress and exacerbations in multiple sclerosis, *BMJ* 328(7434):287, 2004.

62. Haslam C: Managing bladder symptoms in people with multiple sclerosis, *Nursing Times* 101(2):48-52, 2005.

63. Calabresi P: Diagnosis and management of multiple sclerosis, *American Family Physician* 70(10):1-14; 2004.

64. Lee AG, Berlie CL: Multiple sclerosis, *eMedicine* posted June 2, 2005. Available at: www.emedicine.com/oph/ topic179.htm. Accessed November 28, 2005.

65. Scherer K, Bedlack RS, Simel L: Does this patient have myasthenia gravis? *JAMA* 293(15):1906-1914, 2005.

66. Kubis KC, Danesh-Meyer HV, Savino PJ et al: The ice test versus the rest test in myasthenia gravis, *Ophthalmology* 107(11):1995-1998, 2000.

67. Magee DJ: *Orthopedic physical assessment*, ed 4, Philadelphia, 2002, Saunders.

Screening for Cancer

13

A 56-year-old man has come to you for an evaluation without a referral. He has not seen any type of physician for at least 3 years. He is seeking an examination at the insistence of his wife, who has noticed that his collar size has increased two sizes in the last year and that his neck looks "puffy." He has no complaints of any kind (including pain or discomfort), and he denies any known trauma; however, his wife insists that he has limited ability in turning his head when backing the car out of the driveway.

- What questions would be appropriate for your first physical therapy interview with this client?
- What test procedures will you carry out during the first session?
- If you suggest to this man that he should see his physician, how would you make that recommendation? (See the Case Study at the end of the chapter.)

A large part of the screening process is identifying red flag histories and red flag signs and symptoms. Advancing age and previous history of any kind of cancer are two of the most important risk factors for cancer. Following the screening model presented in Chapters 1 and 2, the therapist will use past medical history, clinical presentation, and associated signs and symptoms as the basic tools to screen for cancer.

The client history with interview is the number one tool for cancer screening. Take the client's history, looking for the presence of any risk factors for cancer. Cancer in its early stages is often asymptomatic. Survival rates are increased with early detection and screening, making this element of client management extremely important.

Keep in mind that some cancers such as malignant melanoma (skin cancer) do not have a highly effective treatment. Early detection and referral can make a life and death difference in the final outcome. Morbidity can be reduced and quality of life and function improved with early intervention.

Whether primary cancer, cancer that has recurred locally, or cancer that has metastasized, clinical manifestations can mimic neuromuscular or musculoskeletal dysfunction. The therapist's task is to identify abnormal tissue, not diagnose the lesion.

CANCER STATISTICS

Cancer is the second leading cause of death in the United States in persons under the age of 85 years. Only heart disease claims more lives. There are more than 1 million new cases of cancer in the United States each year; more than half a million will die from cancer this year. One in four deaths in the United States is attributed to cancer.

Predicting lifetime risk of cancer is based on present rates of cancer. Using today's epidemiologic data, 46% of all men and 38% of all

women will develop cancer at some time in their lifetime.[1]

In the past, certain types of cancer were invariably fatal. Today, however, death rates continue to decline for most cancers, and there continues to be a reported reduced mortality from cancer. The percentage of people who have survived longer than 5 years after cancer diagnosis has increased over the past 2 decades.[2]

Fig. 13-1 summarizes current U.S. figures for cancer incidence and deaths by site and sex. Although prostate and breast cancers are the most common malignancies in men and women, respectively, the cancer that most commonly causes death is lung cancer.[1]

Carcinoma in situ is not included in the statistics related to invasive carcinoma or sarcoma as reported by the American Cancer Society (ACS) or the National Cancer Institute (NCI). Carcinoma in situ is considered a premalignant cancer that is localized to the organ of origin. As noted, it is reported separately and primarily relative to breast and skin cancer. Carcinoma in situ of the breast accounts for about 58,490 new cases every year, and in situ melanoma accounts for about 46,170 new cases annually.[1]

Cancer Cure and Recurrence

Cancer is considered cured or in remission when evidence of the disease cannot be found in the individual's body. Early diagnosis and aggressive intervention help people obtain a cure. In general, individuals with no evidence of cancer have the same life expectancy as those who never had

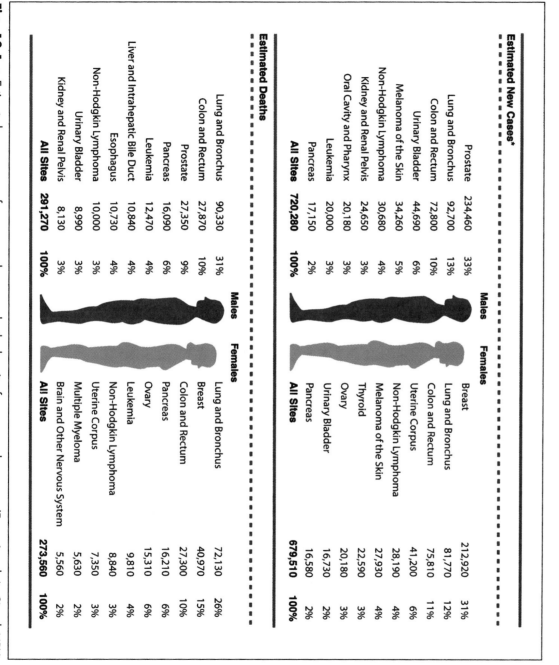

Estimated New Cases*

Males			Females		
Prostate	234,460	33%	Breast	212,920	31%
Lung and Bronchus	92,700	13%	Lung and Bronchus	81,770	12%
Colon and Rectum	72,800	10%	Colon and Rectum	75,810	11%
Urinary Bladder	44,690	6%	Uterine Corpus	41,200	6%
Melanoma of the Skin	34,260	5%	Non-Hodgkin Lymphoma	28,190	4%
Non-Hodgkin Lymphoma	30,680	4%	Melanoma of the Skin	27,930	4%
Kidney and Renal Pelvis	24,650	3%	Thyroid	22,590	3%
Oral Cavity and Pharynx	20,180	3%	Ovary	20,180	3%
Leukemia	20,000	3%	Urinary Bladder	16,730	2%
Pancreas	17,150	2%	Pancreas	16,580	2%
All Sites	**720,280**	**100%**	**All Sites**	**679,510**	**100%**

Estimated Deaths

Males			Females		
Lung and Bronchus	90,330	31%	Lung and Bronchus	72,130	26%
Colon and Rectum	27,870	10%	Breast	40,970	15%
Prostate	27,350	9%	Colon and Rectum	27,300	10%
Pancreas	16,090	6%	Pancreas	16,210	6%
Leukemia	12,470	4%	Ovary	15,310	6%
Liver and Intrahepatic Bile Duct	10,840	4%	Leukemia	9,810	4%
Esophagus	10,730	4%	Non-Hodgkin Lymphoma	8,840	3%
Non-Hodgkin Lymphoma	10,000	3%	Uterine Corpus	7,350	3%
Urinary Bladder	8,990	3%	Multiple Myeloma	5,630	2%
Kidney and Renal Pelvis	8,130	3%	Brain and Other Nervous System	5,560	2%
All Sites	**291,270**	**100%**	**All Sites**	**273,560**	**100%**

Fig. 13-1 • Estimated new cases of cancer and cancer deaths by site for men and women. (From Jemal A, Siegel MPH, Ward E, et al: Cancer statistics 2006, CA: A Cancer Journal for Clinicians 56:106-130, 2006.)

cancer. However, late physical and psychosocial complications of disease and treatment are being recognized.

Cancer recurrence or a new cancer can occur in some individuals with a previous personal history of cancer. Causes of cancer recurrence can include inadequate surgical margin, skip metastases, tumor thrombus, and lymph node metastasis.

Additionally, many of the antineoplastic strategies (e.g., chemotherapy, hormone therapy, radiation therapy) mutate cells further and can initiate or stimulate new malignant tumors. The therapist should consider it a red flag any time a client has a previous history of cancer or cancer treatment.

Childhood Cancers

Cancer is the second leading cause of death in children between the ages of 1 and 14, with accidents remaining the most frequent cause of death in this age group. The most frequently occurring cancers in children are leukemia (primarily, acute lymphocytic leukemia), brain and other nervous system cancers, soft tissue sarcomas, non-Hodgkin's lymphoma, and renal (Wilms') tumor.[1]

Survival rates for childhood cancer have increased to almost 80% now, because of improvements in treatment for many types of cancer over the past 2 decades. The result is an increasing population of long-term cancer survivors. Currently, 1 in 900 young adults is a childhood cancer survivor. Long-term health problems related to the effects of cancer therapy are a major focus of this population group.[3]

It has been shown that, to varying degrees, long-term survivors of childhood cancer are at risk of developing second cancers and of experiencing organ dysfunction, such as cardiomyopathy, joint dysfunction, reduced growth and development, decreased fertility, and early death.[4]

The degree of risk of late effects may be influenced by various treatment-related factors such as the intensity, duration, and timing of therapy. Individual characteristics such as the type of cancer diagnosis, the person's sex, age at time of intervention, and genetic factors as indicated by, for example, family history of cancer may also play a role in cancer recurrence and late effects of treatment.[4,5]

Ethnicity

Racial/ethnic minorities account for a disproportionate number of newly diagnosed cancers. African Americans have a 10% higher incidence rate than whites and a 30% higher death rate from all cancers combined than whites.[1,6]

African Americans have the highest mortality and worst survival of any population. Not only that, but diagnosis occurs at a later stage.[1] The statistics have gotten worse over the past 20 years, and studies have shown that equal treatment yields equal outcomes among individuals with equal disease.[7,8]

Compared with the general population, African Americans die of cancer at a 40% greater rate [they are 30% more likely to die from heart disease]. The Institute of Medicine (IOM) document, *Unequal Treatment, Confronting Racial and Ethnic Disparities in Health Care*, suggests that care providers may be part of the problem.[8]

In terms of risk assessment, therapists must keep these figures in mind when examining and evaluating clients of African American descent. For any ethnic group, the therapist is advised to be aware of cancer and disease demographics and epidemiology for that particular group.

Cancer statistics for Hispanic Americans compared with non-Hispanic Americans are becoming more available.[9,10] There are lower rates of incidence and mortality from the four major cancer killers (breast, prostate, lung, colorectal) but a higher incidence and mortality from cancer with an infectious etiology (stomach, liver, uterine cervix, gallbladder).

The use of cancer screening tests and early detection has been increasing among this group. Mammography among Hispanic women exceeds the national average, but screening for colorectal, cervical, and prostate cancers is below average.

Cancer statistics and epidemiology in this group are problematic. Hispanic people originate from 23 different countries and have enormous diversity among themselves. They are the poorest minority group and have the highest uninsured rate of all groups. The uninsured are less likely to get preventive care such as cancer screening.

The most common cancer among Hispanic women is breast cancer; second is lung cancer. Men are more likely to have prostate cancer but die more often of lung cancer. Hispanics have twice the incidence rate and a 70% higher death rate from liver cancer compared with non-Hispanics. This type of cancer is on the rise in Hispanic women. Cancer is typically diagnosed in Hispanics at a later stage than in non-Hispanic white Americans. Consequently, they have lower cure rates.

Therapists can offer health care education and cancer screening to this unique group of people. This will be increasingly common in our practice as our health care delivery system moves from an illness-based system to a health promotion–based

system. For all groups, high-quality prevention and early detection and intervention can reduce cancer incidence and mortality.[2]

▶ RISK FACTOR ASSESSMENT

Risk factor assessment is a part of the cancer prevention model. Every health care professional has a role and a responsibility to help clients identify risk factors for disease. Knowing the various risk factors for different kinds of cancers is an important part of the medical screening process. Educating clients about their risk factors is a key element in risk factor reduction.

A new branch of medicine called *Preventive Oncology* has developed to address this important area. Preventive oncology or chemoprevention includes primary and secondary prevention. Chemoprevention is based on the hypothesis that certain non-toxic chemicals (e.g., retinoids, cyclooxygenase [COX]-2 inhibitors, hormonal agents) can be given preventatively to interrupt the biological processes involved in carcinogenesis and thus reduce its incidence. Currently, many clinical trials and studies have been devoted to the idea of chemical prevention of cancer development.[11]

Therapists can have an active role in both primary and secondary prevention through screening and education. Primary Prevention involves stopping the processes that lead to the formation of cancer in the first place. According to the *Guide to Physical Therapist Practice*,[12] physical therapists are involved in primary prevention by "preventing a target condition in a susceptible or potentially susceptible population through such specific measures as general health promotion efforts" (*Guide*, p. 41). Risk factor assessment and risk reduction fall under this category.

Secondary Prevention involves regular screening for early detection of cancer and the prevention of progression of known pre-malignant lesions such as skin and colon lesions. This does not prevent cancer but improves the outcome. The *Guide* outlines the physical therapist's role in secondary prevention as "decreasing duration of illness, severity of disease, and number of sequelae through early diagnosis and prompt intervention" (*Guide*, p. 41).

Another way to look at this is through the use of screening and surveillance. *Screening* is a method for detecting disease or body dysfunction before an individual would normally seek medical care. Medical screening tests are usually administered to individuals who do not have current symp-

toms, but who may be at high risk for certain adverse health outcomes.

Surveillance is the analysis of health information to look for problems that may be occurring in the workplace that require targeted prevention. Surveillance has often used screening results from groups of individuals to look for abnormal trends in health status.

Known Risk Factors for Cancer

Certain risk factors have been identified as linked to cancer in general (Table 13-1). More than half of all cancer deaths in the United States could be prevented if Americans adopted a healthier lifestyle and made better use of available screening tests.[13]

According to the NCI, environmental factors, whether linked to lifestyle issues such as smoking and diet or exposure to carcinogens in the air and water, are thought to be linked to an estimated 80% to 90% of cancer cases.[14]

Some of the most common risk factors for cancer include the following:

- Age over 50 (single most important risk factor)
- Ethnicity
- Family history (1st generation)
- Environment and lifestyle

Age

In particular, the therapist must pay close attention to the client's age in correlation with a personal or family history of cancer. Many cancers, such as prostate, colon, ovarian, and some chronic leukemias, have increased incidence in older adults. The incidence of cancer doubles after 25 years of age and increases with every 5-year increase in age until the mid-80s, when cancer incidence and mortality reach a plateau and even decline slightly.

Other cancers occur within very narrow age ranges. Testicular cancer is found in men from about 20 to 40 years of age. Breast cancer shows a sharp increase after age 45. Ovarian cancer is more common in women older than 55. A number of cancers, such as Ewing's sarcoma, acute leukemia, Wilms' tumor, and retinoblastoma, occur mainly in childhood.

Screening for age is discussed more completely in Chapter 2. Please refer to this section for information on screening for this red flag/risk factor.

Ethnicity

As previously mentioned, racial minorities and ethnic groups account for a disproportionate number of newly diagnosed cancers. Screening for ethnicity is discussed more completely in Chapter

TABLE 13-1 ▼ Risk Factors for Cancer

Nonmodifiable risk factors	Modifiable risk factors
Age	Smoking, use of smokeless tobacco
Previous history of cancer	Chemical or other exposure (e.g., paint, cadmium, dye, rubber, arsenic, asbestos, radon, benzene, ionizing radiation, Agent Orange, pesticides, herbicides, organic amines)
Ethnicity	Urban dwelling
Skin color	Alcohol consumption (more than 1-2 drinks per day)
Gender	Sedentary lifestyle; lack of exercise
Heredity (identified oncogenes)	Obesity; diet high in animal fat
Age of menarche, menopause	Radiation/chemotherapy treatment
Adenomatous polyps	Estrogen replacement therapy
Inflammatory bowel disease	Sexually transmitted diseases
Fat distribution patterns	Ionizing radiation
Congenital immunodeficiencies	HTLV-1 (virus, rare in U.S.)
Congenital diseases	Previous lung scarring
Long-term *Helicobacter* infection	Organ transplantation (immunosuppression)
	HIV infection
	Chronic exposure to UV rays
	Geographic location
	Smoked foods, salted fish and meat (nitrates and nitrites)
	Tamoxifen use
	Nulliparity (never having children)
	Vitamin B$_{12}$ deficiency
	Lack of access to or use of health care and screening tests

HTLV-1, Human T lymphotropic virus type 1; *HIV,* human immunodeficiency virus; *UV,* ultraviolet.

2. Please refer to this section for information on screening for this important red flag/risk factor.

Family History and Genetics

Family history is often an important factor in the development of some cancers. This usually includes only first generation family members, including parents, siblings, and children.

Hereditary cancer syndromes account for approximately 5% of breast, ovarian, and colon cancers. Both clients and providers are becoming aware of the potential therapeutic advantages of early identification of hereditary cancer risk.

The hereditary syndromes most frequently identified are hereditary breast and ovarian cancer syndrome (HBOC) due to mutations in BRCA1 and BRCA2 genes; hereditary colon cancer (HCC), specifically, familial adenomatous polyposis (FAP); and hereditary nonpolyposis colorectal cancer.

The small percentage of people who may be suspected of having a hereditary cancer syndrome can be screened regarding personal and family medical history. Critical details such as the cancer site and age at diagnosis are needed for risk assessment. The following are some basic hallmarks of families who could have a hereditary cancer syndrome[15]:

- Diagnosis of cancer in two or more relatives in a family
- Diagnosis of cancer in a family member under the age of 50
- Occurrence of the same type of cancer in several members of a family
- Occurrence of more than one type of cancer in one person
- Occurrence of a rare type of cancer in one or more members of a family[16]

Environment and Lifestyle Factors

It is now apparent that, although genetic predisposition varies, the two key factors determining whether or not people develop cancer are environment and lifestyle. The most important way to reduce cancer risk is to avoid cancer-causing agents.

Obesity, diet, sedentary lifestyle, sexual practices, and the use of tobacco, drugs, and/or alcohol make up the largest percentage of modifiable risk factors for cancer. Current data support the findings that obesity, inappropriate diet, and excess weight cause around one-third of all cancer deaths (Table 13-2).[17,18] Increased body weight and obesity are associated with increased death rates for all cancers and for cancers at specific

TABLE 13-2 ▼ Cancers Linked to Obesity, Diet, and Nutrition

Mouth, pharynx, esophagus	Colon, rectum
Larynx	Breast
Lung	Ovary
Stomach	Endometrium
Pancreas	Cervix
Gallbladder	Prostate
Liver	Kidney
	Bladder
	Uterus

Data from American Institute for Cancer Research (AICR): *Food, nutrition, and the prevention of cancer: a global perspective,* Washington, D.C., 1997. (A second report is due to be published in 2007. Check for updates at www.wcrf.org.)

sites, especially when combined with a sedentary lifestyle.[19-21]

Overweight and obesity may account for 20% of all cancer deaths in U.S. women and 14% in U.S. men.[22] It is estimated that 90,000 cancer deaths could be prevented each year if Americans maintained a healthy body weight.[19]

Excess body weight increases amounts of circulating hormones such as estrogens, androgens, and insulin, all of which are associated with cellular and tumor growth. It has also been shown that physical activity reduces the risk of breast and colon cancers and may reduce the risk of several other types of cancer by decreasing excess body weight and by actually decreasing the circulation of some of the growth-related hormones.[23]

In 1999, the American Institute for Cancer Research (AICR) estimated that at least 20% of all cancers could be prevented if everyone ate at least 5 (½ cup) servings of fruits and vegetables each day.[17] The American Cancer Society offers numerous publications on nutrition and its influence in preventing and treating cancer.[24-26]

Dietary guidelines were updated to 9 servings a day (equal to 4.5 cups) for overall health and chemoprevention in January 2005 by the U.S. Department of Health and Human Services (HHS) in the publication *Dietary Guidelines for Americans 2005.* The *Guidelines* provide authoritative advice for people 2 years of age and older about how good dietary habits can promote health and reduce risks of major chronic diseases.

Specific factors associated with individual cancer types are known in some cases. For example, inadequate hydration is known to increase the risks of colon and bladder cancers. Alcohol consumption is linked with breast, head or neck, and gastrointestinal (GI) cancers. High dietary animal fat intake and tobacco use increase prostate cancer risk. Adenomatous polyps in the colon are known precursors of colorectal cancer.

SEXUALLY TRANSMITTED INFECTIONS

Sexually transmitted diseases (STDs) or sexually transmitted infections (STIs) have been positively identified as a risk factor for cancer. Not all STIs are linked with cancer, but studies have confirmed that human papillomavirus (HPV) is the primary cause of cervical cancer (see Fig. 4-18). With current technology, high-risk HPV DNA can be detected in cervical specimens.[27]

HPV is the leading viral STI in the United States. More than 70 types of HPV have been identified; 23 infect the cervix, and 13 types are associated with cancer (men and women). Infection with one of these viruses does not predict cancer, but the risk of cancer is increased.

In 1970, 1 of every 300 Americans had an STI. Today, 3 million teenagers contract STIs every year; STIs affect about 1 in 4 teens who are sexually active. It is estimated that among women ages 18 to 25 who are sexually active, 4 out of 5 have some form of STI. Nearly 50% of African American teenagers have genital herpes.[28] For every unwed adolescent who gets pregnant this year, 10 teenagers will get an STI.[29,30]

TOBACCO USE

Tobacco and tobacco products are known carcinogens, not just for lung cancer, but also for leukemia and cancers of the cervix, kidney, pancreas, stomach, bladder, esophagus, and oropharyngeal and laryngeal structures. This includes second-hand smoke, pipes, cigars, cigarettes, and chewing (smokeless) tobacco. Combining tobacco with caffeine and/or alcohol brings on additional problems. More people die from tobacco use than from use of alcohol and all the other addictive agents combined.

In any physical therapy practice, clients should be screened for the use of tobacco products (see Fig. 2-2). Client education includes a review of the physiologic effects of tobacco (see Table 2-3). For a more complete discussion of screening for tobacco use, see Chapter 2.

If the client indicates a desire to quit smoking or using tobacco, the therapist must be prepared to help him or her explore options for smoking cessation. Pamphlets and other reading material should be available for any client interested in tobacco cessation. Referral to medical doctors who specialize in smoking cessation may be appropriate for some clients.

OCCUPATION AND LOCAL ENVIRONMENT

Well-defined problems occur in people engaging in specific occupations, especially involving exposure to chemicals and gases. Exposure to carcinogens in the air and water and on our food sources may be linked to cancer. Isolated cases of excessive copy toner dust linked with lung cancer have been reported.[31,32]

Reactions can be delayed up to 30 years, making client history an extremely important tool in identifying potential risk factors. People may or may not even remember past exposures to chemicals or gases. Some may not be aware of childhood exposures. Taking a work or military history may be important (see Chapter 2 and Appendix B-13).

The industrial chemicals people are exposed to vary across the country and will depend on where the individual has lived or where the client lives now. Each state in the United States has its own unique environmental issues. For example, in Montana, there has been a significant chlorine spill, exposure to agricultural chemicals, vermiculite mining, and many other forms of mining.

In New York, Love Canal was the focus of concern in the 1980s and 1990s, when the effects of hazardous wastes dumped in the area were discovered. Alaskan oil spills, air pollution in Los Angeles, and hazardous and radioactive nuclear waste in Washington state burial grounds are a few more examples.

In Utah, Nevada, and Arizona, the Radiation Exposure Compensation Act (RECA) was passed by Congress in 1990, after studies showed a possible link between hundreds of above ground nuclear tests in the late 1950s and early 1960s and various cancers and primary organ diseases.[33-36] Ground-water wells at old open pit copper mines in various states have tested positive for uranium up to 40 times higher than legal limits. Hundreds of active wells tap into groundwater within 5 miles of these sites.

Wherever the therapist practices, it is important to be aware of local environmental issues and the impact these may have on people in the vicinity.

IONIZING RADIATION

Exposure to ionizing radiation is potentially harmful. Ionizing radiation is the result of electromagnetic waves entering the body and acting on neutral atoms or molecules with sufficient force to remove electrons, creating an ion. The most common sources of ionizing radiation exposure in humans are accidental environmental exposure and medical, therapeutic, or diagnostic irradiation.

Nonionizing radiation is electromagnetic radiation that includes radio waves, microwaves, infrared light, and visible light. Nonionizing radiation does not have enough energy to ionize (i.e., break up) atoms. Electronic devices such as laser scanners, high-intensity lamps, and electronic antitheft surveillance devices expose the human to nonionizing radiation. There is not a proven link between exposure to nonionizing radiation and cancer, but there is considerable speculation that long-term exposure to electromagnetic fields may be correlated with the development of various illnesses and diseases.

Some studies have reported the possibility of increased cancer risks, especially of leukemia and brain cancer, for electrical workers and others whose jobs require them to be around electrical equipment. Additional risk factors, however, such as exposure to cancer-initiating agents, may also be involved.[37]

Some researchers have looked at possible associations between electromagnetic exposure and breast cancer, miscarriages, depression, suicides, Alzheimer's disease, and amyotrophic lateral sclerosis (ALS, or Lou Gehrig's disease), but the general scientific consensus is that the evidence is not yet conclusive.[37]

Ultraviolet radiation (UVR), sometimes also called ultraviolet light, is invisible electromagnetic radiation of the same nature as visible light, but having shorter wavelengths and higher energies. The main source of natural ultraviolet radiation is the sun. UVR is conventionally divided into three bands in order of increasing energy: UV-A, UV-B, and UV-C.

In the electromagnetic spectrum, UVR extends between the blue end of the visible spectrum and low-energy x-rays, straddling the boundary between ionizing and nonionizing radiation (which is conventionally set at 100 nm). Because of the different wavelengths and energies, each of the three bands has distinct effects on biologic tissue.

The highest-energy band, UV-C, can damage DNA and other molecules and is used in hospitals for sterilization. UV-C is rapidly attenuated in air and, therefore, it is not found in ground-level solar radiation. Exposure to UV-C, however, can take place close to sources such as welding arcs or germicidal lamps.

UV-B is the most effective UV band in causing tanning and sunburn (erythema), and it can affect the immune system. UV-A penetrates deeper in the skin because of its longer wavelength and plays a role in skin photoaging. UV-A can also affect the immune system. Exposure to UV-A and

UV-B has been attributed to the development of skin cancer.

Tanning lamps emit mostly UV-A radiation with a few percent content of UV-B. Use of tanning lamps and beds can lead to significant exposure to UV-A radiation. Despite known negative health effects from the use of indoor tanning, this practice is still very popular in the United States and Europe, especially among adolescent girls. Therapists have a role in client education, especially concerning reducing modifiable risk factors such as outdoor exposure to the sun without protection and indoor tanning.[38]

MILITARY WORKERS

Survivors of recent wars who have been exposed to chemical agents may be at risk for the development of soft tissue sarcoma, non-Hodgkin's lymphoma, Hodgkin's disease, respiratory and prostate cancers, skin diseases, and many more problems in themselves and their offspring.

Three million Americans served in the armed forces in Vietnam during the 1960s and early 1970s. Large quantities of defoliant agents such as Agent Orange were used to remove forest cover, destroy crops, and clear vegetation from around U.S. military bases.

At least half of the 3 million Americans in Vietnam were there during the heaviest spraying. Many of our military personnel were exposed to this toxic substance. Exposure could occur through inhalation, ingestion, and skin or eye absorption.

In early 2003, the military acknowledged that exposure to Agent Orange is associated with chronic lymphocytic leukemia among surviving veterans. There is also sufficient evidence of an association between Agent Orange and soft tissue sarcoma and non-Hodgkin's lymphoma.[39-41]

Taking an environmental, occupational, or military history may be appropriate when a client has a history of asthma, allergies, or autoimmune disease, along with puzzling, nonspecific symptoms such as myalgias, arthralgias, headaches, back pain, sleep disturbance, loss of appetite, loss of sexual interest, and recurrent upper respiratory symptoms.

The affected individual often presents with an unusual combination of multiorgan signs and symptoms. A medical diagnosis of chronic fatigue syndrome, fibromyalgia, or another more nonspecific disorder is a yellow flag. When and how to take the history and how to interpret the findings are discussed in Chapter 2. The mnemonic CH2OPD2 (Community, Home, Hobbies, Occupation, Personal habits, Diet, and Drugs) can be used as a tool to identify a client's history of exposure to potentially toxic environmental contaminants.[42]

Risk Factors for Cancer Recurrence

As cancer survivors live longer, the chance of recurring cancer increases. Positive lymph nodes, tumor size greater than 2 cm, and a high-grade histopathologic designation, increase a client's risk of cancer recurrence. Recurrence can occur at the original location of the first cancer, in local or distant lymph nodes, or in metastatic sites such as the bone or lung tissues.

Each type of cancer has its own risk factors for cancer recurrence. For example, increased numbers of positive lymph nodes and negative estrogen/progesterone receptor (ER/PGR) status for breast cancer survivors are risk factors (Case Example 13-1). A positive ER/PGR status lowers the risk of breast cancer recurrence because it allows the woman to receive tamoxifen for prevention of recurrence according to age and stage of cancer.

▶ CANCER PREVENTION

Cancer prevention begins with risk factor assessment and risk reduction. The key to cancer prevention lies in minimizing as many of the individual modifiable risk factors as possible. The AICR estimates that recommended diets, together with maintenance of physical activity and appropriate body mass, can in time reduce cancer incidence by 30% to 40%. At current rates, on a global basis, this represents 3 to 4 million cases of cancer per year that could be prevented by dietary and associated means.[18]

There are some simple steps to take in starting this process. The first is to assess personal/family health history. Note any cancers present in first-generation family members. Some helpful tools are available for assessing cancer risk. The Harvard School of Public Health offers an interactive tool to estimate an individual's risk of cancer and offers cancer prevention strategies. Anyone can benefit from it, but accuracy is greatest for adults over age 40 who have never had any type of cancer. It is available at Harvard Center for Cancer Prevention, www.yourcancerrisk.harvard.edu.

Cancer screening is available and widely recommended for the following types of cancer: colorectal, breast, cervix (women), and prostate (men). Early detection at a localized stage is linked with less morbidity and lower mortality.

For example, 90% of colon cancer cases and deaths can be prevented. The American Cancer

CASE EXAMPLE 13-1 Risk Factors for Cancer Recurrence

A 46-year-old woman presented with mid-thoracic back pain present for the past 2 weeks. She described the pain as sharp and rated it as a 7 on the numeric rating scale. The pain was increased when she raised her arms overhead and relieved when she put her arms down. There were no other aggravating or relieving factors.

The client also noted occasional shoulder pain, sometimes with back pain and sometimes by itself. There were no other reported symptoms of any kind.

Past medical history included breast cancer diagnosed and treated 8 years ago with no cancer recurrence. The client had 17 nodes removed (12 were positive) and a mastectomy, followed by chemotherapy (short-term) and

tamoxifen (long-term). The client was estrogen negative.

The clinical presentation was consistent with a posterior rib dysfunction, but there was no identified trauma or cause attributed to the onset of the back pain. The therapist's judgment was that there were enough risk factors in the history for cancer recurrence combined with additional red flags (e.g., age over 40, pain level, insidious onset) to warrant medical evaluation before a plan of care was established.

Results: Client was diagnosed with cancer metastases to the thoracic vertebrae at T4-6. The physician called the therapist to ask what tipped her off to the need for medical referral. Knowing the risk factors for cancer AND for cancer recurrence made a difference in this case.

Society provides a summary of risk factors and early detection screening tests for many types of cancer, including colon cancer. (This information is available at the American Cancer Society Web site, www.cancer.org/colonmd [ACS Colorectal Cancer: Risk & Screening].) The Gail Model Risk Assessment Tool can also be used to assess personal risk for breast cancer. It is available at www.halls.md/breast/riskcom.htm (Breast Cancer Risk [Gail Model] Calculation Methods).

As health care educators, therapists can make use of this information to promote cancer prevention for themselves, their families, and their clients.

Genomics and Cancer Prevention

With the advent of the Genome Project, the sequencing of all genes in humans is nearly completed. Along with this discovery has come the development of a new biology of genetics called genomics. Understanding gene–environment interaction will be a major focus of genomics-based public health.[43]

There are many known or suspected carcinogens that increase an individual's risk of cancer. Different people respond to carcinogens differently. It is still not clear why one person develops cancer and another does not when both have the same risk factors.

Toxicogenomics, the development of molecular signatures for the effects of specific hazardous chemical agents, will bring to our understanding ways to track multiple sources of the same agent, multiple media and pathways of exposures, multiple effects or risks from the same agent, and multiple agents that cause similar effects.[43]

Defects may occur in one or more genes. Damage may occur in genes that involve the metabolism of carcinogens or in genes that deal with the DNA-repair process.[44] An important discovery in the area of gene identification related to cancer suppression is discovery of the p53 suppressor gene. The p53 gene encodes a protein with cancer-inhibiting properties. Loss of p53 activity predisposes cells to become unstable and more likely to take on mutations.[45]

It is possible that genetic defects combined with lifestyle or environmental factors may contribute to the development of cancer. For example, there is a known increase in risk of breast cancer in American women born after 1940 who have BRCA1 or BRCA2 mutation. This suggests that changes in the environment or lifestyle increased the risk already conferred by these genes.[46]

Air pollution is moderately associated with increased lung cancer, but when combined with exposure to tobacco smoke, the risk increases

dramatically. About 50% of all people lack the GSTM1 metabolic gene that can detoxify tobacco smoke and air pollution. People who have this genetic defect and who have heavy exposure to pollution may have a higher risk of developing lung cancer.[44]

Once it is understood how genes and the environment work to contribute to cancer development, this knowledge can be applied to intervention. Anyone with genes that lead to a higher risk of cancer may benefit from chemoprevention.

▶ MAJOR TYPES OF CANCER

There are three major types of cancer: carcinoma, sarcoma, and blood-borne cancers such as lymphoma and the leukemias. *Carcinoma* is a malignant tumor that comprises epithelial tissue and accounts for 85% of all cancers.

Carcinomas affect structures such as the skin, large intestine, stomach, breast, and lungs. These can be fast-growing tumors because they are derived from the epithelial lining of the organ, which grows rapidly and replaces itself frequently.

Carcinomas spread by invading local tissues and by metastasis. Generally, carcinomas tend to metastasize via the lymphatics, whereas sarcomas are more likely to metastasize hematogenously. *Sarcoma* is a fleshy growth and refers to a large variety of tumors arising in the connective tissues that are grouped together because of similarities in pathologic appearance and clinical presentation.

Tissues affected include connective tissue, such as bone and cartilage (discussed subsequently under Bone Tumors), muscle, fibrous tissue, fat, and synovium. The different types of sarcomas are named for the specific tissues affected (e.g., fibrosarcomas are tumors of the fibrous connective tissue; osteosarcomas are tumors of the bone; and chondrosarcomas are tumors arising in cartilage) (Table 13-3).

As a general category, sarcoma differs from carcinoma in the origin of cells composing the tumor (Table 13-4). As mentioned, sarcomas arise in connective tissue (embryologic mesoderm), whereas carcinomas arise in epithelial tissue (embryologic ectoderm) (i.e., cellular structures covering or lining surfaces of body cavities, small vessels, or visceral organs).

Cancers of the blood and lymph system arise from the bone marrow and include leukemia, multiple myeloma, and lymphoma. These cancers are characterized by the uncontrolled growth of blood cells. Metastasis is hematogenous.

▶ METASTASES

Neoplasms are divided into three categories: benign, invasive, and metastatic. Benign neoplasms are non-cancerous tumors that are localized, encapsulated, slow growing, and unable to move or metastasize to other sites.

Invasive carcinoma is a malignant cancer that has invaded surrounding tissue. The spread of cancer cells from the primary site to secondary sites is called *metastasis*. A regional metastasis is the local arrest, growth, and development of a malignant lesion to regional lymph nodes.

A distal or distant metastasis is the distant arrest, growth, and development of a malignant lesion to another organ (e.g., lung, liver, brain). Within the categories of invasive and metastatic tumors, four large subcategories of malignancy have been identified and classified according to the cell type of origin (Table 13-4).

For the therapist, primary cancers arising from specific body structures are not as likely to present with musculoskeletal signs and symptoms. It is more likely that recurrence of a previously treated cancer will have metastasized from another part of the body (secondary neoplasm) with subsequent bone, joint, or muscular presentation.

Metastatic spread can occur as late as 15 to 20 years after initial diagnosis and medical intervention. For this reason, the therapist must take care to conduct a screening interview during the examination, including past medical history of cancer or cancer treatment (e.g., chemotherapy, radiation).

Use the personal/family history form (see Fig. 2-2) in Chapter 2 to assess for a personal or first-degree family history of cancer. When asked about a past medical history of cancer, clients may say "No," even in the presence of a personal history of cancer. This is especially common in those clients who have reached and/or passed the 5-year survival mark.

Always link these two questions together:

Follow-Up Questions

- Have you ever had any kind of cancer?
- If no, have you ever had chemotherapy, radiation therapy, or immunotherapy of any kind?

Mechanisms and Modes of Metastases

Cancer cells can spread throughout the body through the bloodstream (hematogenous or vascular dissemination), via the lymphatic system, or by

TABLE 13-3 ▼ Classification of Soft Tissue and Bone Tumors

Tissue of origin	Benign tumor	Malignant tumor
Connective Tissue		
Fibrous	Fibroma	Fibrosarcoma
Cartilage	Chondroma	Chondrosarcoma
	Enchondroma	
	Chondroblastoma	
Bone	Osteoma	Osteosarcoma
Bone marrow		Leukemia
		Multiple myeloma
		Ewing family of tumors (EFT)
Adipose (fat)	Lipoma	Liposarcoma
Synovial	Ganglion, giant cell of tendon sheath	Synovial sarcoma
Muscle		
Smooth muscle	Leiomyoma	Leiomyosarcoma
Striated muscle	Rhabdomyoma	Rhabdomyosarcoma
Endothelium (Vascular/Lymphatic)		
Lymph vessels	Lymphangioma	Lymphangiosarcoma
		Kaposi's sarcoma
Lymphoid tissue		Lymphosarcoma (lymphoma)
		Lymphatic leukemia
Blood vessels	Hemangioma	Hemangiosarcoma
Neural Tissue		
Nerve fibers and sheaths	Neurofibroma	Neurofibrosarcoma
	Neuroma	Neurogenic sarcoma
	Neurinoma (neurilemmoma schwannoma)	
Glial tissue	Gliosis	Glioma
Epithelium		
Skin and mucous membrane	Papilloma	Squamous cell carcinoma
	Polyp	Basal cell carcinoma
Glandular epithelium	Adenoma	Adenocarcinoma

Data from Purtilo DT, Purtilo RB: *A survey of human disease*, ed 2, Boston, 1989, Little, Brown; Phipps W, et al: *Medical-surgical nursing: concepts and clinical practice*, ed 4, St. Louis, 1990, Mosby.

TABLE 13-4 ▼ Subcategories of Malignancy by Cell Type of Origin

Carcinomas	Sarcomas	Lymphomas	Leukemias
Arise from epithelial cells:	Develop from connective tissues:	Originate in lymphoid tissues:	Cancers of the hematologic system:
Breast	Fat	Lymph nodes	Bone marrow
Colon	Muscle	Spleen	
Pancreas	Bone	Intestinal lining	
Skin	Cartilage		
Large intestine	Synovium		
Lungs	Fibrous tissue		
Stomach			
Metastasize via lymphatics	Metastasize hematogenously	Spread by infiltration	Invasion and infiltration
	Local invasion		

vascular systems have many interconnections that allow tumor cells to pass from one system to the other.

During invasion, tumor cells can easily penetrate small lymphatic vessels and are then transported via the lymph. Tumor emboli may be trapped in the first draining lymph node, or they may bypass these regional lymph nodes (RLNs) to form noncontinuous and distant nodal metastases called "skip metastasis."

The relatively high incidence of anatomic skip metastasis can be attributed to aberrant distribution of lymph nodes.[47] Multiple interconnections between the lymphatic and hematogenous systems may also allow transport of tumor cells via the arterial or venous blood supply, bypassing some lymph nodes while reaching other more distant nodes.[48]

Patterns of blood flow, regional venous drainage, and lymphatic channels determine the distribution pattern of most metastases. For example, breast cancer spreads via the *lymphatics* and via the vertebral venous system to bones in the shoulder, hip, ribs, vertebrae, lungs, and liver.

Primary bone cancer such as osteogenic sarcoma initially metastasizes via *blood* to the lungs. Prostate cancer spreads via *lymphatics* to pelvic and vertebral bones, sometimes appearing as low back and/or pelvic pain radiating down the leg. The more common cancers and their metastatic pathways are provided in Table 13-5.

The high proportion of bone metastases in breast, prostate, and lung cancers is an example of

direct extension into neighboring tissue or body cavities (Fig. 13-2). Once a primary tumor is initiated and starts to move by local invasion, tumor angiogenesis occurs (blood vessels from surrounding tissue grow into the solid tumor). Tumor cells then invade host blood vessels and are discharged into the venous drainage.

Many individuals develop multiple sites of metastatic disease because of the potential of cancers to spread. A metastatic colony is the end result of a complicated series of tumor-host interactions called the *metastatic cascade*.

Metastasis requires a good deal of coordination between cancer cells and the body. Fortunately, many early metastases die in transit for a number of reasons such as blood vessel turbulence and genes that normally suppress growth of micrometastases in new environments. Even so, some metastatic cells do survive and move on to other sites. At secondary sites, the malignant cells continue to reproduce, and new tumors or lesions develop.

Some clients with newly diagnosed cancers have clinically detectable metastases; remaining clients who are clinically free of metastases may harbor occult metastases.

The usual mode of spread and eventual location of metastases vary with the type of cancer and the tissue from which the cancer arises. Early clinical observations led to the idea that carcinomas spread by the lymphatic route, and mesenchymal tumors such as melanoma spread through the bloodstream. We now know that both the lymphatic and

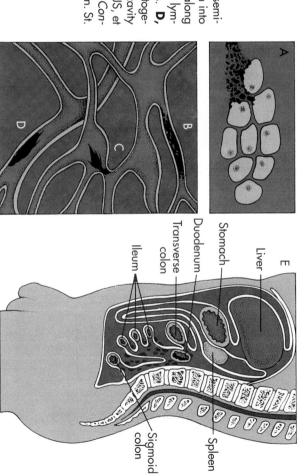

Fig. 13-2 • Some modes of dissemination of cancer. **A,** Direct extension into neighboring tissue. **B,** Permeation along lymphatic vessels. **C,** Embolism via lymphatic vessels to the lymph nodes. **D,** Embolism via blood vessels (hematogenous spread). **E,** Invasion of a body cavity by diffusion. (Modified from Phipps JS, et al, eds: *Medical-surgical nursing: Concepts and clinical practice,* 4th edition. St. Louis, 1991, Mosby.)

TABLE 13-5 ▼ Pathways of Cancer Metastases

Primary cancer	Mode of dissemination	Location of primary metastases
Breast	Lymphatics Blood (vascular or hematogenous)	Bone (shoulder, hips, ribs, vertebrae); CNS (brain, spinal cord) Lung, pleural cavity, liver
Bone	Blood	Lungs, liver, bone, then CNS
Cervical (cervix)	Local extension and lymphatics Blood	Retroperitoneal lymph nodes, bladder, rectum; paracervical, parametrial lymphatics CNS (brain), lungs, bones, liver
Colorectal	Direct extension Peritoneal seeding Blood	Bone (vertebrae) Peritoneum Liver, lung
Ewing's sarcoma	Blood	Lung, bone, bone marrow
Kidney	Lymph Blood	Pelvis, groin Lungs, pleural cavity, bone, liver
Leukemia		Does not really metastasize: causes symptoms throughout body
Liver	Blood	CNS (brain)
Lung (bronchogenic sarcoma)	Blood Blood Direct extension, lymphatics	CNS (brain, spinal cord) Bone Mediastinum (tissue and organs between the sternum and vertebrae such as the heart, blood vessels, trachea, esophagus, thymus, lymph nodes)
Lung (apical or Pancoast's tumors)	Direct extension Blood	8th cervical and 1st and 2nd thoracic nerves within the brachial plexus CNS (brain, spinal cord), bone
Lymphoma	Blood Lymphatics	CNS (spinal cord) Can occur anywhere, including skin, visceral organs
Malignant melanoma	No typical pattern	Mets can occur anywhere; skin and subcutaneous tissue; lungs; CNS (brain); liver; gastrointestinal tract; bone
Nonmelanoma skin cancer	Usually remain local without metastases; local invasion	Bones underlying involved skin; brain
Osteogenic sarcoma (osteosarcoma)	Lymphatics Blood	Lymph nodes, lungs, bone, kidneys, CNS (brain)
Ovarian	Direct extension into abdominal cavity Lymphatics	Nearby organs (bladder, colon, rectum, uterus, fallopian tubes) Liver, lungs; regional and distant
Pancreatic	Blood	Liver
Prostate	Lymphatics	Pelvic and vertebral bones Bladder, rectum Distant organs (lung, liver, brain)
Spinal cord	Local invasion; dissemination through the intervertebral foramina	CNS (brain, spinal cord)
Stomach, gastric	Blood Local invasion	Liver, vertebrae, abdominal cavity (intraperitoneum)
Thyroid	Direct extension Lymphatics Blood	Bone; nearby tissues of neck Regional lymph nodes (neck, upper chest, mediastinum) Distant (lung, bone)

CNS, Central nervous system.

selective movement of tumor cells to a specific organ. For example, in breast cancer, it is thought that the continuous remodeling of bone by osteoclasts and osteoblasts predisposes bone to metastatic lesions.[49] For some cancers, such as malignant melanoma, no typical pattern exists, and metastases may occur anywhere.

Benign Mechanical Transport

Mechanical transport rather than metastasis may be another mechanism of cancer spread. Two potential modes of benign mechanical transport (BMT) have been detected: lymphatic transport of epithelial cells displaced by biopsy of the primary tumor, and breast massage–assisted sentinel lymph node (SLN) localization.[50]

Samples of malignant tissues must be very carefully excised by surgeons who are expert in the biopsy of malignant tissues.[51,52] The risk of local recurrence is increased when intralesional curettage alone is performed.[53]

A second mode of BMT may be the pre-SLN breast massage used to facilitate the localization of SLNs during breast cancer staging. Mechanical transport of epithelial cells to SLNs has been verified. The significance of small epithelial clusters in SLN is unknown; further research is needed before changes are recommended for biopsy and SLN-localizing practices.[50]

The bottom line for the therapist is this: Anyone who has had a recent biopsy (within the past 6 months) must be followed carefully for any signs of local cancer recurrence.

CLINICAL MANIFESTATIONS OF MALIGNANCY

The therapist may be the first to see clinical manifestations of primary cancer but is more likely to see signs and symptoms of cancer recurrence or cancer metastasis. In general, the five most common sites of cancer metastasis are bone, lymph nodes, lung, liver, and brain. However, the therapist is most likely to observe signs and symptoms affecting one of the following systems:

- Integumentary
- Pulmonary
- Neurologic
- Musculoskeletal
- Hepatic

Each of these systems has a core group of most commonly observed signs and symptoms that will be discussed throughout this section (Table 13-6).

Early Warning Signs

For many years, the American Cancer Society has publicized seven warning signs of cancer, the appearance of which could indicate the presence of cancer and the need for a medical evaluation. The following mnemonic is often used as a helpful reminder of these warning signs (Box 13-1).

Bleeding is an important sign of cancer, but a cancer is generally well established by the time bleeding occurs. Bleeding develops secondary to ulcerations in the central areas of the tumor or by pressure on or rupture of local blood vessels. As the tumor continues to grow, it may enlarge beyond its capacity to obtain necessary nutrients, resulting in revitalization of portions of the tumor.

This process of invading and compressing local tissue, shutting off blood supply to normal cells, is called *necrosis*. Tissue necrosis leads ultimately to secondary infection, severe hemorrhage, and the development of pain when regional sensory nerves become involved. Other symptoms can include pathologic fractures, anemia, and thrombus formation.

Awareness of these signals is useful, but it is generally agreed that these symptoms do not always reflect early curable cancer; nor does this list include all possible signs for the different types of cancer.

Lumps, Lesions, and Lymph Nodes

The therapist should take special note of "T" *thickening or lump in breast or elsewhere*. Clients often point out a subcutaneous lesion (often a benign lipoma) and ask us to identify what it is. Baseline examination of a lump or lesion is important. Palpation of skin lesions and lymph nodes is presented in Chapter 4.

Whenever examining a lump or lesion, one should use the mnemonic in Box 4-10 to document and report findings on location, size, shape, consistency, mobility or fixation, and signs of tenderness (see Fig. 4-45). A clinically detectable tumor the size of a small pea already contains billions of cells. Most therapists will be able to palpate a lesion below the skin when it is half that size.[48]

Review Appendix B-19 for appropriate follow-up questions. Keep in mind that the therapist cannot know what the underlying pathology may be when lymph nodes are palpable and questionable. Performing a baseline assessment and reporting the findings are important outcomes of the assessment.

In previous editions of this text, it was noted that any changes in lymph nodes present for longer than 1 month in more than one location was a red flag.

TABLE 13-6 ▼ Signs and Symptoms of Metastases*

Integumentary	Musculoskeletal	Neurologic (CNS)	Pulmonary	Hepatic
Any skin lesion or observable/ palpable skin changes	May present as an asymptomatic soft tissue mass	Drowsiness, lethargy	Pleural pain	Abdominal pain and tenderness
Any observable or palpable change in nailbeds (fingers or toes)	Bone pain	Headaches	Dyspnea	Jaundice
	• Deep or localized	Nausea, vomiting	New onset of wheezing	Ascites (see Fig. 9-8)
Unusual mole (use ABCD method of assessment; see Fig. 4-5)	• Increased with activity	Depression	Productive cough with rust, green, or yellow-tinged sputum	Distended abdomen
	• Decreased tolerance to weight bearing; antalgic gait	Increased sleeping		Dilated upper abdominal veins
		Irritability, personality change		Peripheral edema
Cluster mole formation	• Does not respond to physical agents	Confusion, increased confusion		General malaise and fatigue
Bleeding or discharge from mole, skin lesion, scar, or nipple	Soft tissue swelling	Change in mental status, memory loss, difficulty concentrating		Bilateral carpal/tarsal tunnel syndrome
		Vision changes (blurring, blind spots, double vision)		Asterixis (liver flap) (see Fig. 9-7)
				Palmar erythema (liver palms) (see Fig. 9-5)

Tenderness and soreness around a mole; sore that does not heal

Pathologic fractures
Hypercalcemia (see Table 13-9)
• CNS
• Musculoskeletal
• Cardiovascular
• Gastrointestinal
Back or rib pain

Numbness, tingling
Balance/coordination problems
Changes in deep tendon reflexes
Change in muscle tone for individual with previously diagnosed neurologic condition
Positive Babinski reflex
Clonus (ankle or wrist)
Changes in bowel and bladder function
Myotomal weakness pattern
Paraneoplastic syndrome (see text)

Spider angiomas (over the abdomen) (see Fig. 9-3)
Nailbeds of Terry (see Fig. 9-6)
Right shoulder pain

* Seen most often in a physical therapy practice.
CNS, Central nervous system; *ABCD,* asymmetry, border, color, diameter.

This recommendation is no longer appropriate. The recommendation today, based on an increased understanding of cancer metastases via the lymphatic system and the potential for cancer recurrence, is that all suspicious lymph nodes should be evaluated by a physician (Case Example 13-2).

Supraclavicular lymph nodes that are easily palpable on examination may indicate possible metastatic disease. Any lymph nodes that are hard,

immovable, and nontender raise the suspicion of cancer, especially in the presence of a previous history of cancer.

Keep in mind that lymph nodes can fluctuate over the course of 10 to 14 days. When making the medical referral, look for a cluster of signs and symptoms, recent trauma (including recent biopsy), or a past history of chronic fatigue syndrome, mononucleosis, and allergies. Record and report all findings.

Proximal Muscle Weakness

For the therapist, idiopathic proximal muscle weakness may be an early sign of cancer (Fig. 13-3). This syndrome of proximal muscle weakness is referred to as *carcinomatous neuromyopathy.* It is accompanied by changes in two or more deep tendon reflexes (ankle jerk usually remains intact). Muscle weakness may occur secondary to hypercalcemia, which occurs as an indirect humoral effect on bone (see discussion, Paraneoplastic Syndrome, this chapter). Clients with advanced cancer, multiple myeloma, or breast or lung cancer are affected most often by hypercalcemia.

BOX 13-1 ▼ Early Warning Signs of Cancer

Changes in bowel or bladder habits
A sore that does not heal in 6 weeks
Unusual bleeding or discharge
Thickening or lump in breast or elsewhere
Indigestion or difficulty in swallowing
Obvious change in a wart or mole
Nagging cough or hoarseness

For the physical therapist:

Proximal muscle weakness
Change in deep tendon reflexes

CASE EXAMPLE 13-2 Palpable and Observable Lymph Nodes

A 73-year-old woman was referred to a physical therapy clinic by her oncologist with a diagnosis of cervical radiculopathy. She had a history of uterine cancer 20 years ago and a history of breast cancer 10 years ago.

Treatment included a hysterectomy, left radical mastectomy, radiation therapy, and chemotherapy. She has been cancer free for almost 10 years. When seen by physicians, her family physician, oncologist, and neurologist actually all evaluated her before she was referred to the physical therapist.

Examination by a physical therapist revealed obvious lymphadenopathy of the left cervical and axillary lymph nodes. When asked if the referring physician (or other physicians) saw the "swelling," she told the therapist that she had not disrobed during her medical evaluation and consultation.

The question for us as physical therapists in a situation like this one is how to proceed?

Several steps must be taken. First, the therapist must document all findings. If possible,

photographs of the chest, neck, and axilla should be obtained.

Second, the therapist must ascertain whether or not the physician is already aware of the problem and has requested physical therapy as a palliative measure. Requesting the physician's dictation or notes from the examination is essential.

Contact with the physician will be important soon after the records are obtained, either to confirm the request as palliative therapy or to report your findings and confirm the need for medical reevaluation.

If it turns out that the physician is, indeed, unaware of these physical findings, it is best to send a problem list identified as "outside the scope of a physical therapist" when returning the client to the physician. Be careful to avoid making any statements that could be misconstrued as a medical diagnosis.

We recommend writing a brief letter with the pertinent findings and ending with one of two one-liners:

What do you think?
Please advise.

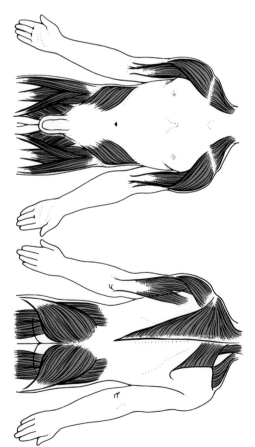

Fig. 13-3 • Proximal muscle weakness can be observed clinically as a positive Trendelenburg test (usually present bilaterally) and abnormal manual muscle testing. It can also be observed functionally when the client has difficulty getting up from sitting or climbing stairs. As the weakness progresses the client may have trouble getting into and out of a vehicle and/or the bathtub. Respiratory muscle weakness may be seen as shortness of breath or reported as altered activity to avoid dyspnea.

Screening for muscle weakness is not always a straightforward process. Sometimes, questions must be directed toward function to find out this information. If a client is asked whether he or she has any muscle weakness, difficulty getting up from sitting, trouble climbing stairs, or shortness of breath, the answer may very well be "No" on all accounts. Consider using the following flow of questions:

Follow-Up Questions

- Do you have any muscle weakness in your arms, legs, back, or chest?
- Do you have any trouble getting into and out of a chair?
- Are there any activities you would like to be able to do that you currently can't do?
- Are there any activities you used to be able to do that you can't do now?
- Are there activities you can do now that used to be much easier?
- Do you have any trouble going up and down stairs without stopping?
- Can you do all your grocery shopping without sitting down or stopping?
- Are you able to complete your household chores (e.g., make a meal, wash and dry clothes) without stopping?

Pain

Pain is rarely an early warning sign of cancer, even in the presence of unexplained bleeding. Night pain that is constant and intense (often rated 7 or higher on the Numeric Rating Scale; see Fig. 3-6) is a red flag symptom of primary or recurring cancer.

Pain is usually the result of destruction of tissue or pressure on tissue due to the presence of a tumor or lesion. The lesion or lesions must be of significant size or location to create pressure and/or occlusion of normal structures; pain will be dependent on the area of the body affected.

Acute and chronic cancer-related pain syndromes can occur in association with diagnostic and therapeutic interventions such as bone marrow biopsy, lumbar puncture, colonoscopy, percutaneous biopsy, and thoracentesis. Chemotherapy and radiation toxicities can result in painful peripheral neuropathies.

Likewise, many different chronic pain syndromes (e.g., tumor-related radiculopathy, phantom breast pain, postsurgical pelvic or abdominal pain, burning perineum syndrome, post-radiation pain syndrome) can occur as a result of tumors or cancer therapy. See further discussion under Oncologic Pain in this chapter.

Change in One or More Deep Tendon Reflexes

When a neurologic screening examination is performed, testing of deep tendon reflexes (DTRs) is usually included. Some individuals have very brisk reflexes under normal circumstances; others are much more hyporeflexive.

Tumors (whether benign or malignant) can also press on the spinal nerve root, mimicking a disc problem. A lesion that is small enough can put just enough pressure to irritate the nerve root, resulting in a hyperreflexive DTR. A large tumor can obliterate the reflex arc, resulting in diminished or absent reflexes.

Either way, changes in DTRs must be considered a red flag sign (possibly of cancer) that should be documented and further investigated. For example, a hyporesponsive patellar tendon reflex that is unchanged with distraction or repeated testing and is accompanied by back, hip, or thigh pain, along with a past history of prostate cancer, presents a different clinical picture altogether. Guidelines for assessing reflexes are discussed in Chapter 4.

Integumentary Manifestations

Internal cancers can invade the skin through vascular dissemination or direct extension. Metastases to the skin may be the first sign of malignancy, especially for breast or upper respiratory tract cancer. Integumentary carcinomatous metastases often present as asymmetrical, firm, skin-colored, red, purple, or blue nodules near the site of the primary tumor (see Fig. 4-24).

Distant cutaneous metastasis can result from leukemia (see Fig. 4-27), multiple myeloma (see Fig. 4-25), and stomach/colon, ovarian, pancreatic, kidney, and breast cancer (Case Example 13-3). The scalp is a common site for such lesions (see Fig. 4-26), which are sometimes accompanied by hair loss called *alopecia neoplastica*.

The integumentary screening examination, including assessment of common skin lesions and nailbed assessment, is presented in Chapter 4. Cancer-related skin lesions (e.g., pinch purpura, renal nodule, local cancer recurrence, Kaposi's sarcoma, xanthomas) are also included in Chapter 4.

During observation and inspection, the therapist should be alert to any potential signs of primary skin cancer or integumentary metastases. When a suspicious skin lesion is noted, the therapist should conduct a risk factor assessment and ask three questions:

CASE EXAMPLE 13-3   Cancer-Related Skin Rash

A 42-year-old woman with a previous history of breast cancer and breast lumpectomy asked a fellow clinician to examine her scar for any sign of cancer recurrence. She had just had her 6-month cancer check-up and was not scheduled to see her oncologist for another 6 months.

In the meantime, she had developed a skin rash over the upper chest wall and axilla of the involved side (upper back and left thigh) (Figs. 13-4 and 13-5). When asked if there were any other symptoms present, she reported feeling feverish and a bit nauseous, and noted slight muscle aching. On examination, the client's vital signs were taken. (See Chapter 2 about the importance of vital signs in the screening process; see also discussion of constitutional symptoms.)

All vital signs were within normal limits for the client's age, except body temperature, which was 102.2°F. The client reported that her normal body temperature was usually 98°F. She was not aware of an elevated body temperature, although she stated she had awakened in the night feeling feverish and took some Tylenol.

Upper quadrant examination was unremarkable, except for skin rash and the presence of bilateral anterior cervical adenopathy. There

was a fullness of lymph node tissue without firmness or distinct nodes palpated in the axilla on the involved side. The clinician was unable to palpate as far into the Zone II space (see Figs. 4-40 and 4-41) as would be expected.

Results: This client had three red flags: recent history of cancer, skin rash, and a constitutional symptom (fever). Even though there was no external sign of local cancer recurrence, and even though she was just seen by her oncologist, these new findings warranted a return visit to her physician.

The skin rash turned out to be Sweet's syndrome, a disorder usually associated with significant constitutional symptoms and involvement of the lungs and joints. Most cases are idiopathic, but some have been associated with malignancies.[54-56]

In this case, no further findings were made despite laboratory and medical tests performed. The use of systemic corticosteroids is usually recommended for Sweet's syndrome, but the client declined and opted to use vitamin supplements, as her symptoms were resolving by that time. She was followed more closely for any cancer recurrence with more frequent testing thereafter.

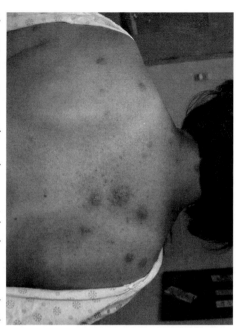

A

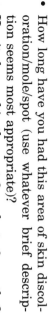

Fig. 13-4 • Day 1. Skin rash on upper back associated with Sweet's syndrome, a disorder usually associated with significant constitutional symptoms and involvement of the lungs and joints. Most cases are idiopathic, but some have been associated with malignancies. (Courtesy Insley Puma Flaig, MD, University of Minnesota Medical Center, Fairview, Minnesota, 2003. Used with permission.)

- How long have you had this area of skin discoloration/mole/spot (use whatever brief description seems most appropriate)?
- Has it changed in the past 6 weeks to 6 months?
- Has your physician examined this area?

No matter what the therapist's own cultural background, as a health care professional, his or her responsibility to screen skin lesions is clear. *How* questions are posed is just as important as *what* is said.

The therapist may want to introduce the subject by saying that as health care professionals, we are trained to observe many body parts (skin, joints, posture, and so on). You notice that the client has an unusual mole (or rash, or whatever has been observed), and you wonder whether this is something that's been there for years. Has it changed in the past 6 weeks to 6 months? Has the client ever shown it to the doctor?

A client with a past medical history of cancer now presenting with a suspicious skin lesion that has not been evaluated by the physician must be advised to have this evaluated as soon as possible.

For any client with a previous history of cancer with surgical removal, it is always a good idea to look at the surgical site(s) for any sign of local cancer recurrence. Start by asking the client if he or she has noticed any changes in the scar. Continue by asking the following:

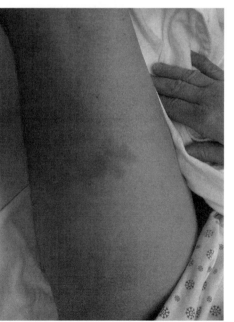

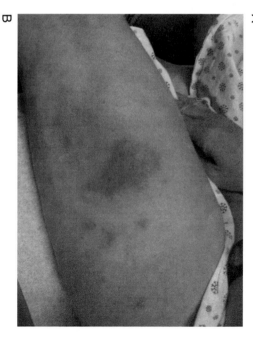

B

Fig. 13-5 • **A,** Day 1 (same client as in Fig. 13-4). Skin rash on upper thigh associated with Sweet's syndrome. **B,** Day 5. Rash progressed quickly to cover large areas of the upper chest wall, axilla, upper back, and left thigh. (Courtesy Insley Puma Flaig, MD, University of Minnesota Medical Center, Fairview, Minnesota, 2003. Used with permission.)

Follow-Up Questions

- Would you have any objections if I looked at (or examined) the scar tissue?

Any suspicious scab or tissue granulation, redness, or discoloration must be noted (photographed, if possible) (see Figs. 4-8 and 17-5). Again, three screening questions apply in this situation. The therapist has a responsibility to report these findings to the appropriate health care professional and to make every effort to ensure client compliance with follow-up.

Skin Cancers

Skin cancers are the most common of all types of cancer and are usually classified as non-melanoma skin cancer (NMSC) and melanoma. Most skin cancers are classified as non-melanoma and are slow growing, easy to recognize, and responsive to intervention, if found early. Non-melanoma skin cancers are further classified as basal cell or squamous cell, depending on the tissue affected. They rarely metastasize to other parts of the body and have a nearly 100% rate of cure.

Melanoma, the most serious of the skin cancers, has a 96% 5-year survival rate if localized, but only a 13% 5-year survival if it is invasive or has spread to other parts of the body. More than 77% of cancer deaths result from invasive melanoma.

The primary warning sign for melanoma is a flat, colored, irregularly shaped lesion that can be mottled with light brown to black colors. It may turn various shades of red, blue, or white or crust on the surface and bleed. A changing mole, the appearance of a new mole, or a mole that is different or growing requires prompt medical attention.[57] The Skin Cancer Foundation advocates use of the ABCD (asymmetry, border irregularity, color variegation, and a diameter of 6 mm or greater) method of early detection of melanoma and dysplastic (abnormal in size or shape) moles (see discussion, Chapter 4; see Fig. 4-5).

Actinic keratosis is a pre-malignant form of skin cancer (see Fig. 4-6). With actinic keratosis, over-exposure to sunlight results in abnormal cell growth, causing a well-defined, crusty patch or bump on sun-exposed parts of the body.

Clients often point out skin lesions or ask the therapist about various lumps and bumps. In addition, the therapist may observe changes in skin, skin lesions, or aberrant tissue during the visual inspection and palpation portion of the examination (see Chapter 4) that need further medical investigation. Mortality is reduced when lesions are found early and treated promptly. Therapists can and should be a part of the screening process for skin cancer.

The cause of skin cancer is well known. Prolonged or intermittent exposure to UV radiation from the sun, especially when it results in sunburn and blistering, damages DNA. The majority of all NMSCs occur on parts of the body unprotected by clothing (i.e., face, neck, forearms, and backs of hands) and in persons who have received considerable exposure to sunlight.

RISK FACTOR ASSESSMENT

All adults, regardless of skin tone and hair color, are at risk for skin cancer; however, some people

---

BOX 13-2 ▼ Risk Factor Assessment for Skin Cancer

- Advancing age
- Personal or family history of skin cancer (particularly melanoma)
- Moles with any of the ABCD features, or moles that are changing in any way
- Complexion that is fair or light with green, blue, or gray eyes
- Skin that sunburns easily; skin that never tans
- History of painful sunburns with blistering during childhood or the adolescent years
- Use of tanning beds or lamps
- Short, intense episodes of sun exposure: the indoor worker who spends the weekend out in the sun without skin protection (or any sporadic exposure to strong sunshine of normally covered skin)
- Transplant recipient

Data from Skin Cancer Foundation, 2005.

---

are at much greater risk than others (Box 13-2). In general, individuals with red, blonde, or light brown hair with light complexion and maybe freckles, many of Celtic or Scandinavian origin, are most susceptible; persons of African or Asian origin are least susceptible.

The most severely affected people usually have a history of long-term occupational or recreational sun exposure. Australia and New Zealand have the highest incidence of melanoma in the world. New Zealand has nearly 5 times the amount of skin cancer that occurs in the United States.

Melanoma occurs in every part of the North American continent. In the United States, the five states with the highest predicted incidence of new cases are California, Florida, Texas, New York, and Pennsylvania. Men are more likely than women to develop non-melanoma and melanoma skin cancers. The rate of melanoma is 10 times higher for whites than blacks because blacks have the protective effects of skin pigment.[58]

Many older adults assume that skin changes are a "normal" sign of aging and do not see a physician when lesions first appear. Early detection and referral is always the key to a better prognosis. In asking the three important questions, the therapist plays an instrumental part in the cancer screening process.

Follow-Up Questions

- How long have you had this?
- Has it changed in the past 6 weeks to 6 months?
- Has your physician seen it?

An increased incidence of skin cancers has been noted after solid organ transplantation, especially liver, heart, and kidney transplants. Squamous and basal cell carcinomas are 250 and 10 times more frequent, respectively, in transplant recipients compared with the general population.[59] Skin cancers developing in transplant recipients are more aggressive, making early detection and intervention imperative. Renal transplant recipients have a cumulative increase that corresponds with the number of years post-transplantation (e.g., 7% after 1 year of immunosuppression, 45% after 11 years, 70% after 20 years).[59]

BASAL CELL CARCINOMA

Basal cell carcinoma involves the bottom layer of the epidermis and occurs mainly on any hair-bearing area exposed to the sun (e.g., face, neck, head, ears, hands). Occasionally, basal cell carcinoma may appear on the trunk, especially the upper back and chest. These lesions grow slowly, attaining a size of 1 to 2 cm in diameter, often after years of growth. Metastases almost never occur, but neglected lesions may ulcerate and produce great destruction, ultimately invading vital structures.

There are a number of common forms of basal cell carcinoma:

• Pearly papule, 2 to 3 mm in diameter and covered by tightly stretched epidermis laced with small delicate, branching vessels (telangiectasia)
• Pearly papule with a small crater in the center
• Scaly, red, sharply outlined plaque
• Ill-defined pale, tough, scarlike tumor

SQUAMOUS CELL CARCINOMA

Squamous cell carcinoma arises from the top of the epidermis and is found on areas often exposed to the sun, typically, the rim of the ear, the face, the lips and mouth, and the dorsa of the hands. These lesions appear as small, red, hard nodules with a smooth or warty surface. The central portion may be scaly, ulcerated, or crusted. Pre-malignant lesions include sun-damaged skin or dysplasias (whitish-discolored areas), scars, radiation-induced keratosis, actinic keratosis (rough, scaly spots), and chronic ulcers.

Metastases are uncommon but are much more likely to occur in lesions arising in chronic leg ulcers, burn scars, and areas of prior x-ray exposure. Although these tumors do not usually metastasize, they are potentially dangerous. They may infiltrate surrounding structures and metastasize to lymph nodes and eventually to distant sites, including bone, brain, and lungs, to become fatal. Invasive tumors are firm and increase in elevation and diameter. The surface may be granular and may bleed easily.

MALIGNANT MELANOMA

Malignant melanoma (MM) is the most serious form of skin cancer. It arises from pigmented cells in the skin called melanocytes. In contrast to basal and squamous cell carcinomas, the majority of MMs appear to be associated with the intensity rather than the duration of sunlight exposure.

The average lifetime risk of developing invasive melanoma is 1 in 65 (a 2000% increase from 1930); the average lifetime risk of developing non-invasive melanoma is 1 in 37.[57] An individual's risk is much greater if any of the risk factors listed in Box 13-2 are present.

Melanoma can appear anywhere on the body, not just on sun-exposed areas. The clinical characteristics of early malignant melanoma are similar, regardless of anatomic site. Unlike benign pigmented lesions, which are generally round and symmetric, the shape of an early MM is often asymmetric.

Whereas benign pigmented lesions tend to have regular margins, the borders of early MM are often irregular (see Fig. 4-5). Round, symmetric skin lesions such as common moles, freckles, and birthmarks are considered "normal." If an existing mole or other skin lesion starts to change and a line drawn down the middle shows two different halves, medical evaluation is needed.

Compared with benign pigmented lesions, which are more uniform in color, MMs are usually variegated, ranging from various hues of tan and brown to black, sometimes intermingled with red and white. The diameters of MM are often 6mm or larger when first identified.

The most common sites of distant metastasis associated with MM are the skin and subcutaneous tissue, lungs, and surrounding visceral pleura, although any anatomic site may be involved. In-transit metastases (unique malignancies that have spread from the primary tumor but may not have reached the regional lymph nodes) typically develop multiple bulky tumors on an arm or leg. Often, these tumors cause pain, swelling, bleeding, ulceration, and decreased mobility.[60]

Other signs that may be important include irritation and itching; tenderness, soreness, or new moles developing around the mole in question; or a sore that keeps crusting and does not heal within 6 weeks. Benign moles tend to be flat, hairless, round or oval, and <6mm in diameter. Pigmentation is generally even. Although there may be color variations, especially in shades of brown, benign moles, freckles, "liver spots," and other

benign skin changes are usually of a single color (most often, a single shade of brown or tan). A single lesion with more than one shade of black, brown, or blue may be a sign of malignant melanoma.

Adolescents frequently have nevi with irregular borders, multiple shades of pigment, or both. Most are normal variations of benign nevi, but a physician should examine any lesion that arouses clinical suspicion or is of concern to the client.

If any of these signs and symptoms is present in a client whose skin lesion has not been examined by a physician, a medical referral is recommended. If the client is planning a follow-up visit with the physician within the next 2 to 4 weeks, the client is advised to point out the mole or skin changes at that time. If no appointment is pending, the client is encouraged to make a specific visit either to the family/personal physician or to a dermatologist.

Clinical Signs and Symptoms of

Early Melanoma

A. Asymmetry: Uneven edges, lopsided in shape, one-half unlike the other half

B. Border: Irregularity, irregular edges, scalloped or poorly defined edges

C. Color: Black, shades of brown, red, white, occasionally blue

D. Diameter: Larger than a pencil eraser

RESOURCES

The Skin Cancer Foundation (www.skincancer.org) has many public education materials available to help the therapist identify suspicious skin lesions. In addition to its Web site, the Skin Cancer Foundation has posters, brochures, videos, and other materials available for use in the clinic. It is highly recommended that these types of education materials be available in waiting rooms as part of a nationwide primary prevention program.

Other Web sites (www.skincheck.com [Melanoma Education Foundation]; www.medicine.usyd.edu.au/melanoma/ [The Melanoma Foundation of the University of Sydney Australia]) provide additional photos of suspicious lesions with additional screening guidelines. Dermik Laboratories offers an excellent encyclopedia of many categories of skin, finger, and nailbed lesions (www.dermnet.com). The therapist must become as familiar as possible with what suspicious skin aberrations may look like in order to refer as early as possible.

Pulmonary Manifestations

Pulmonary metastases are the most common of all metastatic tumors because venous drainage of most areas of the body passes through the superior and inferior venae cavae into the heart, making the lungs the first organ to filter malignant cells. *Primary bone tumors* (e.g., osteogenic sarcoma) metastasize first to the lungs.

Pleural pain and dyspnea may be the first two symptoms experienced by the person (Case Example 13-4). When either or both of these pulmonary symptoms occur, look for increased symptoms with deep breathing and activity. Ask about a productive cough with bloody or rust-colored sputum. Ask about new onset of wheezing at any time or difficulty breathing at night. Symptoms that are relieved by sitting up are indicative of pulmonary impairment and must be reported to the physician.

Symptoms may not occur until tumor cells have expanded and become large enough or invasive enough to reach the parietal pleura, where pain fibers are stimulated. The lining surrounding the lungs allows no pain perception, so it is not until the tumor is large enough to press on other nearby structures or against the chest wall that symptoms may first appear.

Lung cancer is the most common primary tumor to metastasize to the brain. Tumor cells from the lung embolizing via the pulmonary veins and carotid artery can result in metastases to the central nervous system (CNS). Anyone with a history of lung cancer should be screened for neurologic involvement. In any individual, any neurologic sign may be the presentation of a silent lung tumor.[61]

Neurologic Manifestations

As just mentioned, cancer metastasis to the CNS is a common problem. In all, 20% to 40% of individuals with primary sites outside of the CNS will develop brain metastases. The most common primary cancers with metastases to the brain are lung and breast cancer and melanoma. Of all those given a diagnosis of CNS metastasis, 50% have one metastatic lesion, 20% have two, and about 10% have five or more metastatic lesions[62] (Case Example 13-5).

Tumor cells can easily embolize via the pulmonary veins and carotid artery to the brain. The blood–brain barrier does not prevent invasion of the brain parenchyma by circulating metastatic cells. Metastatic brain tumors can increase intracranial pressure, obstruct the normal flow of

cerebrospinal fluid, change mentation, and reduce sensory and motor function.

Whether the pressure-causing lesion is a primary cancer of the brain or spinal cord, or whether it is a cancer that has metastasized to the CNS, clinical signs and symptoms of pressure will be the same because in both cases, the same system is affected.

Clinical Signs and Symptoms

Symptoms of brain tumor are usually general or focal symptoms, depending on the size and location of the lesion. For example, if a tumor is growing in the motor cortex, the client may develop isolated extremity weakness or hemiparesis. If the tumor is developing in the cerebellum, coordination may be affected.

Two of the most common clinical manifestations of brain tumor are headache and personality change, but personality change is often attributed to depression, delaying the diagnosis of brain tumor. Tumors that affect the frontal lobes are most likely to produce personality changes. Seizures occur in approximately one-third of persons with metastatic brain tumors.

Headaches occur in 30% to 50% of persons with brain tumors and are usually bioccipital or bifrontal. They are usually intermittent and of

---

CASE EXAMPLE 13-4   Lung Cancer

A 69-year-old man with a recent total hip replacement (THR) was referred to home health for physical therapy. He did not have a good postoperative recovery and has been slow to regain range of motion, strength, and function.

He experienced dyspnea and chest pain within the first 10 ft of ambulation. He has a past medical history of cancer.

What are the red flags here? How should you proceed?

Red Flags

Age (>40 years old)

Past medical history of cancer

Cardiopulmonary symptoms: shortness of breath and chest pain

How to Proceed: Ask the client how long he has had these symptoms. Take all vital signs as discussed in Chapter 2.

Your next steps may depend, in part, on any procedural instructions you have received from your home health agency. If there is a case manager, contact him or her with your concerns. Ask for a copy of the medical file. Contact the physician's office with your findings.

Difficulty in referral arises when a client has been seen by an orthopedic surgeon but is demonstrating signs and symptoms of possible systemic disease. Diplomacy and communication are the keys to success here.

Document your findings, and make sure these are sent to the primary care physician AND the orthopedic surgeon. The medical record may already indicate awareness of these red flags, and no further follow-up is needed.

If not, then a brief cover letter with your full report should be sent to the physician. The letter should contain the usual "thanks for this referral" kind of introduction with a paragraph about physical therapy intervention.

Then, include a medical problem list such as:

Patient reports shortness of breath and chest pain within the first 3 minutes of ambulation. This has just started in the last few days. His vital signs are: [list these].

Given the patient's age, past medical history of cancer, and new onset of cardiopulmonary symptoms, we would like medical clearance before progressing his exercise and rehab program. Please advise if there are any contraindications for exercise at this time. Thank you.

Make sure you call the physician's office and alert the staff of your concerns and that this letter/fax is on its way. Make telephone contact again within 3 days (sooner if the information is faxed to the doctor's office).

Results: The orthopedic surgeon advised the client to see his primary care physician for follow-up of this problem. After medical examination and testing, the final diagnosis was lung cancer. The medical doctor surmised that the stress of the surgery was enough to advance the cancer from subclinical to clinical status with new onset of symptoms that were not present before the orthopedic surgery.

CASE EXAMPLE 13-5 Bone Metastases and Wrist Sprain

A 75-year-old woman fell and sprained her wrist. Her family doctor sent her to physical therapy. After the interview, her daughter took the therapist aside and commented that her mother seems confused. Other family members are wondering if her fall had anything to do with mental deterioration.

There is a positive personal history for breast cancer. Past medical history included breast cancer, diverticulosis, gallbladder removal, and hysterectomy. There were no current health concerns expressed by the client or her family. She is not taking any medication (prescription or over-the-counter).

Since the wrist was obviously not broken, no x-rays were taken.

What are the red flags in this case? Since she just came to physical therapy from a medical doctor, is follow-up medical attention needed?

Red Flags: Age, confusion, past medical history of cancer, recent loss of balance and fall, lack of diagnostics.

This client actually presents with a cluster of four significant red flags in the screening process. The therapist should carry out a balance and vestibular function screening examination and neurologic screening examination (see Chapter 4). Additional key information may be obtained from this testing.

The next step is to inquire of the client or family member if the doctor is aware of the past history of cancer. Older adults moving closer to family members may give up their lifelong family provider. The new physician may not have all the history compiled. This is especially true when patients visit a "Doc-in-a-Box" at the local mall or convenience care facility.

Likewise, check with the family to see whether the physician has been notified of the client's new onset of confusion.

This is the number one sign of nervous system impairment in older adults.

The therapist is advised to document these findings and report them to the physician. As always, a letter of appreciation for the referral is a good idea. State the physical therapy diagnosis in terms of the musculoskeletal system (see the *Guide to Physical Therapist Practice* and discussion of physical therapy diagnosis in Chapter 1 of this text).

Include a follow-up paragraph with this information: I am concerned that the combination of the patient's age, new onset of confusion as described by her family, and recent history of falls resulting in this episode of care may be an indication of significant underlying pathology.

What do you think? I will treat the musculoskeletal impairment, but please advise if any further follow-up is needed.

Results: Given the client's past history of cancer, and knowing that confusion is not a "normal" sign of aging and that any neurologic sign can be an indicator of cancer, the physical therapist suggested that the family should also talk with the referring physician about these observations.

The client progressed well with the wrist rehabilitation program. The family reported that the physician did not seem concerned about the developing confusion or recent falls. No further medical testing was recommended. Six weeks later, the client fell and broke her hip. At that time, she was given a diagnosis of metastases to the bone and brain (CNS).

during a bowel movement, stooping, lifting heavy objects, or coughing.

Often, the pain can be relieved by taking aspirin, acetaminophen, or other moderate painkillers. Vomiting with or without nausea (unrelated to food) occurs in about 25% to 30% of people with brain tumors and often accompanies headaches when there is an increase in intracra-

increasing duration and may be intensified by a change in posture or by straining.

The headache is characteristically worse on awakening because of differences in CNS drainage in the supine and prone positions; it usually disappears soon after the person arises. It may be intensified or precipitated by any activity that increases intracranial pressure, such as straining

nial pressure. If the tumor invades the meninges, the headaches will be more severe.

Focal manifestations of a space-occupying brain lesion are caused by the local compression or destruction of the brain tissue, as well as by compression secondary to edema. Papilledema (edema and hyperemia of the optic disc) may be the first sign of intracranial tumors. Visual changes do not occur until prolonged papilledema causes optic atrophy.

Nerve and Cord Compression

Symptoms of nerve and/or cord compression may occur when tumors invade and impinge directly on the spinal cord, or more frequently because severe destructive osteolytic lesions of the vertebral bodies from metastases lead to pathologic fracture, fragility, and subsequent deformity of one or more vertebral bodies. Bone collapse can occur spontaneously or following trivial injury, sometimes with bone fragments adding to the compression.[63]

Other (more rare) cancer-related causes of spinal cord compression include radiation myelopathy, malignant plexopathy, and paraneoplastic disorders. Chronic progressive radiation myelopathy can occur in anyone who has received irradiation to the spine or nearby structures. Localized spinal cord dysfunction within the area of the radiation port occurs with numbness and upper motor neuron findings.[64]

Whether from a primary cord tumor or a metastasis, compression of the cord can be the first symptom of cancer. Prostate, lung, and breast cancers are the most common tumors to metastasize to the spine, leading to epidural spinal cord compression, but lymphoma, multiple myeloma, and carcinomas of the colon or kidney and sarcomas can also result in spinal cord and nerve root compression.[65]

Individuals with lymphoma or retroperitoneal tumors may suffer cord compression from tumors that grow through the intervertebral foramen and compress the cord without involving the vertebra.[65] Cord compression is becoming increasingly common, as individuals affected by cancer survive longer with medical treatment.

SIGNS AND SYMPTOMS OF CORD COMPRESSION

Spinal cord compression with resultant quadriplegia, paraplegia, and possible death is the most common pathologic feature of all tumors within the spinal column. Pain and sensory symptoms usually occur in the body below the level of the tumor but not necessarily at predictable levels. For example,

54% of individuals with T1-T6 compression have lumbosacral pain, and a similar number with lumbosacral compression have thoracic pain.[66]

The location of the metastasis is proportionate to the volume or mass of bone in each region: 60% of metastases occur in the thoracic spine, 30% in the lumbosacral spine, and 10% in the cervical spine.[67,68] Compression at the level of the cauda equina is relatively rare (0.7%).[69]

Breast and lung cancers typically cause thoracic lesions, whereas colon and pelvic carcinomas are more likely to affect the lumbosacral spine. In up to one third of affected individuals, spinal cord compression occurs at multiple sites.[65]

Early characteristics of spinal cord compression include pain, sensory loss, muscle weakness, and muscle atrophy. Back pain at the level of the spinal cord lesion occurs in up to 95% of cases, presenting hours to months before the compression is diagnosed.

Pain is caused by the expanding tumor in the bone, bone collapse, and/or nerve damage. Pain is usually described as sharp, shooting, deep, or burning and may be aggravated by lying down, weight bearing, bending, sneezing, or coughing.[65]

Discomfort may occur as thoracolumbar back pain in a beltlike distribution; the pain may extend to the groin or the legs. The pain may be constant or intermittent and occurs most often at rest; pain occurring at night can awaken an individual from sleep; the person reports that it is impossible to go back to sleep.

Symptoms of severe pain preceding the onset of motor weakness generally correlate with epidural compression, whereas muscle weakness and bowel/bladder sphincter dysfunction with very little pain indicates intramedullary metastasis.[70]

Weakness in an individual with cancer may be incorrectly attributed to fatigue, anemia, pain medication, or metabolic derangement. The therapist must remain alert to any subtle signs and symptoms of spinal cord compression as the underlying etiology and report these to the physician immediately.[64]

Over half of individuals present with sensory changes, either starting in the toes and moving caudally in a stocking-like patterns to the level of the lesion, or starting 1 to 5 levels below the level of the actual cord compression.[67]

Less commonly, chest or abdominal pain may occur, caused by nerve root compression from epidural tumor(s). Progressive cord compression is manifested by spastic weakness below the level of the lesion, decreased sensation, and increased

weakness. Bowel and bladder dysfunction are late findings.

CAUDA EQUINA SYNDROME

Cauda equina syndrome is defined as a constellation of symptoms that result from damage to the cauda equina, the portion of the nervous system below the conus medullaris. This syndrome involves peripheral nerves (sensory and motor) within the spinal canal and thecal sac.[71]

Individuals with cauda equina syndrome present differently from those with spinal cord compression. The three most common symptoms of cauda equina syndrome include saddle anesthesia, bowel or bladder dysfunction, and lower extremity weakness.[72]

Diminished sensation over the buttocks and posterior-superior thighs is also common.

Decreased anal sphincter tone, urinary retention, and overflow incontinence occur in 60% to 80% of patients at the time of diagnosis. About half of clients need urinary catheters.[67]

Clinical Signs and Symptoms of Cauda Equina Syndrome

- Low back pain
- Sciatica
- Saddle and/or perinanal hypesthesia or anesthesia
- Decreased rectal tone
- Decreased perineal reflexes
- Bowel and/or bladder changes or dysfunction
- Lower extremity weakness (variable)
- Decreased reflexes (patellar, Achilles)

Individuals with cauda equina syndrome caused by neoplasm may present with a long history of back pain and paresthesias; urinary difficulties are very common.[73] The presentation may mimic a discogenic source, causing a delay in diagnosis, especially in the young adult with a primary tumor. Individuals with metastatic tumors are older with a previous history of cancer.[71]

Associated signs and symptoms of primary or metastatic tumors causing cauda equina syndrome may include abnormal weight loss, hematuria, hemoptysis, melena, and/or constipation.

PERIPHERAL NEUROPATHY

Peripheral neuropathy with loss of vibratory sense, proprioception, and deep tendon reflexes is most often chemotherapy-related (e.g., cisplatin, taxol, vincristine). It is important to differentiate the type and etiology of peripheral neuropathy before planning treatment intervention.

For example, chemotherapy-induced neuropathy is not as likely to respond to lymph drainage and compression bandaging, whereas good results have been seen when this treatment intervention is used for weakness and paresthesias from lymphedema-induced nerve compression (e.g., ovarian cancer, testicular cancer).

In other words, resolution of neuropathy symptoms utilizing principles of manual lymphatic drainage may confirm subclinical lymphedema as the major etiologic factor in some clients.

Paraneoplastic Syndrome

Other neurologic problems occur frequently in individuals with cancer. These may be nonmetastatic and associated with cancer-related opportunistic infections, metabolic disturbances, vascular complications, treatment neurotoxicity, and paraneoplastic syndromes.

When tumors produce signs and symptoms at a distance from the tumor or its metastasized sites, these "remote effects" of malignancy are collectively referred to as *paraneoplastic syndromes*. This can be the first sign of malignancy and may show up months (even years) before the cancer is detected. They are usually caused by one of three phenomena:

- Tumor metastases to the brain
- Endocrine, fluid, and electrolyte abnormalities
- Remote effects of tumors on the CNS

The causes of these syndromes are not well understood. In contrast to the hormone syndromes in which the cancer directly produces a substance that circulates within blood to produce symptoms, the neurologic syndromes are a group of syndromes mediated by the immune response.

Tumors involved in this type of syndrome stimulate the production of immunologically active nervous system proteins. These immune responses are frequently associated with antineuronal antibodies that can be used as diagnostic markers of paraneoplastic disorders. As a result of these immune responses, discrete or multifocal areas of nervous system degeneration can occur, causing diverse symptoms and deficits.[74]

These are not direct effects of either the tumor or its metastases. Cancer cells can acquire new cellular functions uncharacteristic of the originating tissue. Many of these syndromes involve ectopic hormone production by tumor cells. These hormones are distributed by the circulation and act on target organs at a site other than the location of the tumor. Some tumor cells secrete biochemically active substances that can also cause metabolic abnormalities.

Paraneoplastic syndromes are not common, but when they occur, the neuromusculoskeletal system is often affected and the clinical presentation is unusual. The clinical manifestation of paraneoplastic syndrome depends on the tumor effects. The therapist is often the first health care professional to see and/or recognize the incongruence of the signs and symptoms.

In fact, the presentation may confound the medical staff. When the client fails to respond to palliative treatment, physical therapy is recommended. The alert therapist will recognize the unusual presentation and will follow up with a screening examination.

The paraneoplastic syndromes are of considerable importance because they may accompany relatively limited neoplastic growth and provide an early clue to the presence of certain types of cancer (e.g., osteoarthropathy caused by bronchogenic carcinoma, hypercalcemia from osteolytic skeletal metastases). The most common cancer associated with paraneoplastic syndromes is small cell cancer of the lungs (produces adrenocorticotrophic hormone [ACTH] and causes Cushing's syndrome).

CLINICAL SIGNS AND SYMPTOMS OF PARANEOPLASTIC SYNDROMES

Clinical findings of paraneoplastic syndromes may resemble those of primary endocrine, metabolic, hematologic, or neuromuscular disorders. For example, the Lambert-Eaton myasthenic syndrome (LEMS) results in muscle weakness when autoantibodies directed against the presynaptic calcium channels at the neuromuscular junction cause impaired release of acetylcholine from presynaptic nerve terminals.

Gradual, progressive muscle weakness during a period of weeks to months (especially of the pelvic girdle muscles) may occur. Proximal muscles are most likely to be involved (see Fig. 13-3). The weakness does stabilize. Reflexes of the involved extremities are present but diminished. The weakness often improves, and deep tendon reflexes may return with exercise.

In clients who develop myopathies such as dermatomyositis (DM) or polymyositis (PM), the myositis may precede, follow, or arise concurrently with the malignancy. No particular type of cancer has been found to predominate in such cases, but the clients affected are generally older and respond poorly to medical treatment for the myositis.

The course of the paraneoplastic syndrome usually parallels that of the tumor. Therefore, effective medical intervention (rather than physical therapy) should result in resolution of the syndrome. A paraneoplastic syndrome may be the first sign of a malignancy or recurrence of cancer that may be cured if detected early. Paraneoplastic syndromes with musculoskeletal manifestations are listed in Table 13-7.

Even such nonspecific symptoms as anorexia, malaise, weight loss, and fever are truly neoplastic and are probably due to the production of specific factors by the tumor itself. For example, anorexia is a common symptom in clients with cancer that is attributed to tumor production of the protein tumor necrosis factor (TNF), also called cachectin. Fever may be seen in clients with cancer in the absence of infection when it is produced by tumor induction of pyrogen formation by host white cells or by direct tumor production of a pyrogen.

TABLE 13-7 ▼ Paraneoplastic Syndromes Having Musculoskeletal Manifestations

Malignancy	Rheumatic disease	Clinical features
Lymphoproliferative disease (leukemia)	Vasculitis	Necrotizing vasculitis
Plasma cell dyscrasia	Cryoglobulinemia	Vasculitis; Raynaud's phenomenon; arthralgia; neurologic symptoms
Hodgkin's disease	Immune complex disease	Nephrotic syndrome
Ovarian cancer	Reflex sympathetic dystrophy	Palmar fasciitis and polyarthritis
Carcinoid syndrome	Scleroderma	Scleroderma-like changes; anterior tibia
Colon cancer	Pyogenic arthritis	Enteric bacteria cultured from joint
Mesenchymal tumors	Osteogenic osteomalacia	Bone pain; stress fractures
Renal cell cancer (and other tumors)	Severe Raynaud's phenomenon	Digital necrosis
Pancreatic cancer	Panniculitis	Subcutaneous nodules, especially in males

Modified from Gilkeson GS, Caldwell DS: Rheumatologic associations with malignancy, J Musculoskel Med 7(1):72, 1990.

Clinical Signs and Symptoms of
Paraneoplastic Syndromes

* Fever
* Skin rash, pigmentation changes (see Figs. 4-9, 4-10, 4-24)
* Clubbing of the fingers or toes
* Arthralgias
* Paresthesias
* Thrombophlebitis
* Proximal muscle weakness
* Change in deep tendon reflexes (most often hyporeflexia)
* Anorexia, malaise, weight loss
* Signs and symptoms of hypercalcemia (see Tables 13-9 and 13-7)

Rheumatologic Manifestations Rarely, cancer is associated with arthritis and presents as a paraneoplastic syndrome called carcinoma polyarthritis. Polyarthritis has been reported in adults ages 43 to 80 years old when associated with solid tumors and in individuals from 12 to 65 years with hematologic malignancies.[75]

This type of polyarthritis has been associated most often with breast and lung cancers. Palmar fasciitis and polyarthritis have been reported in association with metastatic ovarian carcinoma (Case Example 13-6).[76] Even though cancer polyarthritis is a rare occurrence, the therapist is more likely than most other health care professionals to see this. Timely recognition can reduce morbidity and mortality.

The medical diagnosis can be missed or delayed without careful evaluation. Sometimes, the diagnosis of polymyalgia rheumatica is made in error. Anyone with a sudden onset of rheumatic disease that is seronegative and monarticular and occurs in the presence of a past history of cancer may be demonstrating signs of metastatic cancer or an occult malignancy.

Rheumatologic complaints have a sudden onset and may spare the small joints of the hands and wrists. Clinical features of carcinoma polyarthritis primarily affect asymmetric joints of the lower extremities, often the result of metastasis to the joint or periarticular bone.

Other rheumatologic conditions and muscular disorders can be associated with malignancy (Box 13-3). These conditions often disappear after successful treatment of the underlying malignancy.[75,77]

Digital Clubbing Digital clubbing is another possible sign of paraneoplastic syndrome, especially when associated with pulmonary malignancy

(see Fig. 4-34). Clubbing of the fingers and toes is seen most often with chronic conditions such as congenital heart disease with cyanosis, cystic fibrosis, or chronic obstructive pulmonary disease (COPD). It can also develop with paraneoplastic syndromes and within 10 days of acute systemic illness such as acute pulmonary abscess, heart disease, and ulcerative colitis.

Digital clubbing occurs in the distal phalanx and causes the ends of the digits to become round and wide, like "little clubs." The thumb and index finger are affected first and can be assessed by the Schamroth method (see Fig. 4-35).

Look for recent onset of other signs and symptoms (e.g., pulmonary, hepatic, cardiac, gastrointestinal). For example, digital clubbing accompanied by a recent, unexplained weight loss, hemoptysis, and a significant smoking history may be a red flag sign associated with lung cancer.

Skeletal Manifestations

Primary bone cancer is uncommon; primary cancers of the musculoskeletal system are discussed later in this chapter. The skeleton is, however, the most common organ affected by metastatic cancer. Tumors arising from the breast, prostate, thyroid, lung, and kidney possess a special propensity to spread to bone.

Tumor cells commonly metastasize to the most heavily vascularized parts of the skeleton, particularly the red bone marrow of the long bones (humerus and femur), and the proximal ends of the long bones (humerus and femur), and the vertebral column, pelvis, and ribs (Table 13-8).

Occasionally, a growing bone mass is the first sign of disease. Diagnosis is made by x-ray study and surgical biopsy, requiring immediate attention to suspicious symptoms by referral to the client's physician.

Local swelling can be detected when the lesion protrudes beyond the normal confines of the bone. The swelling of a benign lesion is usually firm and nontender. In the presence of a rapidly growing malignant neoplasm, however, the swelling is more diffuse and frequently tender (Fig. 13-6).

The overlying skin may be warm because of the highly vascularized nature of neoplasms. If the lesion is close to a joint, function in that joint may be disturbed, with painful and restricted range of motion.

Bone Pain

Bone pain, resulting from structural damage, rate of bone resorption, periosteal irritation, and nerve

CASE EXAMPLE 13-6 ▼ Arthritis Associated With Ovarian Carcinoma

A 56-year-old woman was sent to physical therapy by a hand surgeon with a provisional diagnosis of rheumatoid arthritis, pending results of laboratory studies. She described a 3-month history of bilateral finger stiffness with swelling and pain. Most recently, she developed nodules at the proximal interphalangeal joints (PIPs) and thickening of the palms with erythema, both bilaterally.

At the time of her first physical therapy visit, she also reported new onset of right shoulder pain and loss of motion. When asked if she had noticed any symptoms or changes of any kind anywhere else in the body, she mentioned pain and a sense of "fullness" in the left lower abdominal quadrant. She denied having any hip pain on that side or any GI or GU signs and symptoms.

There was no previous history of any significance. When asked about birth histories and deliveries, she reported never being married and never being pregnant. She had her last menstrual period 3 years ago. Her last Papanicolaou (PAP) smear and clinical breast examination were performed 2 years ago, and results were reportedly within normal limits.

During a screening physical examination, the therapist noted visible asymmetry of the lower abdominal quadrant with distention observed on the left compared with the right. There was no warmth or tenderness to abdominal palpation, but an unidentified mass could be felt just to the midline of the left anterior inferior iliac spine (ASIS). Because the client was postmenopausal, there was no need to screen for possible pregnancy.

How would you proceed in a situation like this? Do you suggest the client call and report new onset of shoulder pain and "fullness" to the referring physician? Or, should you suggest she go to her gynecologist for a pelvic examination and updated PAP smear?

The new onset of shoulder pain is important information, given the physician's "provisional diagnosis" while waiting for lab results. Although the apparent pelvic mass is not usually of interest to a hand surgeon, it will be up to the referring physician to decide what further medical testing is needed.

The therapist should provide the physician with the new and additional information obtained, present a plan for physical therapy intervention, and request approval before proceeding, given the new signs and symptoms present. Until a final medical diagnosis is made and cancer ruled out, ultrasound should not be used.

Results: Laboratory tests revealed a normal complete blood count (CBC) and sedimentation rate and routine chemistry results. Special tests for markers to indicate rheumatoid arthritis (rheumatoid factor, antinuclear antibody) were normal.

When this additional information was presented, further tests were ordered. A diagnosis of ovarian cancer (Stage IV) was made, indicating distant metastases. Physical therapy intervention was put on hold until medical treatment (i.e., surgery and chemotherapy) could be completed. She received occupational therapy as an inpatient for home adaptive aids and stretching exercises. Her hand symptoms resolved with medical treatment of the carcinoma.

From Gilkeson GS, Caldwell DS: Rheumatologic associations with malignancy, *J Musculoskel Med* 1990;7:70.

BOX 13-3 ▼ Muscular Disorders Associated With Malignancy

Dermatomyositis and polymyositis
Type II muscle atrophy
Myasthenia gravis
Lambert-Eaton myasthenic syndrome (LEMS)
Metabolic myopathies
Primary neuropathic diseases
Amyotrophic lateral sclerosis
Amyloidosis

TABLE 13-8 ▼ Most Common Sites of Bone Metastases (in order of frequency)

Vertebrae (thoracic 60%/lumbosacral 30%)
Pelvis
Ribs (posterior)
Skull
Femur (proximal)
Others: sternum, cervical spine

Data from Smuckler A, Govindan R: Management of bone metastasis, *Contemp Oncol* 1(13):1-10, 2002.

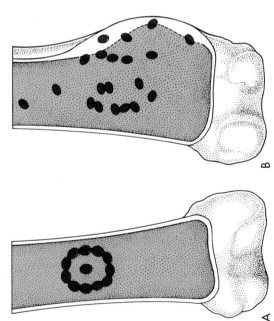

Fig. 13-6 • A, Benign bone tumors have a characteristic sclerotic rim around the periphery of the lesion. The lesion is usually well defined, and there is no evidence of erosion of the cortex or a soft tissue mass. **B,** Malignant bone tumors can have lytic or sclerotic components. It is frequently difficult to know the extent of the lesion within the bone because there is no well-defined sclerotic rim around the tumor. The destructive process is diffuse within the medullary cavity of the bone, and the tumor may break through the cortex of the bone, producing Codman's triangle. Frequently, an associated soft tissue mass is present. Medical differential diagnosis of this lesion is between an osteogenic sarcoma and a chondrosarcoma. (Modified from de Vita VT Jr, Hellman S, eds: *Cancer: Principles and Practice of Oncology.* Philadelphia, 1982, JB Lippincott.)

It is often worse at night, awakening the person; neither sleep nor lying down provides relief. Pain at night that is unrelieved by rest or change in position is a red flag. Assessing night pain is discussed in detail in Chapter 3, under Night Pain and Cancer (see Box 3-7).

Beware of the client who reports disproportionate (excessive) pain relief with aspirin, as this may be a sign of a particular bone cancer called osteoid osteoma. Pain subsiding with salicylates is the hallmark of this entity. Salicylates inhibit the prostaglandins that are produced by osteoid osteomas.

Bone pain associated with skeletal metastases can often be reproduced with a heel strike when an undiagnosed fracture is present in the lower extremities. Watch for pain on weight bearing with a positive heel strike test or reproduced symptoms when hopping on one leg (in the younger client; this is not a likely test to use in the older adult). Perform translational/rotational tests for stress fracture.

The pain does not respond to physical agents or physical therapy intervention. Sometimes, the client may experience some relief after the first few sessions of physical therapy, but pain returns and may even be worse than before. The therapist may think the chosen intervention has been unsuccessful and is at fault. Consider it a red flag whenever a client fails to improve or improves and then gets worse. Further investigation and screening is advised under these circumstances.

Pain may occur around joints because of mechanical, chemical, or bony change; pain and the rate of bone resorption appear to be linked. There is often disturbance of the highly innervated periosteum, giving bone pain its neurogenic-like qualities, especially its unrelenting, intractable quality.

Fracture

Pathologic fractures (e.g., vertebrae, long bones) occur in half of all people with osteolytic mets. In fact, this may be the presenting sign of bone cancer. An injury with subsequent medical evaluation reveals the fracture and the cancer simultaneously.

Back Pain

Neoplastic disease can cause backache, particularly in older adults, or shoulder pain in the presence of breast cancer. Although primary neoplasms of the spine are rare, myeloma and metastatic disease are more common. Malignancy as a cause of low back pain in primary care clients accounts for only 1% of the affected population.[78]

entrapment, is the most common complication of metastatic disease to the skeletal system. A history of sudden onset of severe pain usually indicates the complication of a pathologic fracture (a break in an already weakened bone). Pathologic fractures are the result of metastatic disease of primary cancers most often affecting the lung, prostate, and breast.

Pathologic fractures tend to affect the vertebral body at both the thoracic and lumbar levels. Kyphotic deformity can occur with compression of the cord or cauda equina (see further discussion on Cauda Equina in this chapter).

Bone pain is usually deep, intractable, and poorly localized, sometimes described as burning or aching and accompanied by episodes of stabbing discomfort (Case Example 13-7). The pain may be cyclic and progressive until it becomes constant. The pain is made worse by activity, especially weight bearing. The pain is often associated with trauma during a game or exercise and may be dismissed in children as "growing pains."

CASE EXAMPLE 13-7 Uterine Cancer With Bone Metastasis

A 44-year-old slender, athletic woman with isolated left knee pain of unknown cause was referred to physical therapy by her physician for a "strengthening program." She was actively involved in a variety of physical activities, including a co-ed baseball team, a hiking club, and church basketball intramurals but could not recall any specific injury, fall, or other impact to her leg. She had a pair of shoe orthotics prescribed by a podiatrist 5 years ago "to compensate for my excessive Q-angle."

The physical therapy examination was unremarkable for any joint swelling, redness, or palpable warmth. There was point tenderness along the medial joint line and a palpable though asymptomatic plica. Joint integrity was intact, and all special tests were negative.

A neurologic screening examination was also considered within normal limits, although muscle strength for the quadriceps and hamstrings was diminished by pain. Pain was present on weight-bearing activities but did not prevent the woman from participating in all activities. There was no reported night pain, fever, or other associated signs and symptoms.

Without a definitive physical therapy diagnosis, a treatment plan was outlined to include modalities for pain and a stretching and strengthening program. Within a week's time, this client's pain level escalated on the numeric rating scale (NRS) from 3 to 10 (on a scale from 1 to 10) with constant pain that kept her awake at night for hours. When she returned to the physical therapy clinic, she was using crutches and was not bearing weight on the left leg.

Results: Therapists should be careful about assuming that physical therapy treatment has exacerbated a client's symptoms and instituting a change in program. If the treating therapist decided to continue physical therapy, with the use of some other approach, the physician should have been notified of the change in status.

Given the insidious onset of this joint pain and the rapidly progressive nature of the symptoms, this client was immediately sent back to her physician. A diagnosis of bone metastasis was made, with early stage endometrial carcinoma appearing as an unusual, isolated skeletal lesion.

She was treated with aggressive multidisciplinary therapy, including limb salvage and physical therapy as part of her rehabilitation program. The early referral most likely contributed to her favorable prognosis and cancer-free status 2 years later.

In anyone with a known cancer, the onset of back pain could suggest spinal metastases. An insidious onset of waist-level or midback pain that becomes progressively more severe and more persistent often occurs. The pain is usually unrelieved by lying down and frequently becomes worse at night. Unexplained weight loss with severe back pain aggravated by rest may point to metastatic carcinoma of the spine. Other bone-related cancers such as multiple myeloma can cause severe, unremitting backaches that are present at rest and become worse when lying down.

Hypercalcemia From Skeletal Metastases

Hypercalcemia (greater than normal amounts of calcium in the blood) occurs frequently in clients with metastatic bone disease who have osteolytic lesions (Fig. 13-7). Normal serum calcium levels range between 8.2 and 10.2 mg/dl. Mild hypercal-

cemia occurs when this level drops to around 12 mg/dl; severe hypercalcemia is defined by serum calcium at 14 mg/dl or more.

Hypercalcemia is very common in cases of breast cancer and myeloma, primarily because of an increase in bone resorption, which is caused, in turn, by tumor cell production of parathyroid hormone–related protein that stimulates osteoclastic bone resorption.[68,79]

Other tumors associated with hypercalcemia may include carcinomas of the lung (most commonly, small cell lung cancers), squamous cell carcinoma of the head and neck, renal cell cancer, prostate cancer, lymphoma and leukemia, thyroid cancer, and parathyroid carcinoma (rare). In most cases, hypercalcemia is an indication of progression of disease. Hypercalcemia associated with metastatic breast cancer involving bone may occur with hormone therapy.

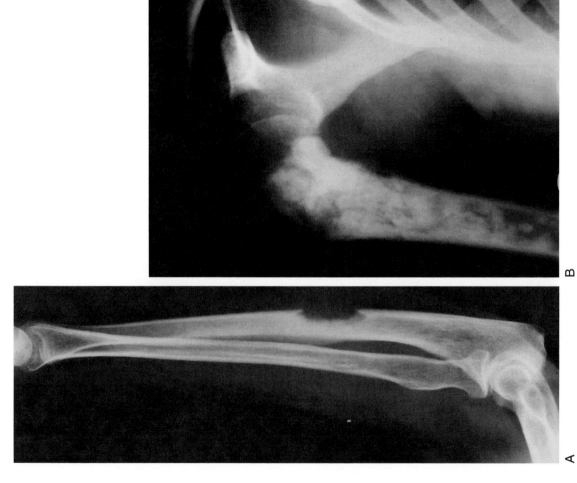

A

B

Fig. 13-7 • Lytic vs. blastic bone: In the following x-rays, you will see a lytic bone lesion on the left from breast cancer. Notice how the bone has distinct punched out segments. This is characteristic of a lytic lesion. On the right, you will see blastic bone lesions from osteosarcoma. The blastic form of bone cancer is a more diffuse pattern of degeneration. (From Dorfman HD, Czerniak B: *Bone tumors.* St. Louis, 1998, Mosby.)

Hypercalcemia is characterized by musculoskeletal, nervous system, cardiovascular/pulmonary, and GI symptoms (Table 13-9). The therapist may see the first signs and symptoms of hypercalcemia in the musculoskeletal system but should watch for others as well.

Signs and symptoms of CNS-related hypercalcemia are similar to other causes of CNS problems and include confusion, drowsiness, lethargy, headache, depression, and irritability. Hypercalcemia can also affect the GI system. The most common hypercalcemia-induced GI signs and symptoms are anorexia, nausea, vomiting, constipation, dehydration, and thirst.

And finally, in the clinical practice of a therapist, hypercalcemia secondary to bone cancer or metastases to the bone may affect the cardiac system. These clients are usually in-patients or are known to have cancer. Hypertension may be the only outward sign of hypercalcemia-induced cardiovascular changes. Vital sign assessment may help identify early signs of cardiac involvement. However, cardiac arrest may present as the first sign of a problem.

TABLE 13-9 ▼ Hypercalcemia

System	Symptom
Central Nervous System (CNS)	Drowsiness, lethargy, coma
	Irritability, personality change
	Confusion, increased confusion
	Headaches
	Depression, memory loss, difficulty concentrating
	Visual disturbances
	Balance/coordination problems
	Changes in deep tendon reflexes (hyporeflexive or hyperreflexive)
	Change in muscle tone for individual with neurologic condition
	Positive Babinski and/or clonus reflex
	Changes in bowel/bladder function
Musculoskeletal	Muscle pain or tenderness and weakness
	Muscle spasms
	Bone pain (worse at night and on weight bearing)
	Pathologic fracture
Cardiovascular	Hypertension
	Arrhythmia
	Cardiac arrest
Gastrointestinal	Anorexia (loss of appetite)
	Nausea
	Vomiting
	Constipation
	Dehydration
	Thirst

Symptoms observed in a physical therapy practice include bilateral carpal/tarsal tunnel syndrome, possibly accompanied by abdominal pain and tenderness with general malaise and fatigue. Right upper quadrant pain with possible referral to the right shoulder may also occur with or without carpal tunnel syndrome (see Table 13-6).

Carpal Tunnel Syndrome

Carpal tunnel syndrome (CTS) can be caused by a wide range of both neuromusculoskeletal and systemic conditions and illnesses (see Table 11-2). Whenever anyone presents with bilateral symptoms of any kind, it is considered a "red flag" symptom. In Chapter 2 of this text, we discussed the various bilateral symptoms the therapist might encounter in a clinical practice.

A common systemic cause of CTS involves the hepatic system (see Chapter 9 for an explanation). Briefly, liver dysfunction results in increased serum ammonia and urea levels. When these toxins are no longer absorbed into the portal vein and removed from the body, they pass directly to the brain.

Ammonia transported to the brain reacts with glutamate (an excitatory neurotransmitter), producing glutamine. The reduction of brain glutamate impairs neurotransmission. This leads to altered CNS metabolism and function. As blood ammonia levels rise, many unusual compounds (e.g., octopamine) form and serve as false neurotransmitters in the CNS. Asterixis (also known as liver flap) and numbness/tingling occur as a result of this ammonia abnormality, causing intrinsic nerve pathology. This can be misinterpreted as CTS (or tarsal tunnel syndrome) (Case Example 13-8).

When screening for bilateral CTS as a result of liver impairment, always ask about the presence of similar symptoms in the feet. Look for a history of alcoholism, cirrhosis, previous cancer, other liver disease, and the use of statins (cholesterol-lowering drugs such as simvastatin [Zocor] and atorvastatin calcium [Lipitor]; liver damage occurs in some people taking these medications).

Ask about the presence of other GI signs and symptoms. A client presenting with shoulder or upper back pain may not think nausea and abdominal bloating are related in any way to the symptoms in the wrists and hands. Perform a quick liver screen and look for signs of liver disease (see Box 9-1 or Appendix B-4).

Hepatic Manifestations

Liver metastases are among the most ominous signs of advanced cancer. The liver filters blood coming in from the GI tract, making it a primary metastatic site for tumors of the stomach, colorectum, and pancreas.

Bisphosphonates (bone resorption inhibitors, such as Fosamax [alendronate], Actonel [risedronate], Evista [raloxifene], and Miacalcin [calcitonin-salmon]) are drugs used to control hypercalcemia and limit or prevent bone loss. In emergent or predictable situations, intravenous use of bisphosphonates (e.g., pamidronate, zoledronic acid) can be used to stabilize and/or prevent hypercalcemia. With their use, health care professionals expect to see fewer cases of hypercalcemia than in the past. These drugs also reduce bone pain, delay skeletally related events (SREs), reduce the number of pathologic fractures, and, in some cases, prolong survival.

CHAPTER 13 SCREENING FOR CANCER ▲ 591

CASE EXAMPLE 13-8 Carpal Tunnel Syndrome Associated With Liver Cancer

A 52-year-old male who was employed as an over-the-road (OTR) trucker was referred by a hand surgeon for bilateral carpal tunnel syndrome (CTS). The client did not want surgery and opted for a more conservative, nonoperative approach.

He was hostile and verbally abusive, refusing to even sit down for his treatment. His wife reported a history of alcohol use/abuse. He was not screened for medical disease, just treated with the CTS protocol in a hand clinic.

During a treatment session, he commented that he had just seen an acupuncturist who told him he has liver disease. Because symptoms of bilateral numbness and tingling in the hands and feet can be a sign of liver impairment, a screening examination was performed.

The client was tested for liver flap and was observed for palmar erythema and nailbed and skin changes. Liver flap was not present, but tremoring of the hands was observed along with palmar erythema. No obvious ascites or angiomas were present.

The client was later given a medical diagnosis of liver cancer.

What are the red flags in this case? How do you return the client to the referring physician for further follow-up?

Red Flags

Age over 50
Reported history of alcohol use/abuse

Bilateral symptoms
Liver impairment diagnosis by acupuncturist
Palmar erythema, motor tremor

Physician Referral: This may depend upon the therapist's relationship with the physician. It may be possible to telephone the physician with exactly what happened and what the therapist sees as "red flags."

If that is not feasible, then a letter (brief and to the point) with a quick summary of the findings and an open-ended question should be faxed or sent. For example,

Date (very important for documentation)
Dear Dr. Lowell,

Thank you for your recent referral of Mr. Smith for hand therapy. We are following our usual protocol for carpal tunnel syndrome. Something has come up that concerns me. Mr. Smith saw Dr. Jyn, the local acupuncturist, who mentioned liver impairment.

Given his age, drinking history, and bilateral CTS, I'm wondering if there isn't something else going on. I noticed a fine tremor in both hands (present at rest and with activity) and color changes in his hands suggestive of palmar erythema.

We will continue treating him, but perhaps an appointment with you sooner than his scheduled 4-week follow-up is in order. What do you think?
(Alternate: Please advise.)
Signature, etc.

▶ ONCOLOGIC PAIN

As mentioned earlier, pain is rarely an early warning sign of cancer and is uncommon in some cancers such as leukemia. However, pain occurs in 60% to 80% of clients with solid tumors.

This pain syndrome has multiple causes, and the therapist must always keep in mind common patterns of referred pain (see Chapter 3; see also Table 3-8). Some pain is caused by pressure on peripheral nerves or displacement of these nerves. Pain may also result from interference with blood supply or from blockage within hollow organs.

A common cause of cancer pain is metastasis of cancer to the bone. This type of pain can occur as a result of pathologic fracture with resultant muscle spasms; if the spine is involved, nerves may be affected. Pain may also result from iatrogenic causes such as surgery, radiation therapy, and chemotherapy. Immobility and inflammation also can lead to pain.

Signs and Symptoms Associated With Levels of Pain

The severity of pain varies from one client to another, but certain signs and symptoms are characteristic of particular levels of pain. For example, in *mild-to-moderate superficial pain*, a sympathetic nervous system response is usually elicited with hypertension, tachycardia, and tachypnea (rapid, shallow breathing).

In *severe or visceral pain,* a parasympathetic nervous system response is more characteristic, with hypotension, bradycardia, nausea, vomiting, tachypnea, weakness, or fainting. Depression and anxiety may increase the client's perception of pain, requiring additional psychologic and emotional support.

Biologic Mechanisms

Five biologic mechanisms have been implicated in the development of chronic cancer pain. The characteristics of the pain depend on tissue structure, as well as on the mechanisms involved.

Bone Destruction

Bone destruction secondary to infiltration by malignant cells or resulting from metastatic lesions is the first and most common of the biologic mechanisms causing chronic cancer pain. Bone metastases cause increased release of prostaglandins and subsequent bone breakdown and resorption.

The client's pain threshold is reduced through sensitization of free nerve endings. Bone pain may be mild to intense. Maladaptive outcomes of bone destruction may include sharp, continuous pain that increases on movement or ambulation. The rich supply of nerves and tension or pressure on the sensitive periosteum or endosteum may cause bone pain.

Other factors contributing to the intense discomfort reported by clients include limited space for relief of pressure, altered local metabolism, weakening of the bone structure, and pathologic fractures ranging in size from microscopic to large.

Visceral Obstruction

Obstruction of a hollow visceral organ and ducts such as the bowel, stomach, or ureters is a second physiologic factor in the development of chronic cancer pain.

Viscus obstruction is most often due to the obstruction of an organ lumen by tumor growth. In the GI or genitourinary tract, obstruction results in either a severe, colicky, crampy pain or true visceral pain that is dull, diffuse, boring, and poorly localized.

If a vein, artery, or lymphatic channel is obstructed, venous engorgement, arterial ischemia, or edema, respectively, will result. In these cases, pain is described as dull, diffuse, burning, and aching. Obstruction of the ducts leading from the gallbladder and pancreas is common in cancer of these organs, although jaundice is more frequently an earlier symptom than pain. Cancer of the throat or esophagus can

obstruct these organs, leading to difficulties in eating or speaking.

Nerve Compression

Infiltration or compression of peripheral nerves is the third physiologic factor that produces chronic cancer pain and discomfort. Pressure on nerves from adjacent tumor masses and microscopic infiltration of nerves by tumor cells result in continuous, sharp, stabbing pain that generally follows the pattern of nerve distribution. The invading cells affect the conduction of impulses by the nervous system and sometimes result in constant, dull, poorly localized pain and altered sensation.

Blockage of the blood in arteries and veins, again both by pressure from tumor masses nearby and by infiltration, can decrease oxygen and nutrient supply to tissues. This deficiency can be perceived as pain that is similar in origin and character to cardiac pain, or angina pectoris, which is chest pain from an insufficient supply of oxygen to the heart. Hyperesthesia or paresthesia may result.

Skin or Tissue Distention

Infiltration or distention of the integument (skin) or tissue is the fourth physiologic phenomenon resulting in chronic, severe cancer pain. This type of pain is secondary to the painful stretching of skin or tissue because of underlying tumor growth. This stretching produces severe, dull, aching, and localized pain, with severity of pain increasing concurrently with increase in tumor size.

Pain associated with headache secondary to brain tumor is thought to be due to traction on pain-sensitive intracranial structures.

Tissue Inflammation, Infection, and Necrosis

Inflammation, infection, and necrosis of tissue may be the fifth and final cause of cancer pain. Inflammation, with its accompanying symptoms of redness, edema, pain, heat, and loss of function, may progress to infection, necrosis, and sloughing of tissue.

If the inflammatory process alone is present, the pain is characterized by a sensitive tenderness. If, however, necrosis and tissue sloughing have occurred, pain may be excruciating.

▶ ## SIDE EFFECTS OF CANCER TREATMENT

Conventional cancer treatment has many side effects because the goal of treatment is to remove

or to kill certain tissues. In any situation, healthy tissue also is usually sacrificed. It is not always possible to differentiate between cancer recurrence and the acute or long-term effects of cancer treatment. For this reason, knowledge of both immediate and delayed side effects of cancer treatment is helpful.

For many years, three basic modalities of cancer treatment have been used, either alone or in combination: surgery, radiation therapy, and chemotherapy. In recent years, immunotherapies involving the use of cells of the immune system to prompt a tumor-killing response have been developed. Immunotherapy may be most effective when combined with conventional treatments, such as chemotherapy and radiation, to improve the success of treatment and decrease the side effects of conventional modalities.

The pharmaceuticals used in chemotherapy are cytotoxic (destructive) and are designed to kill dividing cells selectively by blocking the ability of DNA and RNA to reproduce and by lysing cell membranes. All types of rapidly dividing cells, not just the cancer cells, are affected. Damage to otherwise healthy tissue such as bone marrow, hair follicles, mucosal cells in the mouth, digestive tract, and reproductive system, not just to cancer cells, is the cause of most side effects.

In addition, a combination of drugs (each causing cell death through different pharmacologic mechanisms) is traditionally used for greater efficacy in the systemic treatment of some cancers (e.g., breast cancer). Hence, an overlap of toxicities may result in greater side effects.

Common Physical Effects

The effects of treatment for cancer can be debilitating physiologically, physically, and psychologically. Common physical side effects include bone marrow suppression, severe mucositis, mouth sores, nausea and vomiting, fluid retention, pulmonary edema, cough, headache, CNS effects, peripheral neuropathies, malaise, fatigue, dyspnea, and loss of hair. Emotional and psychologic side effects are present but less evident (Table 13-10).

Bone marrow suppression (myelosuppression) is a common and serious side effect of many chemotherapeutic agents and can be a side effect of radiation therapy in some instances. This condition may lead to significant decreases in production of white blood cells (leukopenia), red blood cells (anemia), and, in some cases, platelets (thrombocytopenia).

Leukopenia (neutropenia) and resultant opportunistic infections have been shown to result in dose reductions, treatment delays, and hospitalizations. People at risk for leukopenia are taught infection prevention techniques and are often supportively or emergently treated with injections of colony stimulating factors such as GCSF (granulocyte colony stimulating factor) or a newer version colony stimulating factor, pegfilgrastim (Neulasta), to stimulate increased production of needed white blood cells.[80]

Another relatively common bone marrow treatment toxicity is *anemia*. A drop in the production of red blood cells and in associated hemoglobin levels causes a loss of oxygenation to many body tissues and results in the many associated symptoms of anemia such as severe fatigue, muscle weakness, dizziness, dyspnea, pallor, and tachycardia.

Red blood cell transfusions and/or the use of injectable epoetin alfa (Epogen), the recombinant form of human erythropoietin, or darbepoetin (Aranesp), a newer version of Epogen, is very useful in the treatment of anemia.

Closely related to anemia is *fatigue*. Cancer-related fatigue is a frequent, difficult, and often debilitating problem. It differs from fatigue of healthy people because it happens independently of rest and activity patterns.[81] Factors contributing to fatigue can include many physical and emotional components of cancer such as anemia, poor nutrition, infection, low thyroid output, tumor breakdown by products, depression, pain, and medications.

Fatigue has been identified as a major determinant of perceived quality of life; it may be temporary, may persist throughout the episode of care, and may even continue many months after treatment has concluded. Adequate hydration, exercise, dietary measures, and treatment of anemia and depression are all measures used to help in the treatment of patients with cancer-related fatigue.[82]

Aggressive chemotherapeutic agents and chest irradiation can cause *cardiopulmonary dysfunction*, especially in the treatment of Hodgkin's disease and breast and lung cancers. High-dose radiation can result in pericardial fibrosis (scarring of the pericardium) and constrictive pericarditis (inflammation of the pericardium). These conditions are usually asymptomatic until the client starts to exercise, and then, exertional *dyspnea* is the first symptom.

Other causes of dyspnea include deconditioning, anemia, peripheral arterial disease, and increased physiologic demand for oxygen because of fever or

TABLE 13-10 ▼ Side Effects of Cancer Treatment

The health care professional must remember that some of the delayed effects of radiation, such as cerebral injury, pericarditis, pulmonary fibrosis, hepatitis, intestinal stenosis, other GI disturbances, and nephritis, may be signs of recurring cancer. The physician must be notified by the affected individual of any new symptoms, change in symptoms, or increase in symptoms.

Surgery	Radiation	Chemotherapy	Biotherapy	Hormonal therapy	Transplant (bone marrow, stem cell)
Disfigurement	Radiation sickness	GI effects	Fever	Nausea	Severe bone marrow suppression
Loss of function	Immunosuppression	Anorexia	Chills	Vomiting	Mucositis
Infection	Decreased platelets	Nausea	Nausea	Hypertension	Nausea and vomiting
Increased pain	Decreased WBCs	Vomiting	Vomiting	Steroid-induced diabetes	Graft vs. host disease (allogenic only)
Deformity	Infection	Diarrhea	Anorexia	Myopathy (Steroid-induced)	Delayed wound healing
Scar tissue	Fatigue	Ulcers	Fatigue	Weight gain	Veno-occlusive disease
Fibrosis	Fibrosis	Hemorrhage	Fluid retention	Altered mental status	Infertility
	Burns	Bone marrow	CNS effects	Hot flashes	Cataract formation
	Mucositis	suppression		Sweating	Thyroid dysfunction
	Diarrhea	Anemia		Impotence	Growth hormone deficiency
	Edema	Leukopenia		Decreased libido	Osteoporosis
	Hair loss	Thrombocytopenia		Morning stiffness	Secondary malignancy
	Delayed wound healing	Skin rashes		Arthralgia, myalgia	
	CNS effects	Neuropathies		Sexual dysfunction	
	Malignancy	Hair loss			
	Osteonecrosis (mandible, clavicle, humerus, femur)	Sterilization			
	Radiation recall	Phlebitis			

Adapted from Goodman CC, Boissonnault WG, Fuller KS: *Pathology: implications for the physical therapist*, ed 2, Philadelphia, 2003, WB Saunders.
GI, Gastrointestinal; *WBC,* white blood cell; *CNS,* central nervous system.

infection. During radiation therapy, the client may be more tired than usual. Resting throughout exercise is important, as are adequate nutrition and hydration.

The skin in the irradiated area may become red or dry and should be exposed to the air but protected from the sun and from tight clothing. Gels, lotions, oils, or other topical agents should not be used over the irradiated skin without a physician's approval. Clients may have other side effects, depending on the areas treated. For example, radiation to the lower back may cause nausea, vomiting, or diarrhea because the lower digestive tract is exposed to the radiation.

Radiation recall is a severe skin reaction that can occur when certain chemotherapy drugs (e.g., Actinomycin, doxorubicin, methotrexate, fluorouracil, hydroxyurea, paclitaxel, liposomal doxorubicin) are given during or soon after radiation treatment.

The skin reaction appears like a severe sunburn or rash on the area of skin where the radiation was previously administered. It can appear weeks to months after the last dose of radiation. It is very important that this reaction be immediately reported because symptoms may be severe enough that chemotherapy must be delayed until the skin has healed.[83]

Bone necrosis and demineralization (*radiation osteonecrosis*) can also result from radiation therapy and are usually not reversible. Individuals with this problem have an increased likelihood of pathologic fractures and need to be carefully handled by the therapist. Any activities, including weight-bearing activities and range of motion, should be addressed prior to the initiation of therapeutic exercise.[84]

Monitoring Laboratory Values

It is very important to review hematologic values in clients receiving these treatment modalities before any type of vigorous physical therapy is initiated. A guideline used by some physical therapy exercise programs is the Winningham Contraindications for Aerobic Exercise. According to these guidelines, aerobic exercise is contraindicated in chemotherapy clients when laboratory values are as follows[85]:

Platelet count	<50,000/mm³
Hemoglobin	<10 g/dl
White blood cell count	<3000/mm³
Absolute granulocytes	<2500/mm³

More specific exercise guidelines for all diseases (and even are available.[86] All treatment facilities

individual physicians within the center) establish their own parameters and protocols. Many centers use hemoglobin levels exclusively as hematocrit is linked with hydration and may not provide the information needed. It does not appear that there is an "industry standard" for these measures.

In an out-patient setting without the benefit of laboratory values for guidance, the therapist is advised to use vital signs as discussed in Chapter 3 of this text, along with rate of perceived exertion (RPE) during exercise. Observe for clinical signs and symptoms of infection and fever, thrombocytopenia, deep vein thrombosis, dehydration, and electrolyte imbalance.

▲ CANCERS OF THE MUSCULOSKELETAL SYSTEM

In addition to increasing age as a red flag and risk factor for cancer, we now add "young age" as a possible red flag factor. Primary bone cancer is more likely to occur in the population under age 25. Both primary bone cancer and cancer that has metastasized to the bone present with the same subset of clinical signs and symptoms because in both cases, the same system (skeletal) is affected.

Sarcoma

Malignant neoplasms or new growths that develop as *primary* lesions in the musculoskeletal tissues are relatively rare, representing less than 1% of malignant disease in all age groups and 15% of annual pediatric malignancies.[87]

Secondary neoplasms that develop in the connective tissues as metastases from a primary neoplasm elsewhere (especially metastatic carcinoma) are common. Fibrosarcomas occurring after radiotherapy can occur usually after a significant latent period (4 years or longer).[88]

High grade (higher grade represents greater likelihood of metastasis based on measures of cell differentiation and growth) and evidence of metastasis are associated with a poor prognosis for all neoplasms of bone or soft tissue. The prognosis for clients with soft tissue sarcoma depends on several factors. Factors associated with a poorer prognosis include age older than 60 years, tumors larger than 5 cm, and histology of high grade.[89]

Soft Tissue Tumors

Soft tissue sarcomas make up a group of relatively rare malignancies. Little is known about important epidemiologic or etiologic factors in clients with soft tissue sarcomas. There is no proven genetic predisposition to the development of soft tissue

sarcomas, but studies do indicate that workers exposed to phenoxyacetic acid in herbicides and chlorophenols in wood preservatives, and radiation to the tonsils, adenoids, and thymus, may have an increased risk of developing soft tissue sarcoma. There are two peaks of incidence in human sarcoma development: early adolescence and the middle decades.

Soft tissue sarcomas can arise anywhere in the body. In adults, most soft tissue sarcomas arise in the extremities (usually the lower extremity, at or below the knee), followed by the trunk and the retroperitoneum. In their early stages, these sarcomas do not usually cause symptoms because soft tissue is relatively elastic, allowing tumors to grow rather large before they are felt or seen.

In contrast, the overwhelming majority of childhood soft tissue sarcomas are rhabdomyosarcomas, and the anatomic distribution of these lesions is entirely different (18% in the extremities, 35% in the head and neck region, and 20% in genitourinary sites).[90] Many of the primary sites in children (e.g., orbit of the eye, paratesticular region, prostate) are never primary sites for soft tissue sarcoma in adults.

RISK FACTORS

Soft tissue sarcomas occur more frequently in persons who have one of the following conditions:

von Recklinghausen's disease
Gardner's syndrome
Werner's syndrome
Tuberous sclerosis
Basal cell nevus syndrome
Li-Fraumen syndrome (*p53* suppressor gene mutations)
Exposure to radiation, herbicides, wood preservatives, vinyl chloride
AIDS (Kaposi's sarcoma)

METASTASES

In children, tumors of the extremities tend to behave relatively aggressively, with a high incidence of nodal spread and distant metastases. In adults, soft tissue sarcomas rarely spread to regional lymph nodes, instead invading aggressively into surrounding tissues with early hematogenous dissemination, usually to the lungs and to the liver.

Even with pulmonary metastases, the survival rate has greatly improved over the past decade with a multidisciplinary approach that includes multiagent chemotherapy and limb-sparing surgery.[90] However, as more people survive for increasingly longer periods, serious and potentially

life-threatening complications of such therapy can develop months to years later.

CLINICAL SIGNS AND SYMPTOMS

Soft tissue sarcomas most often appear as asymptomatic soft tissue masses. Because these lesions arise in compressible tissues and are often far from vital organs, symptoms are few unless they are located close to a major nerve or in a confined anatomic space.

The most common manifestations of these neoplasms are swelling and pain. Pelvic sarcomas may appear with swelling of the leg or pain in the distribution of the femoral or sciatic nerve. Some people attribute swelling to a minor injury, reporting a misleading cause of onset to the therapist. The therapist must always keep this in mind when evaluating a client of any age.

More often, the neoplasm goes unnoticed until some trauma or injury requires medical attention and an x-ray study reveals the lesion. When pain is the most significant symptom, it is usually mild and intermittent, progressively becoming more severe and more constant with rapidly growing neoplasms.

No reliable physical signs are present to distinguish between benign and malignant soft tissue lesions. Consequently, all soft tissue lumps that persist or grow should be reported immediately to the physician.

Clinical Signs and Symptoms of

Soft Tissue Sarcoma

- Persistent swelling or lump in a muscle (most common finding)
- Pain
- Pathologic fracture
- Local swelling
- Warmth of overlying skin

Bone Tumors

Benign and malignant (primary) bone tumors are relatively rare, accounting for 1% of total deaths from cancer. Excluding multiple myeloma, the ratio of benign to malignant bone tumors is approximately 7:1.

Primary bone cancer affects children and young adults most commonly, whereas secondary bone tumors or metastatic neoplasms occur in adults with primary cancer (e.g., cancer of the prostate, breast, lungs, kidneys, thyroid).

Symptoms are not necessarily different between primary and secondary bone cancer, but the *history* is very different. Medical screening with possible

referral is essential for anyone with clinical manifestations discussed in this chapter (see Clinical Manifestations of Malignancy: Skeletal) who also has a past medical history of any kind of cancer.

This text is limited to the most common forms of bone tumors. The two most common childhood sarcomas of the bone are osteosarcoma (osteogenic sarcoma) and Ewing's family of tumors (EFT).

OSTEOSARCOMA

Osteosarcoma (also known as osteogenic sarcoma) is the most common type of bone cancer, occurring between the ages of 10 and 25 years and also in adulthood. It is slightly more common in boys.

Although it can involve any bones in the body, because it arises from osteoblasts, the usual site is the epiphyses of the long bones, where active growth takes place (e.g., lower end of the femur, upper end of the tibia or fibula, upper end of the humerus).

In general, 80% to 90% of osteosarcomas occur in the long bones; the axial skeleton is rarely affected. The growth spurt of adolescence is a peak time for the development of osteosarcoma. Half of all osteosarcomas are located in the upper leg above the knee, where the most active epiphyseal growth occurs.

Risk Factors There appears to be an association between rapid bone growth and risk of tumor formation. Young people previously treated with radiation for an earlier cancer have an increased risk of developing osteosarcoma later.

With chemotherapy given before and after surgical removal, many people can now be cured of osteosarcoma. Survival lessens if metastases are present. Limb sparing surgery rather than amputation is effective in 50% to 80% of people.[91]

Metastases Bone tumors, unlike carcinomas, disseminate almost exclusively through the blood; bones lack a lymphatic system. Metastases to the lungs, pleura, lymph nodes, kidneys, and brain and to other bones are common and occur early in the disease process.

Hematogenous spread occurs to the lungs first and to other bones second. In some cases, surgery can be attempted to remove pulmonary metastases, but survival decreases if metastatic sites are present.

Clinical Signs and Symptoms Osteosarcoma usually appears with pain in a lesional area, usually around the knee in clients with femur or tibia involvement. The pain is initially mild and intermittent but becomes progressive and more severe and more constant over time.

Most lesions produce pain as the tumor starts to expand the bony cortex and stretch the periosteum. A tender lump may develop, and a bone weakened by erosion of the metaphyseal cortex may break with little or no stress. This pathologic fracture often brings the person into the medical system, at which time a diagnosis is established by x-ray study and surgical biopsy. This neoplasm is highly vascularized, so that the overlying skin is usually warm.

Clinical Signs and Symptoms of

Osteosarcoma

- Pain and swelling of the involved body part
- Loss of motion and functional movement of adjacent joints
- Tender lump
- Pathologic fracture
- Occasional weight loss
- Malaise
- Fatigue

EWING'S SARCOMA

Four percent of all childhood tumors are in the Ewing family of tumors (EFT). In the United States, approximately 300 to 400 children and adolescents are diagnosed with a Ewing tumor each year. Almost any bone can be involved, but typically, the pelvis, femur, tibia, ulna, and metatarsus are the most common sites for Ewing's sarcoma.

Risk Factors It is most common between the ages of 5 and 16 years, with a slightly greater incidence in boys than in girls. Most people who have Ewing tumors are of the white race, either Hispanic or non-Hispanic. This tumor is rare in other racial groups.[92] A gene translocation in chromosome 22 has been found with EFT, and there is study in this area. No other risk factors have been identified in the development of Ewing's family of tumors.

Metastases Metastasis is predominantly hematogenous (to lungs and bone), although lymph node involvement may occur. Metastasis usually occurs late in the disease process, but aggressive chemotherapy has increased 5-year survival rates from 10% to 70%.

Clinical Signs and Symptoms Ewing's sarcoma is a rapidly growing tumor that often outgrows its blood supply and quickly erodes the bone cortex, producing a painful, soft, tender, palpable mass. Intramedullary tumors that erode into the periosteum often result in an "onion skin" appearance as the periosteum is elevated and replaced by a new periosteal bone.

The most common symptom of EFT, bone pain, appears in about 85% of people with bone tumors. The pain may be caused by periosteal erosion from a break or fracture of a bone weakened by the tumor.

The pain may be intermittent and may not be accompanied by swelling, resulting in a physical therapy referral. Systemic symptoms such as fatigue, weight loss, and intermittent fever may be present, especially in clients with metastatic disease. Fever may occur when products of bone degeneration enter the bloodstream. In addition, the blood supply to local areas of bone may be compromised, with resultant avascular necrosis of bone.

Ewing's sarcoma occurs most frequently in the long bones and the pelvis, the most common site being the distal metaphysis and the diaphysis of the femur. The next most common sites are the pelvis, tibia, fibula, and humerus (Case Example 13-9). About 30% of the time, the bone tumor may be soft and warm to the touch and the child may have a fever.

Less common presentations of Ewing's sarcoma include primary rib tumor associated with a pleural effusion and respiratory symptoms, mandibular lesions presenting with chin and lip paresthesias, primary vertebral (cervical, lumbar) tumor with symptoms of nerve root or spinal cord compression, and primary sacral tumor with neurogenic bladder. Neurologic symptoms may occur secondary to nerve entrapment by the tumor, and misdiagnosis as lumbar disc disease can occur.[93] If the tumor has spread, the child may feel very tired or may lose weight.

Clinical Signs and Symptoms of Ewing's Family of Tumors (EFT)

- Increasing and persistent pain
- Increasing and persistent swelling over a bone (localized over the area of tumor)
- Decrease in movement if a limb bone is involved
- Fever
- Fatigue
- Weight loss

CHONDROSARCOMA

Chondrosarcoma, the most common malignant cartilage tumor, occurs most often in adults older than 40. However, when it does occur in a younger age group, it tends to be a higher grade of malignancy and capable of metastases.

It occurs most commonly in some part of the pelvic or shoulder girdles or long bones, such as the

---

CASE EXAMPLE 13-9 Back Pain Associated With Ewing's Sarcoma

A 17-year-old male high school athlete noted low back pain 6 weeks ago. He was unable to identify a specific traumatic event or injury but noted that he had been "training pretty hard" the last 2 weeks. Spinal motions were all within normal limits with no apparent step suggestive of spondylolisthesis. There were no obvious postural changes, such as a scoliotic shift or unusual kyphosis/lordosis of the spinal curves.

The only positive evaluation findings included a mild left foot drop and an absent left ankle jerk. Pain was intensified on weight bearing and movement of any kind. Pain was not relieved by rest or aspirin.

There was no fever or recent history of sore throat, upper respiratory or ear infection, and so on. After 1 week in physical therapy, pain began radiating into the posterior aspect of the left thigh. The client had also noted for the first time paresthesias along the lateral side of the left leg. The pain had increased rather markedly over the past 2 weeks.

The therapist might assume that the physical therapy intervention aggravated this client's condition, causing increased symptoms. However, given the unknown cause of pain, symptoms inconsistent with musculoskeletal conditions (e.g., unrelieved by rest), combined with the recent change in symptoms and the presence of positive neurologic symptoms, this client was returned to the physician before continuing further therapy.

Results: A blood test performed at that time indicated that the WBC count was 10,000 mm³ (normal range = 4300 to 10,800 mm³). Further testing, including an x-ray, resulted in a diagnosis of Ewing's sarcoma.

femurs (Fig. 13-8). Chondrosarcomas are the most common malignant tumors of the sternum and scapula.

Chondrosarcoma is usually a relatively slow-growing malignant neoplasm that arises either spontaneously in previously normal bone or as a result of malignant change in a preexisting benign bone tumor (osteochondromas and enchondromas or chondromas).

Risk Factors See information related to soft tissue sarcomas.

Metastases Although slow growing, chondrosarcoma has a high tendency for thrombus formation in the tumor blood vessels, with an increased risk for pulmonary embolism and metastatic spread to the lungs. Metastases develop

late, so the prognosis of chondrosarcoma is considerably better than that of osteosarcoma.

Clinical Signs and Symptoms Clinical presentation of chondrosarcoma varies. *Peripheral chondrosarcomas* (arising from bone surface) grow slowly and may be undetected and quite large. Local symptoms develop only because of mechanical irritation; otherwise, pain is not a prominent symptom.

Pelvic chondrosarcomas are often large and appear with pain referred to the back or thigh, sciatica caused by sacral plexus irritation, urinary symptoms from bladder neck involvement, or unilateral edema caused by iliac vein obstruction.

Conversely, *central chondrosarcomas* (arising within bone) appear with dull pain, and a mass is

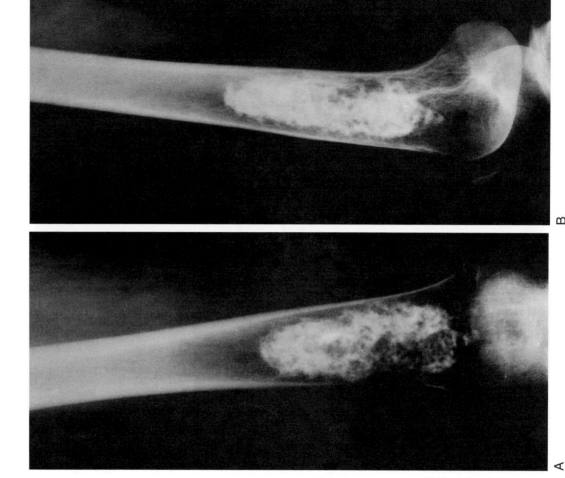

A

B

Fig. 13-8 • Large intramedullary calcified lesion diagnosed as a low-grade chondrosarcoma of the femur. **A,** Anteroposterior radiograph. **B,** Lateral view. (From Dorfman HD, Czerniak B: *Bone tumors.* St. Louis, 1998, Mosby.)

rare. Pain, which indicates active growth, is an ominous sign of a central cartilage lesion.

Clinical Signs and Symptoms of Chondrosarcoma

- Back or thigh pain
- Sciatica
- Bladder symptoms
- Unilateral edema

OSTEOID OSTEOMA

Osteoid osteoma is a non-cancerous osteoblastic tumor that accounts for approximately 10% of benign bone tumors. It occurs predominantly in children and young adults between 7 and 25, affecting males two to three times more often than females.[94]

Osteoid osteoma is a non-cancerous lesion with distinct histologic features, consisting of a central core of vascular osteoid tissue and a peripheral zone of sclerotic bone (Fig. 13-9). This type of tumor commonly occurs in the diaphysis of long bones such as the proximal femur, accounting for more than half of all cases; less often, the hands and feet and posterior elements of the spine are involved.

On x-ray, the lesion is seen as a translucent area representing the nidus, usually measuring less than 1 cm, that is surrounded by bone sclerosis. The nidus may be uniformly radiolucent or may contain variable amounts of calcification. Computed tomography (CT) shows a well-circumscribed small area of low attenuation, representing the nidus, surrounded by a larger area of higher attenuation, representing the reactive bone formation.

Clinical Signs and Symptoms The clinical presentation typically consists of pain, which is often worse at night, increased skin temperature, sweating, and tenderness in the affected region. In many cases, pain is completely relieved by salicylates, which is a hallmark finding for this particular type of bone cancer.

The pathogenesis of this pain may be related to production of prostaglandins by the tumor cells. Prostaglandins can cause changes in vascular pressure, which result in local stimulation of sensory nerve endings. Salicylates in the aspirin inhibit the prostaglandins, reducing painful symptoms.[94]

Clinical Signs and Symptoms of Osteoid Osteoma

- Bone pain (femur, 50% of cases), worse at night; relieved by aspirin
- Warmth and tenderness over the involved site

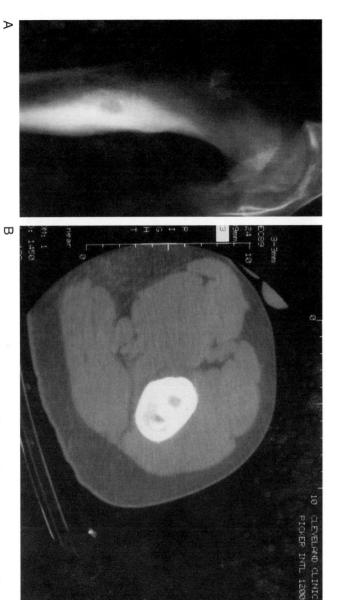

Fig. 13-9 • Osteoid osteoma. **A,** A 15-year-old boy whose pain was worse at night and relieved by aspirin was found to have a well-defined lytic intracortical lesion in the proximal femoral shaft. Note the thickening around and extending above and below the nidus. **B,** Computed tomogram (CT) of the same osteoid osteoma shows marked sclerosis of the bone around the nidus. (From Dorfman HD, Czerniak B: Bone tumors. St. Louis, 1998, Mosby.)

A

B

▼ PRIMARY CENTRAL NERVOUS SYSTEM TUMORS

Primary tumors of the CNS once thought to be rare are now recognized as a significant problem in the United States. The incidence among persons over age 70 has increased sevenfold since 1970, with the incidence in people of all ages rising by 9% in the past three decades.[95] The majority of people who develop primary brain tumors are over the age of 40, but these tumors can cause morbidity and mortality in younger individuals as well.

CNS neoplasms include tumors that lie within the spinal cord (intramedullary), within the dura mater (extramedullary), or outside the dura mater (extradurally). About 80% of CNS tumors occur intracranially, and 20% affect the spinal cord and peripheral nerves. Of the intracranial lesions, about 60% are primary, and the remaining 40% are metastatic lesions, often multiple and most commonly from the lung, breast, kidney, and GI tract.

More common benign tumors are meningiomas (from meninges) and schwannomas (from nerve sheaths), both arising from tissues of origin. These tumors are considered non-cancerous histologically, but sometimes malignant by location, meaning that they can be located in an area where tumor removal is difficult and deficit and death can result.

Any CNS tumor, even if well differentiated and histologically benign, is potentially dangerous because of the lethal effects of increased intracranial pressure and tumor location near critical structures. For example, a small, well-differentiated lesion in the pons or medulla may be more rapidly fatal than a massive liver cancer.

Primary CNS tumors rarely metastasize outside the CNS; there is no lymphatic drainage available, and hematogenous spread is also unlikely. In most cases, CNS spread is contained within the cerebrospinal axis, involving local invasion or CNS seeding through the subarachnoid space and the ventricles.

Whether from primary CNS tumors or cancer that has metastasized to the CNS from some other source, the effects are the same. Clinical manifestations of CNS involvement were discussed earlier in this chapter.

Risk Factors

The incidence of primary CNS lymphoma is increasing among older adults who are immunocompetent and even more so among aging adults who are immunodeficient. The etiology of most primary brain tumors is unknown, although ionizing radiation has been implicated most often.

Children with a history of cranial radiation therapy such as low-dose radiation of the scalp for fungal infection are at significantly greater risk of developing primary brain tumors. However, most radiation-induced brain tumors are caused by radiation to the head used for the treatment of other types of cancer.[96]

Occupational exposure to gases and chemicals has been proposed as a risk factor. Several congenital genetic disorders are directly linked with an increased risk of primary brain tumors (e.g., neurofibromatosis, Turcot's syndrome, tuberous sclerosis). Other potential environmental risk factors such as exposure to vinyl chloride and petroleum products have shown inconclusive results, and no convincing evidence currently links exposure to electromagnetic fields from cell phones or high-tension wires.[97]

Brain Tumors

The incidence of primary brain tumor is increasing in persons of all ages; in children, it is second only to leukemia as a cause of death. Although the causes for this overall increase remain unknown, it is clear that it is not simply a matter of better diagnostic techniques. Adding the number of people who survive other primary cancers but later develop metastatic brain tumors increases the overall incidence dramatically.

Individuals with mental disorders are more likely to be diagnosed with brain tumors and at younger ages than people without mental illness. This increased risk for brain tumors may reflect the early presence of mental symptoms, or there may be a true association between the two conditions. The exact relationship remains unknown at this time.[98]

Primary Malignant Brain Tumors

The most common primary malignant brain tumors are astrocytomas. Low-grade astrocytomas (Grade I), such as juvenile pilocytic astrocytomas, have an excellent prognosis after surgical excision.

At the other extreme is the Grade IV glioma such as glioblastoma multiforme, which is an aggressive, high-grade tumor with a very poor prognosis (usually less than 12 months). There are intermediate histologic grades (II, III) with intermediate survival statistics. Low-grade tumors are more common in children than in adults.[96]

Metastatic Brain Tumors

Cancer can spread through bloodborne metastasis or via cerebrospinal fluid pathways. Therefore, the brain is a common site of metastasis. In fact, metastatic brain tumors are probably the most common form of malignant brain tumors.

The cerebrum is the most common site of metastasis. Cerebellar metastases are less frequent; brain stem metastases are the least common. Approximately two-thirds of people with brain metastases will present with multiple metastases.

Up to 50% of individuals affected with cancers develop neurologic symptoms resulting from brain metastases. Headache, seizures, loss of motor function, and cerebellar signs are the most common early symptoms.

As mentioned previously, any neurologic sign can be the silent presentation of cancer metastasized to the CNS. The most common sources of brain metastases are cancers of the lung and breast, followed by metastases from melanomas and cancers of the colon and kidney.

Clinical Signs and Symptoms of Brain Tumor

- Increased intracranial pressure
- Headache, especially retroorbital; sometimes worse upon awakening, improves during the day
- Vomiting (with or without nausea)
- Visual changes (blurring, blind spots, diplopia, abnormal eye movements)
- Changes in mentation (impaired thinking, difficulty concentrating or reading, memory, or speech)
- Personality change, irritability
- Unusual drowsiness, increased sleeping
- Seizures (without previous history)
- Sensory changes
- Muscle weakness or hemiparesis
- Bladder dysfunction
- Increased lower extremity reflexes compared with upper extremity reflexes
- Decreased coordination, gait changes, ataxia
- Positive Babinski reflex
- Clonus (ankle or wrist)
- Vertigo, head tilt

Spinal Cord Tumors

Spinal tumors are similar in nature and origin to intracranial tumors but occur much less often. They are most common in young and middle-aged adults, and they occur most often in the thoracic spine because of its length, proximity to the mediastinum, and likelihood of direct metastatic extension from lymph nodes involved with lymphoma, breast cancer, or lung cancer.

Metastases

Most metastasis is disseminated by local invasion. Spinal cord tumors account for <15% of brain tumors. As mentioned, 10% of spinal tumors are themselves metastasized neoplasms from the brain.

One other means of dissemination is through the intervertebral foramina. The extradural space communicates through the intervertebral foramina with adjacent extraspinal compartments, such as the mediastinum and retroperitoneal space.

In most cases, extradural tumors are metastatic, reaching the extradural space and then adjacent extraspinal spaces through this foraminal connection. Tumors within the spinal cord (intramedullary) or outside the spinal cord (extramedullary) may metastasize to the dural tube to become intradural tumors.

Clinical manifestations of spinal tumors vary according to their location. See previous discussion in this chapter, Clinical Manifestations of Malignancy: Neurologic. Pain associated with *extramedullary tumors* can be located primarily at the site of the lesion or may refer down the ipsilateral extremity, with radicular involvement from nerve root compression, irritation, or occlusion of blood vessels supplying the cord. Progressive cord compression is manifested by spastic weakness below the level of the lesion, decreased sensation, and increased weakness.

Intramedullary tumors produce more variable signs and symptoms. High cervical cord involvement causes spastic quadriplegia and sensory changes. Tumors in descending areas of the spinal cord produce motor and sensory changes appropriate to functions of that level.

Clinical Signs and Symptoms of Spinal Cord Tumors

- Pain
- Decreased sensation
- Spastic muscle weakness
- Progressive muscle weakness
- Muscle atrophy
- Paraplegia or quadriplegia
- Thoracolumbar pain
- Unilateral groin or leg pain
- Pain at rest and/or night pain
- Bowel/bladder dysfunction (late finding)

CANCERS OF THE BLOOD AND LYMPH SYSTEM

Cancers arising from the bone marrow include acute leukemias, chronic leukemias, multiple myelomas, and some lymphomas. These cancers are characterized by the uncontrolled growth of blood cells.

The major lymphoid organs of the body are the lymph nodes and the spleen (see Fig. 4-39). Cancers arising from these organs are called malignant lymphomas and are categorized as either Hodgkin's disease or non-Hodgkin's lymphoma.

Leukemia

Leukemia, a malignant disease of the blood-forming organs, is the most common malignancy in children and young adults. One-half of all leukemias are classified as *acute*, with rapid onset and progression of disease resulting in 100% mortality within days to months without appropriate therapy.

Acute leukemias are most common in children from 2 to 4 years of age, with a peak incidence again at age 65 years and older. The remaining leukemias are classified as *chronic*, which have a slower course and occur in persons between the ages of 25 and 60 years. From these two broad cat-egories, leukemias are further classified according to specific malignant cell line (Table 13-11).

Leukemia develops in the bone marrow and is characterized by abnormal multiplication and release of white blood cell (WBC) precursors. The disease process originates during WBC development in the bone marrow or lymphoid tissue. In effect, leukemic cells become arrested in "infancy," with most of the clinical manifestations of the disease being related to the absence of functional "adult" cells, which are products of normal differentiation.

With rapid proliferation of leukemic cells, the bone marrow becomes overcrowded with immature WBCs, which then spill over into the peripheral circulation. Crowding of the bone marrow by leukemic cells inhibits normal blood cell production.

Decreased red blood cell (RBC) (erythrocyte) production results in anemia and reduced tissue oxygenation. Decreased platelet production results in thrombocytopenia and risk of hemorrhage. Decreased production of normal WBCs results in increased vulnerability to infection, especially because leukemic cells are functionally unable to defend the body against pathogens.

Leukemic cells may invade and infiltrate vital organs such as the liver, kidneys, lung, heart, or brain.

TABLE 13-11 ▼ Overview of Leukemia

	ALL	ANLL (AML)	CLL	CML
Incidence				
Percentage of all leukemias	20%	20%	25%-40%	15%-20%
Adults	20%	85%	100%	95%-100%
Children	80%-85%	10%-20%	—	3%
Age	Peak: 3-7 years 65+ (older adults)	15-40 years Incidence increases with age from 40-80+	50+	25-60 years
Etiology	Unknown Chromosomal abnormality Environmental factors Down's syndrome (high incidence)	Benzene Alkylating agents Radiation Myeloproliferative disorders Aplastic anemia	Chromosomal abnormalities Slow accumulation of CLL lymphocytes	Philadelphia chromosome Radiation exposure
Prognosis	Adult: Poor Child: 60% with aggressive treatment	Poor even with treatment 10%-15% survival	2-10 years survival Median survival: 6 years	Poor; 2-8 years Median survival: 3-4 years

From Goodman CC, Boissonnault WG, Fuller KS: *Pathology: implications for the physical therapist,* Philadelphia, 2003, WB Saunders, p 519. *ALL,* Acute lymphoblastic leukemia; *ANLL,* acute nonlymphocytic leukemia; *CLL,* chronic lymphocytic leukemia; *CML,* chronic myelogenous leukemia.

Risk Factors

Several predisposing factors for the development of leukemia have been identified. Exposure to ionizing radiation remains the most conclusively identified causative factor in humans. Prior drug therapies, such as chloramphenicol, phenylbutazone, chemotherapy alkylating agents, and benzene, have been implicated in the development of acute leukemia.

Hereditary syndromes associated with development of leukemia include Bloom's syndrome, Down syndrome, Klinefelter's syndrome, neurofibromatosis, and others. In addition, viruses and immunodeficiency disorders have been associated as causative factors.[99]

Clinical Signs and Symptoms

Most of the clinical findings in acute leukemia are due to bone marrow failure, which results from replacement of normal bone marrow elements by malignant cells. Infections are due to a depletion of competent WBCs needed to fight infection. Abnormal bleeding is caused by a lack of blood platelets required for clotting, and severe fatigue is due to a lack of red blood cells. The most common symptoms of leukemia include infection, fever, pallor, fatigue, anorexia, bleeding, anemia, neutropenia, and thrombocytopenia.

For women, the abnormal bleeding may be prolonged menstruation leading to anemia. The Special Questions for Women (see Appendix B-32) may elicit this kind of valuable information, which would then require medical referral. Less common manifestations include direct organ infiltration; clients may experience easy bruising of the skin or abnormal bleeding from the nose, urinary tract, or rectum.

The appearance of a painless, enlarged lymph node or skin lesion (see Fig. 4-27) is followed by weakness, fever, and weight loss. A history of chronic immunosuppression (e.g., anti-rejection drugs for organ transplants, chronic use of immunosuppressant drugs for inflammatory or autoimmune diseases, cancer treatment) in the presence of this clinical presentation is a major red flag.

Clients on immunosuppressants do not usually have an elevated body temperature, so the presence of a fever is a red flag in this group. Significant weight loss with inactivity secondary to pain is another red flag; most inactive individuals experience weight gain, not weight loss. A good rule of thumb to use in recognizing significant weight loss is 10% of the individual's total body weight in 10 to 14 days without trying.

Lymphoproliferative malignancies such as leukemia and lymphoma may also involve extramedullary areas and can present with local-ized or generalized symptoms such as enlarged liver and spleen, bone and joint pain, bone fracture, and parotid gland and testicular infiltration.[99]

Involvement of the synovium may lead to symptoms suggestive of rheumatic disease. A possible presentation in a child with acute lymphoblastic leukemia can be joint pain and swelling that mimics juvenile rheumatoid arthritis (JRA). Leukemic arthritis is present in about 5% of leukemia cases. Acute leukemia can cause joint pain that is severe and episodic and disproportionately severe in comparison to the minimal heat and swelling that are present.[100]

Arthritic symptoms in such a child may be a consequence of leukemic synovial infiltration, hemorrhage into the joint, synovial reaction to an adjacent tumor mass, or crystal-induced synovitis.

Clinical Signs and Symptoms of Acute and Chronic Leukemias

- Infections, fever
- Abnormal bleeding
- Easy bruising of the skin
- Petechiae
- Epistaxis (nosebleeds) and/or bleeding gums
- Hematuria (blood in the urine)
- Rectal bleeding
- Weakness
- Easy fatigability
- Enlarged lymph nodes
- Bone and joint pain
- Weight loss
- Loss of appetite
- Pain or enlargement in the left upper abdomen (enlarged spleen)

Multiple Myeloma

Multiple myeloma is a cancer caused by uncon-trolled growth of plasma cells in the bone marrow. Excessive growth of plasma cells originating in the bone marrow destroys bone tissue and is associated with widespread osteolytic lesions (decreased areas of bone density). Plasma cells are part of the immune system and in multiple myeloma, they grow uncontrolled, forming tumors in the bone marrow.

Bone lesions and hypercalcemia can occur in some hematologic malignancies such as multiple myeloma. Multiple myeloma, to date, is an incur-able disease with a poor prognosis.

Risk Factors

There are no clear predisposing factors, other than exposure to ionizing radiation. This disease can develop at any age from young adulthood to advanced age but peaks among persons between the ages of 50 and 70 years. It is more common in men and African Americans. Molecular genetic abnormalities have been identified in the etiologic complex of this disease. Recent data suggest that a virus (Kaposi-associated herpes virus, HHV-8) may be implicated in AIDS-related cases.[101]

Clinical Signs and Symptoms

Multiple myeloma causes symptoms in many areas of the body. It normally originates in the bone marrow and then causes difficulties in other organs. The onset of multiple myeloma is usually gradual and insidious. Most clients pass through a long presymptomatic period that lasts 5 to 20 years.

Early symptoms involve the skeletal system, particularly the pelvis, spine, and ribs. Some clients have backache or bone pain that worsens with movement (Case Example 13-10). Bone disease is the most common complication and results in severe bone pain, pathologic fractures, hypercalcemia, and spinal cord compression. Renal failure, anemia, cardiac failure, and infection are serious and often fatal complications of this process.[102]

CASE EXAMPLE 13-10   Rib Metastases Associated With Multiple Myeloma

At presentation, a 57-year-old man had rib pain that began 1 month ago. He could not think of any possible cause and denied any repetitive motions, recent trauma, forceful coughing, or history of tobacco use.

Past medical history was significant for hepatitis A (10 years ago) and benign prostatic hyperplasia (BPH). The BPH is reportedly well controlled with medication, but he noticed a decreased need to urinate and mentioned that he has been meaning to have a recheck of this problem.

On examination, there was bilateral point tenderness over the posterior seventh and eighth ribs. Symptoms were not increased by respiratory motions, trunk movements, position, or palpation of the intercostal spaces. Trunk and extremity movements were considered within normal limits, and a neurologic screening examination was unremarkable.

The therapist could not account for the client's symptoms, given the history and clinical presentation. Further screening revealed that the client had noticed progressive fatigue and generalized aching over the previous 2 weeks that he had attributed to the flu. He had lost about 10 pounds during the week of vomiting and diarrhea. Vital signs were taken and were within normal limits. There were no other red flag symptoms to suggest a systemic origin or symptoms.

Results: Without a proper physical therapy diagnosis on which to base treatment, the therapist did not have a clear plan of care. There was no well-defined musculoskeletal problem, but a variety of systemic variables were present (e.g., sudden weight loss and constitutional symptoms accounted for by the flu, oliguria, attributed to BPH, insidious onset of rib pain).

The therapist decided to treat the client for 7 to 10 days and reassess at that time. Intervention consisted of stretching, manual therapy, postural exercises, and Feldenkrais techniques. At the end of the prescribed time, there was no change in clinical presentation.

The therapist asked a colleague in the same clinic for a second opinion at no charge to the client. An ultrasound test for possible rib fracture was performed and was considered negative. No new findings were uncovered, and it was agreed collaboratively (including the client) to request a medical evaluation of the problem from the client's family physician. The client was subsequently given a diagnosis of multiple myeloma and was treated medically.

NOTE: The use of ultrasound over the painful rib was contraindicated in the presence of bone metastases.

Clinical Signs and Symptoms of

Multiple Myeloma

- Recurrent bacterial infections (especially pneumococcal pneumonias)
- Anemia with weakness and fatigue
- Bleeding tendencies
- **Bone destruction**
  - Skeletal/bone pain (especially pelvis, spine, and ribs)
  - Spontaneous fracture
  - Osteoporosis
  - Hypercalcemia (confusion, increased urination, loss of appetite, abdominal pain, vomiting, and constipation)
- **Renal involvement**
  - Kidney stones
  - Renal insufficiency
- **Neurologic abnormalities**
  - Carpal tunnel syndrome
  - Back pain with radicular symptoms
  - Spinal cord compression (motor or sensory loss, bowel/bladder dysfunction, paraplegia)

BONE DESTRUCTION

Bone pain is the most common symptom of myeloma. It is caused by infiltration of the plasma cells into the marrow with subsequent destruction of bone. Initially, the skeletal pain may be mild and intermittent, or it may develop suddenly as severe pain in the back, rib, leg, or arm, often the result of an abrupt movement or effort that has caused a spontaneous (pathologic) bone fracture.

The pain is often radicular and sharply cutting to one or both sides and is aggravated by movement. As the disease progresses, more and more areas of bone destruction and hypercalcemia develop. Symptoms associated with bone pain usually subside within days to weeks after initiation of antiresorptive agents. If left untreated, this disease will result in skeletal deformities, particularly of the ribs, sternum, and spine.

HYPERCALCEMIA

Bone fractures are a result of osteoclast activity and bone destruction. This process results in calcium release from the bone and hypercalcemia. Hypercalcemia is considered an oncologic emergency. To rid the body of excess calcium (hypercalcemia), the kidneys increase the output of urine, which can lead to serious dehydration if there is an inadequate intake of fluids. Vomiting may compound this dehydration. Clients who have symptoms of hypercalcemia (see Table 13-9) should seek immediate medical care because this condition can be life-threatening.

RENAL EFFECTS

Drainage of calcium and phosphorus from damaged bones eventually leads to the development of renal stones, particularly in immobilized clients. Renal insufficiency is the second most common cause of death, after infection, in clients with multiple myeloma.

In addition to bone destruction, multiple myeloma is characterized by disruption of RBC, leukocyte, and platelet production, which results from plasma cells crowding the bone marrow. Impaired production of these cell forms causes anemia, increased vulnerability to infection, and bleeding tendencies.

NEUROLOGIC COMPLICATIONS

Approximately 10% of persons with myeloma have amyloidosis, deposits of insoluble fragments of a monoclonal protein resembling starch. These deposits cause tissues to become waxy and immobile and may affect nerves, muscles, tendons, and ligaments, especially the carpal tunnel area of the wrist. Carpal tunnel syndrome with pain, numbness, or tingling of the hands and fingers may develop. Excess immunoglobulins, caused by multiple myeloma, can cause a hyperviscosity syndrome characterized by changes in mental status, vision, fatigue, angina, and bleeding disorders.[103]

More serious neurologic complications may occur in 10% to 15% of clients with multiple myeloma. Spinal cord compression is usually observed early or in the late relapse phase of disease. Back pain is usually present as the initial symptom, with radicular pain that is aggravated by coughing or sneezing. Motor or sensory loss and bowel/bladder dysfunction are signs of more extensive compression. Paraplegia is a later, irreversible event.

Hodgkin's Disease

Hodgkin's disease is a chronic, progressive, neoplastic disorder of lymphatic tissue characterized by the painless enlargement of lymph nodes with progression to extralymphatic sites such as the spleen and liver.

In Caucasians, Hodgkin's disease demonstrates constant incidence rates, with a first peak occurring in adolescents and young adults and a second peak occurring in older adults. Men are affected more often than women, and boys are affected more often than girls.[104]

Epidemiologic and clinical-pathologic features of Hodgkin's disease suggest that an infectious agent may be involved in this disorder. Recently, accumulated data provide direct evidence supporting a causal role of Epstein-Barr virus in a significant portion of cases, and a greater incidence of Hodgkin's disease has been observed in young individuals who previously had infectious mononucleosis.

Risk Factors

Infection with Epstein-Barr virus and infectious mononucleosis has been associated with Hodgkin's lymphoma. No other risk factors have been identified.

Metastases

The exact mechanism of growth and spread of Hodgkin's disease remains unknown. The disease may progress by extension to adjacent structures or via the lymphatics because lymphoreticular cells inhabit all tissues of the body except the CNS. Hematologic spread may also occur, possibly by means of direct infiltration of blood vessels.

Clinical Signs and Symptoms

Hodgkin's disease usually appears as a painless, enlarged lymph node, often in the neck, underarm, or groin. The therapist may palpate these nodes during a cervical spine, shoulder, or hip examination (see Figs. 4-39 through 4-41).

Lymph nodes are evaluated on the basis of size, consistency, mobility, and tenderness. Lymph nodes up to 1 cm in diameter of soft to firm consistency that move freely and easily without tenderness are considered within normal limits. Lymph nodes >1 cm in diameter that are firm and rubbery in consistency or tender are considered suspicious.

Enlarged lymph nodes associated with infection are more likely to be tender, soft, and movable than slow-growing nodes associated with cancer. Lymph nodes enlarged in response to infections throughout the body require referral to a physician, especially in someone with a current or previous history of cancer. The physician should be notified of these findings, and the client should be advised to have the lymph nodes checked at the next follow-up visit with the physician if not sooner, depending on the client's particular circumstances.

As always, *changes* in size, shape, tenderness, and consistency raise a red flag. Supraclavicular nodes are common metastatic sites for occult lung and breast cancers, whereas inguinal nodes implicate tumors arising in the legs, perineum, prostate, or gonads.

Other early symptoms may include unexplained fevers, night sweats, weight loss, and pruritus (itching). The itching occurs more intensely at night and may result in severe scratches because the client is unaware of scratching during the sleep state. The fever typically peaks in the late afternoon, and night sweats occur when the fever breaks during sleep. Fatigue, malaise, and anorexia may accompany progressive anemia. Some clients with Hodgkin's disease experience pain over the involved nodes after ingesting alcohol.

Symptoms may arise when enlarged lymph nodes obstruct or compress adjacent structures, causing edema of the face, neck, or right arm secondary to superior vena cava compression, or causing renal failure secondary to urethral obstruction.

Obstruction of bile ducts as a result of liver damage causes bilirubin to accumulate in the blood and discolor the skin. Mediastinal lymph node enlargement with involvement of lung parenchyma and invasion of the pulmonary pleura progressing to the parietal pleura may result in pulmonary symptoms, including nonproductive cough, dyspnea, chest pain, and cyanosis.

Dissemination of disease from lymph nodes to bones may cause compression of the spinal cord, leading to paraplegia. Compression of nerve roots of the brachial, lumbar, or sacral plexus can cause nerve root pain.

Clinical Signs and Symptoms of

Hodgkin's Disease

- Painless, progressive enlargement of unilateral lymph nodes, often in the neck
- Pruritus (itching) over entire body
- Unexplained fevers, night sweats
- Anorexia and weight loss
- Anemia, fatigue, malaise
- Jaundice
- Edema
- Nonproductive cough, dyspnea, chest pain, cyanosis
- Nerve root pain
- Paraplegia

Non-Hodgkin's Lymphoma

Non-Hodgkin's lymphoma (NHL) is a group of lymphomas affecting lymphoid tissue and occurring in persons of all ages. It is more common in adults in their middle and older years (40 to 60 years).

Risk Factors

Males are affected more often than females and individuals with congenital or acquired immunodeficiencies (e.g., those undergoing organ transplantation and anyone with autoimmune diseases are all at increased risk for development of NHL).[104,105] In addition some people who have been exposed to large levels of radiation (e.g., nuclear reactor accidents) or extensive radiation and chemotherapy for a different cancer site may be at increased risk for lymphoma.

Individuals infected with the human immunodeficiency virus (HIV) are at increased risk for developing NHL and, to a lesser extent, Hodgkin's disease as well. Acquired immune deficiency syndrome–related lymphoma (ARL) is now the second most common cancer associated with HIV after Kaposi's sarcoma. The relative risk of developing lymphoma within 3 years of an AIDS diagnosis is increased by 165-fold when compared with people without AIDS.[105]

Several possible etiologic mechanisms are hypothesized for NHL. Immunosuppression, possibly in combination with viruses or exposure to certain infectious agents, could be the primary cause. Chemicals, ultraviolet light, blood transfusion, acquired and congenital immune deficiency, and autoimmune disorders increase the risk for NHL.[106]

Other studies link the disease to widespread environmental contaminants, such as benzene found in cigarette smoke, gasoline, automobile emissions, and industrial pollution.

Clinical Signs and Symptoms

NHL presents a clinical picture broadly similar to that of Hodgkin's disease, except that the disease is usually initially more widespread and less predictable. The disease starts in the lymph nodes, although early involvement of the oropharyngeal lymphoid tissue or the bone marrow is common, as is abdominal mass or gastrointestinal involvement with complaints of vague back or abdominal discomfort.[104]

The most common manifestation is painless enlargement of one or more peripheral lymph nodes. Systemic symptoms are not as commonly associated with NHL as with Hodgkin's disease. Clients with non-Hodgkin's lymphomas often have remarkably few symptoms, even though many node areas or extranodal sites are involved.

Most NHLs fall into two broad categories related to their clinical activity: indolent and aggressive lymphomas. Indolent disease may be minimally active and treatable for many years. However, the disease is frequently disseminated at the time of diagnosis. Surgery is usually used only for staging or debulking purposes. Combination chemotherapy, biotherapy (targeted monoclonal antibodies), and radiation therapies are now used as treatment for NHL. Radioactive isotope combinations with monoclonal antibodies are also in use for some types of NHL.[104]

Clinical Signs and Symptoms of Non-Hodgkin's Lymphoma

- Enlarged lymph nodes
- Fever
- Night sweats
- Weight loss
- Bleeding
- Infection
- Red skin and generalized itching of unknown origin

Acquired Immunodeficiency Syndrome–Non-Hodgkin's Lymphoma (AIDS-NHL)

Only recently has AIDS-NHL emerged as a major sequela of HIV infection. It now occurs frequently in clients who survive other consequences of AIDS. The etiologic basis of AIDS-NHL is still under investigation; profound cellular immunodeficiency plays a central role in lymphoma genesis. The molecular pathogenesis is a complex process involving both host factors and genetic alterations.[107]

Nearly 95% of all HIV-associated malignancies are either NHL or Kaposi's sarcoma. People with CNS lymphoma usually have advanced AIDS, are severely debilitated, and are usually thought to be at terminal stages of the disease.[104]

Epstein-Barr virus (EBV) often accompanies NHL. It is generally accepted that EBV acts in the pathogenesis of lymphoma owing to the alteration in balance between host and latent EBV infection in immunodeficiency states, with increased activity of the virus.

Risk Factors

Infection with HIV and related immunodeficiencies resulting from HIV are the primary risk factors for this disease. NHL is more likely to develop among clients who have Kaposi's sarcoma, a history of herpes simplex infection, and a lower neutrophil count.

Clinical Signs and Symptoms

The most common presentations of HIV-related NHL are systemic B symptoms (which may suggest

an infectious process), a rapidly enlarging mass lesion, or both. At the time of diagnosis, approximately 75% of clients will have advanced disease. Extranodal disease frequently involves any part of the body, with the most common locations being the CNS, bone marrow, GI tract, and liver.

Diagnosis of NHL in areas of the body other than the CNS is complicated by a history of fevers, night sweats, and weight loss and loss of appetite, which are also common symptoms related to HIV infection and AIDS.

Although musculoskeletal lesions are not reported as commonly as pulmonary or CNS abnormalities in HIV-positive individuals, a wide variety of osseous and soft tissue changes are seen in this group. Diffuse adenopathy, lower extremity pain and swelling, subcutaneous nodules, and lytic lesions of the extremities are common.[108]

Clinical Signs and Symptoms of
AIDS-NHL

- Painless, enlarged mass
- Subcutaneous nodules
- Constitutional symptoms (fever, night sweats, weight loss)
- Musculoskeletal lesions (lytic bone, pain, swelling)

▶ PHYSICIAN REFERRAL

Early detection of cancer can save a person's life. Any suspicious sign or symptom discussed in this chapter should be investigated immediately by a physician. This is true especially in the presence of a positive family history of cancer, a previous personal history of cancer, and environmental risk factors, and/or in the absence of medical or dental (oral) evaluation during the previous year.

The therapist is not responsible for diagnosing cancer. The primary goal in screening for cancer is to make sure the client's problem is within the scope of a physical therapist's practice. In this regard, documentation of key findings and communication with the physician are both very important.

When trying to sort out neurologic findings, remember to look for changes in DTRs, a myotomal weakness pattern, and changes in bowel/bladder function. These findings will not give you a definitive diagnosis but will provide you with valuable information to offer the physician if further medical testing is advised.

Pain on weight bearing that is unrelieved by rest or change in position and does not respond to treatment, unremitting pain at night, and a history of cancer are all red flags indicating that medical evaluation is needed.

Any recently discovered lumps or nodules must be examined by a physician. Any suspicious finding by report, on observation, or by palpation should be checked by a physician.

If any signs of skin lesions are described by the client, or if they are observed by the therapist, and the client has not been examined by a physician, a medical referral is recommended.

If the client is planning a follow-up visit with the physician within the next 2 to 4 weeks, that client is advised to indicate the mole or skin changes at that time. If no appointment is pending, the client is encouraged to make a specific visit either to the family/personal physician or to a dermatologist.

Guidelines for Immediate Physician Referral

- Presence of recently discovered lumps or nodules or changes in previously present lumps, nodules, or moles, especially in the presence of a previous history of cancer or when accompanied by carpal tunnel or other neurologic symptoms.
- Detection of palpable, fixed, irregular mass in the breast, axilla, or elsewhere requires medical referral or a recommendation to the client to contact a physician for evaluation of the mass. Suspicious lymph node enlargement or lymph node changes; generalized lymphadenopathy.
- Recurrent cancer can appear as a single lump, a pale or red nodule just below the skin surface, a swelling, a dimpling of the skin, or a red rash. Report any of these changes to a physician immediately.
- Notify physician of any suspicious changes in lymph nodes; note the presence of lymphadenopathy, and describe the location and any observed or palpable characteristics.
- Presence of any of the early warning signs of cancer, including idiopathic muscle weakness accompanied by decreased deep tendon reflexes.
- Any unexplained bleeding from any area (e.g., rectum, blood in urine or stool, unusual or unexpected vaginal bleeding, breast, penis, nose, ears, mouth, mole, skin, or scar).
- Any sign or symptom of metastasis in someone with a previous history of cancer (see individual cancer types for specific clinical signs and symptoms; see also Clues to Screening for Cancer).
- Any man with pelvic, groin, sacroiliac, or low back pain accompanied by sciatica and a past history of prostate cancer.

Clues to Screening for Cancer

- Age older than 50 years
- Previous personal history of any cancer, especially in the presence of bilateral carpal tunnel symptoms, back pain, shoulder pain, or joint pain of unknown or rheumatic cause at presentation
- Previous history of cancer treatment (late physical complications and psychosocial complications of disease and treatment can present in a somatic presentation)
- Any woman with chest, breast, axillary, or shoulder pain of unknown cause, especially with a previous history of cancer and/or over the age of 40
- Anyone with back, pelvic, groin, or hip pain accompanied by abdominal complaints, palpable mass
- *For women:* Prolonged or excessive menstrual bleeding (or in the case of the postmenopausal woman who is not taking hormone replacement, breakthrough bleeding)
- *For men:* Additional presence of sciatica and past history of prostate cancer
- Recent weight loss of 10% of total body weight (or more) within 2-week to 1-month period of time without trying; weight gain is more typical with true musculoskeletal dysfunction because pain has limited physical activities
- Musculoskeletal symptoms are made better or worse by eating or drinking (GI involvement)
- Shoulder, back, hip, pelvic, or sacral pain accompanied by changes in bowel and/or bladder function or changes in stool or urine

- Hip or groin pain is reproduced by heel strike/hopping test or translational/rotational stress (bone fracture from metastases)
- When a back "injury" is not improving as expected or if symptoms are increasing
- Early warning signs, including proximal muscle weakness and changes in deep tendon reflexes
- Constant pain (unrelieved by rest or change in position); remember to assess constancy by asking, "Do you have that pain right now?"
- Intense pain present at night (rated 7 or higher on a numeric scale from 0 for "no pain" to 10 for "worst pain")
- Signs of nerve root compression must be screened for cancer as a possible cause
- Development of new neurologic deficits (e.g., weakness, sensory loss, reflex change, bowel or bladder dysfunction)
- Changes in size, shape, tenderness, and consistency of lymph nodes, especially painless, hard, rubbery lymph nodes present in more than one location
- A growing mass, whether painless or painful, is assumed to be a tumor unless diagnosed otherwise by a physician. A hematoma should decrease in size over time, not increase[109]
- Disproportionate pain relieved with aspirin may be a sign of bone cancer (osteoid osteoma)
- Signs or symptoms seem out of proportion to the injury and persist longer than expected for physiologic healing of that type of injury; no position is comfortable (remember to conduct a screening examination for emotional overlay)
- Change in the status of a client currently being treated for cancer

OVERVIEW

CANCER PRESENCE AND PAIN

▼ METASTASES (most commonly seen in a physical therapy setting)

Location:
Integumentary system
Pulmonary system
Neurologic system
Musculoskeletal
Hepatic

Referral:
See Table 13-6

▼ SKIN (MELANOMA ONLY)

Location:
Anywhere on the body
Women: Arms, legs, back, face
Men: Head, trunk
African Americans: Palms, soles, under the nails

Referral:
None

Description:
Usually painless; see ABCD method of detection (text)
Sore that does not heal
Irritation and itching
Cluster mole formation
Tenderness and soreness around a mole

Intensity:
Mild

Duration:
Constant

Associated signs and symptoms:
None

▼ PARANEOPLASTIC SYNDROMES

Location:
Remote sites from primary neoplasm
Organ dependent

Referral

Description:
Asymmetric joint involvement
Lower extremities primarily
Concurrent arthritis and malignancy
Explosive onset at late age
See Tables 13-7 and Box 13-3

Intensity:
Symptom dependent

Duration:
Symptom dependent

Associated signs and symptoms:
Fever
Skin rash
Clubbing of the fingers
Pigmentation disorders
Arthralgias
Paresthesias
Thrombophlebitis
Proximal muscle weakness
Anorexia, malaise, weight loss
Rheumatologic complaints

OVERVIEW   CANCER PRESENCE AND PAIN—cont'd

▼ ONCOLOGIC (CANCER) PAIN

Location: Localized bone pain; referred pain

Referral: May follow nerve distribution

Description: Bone pain: Sharp, intense, constant
    Viscera: Colicky, cramping, dull, diffuse, boring, poorly localized
    Vein, artery, lymphatic channel: Dull, diffuse, burning, aching
    Nerve compression: Sharp, stabbing; follows nerve distribution or dull, poorly localized
    Inflammation: Sensitive tenderness

Intensity: Varies from mild to severe or excruciating
    Bone pain: Increases on movement or weight bearing
    Usually constant; may be worse at night

Duration: With mild to moderate superficial pain: Sympathetic nervous system response (e.g., hypertension, tachycardia, tachypnea)
    With severe or visceral pain: Parasympathetic nervous system response (e.g., hypotension, tachypnea, weakness, fainting)

Associated signs and symptoms: Organ dependent (e.g., esophagus: difficulty eating or speaking; gallbladder: jaundice, nausea; nerve involvement: altered sensation, paresthesia; see individual visceral cancers)

▼ SOFT TISSUE TUMORS

Location: Any connective tissue (e.g., tendon muscle, cartilage, fat, synovium, fibrous tissue)

Referral: According to the tissue involved

Description: Persistent swelling or lump, especially in the muscle

Intensity: Mild, increases progressively to severe

Duration: Intermittent, increases progressively to constant

Associated signs and symptoms: Local swelling with tenderness and skin warmth
    Pathologic fracture

▼ BONE TUMORS

Location: Can affect any bone in the body, depending on the specific type of bone cancer

Referral: According to pattern and location of metastases

Description: Sharp, knifelike, aching bone pain
    Occurs on movement and weight bearing, with pathologic fractures
    Pain at night, preventing sleep

Intensity: Initially mild, progressing to severe

Duration: Usually intermittent, progressing to constant

Associated signs and symptoms: Fatigue and malaise
    Significant unintentional weight loss
    Swelling and warmth over localized areas of tumor
    Soft, tender palpable mass over bone
    Loss of range of motion and joint function if limb bone is involved
    Fever
    Sciatica
    Unilateral edema

OVERVIEW **CANCER PRESENCE AND PAIN—cont'd**

▼ **PRIMARY CENTRAL NERVOUS SYSTEM: BRAIN TUMORS**

Location: Intracranial
Referral: Specific symptoms depend on tumor location
Headaches
Description: Biocipital or bifrontal headache
Intensity: Mild to severe
Duration: Worse in morning on awakening
Diminishes or disappears soon after rising
Aggravating factors: Activity that increases intracranial pressure (e.g., straining during bowel movements, stooping, lifting heavy objects, coughing, bending over)
Prone/supine position at night during sleep
Relieving factors: Pain medications, including aspirin, acetaminophen
Associated signs and
symptoms: Papilledema
Altered mentation:
Increased sleeping
Difficulty in concentrating
Memory loss
Increased irritability
Poor judgment
Vomiting unrelated to food accompanies headaches
Seizures
Neurologic findings:
Positive Babinski reflex
Clonus (ankle or wrist)
Sensory changes
Decreased coordination
Ataxia
Muscle weakness
Increased lower extremity deep tendon reflexes
Transient paralysis

▼ **PRIMARY CENTRAL NERVOUS SYSTEM: SPINAL CORD TUMORS**

Location: Intramedullary (within the spinal cord)
Extramedullary (within the dura mater)
Extradural (outside the dura mater)
Referral: Back pain at the level of the spinal cord lesion
Pain may extend to the groin or legs
Description: Dull ache; sharp, knifelike sensation
Intensity: Mild to severe, progressive; night pain
Duration: Intermittent, progressing to constant, or constant
Aggravating factors: (Back pain) Lying down/rest
Weight bearing
Sneezing or coughing
Associated signs and
symptoms: Muscle weakness
Muscle atrophy
Sensory loss
Paraplegia/quadriplegia
Chest or abdominal pain
Bowel/bladder dysfunction (late findings)

▼ LEUKEMIA

Location: Usually painless; may have pain in the left abdomen; bone and joint pain possible

Referral: None

Description: Dull pain in the abdomen; may occur only on palpation

Intensity: Mild to moderate

Duration: Intermittent (with applied pressure)

Associated signs and symptoms:
Enlarged lymph nodes
Unusual bleeding from the nose or rectum, or blood in urine
Prolonged menstruation
Easy bruising of the skin
Fatigue
Dyspnea
Weight loss, loss of appetite
Fevers and sweats

▼ MULTIPLE MYELOMA

Location: Skeletal pain, especially in the spine, sternum, rib, leg, or arm

Referral: According to the location of the tumor

Description: Sharp, knifelike

Intensity: Moderate-to-severe

Duration: Intermittent, progressing to constant

Associated signs and symptoms:
Hypercalcemia: Dehydration (vomiting), polyuria, confusion, loss of appetite, constipation
Bone destruction with spontaneous bone fracture
Neurologic: Carpal tunnel syndrome; back pain with radicular symptoms; spinal cord compression (motor or sensory loss, bowel/bladder dysfunction, paraplegia)

▼ HODGKIN'S DISEASE

Location: Lymph glands, usually unilateral neck or groin

Referral: According to the location of the metastases

Description: Usually painless, progressive enlargement of lymph nodes

Intensity: Not applicable

Duration: Not applicable

Associated signs and symptoms:
Fever peaks in the late afternoon, night sweats
Anorexia and weight loss
Severe itching over the entire body
Anemia, fatigue, malaise
Jaundice
Edema
Nonproductive cough, dyspnea, chest pain, cyanosis

OVERVIEW   CANCER PRESENCE AND PAIN—cont'd

▼ NON-HODGKIN'S LYMPHOMA (including AIDS-NHL)

Location:	Peripheral lymph nodes
Referral:	Not applicable
Description:	Usually painless enlargement
Intensity:	Not applicable
Duration:	Not applicable
Associated signs and symptoms:	Constitutional symptoms (fever, night sweats, weight loss)
	Bleeding
	Generalized itching and reddened skin
	AIDS-NHL: Musculoskeletal lesions, subcutaneous nodules

🔑 KEY POINTS TO REMEMBER

✓ When put to the task of screening for cancer, always remember our three basic clues:
  ✓ Past Medical History
  ✓ Clinical Presentation
  ✓ Associated Signs and Symptoms

✓ Any suspicious lesions or red flag symptoms, especially in the presence of a past medical history of cancer or risk factors for cancer, should be investigated further. With the increasing number of people diagnosed with cancer, recognizing hallmark findings of cancer is important.

✓ Knowing the systems most often affected by cancer metastasis and the corresponding clinical manifestations is a good starting point. Any time a client reports a past medical history of cancer, we must be alert for signs or indications of cancer recurrence (locally or via metastasis).

✓ Knowing the most common risk factors for cancer in general and risk factors for specific cancers is the next step. Risk factor assessment and cancer prevention are a part of every health care professional's role as educator and in primary prevention.

✓ Whether you are working in an oncology setting or in a general practice with an occasional client, good resource information is available. Thorough, reliable,

and up-to-date information about specific types of cancer, cancer treatments, and recent breakthroughs in cancer research is available from The Abramson Cancer Center of the University of Pennsylvania (Philadelphia, PA) at: http://oncolink.upenn.edu

✓ Spinal malignancy involves the lumbar spine more often than the cervical spine and is usually metastatic rather than primary.

✓ Spinal cord compression from metastases may appear as back pain, leg weakness, and bowel/bladder symptoms.

✓ Fifty percent of clients with back pain from a malignancy have an identifiable preceding trauma or injury to account for the pain or symptoms. Always remember that clients may erroneously attribute symptoms to an event.

✓ Back pain may precede the development of neurologic signs and symptoms in any person with cancer.

✓ The presence of jaundice in association with any atypical presentation of back pain may indicate liver metastasis.

✓ Signs of nerve root compression may be the first indication of cancer, in particular, lymphoma, multiple myeloma, or cancer of the lung, breast, prostate, or kidney.

✎ KEY POINTS TO REMEMBER—cont'd

✓ The five most common sites of metastasis are the lymph nodes, liver, lung, bone, and brain.

✓ Lung, breast, prostate, thyroid, and the lymphatics are the primary sites responsible for most metastatic bone disease.

✓ Monitoring physiologic responses (vital signs) to exercise is important in the immunosuppressed population. Watch closely for early signs (dyspnea, pallor, sweating, and fatigue) of cardiopulmonary complications of cancer treatment.

✓ To determine appropriate exercise levels for clients who are immunosuppressed, review blood test results (WBCs, RBCs, hematocrit, platelets). When these are not available, monitor vital signs and use rate of perceived exertion (RPE) as a guideline.

✓ Besides the seven early warning signs of cancer, the therapist should watch for idiopathic muscle weakness accompanied by decreased deep tendon reflexes.

✓ Changes in size, shape, tenderness, and consistency of lymph nodes raise a red flag. Supraclavicular nodes and inguinal nodes are common metastatic sites for cancer.

✓ No reliable physical signs distinguish between benign and malignant soft tissue lesions. All soft tissue lumps that persist or grow should be reported immediately to the physician.

✓ Malignancy is always a possibility in children with musculoskeletal symptoms.

SUBJECTIVE EXAMINATION

Special Questions to Ask

Special questions to ask will vary with each client and the clinical signs and symptoms presented at the time of evaluation. The therapist should refer to the specific chapter representing the client's current complaints. The case study provided here is one example of how to follow up with necessary questions to rule out a systemic origin of musculoskeletal findings.

A previous history of drug therapy and current drug use may be important information to obtain because prolonged use of drugs such as phenytoin (Dilantin) or immunosuppressive drugs such as azathioprine (Imuran) and cyclosporine may lead to cancer. Postmenopausal use of estrogens has been linked with breast cancer.[110-112]

Past Medical History

A previous personal/family history of cancer may be significant, especially any history of breast, colorectal, or lung cancer that demonstrates genetic susceptibility.

• Have you ever had cancer or do you have cancer now?

  If no, have you ever received chemotherapy, hormone therapy, or radiation therapy?

  If yes, what was the treatment for?

  If yes to previous history of cancer, ask about type of cancer, date of diagnosis, stage (if known), treatment, and date of most recent follow-up visit with oncologist or other cancer specialist.

  Has your physician said that you are cancer-free?

• Have you ever been exposed to chemical agents or irritants, such as asbestos, asphalt, aniline dyes, benzene, herbicides, fertilizers, wood dust, or others? **(Environmental causes of cancer;** see complete environmental/occupational screening survey in Chapter 2 and Appendix B-13):

Clinical Presentation: Early Warning Signs

When using the seven early warning signs of cancer as a basis for screening (see Box 13-1), one or all of the following questions may be appropriate:

• Have you noticed any changes in your bowel movement or in the flow of urination?

  —*If yes,* ask pertinent follow-up questions as suggested in Chapter 10; see also Appendix B-5.

  —*If the client answers no,* it may be necessary to provide prompts or examples of what changes you are referring to (e.g., difficulty in

SUBJECTIVE EXAMINATION—cont'd

starting or continuing the flow of urine, numbness or tingling in the groin or pelvis).

• Have you noticed any sores that have not healed properly?
— If yes, where are they located? How long has the sore been present? Has your physician examined this area?

• Have you noticed any unusual bleeding (for women: including prolonged menstruation or any bleeding for the postmenopausal woman who is not taking hormone replacement) or prolonged discharge from any part of your body?
— If yes, where? How long has this been present? Has your physician examined this area?

• Have you noticed any thickening or lump of any muscle, tendon, bone, breast, or anywhere else?
— If yes, where? How long has this been present? Has your physician examined this area?*
— If no (for women): Do you examine your own breasts? How often do you examine yourself? When was the last time you did a breast self-examination (see Appendix D-6)?

• Do you have any pain, swelling, or unusual tenderness in the breasts? (Pain can be a symptom of cancer; cyclic pain is common with normal breasts, use of oral contraceptives, and fibrocystic disease.)
— If yes, is this pain brought on by strenuous activity? (Spontaneous/systemic or related to specific musculoskeletal cause [e.g., use of one arm])

• Have you noticed any rash on the breast or discharge from the nipple? (Medications such as oral contraceptives, phenothiazines, diuretics, digitalis, tricyclic tranquilizers, reserpine, methyldopa, and steroids can cause clear discharge from the nipple; blood-tinged discharge is always significant.)

• Have you noticed any difficulty in eating or swallowing? Have you had a chronic cough, recurrent laryngitis, hoarseness, or any difficulty with speaking?
— If yes, how long has this been happening? Have you discussed this with your physician?

• Have you had any change in digestive patterns? Have you had increasing indigestion or unusual constipation?
— If yes, how long has this been happening? Have you discussed this with your physician?

• Have you had a recent, sudden weight loss without dieting? (10% of client's total body weight in 10 days to 2 weeks is significant.)

• Have you noticed any obvious change in color, shape, or size of a wart or mole?
— If yes, what have you noticed? How long has this wart or mole been present? Have you discussed this problem with your physician?

• Have you had any unusual headaches or changes in your vision?
— If yes, please describe. (Brain tumors: bioccipital or bifrontal)
— Can you attribute these to anything in particular?
— Do you vomit (unrelated to food) when your headaches occur? (Brain tumors)

• Have you been more tired than usual or experienced persistent fatigue during the last month?

• Can you think of any time during the past week when you may have bumped yourself, fallen, or injured yourself in any way? (Ask when in the presence of local swelling and tenderness.) (Bone tumors)

• Have you noticed any bone pain or problems with any of your bones? Is the pain affected by movement? (Fractures cause sharp pain that increases with movement. Bone pain from systemic causes usually feels dull and deep and is unrelated to movement.)

Associated Signs and Symptoms

• Are you having any symptoms of any kind anywhere else in your body?

---

* An asymptomatic mass that has been present for years and causes only cosmetic concern is usually benign, whereas a painful mass of short duration that has caused a decrease in function may be malignant.

CASE STUDY

REFERRAL

A 56-year-old man has come to you for an evaluation without referral. He has not been examined by a physician of any kind for at least 3 years. He is seeking an evaluation on the insistence of his wife, who has noticed that his neck looks two sizes in the last year and that his neck looks "puffy." He has no complaints of any kind (including pain or discomfort), and he denies any known trauma, but his wife insists that he has limited ability in turning his head when backing the car out of the driveway.

PHYSICAL THERAPY SCREENING INTERVIEW

First, read the client's Family/Personal History form with particular interest in his personal or family history of cancer, presence of allergies or asthma, use of medications or over-the-counter drugs, previous surgeries, available x-ray studies of the neck or spine, and/or history of cigarette smoking (or other tobacco use).

An appropriate lead-in to the following series of questions may be: "Because you have not seen a physician before your appointment with me, I will ask you a series of questions to find out if your symptoms require examination by a physician rather than treatment in this office."

CURRENT SYMPTOMS

What have you noticed different about your neck that brings you here today?

When did you first notice that your neck was changing (in size or shape)?

Can you remember having any accidents, falls, twists, or any other kind of potential trauma at that time?

Do you ever notice any pain, stiffness, soreness, or discomfort in your neck or shoulders?

If yes, please describe (as per the outline in the Core Interview, Chapter 2).

Does this or any pain ever awaken you at night or keep you awake? (**Night pain associated with cancer**)

If yes, follow up with appropriate questions (see the Core Interview, Chapter 2).

ASSOCIATED SYMPTOMS

Have you noticed any numbness or tingling in your arms or hands?

Have you noticed any swollen glands, lumps, or thickened areas of skin or muscle in your neck, armpits, or groin? (**Cancer screen**)

Do you have any difficulty in swallowing? Do you have recurrent hoarseness, flulike symptoms, or a persistent cough or cold that never seems to go away? (**Cancer screen**)

Have you noticed any low-grade fevers or night sweats? (**Systemic disease**)

Have you had any recent unexplained weight gain or loss? (You may need to explain that you mean a gain or loss of 10 to 15 pounds in as many days without dieting.) Have you had a loss of appetite? (**Cancer screen or other systemic disease**)

Do you ever have any difficulty with breathing or find yourself short of breath at rest or after minimal exercise? (**Dyspnea**)

Do you have frequent headaches, or do you experience any dizziness, nausea, or vomiting? (**Systemic disease, carotid artery affected**)

FUNCTIONAL CAPACITY

- What kind of work do you do?
- Do you have any limitations caused by this condition that affects you in any way at work or at home? (**Occupational disease, limitations of activities of daily living [ADL] skills**)

FINAL QUESTIONS

How would you describe your general health?

Have you ever been diagnosed with cancer of any kind?

Is there anything that you would like to tell me that you think is important about your neck or your health in general?

FIRST VISIT: ASSESSING THE MUSCULOSKELETAL SYSTEM

- Observation/Inspection
- Observe for the presence of swelling anywhere, tender or swollen lymph nodes (cervical, supraclavicular, and axillary), changes in skin temperature, and unusual moles or warts. Perform a brief posture screen (general postural observations may be made while you are interviewing the client). Palpate for carotid artery and upper extremity pulses. Check vital signs and **Take the Client's Oral Temperature!**
- Cervical active range of motion (AROM)/passive range of motion (PROM)
- Assess for muscle tightness, loss of joint motion (including accessory movements), if indicated by a loss of passive motion). Assess for compromise of the vertebral artery and, if negative, clear the cervical spine by using a quadrant test with

CASE STUDY—cont'd

overpressure (e.g., Spurling's test) and assess accessory movements of the cervical spine. Perform tests for thoracic outlet syndrome. Palpate the anterior cervical spine for pathologic protrusion while the client swallows.

- Temporomandibular joint (TMJ) screen
  - Clear the joint above (i.e., TMJ) using AROM, observation, and palpation specific to the TMJ.
- Shoulder screen
  - Clear the joint below (i.e., shoulder) by using a screening examination (e.g., AROM/PROM and quadrant testing).
- Neurologic screen (see Chapter 4)

Deep tendon reflexes, sensory screen (e.g., gross sensory testing for light touch), manual muscle test (MMT) screening using break testing of the upper quadrant, grip strength. If test(s) is abnormal, consider further neurologic testing (e.g., balance, coordination, stereognosia, in-depth sensory examination, dysmetria). Ask about the presence of recent visual changes, headaches, numbness, or tingling into the jaw or down the arm(s).

It is always recommended that the therapist give the client ongoing verbal feedback during the examination regarding evaluation results, such as: "I notice you can't turn your head to the right as much as you can to the left—from checking your muscles and joints, it looks like muscle tightness, not any loss of joint movement." . . . or . . . "I notice your reflexes on each side aren't the same (your right arm reacts more strongly than the left)—let's see if we can find out why."

RECOMMENDATION FOR PHYSICIAN VISIT

- I noticed on your intake form that you haven't listed the name of a personal or family physician. Do you have a physician?
- If *yes*, when was the last time you saw your physician? Have you seen your physician for this current problem?

Give the client a brief summary of your findings while making your recommendations, for example, "Mr. X, I notice today that although you don't have any ongoing neck pain, the lymph nodes in your neck and armpit are enlarged but not particularly

tender. Otherwise, all of my findings are negative. Your loss of motion on turning your head is not unusual for a person your age and certainly would not cause your neck to increase in size or shape.

"Given the fact that you have not seen a physician for almost 3 years, I strongly recommend that you see a physician of your choice, or I can give you the names of several to choose from. In either case, I think some medical tests are necessary to rule out any underlying medical problem. For instance, a neck x-ray exam would be recommended before physical therapy treatment is started."

If the client has indicated a positive family history of cancer, it might be appropriate to suggest, "Given your positive family history of previous medical illnesses, the 3 years since you have seen a physician, and the lack of musculoskeletal findings, I strongly recommend . . ." It is important to provide the client with all the information available to you, but without causing undue alarm and emotional stress, which could actually prevent the client from seeking further testing.

If the client does give the name of a physician, you may ask for written permission (disclosure release) to send a copy of your results to the physician. If the client does not have a physician and requests recommendations from you, you may offer to send a copy of your results to the physician with whom the client makes an appointment.

If you think that a problem may be potentially serious and you want this person to receive adequate follow-up without causing alarm, you may offer to let him make the appointment from your office, suggest that your secretary or receptionist make the appointment for him, or even offer to make the initial telephone contact yourself.

RESULTS

This client did comply with the therapist's suggestion to see a physician and was diagnosed as having Hodgkin's disease (a cancer of the lymph system) without constitutional symptoms (i.e., without evidence of weight loss, fever, or night sweats). Medical intervention was initiated, and physical therapy treatment was not warranted.

PRACTICE QUESTIONS

1. Name three predisposing factors to cancer that the therapist must watch for during the interview process as red flags.

2. How do you monitor exercise levels in the oncology patient without laboratory values?

3. In a physical therapy practice, clients are most likely to present with signs and symptoms of metastases to:
   a. Skeletal system, hepatic system, pulmonary system, central nervous system
   b. Cardiovascular system, peripheral vascular system, enteric system
   c. Hematologic and lymphatic systems
   d. None of the above

4. What is the significance of nerve root compression in relation to cancer?

5. Complete the following mnemonic:
   C
   A
   U
   T
   I
   O
   N

6. Whenever a therapist observes, palpates, or receives a client report of a lump or nodule, what three questions must be asked?

7. How can the therapist determine whether a client's symptoms are caused by the delayed effects of radiation as opposed to being signs of recurring cancer?

8. Give a general *description* and *explanation* of the changes seen in deep tendon reflexes associated with cancer.

9. Why is weight loss a significant red flag sign in a physical therapy practice?

10. When tumors produce signs and symptoms at a site distant from the tumor or its metastasized sites, these "remote effects" of malignancy are called:
    a. Bone metastases
    b. Vitiligo
    c. Paraneoplastic syndrome
    d. Ichthyosis

11. A client who has recently completed chemotherapy requires immediate medical referral if he has which of the following symptoms?
    a. Decreased appetite
    b. Increased urinary output
    c. Mild fatigue but moderate dyspnea with exercise
    d. Fever, chills, sweating

12. A suspicious skin lesion requiring medical evaluation has
    a. Round, symmetrical borders
    b. Notched edges
    c. Matching halves when a line is drawn down the middle
    d. A single color of brown or tan

13. What is the significance of Beau's lines in a client treated with chemotherapy for leukemia?
    a. Impaired nail formation from death of cells
    b. Temporary longitudinal groove or ridge through the nail
    c. Increased production of the nail by the matrix as a sign of healing
    d. A sign of local trauma

14. A 16-year-old boy was hurt in a soccer game. He presents with exquisite right ankle pain on weight bearing but reports no pain at night. Upon further questioning, you find he is taking ibuprofen at night before bed, which may be masking his pain.

    What other screening examination procedures are warranted?
    a. Perform a heel strike test.
    b. Review response to treatment.
    c. Assess for signs of fracture (edema, exquisite site tenderness to palpation, warmth over the painful site).
    d. All of the above

15. When is it advised to take a work or military history?
    a. Anyone with head and/or neck pain who uses a cell phone more than 8 hours/day
    b. Anyone over age 50
    c. Anyone presenting with joint pain of unknown cause accompanied by multiple other signs and symptoms
    d. This is outside the scope of a physical therapist's practice

16. A 70-year-old man came to out-patient physical therapy with a complaint of pain and weakness of his fingers and morning stiffness lasting about an hour. He presented with bilateral swelling of the metacarpophalangeal joints of the index and ring fingers.

    He saw his family doctor 4 weeks ago and was given diclofenac, which has not changed his symptoms. Now he wants to try physical therapy. Since he last saw his physician, he has developed additional joint pain in the left knee and right shoulder.

PRACTICE QUESTIONS—cont'd

How can you tell if this is cancer, polyarthritis, or a paraneoplastic disorder?

a. Ask about a previous history of cancer and recent onset of skin rash.

b. You can't. This requires a medical evaluation.

c. Look for signs of digital clubbing, cellulitis, or proximal muscle weakness.

d. Assess vital signs.

17. A 49-year-old man was treated by you for bilateral synovitis of the proximal interphalangeal (PIP) joints in the second, third, and fourth fingers. His symptoms went away with treatment, and he was discharged. Six weeks later, he returned with the same symptoms. There was obvious soft tissue swelling with morning stiffness worse than before.

He also reports problems with his bowels but isn't able to tell you exactly what's wrong. There are no other changes in his health. He is not taking any medications or over-the-counter drugs and does not want to see a doctor.

Are there enough red flags to warrant medical evaluation before resumption of physical therapy intervention?

a. Yes; age, bilateral symptoms, progression of symptoms, report of GI distress

b. No; treatment was effective before—it's likely that he has done something to exac-

erbate his symptoms and needs further education about joint protection.

18. A client with a past medical history of kidney transplantation (10 years ago) has been referred to you for a diagnosis of rheumatoid arthritis. His medications include tacrolimus, methotrexate, Fosamax, and wellbutrin.

During the examination, you notice a painless lump under the skin in the right upper anterior chest. There is a loss of hair over the area. What other symptoms should you look for as red flag signs and symptoms in a client with this history?

a. Fever, muscle weakness, weight loss

b. Change in deep tendon reflexes, bone pain

c. Productive cough, pain on inspiration

d. Nose bleeds or other signs of excessive bleeding

19. A 55-year-old man with a left shoulder impingement also has palpable axillary lymph nodes on both sides. They are firm but movable, about the size of an almond. What steps should you take?

a. Examine other areas where lymph nodes can be palpated.

b. Ask about history of cancer, allergies, or infections.

c. Document your findings and contact the physician with your concerns.

d. All of the above

REFERENCES

1. Jemal A, Murray T, Ward E, Samuels A, et al: Cancer statistics 2005, *CA: A Cancer Journal for Clinicians* 55:10-30, 2005.

2. National Cancer Institute (NCI): Press release. Annual report: the nation finds cancer incidence and death rates on the decline: survival rates show significant improvement, 2004. Available at: www.nci.nih.gov/newcenter/pressreleases/ReportNation2004release. Accessed July 29, 2005.

3. Oeffinger KC, Mertens AC, Hudson MM, et al. Health care of young adult survivors of childhood cancer: a report from the Childhood Cancer Survivor Study, *Ann Fam Med* 2:61-70, 2004.

4. University of Minnesota Cancer Center: Childhood Cancer Survivor Study (CCSS). Available at: http://www.cancer.umn.edu/ltfu. Accessed July 30, 2005.

5. Hawkins M: Long-term survivors of childhood cancers: what knowledge have we gained? Available at www.medscape.com/viewarticle/492506, 2004. Accessed July 30, 2005.

6. Ries LAG, Eisner MP, Kosary CL: *SEER Cancer Statistics Review*, Bethesda, Md, 1973-1999, NCI. Available at: http://seer.cancer.gov/csr/1973_1999/. Accessed September 2002.

7. Bach PB, Schrag D, Brawley OW: Survival of blacks and whites after a cancer diagnosis, *JAMA* 287:2106-2113, 2002.

8. Institute of Medicine (IOM): *Unequal treatment, confronting racial and ethnic disparities in health care*, Washington DC, 2003, IOM. Available at: http://www.iom.edu/ [Click on Reports > select By title > scroll down to "Unequal Treatment. . .]. accessed July 30, 2005.

9. O'Brien K: Cancer statistics for Hispanics, 2003, *CA Cancer J Clinicians* 53:208-226, 2003.

10. Huerta EE: Cancer statistics for Hispanics, 2003: good news, bad news, and the need for a health system paradigm change, *CA Cancer J Clinicians* 53:205-207, 2003.

11. Tsao A, Kim E, Hong W: Chemoprevention of cancer, *CA A Cancer Journal for Clinicians* 54:150-180, 2004.

12. *Guide to Physical Therapist Practice*, 2nd edition. Alexandria, Va, 2003, American Physical Therapy Association.

13. American Cancer Society (ACS). *Cancer Prediction and Early Detection (CPED)*, Atlanta, 2005, ACS. Available at: www.cancer.org. Accessed July 28, 2005.

14. US National Cancer Institute: Cancer Statistics. Available at: http://www.nci.nih.gov/statistics/. Accessed March 27, 2005.

15. Sifri R, Gangadharappa S, Acheson L: Identifying and testing for hereditary susceptibility to common cancers. *CA Cancer J Clinicians* 54:309-326, 2004.

16. National Society of Genetic Counselors (NSGC): *Your Family History. Your Future.* Chicago, Ill: NSGC. Available at: www.nsgc.org. Accessed July 30, 2005.

17. American Institute for Cancer Research (AICR): *Food, Nutrition and the Prevention of Cancer: A Global Perspective.* Washington, DC, 1997, AICR.

18. American Institute for Cancer Research (AICR): *Expert Panel Report: Summary—Food Nutrition and the Prevention of Cancer: A Global Perspective,* Washington, DC, 2005, AICR. Available at: http://www.aicr.org/research/report_summary.lasso. Accessed July 30, 2005.

19. Calle EE, Rodriguez C, Walker-Thurmond K, et al: Overweight, obesity, and mortality from cancer in a prospectively studied cohort of U.S. adults, *N Engl J Med* 348:1625-1638, 2003.

20. Patel AV, Rodriquez C, Bernstein L, et al: Obesity, recreational physical activity, and risk of pancreatic cancer in a large U.S. cohort, *Cancer Epidemiol Biomarkers Prev* 14:459-466, 2005.

21. Key TJ, Schatzkin A, Willett WC, et al: Diet, nutrition, and the prevention of cancer, *Public Health Nutr* 7:187-200, 2004.

22. Mai V, Kant AK, Flood A, et al: Diet quality and subsequent cancer incidence and mortality in a prospective cohort of women, *Int J Epidemiol* 34:54-60, 2005.

23. Eyre H, Kahn R, Robertson RM: Preventing cancer, cardiovascular disease and diabetes: a common agenda for the ACS, American Diabetes Association, American Heart Association, *CA Cancer J Clinicians* 54:190-207, 2004.

24. American Cancer Society (ACS): Nutrition and Cancer Prevention: *A Cancer Journal for Clinicians.* 46(6), November/December 1996.

25. American Cancer Society (ACS): Nutrition and Cancer: Strategy 2000: *A Cancer Journal for Clinicians.* 49(6), November/December 2000.

26. American Cancer Society (ACS): A Nutritional Guide for Cancer Survivors: *A Cancer Journal for Clinicians,* 51(3), May/June 2001.

27. Chen YC, Hunter D: Molecular epidemiology of cancer, *CA: Cancer J Clin* 55:45-54, 2005.

28. Fleming DT: Herpes simplex virus type 2 in the United States, 1976 to 1994. *N Engl J Med* 337:1105-1160, 1997.

29. Center for Disease Control and Prevention, National Center for Health Statistics: *National Vital Statistics Report: Sexually transmitted infections,* Hyattsville, Md, 1999, CDC.

30. Centers for Disease Control and Prevention (CDC): *Tracking the hidden epidemics 2000: Trends in STDs in the United States,* Hyattsville, Md, 2000, CDC. Available at: http://www.cdc.gov/nchstp/od/news/RevBrochure1pdftoc.htm. Accessed July 30, 2005.

31. Armbruster C, Dekan G, Hovorka A: Granulomatous pneumonitis and mediastinal lymphadenopathy due to photocopier toner dust, *Lancet* 348:1518-1519, 1996.

32. Gallardo M, Romero P, Sanchez-Quevedo MC, et al: Siderosilicosis due to photocopier toner dust, *Lancet* 412-413, 1994.

33. US Justice Department: Radiation Exposure Compensation Program. Available at: www.usdoj.gov/civil/torts/const/reca/. Accessed July 30, 2005.

34. National Cancer Institute (NCI): About Radiation Fallout. Report on exposure to iodine 131 from atomic bombs detonated above ground at the Nevada test site: Fact sheets, a dose calculator, and state and county exposures. Available at: rex.nci.nih.gov/INTRFCE_GIFS/radiation_fallout/radiation_131.html. Accessed July 30, 2005.

35. Centers for Disease Control and Prevention (CDC): A Feasibility Study of the Health Consequences to the American Population From Nuclear Weapons Tests Conducted by the United States and Other Nations. Available at: www.cdc.gov/nceh/radiation/fallout/default.htm. Accessed July 30, 2005.

36. United States Department of Energy. DOE Nevada: Detailed, historical reports on nuclear testing at the Nevada test site. Available at: www.nv.doe.gov/news&pubs/publications/historyreports/default.htm. Accessed July 30, 2005.

37. National Safety Council (NSC): Understanding radiation. Sources of Nonionizing Radiation, Posted Dec. 2, 2002. Available at: http://www.nsc.org/issues/rad/nonioniz.htm. Accessed July 30, 2005.

38. Lazovich D, Forster J: Indoor tanning by adolescents: prevalence, practices and policies, *Eur J Cancer* 41:20-27, 2005.

39. Frumkin H: Agent orange and cancer: an overview for clinicians, *CA A Cancer Journal for Clinicians* 53:245-255, 2003.

40. Air Force Research Laboratory: Air Force Health Study. Available at: http://www.brooks.af.mil/AFRL/HED/hedb/afhs/afhs.html. Accessed July 30, 2005.

41. Institute of Medicine (IOM). Reports: Veterans and Agent Orange: Update 2004. Available at: http://www.iom.edu (click on Reports > select by Title > scroll down to: Veterans and Agent Orange). Accessed July 30, 2005.

42. Marshall L: Identifying and managing adverse environmental health effects: taking an exposure history, *Canadian Medical Association Journal* 166:1049-1054, 2002. Available at: www.cmaj.ca/cgi/reprint/166/8/1049.pdf. Accessed July 30, 2005.

43. Omenn GS: Genomics and prevention: a vision for the future, *Medscape Public Health & Prevention* 3(1). Available at: http://www.medscape.com/viewarticle/501299. Accessed April 11, 2005.

44. Lindsey H: Environmental factors & cancer: research roundup, *Oncology Times* 27(4):8-10, 2005.

45. National Cancer Institute (NCI). LHC p53 Resources page. Available at: www.cancer.gov/intra/LHC/p53ref.htm. Accessed July 30, 2005.

46. Couzin J: Choices—and uncertainties—for women with BRCA mutations. *Science* 302:592, 2002.

47. Kitagawa Y, Fujii H, Mukai M, et al: Intraoperative lymphatic mapping and sentinel lymph node sampling in esophageal and gastric cancer, *Surg Oncol Clin N Am* 11:293-304, 2002.

48. McGarvey CL: *Principles of oncology for the physical therapist,* Long Island, NY, 2003, Stony Brook University.

49. Fagan A: Bone metastases in breast cancer, *Rehabilitation Oncology* 22:23-26, 2004.

50. Diaz NM, Vrcel V, Centeno BA, et al: Modes of benign mechanical transport of breast epithelial cells to axillary lymph nodes, *Adv Anat Pathol* 12:7-9, 2005.

51. Mankin HJ, Mankin CJ, Simon MA: The hazards of the biopsy revisited, *J Bone Joint Surg Am* 78:656-663, 1996.

52. Springfield DS, Rosenberg A: Biopsy: complicated, risky (editorial), *J Bone Joint Surg Am* 78:639-643, 1996.

53. Abdu WA, Provencher M: Primary bone and metastatic tumors of the cervical spine, *Spine* 23:2767-2777, 1998.

54. Holden AF: Sweet's syndrome in association with generalized granuloma annulare in a patient with previous breast carcinoma, *Clin Exp Dermatol* 26:668-670, 2001.

55. Bourke JF, Keohane S, Long CC, et al: Sweet's syndrome and malignancy in the UK, *Br J Dermatol* 137:609-613, 1997.

56. Cohen PR, Kurzrock R: Sweet's syndrome revisited: a review of disease concepts, *Int J Dermatol* 42:761-778, 2003.

57. American Academy of Dermatology (ADD). Melanoma Fact Sheet 2005. Available at: www.aad.org. Accessed July 30, 2005.

58. American Cancer Society. Skin Cancer 2002. Available at: www.cancer.org. Accessed July 30, 2005.

59. Chen K, Craig JC, Shumack S: Oral retinoids for the prevention of skin cancers in solid organ transplant recipients: a systematic review of randomized controlled trials, *Br J Dermatol* 152:518-523, 2005.

60. Ross MI: Aid for patients with limb metastases, *World Melanoma Update* 1:15, 1997.

61. Gudas S: The physical therapy challenge in disseminated cancer, *Oncol Sect News APTA* 5:3, 1987.

62. Owens B: Central nervous system cancers. In: Varricchio C, ed. *American Cancer Society, A cancer source book for nurses*, 7th edition, London, 1997, Jones and Bartlett, pp. 349-358.

63. Pigott KH, Baddeley H, Maher EJ: Pattern of disease in spinal cord compression on MRI scan and implications for treatment, *Clin Oncol (R Coll Radiol)* 6:7-10, 1994.

64. Schiff D: Peer viewpoint, *J Support Oncol* 2:398, 401, 2004.

65. Abrahm JL: Assessment and treatment of patients with malignant spinal cord compression, *J Support Oncol* 2:377-401, 2004.

66. Levack P, Graham J, Collie D, et al: Scottish Cord Compression Study Group. Don't wait for a sensory level—listen to the symptoms: a prospective audit of the delays in diagnosis of malignant cord compression, *Clin Oncol (R Coll Radiol)* 14:472-480, 2002.

67. Schiff D: Spinal cord compression, *Neurol Clin* 21:67-86, 2003.

68. Tatu B: Physical therapy intervention with oncological emergencies, *Rehab Oncol* 23:4-6, 2005.

69. Ampil FL, Mills GM, Burton GV: A retrospective study of metastatic lung cancer compression of the cauda equina, *Chest* 120:1754-1755, 2001.

70. Orendacova J, Cizkova D, Kafka J, et al: Cauda equina syndrome, *Prog Neurobiol* 64:613-637, 2001.

71. Bagley CA, Gokaslan ZL: Cauda equina syndrome caused by primary and metastatic neoplasms, *Neurosurg Focus* 16(6), 2004. Available on-line at: http://www.medscape.com/viewarticle/482042_print. Accessed April 18, 2005.

72. Small SA, Perron AD, Brady WJ. Orthopedic pitfalls: cauda equina syndrome, *Am J Emerg Med* 23:159-163, 2005.

73. Uchiyama T, Sakakibara R, Hattori T, et al. Lower urinary tract dysfunctions in patients with spinal cord tumors, *Neurourol Urodyn* 23:68-75, 2002.

74. Bataller A, Dalman J: Paraneoplastic disorders of the central nervous system: update on diagnosis and treatment, *Semin Neurol* 24:461-471, 2004.

75. Stummvoll GH, Aringer M, Machold KP, et al: Cancer polyarthritis resembling rheumatoid arthritis as a first sign of hidden neoplasms. *Scand J Rheumatol* 30:40-44, 2001.

76. Martorell EA, Murray PM, Peterson JJ, et al: Palmar fasciitis and arthritis syndrome associated with metastatic ovarian carcinoma: a report of four cases, *J Hand Surg* 29A:654-660, 2004.

77. Stummvoll GH, Graninger WB: Paraneoplastic rheumatism—musculoskeletal diseases as a first sign of hidden neoplasms, *Acta Med Austriaca* 29:36-40, 2002.

78. Joines JD, McNutt RA, Carey TS, et al: Finding cancer in primary care outpatients with low back pain: a comparison of diagnostic strategies, *J Gen Intern Med* 16:14-29, 2001.

79. Deftos LJ: Hypercalcemia in malignant and inflammatory diseases, *Endocrinol Metab Clin North Am* 31:141-158, 2002.

80. Nirenberg A: Managing hematologic toxicities, *Cancer Nursing* 26:32S-37S, 2003.

81. Barsevick A. Energy conservation and cancer-related fatigue, *Rehabil Oncol* 20:14-17, 2002.

82. National Comprehensive Cancer Network (NCCN). Causes of Cancer Related Fatigue, 2003. Available at: www.nccn.org. Accessed on July 30, 2005.

83. Weaver CG: Cancer Consultants. Radiation recall: managing side effects, treatment & prevention, 2004.

Available at: www.patient.cancerconsultants.com/supportive_treatment.aspx?id=23174. Accessed July 30, 2005.

84. Volk K, Wruble E: Irradiation side effects and their impact on physical therapy, *Acute Care Perspectives* 10:11-13, 2001.

85. Winningham ML, McVicar M, Burke C: Exercise for cancer patients: guidelines and precautions, *Physician Sportsmed* 14:121-134, 1986.

86. Goodman CC, Boissonnault WG, Fuller K: *Pathology: Implications for the physical therapist*, 2nd edition. Philadelphia, 2003, WB Saunders.

87. Mocharnuk R: New perspectives on soft tissue cancers. *Medscape 2002: Clinical Hematology and Oncology.* Available at: http://www.medscape.com/viewarticle/429739. Accessed July 30, 2005.

88. Borman H, Safak T, Ertoy D: Fibrosarcoma following radiotherapy for breast cancer: a case report and review of the literature, *Ann Plast Surg* 41:201-204, 1998.

89. National Cancer Institute (NCI). Treatment statement for health professionals: adult soft tissue sarcoma, *Med News* 2005. Available at: www.meb.unibonn.de/cancer.gov/CDR0000062820.html. Accessed July 30, 2005.

90. Roll L: Cancer in children and adolescents. In: Varricchio C, ed. ACS, *A Cancer Source Book for Nurses*, 8th edition, Boston, 2004, Jones and Bartlett pp. 229-242.

91. American Cancer Society (ACS). Cancer Reference Information. Overview: Osteosarcoma. Available at: http://www.cancer.org/docroot/CRI/CRI_2_1x.asp?dt=52. Accessed July 30, 2005.

92. American Cancer Society (ACS). Cancer Reference Information. Detailed Guide: Ewing's family of tumors. Available at: http://www.cancer.org/docroot/CRI/CRI_2_3x.asp?dt=48. Accessed July 30, 2005.

93. Grubb MR, Currier BL, Pritchard DJ, et al: Primary Ewing's sarcoma of the spine, *Spine* 19:309-313, 1994.

94. Resnick D: *Diagnosis of Bone and Joint Disorders*, 4th edition. Philadelphia, 2002, WB Saunders.

95. Better outlook for people with brain tumors. Johns Hopkins Medical Letter 14:3, 2002.

96. Sagar S, Israel M: Tumors of the nervous system. In: Kasper D, Braunwald E, Fauci A, et al. *Harrison's Principles of Internal Medicine*, 16th edition, New York, 2005, McGraw-Hill.

97. American Cancer Society. Detailed Guide: Brain/CNS tumors in adults, 2005. Available at: http://www.cancer.org/docroot/CRI/CRI_2_3x.asp?dt=3. Accessed July 30, 2005.

98. Carney CP, Woolson RF, Jones L, et al: Occurrence of cancer among people with mental health claims in an insured population, *Psychosom Med* 66:735-743, 2004.

99. Mandrell B: Leukemia. In: Varricchio C, ed: ACS, *A Cancer Source Book for Nurses*, 8th edition. Boston, 2004, Jones and Bartlett pp. 251-264.

100. Abu-Shakra M, Buskila D, Ehrenfeld M, et al: Cancer and autoimmunity: autoimmune and rheumatic features in patients with malignancies, *Ann Rheum Dis* 60:433-441, 2001.

101. Zaidi A, Vesole H: Multiple myeloma: an old disease with new hope for the future, *CA, A Cancer Journal for Clinicians* 51:273-285, 2001.

102. Paulson B, Gudas S: Multiple myeloma, *Rehabilitation Oncology* 21:8-10, 2003.

103. Volker D: Other cancers: multiple myeloma. In: Varricchio C, ed: ACS, *Cancer Source Book for Nurses*, Boston, 2004, Jones and Bartlett pp.324-336.

104. Jones A: Lymphomas. In: Varricchio C, ed: ACS, *A Cancer Source Book for Nurses*, Boston, 2004, Jones and Bartlett Publishers-Hill; pp. 265-276.

105. Lim ST, Levine AM: Recent advances in acquired immunodeficiency syndrome (AIDS)-related lymphoma, *CA Cancer J Clinicians* 55:229-241, 2005.

106. Hardell L, Axelson O: Environmental and occupational aspects on the etiology of non-Hodgkin's lymphoma, *Oncol Res* 10:1-5, 1998.

107. Gaidano G, Carbone A, Dalla-Favera R: Genetic basis of acquired immunodeficiency syndrome–related lymphomagenesis, *J Natl Cancer Inst Monogr* 23:95-100, 1998.

108. Aboulafia AJ, Khan F, Pankowsky D, et al: AIDS-associated secondary lymphoma of bone: a case report with review of the literature, *Am J Orthop* 27:128-134, 1998.

109. Lane JM: When to consider malignant tumor in the differential diagnosis after athletic trauma, Editorial comment, *J Musculoskel Med* 7:16, 1990.

110. Gapstur SM, Morrow M, Sellers TA: Hormone replacement therapy and risk of breast cancer with a favorable histology: results of the Iowa Women's Health Study, *JAMA* 281:2091-2097, 1999.

111. Aubuchon M, Santoro N: Lessons learned from the WHI: HRT requires a cautious and individualized approach, *Geriatrics* 59:22-26, 2004.

112. Rossouw JE, Anderson GL, Prentice RL, et al: Risks and benefits of estrogen plus progestin in healthy postmenopausal women: principal results from the Women's Health Initiative randomized controlled trial, *JAMA* 288:321-333, 2002.

Systemic Origins of Neuromuscular or Musculoskeletal Pain and Dysfunction

The potential for referral of pain from systemic diseases to specific muscles and joints is well documented in the medical literature. These referral patterns most often affect the back and shoulder but may also appear in the chest, thorax, hip, pelvis, groin, sacrum, or sacroiliac joint.

Up to this point the text has focused on each organ system and the pain or other signs and symptoms referred from organs to musculoskeletal sites. In this third section the focus is turned around so that the reader can quickly refer to the site of presenting pain or other symptoms and determine possible systemic involvement.

The therapist may then question the client, as suggested, and determine the possible need for referral to a physician or other appropriate resource. The reader is referred to the individual chapters within this text for an in-depth discussion of the specific visceral or systemic causes of musculoskeletal signs or symptoms.

DECISION-MAKING PROCESS

In Chapter 1, a model for decision making in the screening process was presented including:

• Client history (client demographics, past medical history, personal and family history, psychosocial history)

• Risk-factor assessment
• Clinical presentation, including assessment of pain patterns and pain types and conducting a systems review
• Associated signs and symptoms of systemic diseases
• Review of Systems

The therapist uses this screening model during the screening interview to gather important information and then correlate the subjective findings with the objective findings to recognize presenting conditions that require medical follow-up.

Accordingly, the therapist will want to obtain the client's history, conduct a systems review as outlined in the *Guide*, and remain familiar with types of pain, pain patterns, and signs and symptoms that may suggest systemic origins of problems appearing in the musculoskeletal or neuromuscular system. Taking a step back and looking at the entire case presentation, called the Review of Systems, is often the final step in the screening process.

These guidelines for collecting and correlating subjective and objective information are suggested for any client who demonstrates one or more of the characteristics outlined in Chapter 1.

It is estimated that 80% to 90% of the western population will experience an episode of acute back pain at least once during their lifetime,[1] making it one of the most common problems physical therapists evaluate and treat.[2-4]

Most cases of back pain in adults are related to age-related degenerative processes, physical loading, and musculoligamentous injuries. Many mechanical causes of back pain resolve within 1 to 4 weeks without serious problems.

Sacroiliac (SI) joint dysfunction can mimic low back pain and discogenic disease with pain referred below the knee to the foot. Studies show SI joint dysfunction is the primary source of low back pain in up to 30% of people with low back pain.[5,6] As always, when conducting a physical examination the therapist must consider the possibility of a mechanical problem above or below the area of pain or symptom presentation.

A smaller number of people will develop chronic pain without organic pathology or they may have an underlying serious medical condition. The therapist must be aware that many different diseases can appear as neck pain, back pain, or both at the same time (Table 14-1). For example neck pain to the head, neck, and back. Neck and back pain may arise in the spine from infection, fracture, or inflammatory, metabolic, or neoplastic disorders.

In this chapter general information is offered about back pain with a focus on clinical presentation while keeping in mind risk factors and associated signs and symptoms typical of each visceral system capable of referring pain to the head, neck, and back. Neck and back pain may arise in the spine from infection, fracture, or inflammatory, metabolic, or neoplastic disorders.

Additionally low back pain can be referred from abdominal or pelvic disease. Nonsteroidal antiinflammatory drug (NSAID) use is a typical cause of intraperitoneal or retroperitoneal bleeding causing low back pain. People most often taking NSAIDs have a history of inflammatory conditions such as osteoarthritis.

Although the incidence of back pain from NSAIDs is fairly low (i.e., number of people on NSAIDs who develop GI problems and referred pain), the prevalence (number seen in a physical therapist's practice) is much higher.[8-10] In other words physical therapists are seeing a majority of people with arthritis or other inflammatory conditions who are taking one or more prescription and/or over-the-counter NSAID.[11]

Screening for medical disease is an important part of the evaluation process that may take place more than once during an episode of care (see Fig. 1-4). The clues about the quality of pain, the age of the client, and the presence of systemic complaints or associated signs and symptoms indicate the need to investigate further.

TABLE 14-1 ▼ Viscerogenic Causes of Neck and Back Pain

	Cervical	Thoracic/scapular	Lumbar
Cancer	Metastatic lesions (leukemia, Hodgkin's disease) Cervical bone tumors Cervical cord tumors Lung cancer; Pancoast's tumor Esophageal cancer Thyroid cancer	Mediastinal tumors Metastatic extension Pancreatic cancer Breast cancer	Metastatic lesions Prostate cancer Testicular cancer Pancreatic cancer Colorectal cancer Multiple myeloma Lymphoma
Cardiovascular	Angina Myocardial infarction Aortic aneurysm	Angina Myocardial infarction Aortic aneurysm	Abdominal aortic aneurysm Endocarditis Myocarditis Peripheral vascular: • Post-operative bleeding from anterior spine surgery
Pulmonary	Lung cancer; Pancoast's tumor Tracheobronchial irritation Chronic bronchitis Pneumothorax	Respiratory or lung infection Empyema Chronic bronchitis Pleurisy Pneumothorax Pneumonia	
Renal/Urologic		Acute pyelonephritis Kidney disease	Kidney disorders: • Acute pyelonephritis • Perinephritic abscess • Nephrolithiasis • Ureteral colic (kidney stones) • Urinary tract infection • Dialysis (first-use syndrome) • Renal tumors
Gastrointestinal	Esophagitis Esophageal cancer	Esophagitis (severe) Esophageal spasm Peptic ulcer Acute cholecystitis Biliary colic Pancreatic disease	Small intestine: • Obstruction (neoplasm) • Irritable bowel syndrome • Crohn's disease Colon: • Diverticular disease Pancreatic disease Appendicitis
Gynecologic			Gynecologic disorders: • Cancer • Retroversion of the uterus • Uterine fibroids • Ovarian cysts • Endometriosis • Pelvic inflammatory disease (PID) • Incest/sexual assault • Rectocele, cystocele • Uterine prolapse Normal pregnancy Multiparity

TABLE 14-1 ▼ Viscerogenic Causes of Neck and Back Pain—cont'd

Cervical	Thoracic/scapular	Lumbar
Infection: • Vertebral osteomyelitis • Meningitis • Lyme disease • Retropharyngeal abscess; epidural abscess (post-steroid injection) Osteoporosis Fibromyalgia Psychogenic (nonorganic causes; see chapter 3)	Infection: • Vertebral osteomyelitis • Herpes zoster • HIV Osteoporosis Fibromyalgia Psychogenic (nonorganic) Acromegaly Cushing's syndrome Fracture	Infection: • Vertebral osteomyelitis • Herpes zoster • Spinal tuberculosis • Candidiasis (yeast) • Psoas abscess • HIV Ankylosing spondylitis Fibromyalgia Osteoporosis Psychogenic (nonorganic) Fracture Cushing's syndrome Type III Hypersensitivity disorder (back/flank pain) Post-regional anesthesia
Other Rheumatoid arthritis Fracture Viral myalgias		

USING THE SCREENING MODEL TO EVALUATE THE HEAD, NECK, OR BACK

Past Medical History

A carefully taken, detailed medical history is the most important single element in the evaluation of a client who has musculoskeletal pain of unknown origin or cause. It is essential for the recognition of systemic disease that may be causing integumentary, muscle, nerve, or joint symptoms.

The history combined with the physical examination provides essential clues in determining the need for referral to a physician or other appropriate health care provider. A history of cancer is most important, however long ago. If a client has had a low backache for years, progressive serious disease is unlikely, though the therapist should not be misled by a chronic history of back pain because the client may be presenting with a new episode of serious back pain. Six weeks to 6 months of increasing backache, often in an older client, may be a signal of lumbar metastases, especially in a person with a past history of cancer.

Watch for history of rheumatologic disorders, tuberculosis, and any recent infection (Case Example 14-1). A history of fever and chills with or without previous infection anywhere in the body may indicate a low-grade infection.

Symptoms are likely to appear some time before striking physical signs of disease are evident and before laboratory tests are useful in detecting disordered physiology. Thus an accurate and suffi-

ciently detailed history provides historical clues that can be significant in determining when the client should be referred to a physician or other appropriate health care provider.

The therapist must always ask about a history of motor vehicle accident, blunt impact, repetitive injury, sudden stress caused by lifting or pulling, or trauma of any kind. Even minor falls or lifting when osteoporosis is present can result in severe fracture in older adults (Case Example 14-2).

Risk Factor Assessment

Understanding who is at risk and what the risk factors are for various illnesses, diseases, and conditions will alert the therapist early on as to the need for screening, education, and prevention as part of the plan of care. Educating clients about their risk factors is a key element in risk factor reduction.

Risk factors vary depending on family history, previous personal history, and disease, illness, or condition present. For example, risk factors for heart disease will be different from risk factors for osteoporosis or vestibular/balance problems. When it comes to the musculoskeletal system, risk factors such as heavy nicotine use, injection drug use, alcohol abuse, diabetes, history of cancer, or corticosteroid use may be important.

Always check medications for potential adverse side effects causing muscular, joint, neck, or back pain. Long-term use of corticosteroids can lead to vertebral compression fractures (Case Example 14-3). Fluoroquinolones (antibiotic) can cause neck,

CASE EXAMPLE 14-1 Bilateral Facial Pain

Background: A 79-year-old woman was in a rehabilitation facility following a stroke with resultant left hemiplegia. She told the therapist she was starting to have some new symptoms in her face. She could not smile on her "good" side and was having trouble closing her eyes, which was not a problem after her stroke.

Clinical Presentation: There were no apparent changes in hearing, sensation, or motor control of the right arm. The therapist conducted a new neurologic screening examination and found the following results:

Cranial nerve VII: client was unable to raise and lower either eyebrow or close the eyes tightly; there was bilateral facial drooping; as reported, the client was unable to smile with the right side of her face.

There was no change in sensory or motor findings from the initial evaluation post-CVA. However, deep tendon reflexes were absent in both arms led the therapist to check deep tendon reflexes in the lower extremities, which were also absent. There were no other

significant neurologic changes from the initial evaluation.

The therapist reviewed the Special Questions to Ask: Neck or Back (Pain Assessment and General Systemic) to look for any other screening questions and asked about a recent history of infection. The client reported a mild upper respiratory infection two weeks ago. There were no other obvious red flag findings.

Result: The therapist reported the new episode of signs and symptoms. Red flags observed included bilateral symptoms, absent muscle stretch reflexes, and recent history of infection. A medical evaluation was carried out and a diagnosis of Guillain Barré was made. The client continued to get worse with involvement of the respiratory muscles, foot drop, and numbness in the hands and feet.

A new episode of care was initiated to include physical therapy to strengthen facial musculature and prevent atrophy on the right side and to prevent pneumonia from respiratory muscle involvement.

---

care services intended to prevent health problems or maintain health and by offering wellness screening as part of primary prevention.

Clinical Presentation

During the examination the therapist will begin to get an idea of the client's overall clinical presentation. The client interview, systems review of the cardiopulmonary, musculoskeletal, neuromuscular, and integumentary systems, and assessment of pain patterns and pain types form the basis for the therapist's evaluation and eventual diagnosis.

Assessment of pain and symptoms is often a large part of the interview. In this final section of the text, pain and dysfunction associated with each anatomic part (e.g., back, chest, shoulder, pelvis, sacrum/sacroiliac, hip, and groin) are discussed and differentiated as systemic from musculoskeletal whenever possible.

Characteristics of pain, such as onset, description, duration, pattern, aggravating and relieving factors, and associated signs and symptoms, are presented in Chapter 3 (see Table 3-2; see also

---

chest, or back pain. Headache is a common side effect of many medications.

Keep in mind that physical and sexual abuse are risk factors for chronic head, neck, and back pain for men, women, and children (see Appendix B-3).

Age is a risk factor for many systemic and viscerogenic problems. The risk of certain diseases associated with back pain increases with advancing age (e.g., osteoporosis, aneurysm, myocardial infarction, cancer). Under the age of 20 or over the age of 50 are both red flag ages for serious spinal pathology.

As with all decision-making variables, a single risk factor may or may not be significant and must be viewed in context of the whole patient/client presentation. See Appendix A-2 for a list of some possible health risk factors.

Routine screening for osteoporosis, hypertension, incontinence, cancer, vestibular or balance problems, and other potential problems can be a part of the physical therapist's practice. Therapists can advocate disease prevention, wellness, and promotion of healthy lifestyles by delivering health

CASE EXAMPLE 14-2 Minimal Trauma

Background: An in-patient acute care therapist was working with a 75-year-old woman who was 1-day status post right total hip replacement (THR). The patient reported getting out of bed by herself early in the morning and falling against the night stand. She complained of low back pain when the therapist arrived to help her sit up in bed and stand. The pain was in the left lumbar area without radiation.

Past Medical History: Past medical history included osteoporosis (treated with bisphosphonate medication, calcium, and vitamin D), breast cancer with mastectomy 30 years ago, and hypothyroidism treated with medication (Synthroid).

Clinical Presentation: No pre-operative baseline information was available regarding the client's physical function, gait pattern, or range of motion for the spine or hips. There was moderate tenderness to palpation and percussion of the sacrum on the left side. Mild tenderness was reported with percussion to the upper and lower lumbar spine. There were no apparent skin changes, bruising, warmth, or swelling.

The patient could ambulate slowly with a walker but reported pain in both hips with each step. She could only take small steps moving approximately 2 to 4 inches forward with each step. Lumbar range of motion was very limited in flexion, side bending, and extension. She was unable to straighten up to a fully upright standing position due to her low back/sacral pain.

Outcome: The therapist filed an incident report with the hospital unit clerk and spoke directly with the nursing supervisor requesting an ortho consult before continuing with the standard THR rehabilitation protocol.

The patient was diagnosed with a sacral insufficiency fracture on the left at S3. X-rays and MRI also revealed scoliosis of the lumbosacral spine, moderate degenerative arthritis, and marked narrowing of the intervertebral disc spaces throughout the lumbar spine, and old compression fractures at T11 and T12. There was no evidence of bone lesions suggestive of breast cancer metastasis. Moderate foraminal stenosis was observed at the right L3 nerve root.

The client returned to physical therapy with an altered rehabilitation program consisting of weight-bearing exercises on the left (to stimulate osteoblastic bone formation) as tolerated given the compromise on both sides. She had a minimally invasive hip procedure so aquatic therapy was approved when there were no openings in the skin at the incision site (1 week later).

Appendix C-4). Reviewing the comparison in Table 3-2 will assist the therapist in recognizing systemic versus musculoskeletal presentation of signs and symptoms.

Effect of Position

When seen early in the course of symptoms, neck or back pain of a systemic or viscerogenic origin is usually accompanied by full and painless range of motion without limitations. When the pain has been present long enough to cause muscle guarding and splinting, then subsequent biomechanical changes occur.

Typically systemic back pain is not relieved by recumbency. In fact the bone pain of metastasis or myeloma tends to be more continuous, progressive, and prominent when the client is recumbent.

Beware of the client with acute backache who is unable to lie still. Almost all clients with regional or nonspecific backache seek the most comfortable position (usually recumbency) and stay in that position. In contrast, individuals with systemic backache tend to keep moving trying to find a comfortable position.

In particular, visceral diseases, such as pancreatic neoplasm, pancreatitis, and posterior penetrating ulcers, often have a systemic backache that causes the client to curl up, sleep in a chair, or pace the floor at night.

Back pain that is unrelieved by rest or change in position, or pain that does not fit the expected mechanical or neuromusculoskeletal pattern, should raise a red flag. When the symptoms cannot be reproduced, aggravated, or altered in any way

CASE EXAMPLE 14-3   Corticosteroid Use

Referral: A 73-year-old man was referred to a physical therapist by his family practitioner for evaluation of middle to low back pain that started when he stepped down from a curb. He was not experiencing radiating pain or sciatica and appeared to be in good general health. His medical history included bronchial asthma treated with oral corticosteroids and an abdominal hernia repaired surgically 10 years ago.

Clinical Presentation: Vital signs were measured and appeared within normal limits for the client's age. There were no constitutional symptoms, no fever present, and no other associated signs or symptoms reported.

There was a marked decrease in thoracic and lumbar range of motion from T10 to L1 and tenderness throughout this same area. No other objective findings were noted despite a careful screening examination.

The client was treated conservatively over a 2-week period but without change in his painful symptoms and without improvement in spinal movement. A second therapist in the same clinic was consulted for a reevaluation without significant differences in findings. Several suggestions were made for alternative treatment techniques. After 1 more week without change in client symptoms, the client was reevaluated. **What is the next step in the screening process?**

Using Table 14-1 the therapist can scan down the Thoracic/Scapular and Lumbar columns for any screening clues. Prostate and testicular cancers are listed along with metastatic lesions. Given the client's age, questions should be asked

about a past history of cancer and any associated urinary signs and symptoms.

Given his age, cardiovascular causes of back pain are also possible. Review past medical history, risk factors, and ask about signs and symptoms associated with angina, myocardial infarction, and aneurysm.

The therapist can continue to review Table 14-1 for potential pulmonary and gastrointestinal causes of this client's back pain and ask any further questions regarding possible risk factors and past history. Record all positive findings and conduct a final Review of Systems.

Use the Special Questions to Ask: Neck or Back at the end of this chapter to reassess the client's general health and clinical presentation. Not all questions must be asked; the therapist will use his or her judgment based on known history for this client and current clinical findings.

Result: In this case the client's age, lack of improvement with a variety of treatment techniques, and history of long-term corticosteroid use necessitated a return to the referring physician for further medical evaluation.

Long-term corticosteroid therapy and radiation therapy for cancer are risk factors for ischemic or avascular necrosis. Hip or back pain in the presence of these factors should be examined carefully.

Radiographic testing demonstrated ischemic vertebral collapse secondary to chronic corticosteroid administration. Diffuse osteopenia and a compression fracture of the tenth thoracic vertebral body were also mentioned in the medical report.

during the examination, additional questions to screen for medical disease are indicated.

Night Pain

Pain at night can signal a serious problem such as tumor, infection, or inflammation. Long-standing night pain unaltered by positional change suggests a space-occupying lesion, such as a tumor.

Systemic back pain may get worse at night, especially when caused by vertebral osteomyelitis,

septic discitis, Cushing's disease, osteomalacia, primary and metastatic cancer, Paget's disease, ankylosing spondylitis, or tuberculosis (of the spine) (see Chapter 3 and Appendix B-22).

Associated Signs and Symptoms

After reviewing the client history and identifying pain types or pain patterns, the therapist must ask the client about the presence of additional signs and symptoms. Signs and symptoms associated

with systemic disease are often present but go unidentified either because the client does not volunteer the information or the therapist does not ask. To assess for associated signs and symptoms, the therapist can end the client interview with the following question:

Follow-Up Questions

• Are there any other symptoms anywhere else in your body that you haven't told me about or we haven't discussed? They do not have to be related to your back pain or symptoms.

The client with back pain and bloody diarrhea or the person with mid-thoracic or scapular pain in the presence of nausea and vomiting may not think the two symptoms are related. If the therapist only focuses on the chief complaint of back, neck, shoulder, or other musculoskeletal pain and does not ask about the presence of symptoms anywhere else, an important diagnostic clue may be overlooked.

Other possible associated symptoms may include fatigue, dyspnea, sweating after only minor exertion, and GI symptoms (see also Appendix A-2 for a more complete list of possible associated signs and symptoms).

If the therapist fails to ask about associated signs and symptoms, the Review of Systems offers one final step in the screening process that may bring to light important clues.

Review of Systems

Clusters of these associated signs and symptoms usually accompany the pathologic state of each organ system (see Box 4-17). As part of the physical assessment, the therapist must conduct a Review of Systems. General questions about fevers, excessive weight gain or loss, and appetite loss should be followed by questions related to specific organ systems. Medications should be reviewed for possible adverse side effects.

Throughout the interview the therapist must remain alert to any yellow (cautionary) or red (warning) flags that may signal the need for further screening. Review of Systems is important even for clients who have been examined by a medical doctor. It has been reported that only 5% of physicians assess patients for "red flags."[12]

During the Review of Systems a pattern of systemic or viscerogenic origin may be seen as the therapist combines information from the client history, risk factors present, associated signs and symptoms, and yellow or red flag findings.

Red Flag Signs and Symptoms

Watch for the most common red flags associated with back pain of a systemic origin (Box 14-1). Individuals with serious spinal pathology almost always have one or more of these red flags; they can be missed when the clinician (physician or therapist) assumes the client's symptoms are the result of mechanical-induced back pain. See also Appendix A-2.

Key findings are age older than 50, significant recent weight loss, previous malignancy, and constant pain that is not relieved by positional change or rest and is present at night, disturbing the person's sleep.

Back pain in children is always a red flag especially if it has been present for more than 6 weeks. Children are less likely to report associated signs and symptoms and must be interviewed carefully. Ask about any other joint involvement, swelling anywhere, changes in range of motion, and the presence of any constitutional and GI symptoms. A recent history of viral illnesses may be linked to myalgias and discitis. Most common causes of back pain in children are listed in Table 14-2. Red flags requiring medical evaluation or reevaluation include back pain or symptoms that

---

BOX 14-1 ▼ **Most Common Red Flags Associated with Back Pain of Systemic Origin**

• Age less than 20 or over 50
• Previous history of cancer
• Constitutional symptoms (e.g., fever, chills, unexplained weight loss)
• Recent urinary tract infection
• History of injection drug use
• Immunocompromised condition (e.g., prolonged use of corticosteroids, transplant recipient, autoimmune diseases)
• Failure to improve with conservative care (usually over 4 to 6 weeks)
• Pain is not relieved by rest or recumbency
• Severe, constant nighttime pain
• Progressive, neurologic deficit; saddle anesthesia
• Back pain accompanied by abdominal, pelvic, or hip pain
• History of falls or trauma (screen for fracture, osteoporosis, domestic violence, alcohol use)
• Significant morning stiffness with limitation in all spinal movements (ankylosing spondylitis or other inflammatory disorder)
• Skin rash (inflammatory disorder, e.g., Crohn's disease, ankylosing spondylitis)

TABLE 14-2 ▼ Causes of Back Pain in Children

Inflammatory conditions	Developmental conditions	Trauma	Neoplastic disease	Other
Discitis	Spondylolysis	Muscle strain	Leukemia	Mechanical
Vertebral osteomyelitis	Spondylolisthesis	Stress fracture	Hodgkin's disease	Psychosomatic
Spinal abscess	Scheuermann's syndrome	Overuse	Non-Hodgkin's	
Non-spinal infections (e.g.,	Scoliosis	syndrome	lymphoma	
pancreatitis, pyelonephritis)		Physical	Ewing's sarcoma	
Rheumatoid arthritis (cervical		abuse	(primary)	
spine involved most often)			Osteogenic sarcoma	
Ankylosing spondylitis			(osteosarcoma)[primary]	
(presents during			Rhabdomyosarcoma	
adolescence)			(rare; skeletal	
			metastasis)	

Behrman RE, editor: *Nelson's textbook of pediatrics*, ed 17, Philadelphia, 2004, WB Saunders. Used with permission.

are not improving as expected, steady pain irrespective of activity, symptoms that are increasing, or the development of new or progressive neurologic deficits, such as weakness, sensory loss, reflex changes, bowel or bladder dysfunction, or myelopathy.

Use the Quick Screen Checklist (see Appendix A-1) to conduct a consistent and complete screening examination.

A few key screening questions might include:

Follow-Up Questions

- Have you had an injury or trauma to your head, face, neck, or back?
- Do you have (or have you recently had) a fever? Headache? Sore throat? Skin rash?
- Have you ever had cancer of any kind? Ever been treated with chemotherapy or radiation therapy?
- Are you taking any medications?
- Have you had any problems with your bowels or bladder?

▶ LOCATION OF PAIN AND SYMPTOMS

There are many ways to examine and classify head, neck, and back pain. Pain can be divided into anatomic location of symptoms (where is it located?); cervical, thoracic, scapular, lumbar, and sacroiliac joint/sacral (as shown in Table 14-1). For example, intrathoracic disease refers more often to the neck, midthoracic spine, shoulder, and upper

trapezius areas. Visceral disease of the abdomen and/or pelvis is more likely to refer pain to the low back region. Later in this section spine pain is presented by the source of symptoms (what is causing the problem?).

Whenever faced with the need to screen for medical disease the therapist can review Table 14-1. First identify the location of the pain. Then scan the list for possible causes. Given the client's history, risk factors, clinical presentation, and associated signs and symptoms, are there any conditions on this list that could be the possible cause of the client's symptoms? Is age or gender a factor? Is there a positive family or personal history?

Sometimes reviewing the possible causes of pain based on location gives the therapist a direction for the next step in the screening process. What other questions should be asked? Are there any tests that will help differentiate symptoms of one anatomical area from another? Are there any tests that will help identify symptoms that point to one system versus another?

Head

The therapist may evaluate pain and symptoms of the face, scalp, or skull. Headaches are a frequent complaint given by adults and children. It may not be the primary reason for seeing a physical therapist but is often mentioned when asked if there are any other symptoms of any kind anywhere else in the body.

The brain itself does not feel pain because it has no pain receptors. Most often the headache is caused by an extracranial disorder and is consid-

ered "benign." Headache pain is related to pressure on other structures such as blood vessels, cranial nerves, sinuses, membrane surrounding the brain. Serious causes have been reported in 1% to 5% of the total cases, most often attributed to tumors and infections of the central nervous system.[1,13] In the past, headache was viewed as many disorders along a continuum. Better headache classifications have brought about the development of many discrete entities among these disorders.[14,15] The International Headache Society (HIS) has published commonly used *International Classification of Headache Disorders* (edition 2, revised), which divides headaches into three parts: primary headache, secondary headache, and cranial neuralgias.[16,17]

Primary headache includes migraine, tension-type headache, and cluster headache. Secondary headaches, of which there is a large number, are attributed to some other causative disorder specified in the diagnostic criteria attached to them.

The therapist often provides treatment for secondary headache called cervicogenic headache (CGH). This type of headache is defined as referred pain in any part of the head caused by musculoskeletal tissues innervated by cervical nerves (C1-C4).[18] CGHs are frequently associated with chronic tension or acute whiplash injury, intervertebral disc disease, or progressive facet joint arthritis (e.g., cervical spondylosis, cervical arthrosis) (Table 14-3).

Causes of Headaches

Headache can be a symptom of neurologic impairment, hormonal imbalance, neoplasm, side effect of medication,[15] or other serious condition (Box 14-2). Headache may be the only symptom of hypertension, cerebral venous thrombosis, or impending stroke.[19] Sudden, severe headache is a classic symptom of temporal vasculitis (arteritis), a condition that can lead to blindness if not recognized and treated promptly.

TABLE 14-3 ▼ Clinical Signs and Symptoms of Major Headache Types

Migraine	Tension	Cervicogenic
Can be headache-free	Described as dull pressure	Pain starts in the occipital region and spreads anteriorly toward the frontal area
Migraines with headache are often described as throbbing or pulsating	Sensation of band or vise around the head	Usually bilateral
Often one-sided (unilateral); often around or behind one eye	Headache pain is bilateral or global (entire head)	Pain intensity fluctuates from mild to severe
Associated with nausea, vomiting	Muscular tenderness or soreness in soft tissues of the upper cervical spine	Often made worse by neck movements or sustained postures
Common triggers:	Not usually accompanied by associated signs and symptoms	Can resemble migraines with throbbing pain, nausea, phonophobia, photophobia
• Alcohol	May get worse with loud sounds or bright lights	History of trauma (e.g., whiplash), disc disease, or arthritis may be helpful
• Food	Current diagnosis or history of anxiety, depression, or panic disorder	
• Hormonal changes		
• Hunger		
• Lack of sleep		
• Perfume		
• Stress		
• Medications		
• Environmental factors (e.g., pollutants, air pressure changes, temperature)		
May be preceded by prodromal symptoms:		
• Visual changes (aura)		
• Motor weakness		
• Dizziness		
• Paresthesias		
Facial pallor, cold hands and feet		
History of headaches in childhood; family history of migraines		

Recognizing associated signs and symptoms and performing vital sign assessment, especially blood pressure monitoring, are important screening tools for vascular-induced headaches (see Chapter 4 for information on monitoring blood pressure).

Stress and inadequate coping are risk factors for persistent headache. Headache can be part of anxiety, depression, panic disorder, and substance abuse.[20] Headaches have been linked with excessive caffeine consumption or withdrawal in children, adolescents, and adults.[21]

Therapists often encounter headaches as a complaint in clients with post-traumatic brain injury, post-whiplash injury, or post-concussion injury. A constellation of other symptoms are often present such as dizziness, memory problems, difficulty concentrating, irritability, fatigue, sensitivity to noise, depression, anxiety, and problems with making judgments. Symptoms may resolve in the first 4 to 6 weeks following the injury but can persist for months to years causing permanent disability.[22]

CANCER

The greatest concern is always whether or not there is brain tumor causing the headaches. Only a minority of individuals who have headaches have brain tumors. Risk factors include occupational exposure to gases and chemicals and history of cranial radiation therapy for fungal infection of the scalp or for other types of cancer.

A previous history of cancer, even long past history, is a red flag for insidious onset of head and occipital neck pain. Metastatic lesions of the upper cervical spine are difficult to diagnose. Plain radiographs generally appear negative, which can delay diagnosis of clients with C1-C2 metastatic disease.[23]

The alert therapist may recognize the need for further imaging studies or medical evaluation. Persistent documentation of clinical findings and nonresponse to physical therapy intervention with repeated medical referral may be required.

Although primary head and neck cancers can cause headaches, neck pain, facial pain, and/or numbness in the face, ear, mouth, and lips are more likely. Other signs and symptoms can include sore throat, dysphagia, a chronic ulcer that does not heal, a lump in the neck, and persistent or unexplained bleeding. Color changes in the mouth known as leukoplakia (white patches) or erythroplakia (red patches) may develop in the oral cavity as a premalignant sign.[24]

Cancer recurrence is not uncommon within the first 3 years after treatment for cancers of the head and neck; often these cancers are not diagnosed

---

BOX 14-2 ▼ Systemic Origins of Headache

Cancer
Primary neoplasm
Chemotherapy; brain radiation

Cardiovascular
Migraine
Ischemia (atherosclerosis; vertebrobasilar insufficiency)
Cerebral vascular thrombosis
Arteriovenous malformation
Subarachnoid hemorrhage
Giant cell arteritis; vascular arteritis; temporal vasculitis
Hypertension
Febrile illnesses
Hypoxia
Systemic lupus erythematosus

Pulmonary
Obstructive sleep apnea
Hyperventilation (e.g., associated with anxiety or panic attacks)

Renal/Urologic
Kidney failure; renal insufficiency
Dialysis (first-use syndrome)

Gynecologic
Pregnancy
Dysmenorrhea

Neurologic
Post-seizure
Disorder of cranium, cranial structures (e.g., nose, eyes, ears, teeth, neck)
Cranial neuralgia (e.g., trigeminal, Bell's palsy, occipital, Herpes zoster, optic neuritis)
Brain abscess
Hydrocephalus

Other
History of physical or sexual abuse
Side effect of medications
Allergens (environmental or food)
Overuse of medications (analgesic rebound effect)
Psychogenic/psychiatric disorder
Substance abuse/withdrawal (drugs and/or alcohol)
Caffeine use/withdrawal
Candidiasis (yeast)
Trauma (e.g., cervicogenic headache, fracture, eating disorders with forced vomiting)
Infection (e.g., meningitis, sinusitis, syphilis, tuberculosis, sarcoidosis, herpes)
Post-dural puncture
Scuba diving
Hantavirus
Paget's disease (when skull is affected)
Hypoglycemia
Fibromyalgia

until an advanced stage due to neglect on the part of the affected individual. Cervical spine metastasis is most common with distant metastases to the lungs, although any part of the body can be affected.[25] Anyone with a history of head and neck cancer should be screened for cancer recurrence when seen by a therapist for any problem.

As always, prevention and early detection improve survival rates. Education is important because most of the risk factors (tobacco and alcohol use, betel nut, syphilis, nickel exposure, woodworking, sun exposure, dental neglect) are modifiable.[26]

Tension-type or migraine headaches can occur with tumors. Rapidly growing tumors are more likely to be associated with headache and will eventually present with other signs and symptoms such as visual disturbances, seizures, or personality changes.[26] Headaches associated with brain tumors are usually bioccipital or bifrontal, intermittent, and of increasing duration.

The headache is worse on awakening because of differences in CNS drainage in the supine and prone positions and usually disappears soon after the person arises. It may be intensified or precipitated by any activity that increases intracranial pressure, such as straining during a bowel movement, stooping, lifting heavy objects, or coughing.

Often, the pain can be relieved by taking aspirin, acetaminophen, or other moderate painkillers. Vomiting with or without nausea (unrelated to food) occurs in about 25% to 30% of people with brain tumors and often accompanies headaches when there is an increase in intracranial pressure. If the tumor invades the meninges, the headaches will be more severe.

Recognizing the need for medical referral for the client with complaints of headaches can be difficult. Past medical history can be complex in adults and screening clues are often confusing. Careful review of the clinical presentation is required. For example, although pain associated with the CGH can be constant (a red flag symptom) the intensity often varies with activity and postures. Sustained posture consistently increases intensity of painful symptoms.

MIGRAINES

Migraine headaches are often accompanied by nausea, vomiting, and visual disturbances, but the pain pattern is also often classic in description. Age is a yellow flag because migraines generally begin in childhood to early adulthood. Migraines can first occur in an individual beyond the age of 50 (especially in peri-menopausal or menopausal women); advancing age makes other types of headaches more likely. A family history is usually present, suggesting a genetic predisposition in migraine sufferers. In addition to the typical clinical presentation there are usually normal examination results.

Migraines can present with paralysis or weakness of one side of the body mimicking a stroke. A medical examination is required to diagnose migraine, especially in cases of hemiplegic migraines. Medical evaluation and treatment for migraines in general is recommended.

There is a role for the physical therapist because the beneficial effects of exercise on migraine headaches has been documented.[27,28] Physical therapy is most effective for the treatment of migraine when combined with other treatments such as thermal biofeedback and relaxation training.[29]

When present, associated signs and symptoms offer the best yellow or red flag warnings. For example, throbbing headache with unexplained diaphoresis and elevated blood pressure may signal a significant cardiovascular event. Daytime sleepiness, morning headache, and reports of snoring may point to obstructive sleep apnea. Headache-associated visual disturbances or facial numbness raises the suspicion of a neurologic origin of symptoms. Other red flags are listed in Box 14-3.

The therapist is advised to follow the same screening decision-making model introduced in Chapter 1 (see Box 1-7) and reviewed briefly at the beginning of this chapter. Physical examination should include measurement of vital signs, a general assessment of cardiac and vascular signs, and a thorough head and neck examination. A screening neurologic examination should address mental status (including pain behavior), cranial nerves, motor function, reflexes, sensory systems, coordination, and gait (see Chapter 4). Special Questions to Ask: Headache are listed at the end of this chapter and in Appendix B-15.

Cervical Spine

Neck pain is very common and has many mechanical and systemic causes. Neck and shoulder pain and neck and upper back pain often occur together making the differential diagnosis more difficult.

Traumatic and degenerative conditions of the cervical spine, such as whiplash syndrome and arthritis are the major primary musculoskeletal causes of neck pain.[30] The therapist must always ask about a history of motor vehicle accident or trauma of any kind, including domestic violence.

reduced spontaneously. Symptoms of cervical radiculopathy are common with A-A joint involvement.[7]

Radicular symptoms accompanied by weakness, coordination impairment, gait disturbance, bowel or bladder retention or incontinence, and sexual dysfunction can occur whenever cervical myelopathy occurs, whether from a mechanical or medical cause. An imaging study is usually needed to differentiate biomechanical from medical cause of radicular pain, especially when conservative care fails to bring about improvement.[31]

Clinical Signs and Symptoms of
Cervical Myelopathy

- Wide-based spastic gait
- Clumsy hands
- Visible change in handwriting
- Difficulty manipulating buttons or handling coins
- Hyperreflexia
- Positive Babinski test
- Positive Hoffman sign
- Lhermitte's sign
- Urinary retention followed by overflow incontinence (severe myelopathy)

Cervical or neck pain with or without radiating arm pain or symptoms may be caused by a local biomechanical dysfunction (e.g., shoulder impingement, disc degeneration, facet dysfunction) or a medical problem (e.g., infection, tumor, fracture). Referred pain presenting in these areas from a systemic source may occur from infectious disease, such as vertebral osteomyelitis, or from cancer, cardiac, pulmonary, or abdominal disorders (see Table 14-1).

Rheumatoid arthritis is often characterized by polyarthritic involvement of the peripheral joints but the cervical spine is often affected early on (first 2 years) in the course of the disease. Deep aching pain in the occipital, retroorbital, or temporal areas may be present with pain referred to the face, ear, or subocciput from irritation of the C2 nerve root. Some clients may have atlantoaxial subluxation and report a sensation of the head falling forward during neck flexion or a clunking sensation during neck extension as the A-A joint is

Torticollis of the sternocleidomastoid muscle may be a sign of underlying thyroid involvement. Anterior neck pain that is worse with swallowing and turning the head from side to side may be present with thyroiditis. Ask about associated signs and symptoms of endocrine disease (e.g., temperature intolerance; hair, nail, skin changes; joint or muscle pain; see Box 4-17) and a previous history of thyroid problems.[32]

Palpate the anterior spine and have the client swallow during palpation. Palpation of a soft tissue mass or lump should be noted. See guidelines for palpation in Chapter 4. Palpation of a firm, fixed, and immoveable mass raises a red flag of suspicion for neoplasm. Visually inspect and palpate the trachea for lateral deviation to either side.[33]

Anterior disc bulge into the esophagus or pharynx and/or anterior osteophyte of the vertebral body may give the sensation of difficulty swallowing or feeling a lump in the throat when swallowing. Anxiety can also cause a sensation of difficulty swallowing with a lump in the throat. Conduct a cranial nerve assessment for cranial nerves V and VII (see Table 4-9). See also Appendix B-8.

Vertebral artery syndrome caused by structural changes in the cervical spine is characterized by the client turning the whole body instead of turning the head and neck when attempting to look at something beyond his or her peripheral vision. Combined cervical motions such as extension, rotation, and side bending cause dizziness, visual disturbances, and nystagmus.

Decreased blood flow to the brain, referred to as cerebral ischemia, may be caused by vertebrobasilar insufficiency (VBI) and occurs when decreased vertebral height, osteophyte formation, postural changes, and ligamentous changes reduce the foraminal space and encroach on the vertebral artery. Tests for vertebral artery patency may help identify the underlying cause of neck pain; these tests must be carried out carefully especially with older adults.

Thoracic Spine

As with the cervical spine and any musculoskeletal part of the body, the therapist must look for the cause of thoracic pain at the level above and below the area of pain and dysfunction. Shoulder impingement and mechanical problems in the cervical spine can refer pain to the thoracic spine.

Systemic origins of musculoskeletal pain in the thoracic spine (Table 14-4) are usually accompa-

nied by constitutional symptoms and other associated symptoms. Often these additional symptoms develop after the initial onset of back pain, and the client may not relate them to the back pain and therefore may fail to mention them.

The close proximity of the thoracic spine to the chest and respiratory organs requires careful screening for pleuropulmonary symptoms in anyone with back pain of unknown cause or past medical history of cancer or pulmonary problems. Thoracic pain can also be referred from the kidney, biliary duct, esophagus, stomach, gallbladder, pancreas, and heart.

Thoracic aortic aneurysm, angina, and acute myocardial infarction are the most likely cardiac causes of thoracic back pain. Usually, there is a cardiac history and associated signs and symptoms, such as weak or thready pulse, extremely high or extremely low blood pressure, or unexplained perspiration and pallor.

Tumors occur most often in the thoracic spine because of its length, the proximity to the mediastinum, and direct metastatic extension from lymph nodes with lymphoma, breast, or lung cancer. The client may report symptoms typical of cancer. Tumor involvement in the thoracic spine may produce ischemic damage to the spinal cord or early cord compression since the ratio of canal

---

TABLE 14-4 ▼ Location of Systemic Thoracic/Scapular Pain

Systemic origin	Location
Cardiac	
Myocardial infarct	Midthoracic spine
Aortic aneurysm	Thoracic spine; thoracolumbar spine
Pulmonary	
Basilar pneumonia	Right upper back
Empyema	Scapula
Pleurisy	Scapula
Pneumothorax	Ipsilateral scapula
Renal	
Acute pyelonephritis	Costovertebral angle (posteriorly)
Gastrointestinal	
Esophagitis	Midback between scapulae
Peptic ulcer: stomach/duodenal	Sixth through tenth thoracic vertebrae
Gallbladder disease	Midback between scapulae; right upper scapula or subscapular area
Biliary colic	Right upper back; midback between scapulae; right interscapular or subscapular areas
Pancreatic carcinoma	Midthoracic or lumbar spine
Other	
Acromegaly	Midthoracic or lumbar spine
Breast cancer	Midthoracic spine or upper back

diameter to cord size is small, resulting in rapid deterioration of neurologic status (Case Example 14-4).

Peptic ulcer can refer pain to the midthoracic spine between T6 and T10. The therapist should look for a history of NSAID use and ask about blood in the stools and the effect of eating food on pain

and bowel function (see further discussion, Chapter 2).

Scapula

Most causes of scapular pain occur along the vertebral border and result from various primary musculoskeletal lesions. However, cardiac, pul-

---

CASE EXAMPLE 14-4   Midthoracic Back Pain

Background: A 55-year-old woman presents with sharp pain in the midback region around T5 to T6. The pain started after vacuuming her house last week. She has been taking Tylenol, but the pain is unrelieved. She reports being unable to find a comfortable position; the pain is keeping her awake at night.

History reveals a previous episode of pain in the same area two months ago. The pain started after she went grocery shopping and carried the heavy bags into her house. At that time, Tylenol quickly relieved her symptoms. The pain from the previous episode was described as "aching," not sharp like today.

Past Medical History: Past medical history includes breast cancer 15 years ago, surgical hysterectomy 10 years ago, and hypothyroidism. She does not remember what kind of breast cancer she had. She was treated with a lumpectomy and radiation. She has not had a mammography or clinical breast exam in the past five years. She does not perform self-breast examination on a regular or consistent basis.

She takes Synthroid for her thyroid problem, but is not taking any other prescription medication. She takes a daily vitamin and 1200 mg of calcium, but no other supplements. Tylenol is the only other over-the-counter product.

She does not smoke or drink, even socially. She does not use any other substances of any kind. She reports there are no other symptoms of any kind anywhere else in her body.

Clinical Presentation: Vital signs are normal. There are no visible or palpable lesions in the upper quadrant on either side. Axillary and supraclavicular lymph nodes are not enlarged or palpable. Submandibular lymph nodes are palpable, but not tender or hard.

Neurologic screening exam is normal including bowel and bladder function, although the client reports a sensation of intermittent "weakness" in her left arm. There is exquisite pain on palpation of the thoracic spine from T4 to T6. There was no apparent movement dysfunction observed.

How can you differentiate between a disc problem and bony metastases?

A differential diagnosis of this type is outside the scope of the physical therapist's practice and requires a medical evaluation. The physician's differential diagnosis may include mammography, x-rays, and CT scan or MRI to assist in the diagnosis.

Severe back pain that is unrelieved by rest or change of position and present at night in a woman with a past history of breast cancer requires immediate referral. Breast cancer has a predilection for axial skeletal bony metastases. Metastases can also occur hematogenously to the lungs (see Table 13-5). The therapist can perform a pulmonary system screening examination and ask about specific pulmonary signs and symptoms.

Reviewing Table 14-1 for possible viscerogenic causes of midthoracic back pain in a 57 year old, the screening process can also include a brief cardiovascular examination and questions about GI function. Baseline information of this type can be extremely helpful later when documenting change in status or condition.

Rather than provide physical therapy intervention and assessing the results, immediate medical evaluation is in the best interest of this client. If the medical tests come back negative or if there is a disc problem, then the appropriate physical therapy intervention can be prescribed.

monary, renal, and GI disorders can cause scapular pain.

Specific questions to rule out potential systemic origin of symptoms are listed in each individual chapter. For example, if the client reports any renal involvement, the therapist can use the questions at the end of Chapter 10 to screen further for urologic involvement. Appendix A contains a series of screening questions based on the presence of specific factors (e.g., gender, joint pain, night pain, shortness of breath).

Lumbar Spine

Low back pain (LBP) is very prevalent in the adult population, affecting up to 80% of all adults sometime in their lifetimes. In most cases, acute symptoms resolve within a few weeks to a few months. Individuals reporting persistent pain and activity limitation must be given a second screening examination.

As Table 14-1 shows, there is a wide range of potential systemic causes of low back pain. Older adults with more comorbidities are at increased risk for LBP. Bone and joint diseases (inflammatory and non-inflammatory), lung and heart diseases, and enteric diseases top the list of conditions contributing to LBP in older adults.[34]

Sacrum/Sacroiliac

Sacral or sacroiliac pain in the absence of trauma and in the presence of a negative spring test (posterior-anterior glide of sacrum between the innominates) must be evaluated more closely. The most common etiology of serious pathology in this anatomic region comes from the spondyloarthropathies (disease of the joints of the spine) such as ankylosing spondylitis, Reiter's syndrome, psoriatic arthritis, and arthritis associated with chronic inflammatory bowel (enteropathic) disease.

Spondyloarthropathy is characterized by morning pain accompanied by prolonged stiffness that improves with activity. There is limitation of motion in all directions and tenderness over the spine and sacroiliac joints. The most significant finding in ankylosing spondylitis is that the client has night (back) pain and morning stiffness as the two major complaints, but asymmetric sacroiliac involvement with radiation into the buttock and thigh can occur.

In addition to back pain, these rheumatic diseases usually include a constellation of associated signs and symptoms, such as fever, skin lesions, anorexia, and weight loss that alert the therapist to the presence of systemic disease. Such symptoms present a red flag identifying clients who should be referred to a physician.

Age, gender, and risk factors are important in assessing for systemic origin of symptoms associated with any of these inflammatory conditions. Clients with these diseases have a genetic predisposition to these arthropathies, which are triggered by a number of environmental factors such as trauma and infection. Each of these clinical entities has been discussed in detail in Chapter 12.

Polymyalgia rheumatica and fibromyalgia syndrome are muscle syndromes associated with lumbosacral pain. Fibromyalgia syndrome refers to a syndrome of pain and stiffness that can occur in the low back and sacral areas with localized tender areas. Both these disorders are also discussed in Chapter 12.

▶ SOURCES OF PAIN AND SYMPTOMS

Pain can be evaluated by the source of symptoms (what is causing the problem?). It could be visceral, neurogenic, vasculogenic, spondylogenic, or psychogenic in origin. Specific symptoms and characteristics of pain (frequency, intensity, duration, description) help identify sources of back pain (Table 14-5).

The therapist must look at the history and risk factors, too. Any associated signs and symptoms that might reflect any one (or more) of these sources should be identified. Again, the therapist can use the tables in this chapter along with screening questions provided in Appendix A to help guide the screening process.

Viscerogenic

Visceral pain is not usually confused with pain originating in the head, neck, and back because sufficient specific symptoms and signs are often present to localize the problem correctly. It is the unusual presentation of systemic disease in the therapist's practice that will make it more difficult to recognize.

Low back pain is more likely to result from disease in the abdomen and pelvis than from intrathoracic disease, which usually refers pain to the neck, upper back, and shoulder. Disorders of the GI, pulmonary, urologic, and gynecologic systems can cause stimulation of sensory nerves supplied by the same segments of the spinal cord, resulting in referred back pain.[35] As discussed in Chapter 3, the central nervous system may not be able to distinguish which part of the body is responsible for the input into common neurons.

TABLE 14-5 ▼ Neck and Back Pain: Symptoms and Possible Causes

Symptom	Possible cause
Night pain unrelieved by rest or change in position; made worse by recumbency	Tumor
Fever, chills, sweats	Infection
Unremitting, throbbing pain	Aortic aneurysm
Abdominal pain radiating to midback; symptoms associated with food; symptoms worse after taking NSAIDs	Pancreatitis, gastrointestinal disease, peptic ulcer
Morning stiffness that improves as day goes on	Inflammatory arthritis
Leg pain increased by walking and relieved by standing	Vascular claudication
Leg pain increased by walking, unaffected by standing, but sometimes relieved by sitting or prolonged rest	Neurogenic claudication
"Stocking glove" numbness	Referred pain, nonorganic pain
Global pain	Nonorganic pain
Long-standing back pain aggravated by activity	Deconditioning
Pain increased by sitting	Discogenic disease
Sharp, narrow band of pain radiating below the knee	Herniated disc
Chronic spinal pain	Stress/psychosocial factors (unsatisfying job, fear-avoidance behavior)
Back pain dating to specific injury	Strain or sprain, fracture
Back pain in athletic teenager	Epiphysitis, juvenile discogenic disease, spondylolysis, or spondylolisthesis
Exquisite tenderness over spinous process	Tumor, fracture, infection
Back pain preceded or accompanied by skin rash	Inflammatory bowel disease

Modified from Nelson BW: A rational approach to the treatment of low back pain, *J Musculoskel Med 10*(5):75, 1993.

Back pain can be associated with distention or perforation of organs, gynecologic conditions, or gastroenterologic disease. Pain can occur from compression, ischemia, inflammation, or infection affecting any of the organs (Fig. 14-1).

Referred pain can also originate in organs that share pain innervation with areas of the lumbosacral spine. Colicky pain is associated with spasm in a hollow viscus. Severe, tearing pain with sweating and dizziness may originate from an expanding abdominal aortic aneurysm. Burning pain may originate from a duodenal ulcer.

Muscle spasm and tenderness along the vertebrae may be elicited in the presence of visceral impairment. For example spasm on the right side at the 9th and 10th costal cartilages can be a symptom of gallbladder problems. The spleen can cause tenderness and spasm at the level of T9 through T11 on the left side. The kidneys are more likely to cause tenderness, spasm, and possible cutaneous pain or sensitivity at the level of the 11th and 12th ribs.

Most often, past medical history, clinical presentation, and associated signs and symptoms will alert the therapist to an underlying systemic origin of musculoskeletal symptoms. Any client older than 50 with back pain, especially with insidious

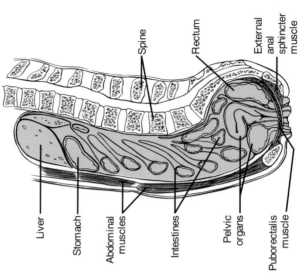

Fig. 14-1 ● Sagittal view of abdominal and pelvic cavities to show the proximity of viscera to the spine. The abdominal muscles and muscles of the pelvic floor provide anterior and inferior support, respectively. Any dysfunction of the musculature can alter the relationship of the viscera; likewise anything that impacts the viscera can affect the dynamic tension and ultimately the function of the muscles. Pathology of the organs can refer pain through shared pathways or by direct distention as a result of compression from inflammation and tumor.

onset or unknown cause, must have vital signs taken, including body temperature.

Careful questioning can elicit important information that the client withheld, thinking it was irrelevant to the problem, such as low back pain alternating with abdominal pain at the same level or back pain alternating with bouts of bloody diarrhea.

The therapist should look for clusters of signs and symptoms that may suggest involvement of a particular system. Using the Systems Review chart in Chapter 4 (see Box 4-17) can be very helpful in identifying visceral sources of symptoms.

Neurogenic

Neurogenic pain is not easily differentiated. Radicular pain results from irritation of axons of a spinal nerve or neurons in the dorsal root ganglion whereas referred pain results from activation of nociceptive free nerve endings (nociceptors) in somatic or visceral tissue.

Neurologic signs are produced by conduction block in motor or sensory nerves, but conduction block does not cause pain. Thus, even in a client with back pain and neurologic signs, whatever causes the neurologic signs is not causing the back pain by the same mechanism. Therefore, finding the cause of the neurologic signs does not always identify the cause of the back pain.[36] The therapist must look further.

Conditions such as radiculitis may cause both pain and neurologic signs but in that case the pain occurs in the lower limb, not in the back or in the upper extremity, not in the neck. If root inflammation also happens to involve the nerve root sleeve, neck or back pain might also arise. In such a case the individual will have three problems each with a different mechanism: neurologic signs due to conduction block, radicular pain due to nerve-root inflammation, and neck or back pain due to inflammation of the dura.[36]

Identifying a mechanical cause of pain does not always rule out serious spinal pathology. For example neurogenic pain can be caused by a metastatic lesion applying pressure or traction on any of the neural components. The therapist must rely on history, clinical presentation, and the presence of any associated signs and symptoms to make a determination about the need for medical referral.

Sciatica alone or sciatica accompanying back pain is an important but unreliable symptom. For example, diabetic neuropathy can cause nerve root irritation. Prostatic metastases to the lumbar and pelvic regions or other neoplasms of the spine can create a clinical picture that is indistinguishable from sciatica of musculoskeletal origin (see Table 16-1 Sciatica). This similarity may lead to long and serious delays in diagnosis. Such a situation may require persistence on the part of the therapist and client in requesting further medical follow up.

Spinal stenosis caused by a narrowing of the spinal canal, nerve root canals, or intervertebral foramina may produce neurogenic claudication (Fig. 14-2). The canal tends to be narrow at the lumbosacral junction, and the nerve roots in the cauda equina are tightly packed. Pressure on the cauda equina from tumor, disc protrusion, infection, or inflammation can result in cauda equina syndrome, which is a medical emergency.

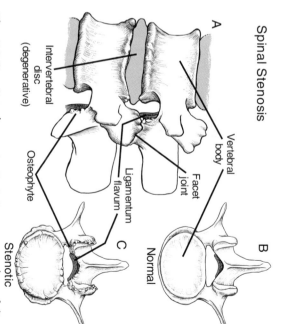

Fig. 14-2 • Spinal stenosis. **A,** Aging causes a loss of disc height and compression of the vertebral body. The bone attempts to cushion itself by forming a lip or extra rim around the periphery of the endplates. This lipping can extend far enough to obstruct the opening to the vertebral canal. At the same time, the ligamentum flavum begins to hypertrophy or thicken and osteophytes (bone spurs) develop. Degenerative disease can cause the apophyseal (facet) joints to flatten out or become misshapen. Any or all of these variables can contribute to spinal stenosis. **B,** Normal, healthy vertebral body with a widely open vertebral canal. **C,** Stenotic spine from a variety of contributing factors. Many clients have all of these changes, but some do not. The presence of pathologic changes is not always accompanied by clinical symptoms.

Spinal Stenosis

A
Intervertebral disc (degenerative)
Vertebral body
Osteophyte
Facet joint
Ligamentum flavum

B
Normal

C
Stenotic

Clinical Signs and Symptoms of
Cauda Equina Syndrome

• Low back pain
• Unilateral or bilateral sciatica
• Saddle anesthesia; perineal hypoesthesia

Continued on p. 646

- Change in bowel and/or bladder function (e.g., difficulty initiating flow of urine, urine retention, urinary or fecal incontinence, constipation, decreased anal tone and sensation)
- Lower extremity motor weakness and sensory deficits
- Diminished or absent lower extremity deep tendon reflexes

The emerging nerve root exits through a shallow lateral recess and also may be compressed easily. Any combination of degenerative changes, such as disc protrusion, osteophyte formation, and ligamentous thickening, reduces the space needed for the spinal cord and its nerve roots (see Fig. 14-2).

Confusion with spinal stenosis syndromes may occur when atheromatous change in the internal iliac artery results in ischemia to the sciatic nerve. The subsequent sciatic pain with vascular claudication-like symptoms may go unrecognized as a vascular problem. The therapist may be able to recognize the need for medical intervention by combining a careful subjective and objective examination with knowledge of vascular and neurogenic pain patterns (Table 14-6). This is especially true in the treatment of unusual cases of sciatica or back pain with leg pain.

The client with a neurogenic source of back pain may develop a characteristic pattern of symptoms, with back pain, discomfort in the buttock, thigh, or leg and numbness and paresthesia in the leg developing after the person walks a few hundred yards (neurogenic claudication). The person may be forced to stop walking and obtains relief after long periods of rest. The pattern of symptoms is similar to that of intermittent claudication associated with vascular insufficiency, the major differences being immediate response to rest and position of the spine (see Fig. 14-4; see also Fig. 14-2).

The vertebral canal is wider when the spine is flexed, so relief from neurogenic pain may be obtained when the spine is flexed forward. Some individuals will bend over or squat as if to tie their shoelaces to assume a flexed spine position in public situations. Position of the spine (e.g., flexion or extension) does not affect symptoms of a vascular origin.

Vasculogenic

Pain of a vascular origin may be mistaken for pain from a wide variety of musculoskeletal, neurologic, and arthritic disorders. Conversely, in a client with known vascular disease, a primary musculoskeletal disorder may go undiagnosed (e.g., discogenic disease, spinal cord tumor, peripheral neuritis, arthritis of the hip) because all symptoms are attributed to cardiovascular insufficiency.

Vasculogenic pain can originate from both the heart (viscera) and the blood vessels (soma), primarily peripheral vascular disease. Back pain has been linked to atherosclerotic changes in the posterior wall of the abdominal aorta in older adults.[37] The therapist can rely on special clues regarding vasculogenic-induced pain in the screening process (Box 14-4).

Vascular injury to the great vessels, which are in proximity to the vertebral column, can occur during lumbar disc surgery or can present as a complication post-operatively. In rare cases severe bleeding can result in back pain and hypotension in the acute care phase. Late complications of back pain from pseudoaneurysms can occur years after spine surgery.[38]

Once the history has been reviewed, the therapist assesses the pain pattern present on clinical examination, asks about associated signs and symptoms, and conducts a review of systems.

Vascular back pain may be described as "throbbing" and almost always is increased with any activity that requires greater cardiac output and diminished or even relieved when the workload or

---

TABLE 14-6 ▼ Back Pain: Vascular or Neurogenic?

Vascular	Neurogenic
Throbbing	Burning
Diminished, absent pulses	No change in pulses
Trophic changes (skin color, texture, temperature)	No trophic changes; look for subtle strength deficits (e.g., partial foot drop, hip flexor or quadriceps weakness; calf muscle atrophy)
Pain present in all spinal positions	Pain increases with spinal extension, decreases with spinal flexion
Symptoms with standing: no	Symptoms with standing: yes
Pain increases with activity; promptly relieved by rest or cessation of activity	Pain may respond to prolonged rest

---

BOX 14-4 ▼ Clues to Vasculogenic Pain

Pain of a vascular origin may be:

Described as "throbbing"

Accompanied by leg pain that is relieved by standing still or rest

Accompanied by leg pain that is described as "aching, cramping or tired"

Present in all spinal positions and increased by exertion

Accompanied by a pulsing sensation in abdomen or palpable abdominal pulse

Caused by a back injury (lifting) in someone with known heart disease or past history of aneurysm

Accompanied by pelvic pain, leg pain, or buttock pain

Presented as arm pain when working with the arms overhead

Accompanied by temperature changes in the extremities

An early or late complication of lumbar surgery; ask about a history of previous spine surgery

---

activity is stopped. A "throbbing" headache may be a vascular headache from a variety of causes.

Women in the peri- and menopausal states may experience vascular headaches from fluctuating hormonal levels. Clients on cardiac medication such as glyceryl trinitrate, which relaxes smooth muscle especially blood vessels and is used to prevent angina, may also report episodes of throbbing headaches. Vascular symptoms of this kind require medical evaluation.

Atherosclerosis and the resulting peripheral arterial disease are the underlying causes of most vascular back pain. Often the client history will reveal significant cardiovascular risk factors such as smoking, hypertension, diabetes, advancing age, or elevated serum cholesterol (see Table 6-3 and discussion of peripheral vascular disease in Chapter 6).

Older age is an important red flag when assessing for pain of a vasculogenic origin. Most often, clients with back pain and any of the vascular clues listed are middle-aged and older. A personal or family history of heart disease is a second red flag. Continuous midthoracic pain can be a symptom of myocardial infarction, especially in a postmenopausal woman with a positive family history of heart disease.

Older clients with long-term nonspecific lower back pain may have occluded lumbar/middle sacral arteries associated with disc degeneration. Back

pain and neurogenic symptoms in the presence of high serum LDL cholesterol levels raises a red flag.[39]

Spondylogenic

Bone tenderness and pain on weight bearing usually characterize spondylogenic back pain (or the symptoms produced by bone lesions). Associated signs and symptoms may include weight loss, fever, deformity, and night pain. There are numerous conditions capable of producing bone pain, but the most common pathologic disorders are fracture from any cause, osteomalacia, osteoporosis, Paget's disease, infection, inflammation, and metastatic bone disease (Case Example 14-5).

The acute pain of a compression fracture superimposed on chronic discomfort, often in the absence of a history of trauma, may be the only presenting symptom. The client may recall a "snap" associated with mild pain, or there may have been no pain at all after the "snap." More intense pain may not develop for hours or until the next day.

Back pain over the thoracic or lumbar spine that is intensified by prolonged sitting, standing, and the Valsalva maneuver may resolve after 3 or 4 months as the fractures of the vertebral bodies heal. Clients who undergo kyphoplasty or vertebroplasty often have immediate pain relief.

The pain of untreated vertebral compression fractures may persist because of microfractures of biomechanical effects from deformity. Other symptoms include pain on percussion over the fractured vertebral bodies, paraspinal muscle spasms, loss of height, and kyphoscoliosis.

When asking about the presence of any associated symptoms the therapist must keep in mind that older adults with vertebral compression fractures or kyphotic posture for any reason may report other pulmonary, digestive, and skeletal problems. These symptoms may not be indicative of back pain from a systemic cause but rather organic dysfunction from a skeletal cause (i.e., somatic-visceral response from the effects of a forward bent, kyphotic posture on the viscera).[43]

Sacral stress fractures should be considered in low back pain of postmenopausal women with risk factors and athletes, particularly runners, volleyball players, and field hockey players (see further discussion on spondylogenic causes of sacral pain in Chapter 15).

Psychogenic

Psychogenic pain is observed in the client who has anxiety that amplifies or increases the person's perception of pain. Depression has been implicated

CASE EXAMPLE 14-5 Osteoporosis

A 59-year-old man came to physical therapy for midthoracic back pain that seemed to come on gradually over the last few weeks and was starting to make his job as a janitor more difficult. There were no other symptoms to report: no neck, chest, or arm pain.

Past medical history was without incident. The client had never missed a day of work due to illness, never been hospitalized, had no previous history of surgery. He has a 40-pack year history of smoking and "throws back a few beers" every night (six-pack daily for the last 15 years).

Clinical Presentation: Postural examination revealed a significant thoracic kyphosis with limited passive and active extension to neutral. Range of motion in the lumbar spine was within normal limits. Range of motion in the hip and knee was also normal.

The client could take a deep breath without increasing his pain but not without setting off a long series of coughing. There was local tenderness palpable in the midthoracic paraspinal, and rhomboid muscles without evidence of erythema, swelling, or other skin changes.

Neurologic screening examination was normal.

What are the red flags? Is a medical referral needed before initiating treatment?

Red flags include age and a significant history of tobacco and alcohol abuse. All three are risk factors for reduced bone mass and fracture. Osteopenia and osteoporosis are often overlooked in men and occur more often than previously appreciated.[40,41] Thirty percent of osteoporotic fractures occur in men.[42]

An x-ray would be a good idea in this case before beginning a program of back extension exercises or applying any manual therapy.

---

in many painful conditions as the primary underlying problem.

Anxiety, depression, and panic disorder (see Chapter 3 for further discussion of anxiety, depression, and panic disorder) can lead to muscle tension, more anxiety, and then to muscle spasm. Signs and symptoms of these conditions are listed in Tables 3-9 and 3-10. Other signs of psychogenic-induced back pain may be:
• Paraplegia with only stocking glove anesthesia
• Reflexes inconsistent with the presenting problem or other symptoms present
• Cogwheel motion of muscles for weakness
• SLR in the sitting versus the supine position (person is unable to complete SLR in supine but can easily perform an SLR in a sitting position)
• SLR supine with plantar flexion instead of dorsiflexion reproduces symptoms

The client may use words to describe painful symptoms characterized as "emotional." Recognizing these descriptors will help the therapist identify the possibility of an underlying psychologic or emotional etiology. An "exploding" or "vicious" headache, "agonizing" neck pain, or "punishing" backache are all red flag descriptors of psychogenic origin (see Table 3-1).

The client who is unable to concentrate on anything except the symptoms and who reports the symptoms interfere with every activity may need a psychologic/psychiatric referral. The therapist can screen for illness behavior as described in Chapter 3. Recognizing illness behavior helps the therapist clarify the physical assessment and alerts the therapist to the need for further psychologic assessment.[1]

Many studies have now shown a link between psychosocial distress and chronic neck or back pain.[44-46] Factors associated with chronic low back pain may include job dissatisfaction, depression, fear-avoidance behavior, and compensation issues.[47,48] It may be necessary to conduct a social history to assess the client's recent life stressors and history of depression, drug, or alcohol abuse.

The presence of psychosocial risk factors does not mean the pain is any less real nor does it reduce the need for symptom control. The therapist concentrates on pain management issues and improving function. Tools to screen for emotional overlay and fear-avoidance behavior are available in Chapter 3 of this text.

► SCREENING FOR ONCOLOGIC CAUSES OF BACK PAIN

Cancer is a possible cause of referred pain. Head and neck pain from cancer is discussed earlier in this chapter (see Causes of Headache).

Multiple myeloma is the most common primary malignancy involving the spine often resulting in diffuse osteoporosis and pain that is not relieved while the person is recumbent. For most oncologic causes of back pain, the thoracic and lumbosacral areas are affected. As a general rule thoracic pain must be screened for metastatic carcinoma.

Pain and dysfunction in the lumbosacral area may be caused by direct spread of cancer from the abdomen or pelvic areas. When the lumbar spine is affected by metastases it is usually from breast, lung, prostate, or kidney neoplasm. GI cancer, myelomas, and lymphomas can also spread to the spine via the paravertebral venous plexus. This thin-walled and valveless venous system probably accounts for the higher incidence of metastases in the thoracic spine from breast carcinoma and in the lumbar region from prostatic carcinoma.

Past Medical History

Prompt identification of malignancy is important, starting with knowledge of previous cancers. Past history of cancer anywhere in the body is a red flag warning that careful screening is required. Always ask clients who deny a previous personal history of cancer about any previous chemotherapy or radiation therapy.

Early recognition and intervention does not always improve prognosis for survival from metastatic cancer, but it does reduce the risk of cord compression and paraplegia. It is important to remember that the history can be misleading. For example, almost 50% of clients with back pain from a malignancy have an identifiable (or attributable) antecedent injury or trauma[49] (Case Example 14-6).

It is unclear if this is a coincidence or merely reflective of weakness in the musculoskeletal system leading to loss of balance and strength and, ultimately, an injury. If the trauma results in significant injury (e.g., fracture), then the underlying cancer is usually identified right away. But if soft tissue injury does not necessitate an x-ray or other imaging study, then the underlying oncologic cause

---

Background: A 41-year-old woman presented with low back pain (LBP) after a skiing accident 6 months ago. She continued skiing, but reinjured her back a month later while loading bicycles onto a car.

She did not seek help at that time, thinking the pain would resolve with healing and time. She took acetaminophen and over-the-counter NSAIDs but did not think these helped with her symptoms.

She reports her stress level as "high" due to family problems. She reports her fatigue level to be "high" also because of caring for four preschool aged children and a sick husband. She has lost 6 pounds in the last month trying to keep up with work and home activities. She currently reports her height and weight as 5 feet 4 inches tall and 108 pounds.

She reports her LBP is "always there," but gets worse with activity or movement. There is no numbness or tingling, but the pain does radiate into the buttocks on both sides. When asked if there were any symptoms anywhere else in her body, she mentioned a mild discomfort in the lower thorax/chest that gets worse when she coughs or takes a deep breath.

She has seen her family physician and told that the LBP is post-repetitive trauma and that she needs to give it time to heal. She was advised to avoid activities that could strain her back. She decided to see a physical therapist for exercises.

Past Medical History

- Benign breast cyst reported as negative 5 months ago
- Cesarean section delivery of all four children without complications

Clinical Presentation

Posture: Standing and sitting postures appeared natural; normal lumbar lordosis
Thin and pale, but in no acute distress
Vital signs: all normal
Alert and oriented to time, place, and person

Neurologic screen

Cranial nerves	WNL
MMT	WNL (5/5 all extremities)
Sensory exam	WNL (light touch, pinprick)
DTR	Brisk 3+, equal in all 4 extremities

CASE EXAMPLE 14-6　Multiple Myeloma Presenting as Back Pain—cont'd

SLR　Limited to 25 degrees, bilaterally because of back pain and apprehension

Romberg　WNL

Unable to test physiologic (accessory, joint play) motions of the spine due to painful response

Unable to test for hip motion or overpressure of the sacroiliac joint because of pain

Positive tapping test (percussion over spinous processes) from L4 to SI

Walking pattern unremarkable; no antalgic gait

Able to walk in tandem and squat

Able to stand and walk on both heels and toes, bilaterally

Associated Signs and Symptoms

No report of fever, chills, night sweats, or night pain

No report of GI or GU dysfunction

Mild discomfort in the lower thorax/chest that gets worse when she coughs or takes a deep breath

What else do you need to know in the screening process?

Past history of infections of any kind? Cancer?

Recent or current medications besides over-the-counter NSAIDs?

Tobacco use? Substance use (especially injection drugs with back pain)?

Did the physician examine your spine?

Were any x-rays or other imaging studies done?

Did you have a urinalysis or blood test done?

Recheck her vital signs on another day. Ask her to report any sweats, chills, or fever over the next 24 to 72 hours.

Any cough or shortness of breath? (Remember to ask about any functional limitations, not just ask if the client is having these symptoms.)

Any other respiratory signs and symptoms or red flags?

Take a more detailed birth/delivery history.

Type of birth control used (intrauterine contraceptive device?)

Date of last pap smear and mammogram.

Has she had a hysterectomy (consider surgical menopause and osteoporosis)? Ask about sexually transmitted infections or the possibility of physical or sexual assault.

Any pelvic symptoms? Vaginal discharge? Unusual bleeding? Missed menses?

What other steps can you take in the screening process?

Turn to Table 14-1. As you look this over, does anything else come to mind given the client's age, gender, and history? Vertebral osteomyelitis is one possibility. Review the risk factors for this condition. Making a diagnosis of vertebral osteomyelitis would be outside the scope of a physical therapist's practice but identifying risk factors and associated signs and symptoms aids the therapist in making a referral decision.

Review Clues Suggesting Systemic Head, Neck, or Back Pain at the end of this chapter. After looking this list over, the therapist may be prompted to ask if there are any other painful or symptomatic joints anywhere else in the body.

The therapist can scan the Special Questions to Ask: Back to see if there have been any questions left out or that now seem appropriate to ask based on the information gathered so far. Review Special Questions for Women.

Given the information you have, would you treat or refer this client?

Even though the vital signs are unremarkable and the neurologic screen appears negative, there are plenty of red flags here. Weight loss of 6 pounds even with emotional or psychologic stress in a thin person must be considered significant until proven otherwise.

Her age is borderline at 41 but there is an increased risk for diseases and illnesses with increasing age. Her pain appears to be constant, but can be made worse with activity or movement. The fact that she injured her back 6 months ago, but is too acute to still examine today is a red flag for possible orthopedic involvement that requires additional medical testing. This is not the expected clinical picture. The positive tapping test with percussion over the spine is another orthopedic red flag.

Radiating pain into the buttocks on both sides (bilateral) raises a red flag. It may be neurologic from a disc problem. There is also a possibility of vascular cause of bilateral buttock pain. The client is not as old as one might expect with vascular claudication but at age 41 it still must be considered. Palpate for abdominal pulse (possi-

CASE EXAMPLE 14-6 Multiple Myeloma Presenting as Back Pain—cont'd

ble aneurysm). Check the width of the aortic pulse.

Pain on inspiration should prompt auscultation of respiratory sounds.

Screening for psychogenic or emotional overlay may be appropriate. If the therapist decides to treat the client as part of the diagnostic process without the aid of imaging studies, caution is advised with any intervention. Obtaining the medical records is important, especially the physician's notes from the client's most recent visit.

Do not hesitate to contact the physician with your findings first and wait for agreement with your treatment plan. What the therapist observes during the examination may not be what the physician saw (e.g., acute presentation, positive tapping test, bilateral buttock pain).

If the client does not respond to physical therapy intervention, consider it the final red flag and refer immediately.

Result: The therapist made a judgment for immediate medical consultation by phone and by sending a faxed copy of the physical therapy evaluation. After conferring with the physician, an MRI scan was requested along with a com-

plete blood cell count. The client had a compression fracture involving the central aspect of both the superior and inferior endplates of L5.

Blood cell counts were significantly decreased below normal (WBC, hemoglobin, hematocrit, and platelets). Erythrocyte sedimentation rate (ESR or sed rate) and total protein levels were elevated.

Further diagnostic testing revealed a diagnosis of multiple myeloma. The diagnosis was confirmed with bone marrow biopsy, which showed infiltration of plasma cells. Further radiologic imaging revealed metastatic involvement of several ribs on both sides of the thoracic cage, right tibial head, and left ulna.

Physical therapy intervention was not appropriate in this case. A 41-year-old woman with LBP following repetitive injuries can be very deceiving. Multiple myeloma is unusual in people younger than 40 years and affects more men than women and more blacks than whites.

Exposure to radiation, wood dust, or pesticides can contribute to the development of multiple myeloma. The therapist did not ask any questions about occupational or environmental exposures because there was nothing in the history or clinical presentation to suggest it.

Data from: Dajoyag-Mejia MA, Cocchiarella A: Multiple myeloma presenting as low back pain, *J Musculoskel Med* 21(4):229-232, 2004.

may go undetected. Once again the therapist may be the first to recognize the cluster of clinical signs and symptoms and/or red flag findings to suggest a more serious underlying pathology.

Risk Factors

As mentioned, a previous history of cancer is a primary risk factor for cancer recurrence with metastases to the spine. Until now there has been an emphasis on advancing age as a key red flag. Back pain at a young age is a red flag as well.

As a general rule, persistent backache due to extraspinal causes is rare in children. However, primary bone cancer occurs most often in adolescents and young adults, hence the new red flag: age younger than 20 years. The axial skeleton is affected more than the spine in this age group, but metastases to the vertebrae can occur.

Clinical Signs and Symptoms of
Oncologic Spine Pain

- Severe weakness without pain
- Weakness with full range
- Sciatica caused by metastases to bones of pelvis, lumbar spine, or femur
- Pain does not vary with activity or position (intense, constant); night pain
- Skin temperature differences from side to side
- Progressive neurologic deficits
- Positive percussive tap test to one or more spinous process
- Occipital headache, neck pain, palpable external mass in neck or upper torso
- Cervical pain or symptoms accompanied by urinary incontinence
- Look for signs and symptoms associated with other visceral systems (e.g., GI, GU, pulmonary, gynecologic)

Clinical Presentation

Back pain associated with cancer is usually constant, intense, and worse at night or with weight-bearing activities, although vague, diffuse back pain can be an early sign of non-Hodgkin's lymphoma and multiple myeloma. Pain with metastasis to the spine may become quite severe before any radiologic manifestations appear.

Back pain associated with malignant retroperitoneal lymphadenopathy from lymphomas or testicular cancers is characterized as persistent, poorly localized low back pain present at night but relieved by forward flexion. Pain may be so excruciating while lying down that the person can sleep only while sitting in a chair hunched forward over a table.

Palpate the midline of the spinous processes for any abnormality or tenderness. Perform a tap test (percussion over the involved spinous process).[50] Reproduction of pain or exquisite tenderness over the spinous process(es) is a red flag sign requiring further investigation and possible medical referral.

Neoplasm (whether primary or secondary) may interfere with the sympathetic nerves; if so, the foot on the affected side is warmer than the foot on the unaffected side. Paresis in the absence of nerve root pain suggests a tumor. Severe weakness without pain is very suggestive of spinal metastases. Gross muscle weakness with a full range of straight leg raise (SLR) and without a history of recent acute sciatica at the upper two lumbar levels is also suggestive of spinal metastases.

A short period of increasing central backache in an older person is always a red flag symptom, especially if there is a previous history of cancer. The pain spreads down both lower limbs in a distribution that does not correspond with any one nerve root level. Bilateral sciatica then develops, and the back pain becomes worse.

X-rays do not show bone destruction from metastatic lesions until the lytic process has destroyed 30% to 50% of the bone. The therapist cannot assume metastatic lesions do not exist in the client with a past medical history of cancer now presenting with back pain and "normal" x-rays.[51-53]

Associated Signs and Symptoms

Clinical signs and symptoms accompanying back pain from an oncologic cause may be system related (e.g., GI, GU, gynecologic, spondylogenic) depending on where the primary neoplasm is located and the location of any metastases (Case Example 14-7).

The therapist must ask about the presence of constitutional symptoms, symptoms anywhere else in the body, and assess vital signs as part of the screening process. Review the red flags in Box 14-1 and conduct a Review of Systems to identify any clusters of signs and symptoms.

▶ SCREENING FOR CARDIAC CAUSES OF NECK AND BACK PAIN

Vascular pain patterns originate from two main sources: cardiac (heart viscera) and peripheral vascular (blood vessels). The most common referred cardiac pain patterns seen in a physical therapy practice are angina, myocardial infarction, and aneurysm.

Pain of a cardiac nature referred to the soma is based on multisegmental innervation. For example, the heart is innervated by the C3 through T4 spinal nerves. Pain of a cardiac source can affect any part of the soma (body) also innervated by these levels. This is why someone having a heart attack can experience jaw, neck, shoulder, arm, upper back, or chest pain. See Chapter 3 for an in-depth discussion of the origins of viscerogenic pain patterns affecting the musculoskeletal system.

On the other hand, pain and symptoms from a peripheral vascular problem are determined by the location of the underlying pathology (e.g., aortic aneurysm, arterial or venous obstruction). Peripheral vascular patterns will be reviewed later in this chapter.

Angina

Angina may cause chest pain radiating to the anterior neck and jaw, sometimes appearing only as neck and/or jaw pain and misdiagnosed as temporomandibular joint (TMJ) dysfunction. Postmenopausal women are the most likely candidates for this type of presentation.

Angina and/or myocardial infarction can appear as isolated midthoracic back pain in men or women (see Figs. 6-4 and 6-8). There is usually a lag time of 3 to 5 minutes between increase in activity and onset of musculoskeletal symptoms caused by angina.

Myocardial Ischemia

Heart disease and myocardial infarction (MI), in particular, can be completely asymptomatic. In fact, sudden death occurs without any warning in 50% of all MIs. Back pain from the heart (cardiac pain pattern) can be referred to the ante-

A 52-year-old woman presented in physical therapy with low back pain radiating down the right leg to the knee. She had recently completed chemotherapy for acute myelocytic leukemia and was referred to physical therapy by the oncology nurse. Bone marrow biopsy one month ago was negative for leukemic cells.

Clinical Presentation: The client presented with acute low back pain described as "going across my low back area." She had a normal gait pattern but decreased lumbar motions in forward bending, right side bending, and left rotation.

Her pain was relieved by forward bending. Pain was too intense to conduct accessory motion testing because the client was unable to lie down for more than a minute before having to sit up.

Neurologic screen revealed a positive straight-leg raise on the right, intact sensation, and decreased ankle reflex on the right (patellar tendon reflex was assessed as normal). Manual muscle strength testing was deferred due to the client's extreme agitation during testing. There were no reported changes in bowel or bladder.

When asked if there were any other symptoms of any kind anywhere else, the client raised her shirt and showed the therapist several

nodules on her skin. They were not tender or oozing any discharge. The client reported she first noticed them about a week before her back pain started. She had not remembered to tell the nurse or her doctor about them.

Outcome: This is a good case to point out that even though the client has a known condition such as cancer and the referral comes from a health care professional, screening for medical disease as the cause of the pain or symptoms is still very important.

The therapist made phone contact with the referring nurse and reported findings from the evaluation. Of particular concern were the skin lesions and neurologic changes. The nurse was unaware of these changes. The therapist requested a medical evaluation before starting a physical therapy program.

The client was diagnosed with cancer metastases to the spine and cauda equina syndrome. Cauda equina syndrome caused by mechanical compression of the spinal nerve roots by tumor (or infection) requires immediate medical attention.

The client underwent urgent total spine irradiation, which did relieve her back pain. She declined further medical care (i.e., chemotherapy) and decided to continue with physical therapy to regain motion and strength.

Abdominal Aortic Aneurysm (AAA)

On occasion, an abdominal aortic aneurysm (see Fig. 6-11) can cause severe back pain. An aneurysm is an abnormal dilation in a weak or diseased arterial wall causing a sacklike protrusion. Prompt medical attention is imperative because rupture can result in death. Aneurysms can occur anywhere in any blood vessel, but the two most common places are the aorta and cerebral vascular system. AAA occurs most often in men in the sixth or seventh decade of life.

Risk Factors

The major risk factors for AAA include age, male gender, smoking, and family history.[54] Although the underlying cause is most often atherosclerosis, the therapist should be aware that aging athletes involved in weight lifting are at risk for tears in the arterial wall, resulting in an aneurysm. There is often a history of intermittent claudication and decreased or absent peripheral pulses. Other risk factors include congenital malformation and

rior neck and/or midthoracic spine in both men and women.

When pain does present, it may look like one of the patterns shown in Fig. 6-9. There are usually some associated signs and symptoms such as unexplained perspiration (diaphoresis), nausea, vomiting, pallor, dizziness, extreme anxiety, and/or abnormal vital signs.

Age and past medical history are important when screening for angina or MI as possible causes of musculoskeletal symptoms. Vital sign assessment is a key clinical assessment (Case Example 14-8).

CASE EXAMPLE 14-8   Back Pain and Dizziness after Colonoscopy

An 87-year-old woman visiting her daughter from out of town fell and suffered a compression fracture of L1. She reported having "heart problems" during a colonoscopy several weeks before this fall. She has had extreme back pain and is being given Vicodin (opioid analgesic for mild pain).

She is nauseated and attributes this to the pain medication. Blood pressure is 200/90 with pulse in the low 80s. There is no respiratory distress, no heart palpitations and no fever. She reports being on many blood pressure and heart medications and thyroid meds.

The family reports she has dizzy spells and is weak. She frequently loses her balance, but does not fall. She is extremely tired and the family reports she sleeps much during the day.

She has been referred to physical therapy through a home health agency. Since she is from out of town, she does not have a primary care physician. The daughter took her to a local walk-in clinic. The nurse practitioner then referred her to home health. Physical therapy was prescribed for the dizziness and falling.

You suspect the symptoms of dizziness, drowsiness, and weakness may be drug-induced. What do you do in a case like this?

Conduct an evaluation and gather as much information as you can from the client and family members. Use the Quick Screen Checklist and complete a Review of Systems. Organize the information you obtain from the evaluation so that the need for any other screening questions can be identified.

Look up potential side effects of Vicodin and ask the client about the presence of any other symptoms of any kind. See if any of the reported signs and symptoms point to side effects of medication. Conduct a cardiovascular screening examination (see Chapter 4).

Do not hesitate to contact the local clinic/nurse practitioner and ask if the client's symptoms could be cardiac or drug-induced. Report the abnormal vital signs. There may be a change in drug dosage, suggested drug administration (with or without food, time of day), or change in prescribed drug that can alleviate symptoms while still controlling pain. Vital signs may return to normal with better pain control unless there is an underlying cardiovascular reason for her symptoms.

Assess muscle weakness, vestibular function, and balance. Look for modifiable risk factors. Offer as much intervention as possible, given the temporary visiting situation and short-term episode of care.

Document findings, problem list, and plan of care and communicate these results with the referring agency. Medical referral may be advised given the client's age, vital signs, history of heart disease, and use of multiple medications.

vasculitis. Often the presence of these risk factors remains unknown until an aneurysm becomes symptomatic.

Clinical Presentation

Pain presents as deep and boring in the midlumbar region. The pattern is usually described as sharp, intense, severe or knifelike in the abdomen, chest, or anywhere in the back (including the sacrum). The location of the symptoms is determined by the location of the aneurysm (Fig. 6-11).

Most aortic aneurysms (95%) occur just below the renal arteries. An objective examination may reveal a pulsing abdominal mass or abnormally widened aortic pulse width (see Fig. 4-52).

Obesity and abdominal ascites or distention makes this examination more difficult. The thera-

pist can also listen for bruits. Bruits are abnormal blowing or swishing sounds heard on auscultation of the arteries.

Bruits with both systolic and diastolic components suggest the turbulent blood flow of partial arterial occlusion. The client will be hypertensive if the renal artery is occluded as well. Peripheral pulses may be diminished or absent. Other historical clues of coronary disease or intermittent claudication of the lower extremities may be present.

Monitoring vital signs is important, especially among exercising senior adults. Teaching proper breathing and abdominal support without using a Valsalva maneuver is important in any exercise program, but especially for those clients at increased risk for aortic aneurysm.

Clinical Signs and Symptoms of

Impending Rupture or Actual Rupture of the Aortic Aneurysm

- Rapid onset of severe neck or back pain
- Pain may radiate to chest, between the scapulae, or to posterior thighs
- Pain is not relieved by change in position
- Pain is described as "tearing" or "ripping"
- Other signs: cold, pulseless lower extremities, blood pressure differences between arms (more than 10 mmHg diastolic)

The U.S. Preventive Services Task Force (USPSTF) updated its guidelines for medical screening for AAA in 2005. The new guidelines recommend ultrasound screening for men aged 65 to 75 years old who are current or former smokers. Only one study of AAA screening in women has been done and showed no significant reduction in AAA-related mortality with routine screening.[54] The therapist should advise men in this age group who have ever smoked to discuss their risk for AAA with a medical doctor. Any male with these two risk factors especially presenting with any of these signs or symptoms must be referred immediately.

The orthopedic or acute care therapist must be aware that aortic damage (not an aneurysm but sometimes referred to as a pseudo-aneurysm) can occur with any anterior spine surgery (e.g., spinal fusion, spinal fusion with cages). Blood vessels are moved out of the way and can be injured during surgery. If the client (usually a postoperative inpatient) has internal bleeding from this complication there may be:

- Distended abdomen
- Changes in blood pressure
- Changes in stool
- Possible back and/or shoulder pain

In such cases, the client's recent history of anterior spinal surgery accompanied by any of these symptoms is enough to notify nursing or medical staff of concerns. Monitoring post-operative vital signs in these clients is essential.

SCREENING FOR PERIPHERAL VASCULAR CAUSES OF BACK PAIN

Most physical therapists are very familiar with the signs and symptoms of peripheral vascular disease (PVD) affecting the extremities, including both arterial and venous disease (see previous discussion, Chapter 6).

When assessing back pain for the possibility of a vascular cause, remember peripheral vascular disease can cause back pain. The location of the pain or symptoms is determined by the location of the pathology (Fig. 14-3).

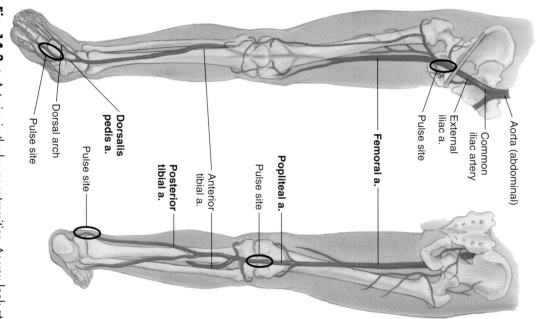

Aorta (abdominal)

Common iliac a.

External iliac artery

Pulse site

Femoral a.

Popliteal a.

Pulse site

Anterior tibial a.

Posterior tibial a.

Dorsalis pedis a.

Pulse site

Dorsal arch

Pulse site

Fig. 14-3 • Arteries in the lower extremities. As you look at this illustration, note the location of the arteries in the lower extremities starting with the aorta branching into the common iliac artery, which descends on both sides into the legs. Once the common iliac artery passes through the pelvis to the femur, it becomes the femoral artery and then the popliteal artery behind the knee before branching into the popliteal artery. The final split comes as the popliteal artery divides to form the anterior tibial artery down the front of the lower leg and the posterior tibial artery down the back of the lower leg. The anterior tibial artery also becomes the dorsalis pedis artery. Note the pulse points shown with bold, black ovals and remember that distal pulses disappear with aging and the presence of atherosclerosis causing peripheral vascular disease. (From Jarvis C: *Physical examination and health assessment*, ed 4. Philadelphia, 2004, WB Saunders; Fig 20-2, pg 535.)

With obstruction of the aortic bifurcation, the client may report back pain alone, back pain with any of the following features, or any of these signs and symptoms alone (Table 14-7):

- Bilateral buttock and/or leg pain or discomfort
- Weakness and fatigue of the lower extremities
- Atrophy of the leg muscles
- Absent lower extremity pulses
- Color and/or temperature changes in the feet and lower legs

Symptoms are often (but not always) bilateral because the obstruction occurs before the aorta divides (i.e., before it becomes the common iliac artery and supplies each leg separately). Frequently, someone with symptomatic atherosclerotic disease in one blood vessel has similar pathology in other blood vessels as well. Over time, there may be a progression of symptoms as the disease worsens and blood vessels become more and more clogged with plaque and debris.

With obstruction of the iliac artery the client is more likely to present with pain in the low back, buttock, and/or leg of the affected side and/or numbness in the same area(s). Obstruction of the femoral artery can result in thigh and/or calf pain, again with distal pulses diminished or absent.

Ipsilateral calf/ankle pain or discomfort (intermittent claudication) occurs with obstruction of the popliteal artery and is a common first symptom of PVD.

Adults over the age of 50 presenting with back pain of unknown cause and mild to moderate elevation of blood pressure should be screened for the presence of peripheral vascular disease.

Back Pain: Vascular or Neurogenic?

The medical differential diagnosis is difficult to make between back pain of a vascular versus neurogenic origin. Frequently, vascular and neurogenic claudication occurs in the same age group (over 60 and even more often, after age 70). Sometimes clients are referred to physical therapy to help make the differentiation (Case Example 14-9).

Vascular and neurogenic disease often coexists in the same person with an overlap of symptoms of each. There are several major differences to look for but especially response to rest (i.e., activ-

TABLE 14-7 ▼ Back and Leg Pain from Arterial Occlusive Disease

The location of discomfort, pain, or other symptoms is determined by the location of the pathology (arterial obstruction).

Site of occlusion	Signs and symptoms

Aortic bifurcation	• Sensory and motor deficits
	  • Muscle weakness and atrophy
	  • Numbness (loss of sensation)
	  • Paresthesias (burning, pricking)
	  • Paralysis
	• Intermittent claudication (pain or discomfort relieved by rest): bilateral buttock and/or leg, low back, gluteal, thigh, calf
	• Cold, pale legs with decreased or absent peripheral pulses

Iliac artery	• Intermittent claudication (pain or discomfort in the buttock, hip, thigh of the affected leg; can be unilateral or bilateral; relieved by rest) • Diminished or absent femoral or distal pulses • Impotence in males
Femoral and popliteal artery	• Intermittent claudication (pain or discomfort; calf and foot; may radiate) • Leg pallor and coolness • Dependent rubor • Blanching of feet on elevation • No palpable pulses in ankles and feet • Gangrene
Tibial and common peroneal artery	• Intermittent claudication (calf pain or discomfort; feet occasionally) • Pain at rest (severe disease); possibly relieved by dangling leg • Same skin and temperature changes in lower leg and foot as described above • Pedal pulses absent; popliteal pulses may be present

From Goodman CC, Fuller K, Boissonnault WG: *Pathology: implications for the physical therapist*, ed 2, Philadelphia, 2003, WB Saunders.

CASE EXAMPLE 14-9 Spinal Stenosis

Background: A 68-year-old woman with a long history of degenerative arthritis of the spine was referred to physical therapy for conservative treatment toward a goal of improving function despite her painful symptoms. She was a nonsmoker with no other significant previous medical history.

Her symptoms were diffuse bilateral lumbosacral back pain into the buttocks and thighs, which increased with walking or any activity and did not subside substantially with rest (except for prolonged rest and immobility).

Clinical Presentation: On examination, this client moved slowly and with effort, complaining of the painful symptoms described. There was no tenderness of the sacroiliac joint or sciatic notch but a subjective report of tenderness over L4 to L5 and L5 to S1. Tap test was negative; the client reported mild diffuse tenderness. There was no palpable step-off or dip of the spinous processes for spondylolisthesis and no paraspinal spasm, but a marked right lumbar scoliosis was noted. The client reported knowledge of scoliosis since she was a child.

A neurologic screening examination revealed normal straight leg raise and normal sensation and reflexes in both lower extremities. Motor examination was unremarkable for an inactive 68-year-old woman. Dorsalis pedis and posterior tibialis pulses were palpable but weak bilaterally.

Despite physical therapy treatment and compliance on the part of the client with a home program, her symptoms persisted and progressively worsened.

What is the Next Step in the Screening Process?

Re-evaluate the client's movement dysfunction and the selected intervention to date. Was the right treatment approach taken? Reassess red flag findings (age, lack of improvement with intervention) and conduct a review of systems (if this has not already been done).

In this case the client's age, negative neurologic screening examination, and diminished lower extremity pulses suggested a second look for vascular cause of symptoms.

Vital signs were assessed along with a peripheral vascular screening examination. The Bike Test was administered but the results were unclear with increased pain reported in both extension and flexion.

Result: She returned to her physician with a report of these findings. Further testing showed that in addition to degenerative arthritis of the lumbosacral spine, there was secondary stenosis and marked aortic calcification, indicating a vascular component to her symptoms.

Surgery was scheduled: an L4 to L5 laminectomy with fusion, iliac crest bone graft, and decompression foraminotomies. Postoperatively, the client subjectively reported 80% improvement in her symptoms with an improvement in function, although she was still unable to return to work.

1. Vascular-induced back and/or leg pain or discomfort is alleviated by rest and usually within 1 to 3 minutes. Conversely, activity (usually walking) brings the symptoms on within 1 to 3, sometimes 3 to 5 minutes. Neurogenic-induced symptoms often occur immediately with use of the affected body part and/or when adopting certain positions. The client may report the pain is relieved by prolonged rest or not at all.

What is the effect of changing the position of the spine on pain of a vascular nature? Are the vascular structures compromised in any way by forward bending, side bending, or backward bending (Fig. 14-4)? Are we asking the diseased heart or compromised blood vessels to supply more blood to this area?

It is not likely that movements of the spine will reproduce back pain of a vascular origin. What about back pain of a neurogenic cause? Forward bending opens the vertebral canal (vertebral foramen) giving the spinal cord (through L1) additional space. This is important in preventing painful symptoms when spinal stenosis is present bilaterally.

2. Given the presence of low back and/or leg (neurogenic or vascular) pain), position of the spine, and the presence of any trophic (skin) changes (see Table 14-6).

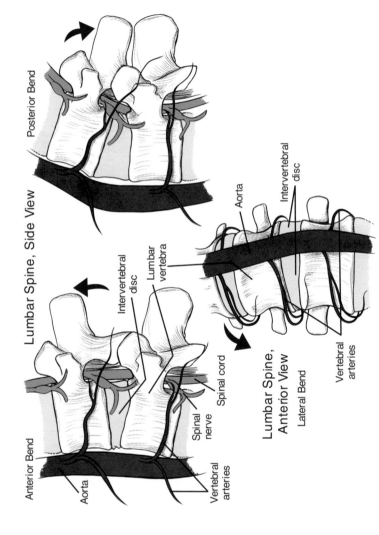

Lumbar Spine, Side View

Posterior Bend

Anterior Bend

Intervertebral disc

Lumbar vertebra

Spinal nerve

Spinal cord

Vertebral arteries

Aorta

Lumbar Spine, Anterior View

Lateral Bend

Aorta

Intervertebral disc

Vertebral arteries

Fig. 14-4 • Vascular supply is not compromised by position of the spine so there is usually no change in back pain that is vascular-induced with change of position. Forward bend, extension, and side bending do not aggravate or relieve symptoms. Rather, increased activity requiring increased blood supply to the musculature is more likely to reproduce symptoms; likewise, rest may relieve the symptoms. Watch for a lag time of 3 to 5 minutes after the start of activity or exercise before symptoms appear or increase as a sign of a possible vascular component.

Unless there is a spinal neuroma, a true stenosis with spinal cord pressure does not occur in the lumbar region since the spinal cord ends at L1 in most people. Neural symptoms at L1 to L3 are rare and more likely indicate a spinal tumor rather than disc or facet pathology. Nerve pressure leading to radicular symptoms (e.g., pain, numbness, myotomal weakness) below L2 is not true stenosis of the vertebral canal, but rather intervertebral foraminal stenosis with encroachment of the peripheral nerve as it leaves the spinal canal through the neural foramina.

The position of comfort for someone with back pain associated with spinal stenosis is usually lumbar flexion. The client may lean forward and rest the hands on the thighs or lean the upper body against a table or cupboard.

The Bike Test

The van Gelderen Bicycle Test is one way to assess the cause of back pain (Fig. 14-5). It offers clues to the source (neurogenic or vascular), but it is not a definitive test by itself. The Bike Test is based on two of the three variables listed earlier:

(1) response to rest, and (2) position of the spine. Trophic (skin) changes are assessed separately.

In theory, if someone has back pain of a vascular origin, what is the effect of peddling a stationary bicycle? Increased demand for oxygen can result in back pain when the cardiac workload/oxygen need is greater than the ability of the affected coronary arteries to supply the necessary oxygen.

Normally, the response would be angina (chest pain or discomfort or whatever pattern the client typically experiences). In the case of referred pain patterns, the client may experience midthoracic or even lumbar pain. How soon do these symptoms appear? With musculoskeletal pain of a cardiac origin, there is a 3- to 5-minute lag time before the onset of symptoms. Immediate reproduction of painful symptoms is more indicative of neuromusculoskeletal involvement.

After peddling for 5 minutes and observing the client's response, ask him or her to lean forward and continue peddling. What is the expected response if the back, buttock, or leg pain is vascular-induced? In other words, what is the response

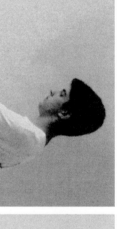

A

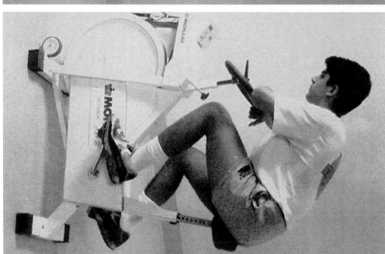

B

Fig. 14-5 • Bicycle test. Assessing the underlying cause of intermittent claudication: Vascular or neurogenic? The effect of stooping over while pedaling on vascular claudication is negligible, whereas a change in spine position can aggravate or relieve claudication of a neurogenic origin. **A,** The client is seated on an exercise bicycle and asked to pedal against resistance without using the upper extremities except for support. If pain into the buttock and posterior thigh occurs, followed by tingling in the affected lower extremity, the first part of the test is positive, but whether it is vascular or neurogenic remains undetermined. **B,** While pedaling, the client leans forward. If the pain subsides over a short time, the second part of the test is positive for neurogenic claudication but negative for vascular-induced symptoms. The test is confirmed for neurogenic cause of symptoms when the client sits upright again and the pain returns. (From Magee DJ: *Orthopedic physical assessment,* ed 4, Philadelphia, 2002, WB Saunders.)

to a change in position when someone has back pain of a vascular origin?

Typically there is no change because a change in position does not reproduce or alleviate vascular symptoms. The therapist can palpate pulses before and after the test to confirm the presence of vascular symptoms. What about neurogenic impairment? The client with neurogenic back pain may report a decrease in pain intensity or duration with forward flexion. Leaning forward (spinal flexion) can increase the diameter of the spinal canal, reducing pressure on the neural tissue.

When using the bike test to look for neurogenic claudication, the client starts pedaling while leaning back slightly. This position puts the lumbar spine in a position of extension. If the pain is reproduced, the first part of the test is positive for a neurogenic source of symptoms. The client then leans forward while still pedaling. If the pain

is less or goes away, the second part of the test is positive for neurogenic claudication. With neurogenic claudication, the pain returns when the individual sits upright again.

There is one major disadvantage to this test. Many clients in their sixth and seventh decades have both spinal stenosis and atherosclerosis contributing to painful back and/or leg symptoms. What if the client has back pain before even getting on the bicycle that is not relieved when bending forward? What diagnostic information does that provide?

The client could be experiencing neurogenic back pain that would normally feel better with flexion, but now while pedaling vascular compromise occurs. In some cases neurogenic pain lasts for hours or days despite change in position because once the neurologic structures are irritated, pain signals can persist.

The bike test has its greatest use when only one source of back pain is present: either vascular or neurogenic and even then, chronic neurogenic pain may not be modulated by change in position.

The therapist must rely on results of the screening interview and examination, taking time to perform a Review of Systems to identify clients who may need further medical evaluation. In some cases medical referral is not required. Identifying the underlying pathologic mechanism directs the therapist in choosing the most appropriate intervention.

▶ SCREENING FOR PULMONARY CAUSES OF NECK AND BACK PAIN

There are many potential pulmonary causes of back pain. The lungs occupy a large area of the upper trunk (see Fig. 7-1), with an equally large anterior and posterior thoracic area where pain can be referred. The most common conditions known to refer pulmonary pain to the somatic areas are pleuritis, pneumothorax, pulmonary embolus, cor pulmonale, and pleurisy.

Past Medical History

A recent history of one of these disorders in a client with neck, shoulder, chest or back pain raises a red flag of suspicion. In keeping with model for screening the therapist should review (1) past medical history, (2) risk factors, (3) clinical presentation, and (4) associated signs and symptoms (Box 14-5).

Clinical Presentation

Pulmonary pain patterns vary in their presentation based, in part, by the lobe(s) or segment(s) involved and by the underlying pathology. Several different pain patterns are presented in Chapter 7 (see Fig. 7-10).

Autosplinting is considered a valuable red flag of possible pulmonary involvement. Autosplinting occurs when the client prefers to lie on the involved side. Because pain of a pulmonary source is referred from the ipsilateral side, putting pressure on the involved lung field reduces respiratory movements and therefore reduces pain. It is uncommon for a person with a true musculoskeletal problem to find relief from symptoms by lying on the involved side.

The therapist should perform the following tests for clients with back pain who have a suspicious history or concomitant respiratory symptoms:
- Vital sign assessment
- Auscultation

BOX 14-5 ▼ Screening for Pulmonary-Induced Neck or Back Pain

History:

Previous history of cancer (any kind, but especially lung, breast and bone cancer)
Previous history of recurrent upper respiratory infection (URI) or pneumonia
Recent scuba diving, accident, trauma or overexertion (pneumothorax)

Risk Factors:

Smoking
Trauma (e.g., rib fracture, vertebral compression fracture)
Prolonged immobility
Chronic immunosuppression (e.g., corticosteroids, cancer chemotherapy)
Malnutrition, dehydration
Chronic diseases: diabetes mellitus, chronic lung disease, renal disease, cancer
Upper respiratory infection or pneumonia

Pain pattern:

Sharp, localized
Aggravated by respiratory movements
Prefer to sit upright
Autosplinting decreases the pain
ROM does not reproduce symptoms (e.g., shoulder and/or trunk movements)

Associated Signs and Symptoms

Dyspnea
Persistent cough
Constitutional symptoms: fever, chills
Weak and rapid pulse with concomitant fall in blood pressure (e.g., pneumothorax)

- Assess the effect of reproducing respiratory movements on symptoms (e.g., does deep breathing, laughing, or coughing reproduce the painful symptoms?)
- ROM: assess active trunk side bending and rotation
- Can pain or symptoms be reproduced with palpation (e.g., palpate the intercostals)?

Although reproducing pain or increased pain on respiratory movements is considered a hallmark sign of pulmonary involvement, symptoms of pleural, intercostal, muscular, costal, and dural origin all increase with coughing or deep inspiration.

Only pain of a cardiac origin is ruled out when symptoms increase in association with respiratory movements. For this reason the therapist must always carefully correlate clinical presentation

with client history and associated signs and symptoms when assessing for pulmonary disease.

Forceful coughing from an underlying pulmonary problem can cause an intercostal tear, which can be palpated. Even if some symptoms can be reproduced with palpation, the problem may still be pulmonary-induced, especially if the cause is repeated, forceful coughing from a pulmonary etiology.

Pancoast's tumors of the lung may invade the roots of the brachial plexus as they enlarge, appearing as pain in the C8 to T1 region. Other signs may include wasting of the muscles of the hand and/or Horner's syndrome with unilateral constricted pupil, ptosis, and loss of facial sweating (see the section on Lung Cancer in Chapter 7). *Tracheobronchial irritation* can cause pain to be referred to sites in the neck or anterior chest at the same levels as the points of irritation in the air passages (see Fig. 7-2). This irritation may be caused by inflammatory lesions, irritating foreign materials, or cancerous tumors.

Associated Signs and Symptoms

Assessing for associated signs and symptoms will usually bring to light important red flags to assist the therapist in recognizing an underlying pulmonary problem. Neck or back pain that is reproduced, increased with inspiratory movements, or accompanied by dyspnea, persistent cough, cyanosis, or hemoptysis must be evaluated carefully. Clients with respiratory origins of pain usually also show signs of general malaise or constitutional symptoms.

▶ SCREENING FOR RENAL AND UROLOGIC CAUSES OF BACK PAIN

When considering the possibility of a renal or urologic cause of back pain, the therapist can use the same step-by-step approach of looking at the history, risk factors, clinical presentation, and associated signs and symptoms.

For example, in anyone with back pain reported in the T9 to L1 area corresponding to pain patterns from the kidney or urinary tract (see Figs. 10-7 and 10-8), ask about a history of kidney stones, urinary tract infections (UTIs), and trauma (fall, blow, lift).

Origin of Pain Patterns

As discussed in Chapter 3 there can be at least three possible explanations for visceral pain patterns including embryologic development, multi-segmental innervation, and direct pressure on the diaphragm.

All three of these mechanisms are found in the urologic system. The *embryologic* origin of urologic pain patterns begins with the testicles and ovaries. These reproductive organs begin in utero where the kidneys are in the adult and then migrate during fetal development following the pathways of the ureters. A kidney stone down the pathway of the ureter causes pain in the flank radiating to the scrotum (male) or labia (female).

Evidence of the influence of *multisegmental innervation* is observed when skin pain over the kidneys is reported. Visceral and cutaneous sensory fibers enter the spinal cord close to each other and converge on the same neurons. When visceral pain fibers are stimulated, cutaneous fibers are stimulated, too. Thus, visceral pain can be perceived as skin pain.

None of the components of the lower urinary tract comes in contact with the diaphragm, so the bladder and urethra are not likely to refer pain to the shoulder. Lower urinary tract impairment is more likely to refer pain to the low back, pelvic, or sacral areas. However, the upper urinary tract can impinge the diaphragm with resultant referred pain to the costovertebral area or shoulder.

Past Medical History

Kidney disorders such as acute pyelonephritis and perinephric abscess of the kidney may be confused with a back condition. Most renal and urologic conditions appear with a combination of systemic signs and symptoms accompanied by pelvic, flank, or low back pain.

The client may have a history of recent trauma or a past medical history of urinary tract infections to alert the clinician to a possible renal origin of symptoms.

Clinical Presentation

Acute pyelonephritis (see Fig. 7-4) and other kidney conditions appear with aching pain at one or several costovertebral areas, posteriorly, just lateral to the muscles at T12 to L1, from acute distention of the capsule of the kidney.

The pain is usually dull and constant, with possible radiation to the pelvic crest or groin. The client may describe febrile chills, frequent urination, hematuria, and shoulder pain (if the diaphragm is irritated). Percussion to the flank areas reveals tenderness; the therapist should perform Murphy's percussion test (see Fig. 4-51).

Nephrolithiasis (kidney stones) may appear as back pain radiating to the flank or the iliac crest

(see Fig. 7-4) (Case Example 14-10). Kidney stones may occur in the presence of diseases associated with hypercalcemia (excess calcium in the blood), such as hyperparathyroidism, metastatic carcinoma, multiple myeloma, senile osteoporosis, specific renal tubular disease, hyperthyroidism, and Cushing's disease. Other conditions associated with calculus formation are infection, urinary stasis, dehydration, and excessive ingestion or absorption of calcium.

Ureteral colic, caused by passage of a kidney stone (calculus), appears as excruciating pain that radiates down the course of the ureter into the urethra or groin area. The pain is unrelieved by rest or change in position. These attacks are intermittent and may be accompanied by nausea, vomiting, sweating, and tachycardia. Localized abdominal muscle spasm may be present. The urine usually contains erythrocytes or is grossly bloody.

Urinary tract infection affecting the lower urinary tract is related directly to irritation of the bladder and urethra. The intensity of symptoms depends on the severity of the infection. Although low back pain may be the client's chief complaint, further questioning usually elicits additional urologic symptoms. The therapist should ask about

- Urinary frequency, urgency, dysuria (burning pain on urination), nocturia (frequency at night)
- Constitutional symptoms (fever, chills, nausea, vomiting)
- Blood in urine
- Testicular pain

Clients can be asymptomatic with regard to urologic symptoms, making the physical therapy diagnosis more difficult.

Screening Questions: Renal and Urologic System

It is important to ask questions about the presence of urologic symptoms (see Appendix B-5). Many people (therapists and clients alike) are uncomfortable discussing the details of bladder (or bowel)

CASE EXAMPLE 14-10   Back and Flank Pain

Background and Description of Client:
JH is a 57-year-old male with a history of mild mental retardation, seizure disorder, obesity, osteoarthritis, hypertension, and cervical disc disease (MRI reveals herniation at C7-T1 and spondylosis at C5-C6). He resides at a residential facility and is well known to PT over the past 6 years because of 5 separate PT examinations related to complaints of insidious onset of back pain.

These previous episodes of back pain resolved without PT intervention. JH presented in physical therapy this time with complaints of low back and right hip pain that he and his primary physician attributed to a minor fall 2 months prior to the PT examination. PT was not consulted during the initial period after the fall, because x-rays were unremarkable and JH had not complained of any symptoms at that time.

When asked to point to the area of pain, JH indicated his right lower lumbar area and along the right hip and flank. He was unable to describe the pain due to some cognitive limitations, but he did report that it was unrelieved with rest and occurred intermittently.

JH works full-time in a sheltered workshop doing piecework. He reported that the pain kept him from performing his job fully, and he found that lifting boxes was particularly difficult due to the bending. He also reported that prolonged ambulation or exercise caused an increase in the flank pain. He was taking over-the-counter ibuprofen for his pain; however, it was not effective.

JH is on the following medications: Colace (for constipation), Allegra (for allergy), Tegretol (for seizures), Zoloft (for obsessive-compulsive disorder), Risperdal (for psychosis), Buspar (for anxiety), and ibuprofen (PRN for pain).

Clinical Presentation: Vital signs were as follows: HR: 65; BP: 130/70; RR: 12; Temp: 99°. These were not significantly different from JH's normal vital signs.

Gait analysis was significant for an antalgic gait, slight increase in base of support, decreased trunk and pelvic rotation, significant ankle pronation, and pes planus bilaterally (JH does not like to wear his orthotics). He is an independent ambulator on all surfaces without the use of an assistive device. He lives in a 2-

CASE EXAMPLE 14-10 Back and Flank Pain—cont'd

story home and is able to ascend and descend stairs independently without complaints of pain.

Posture in standing was significant for decreased lumbar lordosis, rounded shoulders, and forward head, left shoulder mildly depressed.

Strength testing revealed strength of 4+/5 throughout upper extremities, trunk, and left lower extremity. JH was very hesitant with resisted strength testing on his right lower extremity for fear of pain; therefore no formal data was obtained. JH did report pain upon mildly resisted right hip flexion, abduction, and adduction.

PROM was all within functional limits. There was no apparent evidence of inflammation in bilateral knees or hips. PT was unable to reproduce symptoms with palpation along spine and bilateral hips and knees.

Right knee extension AROM in sitting revealed pain in right flank. Right SLR test in supine also revealed similar pain in right flank. Right side bending produced right flank pain. Left side bending produced no symptoms.

Neurologic examination revealed intact sensation to light touch along dermatomal pattern. DTR's were 1+ throughout.

Evaluation: JH's symptoms appeared inconsistent and dependent upon level of physical activity. It seemed counterintuitive that a minor fall 2 months prior to this examination could cause the current symptoms. The location of the pain also raised some concerns, because JH had never before complained of flank pain.

PT did not have access to the prior x-rays taken at the time of the fall. Therefore, PT requested further x-rays of JH's hip and spine from the orthopedic surgeon serving as consultant to rule out a more serious orthopedic or systemic issue. Physical therapy was deferred until the x-ray results were examined and reviewed by the orthopedic consultant and PT.

Outcome and Discussion: AP pelvis and frog view x-rays of hips were reviewed by the orthopedic consultant and PT, and it was

concluded that the x-rays were unremarkable. AP and lateral x-rays of JH's TLS spine at first glance also appeared to be unremarkable, and the x-ray report agreed with our initial assessment.

However, upon closer inspection, there was a circular 2-cm suspicious area that appeared on film at the level and location of JH's right kidney. The orthopedic surgeon ordered further imaging to confirm a diagnosis of kidney stone. An intravenous pyelogram (IVP) did confirm the diagnosis. After appropriate treatment for the kidney stones, JH reported that the pain on his right side had resolved.

JH was well known to the physical therapy department due to his previous examinations. JH was a challenging case because of the previous "false alarms" and because he does not always accurately communicate his symptoms due to his mild cognitive limits.

He also has comorbidities that warrant a more cautious approach in treating and assessing his complaints. These include hypertension and a seizure disorder and the multitude of medication that he takes.

It is up to the physical therapist to understand him and try to interpret his meanings as closely as she/he can. Fortunately in this case, JH's chief complaint of flank pain was different enough from previous complaints, and the films clearly showed a systemic cause of JH's symptoms.

Instructor's Comments: Some additional screening questions/information that might help with a case like this:

1. Did he have any symptoms of genitourinary distress (pain on urination? blood in the urine? difficulty starting or continuing a flow of urine? nocturia? frequency? or changes in bladder function)?
2. Did he have a past medical history of kidney stones?
3. Was Murphy's percussion test positive?
4. Was there a report of any constitutional symptoms (night sweats? spiked temps? flulike symptoms)?

Used with permission. Josephine Yee, DPT: Case report submitted as part of course requirements in fulfillment of DPT 910, New York, 2002, Stony Brook.

function. If presented in a professional manner with a brief explanation, both parties can be put at ease. For example, the interview may go something like this:

"I'm going to ask a few other questions that may not seem like they fit with the back pain (shoulder pain, pelvic pain) you're having. There are many possible causes of back pain and I want to make sure I don't leave anything out.

If I ask you anything you don't know, please pay attention over the next few days and see if you notice something. Don't hesitate to bring this information back to me. It could be very important."

To the therapist: The important thing to look for is CHANGE. Many people have problems with incontinence, nocturia, or frequency. If someone has always experienced a delay before starting a flow of urine, this may be normal for him (or her).

Many women have nocturia after childbirth but most men do not get up at night to empty their bladders until after age 65. They may not even be aware that this has changed for them. Often, it is the wife or partner who answers the question about getting up at night as "yes!" Likewise if a man has always had a delay in starting a flow of urine, he may not be aware that the delay is now twice as long as before. Or he may not recognize that being unable to continue a flow of urine is not "normal" and in fact, requires medical evaluation.

Pseudorenal Pain

Sometimes clients appear to have classic symptoms of a kidney problem, but without any associated signs and symptoms. Such a situation can occur with someone who has a mechanical derangement of the costovertebral or costotransverse joint or irritation of the costal nerve (radiculitis, T10-T12).

What does this look like in the clinic? How does the therapist make the differentiation? Use the same guidelines for decision making in the screening process presented throughout this text (e.g., history, risk factors, associated signs, and symptoms).

History

Trauma is often the underlying etiology. The client may or may not report assault. The individual may not remember any specific trauma or accident. Pseudorenal pain can occur when floating ribs become locked with the ribs above, but this is a rare cause of these symptoms. Radiculitis or mechanical derangement of the T10 to T12 costovertebral or costotransverse joint(s) is more likely.

Risk Factors

Unknown or none for this condition.

Clinical Presentation

Pain pattern is affected by change in position:

• Lying on that side increases pain (remember clients with renal pain prefer pressure on the involved side; musculoskeletal symptoms are often made worse by lying on the affected side).

• Prolonged sitting increases pain; slumped sitting especially increases pain; the therapist can have the client try this position and see what effect it has on symptoms.

• Symptoms are reproduced with movements of the spine (especially forward flexion and side bending).

• Presence of costovertebral angle tenderness: the therapist may be able to reproduce pain with palpation; Murphy's sign is negative (see Fig. 4-51).

A positive Murphy's test for renal involvement elicits kidney pain or reproduces the referred back pain and must be reported to the physician. A negative response occurs when there is no discomfort or pain or pain that can be reproduced by local palpation at the costovertebral angle. The therapist must ask about the presence of signs and symptoms associated with renal disease.

One final note about pseudorenal back pain: thoracic disc disease can mimic kidney disease and presents with flank, buttock, and/or leg pain. MRIs are negative, but may show only the lumbar spine.[55]

In the case of a possible thoracic disc mimicking renal involvement, the therapist can provide the physician with clinical findings and the reason for the referral. Look for a history of straining, lifting, accident, or other mechanical injury to the thoracic spine.

The therapist must look carefully for evidence of neurologic involvement. Perform a screening neurologic assessment as outlined in Chapter 4. There may be bladder changes, which can be confusing; are these urologic-induced or disc-related? Report any suspicious symptoms.

Associated Signs and Symptoms

Usually none when pseudorenal pain is present.

▲ SCREENING FOR GASTROINTESTINAL CAUSES OF BACK PAIN

Back pain of a visceral origin occurs most often as a result of gastrointestinal (GI) problems. Pain patterns associated with the GI system can present as sternal, shoulder, scapular, midback, low back, or hip pain and dysfunction. If the client had primary symptoms of GI impairment (abdominal pain, nausea, diarrhea, or constipation; see Fig. 8-16), he or she would see a medical doctor.

As it is, the referred pain patterns are quite convincing that the musculoskeletal region described is the problem. Referred pain patterns for the GI system are presented in Fig. 8-17 (anterior and posterior). These are the pain patterns the therapist is most likely to see.

Past Medical History and Risk Factors

Taking a closer look at past medical history, risk factors, and clinical presentation and asking about associated signs and symptoms may reveal important red flags and clues pointing to the GI system. The most significant and common history is one of long-term or chronic use of nonsteroidal antiinflammatory drugs (NSAIDs). Risk factors and assessment of risk for NSAID-induced gastropathy are discussed in detail in Chapter 8.

Other significant risk factors in the history include the long-term use of immunosuppressants, past history of cancer, history of Crohn's disease (also known as regional enteritis), or previous bowel obstruction.

Signs and Symptoms of GI Dysfunction

The most common signs and symptoms associated with the GI system are listed in Box 14-6 and discussed in greater detail in Chapter 8. Back pain (as well as hip, pelvic, sacral, and lower extremity pain) with any of these accompanying features should be considered a red flag for the possibility of GI impairment.

Anterior neck (esophageal) pain may occur, usually with a burning sensation ("heartburn") or other symptoms related to eating or swallowing (e.g., dysphagia, odynophagia). Esophageal varices associated with chronic alcoholism may appear as anterior neck pain but usually occur at the xiphoid process and are recognized as heartburn.

Anterior neck pain can also occur as a result of a discogenic lesion requiring a careful history and neurologic screening to document findings. Clients with eating disorders who repeatedly binge and then purge by vomiting may report anterior neck pain without realizing the correlation between eating behaviors and symptoms.

When assessing neck pain, the therapist should look for other associated signs and symptoms, such as sore throat; pain that is relieved with antacids, the upright position, fluids, or avoidance of eating; and pain that is aggravated by eating, bending, or recumbency.

Dysphagia or difficulty swallowing, *odynophagia* (painful swallowing), and *epigastric pain* are indicative of esophageal involvement. Certain types of drugs (e.g., antidepressants, antihypertensives, asthma medications) can make swallowing difficult, requiring a careful evaluation during the client interview.

Early satiety (the client takes one or two bites of food and is no longer hungry) is another red flag symptom of the GI system (Case Example 14-11-Early Satiety and Weight Loss). In general back pain made better, worse, or altered in any way by eating is a red flag symptom. If the change in symptom(s) occurs immediately to within 30 minutes of eating, the upper gastrointestinal tract or stomach/duodenum may be a possible cause. Change in symptoms 2 to 4 hours *after* eating is more indicative of the lower GI tract (intestines/colon).

Bloody diarrhea, fecal incontinence, and *melena* are three additional signs of lower GI involvement. It is important to ask the client about the presence of specific signs that may be too embarrassing to mention (or the client may not see the connection between back pain and bowel smears on the underwear). Asking someone with back pain about bowel function can be accomplished in a very professional manner. The therapist may tell the client:

"I am going to ask you a series of questions about your bowels. This may not seem like it is connected to your current problem, so just bear with me. These are important questions to make sure we have covered every possibility. If you do not know the answer to the question, pay attention over the next day or two to see how everything is working. If you notice anything unusual or different, please let me know when you come in next time."

Follow-Up Questions

- When was your last bowel movement? (Look for a change of any kind in the client's normal elimination pattern. Additionally, failure to have a bowel movement over a much longer period of time than expected for that client may be a sign of impaction/obstruction/obstipation.)
- Are you having any diarrhea?
- Is there any blood in your stool?
- Have you ever been told you have hemorrhoids or do you know that you have hemorrhoids?
- Do you have difficulty wiping yourself clean?
- Do you find smears on your underwear later after a bowel movement?
- Do you have small amounts of stool leakage?

Again, when it comes to something like bowel smears on the underpants, it is important to distinguish between pathology and poor hygiene. The key to look for is change such as the new appearance of a problem that was not present before the onset of back pain or other symptoms. With blood in the stools, a medical doctor must differentiate between internal versus external bleeding.

Melena is a dark, tarry stool caused by oxidation of blood in the GI tract (usually the upper GI tract, but it can be the lower GI tract). The most common causes of abdominal bleeding are chronic use of NSAIDs leading to ulceration, Crohn's disease, or ulcerative colitis, and diverticulitis or diverticulosis. Anyone with a history of these problems presenting with new onset of back pain must be screened for medical disease.

Hemorrhage or visible blood in the toilet may be a sign of anal fissures, hemorrhoids, or colon cancer. The etiology must be determined by a medical doctor. Be aware that there is an increased incidence of rectal bleeding from anal fissures and local tissue damage associated with anal intercourse. This occurs predominantly in the male homosexual or bisexual population, but can be seen

in heterosexual partners who engage in anal intercourse. There are also increasing reports of adolescents engaging in oral and anal intercourse as a form of birth control.

It may be necessary to take a sexual history. The therapist should offer the client a clear explanation for any questions concerning sexual activity, sexual function, or sexual history. There is no way to know when someone will be offended or claim sexual harassment. It is in the therapist's best interest to maintain the most professional manner possible.

There should be no hint of sexual innuendo or humor injected into any of the therapist's conversations with clients at any time. The line of sexual impropriety lies where the complainant draws it and includes appearances of misbehavior. This perception differs broadly from client to client.[50]

You may need to include the following questions (see also Appendix B-29). Always offer an explanation for taking a sexual history. For example, *"There are a few personal questions I'll need to ask that may help sort out where your symptoms are coming from. Please answer these as best you can."*

Follow-Up Questions

- Are you sexually active?
  "Sexually active" does not necessarily mean engaging in sexual intercourse. Sexual touch is enough to transmit many sexually transmitted infections. The therapist may have to explain this to the client to clarify this question. Oral and anal intercourse are often not viewed as "sexual intercourse" and will result in the client answering the question with "No" when, in fact, for screening purposes, the answer is "Yes."
- Have you had more than one sexual partner (one at a time or during the same time period)?
- Have you ever been told you have a sexually transmitted infection or disease such as herpes, chlamydia, gonorrhea, venereal, HIV, or other disease?
- Is there any chance the bleeding you are having could be related to sexual activity?

For women:

- What form of birth control are you using? (Risk factor: IUCD)
- Is there any possibility you could be pregnant?
- Have you ever had an abortion?

CASE EXAMPLE 14-11 Early Satiety and Weight Loss

Background: A 78-year-old female was referred to physical therapy by her orthopedic surgeon 6 weeks status post total knee replacement (TKR). Her active knee flexion was 70 degrees; passive knee flexion was only 86 degrees. There was a 15-degree extensor lag.

During the course of her rehabilitation program, her adult daughters took turns bringing her to the clinic. They all commented on how much weight she had lost, though to the therapist she looked quite obese.

When asked about the weight loss, she replied, "Oh, I take a bite or two and then I'm not very hungry." This symptom (early satiety with weight loss) had been present for the last 2 months (starting prior to the TKR).

She did not have any other signs or symptoms associated with the GI system. There were no reported changes in bowel function or the appearance of her stools, no blood in the stools, no back or sacral pain, no night pain that was not directly related to her knee, and no other changes in her health.

Her social history included the recent death of a spouse. She had taken care of her husband at home for the last 3 years after he had a severe stroke. She knew she needed a knee replacement, but put it off because of her husband's poor health. Within 6 weeks of his death, she scheduled the needed operation.

Could her weight loss be a delayed grieving reaction? Emotional overlay? How can you tell?

The screening process often begins with the recognition and categorization of red flags. It is not within the scope of a physical therapist's practice to diagnose psychologic or emotional problems. Clearly, many of the clients and patients in our clinics have significant psychologic needs and emotional responses to their illnesses, injuries, or conditions.

Identifying a cluster of signs and symptoms suggestive of a psychologic or behavioral component may help determine the need for behavioral counseling or a psych consult. However, the therapist's plan of care may include the use of specific client management skills based on observation of particular behavioral patterns.

What do you see in the history, clinical presentation, and associated signs and symptoms as they are presented here that raise a red flag?

• History: age and positive social history for recent personal loss

• Clinical Presentation: unremarkable; consistent with orthopedic diagnosis

• Associated Signs and Symptoms: early satiety with weight loss

Viewing the whole client or patient and identifying the presence of emotional overlay to symptoms can be accomplished using the McGill Pain questionnaire, Waddell's nonorganic signs adapted for the knee, and listening to the client's response to her condition and the rehabilitation program (symptom magnification). These 3 assessment tools are discussed in Chapter 3.

There are really only 2 red flags here (age and early satiety with weight loss), but they are significant enough to warrant contact with her physician. The next question is: to whom do you send her? The referring orthopedist or her family doctor (if she has one)?

It may be best to communicate all findings with the referring physician or health care provider. The therapist can leave the door open by asking any one of the following questions:

• Do you want to see Mrs. So-and-So back in your office or shall I send her to her family physician?

• Do you want Mr. X/Mrs. Y to check with his/her family doctor or do you prefer to see him/her yourself?

• How do you want to handle this? or How do you want me to handle this?

Outcome: The orthopedic surgeon recommended referral to her primary care physician. Examination and diagnostic tests resulted in a diagnosis of esophageal cancer (early stage). The client was treated successfully for the cancer while completing her rehabilitation program.

—*If yes,* follow up with careful (sensitive) questions about how many, when, where, and any immediate or delayed complications (physical or psychologic).

Back pain from any cause may impair sexual function. Many health care professionals do not address this issue; the therapist can offer much in the way of education, pain management, improved function, and proper positioning for work and recreation. Some publications are available to assist therapists discuss sexual function and pain control for the client with back pain.[56,57]

Esophagus

Esophageal pain will occur at the level of the lesion and is usually accompanied by epigastric pain and heartburn. Severe esophagitis (see Fig. 8-11) may refer pain to the anterior cervical or more often, the midthoracic spine.

The pain pattern will most likely present in a band of pain starting anteriorly and spreading around the chest wall to the back. Rarely, pain will begin in the midback and radiate around to the front. Referred pain to the midthoracic spine occurs around T5-6.

As with cervical pain of GI origin, there may be a history of alcoholism with esophageal varices, cirrhosis, or an underlying eating disorder. If liver impairment is an underlying factor, there may be signs such as asterixis (liver flap or flapping tremor), palmar erythema, spider angiomas, and carpal (tarsal) tunnel syndrome (see discussion, Chapter 9).

Keep in mind that this same type of midthoracic back pain can occur with thoracic disc disease. Look for a history of trauma and neurologic changes typically associated with disc degeneration (e.g., bowel and bladder changes, numbness and tingling or paresthesias in the upper extremities); these are not usually present with esophageal impairment. Lower thoracic disc herniation can cause groin pain, leg pain, or mimic kidney pain.

Stomach and Duodenum

Long-term use of NSAIDs is the most common cause of back pain referred from the stomach or duodenum. Ulceration and bleeding into the retroperitoneal area can cause pain in the back or shoulder. The primary and referred pain patterns for pain of a stomach or duodenal source are shown in Fig. 8-12.

The referred pain to the back is at the level of the lesion, usually between T6 and T10. For the client with midthoracic spine pain of unknown cause or which does not fit the expected musculoskeletal presentation, ask about associated signs and symptoms such as

- Blood in the stools
- Symptoms associated with meals
- Relief of pain after eating (immediately or 2 hours later)
- Increased symptoms with or during a bowel movement
- Decreased symptoms after a bowel movement

The pain of peptic ulcer (see Figs. 8-7 and 8-12) occasionally occurs only in the midthoracic back between T6 and T10, either at the midline or immediately to one side or the other of the spine. Posterior penetration of the retroperitoneum with blood loss and resultant referred thoracic pain is most often caused by long-term use of nonsteroidal antiinflammatory drugs (NSAIDs). The therapist should look for a correlation between symptoms and the timing of meals, as well as the presence of blood in the feces or relief of symptoms with antacids.

Small Intestine

Diseases of the small intestine (e.g., Crohn's disease, irritable bowel syndrome, obstruction from neoplasm) usually produce mid-abdominal pain around the umbilicus (see Fig. 8-2), but the pain may be referred to the back if the stimulus is sufficiently intense or if the individual's pain threshold is low (see Fig. 8-13) (Case Example 14-12).

For the client with low back pain of unknown cause or suspicious presentation, ask if there is ever any abdominal pain present. Alternating abdominal/low back pain at the same level is a red flag that requires medical referral. Since both symptoms do not always occur together, the client may not recognize the relationship or report the symptoms. The therapist must be sure and ask appropriate screening questions (Case Example 14-13).

Look for a known history of Crohn's disease (regional enteritis), irritable bowel syndrome, bowel obstruction, or cancer. Low back, sacral, or hip pain may be a new symptom of an already established disease. The client may not be aware that 25% of the people with GI disease have concomitant back or joint pain.

Enteric-induced arthritis can be accompanied by a skin rash that comes and goes. A flat red or purple rash or raised skin lesion(s) is possible, usually preceding the joint or back pain. The therapist must ask the client if he/she has had any skin rashes in the last few weeks.

CASE EXAMPLE 14-12 Crohn's Disease and Back Pain

A 23-year-old ballet dancer with "shin splints" comes to you from a sports medicine doctor. Beside anterior lower leg pain, she also reports low back pain that seems to come and go with overuse. She has a history of Crohn's disease.

Can symptoms of anterior compartment syndrome be caused by Crohn's disease?

It is very unlikely. There are no reported cases to date. Crohn's disease is linked with low back, hip, and sometimes knee pain (knee pain is usually associated with hip pain and usually does not occur alone).

Anterior compartment syndrome is easily reproducible with tenderness on palpation of the anterior tibial region. The pain pattern and etiology is fairly typical and symptoms respond to treatment. If the soft tissues are acutely inflamed, surgical intervention may be required.

What questions can you ask to rule out a GI cause for her back pain?

• Ask about the presence of GI signs and symptoms:

Are you having any nausea, vomiting, diarrhea, or constipation?

Any change in your bowel movements? Any trouble wiping yourself clean after a bowel movement?

Any blood in the stools?

• Any other symptoms of any kind? (headaches, sweats, fever)

• Is there abdominal pain and is it at the same level as the back pain?

• Does the abdominal and/or back pain change with food intake (assess from 30 minutes to 2 hours after eating)?

• Is there relief of back pain with passing gas or having a bowel movement?

• Is there a recent (chronic) history of antibiotic and/or NSAID use?

• Has the client experienced any joint pain anywhere else in the body?

Any skin rashes anywhere?

A "yes" answer to any of these questions is a significant red flag and must be evaluated in context of the overall clinical presentation and findings from the Review of Systems.

The therapist may treat joint or back pain when there is an unknown or unrecognized enteric cause. Palliative intervention for musculoskeletal symptoms or apparent movement impairment can make a difference in the short-term, but does not affect the final outcome.

Eventually the GI symptoms will progress; symptoms that are unrelieved by physical therapy intervention are red flags. Medical treatment of the underlying disease is essential to correcting the musculoskeletal component.

▲ SCREENING FOR LIVER AND BILIARY CAUSES OF BACK PAIN

The primary pain pattern for liver disease is right over the liver. In primary liver pathology, palpation of the organ will reproduce the symptoms and the examiner can feel the liver distention. The normal, healthy liver is located up under the right side of the diaphragm and ribs. The gallbladder is tucked up under the liver (see also Fig. 9-2).

When a referred pain pattern occurs, there may be pain on palpation of the liver, but the primary complaint is of back pain. There is no report of anterior pain to alert the examiner to the need for liver palpation. In anyone with the referred pain patterns depicted and described in Fig. 9-10, liver palpation may be required as part of the physical assessment (see Figs. 4-48 and 4-49). In addition to a painful and distended liver, the client may report

• Pain/nausea 1 to 3 hours after eating (gallstones)

• Pain immediately after eating (gallbladder inflammation)

• Muscle guarding/tenderness and fever/chills in the right upper quadrant (posterior)

Other signs and symptoms associated with liver impairment are discussed in detail in Chapter 9 and include

• Liver flap (asterixis)

• Nail bed changes (Nail of Terry)

• Palmer erythema (liver palms)

• Spider angiomas

• Ascites, jaundice

Gallbladder and biliary disease may also refer pain to the interscapular or right subscapular area.

CASE EXAMPLE 14-13 Abdominal and Back Pain at the Same Level

Background: A 68-year-old accountant came to physical therapy as a self-referral for low back pain. He reported slipping on a patch of ice as the mechanism of injury.

Symptoms were mild, but distressing to this gentleman. He reported pain as "sore" and "aching," with any spinal twisting or side bending to the right. The pain was present across the low back on both sides.

The client reported symptoms of stomach distress from time to time. He attributed this to his trips overseas, eating foods from Ireland, Scotland, Germany, and the Netherlands.

Lumbar range of motion was fairly typical of a nearly 70 year old with most of his functional forward flexion from the hips and thoracic spine. True physiologic motion in the lumbar spine was negligible. Accessory spinal motions were also limited globally. Active rotation and side bending were stiff and limited to both sides, but only painful to the right.

Neurologic screening exam was negative. The therapist did not ask about the presence of any other symptoms of any kind anywhere else in his body. No questions were asked about changes in the pattern of his bowel movements or appearance of his stools.

Given the examination results as tested, a conditioning exercise program seemed most appropriate. The client began a stationary bicycling program alternating with walking when the weather permitted. He reported gradual relief from his symptoms and return of motion and function to his previous levels.

Four months later this same client reported another injury while walking with subsequent back pain.

What are the red flag findings? What is the next step in the screening process?

The client's age (over 50) is the first red flag. Back pain across both sides can be considered bilateral and therefore a red flag until further assessment is completed. The presence of back pain and abdominal pain or discomfort warrants some additional questions.

The therapist should conduct a more thorough pain assessment and ask about the location of the symptoms as well as the presence of any additional GI symptoms. Back pain and abdominal pain at the same level is always a red flag.

Screening questions related to the back and GI dysfunction are available at the end of this chapter. Questions about changes in bowel function may reveal some important clues. A screening physical assessment of the abdomen including visual inspection, palpation, and auscultation as described in Chapter 4 may be helpful. Vital sign assessment is always recommended.

Result: The key red flag in this case was alternating back and abdominal pain at the same level. The client did not see a connection between these two episodes of pain. When his back hurt he did not have any abdominal pain and vice versa.

The client was advised to see his regular physician for an evaluation. He was diagnosed with colon cancer in advanced stages and died 6 weeks later. Earlier detection may have made a difference in this case but the cyclical nature of his presentation masked the true significance of his symptoms.

The Pancreas

Acute pancreatitis may appear as epigastric pain radiating to the midthoracic spine (see Fig. 8-15). Pain from the head of the pancreas is felt to the right of the spine, whereas pain from the body and tail is perceived to the left of the spine. More rarely, pain may be referred to the upper back and midscapular areas.

The therapist should be observant for any report of fever and chills, nausea and indigestion, changes in urine or stool, or signs of jaundice. The client may not associate GI symptoms with the scapular pain or discomfort. The therapist can use specific questions to rule out potential GI problems (see Special Questions to Ask in this chapter and in greater detail in Chapter 8).

may be experiencing back pain from a gynecologic cause?

As always, the model for screening includes history, presence of any risk factors, clinical presentation, and associated signs and symptoms. Obviously, gender is a clear red flag of possible gynecologic involvement in the case of back (or pelvic, groin, hip, sacral or SI) symptoms.

Whenever there is an absence of objective musculoskeletal findings, a history of gynecologic involvement, or associated signs and symptoms of gynecologic disorders, the therapist is encouraged to ask appropriate questions to determine the need for a gynecologic evaluation (Case Example 14-14).

The therapist must determine what phase the woman is in her reproductive life cycle (see previous discussions of Life Cycles and Menopause in Chapter 2). If the client is an adolescent, has she begun her menstrual cycle (menses)? If a young to middle-aged adult, is she menstruating, or has she

▶ SCREENING FOR GYNECOLOGIC CAUSES OF BACK PAIN

Gynecologic disorders can cause midpelvic or low back pain and discomfort. Gynecologic-induced back pain occurs most often in women of childbearing ages (commonly between ages 20 and 45). How can the therapist recognize when a woman

There may be a history of alcohol and tobacco use. Associated symptoms, which are usually GI related, may include diarrhea, anorexia, pain after a meal, and unexplained weight loss. The pain is relieved initially by heat, which decreases muscular tension, and may be relieved by leaning forward, sitting up, or lying motionless.

The therapist should remain alert for the client with low back pain who seems to benefit from heat modalities but then suddenly gets worse and does not improve with physical therapy intervention.

Data from: Requejo, SM, Barnes R, Kulig K, et al: The use of a modified classification system in the treatment of low back pain during pregnancy: a case report, *JOSPT* 32(7):318-326, 2002.

CASE EXAMPLE 14-14   Movement Disorder

A 28-year-old woman in the twentieth week of her first pregnancy reported low back pain of approximately 2 weeks' duration. She could not recall any injury or cause for her pain and attributed it to her pregnancy. She did report a 6-year history of back pain caused by exercise (military press); prior to this episode her back pain could be relieved by rest, heat, and massage therapy.

The current back pain was located bilaterally in the thoracolumbar paraspinal region and described as a "nagging ache." The client rated her pain as a 7 to 9 on the Numeric Rating Scale (NRS; see Fig. 3-6), worse in the afternoon and evening. Pain was aggravated by sitting more than 20 minutes and bending forward. She reported episodes of night pain that could be relieved by a change in position.

There were no other symptoms anywhere in her body; she was not taking any medications except for prenatal vitamins. She reported her pregnancy was "normal" with appropriate weight gain. There has been no spotting or vaginal bleeding during the pregnancy. Vital signs were within normal limits (WNL).

Is a Medical Screening Examination Needed?

The client's age is not a red flag at this time. Although she reports an insidious onset for her symptoms, the pain is not constant and can be relieved with a change in position. The pain wakes her up at night but she is able to get back to sleep by getting up and walking or by changing position. Vital signs were normal and there were no constitutional symptoms.

At this point the evaluation can proceed as usual. The therapist should include a screening neurologic assessment as part of the examination. Movement testing further confirmed an extension syndrome with worse symptoms during trunk flexion and improved pain after repetitive trunk extension.

No further medical screening is required unless additional red flag symptoms develop. The client's improvement with physical therapy intervention confirmed the decision that medical referral was not necessary.

had a hysterectomy and experienced surgically induced menopause?

Past Medical History

Gynecologic conditions causing back pain can include retroversion (tipping back) of the uterus, ovarian cysts, uterine fibroids, endometriosis, pelvic inflammatory disease, or normal pregnancy (Case Example 14-15).

Usually, there is a history of a chronic or long-standing gynecologic disorder, and the association between back pain and gynecologic disorder has been established. There may be a history of sexual assault, incest, sexually transmitted disease, ectopic pregnancy, use of an intrauterine contraceptive device, dysuria, or abortion.

Risk Factors

Often the history and risk factors for back or pelvic pain are synonymous, especially multiple pregnancies and births, with administration of an epidural during delivery, prolonged pushing, and/or use of forceps. Other risk factors include abnormal uterine position, endometriosis, ovarian cysts and uterine fibroids, ectopic pregnancy, and

the use of an intrauterine contraceptive device (IUCD).

Back pain is common during pregnancy beginning most often during the second trimester between the fifth and seventh months of gestation.[58,59] Women who have had multiple pregnancies or births may have sacroiliac or low back pain associated with poor abdominal tone and ligamentous laxity. The risk of developing chronic postpartum back pain may be doubled among women who received epidural anesthesia during labor.[60]

Additionally, women who have had one or more abortions may seek health care months to years later with a variety of physical and psychologic symptoms referred to as post-abortion syndrome or post-abortion survivor's syndrome. This condition has not been classified in the *Diagnostic and Statistical Manual* and its existence remains controversial.

Multiple Pregnancies and Births

Even though pregnancy and childbirth are natural physiologic processes, these events can be traumatic to the soft tissues of the pelvic floor. Referred pain to the low back from the consequences of this

---

CASE EXAMPLE 14-15   Back Pain During Pregnancy

A 32-year-old Native American woman in the third trimester of her second pregnancy presented with acute onset of mid- to right-sided lumbar pain. She reported pain radiating around to the right side. An abdominal sonogram was negative and all lab values were within normal limits. The client declined any further imaging studies and requested a referral to physical therapy.

What will you need to do to make sure this client's problem is within the scope of a physical therapy practice?

Take a thorough history (including childbirth histories) and evaluate pain pattern(s) carefully.

Screen for domestic abuse sometime during the evaluation or early treatment intervention.

Ask about the presence of any other symptoms, even if they seem unrelated to her pregnancy or back pain.

See if you can reproduce the symptoms by palpation or through position or movement; assess for trigger points.

Take all vital signs and ask about the presence of constitutional symptoms.

Assess for rectus abdominis diastasis (separation of the rectus abdominal muscles) as a possible contributing factor.

Outcome: During palpation of the ribs, the therapist noted an outward flaring of the lower ribs. There were pain and tenderness at the interchondral junctions between the eighth and tenth ribs.

The history was significant for chronic cough from smoking. The woman reported feeling the child in a horizontal position pushing against the lower ribs.

Based on these findings, the therapist telephoned the physician and asked if there was any chance a rib fracture could be causing the painful symptoms. The client agreed to an x-ray and the radiograph showed a fracture of the right tenth rib.

event is possible. If the woman's history includes a recent birth or multiple previous births, she may not recognize the association between her current symptoms and her pregnancy/delivery history.

Abnormal Uterine Positions

Having an understanding of the normal female reproductive anatomy (see Fig. 15-4) can help the therapist better appreciate musculoskeletal pain and dysfunction that can occur with abnormal uterine positions (see Fig. 15-5).

Taking a careful history and correlating symptoms with a woman's monthly cycle can help the therapist determine when to refer a client for a possible gynecologic cause of back, pelvic, or sacral pain/symptoms. Many problems affecting the pelvic floor musculature can be treated successfully by a physical therapist and do not require medical referral.

Endometriosis

Endometriosis is an estrogen-dependent disorder defined by the presence of endometrial tissue (lining of the uterus) outside of the uterus. Each month as the woman's body prepares for a fertilized egg, the uterus becomes engorged with blood, providing a fertile place for the egg to attach and begin growing. If and when the unfertilized egg passes out of the body, the uterus sloughs off the lining of blood and the woman has a flow of menstrual blood for about 3 to 5 days.

Endometriosis occurs when the uterus sheds this blood up into the body, rather than down and out through the vagina. Endometrial tissue found outside of the uterus on other organs or structures within the pelvic cavity and the body responds each month the same way as the endometrium during the menstrual cycle. The misplaced tissue engorges with blood just as it would when lining the uterus. The blood cannot drain out of the body and the result is lesions or "chocolate cysts" wherever the endometrial tissue is located, with subsequent swelling, bleeding, and scarring.[61]

These pockets of blood can be deposited anywhere in the body. Whereas it was once thought that the blood just reached the pelvic and abdominal cavities, coating the viscera contained within, it is clear now that endometrial tissue migrates throughout the body. It has been recovered from bone, lungs, and even the brain.[62]

Pain can occur anywhere, but often the woman experiences back, pelvic, hip, and/or sacral pain that can be mistaken for a musculoskeletal, musculoligamentous, or neuromuscular impairment of the lumbar spine (Case Example 14-16).

The key to recognizing this condition is that often it is cyclical. Symptoms come and go with the menstrual cycle. After menopause pain can persist from scar tissue. There may be urinary tract and bowel involvement with associated symptoms ranging from urinary frequency, intermittent dysuria, and bloody stools to ureteral or bowel obstruction.

This condition is more common than previously thought. It is estimated that up to 50% of the female population who are infertile are affected by endometriosis.[62] It is not clear what, if any, risk factors increase a woman's risk of developing endometriosis. Endometriosis has been linked with other health problems such as chronic fatigue syndrome, hypothyroidism, fibromyalgia, rheumatoid arthritis, multiple sclerosis, and systemic lupus erythematosus.[63] Endometriosis is a risk factor for ovarian and breast cancer.[62]

A cure has not been found at the present time but for many women it can be managed with medications and/or surgery. The therapist can be helpful in providing pain management strategies that can reduce sick leave and improve daily function. See Box 15-5 for more information on this condition.

Clinical Signs and Symptoms of
Endometriosis

- Intermittent, cyclical, or constant pelvic and/or back pain (unilateral or bilateral)
- Pain during or after sexual intercourse
- Painful bowel movements or painful urination during menstrual period
- Small blood loss (spotting) before or between periods
- Heavy or irregular menstrual bleeding
- Bleeding anywhere else (nose bleeds, coughing up blood, blood in urine or stools)
- Fatigue
- History of ectopic pregnancy, miscarriage, infertility
- GI problems (abdominal bloating and cramping, nausea, diarrhea, constipation)

Ovarian Cysts and Uterine Fibroids

Ovarian cysts are often asymptomatic until they grow large enough to pull the ovary out of its normal position, sometimes cutting off the blood supply to the ovary. As the weight of the ovary causes a change in position, pressure is exerted against the uterus, bladder, intestines, or vagina causing a variety of symptoms.

CASE EXAMPLE 14-16   Endometriosis

Case Description: A 25-year-old female was referred for physical therapy with a diagnosis of nonspecific low back pain. She presented with the sudden onset of pain in the left lumbosacral region, left lower abdominal quadrant, and left buttock and anterior thigh which was constant and severe.

Medical examination ruled out a renal source of pain and diagnosed the client with a low back sprain. X-rays and MRIs were negative and ruled out a spondylogenic, oncologic, or discogenic lesion. She was given an injection of Demerol and prescription for non-steroidal anti-inflammatory drugs and anti-spasmodics and referred to physical therapy.

Past Medical History and Risk Factors: The client was a nonsmoker and consumed alcohol only on occasion. Personal family history was unremarkable; she reported that her mother had rheumatoid arthritis and hypothyroidism.

Clinical Presentation: The client was seen in physical therapy 3 weeks after the initial painful episode. She presented with a chief complaint of sharp, constant pain in the left lumbosacral region, which occasionally radiated into the left lower abdominal quadrant and into the left buttock and the anterior thigh as far distally as the knee.

The pain was worse when sitting or walking. She was only able to sleep 1 to 2 hours at a time because of the severity of the pain. There was no report of bowel or bladder changes. The hip and sacroiliac joint were ruled out as the sources of pain. A neurologic screening examination was negative.

Trunk motions were mildly restricted with increased pain during forward flexion. There was a positive left straight-leg raise test at 60 degrees. The client appeared to have a musculoskeletal based movement impairment.

Physical examination determined the most significant clinical finding to be exquisite tenderness in the left lower abdominal quadrant. The client reported marked tenderness with palpation over the left lower abdominal quadrant just proximal to the ASIS. She also reported tenderness with palpation directly over the left lumbar paraspinal region just superior to the iliac crest.

Red Flags: The sudden onset, intensity, severity, and duration of the client's back pain raised a red flag. The left lower quadrant was the location of greatest tenderness and severe subjective pain, both experienced at rest and with activity. The client's gender and childbearing age raise yellow warning flags.

Should the therapist treat this client and reassess symptoms and clinical presentation in 2 weeks or refer immediately?

Once again, the decision to carry out a physical therapy plan of care with direct intervention versus making a medical referral is based on clinical judgment. Given the presentation of this case, either decision could be justified.

Since she was evaluated by a medical doctor who sent her to physical therapy, a telephone call would be more appropriate than suggesting the client go back to her doctor.

In this case the therapist made the decision not to treat the client given the fact that a delay in diagnosis with risk for increased morbidity and possible mortality is possible with low back pain from serious pelvic pathology.

Outcomes: The therapist conferred with the referring orthopedic surgeon and a referral was made to a gynecologist. Further testing provided a diagnosis of endometriosis and ovarian cyst. The client underwent laparoscopy; the diagnosis of endometriosis was confirmed.

Following medical and surgical intervention, the lower quadrant pain was abolished, and the low back pain and leg pain significantly diminished in frequency and intensity, enabling the client to return to her normal activities.

Discussion: Given the prevalence of endometriosis, physical therapists are likely to encounter clients with this disorder in orthopedic physical therapy practice. Proper differential diagnosis is necessary to identify the risk factors and physical findings that would provide early diagnosis of endometriosis and avoid the morbidity associated with this and other pelvic disorders.

From Troyer, MR: Differential diagnosis of endometriosis in a patient with nonspecific low back pain. Case report presented in partial fulfillment of DPT 910, Principles of Differential Diagnosis, Institute for Physical Therapy Education, Widener University, Chester, Pennsylvania, 2005. Used with permission.

Lower abdominal or pelvic pain is most common but back pain associated with ovarian cysts and uterine fibroids can occur, usually presenting in a cyclical pattern associated with the menstrual cycle similar to endometriosis. A physician must determine the underlying gynecologic cause of back (hip, pelvic, sacral) pain or symptoms.

In a screening context, we look for red flag histories, clinical presentation, risk factors, and associated signs and symptoms. Obesity may be a risk factor because more than half of the women affected by this disorder are obese but other risk factors remain unknown. Ovarian cysts present as part of the polycystic ovarian syndrome put the woman at increased risk for insulin resistance and potentially at increased risk for cardiovascular disease as a result.[64,65]

If the Review of Systems points to a gynecologic source of pain/symptoms, further questions can be asked and a referral made if appropriate. Low back pain is a late finding for some women with ovarian cancer (see Chapter 15).

Clinical Signs and Symptoms of
Ovarian Cysts

- Abdominal pressure, pain, or bloating
- Discomfort during urination, bowel movements, or sexual intercourse
- Irregular menses, infertility
- Dull aching low back, buttock, pelvic, or groin pain
- Sudden, sharp pain with rupture or hemorrhage

Ectopic Pregnancy

An ectopic pregnancy is a live pregnancy that takes place outside the uterus. As shown in Fig. 15-6, this may occur in a variety of places such as the ovary, the tube (tubal pregnancy), outside lining of the uterus, or along the peritoneal cavity. None of these locations can sustain a viable ovum and the woman will have a spontaneous abortion (miscarriage).

Risk factors include sexually transmitted diseases, prior tubal surgery, and current use of an intrauterine contraceptive device. Depending on the location of the ectopic pregnancy, symptoms can include back, hip, sacral, abdominal, pelvic, and/or shoulder pain. Shoulder pain is more likely to occur if there is retroperitoneal bleeding when rupture of the developing embryo and hemorrhage occurs with pressure on the diaphragm.

It is usually unilateral on the same side as the bleeding, but can cause bilateral shoulder pain if

the hemorrhage is significant enough to impinge both sides of the diaphragm. The pain is usually of a sudden onset (when rupture and hemorrhage occur) with intense, constant pain. Situations of this type represent a medical emergency. Most likely the client did not come to the therapist for this problem but may develop emerging symptoms while being treated for some other orthopedic or neurologic problem.

Consider it a red flag when any woman of child-bearing age who is sexually active has sudden, intense pain as described. Take her blood pressure and other vital signs while asking appropriate screening questions. Seek immediate medical assistance.

Clinical Signs and Symptoms of
Ectopic Pregnancy

- Amenorrhea or irregular bleeding and spotting
- Diffuse, aching lower abdominal quadrant or low back pain; can cause ipsilateral shoulder pain
- May progress to a sharper, intermittent type of pain

Intrauterine Contraceptive Device (IUCD)

The intrauterine contraceptive device (IUCD is the current medical term; known by most women as an IUD) has become popular once again, having gone out of favor in the 1970s when the copper T caused so many problems. Although this contraceptive device has been improved, there are still potential problems (Fig. 14-6). The body may recognize this as a foreign object and set up an immune response

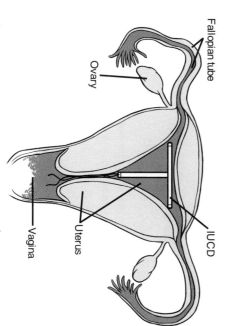

Fallopian tube

Ovary

Uterus

Vagina

IUCD

Fig. 14-6 • Intra-uterine contraceptive device (IUCD or IUD) a potential source of low back, pelvic, sacral, or even hip pain in any woman of reproductive age who is using this form of birth control.

or try to wall it off. The IUCD can become embedded in the tissue of the uterus, causing inflammation, infection and scarring.

For any woman with low back, pelvic, sacral or hip pain who is in the reproductive age range it may be necessary to ask about her method of birth control: Are you using an IUD for birth control?

Clinical Presentation

Back pain that is associated with the menstrual cycle occurs most often at or around the point of ovulation (between day 10 and day 14 for most women) and again just prior to or during menstrual flow (between days 23 and 28 for most women). Day 1 is counted as the first day the woman experiences bleeding with her menstrual cycle.

Back pain associated with the menstrual cycle may be a regular feature for a woman, it may occur intermittently, or it may be new onset, and the woman is unaware of the link between the two until she charts her monthly cycle and correlates it with her back pain.

A woman may have back pain accompanied by or alternating with sharp, bilateral, and cramping pain in the lower abdominal and/or pelvic quadrants. Menstrual pain can be referred to the rectum, lower sacrum, or coccyx. Tumors, masses, or even endometriosis may involve the sacral plexus or its branches, causing severe, burning pain.

Associated Signs and Symptoms

After gathering information during the examination, the therapist performs a Review of Systems looking for clusters of signs and symptoms suggesting a gynecologic cause of low back pain. If appropriate, the next step is to ask a few final screening questions.

Clinical Signs and Symptoms of Gynecologic Disorders

- Missed menses, irregular menses, history of menstrual disturbances, painful menstruation
- Tender breasts
- Nausea, vomiting
- Chronic constipation (with laxative and enema dependency)
- Pain on defecation
- Fever, night sweats, chills
- Low blood pressure (hemorrhaging with ectopic pregnancy)
- Vaginal discharge

- Abnormal vaginal bleeding
  - Late menstrual periods with persistent bleeding periods
  - Spotting before period or between periods
  - Irregular, longer, heavier menstrual periods, no specific pattern
  - Any postmenopausal bleeding
- Urinary problems (intermittent dysuria, frequency, urgency, hematuria)

▶ SCREENING FOR MALE REPRODUCTIVE CAUSES OF BACK PAIN

Men can experience back pain (as well as hip, groin, SI, and sacral pain) caused by referred pain from the male reproductive system. Prostate cancer is the second most common cancer in males over the age of 60 in the United States.[66]

The incidence of prostate cancer has risen 60% to 75% in the Western world in the last 15 years and is expected to continue to rise over the next 20 years, making it very likely that the therapist will treat clients with prostate pathology.[67]

Testicular cancer, though relatively rare, is the most common cancer in males ages 15 to 35 years and on the rise. Details of both conditions are discussed in Chapter 10. Benign prostatic hyperplasia (BPH) is one of the most common disorders of the aging male population affecting 50% of men over age 50.

Risk Factors

Risk factors for prostate dysfunction include advancing age, family history, ethnicity (greater risk for African American men), diet, and possibly exposure to chemicals. Not all disorders of this system occur with aging, so the therapist must remain alert for red flag symptoms in males of any age.

Clinical Presentation

Back pain, changes in bladder function, and sexual dysfunction are the most common symptoms associated with male reproductive disorders. Any obstruction, growth, or inflammation of the prostate can directly affect the urethra, resulting in difficulty starting a flow of urine, continuing a flow of urine, frequency, and/or nocturia.

Prostate cancer is often asymptomatic and only diagnosed when the man seeks medical assistance because of symptoms of urinary obstruction or sciatica. Sciatic pain affects the low back, hip, and leg and is caused by metastasis to the bones of the pelvis, lumbar spine, or femur.

Associated symptoms may include melena, sudden and moderate to high fever, chills, and changes in bowel or bladder function. Men who have reached the fifth decade or more are most commonly affected.

Testicular cancer presents most often as a painless swelling nodule in one gonad, noted incidentally by the client or his sexual partner. This is described as a lump or hardness of the testis, with occasional heaviness or a dull, aching sensation in the lower abdomen or scrotum. Acute pain is the presenting symptom in about 10% of affected men.

Involvement of the epididymis or spermatic cord may lead to pelvic or inguinal lymph node metastases, although most tumors confined to the testis itself will spread primarily to the retroperitoneal lymph nodes. Subsequent cephalad drainage may be to the thoracic duct and supraclavicular nodes. Hematogenous spread to the lungs, bone, or liver may occur as a result of direct tumor invasion.

In about 10% of affected individuals, dissemination along these pathways results in thoracic, lumbar, supraclavicular, neck, or shoulder pain or mass as the first symptom. Other symptoms related to this pathway of dissemination may include respiratory symptoms or GI disturbance.

As discussed earlier, back pain caused by neoplasm is typically progressive, is more pronounced at night, and may not have a clear association with activity level (as is more characteristic of mechanical back pain). The usual progression of symptoms in clients with cord compression is back pain followed by radicular pain, lower extremity weakness, sensory loss, and, finally, loss of sphincter (bowel and bladder) control.

Associated Signs and Symptoms

Besides changes in urinary patterns, the therapist must ask about discharge from the penis, constitutional symptoms, and pain in any of the nearby soft tissue areas (groin, rectum, scrotum). Is there any blood in the urine (or change in color from yellow to orange or red)? Recurrent urinary tract infection is common in prostatitis, but does not lead to prostate cancer.

Because the therapist is not going to be treating any of these problems, any red flags should be reported to the physician. A rectal exam may be needed. Access to the prostate is easiest through this type of exam. By pressing on the prostate, the physician can reproduce painful symptoms as part of the differential diagnosis (see Fig. 10-5).

Many men are reluctant to pursue diagnosis and treatment whenever the male reproductive system is involved. Early detection and treatment of these conditions can result in a good outcome. Screening questions for men are a good way to elicit red flag history, risk factors, and signs or symptoms. The therapist must follow up with the client and make sure contact is made with the appropriate health care professional.

Clinical Signs and Symptoms of Prostate Pathology

- May be asymptomatic early on
- Urinary dysfunction (hesitancy, frequency, urgency, nocturia, dysuria)
- Low back, inner thigh, or perineal pain or stiffness
- Suprapubic or pelvic pain
- Testicular or penis pain
- Sciatica (prostate cancer metastases)
- Bone pain, lymphedema of the groin, and/or lower extremities (prostate cancer metastases)
- Neurologic changes from spinal cord compression (prostate cancer metastases to the vertebrae)
- Sexual dysfunction (difficulty having an erection, painful ejaculation, cramping/discomfort after ejaculation)
- Constitutional symptoms with prostatitis
- Blood in urine or semen

SCREENING FOR INFECTIOUS CAUSES OF BACK PAIN

Drug abuse, immune suppression, and human immunodeficiency virus (HIV) may predispose to infection. Fever in anyone taking immunosuppressants is a red flag symptom indicating a possible underlying infection. Many people with a spinal infection do not have a fever; they are more likely to have a red flag history or risk factors.[1]

Vertebral Osteomyelitis

Vertebral osteomyelitis is a bone infection most often affecting the first and second lumbar vertebrae, causing low back pain. There are many causative factors. Osteomyelitis may occur in diabetics, injection drug users (IDUs), alcoholics, clients taking corticosteroid drugs, clients with spinal cord injury and neurogenic bladder, and otherwise debilitated or immune-suppressed clients. Older children can be affected although the most common peak is after the third decade of life.

Vertebral osteomyelitis is increasingly being reported as a complication of nosocomial bacteremia. *Staphylococcus aureus*, often methicillin-resistant (MRSA), is the most common causative organism. Osteomyelitis also can occur after surgery, open fractures, penetrating wounds, skin breakdown and ulcers, and systemic infections. It may result from a hematogenous spread through arterial and venous routes secondary to surgically implanted hardware for internal fixation of the spine, pelvic inflammatory disease, or genitourinary tract infection.

A physician should evaluate new onset of back pain in anyone who has been treated with vancomycin therapy for MRSA. Vancomycin therapy may give the appearance of being effective with resolution of fever and the return of white blood cell counts to normal ranges but in fact be insufficient to prevent or reverse the progression of hematogenous MRSA vertebral osteomyelitis.[68]

In the adult, usually two adjacent vertebrae and their intervening disc are involved, and the vertebral body(ies) may undergo destruction and collapse. Abscess formation may result, with possible neurologic involvement. The abscess can advance anteriorly to produce an abscess that can extend to the psoas muscle producing hip pain.

The most consistent clinical finding is marked local tenderness over the spinous process of the involved vertebrae with "nonspecific backache." The classic history describes pain that has been increasing in severity over a period of 1 to 3 weeks. Movement is painful, and there is marked muscular guarding and spasm of the paravertebral muscles and the hamstrings. The involved vertebrae are usually exquisitely sensitive to percussion, and pain is more severe at night.

There may be no rise in temperature or abnormality in white blood cell count because generalized sepsis is not present, but an elevated erythrocyte sedimentation rate is likely. A low-grade fever is most common in adults when body temperature changes do occur.

Children are more likely to present with acute, severe complaints including high fever, intense pain, and localized manifestations such as edema, erythema, and tenderness. Acute hematogenous osteomyelitis seen in children usually originates in the metaphysis of a long bone. Precipitating trauma is often present in the history, and well-localized, acute bone pain of 1 day to several days' duration is the primary symptom. The pain is most commonly severe enough to limit or restrict the use of the involved extremity, and fever and malaise consistent with sepsis are usual.

Clinical Signs and Symptoms of
Vertebral Osteomyelitis

- Pain and local tenderness over the involved spinous process(es); possible swelling, redness, and warmth in the affected area
- Night pain
- Stiff back with difficulty bearing weight, moving, walking
- Paravertebral muscle guarding or spasm
- Positive straight leg raise (SLR)
- Hip pain if infection spreads to the psoas muscle
- May be constitutional symptoms (fever, malaise)
- Recent history of bacterial infection (e.g., pharyngitis, otitis media in children)

Disc Space Infection

Disc space infection is a form of subacute osteomyelitis involving the vertebral end-plates and the disc in both children and adults. The lower thoracic and lumbar spines are the most common sites of infection.

Symptoms associated with postoperative disc space infection occur 2 to 8 weeks after discectomy. Discitis of an infectious type occurs following bacteremia secondary to urinary tract infection, with or without instrumentation (e.g., catheterization or cystoscopy). Low-grade viral or bacterial infection (e.g., gastroenteritis, upper respiratory infection, urinary tract infection) is most often implicated in young children with discitis (4 years old and younger). Ask the parent, guardian, or caretaker of any young child with back pain if there has been a recent history of sore throat, cold, ear infection, or other upper respiratory illness.

Adults with disc space infection often complain of low back pain localized around the disc area. The pain can range from mild to "excruciating" sometimes described as "knifelike." Such severe pain is accompanied by restricted movement and constant pain, present both day and night. The pain is usually made worse by activity, but unlike most other causes of back pain, it is *not* relieved by rest. If the condition becomes chronic, pain may radiate into the abdomen, pelvis, and lower extremities.

Children present with a history of increasingly severe localized back pain often accompanied by a limp or refusal to walk. There may be an increased lumbar lordosis. Pain may occur in the flank, abdomen, or hip. Symptoms may get worse with passive straight leg raise testing or other hip motion. A neurologic screening examination is usually negative.

Physical examination may reveal localized tenderness over the involved disc space, paraspinal muscle spasm, and restricted lumbar motion. A straight-leg raise (SLR) may be positive, and fever is common (Case Example 14-17).

Bacterial Endocarditis

Bacterial endocarditis often presents initially with musculoskeletal symptoms, including arthralgia, arthritis, low back pain, and myalgias. Half of these clients will have only musculoskeletal symptoms, without other signs of endocarditis.

The early onset of joint pain and myalgia is more likely if the client is older and has had a previously

diagnosed heart murmur or prosthetic valve (risk factors). Other risk factors include injection drug use, previous cardiac surgery, recent dental work, and recent history of invasive diagnostic procedures (e.g., shunts, catheters).

Almost one third of clients with bacterial endocarditis have low back pain. In many persons it is the principal musculoskeletal symptom reported. Back pain is accompanied by decreased range of motion and spinal tenderness. Pain may affect only one side, and it may be limited to the paraspinal muscles.

Endocarditis-induced low back pain may be very similar to the pain pattern associated with a

---

CASE EXAMPLE 14-17 Septic Discitis

Background: A 72-year-old man with leg myalgia and stabbing back pain of 2 weeks' duration was referred to physical therapy for evaluation by a rural nurse practitioner. When questioned about past medical history, the client reported a prostatectomy 22 years ago with no further problems. He was not aware of any other associated signs and symptoms but reported a recurring dermatitis that was being treated by his nurse practitioner. There were no skin lesions associated with the dermatitis present at the time of the physical therapist evaluation.

Clinical Presentation: The examination revealed spasm of the thoracolumbosacral paraspinal muscles bilaterally. The client reported extreme sensitivity to palpation of the spinous processes at L3 and L4; tap test reproduced painful symptoms. Spinal accessory motions could not be tested because of the client's state of acute pain and immobility.

Hip flexion and extension reproduced the symptoms and produced additional radiating flank pain. A straight-leg raise (SLR) caused severe back pain with each leg at 30 degrees on both sides. A neurologic examination was otherwise within normal limits. Vital signs were taken: blood pressure of 180/100 mm Hg; heart rate of 100 beats/min; temperature of 101°F.

What are the red flags in this case?

- Age
- Recurring dermatitis

- Positive tap test
- Bilateral SLR
- Vital signs

Result: The therapist contacted the nurse practitioner by telephone to report the findings, especially the vital signs and results of the SLR. It was determined that the client needed a medical evaluation, and he was referred to a physician's center in the nearest available city. A summary of findings from the physical therapist was sent with the client along with a request for a copy of the physician's report.

The client returned to the physical therapist's clinic with a copy of the physician's report with the following diagnosis: *Clostridium perfringens* septic discitis (made on the basis of blood culture). The prescribed treatment was intravenous antibiotic therapy for 6 weeks, progressive mobilization, and a spinal brace to be provided and fitted by the physical therapist. The client's back pain subsided gradually over the next 2 weeks, and he was followed up at intervals until he was weaned from the brace and resumed normal activities.

Septic discitis may occur following various invasive procedures, or it may be related to occult infections, urinary tract infections, septicemia, and dermatitis. Contact dermatitis was the most likely underlying cause in this case.

herniated lumbar disc; it radiates to the leg and may be accentuated by raising the leg, coughing, or sneezing. The key difference is that neurologic deficits are usually absent in clients with bacterial endocarditis. The therapist can review history and risk factors and conduct a Review of Systems to help in the screening process.

PHYSICIAN REFERRAL

Most adults with an episode of acute back pain experience recovery within 1 to 4 weeks. As many as 90% of affected individuals resume normal activity levels during this time.[69]

All clients who have not regained usual activity after 4 weeks should be formally reassessed including a review of the history and examination, looking for yellow or red flags, testing for any neurologic deficit, and conducting a review of systems to identify any evidence of systemic disease.

Reassessment of movement dysfunction is critical at this stage to look for alternate impairments not previously observed or identified. The therapist must consider whether the underlying primary problem is spinal or nonspinal, mechanical or medical, and what specific structures are involved.

Review concepts from the screening physical assessment in Chapter 4 to make sure the evaluation is complete. Inspection, palpation, and auscultation may reveal key findings previously missed. Assessment of fear-avoidance may be needed as discussed in Chapter 3.

Medical referral is made on the basis of a comparison of baseline data with findings upon reassessment. Providing the physician with concise but comprehensive information about findings and concerns is a helpful part of the medical differential diagnostic process.

Guidelines for Immediate Medical Attention

Immediate medical referral is not always required when a client presents with any one of the red flags listed in Box 14-1. When viewed as a whole, the history, risk factors, and any cluster of red flag findings will guide the therapist in making a final intervention versus referral decision.

• Neck pain with evidence of vertebrobasilar insufficiency (VBI) (e.g., reproduction of symptoms with vertebral artery testing such as vertigo, visual changes, headaches, nausea) requires medical attention. VBI can develop into cerebral or brainstem ischemia, leading to severe morbidity or death.[70]

• Immediate medical attention is required when anyone with low back pain (LBP) presents with symptoms of cauda equina (e.g., saddle anesthesia, fecal incontinence, motor weakness of the legs, radiculopathy, unable to heel or toe walk, altered knee or ankle deep tendons reflexes). Acute mechanical compression of nerves in the lower extremities, bowel, and bladder as they pass through the caudal sac may be a surgical emergency.

• Massive midline rupture of a disk in the lower lumbar levels can lead to LBP, rapidly progressive bilateral motor weakness and sciatica, saddle anesthesia (buttock and medial and posterior thighs; the area that would come in contact with a saddle when sitting on a horse), and bowel and bladder incontinence or urinary retention.[71]

• Men between the ages of 65 and 75 who ever smoked should undergo medical screening for abdominal aortic aneurysm. Any male with these two risk factors, especially presenting with signs or symptoms of AAA must be referred immediately.

• Sudden, intense back and/or shoulder pain in a sexually active woman of childbearing age may signal the end of an ectopic pregnancy. Sudden change in blood pressure, pallor, pain, and dizziness will alert the therapist to the need for immediate medical attention.

Guidelines for Physician Referral

• Red flags requiring physician referral or reevaluation include back pain or symptoms that are not improving as expected, steady pain irrespective of activity, symptoms that are increasing, or the development of new or progressive neurologic deficits, such as weakness, sensory loss, reflex changes, bowel or bladder dysfunction, or myelopathy.

• A positive Sharp-Purser test for atlantoaxial subluxation in the client with rheumatoid arthritis (sensation of head falling forward during neck flexion and clunking during neck extension) must be evaluated by an orthopedic surgeon.[7]

• The erythrocyte sedimentation rate, serum calcium level, and alkaline phosphatase level are usually elevated if cancer is present.[72]

• Reproduction of pain or exquisite tenderness over the spinous process(es) is a red flag sign requiring further investigation and possible medical referral.

Clues to Screening Head, Neck, or Back Pain

General

- Age younger than 20 and older than 50 with no history of a precipitating event
- Back pain in children is uncommon and constitutes a red flag finding, especially back pain that lasts more than 3 weeks
- Nocturnal back pain that is constant, intense, and unrelieved by change in position
- Pain that causes constant movement or makes the client curl up in the sitting position
- Back pain with constitutional symptoms: fatigue, nausea, vomiting, diarrhea, fever, sweats
- Back pain accompanied by unexplained weight loss
- Back pain accompanied by extreme weakness in the leg(s), numbness in the groin or rectum, or difficulty controlling bowel or bladder function (**cauda equina syndrome;** rare but requires immediate medical attention)
- Back pain that is insidious in onset and progression (remember to assess for unreported sexual assault or physical abuse)
- Back pain that is relieved by sitting up and leaning forward (**pancreas**)
- Back pain that is unrelieved by recumbency
- Back pain that does not vary with exertion or activity
- Back pain that is accompanied by multiple joint involvement (**gastrointestinal, rheumatoid arthritis, fibromyalgia**) or by sustained morning stiffness (**spondyloarthropathy**)
- Severe, persistent back pain with full and painless movement of the spine
- Sudden, localized back pain that does not diminish in 10 days to 2 weeks in postmenopausal women or osteoporotic adults (**osteoporosis with compression fracture**)

Past Medical History

- Previous history of cancer, Crohn's disease, or bowel obstruction
- Long-term use of nonsteroidal antiinflammatory drugs (**gastrointestinal bleeding**), steroids, or immunosuppressants (**infectious cause**)
- Recent history or previous history of recurrent upper respiratory infection or pneumonia
- Recent history of surgery, especially back pain 2 to 8 weeks after discectomy (**infection**)
- History of osteoporosis and/or previous vertebral compression fracture(s) (**fracture**)

- History of heart murmur or prosthetic valve in an older client who currently has low back pain of unknown cause (**bacterial endocarditis**)
- History of intermittent claudication and heart disease in a man with deep midlumbar back pain; assess for pulsing abdominal mass (**abdominal aortic aneurysm**)
- History of diseases associated with hypercalcemia, such as hyperparathyroidism, multiple myeloma, senile osteoporosis, hyperthyroidism, Cushing's disease, or specific renal tubular disease not appearing with back pain radiating to the flank or iliac crest (**kidney stone**)

Oncologic

- Back pain with severe lower extremity weakness without pain, with full range of motion and recent history of sciatica in the absence of a positive straight leg raise
- Bilateral leg pain with motor and reflex impairments
- Bone tenderness over the spinous processes when tumor interferes with sympathetic nerves
- Temperature differences: involved side warmer (**infection or neoplasm**)
- Associated signs and symptoms: significant weight loss; night pain disturbing sleep; extreme fatigue; constitutional symptoms such as fever, sweats; other organ/system-dependent symptoms such as urinary changes (urologic), cough, and dyspnea (pulmonary); abdominal bloating or bloody diarrhea (gastrointestinal)

Cardiovascular

- Back pain that is described as "throbbing"
- Back pain accompanied by leg pain that is relieved by standing still or rest
- Back pain that is present in all spinal positions and increased by exertion
- Back pain accompanied by a pulsating sensation or palpable abdominal pulse
- Low back, pelvic, and/or leg pain with temperature changes from one leg to the other (involved side warmer: venous occlusion or tumor; involved side colder: arterial occlusion)
- Back injury occurred during weight lifting in someone with known heart disease or past history of aneurysm

Pulmonary

- Associated signs and symptoms (dyspnea, persistent cough, fever and chills)
- Back pain aggravated by respiratory movements (deep breathing, laughing, coughing)

- Back pain relieved by breath holding or Valsalva maneuver
- Autosplinting by lying on the involved side or holding firm pillow against the chest/abdomen decreases the pain
- Spinal/trunk movements (e.g., trunk rotation, trunk side bending) do not reproduce symptoms (exception; an intercostal tear caused by forceful coughing from underlying diaphragmatic pleurisy can result in painful movement but is also reproduced by local palpation)
- Weak and rapid pulse accompanied by fall in blood pressure (pneumothorax)

Renal/Urologic

- Renal and urethral pain is felt throughout T9 to L1 dermatomes; pain is constant but may crescendo (kidney stones)
- Kidney pain of an inflammatory nature can be relieved by a change in position. However, renal colic (e.g., infection) remains unchanged by a change in position. But there are usually constitutional symptoms associated with either inflammation or infection to tip off the alert therapist.
- Back pain at the level of the kidneys can be caused by ovarian or testicular cancer
- Back pain and shoulder pain, either simultaneously or alternately, may be renal/urologic in origin
- Side bending to the same side and pressure placed along the spine at that level is "more comfortable;" pain may be reduced, but it is not eliminated when the kidney is involved. The client with kidney disease/disorder may prefer this position because it moves the kidney out away from the spine and away from any compressive forces causing painful symptoms.
- Associated signs and symptoms (blood in urine, fever, chills, increased urinary frequency, difficulty starting or continuing stream of urine, testicular pain in men)
- Assess for costovertebral angle tenderness; pain is affected by change of position (**pseudorenal pain**)
- History of traumatic fall, blow, lift (**musculoskeletal**)

Gastrointestinal

- Back and abdominal pain at the same level (may occur simultaneously or alternately); check for gastrointestinal history or associated signs and symptoms
- Back pain with abdominal pain at a lower level than the back pain; look for its source in the back

- Back pain associated with food or meals (increase or decrease in symptoms)
- Back pain accompanied by heartburn or relieved by antacids
- Associated signs and symptoms (dysphagia, odynophagia, melena, early satiety with weight loss, tenderness over McBurney's point, positive iliopsoas or obturator sign, bloody diarrhea)
- Sacral pain occurs when the rectum is stimulated, such as during a bowel movement or when passing gas and relieved after each of these events

Gynecologic

- History or current gynecologic disorder (e.g., uterine retroversion, ovarian cysts, uterine fibroids, endometriosis, pelvic inflammatory disease, sexual assault/incest, intrauterine contraceptive device, multiple births with prolonged labor or forceps use)
- Associated signs and symptoms (missed or irregular menses, tender breasts, cyclic nausea and vomiting, chronic constipation, vaginal discharge, abnormal uterine bleeding or bleeding in a postmenopausal woman)
- Low back and/or pelvic pain developing soon after a missed menstrual cycle; blood pressure may be significantly low, and there may be concomitant shoulder pain when hemorrhaging occurs (**ectopic pregnancy**)
- Low back and/or pelvic pain occurring intermittently but with regularity in response to menstrual cycle (e.g., ovulation around days 10 to 14 and onset of menses around days 23 to 28)

Nonorganic (Psychogenic) (see discussion, Chapter 3)

- Widespread, nonanatomic low back tenderness with overreaction to superficial palpation
- Assess for nonorganic signs such as axial loading (downward pressure on the top of the head) or shoulder-hip rotation (client rotates shoulder and hips with feet planted); Waddell's nonorganic signs (see Table 3-12)
- Regional (whole leg) pain, numbness, weakness, sensory disturbances
- Chronic use of (or demand for) narcotics

Pediatrics

- Children presenting with back pain are very different from adults with the same problem; children are less likely than adults to report

symptoms when there is no organic cause for the complaint[73]

- Eighty-five percent (85%) of children with back pain lasting more than 2 months have a diagnosable lesion[74]

- Children with persistent reports of low back pain must be evaluated and reevaluated until a diagnosis is reached; X-rays and laboratory values are needed

OVERVIEW (FIGURE 14-7)

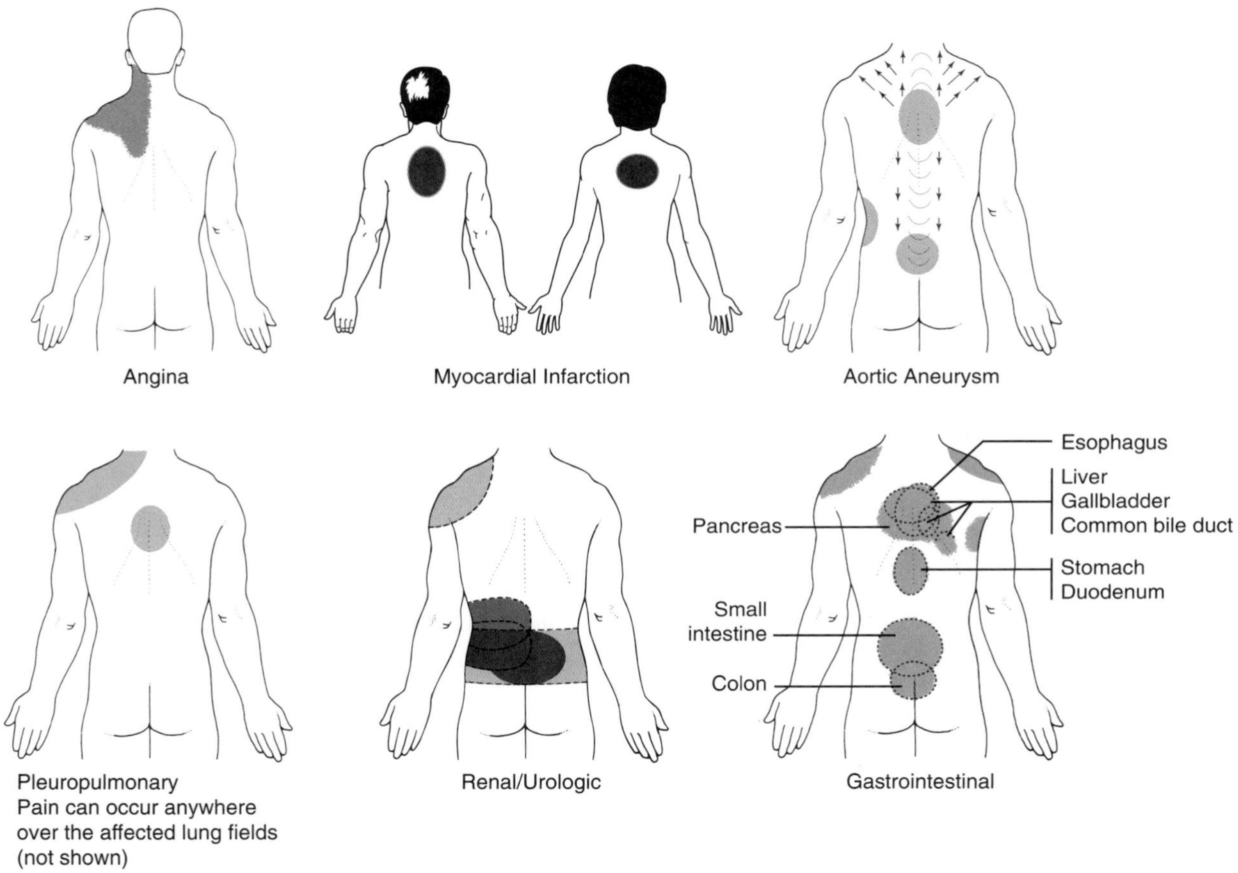

Angina

Myocardial Infarction

Aortic Aneurysm

Renal/Urologic

Gastrointestinal

Colon
Small intestine
Pancreas
Esophagus
Liver
Gallbladder
Common bile duct
Stomach
Duodenum

Pleuropulmonary
Pain can occur anywhere over the affected lung fields (not shown)

Fig. 14-7 • Composite picture of referred back pain patterns. Not pictured: gynecologic pain patterns.

🔑 KEY POINTS TO REMEMBER

✔ Clients may inaccurately attribute symptoms to a particular incident or activity, or they may fail to recognize causative factors.

✔ At presentation, any person with musculoskeletal pain of unknown cause and/or a past medical history of cancer should be screened for medical disease. Special Questions for Men and Women may be helpful in this screening process.

✔ Consider visceral origin of back pain in the absence of muscular spasm, tenderness, and impaired movement.[50]

✔ Perform a breast exam on any woman with upper back pain, especially women with a history of cancer.

✔ Backache may be the earliest and only manifestation of visceral disease.[50]

✔ Neck or back pain in the presence of normal range of motion and strength is a yellow flag symptom.

✔ Persistent backache due to extraspinal pathology is rare in children but common in adults.[50]

✔ Children, adolescents, and especially athletes reporting back pain of more than 3 weeks duration may need medical referral, depending on the history and clinical presentation.[75]

✔ Lumbar spasm (not hypertonus) may occur in the presence of severe pain from retroperitoneal diseases (e.g., renal tumors, abscesses, appendicitis, kidney stones, lymphoma)[50]

✔ Back pain accompanied by recent history of infection (especially urinary tract infection) or in the presence of constitutional symptoms (e.g., fever, chills, nausea; see Box 1-3) must be screened more carefully.

✔ Nonpainful paresthesias can be the result of neural compression but also occur from ischemia (atherosclerosis, tumor, prodromal sign of a migraine headache); painful paresthesias are more likely indicative of an inflammatory or mechanical process.

✔ When symptoms seem out of proportion to the injury, or if they persist beyond the expected time for the nature of the injury, medical referral may be indicated.

✔ Pain that is unrelieved by rest or change in position or pain/symptoms that do not fit the expected mechanical or neuromusculoskeletal pattern should serve as red flag warnings.

✔ When symptoms cannot be reproduced, aggravated, or altered in any way during the examination, additional questions to screen for medical disease are indicated.

✔ Always rule out trigger points as a possible cause of musculoskeletal symptoms before referring the client elsewhere.

✔ Postoperative infection of any kind may not appear with any clinical signs/symptoms for weeks or months.

✔ Muscle weakness without pain, without history of sciatica, and without a positive straight leg raising is suggestive of spinal metastases.

✔ Sciatica may be the first symptom of prostate cancer metastasized to the bones of the pelvis, lumbar spine, or femur.

✔ Back pain may be a symptom of depression.

✔ Urinary incontinence concomitant with cervical spine pain requires a neurologic screening examination and possible medical referral.

✔ Anterior neck pain, movement dysfunction, and torticollis of the sternocleidomastoid muscle may be a sign of underlying thyroid involvement.

✔ The therapist may need to screen for illness behavior and the need for psychologic evaluation. Many clients with chronic back pain have both a physical problem and varying degrees of illness behavior. A single behavioral sign or symptom may be normal; multiple findings of several different kinds are much more significant.[1]

SUBJECTIVE EXAMINATION

Special Questions to Ask: Headache

See Appendix C-4 for a complete pain assessment.

History

- Do other family members have similar headaches?
- What major life changes or stressors have you had in the last six months?
- Have you ever had a head injury? Cancer of any kind? A hysterectomy? High blood pressure? A stroke? Seizures?
- Have you been hit or kicked in the head, neck, or face? Pushed against a wall or other object? Pulled or thrown by the hair?
- For women of childbearing age: Is it possible you are pregnant?

Site

- Where do you feel the headache? Can you point to it with one finger (localized vs. diffuse)? Does it move?

Onset

- Do you recall your first headache of this type?
- Was it caused by a fall or trauma? (Therapist may have to screen for trauma associated with domestic violence as a potential cause)

Frequency

- How often do you have this type of headache?

Intensity

- On a scale from 0 (no pain) to 10 (worst pain), how would you rate your headache now? Worst it has been?
- Does the pain keep you from your daily activities? From exercise or recreation? From work?

Duration

- How long do your headaches last?

Description

- What do your headaches feel like? (The client may have more than one type of headache.)
- Alternate question: What words would you use to describe the pain?

Pattern

- Is there a pattern to your headaches (e.g., weekly? Monthly? Morning to evening?)
- Do you wake up in the early morning hours with a headache? (occipital pain: hypertension)

- For women who are perimenopausal or menopausal (natural or surgically induced): Are the headaches cyclical? (Monthly? Right before or right after the menstrual flow?)

Aggravating Factors

- What makes the headache worse?
- Are you aware of any triggers that can bring the headache on? (Alcohol, noise, lights, food, coughing or sneezing, fatigue or lack of sleep, stress, caffeine withdrawal; for women: menstrual cycle)
- Do you grind your teeth during the day or at night?

 —If yes, assessment of the cervical spine and temporomandibular joints is indicated. Referral to a dentist may be required.

- Are you taking any medications? (Headache can be a side effect of many different medications, but especially NSAIDs, muscle relaxants, antianxiety and antidepressant agents, food and drugs containing nitrates, calcium, and beta blockers.)

Relieving Factors

- Is there anything you can do to make the headache better?

 —If yes, how? (caffeine, medications, sleep, avoid certain foods, alcohol, cigarettes) [Ask follow up questions about use of over-the-counter or prescription drugs and/or herbs or pharmaceuticals.]

 How does rest affect your symptoms?

Associated Symptoms

- Do you have any symptoms of any kind anywhere else in your head or body? (Follow up with questions about vision changes, dizziness, ringing in the ears, mood changes, nausea, vomiting, nasal congestion, nose bleeds, light or sound sensitivity, paresthesias such as numbness and tingling of the face or fingers, difficulty swallowing, hoarseness, fever, chills.)

For the therapist

- Take the client's blood pressure and pulse and assess for cardiovascular risk factors.
- Auscultate for bruits in the temporal and carotid arteries (temporal arteritis, carotid stenosis).
- Headaches that cannot be linked to a neuromuscular or musculoskeletal cause (e.g., dys-

SUBJECTIVE EXAMINATION—cont'd

function of the cervical spine, thoracic spine, or temporomandibular joints; muscle tension, poor posture, nerve impingement) may need further medical referral and evaluation.

Special Questions to Ask: Neck or Back

To the therapist: If a more complete screening interview is required, see *Special Questions to Ask* at the end of each chapter for further questions related to the individual organ systems.

Pain Assessment (See also Appendix C-4)

- When did the pain or symptoms start?
- Did it (they) start gradually or suddenly? **(Vascular versus trauma problem)**
- Was there an illness or injury before the onset of pain?
- Have you noticed any changes in your symptoms since they first started to the present time?
- Is the pain aggravated or relieved by coughing or sneezing? **(Nerve root involvement, muscular)**
- Is the pain aggravated or relieved by activity?
- Are there any particular positions (sitting, lying, standing) that make your back pain feel better or worse?
- Does the pain go down the leg? *If so,* how far does it go?
- Have you noticed any muscular weakness?
- Have you been treated previously for back disorders?
- How has your general health been both before the beginning of your back problem and today?
- How does rest affect the pain or symptoms?
- Do you feel worse in the morning or evening . . . **OR** . . . What difference do you notice in your symptoms from the morning when you first wake up until the evening when you go to bed?

General Systemic

Most of these questions may be asked of clients who have pain or symptoms anywhere in the musculoskeletal system.

- Have you ever been told that you have osteoporosis or brittle bones?
- Have you ever fractured your spine?
- Have you ever been diagnosed or treated for cancer in any part of your body?

If no, have you ever had chemotherapy or radiation therapy for anything? **(Rectal bleeding is a sign of radiation proctitis.)**

- Do you ever notice sweating, nausea, or chest pains when your current symptoms occur?
- What other symptoms have you had with this problem? For example, have you had:

  Numbness
  Burning, tingling
  Nausea, vomiting
  Loss of appetite
  Unexpected or significant weight gain or loss
  Diarrhea, constipation, blood in your stool or urine
  Difficulty in starting or continuing the flow of urine or incontinence (inability to hold your urine)
  Hoarseness or difficulty in swallowing
  Heart palpitations or fluttering
  Difficulty in breathing while just sitting or resting or with mild effort (e.g., when walking from the car to the house)
  Unexplained sweating or perspiration
  Night sweats, fever, chills
  Changes in vision: blurred vision, black spots, double vision, temporary blindness
  Fatigue, weakness, sudden paralysis of one side of your body, arm, or leg **(Transient ischemic attack)**
  Headaches
  Dizziness or fainting spells

- Have you had a recent cold, sore throat, upper respiratory infection, or the flu? Have you ever been diagnosed with HIV?

Cardiovascular

- Have you ever been told you have high blood pressure or heart trouble?
- Do you ever have chest pain or discomfort when your back hurts or just before your back starts hurting?
- Do you ever have swollen feet or ankles? *If yes,* are they swollen when you get up in the morning? **(Edema/congestive heart failure)**
- Do you ever get cramps in your legs if you walk for several blocks? **(Intermittent claudication)**
- Do you ever have bouts of rapid heart action, irregular heartbeats, or palpitations of your heart?
- Have you ever felt a "heartbeat" in your abdomen when you lie down?

SUBJECTIVE EXAMINATION—cont'd

—If *yes*, is this associated with low back pain or left flank pain? (**Abdominal aneurysm**)

• Do you ever notice sweating, nausea, or chest pain when your current symptoms (e.g., head, neck, jaw, back pain) occur?

Pulmonary

• Are you able to take a deep breath?

• Do you ever have shortness of breath or breathlessness with your back pain?

—How far can you walk before you feel breathless?

—What symptoms stop your walking (e.g., shortness of breath, heart pounding, chest tightness, or weak legs)?

• Have you had any trouble with coughing lately?

—If *yes*, have you strained your back from coughing?

Renal/Urologic

• Have you noticed any changes in the flow of urine since your back/groin pain started?

—If *no*, it may be necessary to provide prompts or examples of what changes you are referring to (e.g., difficulty in starting or continuing the flow of urine, numbness or tingling in the groin or pelvis, increased frequency, getting up at night)

• Have you had burning with urination during the last 3 to 4 weeks? Fever and/or chills?

• Do you ever have blood in your urine or notice blood in the toilet going to the bathroom?

• Do you have any problems with your kidneys or bladder? If *so*, describe.

• Have you ever had kidney or bladder stones? If *so*, how were these stones treated?

• Have you ever had an injury to your bladder or to your kidneys? If *so*, how was this treated?

• Have you had any infections of the bladder, and how were these infections treated?

—Were they related to any specific circumstances (e.g., pregnancy, intercourse)?

• Have you had any kidney infections, and how were these treated?

—Were they related to any specific circumstances (e.g., pregnancy, after bladder infections, a strep throat, or strep skin infections)?

• Do you ever have pain, discomfort, or a burning sensation when you urinate? (**Lower urinary tract irritation**)

• Have you noticed any changes in color or blood in your urine?

Gastrointestinal

• Are you having any stomach or abdominal pain either at the same time as the back pain or at other times?

—If *yes*, assess the location and the presence of any GI symptoms.

• Have you noticed any association between when you eat and when your symptoms increase or decrease?

—Do you notice any change in your symptoms 1 to 3 hours after you eat?

—Do you notice any pain beneath the breastbone (epigastric) or just beneath the wing bone (subscapular) 1 to 2 hours after eating?

• Do you have a feeling of fullness after only one or two bites of food? (**Early satiety**)

• Is your back pain relieved after having a bowel movement? (**Gastrointestinal obstruction**)

• Do you have rectal, low back, or sacroiliac pain when passing stool or having a bowel movement?

• Do you have any blood in your stools or change in the normal color of your bowel movements (e.g., black, red, mahogany color, gray color)? (**Hemorrhoids, prostate problems, cancer**)

• Are you having any diarrhea, constipation, or other changes in your bowel function?

• Do you have frequent heartburn or take antacids to relieve heartburn or acid indigestion?

• Have you had any skin rashes or skin lesions in the last 6 weeks (**Regional enteritis or Crohn's disease**)

To the therapist: It may be necessary to conduct a risk factor assessment for NSAID-induced back pain (see discussion Chapter 8) or screen for eating disorders (see Appendix B-12)

Special Questions to Ask: Sexual History

There are a wide range of reasons why it may be necessary to ask questions about sexual function, birth control, and sexually transmitted diseases. For example, joint pain can be caused by sexually transmitted infections. Low back, sacral, and pelvic pain can be caused by sexual trauma or sexual violence. Sciatica accompanied by unreported impotence can be caused by prostate cancer metastasized to the skeletal system.

Whenever taking a sexual history seems appropriate, remember to offer your clients a clear explanation for any questions asked concerning sexual history. The therapist may want to introduce the series of

SUBJECTIVE EXAMINATION—cont'd

questions by saying, "When evaluating low back pain sometimes it's necessary to ask some more personal questions. Please answer as accurately as you can."

The personal nature of some questions sometimes leads clients to feel embarrassed. It is important to assure them that they will not be judged and that providing accurate information is crucial to providing good care. Investing in good history taking can lead to early detection and early treatment with less morbidity and better outcomes.[76]

Try to avoid medical terminology and jargon—a common pitfall among healthcare providers when they feel embarrassed. Listen to the words the clients use to describe sexual activities and practices and then use their preferred words when appropriate.

Men who have sex with men may identify themselves as homosexual, bisexual, or heterosexual. No matter what label is used, these men are at increased risk for sexually transmitted diseases (STDs) as well as psychologic and behavioral disorders, drug abuse, and eating disorders. Avoid terms such as "gay," "queer," and "straight" when talking about sexual practices or sexual identity.[77]

There is no way to know when someone will be offended or claim sexual harassment. It is in your own interest to behave in the most professional manner possible. There should be no hint of sexual innuendo or humor injected into any of your conversations with clients at any time. The line of sexual impropriety lies where the complainant draws it and includes appearances of misbehavior. This perception differs broadly from client to client.[50]

It is also true that clients sometimes behave inappropriately; there may be times when the therapist must remind clients of appropriate personal boundaries. At the same time, the therapist must be prepared to hear just about anything if and when it is necessary to ask questions about sexual history or sexual practices. Be aware of your facial expressions, body language, and verbal remarks in response to a client's answers to these questions.

What if a man or woman with pelvic or sacral pain tells you he or she has been the victim of repeated violent sexual acts? What if a client admits to being the victim of physical or emotional assault? The therapist must be prepared to respond in a professional and responsible way. Additional training in this area may be helpful. Many local organizations such as Planned Parent-

hood, Lambda Alliance, and AIDS Council may offer helpful information and/or training.

> The therapist may want to introduce the series of questions by saying, "When evaluating low back pain sometimes it's necessary to ask some more personal questions. Please answer as accurately as you can."

- Are you sexually active?
  Follow up question: How does sexual activity affect your symptoms?

"Sexually active" does not necessarily mean engaging in sexual intercourse. Sexual touch is enough to transmit many sexually transmitted infections. You may have to explain this to your client to clarify this question. Oral and anal intercourse are often not viewed as "sexual intercourse" and will result in the client answering the question with "No" when, in fact, for screening purposes, the answer is "Yes."

- Do you have pain with certain positions? (e.g., For the therapist: a position with the woman on top can be more difficult with **prolapsed uterus; the penis or other object touching inflamed cervix also can cause pain**)

- Have you had more than one sexual partner? **(increases risk of sexually transmitted diseases)**

- Have you ever been told you have a sexually transmitted infection or disease such as herpes, genital warts, Reiter's disease, syphilis, "the clap," chlamydia, gonorrhea, venereal, HIV or other disease?

- Have you ever had sexual intercourse without wanting to? Alternate: Have you ever been raped?

- Do you have any blood in your urine or your stools? Alternate question: Do you have any bleeding when you go to the bathroom?
  - What do you think could be causing this?
  - *If yes*, do you have a history of hemorrhoids?

Special Questions to Ask: Women Experiencing Back, Hip, Pelvic, Groin, Sacroiliac (SI), or Sacral Pain

Not all these questions will need to be asked. Use your professional judgment to decide what to ask based on what the woman has told you and what you have observed during the examination.

SUBJECTIVE EXAMINATION—cont'd

Past Medical History

Have you ever been told that you have:

- Retroversion of the uterus (tipped back)
- Ovarian cysts
- Fibroids or tumors
- Endometriosis
- Cystocele (sagging bladder)
- Rectocele (sagging rectum)
- Pelvic inflammatory disease (PID)?
- Have you had vaginal surgery or a hysterectomy? **(Hysterectomy: joint pain and myalgias may occur; vaginal surgery: incontinence)**
- Have you had a recent history of bladder or kidney infections? **(Referred back pain)**
- Have you ever been told you have "brittle bones" or osteoporosis?
- Have you ever had a compression fracture of your back?

Menstrual History

A menstrual history may be helpful when evaluating back or shoulder pain of unknown cause in a woman of reproductive age. Not all these questions will need to be asked. Use your professional judgment to decide what to ask based on what the woman has told you and what you have observed during the examination.

- Is there any connection between your (back, hip, sacroiliac) pain/symptoms and your menstrual cycle (related to either ovulation, midcycle, or menses)?
- Since your back/sacroiliac (or other) pain/symptoms started, have you seen a gynecologist to rule out any gynecologic cause of this problem?
- Where were you in your menstrual cycle when your injury or illness occurred?
- Where are you in your menstrual cycle today (premenstrual/midmenstrual/postmenstrual)? **(Appropriate question for shoulder or back pain of unknown cause)**
- Please describe any other menstrual irregularity or problems not already discussed.

For the Young Female Adolescent/Athlete

- Have you ever had a menstrual period?
  If yes, do you have a menstrual period every month? (amenorrhea or irregular cycles can be a natural part of development but also the result of an eating disorder)

- Have you ever gone 3 months without having a period?
  If yes, please describe.
- Do your periods change with your training regimen?
- Are you taking birth control pills or using a patch or injection?
  If yes, are you using them for birth control, to regulate your menstrual cycle, or both? (Assess risk factors and monitor blood pressure.)
- How long have you been on birth control?
- When was the last time you saw the doctor who prescribed birth control for you?
- Please describe any other menstrual irregularity or problems not already discussed.

Reproductive History

- Is there any possibility you could be pregnant?
- Was your last period normal for you?
- What form of birth control are you using? (If the client is using birth control pills, patches, or injections check her blood pressure.)
- Do you have an intrauterine coil or loop contraceptive device (IUD or IUCD)? **(PID and ectopic pregnancy can occur.)**
- **For the pregnant woman:** Are you under the care of a physician? Have you had any spotting or bleeding during your pregnancy?
- Have you recently had a baby? **(Birth trauma)**
  If yes: Did you have an epidural (anesthesia)? **(Postpartum back pain)**
  If yes, Did you have any significant medical problem during your pregnancy or delivery?
- Have you ever had a tubal or ectopic pregnancy? Is it possible that you may be pregnant now?
- How many pregnancies have you had?
- How many live births have you had?
- Have you ever had an abortion or miscarriage?
  If yes, follow up with careful (sensitive) questions about how many, when, where, and any immediate or delayed complications (physical or psychologic). (Weakness secondary to blood loss, infection, scarring; blood in **peritoneum irritating diaphragm causing lumbar and/or shoulder pain**); ask about the onset of symptoms in relation to the incident.
- Do you ever experience a "falling out" feeling or pelvic heaviness after standing for a long time? **(Uterine prolapse; pelvic floor weakness; incontinence)**

SUBJECTIVE EXAMINATION—cont'd

- Do you ever leak urine with coughing, laughing, lifting, exercising, or sneezing? **(Stress incontinence; tension myalgia of pelvic floor)**

  If yes to incontinence: Ask several additional questions to determine the frequency, the amount of protection needed (as measured by the number and type of pads used daily), and how much this problem interferes with daily activities and lifestyle. See also Appendix B-5.

- Do you have an unusual amount of vaginal discharge or vaginal discharge with an obvious odor? **(Referred back pain)**

  If yes, do you know what is causing this discharge? Is there any connection between when the discharge started and when you first noticed your back/sacroiliac (or other) symptoms?

- For the postmenopausal woman: Are you taking hormone replacement therapy (HRT) or any natural hormone products?

Special Questions to Ask: Men Experiencing Back, Hip, Pelvic, Groin, or Sacroiliac Pain

- Have you ever had prostate problems or been told you have prostate problems?

- Have you ever been told you have a hernia? Do you think you have one now?

  If yes, follow up with medical referral. Strangulation of the bowel can lead to serious compli-

cations. If the client has been evaluated by a physician and has declined treatment (usually surgery), encourage him to follow up on this recommendation.

- Have you recently had kidney stones, bladder or kidney infections?

- Have you had any changes in urination recently?

- Do you ever have blood in your urine?

- Do you ever have pain, burning, or discomfort on urination?

- Do you urinate often, especially during the night?

- Can you easily start a flow of urine?

- Can you keep a steady stream without stopping and starting?

- When you are done urinating, does it feel like your bladder is empty or do you feel like you still have to go, but you can't get any more out?

- Do you ever dribble or leak urine?

- Do you have trouble getting an erection?

- Do you have trouble keeping an erection?

- Do you have trouble ejaculating? (Therapists beware; this term may not be understood by all clients.)

- Any unusual discharge from your penis?

- **To the therapist:** If the client is having difficulty with sexual function, it may be necessary to conduct a screening examination for bladder or prostate involvement. See Appendix B-5.

CASE STUDY: STEPS IN THE SCREENING PROCESS

REFERRAL

A 47-year-old man with low back pain of unknown cause has come to you for exercises. After gathering information from the client's history and conducting the interview, you ask him:

Follow-Up Questions

• Are there any other symptoms of any kind anywhere else in your body?

The client tells you he does break out into an unexpected sweat from time to time, but does not think he has a temperature when this happens. He has increased back pain when he passes gas or a bowel movement, but then the pain goes back to the "regular" pain level [reported as 5 on a scale from 0 to 10]. Other reported symptoms include

• Heartburn and indigestion
• Abdominal bloating after meals
• Chronic bronchitis from smoking [3 packs/day]
• Alternating diarrhea and constipation

Use the list of signs and symptoms in Box 4-17 to review this case.

Do these symptoms fall into any one category?

It appears that many of the symptoms may be gastrointestinal in nature.

What is the next step in the screening process?

Since the client has mentioned unexplained sweating but no known fevers, take the time to measure all vital signs, especially body temperature. Turn to Special Questions to Ask at the end of Chapter 8 and scan the list of questions for any that might be appropriate for this client.

For example, find out about the use of non-steroidal antiinflammatories (prescription and over-the-counter; be sure to include aspirin). Follow up with:

Follow-Up Questions

• Have you ever been treated for an ulcer or internal bleeding while taking any of these pain relievers?
• Have you experienced any unexpected weight loss in the last few weeks?
• Have you traveled outside the United States in the last year?
• What is the effect of eating or drinking on your abdominal pain? Back pain?
• Have the client pay attention to his symptoms over the next 24 to 48 hours:
  —Immediately after eating
  —Within 30 minutes of eating
  —One to two hours later
• Do you have a sense of urgency so that you have to find a bathroom for a bowel movement or diarrhea right away without waiting?

Ask any further questions that may be appropriate as listed in this chapter or from the more complete *Special Questions to Ask* section of Chapter 8 (see the subsection: Associated Signs and Symptoms: Change in bowel habits).

You will make your decision to refer this client to a physician depending on your findings from the clinical examination and the client's responses to these questions. Use the Quick Screen Checklist in Appendix A-1 to see if you have left anything out that might be important.

This does not appear to be an emergency since the client is not in acute distress. An elevated temperature or other unusual vital signs might speed the referral process along.

PRACTICE QUESTIONS

1. The most common sites of referred pain from systemic diseases are:
   a. Neck and back
   b. Shoulder and back
   c. Chest and back
   d. None of the above

2. To screen for back pain caused by systemic disease:
   a. Perform special tests (e.g., Murphy's percussion, Bike test)
   b. Correlate client history with clinical presentation and ask about associated signs and symptoms
   c. Perform a Review of Systems
   d. All of the above

3. What are two ways of classifying back pain (as presented in the text)?

4. Which statement is the most accurate?
   a. Arterial disease is characterized by intermittent claudication, pain relieved by elevating the extremity, and history of smoking.
   b. Arterial disease is characterized by loss of hair on the lower extremities, throbbing pain in the calf muscles that goes away by using heat and elevation.
   c. Arterial disease is characterized by painful throbbing of the feet at night that goes away by dangling the feet over the bed.
   d. Arterial disease is characterized by loss of hair on the toes, intermittent claudication, and redness or warmth of the legs that is accompanied by a burning sensation.

5. Pain associated with pleuropulmonary disorders can radiate to:
   a. Anterior neck
   b. Upper trapezius muscle
   c. Ipsilateral shoulder
   d. Thoracic spine
   e. All of the above

6. Which of the following are clues to the possible involvement of the GI system?
   a. Abdominal pain alternating with TMJ pain within a 2-week period of time
   b. Abdominal pain at the same level as back pain occurring either simultaneously or alternately
   c. Shoulder pain alleviated by a bowel movement
   d. All of the above

7. Percussion of the costovertebral angle resulting in the reproduction of symptoms signifies:

   a. Radiculitis
   b. Pseudorenal pain
   c. Has no significance
   d. Medical referral is advised

8. A 53-year-old woman comes to physical therapy with a report of leg pain that begins in her buttocks and goes all the way down to her toes. If this pain is of a vascular origin she will most likely describe it as
   a. Sore, hurting
   b. Hot or burning
   c. Shooting or stabbing
   d. Throbbing, "tired"

9. Twenty-five percent of the people with GI disease such as Crohn's disease (regional enteritis), irritable bowel syndrome, or bowel obstruction have concomitant back or joint pain.
   a. True
   b. False

10. Skin pain over T9 to T12 can occur with kidney disease as a result of multisegmental innervation. Visceral and cutaneous sensory fibers enter the spinal cord close to each other and converge on the same neurons. When visceral pain fibers are stimulated, cutaneous fibers are stimulated, too. Thus, visceral pain can be perceived as skin pain.
   a. True
   b. False

11. Autosplinting is the preferred mechanism of pain relief for back pain caused by kidney stones.
   a. True
   b. False

12. Back pain from pancreatic disease occurs when the body of the pancreas is enlarged, inflamed, obstructed or otherwise impinging on the diaphragm.
   a. True
   b. False

13. A 53-year-old postmenopausal woman with a history of breast cancer 5 years ago with mastectomy presents with a report of sharp pain in her midback. The pain started after she lifted her 2-year-old granddaughter 3 days ago. Tylenol seems to help but the pain is keeping her awake at night. Once she wakes up, she cannot find a comfortable position to go back to sleep.

    What are the red flags? What will you do to screen for a medical cause of her symptoms?

REFERENCES

1. Waddell G: *The back pain revolution*, ed 2, Edinburgh, 2004, Churchill Livingstone.
2. Jette AM, Davis KD: A comparison of hospital-based and private outpatient physical therapy practices, *Phys Ther* 71(6):366-381, 1991.
3. Jette AM, Smith K, Haley SM et al: Physical therapy episodes of care for patients with low back pain, *Physical Therapy* 74(2):101-115, 1994.
4. Freburger JK, Carey TS, Holmes GM: Management of back and neck pain: who seeks care from physical therapists? *Physical Therapy* 85(9):872-886, 2005.
5. Bernard TN Jr, Kirkaldy-Willis WH: Recognizing specific characteristics of nonspecific low back pain, *Clin Orthop* 217:266-280, 1987.
6. Shaw JA: The role of the sacroiliac joint as a cause of low back pain and dysfunction. In Vleeming A, Mooney V, Snijders C, et al, editors: *The First Interdisciplinary World Congress on low back pain and its relation to the sacroiliac joint*, Rotterdam, the Netherlands, 1992, ECO, pp 67-80.
7. Kim DH, Hilibrand AS: Rheumatoid arthritis in the cervical spine, *J Am Acad Orthop Surg* 13(7):463-474, 2005.
8. Boissonnault WG, Koopmeiners MB: Medical history profile: orthopaedic physical therapy outpatients, *JOSPT* 20:2-10, 1994.
9. Boissonnault WG: Prevalence of comorbid conditions, surgeries, and medication use in a physical therapy outpatient population: a multi-centered study, *JOSPT* 29:506-519; discussion 520-525, 1999.
10. Boissonnault WG, Meek PD: Risk factors for antiinflammatory drug or aspirin induced gastrointestinal complications in individuals receiving outpatient physical therapy services, *JOSPT* 32:510-517, 2002.
11. Biederman RE: Pharmacology in rehabilitation: nonsteroidal antiinflammatory agents, *JOSPT* 35:356-367, 2005.
12. Bishop PB, Wing PC: Compliance with clinical practice guidelines in family physicians managing worker's compensation board patients with acute lower back pain, *Spine Journal* 3(6):442-450, 2003.
13. Leon-Diaz A, Gonzalez-Rabelino G, Alonso-Cervino M: Analysis of the etiologies of headaches in a pediatric emergency service, *Rev Neurol* 39(3):217-221, 1-15, 2004.
14. Olesen J, Steiner TJ: The international classification of headache disorders, ed 2 (ICDH-II), *J Neurol Neurosurg Psychiatry* 75(6):808-811, 2004.
15. Silberstein SD, Olesen J, Bousser MG, et al: The international classification of headache disorders, ed 2 (ICHD-II)—revision of criteria for 8.2 medication overuse headache, *Cephalalgia* 25(6):460-465, 2005.
16. Headache Classification Committee of the International Headache Society: Classification and diagnostic criteria for headache disorders, cranial neuralgias, and facial pain, *Cephalalgia* 8(Suppl 7):1-96, 1988.
17. Headache Classification Committee of the International Headache Society: *Classification and diagnostic criteria for headache disorders, cranial neuralgias and facial pain*, ed 2 (revised), *Cephalalgia* 25(12):460-465, 2004.
18. Petersen SM: Articular and muscular impairments in cervicogenic headache, *JOSPT* 33(1):21-30, 2003.
19. Agostoni E: Headache in cerebral venous thrombosis, *Neurol Sci* 25(Suppl 3):S206-S210, 2004.
20. Jacobson SA, Folstein MF: Psychiatric perspectives on headache and facial pain, *Otolaryngol Clin North Am* 36(6):1187-1200, 2003.
21. Hering-Hanit R, Gadoth N: Caffeine-induced headache in children and adolescents, *Cephalalgia* 23(6):332-335, 2003.
22. Ryan LM, Warden DL: Post concussion syndrome, *Int Rev Psychiatry* 15(4):310-316, 2003.
23. Phillips E, Levine AM: Metastatic lesions of the upper cervical spine, *Spine* 14(10):1071-1077, 1989.

24. O'Reilly MB: Nonresectable head and neck cancer, *Rehab Oncology* 22(2):14-16, 2004.
25. Neville BW, Day TA: Oral cancer and precancerous lesions, *CA J Clin* 52(4):195-215, 2002.
26. Purdy RA, Kirby S: Headaches and brain tumors, *Neurol Clin* 22(1):39-53, 2004.
27. Narin SO, Pinar L, Erbas D, et al: The effects of exercise and exercise-related changes in blood nitric oxide level on migraine headache, *Clin Rehabil* 17(6):624-630, 2003.
28. Sandor PS, Afra J: Nonpharmacologic treatment of migraine, *Curr Pain Headache Rep* 9(3):202-205, 2005.
29. Biondi DM: Physical treatments for headache: a structured review, *Headache* 45(6):738-746, 2005.
30. Gorski JM, Schwartz LH: Shoulder impingement presenting as neck pain, *JBJS* 85-A(4):635-638, 2003.
31. Slipman CW, Issac Z, Patel R, et al: Chronic neck pain: the specific syndromes, *J Musculoskel Med* 20(1):24-33, 2003.
32. Koopmeiners MB: Personal communication, 2003.
33. Boissonnault WG: Personal communication, 2003.
34. Hartvigsen J, Christensen K, Frederiksen H: Back pain remains a common symptom in old age. A population-based study of 4,486 Danish twins aged 70-102, *Eur Spine J* 12(5):528-534, 2003.
35. O'Neill CW, Kurgansky ME, Derby R, et al: Disc stimulation and patterns of referred pain, *Spine* 27(24):2776-2781, 2002.
36. Bogduk N: Evidence-based clinical guidelines for the management of acute low back pain, *The National Musculoskeletal Medicine Initiative*, 2002. Available online: http://www.emia.com.au/MedicalProviders/Evidence-BasedMedicine/afnm/ch1.html. Accessed September 15, 2005.
37. Kauppila LI, McAlindon T, Evans S, et al: Disc degeneration/back pain and calcification of the abdominal aorta. A 25-year follow-up study in Framingham, *Spine* 22:1642-1647, 1997.
38. Bingol H, Cingoz F, Yilmaz AT et al: Vascular complications related to lumbar disc surgery, *J Neurosurg: Spine* 100(3):249-253, 2004.
39. Kauppila LI, Mikkonen R, Mankinen P, et al: MR aortography and serum cholesterol levels in patients with long-term nonspecific lower back pain, *Spine* 29(19):2147-2152, 2004.
40. Seeman E: The dilemma of osteoporosis in men, *Am J Med* 98(2A):76SS-88S, 1995.
41. Orwoll ES, Klein RF: Osteoporosis in men, *Endocr Rev* 16:87-116, 1995.
42. Blain H: Osteoporosis in men: epidemiology, physiopathology, diagnosis, prevention, and treatment, *Rev Med Interne* 25(Suppl 5):S552-S559, 2005.
43. Silverman SL: The clinical consequences of vertebral compression fracture, *Bone* 13:S27-S31, 1992.
44. Hoogendoorn WE, van Poppel MN, Bongers PM, et al: Systematic review of psychosocial factors at work and private life as risk factors for back pain, *Spine* 25:2114-2125, 2000.
45. Marras WS, Davis KG, Heaney CA, et al: The influence of psychosocial stress, gender, and personality on mechanical loading of the lumbar spine, *Spine* 25(23):3045-3054, 2000.
46. Thorbjornsson CO, Alfredsson L, Fredrikson K, et al: Physical and psychosocial factors related to low back pain during a 24-year period, *Occup Environ Med* 55(2):84-90, 1998.
47. Kendall NAS, Linton SJ, Main CJ: *Guide to assessing psychological yellow flags in acute low back pain: risk factors for long-term disability and work loss*, Wellington, New Zealand, 1997, Accident Rehabilitation and Compensation Insurance Corporation of New Zealand and the National Health Committee.
48. Borkan J, Van Tulder M, Reis S, et al: Advances in the field of low back pain in primary care. A report from the Fourth International Forum, *Spine* 27(5):E128-E132, 2002.

49. Mazanec DJ, Segal AM, Sinks PB: Identification of malignancy in patients with back pain: red flags, *Arthritis Rheum* 36(suppl):S251-S258, 1993.

50. Rex L: *Evaluation and treatment of somatovisceral dysfunction of the gastrointestinal system*, Edmonds WA, 2004, URSA Foundation.

51. Deyo RA, Diehl AK: Cancer as a cause of back pain: frequency, clinical presentation, and diagnostic strategies, *J Gen Intern Med* 3(3):230-238, 1988.

52. Wong DA, Fornasier VL, MacNab I: Spinal metastases: the obvious, the occult, and the imposters, *Spine* 15(1):1-4, 1990.

53. Ross MD, Bayer E: Cancer as a cause of low back pain in a patient seen in a direct access physical therapy setting, *JOSPT* 35(10):651-658, 2005.

54. Fleming C, Whitlock EP, Beil TL, et al: Screening for abdominal aortic aneurysm: a best evidence systematic review for the U.S. Preventive Services Task Force, *Ann Intern Med* 142(3):203-211, 2005.

55. Herkowitz HN, editor: *The spine*, Philadelphia, 1999, WB Saunders.

56. *Sex and Back Pain Video*, Dixfield, Maine, IMPACC, Inc. Available at: www.impaccusa.com. Accessed September 21, 2005.

57. *Sex and Back Pain Patient Manual*, Dixfield, Maine, IMPACC, Inc. Available at: www.impaccusa.com. Accessed September 21, 2005.

58. Padua L, Caliandro P, Aprile I, et al: Back pain in pregnancy, *Eur Spine J* 14(2):151-154, 2005.

59. Borg-Stein J, Dugan SA, Gruber J: Musculoskeletal aspects of pregnancy, *Am J Phys Med Rehabil* 84(3):180-192, 2005.

60. Pauls J: Physical therapy for women, *PT Magazine* 1(2):64-67, 1993.

61. Deevey S: Endometriosis: Internet resources, *Medical Ref Serv Quart* 24(1):67-77, 2005.

62. Giudice LC, Kao LC: Endometriosis, *The Lancet* 364(9447):1789-1799, 2004.

63. Sinaii N, Cleary SD, Ballweg ML, et al: High rates of autoimmune and endocrine disorders, fibromyalgia, chronic fatigue syndrome, and atopic diseases among women with endometriosis: a survey analysis, *Hum Reprod* 17(10):2715-2724, 2002.

64. Svendsen PF, Nilas L, Norgaard K, et al: Polycystic ovary syndrome. New pathophysiological discoveries, *Ugeskr Laeger* 167(34):3147-3151, 2005.

65. Dokras A, Bochner M, Hollinrake E, et al: Screening women with polycystic ovary syndrome for metabolic syndrome, *Obstet Gynecol* 106(1):131-137, 2005.

66. Jemal A, Murray T, Ward E, et al: Cancer statistics 2005, *CA A Cancer J Clin* 55(1):10-30, 2005.

67. Siddiqui E, Mumtaz FH, Gelister J: Understanding prostate cancer, *J R Soc Health* 124(5):219-221, 2004.

68. Gelfand MS, Cleveland KO: Vancomycin therapy and the progression of methicillin-resistant *Staphylococcus aureus* vertebral osteomyelitis, *South Med J* 97(6):593-597, 2004.

69. Patel RK, Everett CR: Low back pain: 20 clinical pearls, *J Musculoskel Med* 20(10):452-460, 2003.

70. Asavasopon S, Jankoski J, Godges JJ: Clinical diagnosis of vertebrobasilar insufficiency: resident's case problem, *JOSPT* 35(10):645-650, 2005.

71. Wiesel BB, Wiesel SW: Radiographic evaluation of low back pain: a cost-effective approach, *J Musculoskel Med* 21(10):528-538, 2004.

72. Mazanec DJ: Recognizing malignancy in patients with low back pain, *J Musculoskel Med* 13(1):24-31, 1996.

73. King H: Evaluating the child with back pain, *Pediatric Clinics of North America* 33(6):1489-1493, 1986.

74. Behrman R, Kliegman RM, Arvin AM, editors: *Nelson's textbook of pediatrics*, ed 17, Philadelphia, 2004, WB Saunders.

75. McTimoney CA, Micheli LJ: Managing back pain in young athletes, *J Musculo Med* 21(2):63-69, 2004.

76. Goode B: Personal communication, Centers for Disease Control and Prevention, Raleigh, North Carolina, 2006.

77. Knight D: Health care screening for men who have sex with men, *Amer Fam Phys* 69(9):2149-2156, 2004.

Screening the Sacrum, Sacroiliac, and Pelvis

Following the model for decision-making in the screening process outlined in Chapter 1 (see Box 1-7), we now turn our attention to pain from medical conditions, illnesses, and diseases referred to the sacrum, sacroiliac (SI), and pelvic regions.

The basic premise is that physical therapists must be able to identify signs and symptoms of systemic origin that can mimic neuromuscular or musculoskeletal (neuromusculoskeletal, or NMS) dysfunction in these areas.

In the screening process, therapists will watch for yellow (caution) or red (warning) flags to direct them. Clinicians rely on special questions to ask men and women with significant risk factors, significant past medical history, suspicious clinical presentation, or associated signs and symptoms.

With a careful interview and the right screening questions, the therapist can identify clues suggestive of a problem outside the scope of a physical therapist's practice that may require medical referral. Specific tests to screen for an underlying infectious or inflammatory source of pelvic or abdominal pain are also presented with a suggested order of testing.

When dealing with painful symptoms of the sacral and pelvic areas, the therapist may need to ask questions about sexual history or sexual practices. The therapist must remain aware of facial expressions, body language, and verbal remarks in response to a client's answers to these questions.

The therapist must be prepared to respond in a professional and responsible way if a man or woman with pelvic or sacral pain reports that he or she has been the victim of repeated violent sexual acts, or if a client admits to physical or emotional assault. More about the client interview, the screening interview, and screening for assault and domestic (intimate partner) violence is included in Chapter 2 (see also Appendix B-29).

▶ THE SACRUM AND SACROILIAC JOINT

Evaluating the sacroiliac (SI) joint can be difficult in that no single physical examination finding can predict a disorder of the SI joint. Pain originating from the SI joint can mimic pain referred from lumbar disc herniation, spinal stenosis, facet joint dysfunction, or even a disorder of the hip.[1]

The most common clinical presentation of sacroiliac pain is associated with a memorable *physical event* that initiated the pain, such as a misstep off a curb, a fall on the hip or buttocks, lifting of a heavy object in a twisted position, or childbirth (Case Example 15-1). A history of previous spine surgery is very common in clients with SI intra-articular pain.[1]

The most typical *systemic diseases* that refer pain to the sacrum and sacroiliac joint include endocarditis, prostate cancer or other neoplasm,

CASE EXAMPLE 15-1   Sacroiliac Pain Caused by Pelvic Floor Dysfunction

Background: A 33-year-old woman referred by her orthopedic surgeon presented with low back pain centered over the sacroiliac (SI) region. She described it as "sharp" and "knife-like." It comes and goes with no warning. Sometimes, it is so severe she cannot catch her breath and falls to her knees. After that, she cannot stand up straight for several hours and walks "hunched over."

The pain presented on both sides intermittently, but the primary pain pattern was localized in the left SI area. Heat seems to help for a short time, but nothing brings complete relief all the time.

She has a previous history of disc herniation with discectomy and laminectomy and complete resolution of symptoms. No cause is known for this new onset of SI symptoms. No radiating symptoms are apparent, and recent magnetic resonance imaging shows no sign of disc protrusion at this time. (She tried doing her previous program of McKenzie exercises, but no change in symptoms occurred.)

Clinical Presentation: Physical therapy examination reveals the following: Antalgic gait secondary to pain. Trendelenburg sign: negative. Slight left lumbar lateral shift; posture within normal limits otherwise. Active lumbar motions are full, with a normal capsular end feel and no reproduction of symptoms. Repeated trunk and lumbar motions do not elicit painful symptoms. Neurologic screen: negative for abnormal reflexes, abnormal sensation, decreased strength, or altered neural tension. Hamstrings are tight bilaterally, but a straight leg raise does not increase symptoms. In fact, it is the only time in the assessment when the client reports a slight decrease in pain.

Examination of the SI area revealed an upslip on the left (anterior superior iliac spine [ASIS] and posterior superior iliac spine [PSIS] on the left are higher than ASIS and PSIS on the right, indicating an upward movement of the ilium on the sacrum on the high side; leg length discrepancy or muscle spasm from a disc lesion can also cause an upslip). Given her past history of discogenic lesion, it is possible that altered muscle acti-

vation is the cause. This will have to be examined further.

Is a screening examination for systemic origin of symptoms warranted? Why, or why not? Using our screening model, review the past medical history. Are there any red flags here? No, but the history is very incomplete. We know she had a previous discogenic lesion treated operatively. Nothing of her personal or family history is included.

Even in a musculoskeletal assessment, we will want to know about pregnancy and birth histories; use of medications, over-the-counter drugs, and illicit drugs; smoking and drinking history or current use; levels of activity before the onset of symptoms; correlation of symptoms with menses or births; occupation and work-related activities; and history of cancer.

A general screening interview will ask about recent history of infection, the presence of joint pain or skin rash anywhere else, and the presence of any constitutional or other symptoms.

Next, review the clinical presentation. Are there any red flags here? Not really. There is no night pain. There is the fact that nothing seems to make it better or worse, but one red flag by itself usually is not highly significant. We will tuck that bit of information in the back of our minds as we continue the evaluation process.

Hamstring stretching brings some mild, temporary relief. This suggests a muscular component, but that has to be further evaluated. The SI upslip could be the cause of the symptoms, but this will not be determined until the alignment and cause of the upslip are corrected.

A trigger point assessment may be needed as well.

Step three involves a review of associated signs and symptoms. We do not know about constitutional symptoms, relationship of SI pain to menses, or the presence of any other symptoms associated with the viscera (e.g., gastrointestinal, urologic). It is always recommended to take the client's temperature in the presence of pain of unknown cause.

What to Do: Several strategies are presented here. Intervention for the upslip may be the first step with reassessment of symptoms. If a lack of progress occurs, the therapist can go back and ask more specific questions. Or, the therapist

---

CASE EXAMPLE 15-1 Sacroiliac Pain Caused by Pelvic Floor Dysfunction—cont'd

can treat the upslip while continuing to interview the client each day, obtaining additional pertinent information before making a final decision.

Result: In the end, it was discovered that the client had significant pelvic floor dysfunction with levator ani spasm and detrusor imbalance with urinary incontinence. She reported a complicated birth history with her first child, which was repeated with less severity during the births of her second and third children.

Intercourse was extremely painful, but the client was too embarrassed to bring this up until the therapist asked directly about sexual activity. The client finally described a sensation as if "trying to deliver a baby through my rectum" during intercourse (a sign of levator ani dysfunction).

Once all the additional information had been brought out and organized, the client shared the signs and symptoms with her gynecologist. An internal vaginal examination reproduced her symptoms exactly. The evaluating therapist was not trained in pelvic floor assessment and did not make this finding directly.

In looking back, it is likely that development of the discogenic lesion was linked to birth/delivery problems (or perhaps, vice versa; it was never known for sure). Closer examination

revealed a loss of lumbar stabilization because of multifidus impairment. Muscle impairment at the time of the disc lesion and births probably contributed to the gradual development of pelvic floor dysfunction.

Changes were also noted in the abdominal muscles with a loss of co-contraction between the multifidus and the transversus abdominis. The levator ani and pelvic floor muscles were in a contract-hold pattern, contributing to the painful symptoms described.

Heat relaxed the muscles, but only for a short time. Hamstring stretching may have brought about an inhibition to the pelvic floor muscles, reducing pain.

A program directed at restoring normal muscle tone and function in the lumbar spine, abdominal muscles, and pelvic floor resulted in immediate reduction and eventual elimination of painful symptoms and return of comfortable coitus. Symptoms of urinary incontinence also were resolved.

Although the SI upslip could be corrected, the client could not maintain the correction. Because she was pain free, she did not return to physical therapy for further evaluation of the underlying biomechanics around the SI upslip.

---

gynecologic disorders, rheumatic diseases that target the sacroiliac area (e.g., spondyloarthropathies such as ankylosing spondylitis, Reiter's syndrome, or psoriatic arthritis), and Paget's disease (Table 15-1).[2]

Disorders of the large intestine and colon, such as ulcerative colitis, Crohn's disease (regional enteritis), carcinoma of the colon, and irritable bowel syndrome, can refer pain to the sacrum when the rectum is stimulated.

A medical differential diagnosis may be needed to exclude fracture, infection, or tumor. Insufficiency fractures of the sacrum are not uncommon and usually occur in osteoporotic bone with minimal or unremembered trauma.[3] (See further discussion in this chapter on spondylogenic causes of sacral pain.)

Using the Screening Model to Evaluate Sacral/SI Symptoms

The principles guiding evaluation of sacroiliac joint or sacral pain are consistent with the information presented throughout this text and, in particular, in the chapter on back pain (see Chapter 14).

Each of the disorders listed in Table 15-1 usually has its own unique *clinical presentation* with clues available in the *past medical history*. The presence of *associated signs and symptoms* is always a red flag. Most of these conditions have clear red flag clues that come to light if the client is interviewed carefully.

Clinical Presentation

Insidious onset or unknown cause is always a red flag. Without a clear cause, the therapist looks for

TABLE 15-1 ▼ Causes of Sacral and Sacroiliac (SI) Pain

Systemic	Neuromuscular/musculoskeletal[8]

Infectious/Inflammatory

Spondyloarthropathy:
Ankylosing spondylitis
Reiter's syndrome
Psoriatic arthritis
Inflammatory bowel disease (arthritis associated with IBD)
Vertebral osteomyelitis
Endocarditis
Tuberculosis (uncommon)

Spondylogenic

Fracture (traumatic, insufficiency, pathologic), metabolic
bone disease
• Osteoporosis (insufficiency fractures)
• Paget's disease
• Osteodystrophy
• Osteoarthritis

Gynecologic

Reproductive cancers
Retroversion of the uterus
Uterine fibroids
Ovarian cysts
Endometriosis
Pelvic inflammatory disease (PID)
Incest/sexual assault
Rectocele, cystocele
Uterine prolapse
Normal pregnancy; multiparity (more than one pregnancy)

Gastrointestinal

Ulcerative colitis
Colon cancer
Irritable bowel syndrome
Crohn's disease (regional enteritis)

Cancer

Primary tumors (rare: giant cell, chondrosarcoma, synovial
villoadenoma)
Metastatic lesions (history of cancer)
• Prostate cancer
• Colorectal cancer
• Multiple myeloma

Other

Fibromyalgia
Genital herpes simplex virus (rare)[2]

Idiopathic (unknown)
Trauma
Myofascial or kinetic chain imbalance
Enthesis (tendon insertion)/ligamentous sprain
Degenerative joint disease
Bone harvesting for grafts (may cause secondary instability)
Lumbar spine fusion or hip arthrodesis
Myofascial syndromes (mimics SI joint pain)
Discogenic disease (mimics SI joint pain)
Nerve root compression (mimics SI joint pain)
Zygapophyseal joint pain (mimics SI joint pain)

something else in the history or accompanying signs and symptoms. Even with a known or assigned cause, it is important to keep other possibilities in mind and to watch for red flags (Box 15-1). Sacral pain in the absence of a history of trauma or overuse is a clue to the presentation of systemic backache.

The amount and direction of pain radiation can offer helpful clues. Low back or sacral pain radiating around the flank suggests the renal or urologic system. In such cases, the therapist is likely to ask questions about bladder or urologic function.

Low back or sacral pain radiating to the buttock or legs may be vascular. Questions about the effects of activity on symptoms and history of cardiovascular or peripheral vascular diseases are important (see discussion, Chapter 14). Sorting out pain of a vascular versus neurogenic cause is also discussed in Chapter 14.

Most commonly, unless pain causes muscle spasm, splinting, and subsequent biomechanical changes, clients affected by systemic or viscerogenic causes of sacral or SI pain demonstrate a remarkable lack of objective findings to implicate the sacroiliac joint or sacrum as the causative factor for the presenting symptoms. Pain elicited

BOX 15-1 ▼ Red Flags Associated With Sacroiliac/Sacral Pain or Symptoms

History

- Sacroiliac/sacral pain without a history of trauma or overuse (rule out assault, anal intercourse)
- Previous history of cancer
- Previous history of gastrointestinal disease (ulcerative colitis, Crohn's disease, irritable bowel syndrome)

Risk Factors

- Osteoporosis
- Sexually transmitted infection
- Long-term use of antibiotics (colitis)

Clinical Presentation

- Lack of objective findings
- Anterior pelvic, suprapubic, or low abdominal pain at the same level as the sacrum

Associated Signs and Symptoms

- Pain relieved by passing gas or having a bowel movement
- Presence of gastrointestinal, gynecologic, or urologic signs and symptoms

by pressing on the sacrum with the client in a prone position suggests sacroiliitis (inflammation of the sacroiliac joint) or mechanical derangement.

SI JOINT PAIN PATTERN

Whether from a mechanical or a systemic origin, the patient usually experiences pain over the posterior SI joint and buttock, with or without lower extremity SI joint pain. Pain may be unilateral or bilateral (Fig. 15-1)[4] and can be referred to a wide referral

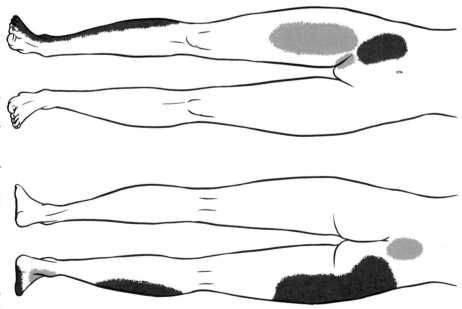

Fig. 15-1 • Unilateral sacroiliac (SI) pain pattern. Pain coming from the sacroiliac joint is usually centered over the area of the posterior superior iliac spine (PSIS), with tenderness directly over the PSIS. Lower lumbar pain occurs in 72% of cases; it rarely presents as upper lumbar pain above L5 (6%). It may radiate over the buttocks (94%), down the posterior-lateral thigh (50%), and even past the knee to the ankle (14%) and lateral foot (8%). Paresthesias in the leg are not a typical feature of SI joint pain. The affected individual may report abdominal (2%), groin or pubic (14%), or anterior thigh pain (10%). Anterior symptoms may occur alone or in combination with posterior symptoms. Occasionally, a client will report bilateral pain. (Data from Slipman CW, Jackson HB, Lipetz JS, et al: Sacroiliac joint pain referral zones. Arch Phys Med Rehab 81:334-338, 2000.)

zone, including the lumbar spine, abdomen, groin, foot, and ankle.[1,5]

Clients with SI joint pain rarely have pain at or above the level of the L5 spinous process, although it is possible. The presence of midline lumbar pain tends to exclude the SI joint as a potential pain generator.[6]

A wide range of SI joint–referred pain patterns occur because innervation is highly variable and complex, or because pain may be somatically referred, as discussed in Chapter 3. Adjacent structures, such as the piriformis muscle, sciatic nerve, and L5 nerve root, may be affected by intrinsic joint disease and can become active nociceptors. Pain referral patterns also may be dependent on the distinct location of injury within the SI joint.[7]

SI pain can mimic discogenic disease with radicular pain down the leg to the foot. People who report midline lumbar pain when they rise from a sitting position are likely to have discogenic pain. Clients with unilateral pain below the level of the L5 spinous process and pain when they rise from sitting are likely to have a painful SI joint.[6]

Pain from SI joint syndrome may be aggravated by sitting or lying on the affected side. Pain gets worse with prolonged driving or riding in a car, weight bearing on the affected side, the Valsalva maneuver, and trunk flexion with the legs straight.[7]

SI pain can also mimic the pain pattern of kidney disease with anterior thigh pain, but with SI dysfunction, no signs and symptoms (e.g., constitutional symptoms, bladder dysfunction) are associated, as would be the case with thigh pain referred from the renal system.

Screening for Infectious/Inflammatory Causes of Sacroiliac Pain

Joint infections spread hematogenously through the body and can affect the sacroiliac joint. Usually, the infection is unilateral and is caused by *Pseudomonas aeruginosa*, *Staphylococcus aureus*, *Cryptococcus* organisms, or *Mycobacterium tuberculosis*.

Risk factors for joint infection include trauma, endocarditis, intravenous drug use, and immunosuppression. Postoperative infection of any kind may not appear with any clinical signs or symptoms for weeks or months.

Infection can cause distention of the anterior joint capsule, irritating the lumbrosacral nerve roots.[8] Inflammation of the sacroiliac joint may result from metabolic, traumatic, or rheumatic causes. Sacroiliitis is present in all individuals with ankylosing spondylitis.[9]

Rheumatic Diseases as a Cause of Sacral or SI Pain

The most common systemic causes of sacral pain are noninfected, inflammatory erosive rheumatic diseases that target the SI, including ankylosing spondylitis, Reiter's syndrome, psoriatic arthritis, and arthritis associated with inflammatory bowel disease (IBD) such as regional enteritis (Crohn's disease).

Reiter's syndrome (see Chapter 12) occurs most often in young men with venereal disease. Reiter's syndrome often presents as a triad of symptoms, including arthritis, conjunctivitis, and urethritis. These three symptoms in the presence of sacral pain raise a red flag. The therapist must ask about pain in other joints, urologic symptoms, and a recent (or current) history of conjunctivitis (red, painful inflammation of the eye).

A positive sexual history or known diagnosis of venereal disease is helpful information. With sacral or SI pain, the therapist should always consider taking a sexual history (see Special Questions to Ask, Chapter 14 or Appendix B-29).

Crohn's disease (see Chapter 8) may be accompanied by skin rash and joint pain. This enteric condition is well known for its arthritic component, which is present in up to 25% of all cases. The client may have had Crohn's disease for years and may not recognize the onset of these new symptoms as part of that condition. Skin rash may precede joint pain by days or weeks. The hips, thighs, and legs are affected most often; the rash may be raised or flat, purple or red. Knowing the history and association between skin lesions and joint pain can help the therapist direct screening questions and make a reasonable decision about referral.

Screening for Spondylogenic Causes of Sacral/Sacroiliac Pain

Metabolic bone disease (MBD) such as osteoporosis, Paget's disease, and osteodystrophy can result in loss of bone mineral density and deformity or fracture of the sacrum. The therapist should review cases of sacral pain for the presence of risk factors for any of these metabolic bone diseases (see the discussion on metabolic bone disease in Chapter 11). Neoplasm and fracture are two other possible bony causes of sacral pain. Neoplasm is discussed separately in this chapter.

Metabolic Bone Disease

Mild to moderate MBD may occur with no visible signs. Advanced cases of MBD include constipation, anorexia, fractured bones, and deformity.

OSTEOPOROSIS

Osteoporosis can cause insufficiency fractures of the sacrum. The therapist must assess for risk factors (see Boxes 15-2 and 11-3) in anyone with sacral pain, especially those in whom pain has an unknown cause, postmenopausal women, older men (over 65), and anyone with a known history of osteoporosis or Paget's disease. See further discussion, Osteoporosis, in Chapter 11, and Fractures, at the end of this section.

PAGET'S DISEASE

Paget's disease as a cause of lumbar, sacral, sacroiliac (SI), or pelvic pain occurs most commonly in men over 70 years of age (although it can occur earlier and in women). It is the second most common metabolic bone disease after osteoporosis.

Characterized by slowly progressive enlargement and deformity of multiple bones, it is associated with unexplained acceleration of bone deposition and resorption. The bones become weak, spongy, and deformed. Redness and warmth may be noted over involved areas, and the most common symptom is bone pain (see further discussion, Chapter 11, Paget's disease; see also excellent online article).[10]

Fracture

Three types of fractures affect the sacrum: traumatic, insufficiency, and pathologic. Trauma resulting in fracture occurs most often with lateral compression injuries seen in motor vehicle accidents or vertical shear injuries resulting from a fall from height onto the lower limbs. Less commonly, direct stress to the sacrum from a high fall landing on the buttocks can cause traumatic sacral fracture.[11] Other risk factors for sacral fracture are listed in Box 15-2.

BOX 15-2 ▼ **Risk Factors for Sacral Fractures**

- Osteoporosis (see also Box 11-3)
- Paget's disease
- Gender (female)
- Athletes, military personnel (overuse, overtraining, improper footwear or training surface)
- Athletic pregnant or postpartum women
- Pelvic radiation
- Lumbar-sacral fusion (early postoperative)
- Osteomyelitis
- Multiple myeloma
- Trauma (motor vehicle accident, fall, assault)
- Prolonged use of corticosteroids

Trauma-related fatigue or stress fracture of the sacrum occurs most often in young active persons and older adults with osteoporosis. Fatigue or stress fractures can develop as a result of submaximal repetitive forces over time such as occur with overuse or overtraining in military personnel and athletes (e.g., runners, volleyball and field hockey players). Less often, pregnant or postpartum women experience sacral stress fractures, especially if they are participating in athletic training activities or running.[12]

Insufficiency fractures of the sacrum result from a normal stress acting on bone with deficient elastic resistance. Reduced bone integrity is most often associated with postmenopausal or corticosteroid-induced osteoporosis and radiation therapy.[11] Insufficiency fractures occur insidiously or as a result of minor trauma, possibly even from weight bearing transmitted through the spine.[13]

Pathologic fracture describes fractures that occur as a result of bone weakened by neoplasm or other disease conditions (e.g., osteomyelitis, giant cell tumor, chordoma, Ewing's sarcoma, multiple myeloma). Insufficiency fractures are actually a subset of pathologic fractures confined to bones with structural alterations due to metabolic bone disease.[11]

Clinical manifestations of sacral fractures can present with a wide range of signs and symptoms, many of which are present inconsistently and are considered nonspecific.[14] Bilateral or multiple stress fractures of the sacrum or pelvis have been reported.[15]

The client may report or demonstrate localized pain, tenderness with palpation, antalgic gait, and leg length discrepancy. With all sacral fractures, hip, low back, sacral, groin, or buttock pain may occur, especially with multiple stress fractures of the pelvic and sacral bones. Symptoms may mimic other conditions such as disc disease, recurrence of a local tumor, or metastatic disease.[11]

Diagnostic imaging may be needed to make the final medical diagnosis. Radiographic studies (x-rays) are often negative in the early phases of stress reactions or fractures. More advanced diagnostic bone imaging may show changes when the client becomes symptomatic.

New onset of sacral or buttock pain 1 to 2 weeks after multilevel lumbosacral fusion with instrumentation should be evaluated for sacral insufficiency fractures, especially if the patient has a recent history of prolonged sitting.[16]

Screening for Gynecologic Causes of Sacral Pain

See discussion, Gynecologic Causes of Pelvic Pain, this chapter.

Screening for Gastrointestinal Causes of Sacral/Sacroiliac Pain

The *primary* pain pattern for gastrointestinal (GI) disease involves the midabdominal region around the umbilicus. It is not likely that the therapist will see clients with this chief complaint; they are more likely to see a doctor or go to the emergency department.

However, the therapist may be evaluating or treating a client for an orthopedic or neurologic problem who reports GI symptoms. When a client relates symptoms associated with the viscera or abdomen, the therapist must think in terms of screening questions to discern whether these symptoms require immediate medical assessment and intervention.

The therapist is more likely to see clients with *referred* low back or sacral pain from the small or large intestine as it presents in the low back or sacral area (see Figs. 8-13 and 8-14). Although these illustrations depict the pain in small, very round areas, actual pain patterns can vary quite a bit. The location will be approximately the same, but individual variation does occur.

The therapist must ask about the presence of abdominal pain or GI symptoms, occurring either simultaneously or alternating but at the same anatomic level as back or sacral pain. See Case Example 14-13 to review the importance of looking for this particular red flag.

Sacral pain from a GI source may be reduced or relieved after the person passes gas or completes a bowel movement. It may be appropriate to ask a client the following:

Follow-Up Questions

- Is your pain relieved by passing gas or having a bowel movement?

The patient may have a history of GI disease or medication use to treat conditions such as

- Ulcerative colitis
- Crohn's disease
- Irritable bowel syndrome (IBS)
- Colon cancer
- Long-term use of antibiotics (colitis)

Keep these conditions in mind when asking questions about past medical history of anyone with lumbar spine or sacral pain patterns.

Screening for Tumors as a Cause of Sacral/Sacroiliac Pain

Primary sacral tumors include benign and malignant growths. Benign neoplasms include osteochondroma, giant cell tumor, and osteoid osteoma. The more common primary malignant lesions directly affecting the sacrum include chordoma, osteosarcoma, and myeloma.

Metastatic bone disease to the sacrum from primary breast, lung, and prostate is far more common. Sacral insufficiency fractures after pelvic radiation for rectal carcinoma can occur, although these are rare.[17]

Although rare, sacral neoplasms usually are not diagnosed early in the disease course because of mild symptoms resembling low back pain or sciatica.[18] Referral to a physical therapist before a correct medical diagnosis is made is not unusual.

Giant cell tumor is a highly aggressive local tumor of the bone. The sacrum is the third most common site of involvement. Clients present with localized pain in the lower back and sacrum that may radiate to one or both legs. Swelling may be noted in the involved area. When asked about the presence of other symptoms anywhere in the body, the client may report abdominal complaints and neurologic signs and symptoms (e.g., bowel and bladder or sexual dysfunction, numbness and weakness of the lower extremity).[19,20]

Colorectal or anorectal cancer as a cause of sacral pain is possible as the result of local invasion. Severe sacral pain in the presence of a previous history of uterine, abdominal, prostate, rectal, or anal cancer requires immediate medical referral.

Prostatic (males) *or reproductive cancers* in men and women can result in sacral pain. See further discussion under Testicular Cancer (see Chapters 10 and 14), Prostate Cancer (see Chapter 10), and Gynecologic Conditions (this chapter).

▶ THE COCCYX

The coccyx or tailbone is a small triangular bone that articulates with the bottom of the sacrum at the sacrococcygeal joint. Injury or trauma to this area can cause coccygeal pain called coccygodynia.

Coccygodynia

Most cases of coccygodynia or coccydynia (pain in the region of the coccyx) seen by the physical therapist occur as a result of trauma such as a fall directly on the tailbone or events associated with childbirth.

Symptoms include localized pain in the tailbone that is usually aggravated by direct pressure such as that caused by sitting, passing gas, or having a bowel movement. Moving from sitting to standing may also reproduce or aggravate painful symptoms.

Coccygodynia is reproduced on bidigital manipulation of the coccyx. A medical diagnosis is confirmed when at least 75% relief of coccygeal pain results from injection of local anesthetic into the sacrococcygeal joint on two separate occasions.[21]

In the case of *persistent* coccygodynia with a history of trauma, the therapist must keep in mind the possibility of rectal or bladder lesions (Box 15-3). When asked about the presence of other symptoms, clients with coccygodynia after a traumatic fall may also report bladder, bowel, or rectal symptoms. The therapist must ask whether bladder, bowel, or rectal symptoms were present before the fall. Because 50% of all clients with back or sacral pain from a malignancy have preceding trauma or injury, the apparent trauma (especially if the client reports associated symptoms that were present before the trauma) may be something more serious.

For possible clues to treating a client with coccygodynia, the therapist should review Box 15-3, keeping in mind the risk factors for each of these conditions. The therapist should also conduct a neurologic screening examination to identify any signs or symptoms of disc disease. Past history of any of the problems listed is a yellow (warning) flag. Blood in the toilet after a bowel movement may be a sign of anal fissures, hemorrhoids, or colorectal cancer and requires medical evaluation.

BOX 15-3 ▼ Causes of Coccygeal Pain

- Discogenic disease (herniation)
- Degenerative spondylolysis or spondylolisthesis
- Lumbar spinal stenosis
- Sacroiliac joint dysfunction
- Anal fissures
- Inflammatory cysts
- Prostatitis
- Thrombosed hemorrhoids
- Chordoma (neoplasm)
- Pilonidal cysts
- Trauma (fall, childbirth, anal intercourse)
- Nonunion fracture (sacrum, coccyx)
- Coccygeal disc injury (rare)

Data from Wood KB, Mehbod AA: Operative treatment for coccygodynia. *J Spinal Disord Tech* 17(6):511-515, 2004.

▲ THE PELVIS

Once again, the principles used in screening for systemic or viscerogenic causes of back, sacral, and SI pain also apply to pelvic pain. The history and associated signs and symptoms may vary somewhat according to the cause, but many of the causes are the same (e.g., cancer, GI, vascular, urogenital) (Table 15-2).

The most common primary causes of pelvic pain seen in a physical therapy practice are musculoskeletal, neuromuscular, gynecologic, infectious, vascular, cancer, and gastrointestinal (in descending order). Infectious disease is the most common systemic cause of pelvic pain. Chronic pelvic pain is most commonly associated with endometriosis, adhesions, IBS, and interstitial cystitis.[22,23]

The therapist must keep in mind that pelvic pain and symptoms can be referred to the pelvis from the hip, sacrum, SI area, or lumbar spine. At the same time, pelvic diseases can refer pain or symptoms to the abdomen, low back, buttocks, groin, and thigh. This means that anytime a client presents with pain or dysfunction in any of these areas, pelvic disease must be considered as a possible cause.

The anterior pelvic wall is part of the musculature of the abdominal cavity. The lateral walls are covered by the iliopsoas and obturator muscles, and inferiorly, the outlet is guarded by the levator ani and pubococcygeus muscles, with which the corresponding muscles of the opposite side form the pelvic diaphragm.

These two anatomic regions are separated only by walls of muscle. Because the pelvic cavity is in direct communication with the abdominal cavity (see Fig. 14-1), any organ disease or systemic condition of the pelvic or abdominal cavity can cause primary pelvic pain or referred musculoskeletal pain, as is described in this section.

The therapist should keep in mind that pelvic pain and low back pain often occur together or alternately. Whenever discussing pelvic pain, the therapist should ask about the presence of unreported low back pain.

Using the Screening Model to Evaluate the Pelvis

When our screening model is followed, the same steps are always taken. A personal or family history is obtained, and risk factor assessment is performed. Once the history has been established, the pelvic pain pattern is reviewed. The therapist looks for red flags that may suggest systemic or viscerogenic causes. Additional questions may be

TABLE 15-2 ▼ Causes of Pelvic Pain

Systemic	Neuromuscular/musculoskeletal
Gynecologic	Hip, sacroiliac joint, low back, sacral, or coccyx dysfunction*
Pregnancy (including ectopic, ruptured or unruptured)	Muscle impairment (hamstrings, abdominals, rectus femoris,
Uterovaginal prolapse	adductor muscles, pelvic floor muscles, levator ani)†
Vulvodynia	Psoas abscess (abdominal or pelvic infectious process)
Dysmenorrhea	Stress reactions/fractures
Endometriosis	Pubic strain/sprain/separation
Premenstrual tension	Sexual, birth, or activity-related trauma or injury:
Tumors, fibroids, adhesions, polyps	Levator ani syndrome
Ovarian cysts, varicosities, or torsion	Tension myalgia
Gynecalgia	Coccygodynia
Intrauterine contraceptive device (IUCD)	Neurologic disorders
Adnexal torsion (ovaries, fallopian tubes twisted) (rare)	Nerve entrapment
	Incomplete spinal cord lesion
Infection/Inflammation	Multiple sclerosis
Spontaneous, therapeutic, or incomplete	Pudendal neuralgia
abortion; postabortion syndrome	Scoliosis
Septic arthritis	Osteoporosis
Ankylosing spondylitis	Somatization disorders
Ileal Crohn's disease	
Acute or chronic appendicitis	
Herpes zoster	
Osteomyelitis	
Pelvic inflammatory disease (PID)	
Sexually transmitted infection	
Postpartum infection	
Vascular Disorders	
Arterial occlusion; ischemia	
Abdominal angina	
Abdominal aneurysm	
Pelvic congestion	
Varicosities or pelvic thrombophlebitis	
Cancer	
Gastrointestinal Disorders	
Inflammatory bowel disease (IBD)	
Crohn's disease	
Ulcerative colitis	
Irritable bowel syndrome (IBS)	
Diverticular disease	
Constipation (common in older adults)	
Neoplasm	
Hernia	
Urogenital	
Chronic urinary tract infection	
Interstitial cystitis	
Acute pyelonephritis	
Kidney stones (ureteric calculus)	
Chronic prostatitis, prostate cancer	

* The combined medical and physical therapy differential diagnosis includes many origins of pathokinesiologic conditions, including joint laxity; subluxations or displacements; thoracolumbar hypermobility; bursitis; osteoarthritis; spondyloarthropathy; fracture; and postural, ligamentous, or osteoporosis/osteomalacia. (This list is not exhaustive.)

† As with joint dysfunction, the differential diagnosis of muscle pathokinesiologic conditions can include many origins (e.g., trigger points, tendinous avulsion, strain/sprain/tear, weakness, loss of flexibility, hypertonus or hypotonus, diastasis recti).

TABLE 15-2 ▼ Causes of Pelvic Pain—cont'd

Systemic	Neuromuscular/musculoskeletal

Other
Psychogenic; somatization disorder
Trauma/sexual assault
Surgery (abdominal/laparoscopic, tubal, pelvic)
Fibromyalgia
Autonomic nervous system dysfunction
Paget's disease
Lead or mercury toxicity
Substance abuse (cocaine)
Sickle cell anemia

needed to complete the screening process. These questions are presented for all causes of pelvic pain at the end of this chapter.

History Associated With Pelvic Pain

With so many possible causes of pelvic pain, many different factors in the past medical history can raise a red flag. Pelvic pain is a very complex problem. Many medical texts are written about just this one anatomic area.

This text does not attempt to explain or discuss all the possible causes of pelvic pain. Rather, the intent is for the Reader to learn how to screen for the possibility of systemic or viscerogenic sources of pelvic pain or symptoms. With a good understanding of what is important in the history and a list of possible follow-up questions, the therapist assesses each client, keeping in mind that medical referral may be needed.

Some of the more common red flag histories associated with pelvic pain are listed in Box 15-4. With the use of categories from the medical screening model, risk factors, clinical presentation, and associated signs and symptoms also are listed.

Most conditions that affect the pelvic structures are found in women, but men may also experience pelvic floor dysfunction and pain. Sexual assault, anal intercourse, prostate or colon cancer, and sexually transmitted disease are the most common causes for men. Prostate problems such as benign prostatic hyperplasia (BPH) or prostatitis can cause lower abdominal, back, thigh, or pelvic pain.

Clinical Presentation

In the screening process, clinical presentation and especially pain patterns are very important. Mech-anisms of viscerogenic pain (i.e., how these patterns develop) are discussed in Chapter 3.

Pelvic pain may be visceral pain, caused by stimulation of autonomic nerves (T11 to S3); somatic pain, caused by stimulation of sensory nerve endings in the pudendal nerves (S2, S3); or peritoneal pain (pressure from inflammation, infection, or obstruction of the lining of the pelvic cavity).

Peritoneal pain may be caused by disruption of the autonomic nerve supply of the visceral pelvic peritoneum, which covers the upper third of the bladder, the body of the uterus, and the upper third of the rectum and the rectosigmoid junction. It is insensitive to touch but responds with pain on traction, distention, spasm, or ischemia of the viscus.

Peritoneal pain may also occur in relation to the parietal pelvic peritoneum, which covers the upper half of the lateral wall of the pelvis and the upper two thirds of the sacral hollow—all supplied by somatic nerves. These somatic nerves also supply corresponding segmental areas of skin and muscles of the trunk and the anterior abdominal wall. Painful stimulation of the parietal pelvic peritoneum may cause referred segmental pain and spasm of the iliopsoas muscle and muscles of the anterior abdominal wall.

Knowing the characteristics of pain patterns typical of each system is essential. When the client describes these patterns, it is possible for the therapist to recognize them for what they are and to see how the clinical presentation differs from neuromuscular or musculoskeletal impairment and dysfunction.

Pelvic disease may cause primary pelvic pain and may also refer pain to the low back, thigh,

BOX 15-4 ▼ Red Flags Associated with Pelvic Pain or Symptoms

History*

- History of reproductive, colon, or breast cancer
- History of dysmenorrhea, ovarian cysts, pelvic inflammatory disease, sexually transmitted disease
- Endometriosis
- Chronic bladder or urinary tract infections
- Chronic irritable bowel syndrome
- Previous history of pelvic/bladder surgeries, especially hysterectomy
- Recent abortion or miscarriage
- History of assault, incest, trauma
- History of prolonged labor; use of forceps or vacuum extraction during delivery
- History of multiple births
- Chronic yeast/vaginal infections
- History of varicose veins in the lower extremities (risk factor for pelvic congestion syndrome)

Risk Factors

- Recent intrauterine contraceptive device (rejection) or long-term use, especially without medical follow-up (scar tissue)
- Perimenopause, menopause (vaginitis)
- Sexual activity without use of a condom
- Multiple sexual partners
- Childbirth, recent abortion, multiple abortions

Clinical Presentation

- Poorly localized, diffuse; client unable to point to one spot
- Aggravated by increased intra-abdominal pressure (e.g., standing, walking, sexual intercourse, coughing, constipation, Valsalva's maneuver)
- Pelvic pain is not affected by specific movements but gets worse toward the end of the day or after standing for a long time
- May be temporarily relieved by position change (e.g., getting off feet, resting or elevating the legs, putting the feet up)
- Pelvic pain is not reduced or eliminated by scar or soft tissue mobilization or by trigger point release of myofascial structures in the pelvic cavity
- Positive McBurney's, Blumberg's, or iliopsoas/obturator sign (see Chapter 8)

Associated Signs and Symptoms

- Discharge from vagina or penis
- Urologic signs or symptoms
- Unreported abdominal pain
- Dyspareunia (painful or difficult intercourse)
- Constitutional symptoms
- Missed menses or unexplained/unexpected spotting (light staining of blood) (e.g., ectopic pregnancy) ask about shoulder pain
- Headache, fatigue, irritability

*Many of the histories listed here are also *risk factors* for pelvic pain.

groin, and rectum. Usually, pelvic disease appears as acute illness with sudden onset of severe pain accompanied by nausea and vomiting, fever, and abdominal pain. Mild to moderate back or pelvic pain that gets worse as the day progresses may be associated with gynecologic disorders. The therapist is more likely to see the atypical presentation of systemically related central lumbar and sacral pain, which is easily mistaken for mechanical pain.

Associated Signs and Symptoms

While collecting pertinent personal and family history, conducting a risk factor assessment, and evaluating the client's pain pattern, the therapist listens and looks for any yellow or red flags. From there, the therapist formulates any additional questions that may be appropriate on the basis of data collected so far. Before leaving the screening task, the therapist asks a few final questions. The first is about the presence of any associated signs and symptoms.

For example, perhaps the client has pelvic pain and unreported shoulder pain. She may not think her previously unreported shoulder pain has any connection with the current pelvic pain. Or, she may not see that the presence of a vaginal discharge is linked in any way to her low back and pelvic pain. Discharge from the vagina or penis (yellow or green, with or without an odor) in the presence of low back, pelvic, or sacral pain may be a red flag.

To bring this information out and make any of these connections, the therapist must ask about the presence of any associated signs and symptoms. Ask the client the following:

Follow-Up Questions

- Do you have any symptoms anywhere else in your body? Tell me even if you don't think they are related to your pelvic pain.

If the client says "No," then ask about the presence of urologic symptoms and constitutional symp-

toms, and look for a connection between the menstrual cycle and symptoms. If it appears that there may be a gynecologic basis for the client's symptoms, the therapist may want to ask some additional questions about missed menses, shoulder pain, and spotting or bleeding.

The therapist should assess for the presence of dysmenorrhea, defined as painful cramping during menstruation. Dysmenorrhea may be primary (of unknown cause) or secondary as a result of a pelvic pathologic condition related to endometriosis, intrauterine tumors or polyps (myomas), uterine prolapse, pelvic inflammatory disease, cervical stenosis, and adenomyosis (benign invasive growths of the endometrium into the muscular layers of the uterus).

Dysmenorrhea is characterized by spasmodic, cramp-like pain that comes and goes in waves and radiates over the lower abdomen and pelvis, thighs, and low back, sometimes accompanied by headache, irritability, mental depression, fatigue, and GI symptoms.

Screening for Neuromuscular and Musculoskeletal Causes of Pelvic Pain

The therapist is most likely to see pelvic pain caused by a neuromuscular or musculoskeletal problem. The therapist must remember that pelvic pain or symptoms may be referred from systemic or neuromusculoskeletal origins from the hip, SI joint, sacrum, or low back.

Likewise, pelvic diseases can refer pain and symptoms to the low back, groin, and thigh. When evaluating low back or pelvic pain, the therapist must assess for pelvic floor laxity or tension, psoas abscess, trigger points, history of birth or sexual trauma, and the presence of any associated signs and symptoms.

Neurologic disorders (e.g., nerve entrapment, incomplete spinal cord lesion, multiple sclerosis, Parkinson's, stroke, pudendal neuralgia) can cause pelvic pain and dysfunction. Pudendal nerve entrapment is characterized by pain relief when one is sitting on a toilet seat or standing; elimination of symptoms after a pudendal nerve block is diagnostic.

Pregnancy-related low back pain and pelvic pain are also common and have an impact on daily life for many women. Prevention and treatment of symptoms is an important issue for therapists who work in the area of women's health.[24]

Musculoskeletal dysfunction of the pelvic girdle and low back may manifest as dyspareunia (painful intercourse). Hypertonus of the pelvic floor and pelvic floor trigger points can contribute to entrance dyspareunia. Deep thrust dyspareunia may be related to SI or low back dysfunction. Dyspareunia symptoms that are reduced in alternate positions may indicate a musculoskeletal component, especially when other signs and symptoms characteristic of musculoskeletal dysfunction are also present.[25]

One of the most common musculoskeletal sources of pelvic pain is the trigger point. Muscles most likely to refer pain to the pelvic area include the abdominals, quadratus lumborum, and iliopsoas.[26]

Typical aggravating and relieving factors for pain from a neuromuscular or musculoskeletal source include the following:

• Aggravated by exercise, weight bearing
• Aggravated by trunk/lumbar rotation
• Relieved by rest or stretching
• Pain or altered movement pattern produced by trunk and lumbar rotation
• Eliminated by trigger point therapy

The therapist looks for a contributing history such as a fall on the buttocks, pregnancy, or trauma. Avulsion of hamstrings from a sports injury may be reported. Trauma from physical or sexual assault may remain unreported. Screening for assault is an important part of many evaluations (see Chapter 2).

The therapist also looks for muscle impairment. For therapists trained in pelvic floor palpation, external and internal palpation of the pelvic floor musculature is helpful.[27] Examination includes observation for varicosities and assessment of muscle tone and the presence of trigger points.[26,28,29] Many clients who experience low back, pelvic, SI, sacral, or groin pain have unrecognized pelvic floor dysfunction.

Fig. 15-2 gives a simple representation of how the puborectalis muscle acts as a sling around various structures of the pelvis. The condition and position of the pelvic sling are very important in the maintenance of normal pelvic floor health.

Fig. 14-1 provides a visual reminder that the muscles of the pelvic floor support the reproductive organs and the viscera in the peritoneum. Any impairment of these organs may cause dysfunction of the pelvic floor and vice versa. Any weakness or dysfunction of the pelvic floor can lead to problems with the viscera located in the abdominal or pelvic cavities.

Anterior Pelvic Pain

Anterior pelvic pain occurs most often as a result of any disorder that affects the hip joint, including inflammatory arthritis; upper lumbar vertebrae

cygeal regions usually appears as localized pain in the lower lumbar spine and over the sacrum, often radiating over the sacroiliac ligaments. Pain radiating from the sacroiliac joint can commonly be felt in both the buttock and the posterior thigh and is often aggravated by rotation of the lumbar spine on the pelvis. A proximal hamstring injury, including avulsion of the ischial epiphysis in the adolescent, may also cause posterior pelvic and buttock pain.

Coccydynial and sacrococcygeal pain is a common presentation in women and is often associated with a fall on the buttocks or traumatic childbirth. It manifests with the person having difficulty sitting on firm surfaces and having pain in the coccygeal region on defecation or straining.

Levator ani syndrome and tension myalgia may produce symptoms of pain, pressure, and discomfort in the rectum, vagina, perirectal area, or low back and can mimic a discogenic problem. Spasm and tenderness in the levator ani may occur in men and women and may be caused by birthing trauma (women), neurologic abnormalities in the lumbosacral spine, sexual assault or sexual trauma, or anal fissures from anal intercourse. Pain or rectal pressure may occur during sexual intercourse, as may throbbing pain during bowel movement with accompanying constipation and impaired bowel and bladder function.

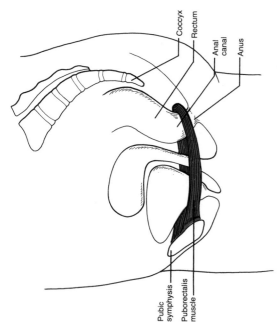

Fig. 15-2 • Pelvic sling. Puborectalis muscle forms a U-shaped sling encircling the posterior aspect of the rectum and returns along the opposite side of the levator hiatus to the posterior surface of the pubis. This shows how the condition and position of the pelvic sling contribute to the function of the pelvic floor and the encircled viscera. Obesity, multiparity, and prolonged pushing during labor and delivery are just a few of life's events that can disrupt the integrity of the pelvic sling and the pelvic floor. (From Myers RS: *Saunders manual of physical therapy practice*, Philadelphia, 1995, WB Saunders.)

Posterior Pelvic Pain

Posterior pelvic pain originating in the lumbosacral, sacroiliac, coccydynial, and sacrococ-

(disc disease is rare at these segments); pregnancy with separation of the symphysis pubis; local injury to the insertion of the rectus abdominis, rectus femoris, or adductor muscle; femoral neuralgia; and psoas abscess.

Stress reactions of the pubis or ilium, sometimes called stress fractures, can occur during traumatic labor and delivery, but they are more common in osteomalacia and Paget's disease and produce anterior pelvic pain. Traumatic stress reactions may also occur in joggers, military personnel, athletes, and pregnant women during delivery. Symptoms may include pain in the involved areas that is aggravated by active motion of the limb or deep pressure and weight bearing during ambulation.

Femoral hernia, which accounts for 20% of hernias in women, may cause lateral wall pelvic pain when the hernia strangulates. The referred pain pattern is located down the medial side of the thigh to the knee; inguinal hernias are likely to cause groin pain. Immediate surgical repair is indicated.

Screening for Gynecologic Causes of Pelvic Pain

Pregnancy, multiparity, and prolonged labor and delivery (especially combined with obesity) are risk factors for gynecologic conditions that can alter the normal position of the bladder, uterus, and rectum in relation to one another (Fig. 15-3), resulting in problems such as rectocele, cystocele, and prolapsed uterus with concomitant pelvic floor pain and dysfunction.

Gynecologic causes of pelvic pain are most often produced by congenital anomaly, inflammatory processes (including infection), neoplasia, or trauma. In addition, pelvic pain may be associated with pregnancy, endometriosis, and altered uterine position (Fig. 15-4). Variations in the angle and position of the uterus occur from woman to woman. Many women are unaware of their uterine position. Only if the physician tells her, "You have a tipped uterus," or "You have a retroverted uterus," will she know whether any change from the normal position of the uterus has occurred. Other women experience extreme pain associated with the menstrual cycle, which may be linked with uterine position.

Children younger than 14 years rarely experience pelvic pain of gynecologic origin. Infection is the most likely cause and is limited to the vulva and vagina. Theoretically, infection can ascend to involve the peritoneal cavity, causing iliopsoas abscess and pelvic, hip, or groin pain, but this rarely happens in this age group.

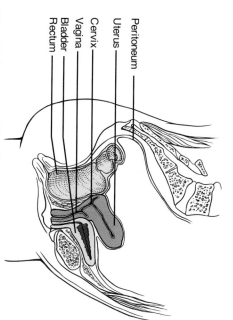

Fig. 15-3 • Normal female reproductive anatomy (sagittal view). Locate the rectum, uterus, bladder, vagina, and cervix in this illustration. Note the size, shape, and orientation of each of these structures. The rectum turns away from the viewer in this sagittal section, giving it the appearance of ending with no connection to the intestines. Understanding the normal orientation of these structures will help when each of the diseases that can cause low back pain is considered.

Peritoneum
Uterus
Cervix
Vagina
Bladder
Rectum

Pregnancy

Pelvic pain associated with normal pregnancy is similar to low back pain, as was discussed earlier in Chapter 14. About 1% of all pregnancies take place outside the endometrium (or ectopic), with most ectopic implantations occurring in the fallopian tube (Fig. 15-5). Risk factors include tubal ligation; sexually transmitted disease; pelvic inflammatory disease; infertility or infertility treatment; previous tubal, pelvic, or abdominal surgery; or the use of an intrauterine contraceptive device (IUCD; rings, loops, coils, or Ts) (see Fig. 14-6).

Symptoms of ectopic pregnancy most often include unexplained vaginal spotting, bursts of bleeding, and sudden lower abdominal and pelvic cramping shortly after the first missed menstrual period. At first, the pain may be a vague "twinge" or soreness on the affected side; later it can be sharp and severe.

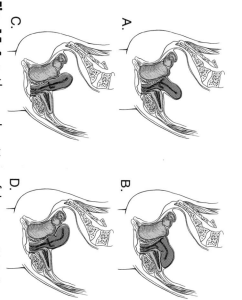

Fig. 15-4 • Abnormal positions of the uterus. Variations in the angle and position of the uterus occur from woman to woman. Each illustration depicts a slightly different anatomic position of the uterus. **A**, Midline position. Usually, the uterus is above and parallel to the bladder. In the midline position, the uterus is more vertical. **B**, Anteflexed uterus. The uterus is in its proper position above the bladder, but the upper one-third to one-half of the body is flexed forward. **C**, Retroverted uterus. About 20% of American women have a tilted, or retroverted, uterus. The top of the uterus naturally slants toward the spine rather than toward the umbilicus. An extremely tilted uterus called retroflexion may even bend down toward the tailbone. A woman with a retroflexed uterus may be unable to use a tampon or a diaphragm. Back pain is more likely to occur with pregnancy and labor for the woman with a retroverted or retroflexed uterus.

A.

B.

C.

D.

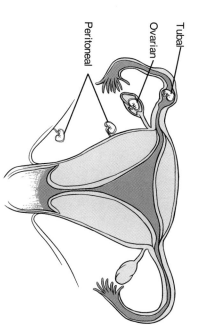

Fig. 15-5 • Ectopic pregnancy. An ectopic pregnancy can occur when the egg is fertilized and implanted outside the uterus. The ovum can be embedded inside the ovary (ovarian pregnancy), inside the fallopian tube (tubal pregnancy), or anywhere between the ovary and the uterus, including along the outside lining of the uterus (extrauterine) or inside the abdominal cavity along the peritoneum as shown. Rupture of the ovum and hemorrhage is the usual result. If this occurs early in the menstrual cycle, the woman may experience heavier bleeding than usual but remain unaware of the failed pregnancy.

Tubal
Ovarian
Peritoneal

Gradual hemorrhage causes pelvic (and sometimes low back or shoulder) pain and pressure, but rapid hemorrhage results in hypotension or shock. Tubal rupture is common and requires medical attention and diagnosis.

Clinical Signs and Symptoms of
Ectopic Pregnancy

- Unexplained vaginal bleeding (spotting), missed menses
- Sudden, unexplained lower abdominal and pelvic cramping (especially after first missed menstrual period); usually unilateral
- Pain may be mild, progressing to severe over a matter of hours to days
- Low back (unilateral or bilateral) or shoulder pain (unilateral)
- Hypotension (low blood pressure and pulse rate), shock (tubal rupture)

Prolapsed Conditions

Prolapse is the collapse, falling down, or downward displacement of structures such as the uterus, bladder, or rectum. A pelvic examination is performed by a physician or other trained professional, such as a physical therapist, to identify prolapse (Fig. 15-6).

Uterovaginal prolapse can cause low-grade and persistent pelvic pain. Prolapse may result from a combination of basic anatomic structure, effects of pregnancy and labor, postmenopausal hormone deficiency, and poor general muscular fitness. Pelvic floor tension myalgia and prolapse often occur together. Obesity combined with chronic cough, constipation, and multiparity is a common contributing factor to pelvic floor problems.

UTERINE PROLAPSE

Uterine prolapse occurs most often after childbirth and is graded as first, second, or third degree prolapse (Fig. 15-7). Secondary prolapse may occur with prolonged pushing during labor and delivery, large intrapelvic tumors, or sacral nerve disorders, or it may follow surgical resection.

The pain of prolapse is central, suprapubic, and dragging in the groin, and a sensation of a lump at the vaginal opening is noted. Pain is primarily due to stretching of the ligamentous supports and secondarily to excoriation (scratch or abrasion) of the prolapsed cervical or vaginal tissue, which may occur.

Third degree prolapse is often accompanied by low back pain with or without pelvic, sacral, or abdominal cramping and heaviness. Symptoms are relieved by rest and lying down and are often aggravated by prolonged standing, walking, coughing, sexual intercourse, or straining. Urinary incontinence is commonly associated with uterine prolapse.

Sexual intercourse is possible because the soft tissues of the uterus and vagina can be pushed or pressed out of the way. However, excoriation (scratching or abrasion) of the tissue may occur, accompanied by bleeding and local pain. Care must be taken when anything is inserted into the vagina. Excessive, repetitive force should be avoided.

Some women use a removable device called a pessary for a prolapsed uterus or rectum. It is placed in the vagina to support the prolapsed structure. These devices are usually considered temporary and should be used in conjunction with a program to rehabilitate the pelvic floor dysfunction.

Identifying the presence of uterine prolapse does not necessarily require medical referral. Conservative care such as a program of pelvic floor recovery and management of sexual intercourse can be very helpful for the woman and may be the first step in treatment. Client education about positions in which gravity is used to assist the uterus in resuming its normal position can be very helpful.

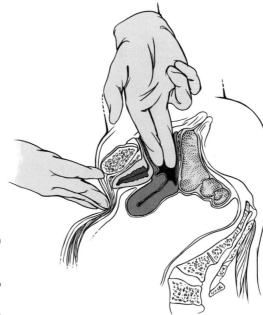

Fig. 15-6 • Pelvic examination. With the woman in the lithotomy position (supine with hips and knees flexed and feet in stirrups), the examiner inserts one or two gloved fingers into the vaginal canal up to the point of the cervix or soft tissue obstruction. The examiner applies firm pressure in the lower abdomen above the bladder while the woman bears down slightly as if performing a Valsalva maneuver. The examiner evaluates the tone of the pelvic floor and the position of the uterus during this test. Integrity of the pelvic floor (e.g., muscle tone, laxity, trigger points) can also be tested.

For example, supine with a pillow or wedge support under the pelvis is a helpful rest position and can be used while the patient is doing pelvic floor exercises. It is also a more comfortable position for sexual intercourse for some women.

Clinical Signs and Symptoms of
Uterine Prolapse

* Lump in vaginal opening
* Pelvic discomfort, backache
* Abdominal cramping
* Symptoms relieved by lying down
* Symptoms made worse by prolonged standing, walking, coughing, or straining
* Urinary incontinence

CYSTOCELE AND RECTOCELE

Cystocele is the protrusion or herniation of the urinary bladder against the wall of the vagina. Rectocele is a protrusion or herniation of the rectum and posterior wall of the vagina into the vagina (Fig. 15-8).

Similar to the prolapsed uterus, these two pelvic floor disorders occur most often after pregnancy and childbirth but may also be associated with surgery and obesity (especially obesity combined with multiple pregnancies and births). These conditions are the result of pelvic floor relaxation or structural overstretching of the pelvic musculature or ligamentous structures. Patient history may include prolonged labor, bearing down before full dilation, forceful delivery of the placenta, instrument delivery (e.g., forceps, vacuum suction), chronic cough, or lifting of heavy objects.

Trauma to the pudendal or sacral nerves during birth and delivery is an additional risk factor. Decreased muscle tone due to aging, complications of pelvic surgery, or excessive straining during bowel movements may also result in prolapse. Pelvic tumors and neurologic conditions such as spina bifida and diabetic neuropathy, which interrupt the innervation of pelvic muscles, can also increase the risk of prolapse.

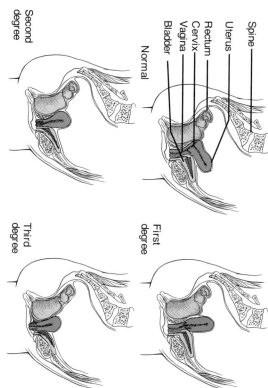

Fig. 15-7 • Uterine prolapse. First-degree *prolapse* (in vagina): the uterus has dropped up to one-third of the way into the vaginal canal. *Second-degree prolapse* (vaginal introitus): the uterus has descended fully into the vaginal canal, right down to the vaginal opening. Third-degree *prolapse* (outside vagina): the uterus is displaced downward even further and bulges outside the vaginal opening.

Spine
Uterus
Rectum
Cervix
Vagina
Bladder

Normal
First degree
Second degree
Third degree

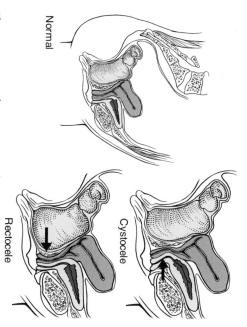

Normal
Rectocele
Cystocele

Fig. 15-8 • Pelvic organ prolapse. Cystocele. The arrow shows displacement of the bladder against the vaginal canal. Rectocele. The uterus and bladder are in their proper anatomic place, but the rectum has prolapsed and is compressing against the vaginal canal. Many women have both conditions at the same time as a result of pregnancy and childbirth.

Clinical Signs and Symptoms of

Cystocele

- Urinary frequency and urgency
- Difficulty emptying the bladder
- Cystitis (bladder infection)
- Painful lump or bearing down sensation in the perineal area
- Urinary stress incontinence

Rectocele

- Pelvic, perineal pain and difficulty with defecation
- Feeling of incomplete rectal emptying
- Constipation
- Painful intercourse
- Aching or pressure after a bowel movement

Endometriosis

Endometriosis (see Chapter 14) is a pathologic condition of retrograde menstruation. Tissue resembling the mucous membrane lining the uterus occurs outside the normal location in the uterus but within the pelvic cavity, including the ovaries, pelvic peritoneum, bowel, and diaphragm. It occurs most often during the reproductive years and in up to 50% of women with infertility.[30,31] Severity of pain is related more to the site than to the extent of disease.

Pelvic pain associated with endometriosis can be referred to the low back, rectum, and lower sacral or coccygeal region, starting before or after the onset of menstruation and improving after cessation of menstrual flow, with cyclic recurrence. As the condition progresses, pain continues throughout the cycle, with exacerbation at menstruation and, finally, constant severity.

Other symptoms may include rectal discomfort during bowel movements, diarrhea, constipation, recurrent miscarriage, and infertility. See Box 15-5 for more information on this condition.

Gynecalgia

Although a pathologic cause can be identified for most cases of chronic pelvic pain, a small percentage remains for which no physical cause can be determined, and the term gynecalgia is used. Women with gynecalgia syndrome are usually 25 to 40 years of age and have at least one child. The symptoms are of at least 2 years' duration (and often many more), with acute exacerbation from time to time.

Pain associated with gynecalgia is vague and poorly localized, although it is usually confined to the lower abdomen and pelvis, radiating to the groin and upper and inner thighs. Other symptoms include dyspareunia, menstrual changes, low back pain, urinary and bowel changes, fatigue, and obvious anxiety and depression.

Screening for Infectious Causes of Pelvic Pain

Infection is the most common cause of systemically induced pelvic pain. Infection or inflammation within the pelvis from acute appendicitis, diverticulitis, Crohn's disease, osteomyelitis, septic arthritis of the SI joint, urologic disorders, sexually transmitted infection (e.g., *Chlamydia* trachomatis), and salpingitis (inflammation of the fallopian tube) can produce visceral and somatic pelvic pain because of the involvement of the parietal peritoneum.

Secondary pelvic infection may follow surgery, septic abortion, pregnancy, or recent birth as a result of the entry of endogenous bacteria into the damaged pelvic tissues. Pelvic inflammatory disease (PID) and sexually transmitted infection are the most common causes of infection in women.

All these disorders have similar signs and symptoms during the acute phase. The client may not have any pain but will report low back or pelvic "discomfort," or there may be a report of acute, sharp, severe aching on both sides of the pelvis. Accompanying groin discomfort may radiate to the inner aspects of the thigh.

Keep in mind that in the older adult, the first sign of any infection might not be an elevated temperature, but rather, confusion, increased confusion, or some other change in mental status.

Right-sided abdominal or pelvic inflammatory pain is often associated with appendicitis, whereas left-sided pain is more likely associated with diverticulitis. Bilateral pain may indicate infection. The pain may be aggravated by increased abdominal pressure (e.g., coughing, walking). Knowing these pain patterns helps the therapist quickly decide what questions to ask and which associated signs and symptoms to look for. The therapist should test for iliopsoas or obturator abscesses (see Chapter 8).

Other red flag symptoms may be reported in response to specific questions about disturbances in urination, odorous vaginal discharge, tachycardia, dyspareunia (painful or difficult intercourse), or constitutional symptoms such as fever, general malaise, and nausea and vomiting.

Pelvic Inflammatory Disease

PID consists of a variety of conditions (i.e., it is not a single entity), including endometritis, salpingitis,

BOX 15-5 ▲ Resources

Endometriosis*

- Endometriosis Zone, a service of The Universe of Women's Health—a commercial organization directed by a board of obstetricians and gynecologists. Information is directed at medical professionals, the medical industry, and women. The Endometriosis Zone is found at both of the following Web links:
  http://www.endozone.org
  http://www.endometriosiszone.org

- Endometriosis Research Center was started as a lobbying organization. The goal of the ERC is to bring science and support together through education.
  http://www.endocenter.org or call (800) 239-7280.

- The International Endometriosis Association (IEA)
  The IEA was established by Mary Lou Ballweg, RN, PhD, as an advocacy organization for endometriosis; offers online support for women diagnosed with endometriosis.
  http://www.endometriosisassn.org

- The National Library of Medicine offers an interactive tutorial about endometriosis in both English and Spanish at:
  http://www.nlm.nih.gov/medlineplus/tutorials/endometriosis

Pelvic Inflammatory Disease (PID)

- The National Women's Health Information Center (NWHIC) offers information on all aspects of women's health, including PID; (1-800-994-9662) or online at:
  http://www.4woman.gov/

- Centers for Disease Control and Prevention provides a PID Fact Sheet:
  http://www.cdc.gov/std/PID/STDFact-PID.htm

- Mount Auburn Obstetrics & Gynecologic Associates, Cincinnati, Ohio, a group of obstetric and gynecologic (OBGYN) professionals; offering online education about endometriosis and other OBGYN topics:
  http://www.mtauburnobgyn.com/pid.html

Pelvic Pain

- The American College of Obstetricians and Gynecologists (ACOG) offers information, education, and publications related to a wide variety of women's health issues:
  http://www.acog.org/
  The ACOG has recently issued a new practice bulletin on chronic pelvic pain in women. The guidelines were published as: ACOG Practice Bulletin No. 51. Chronic Pelvic Pain in Obstetrics and Gynecology 103(3):589-605, 2004. To read more about these guidelines, go to:
  http://www.medscape.com/viewarticle/471545
  The International Pelvic Pain Society is a professional organization with the goal to enhance and improve the treatment of diseases that cause pelvic pain in men and women. Education for health care professionals is a major focus of this organization, which can be reached at:
  http://www.pelvicpain.org/

* Data from Deevey S: Endometriosis: Internet resources. Med Ref Serv Q 24(1):67-77, Spring 2005.

---

tubo-ovarian abscess, and pelvic peritonitis. Any inflammatory condition that affects the female reproductive organs (uterus, fallopian tubes, ovaries, cervix) may come under the diagnostic label of PID.

PID is a bacterial infection that occurs whenever the uterus is traumatized; it is often associated with sexually transmitted infection/disease (STI/STD) and may occur after birth or after an abortion. Infection can be introduced from the skin, vagina, or GI tract. It can be an acute, one-time episode or may be chronic with multiple recurrences.

It is estimated that two-thirds of all cases are caused by STIs such as *chlamydia* and *gonorrhea*.[32] *Chlamydia* is a bacterial sexually transmitted infection that is acquired through vaginal, oral, or anal intercourse. It is often asymptomatic but can present with vaginal bleeding and discharge and burning during urination. Pelvic pain does not occur until *chlamydia* leads to PID. When detected and treated early, *chlamydia* is relatively easy to cure.

A direct relationship has been observed between early age of first sexual intercourse, the number of sexual partners a woman has, and the risk of STD (especially human papillomavirus, or HPV, a risk factor for cervical cancer).[33,34] PID may occur if *chlamydia* is not treated; even if it is treated, damage to the pelvic cavity cannot be reversed. The more partners a woman has, the greater is the risk of PID.

If it progresses to PID, scarring in the pelvic organs, including the ovaries, fallopian tubes, bowel, and bladder, may cause chronic pain. Women can be left infertile because of damage and scarring to the fallopian tubes. After a single episode of PID, a woman's risk of ectopic pregnancy

increases sevenfold compared with the risk for women who have no history of PID.[35,36]

Clinical Signs and Symptoms of
Pelvic Inflammatory Disease

- Often asymptomatic
- Vaginal discharge or bleeding
- Burning on urination (dysuria)
- Moderate (dull aching) to severe abdominal and/or pelvic pain; back pain is possible
- Painful intercourse (dyspareunia)
- Painful menstruation
- Constitutional symptoms (fever, chills, nausea, vomiting)

STIs such as *chlamydia* and *syphilis* are on the rise among America's sexually active young adult population (ages 18 to 25). In fact, *chlamydia* was the most commonly reported infectious disease in the United States in 2004. According to the Centers for Disease Control (CDC) annual report, the highest rates of *chlamydia* occur in sexually active women ages 15 to 19. Syphilis predominates in homosexual men (men having sex with men) who engage in risky sexual behavior (e.g., unprotected oral sex).[36-38]

It does not happen often, but there may be times when the therapist must ask about the possibility of an STI. Sexually active women with vague symptoms are the most likely group to be interviewed about STIs/STDs. See specific screening questions in Chapter 14 and Appendix B-29.

Any of the red flags listed in Box 15-4 in the presence of pelvic pain raises the suspicion of a medical problem. Medical referral must be made as quickly as possible. Early medical intervention can prevent the spread of infection and septicemia, and can preserve fertility. Damage to the pelvic floor from any of these conditions can result in pelvic floor dysfunction that is within the scope of a physical therapist's practice. See Box 15-5 for resources that can provide more information on this and other conditions.

Screening for Vascular Causes of Pelvic Pain

Vascular problems that affect the pelvic cavity and pelvic floor musculature have two primary causes. The first is the general condition of peripheral vascular disease (PVD); the second is a specific example of PVD called pelvic congestion syndrome from ovarian varicoceles. Other conditions such as abdominal angina and abdominal aneurysm are less common vascular causes of pelvic pain; these

conditions are discussed in greater detail in Chapter 6.

Peripheral Vascular Disease

The iliac arteries may become gradually occluded by atherosclerosis or may be obstructed by an embolus. The resultant ischemia produces pain in the affected limb but may also give rise to pelvic pain. Whether the occlusion is thrombotic or embolic, the client may report pain in the pelvis, affected limb, and possibly the buttocks.

The pain is characteristically aggravated by exercise (claudication). Typically, symptoms develop 5 or 10 minutes after the client has started the activity. This lag time is characteristic of a vascular pain pattern associated with atherosclerosis or blood vessel occlusion.

Musculoskeletal causes of pelvic pain are also made worse by activity and exercise, especially weight-bearing exercise, but the timing is not as predictable as with pain from vascular causes. Musculoskeletal conditions may cause pain immediately (e.g., with muscle strain or trigger points) or, more likely, after prolonged activity or exercise. The affected limb becomes colder and paler. In sudden occlusion, diminished sensation to pinprick may be observed on examination. Femoral and distal arteries should be palpated for pulsation.

Thrombosis of the large iliac veins may occur spontaneously after injury to the lower limb and pelvis, or it may appear after pelvic surgical procedures. An estimated 30% of clients have asymptomatic deep vein thrombosis after major surgery. Thrombosis that occludes the iliac vein produces an enlarged, warm, and painful leg; occasionally, discomfort in the pelvis is noted.

Anyone with PVD can demonstrate the same kind of symptoms in the pelvic floor structures. The most likely age group to be affected by vascular disease is adults over 60, especially women who are postmenopausal.

Watch for a history of heart disease with a clinical presentation of pelvic, buttock, and leg pain that is aggravated by activity or exercise (claudication). Look for changes in skin and temperature on the affected side (arterial occlusion or venous thrombosis), especially in the presence of known heart disease or recent pelvic surgery (see Box 4-12; see Case Example 15-2).

Pelvic Congestion Syndrome

Varicose veins of the ovaries (varicosities) cause the blood in the veins to flow downward rather than up toward the heart. They are a manifesta-

CASE EXAMPLE 15-2 Pelvic and Buttock Pain

A 34-year-old man with leukemia had a routine bone marrow biopsy near the left posterior superior iliac crest. No problems were noted at the time of biopsy, but 2 days later, the man came into physical therapy complaining of pelvic pain.

He said his platelet count was 50,000/uL and international normalized ratio (INR, a measure of clotting time) was "normal." Laboratory values were recorded on the day of the biopsy.

The only clinical findings were a positive Faber's (Patrick's) test on the left and tenderness to palpation over the left sciatic notch, about an inch below the biopsy site. No abnormal neurologic signs were observed.

What are the red flags in this scenario?
Use the screening model to find the red flags and decide what to do.

History: Current history of cancer; recent history of biopsy

Clinical Presentation: Reduced platelet count (normal is >100,000); new onset of painful symptoms within 48 hours of biopsy; tenderness to palpation in left buttock

Associated Signs and Symptoms: None. Client had no other signs and symptoms.

The therapist has to make a clinical judgment in a case like this. The platelet level is low, putting the client at risk for poor clotting and spontaneous bleeding, but the INR suggests that the body is able to initiate the coagulation cascade.

Given the timing between the biopsy and the symptoms, it is likely that the procedure caused an intramuscular hematoma. The diagnosis can be made with a computed tomography scan. The location of biopsy needle entry indicates that the gluteus medius was punctured. No major blood vessel is located in this area, so the problem is rare.

Pain after bone marrow biopsy is usually mild to moderate and gradually gets better. The use of ice, massage, and, later, moist heat is safe when properly applied. Worsening buttock pain over the next 24 to 48 hours would necessitate a medical referral.

It is always a good idea to contact the primary care physician and report your findings and intended intervention. This gives the doctor the option of following up with the client immediately if he or she thinks it is warranted.

---

tion of PVD and a potential cause of chronic pelvic pain. The condition has been called pelvic congestion syndrome (PCS) or ovarian varicocele.

The specific impairment associated with PCS is an incompetent and dilated ovarian vein with retrograde blood flow (Fig. 15-9). Venous stasis produces congestion and pelvic pain. Imaging studies have verified the fact that very few venous valves are found in the blood vessels of the pelvic area.[39-41]

Any compromise of the valves (or blood vessels) in the area can lead to this condition. It can also occur as the result of kidney removal or donation because the ovarian vein is cut when the kidney is removed. Varicosity of the gonadal venous plexus can occur in men and is more readily diagnosed by the presentation of observable varicosities of the scrotum.

Many women are unaware that they have this problem and remain asymptomatic. Women of childbearing age are affected most often. Many have had three or four (or more) pregnancies and are 40 years old or older.

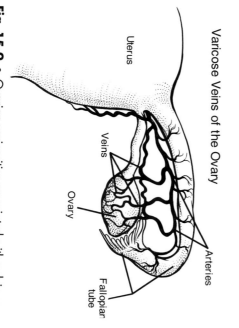

Varicose Veins of the Ovary

Uterus

Veins

Ovary

Arteries

Fallopian tube

Fig. 15-9 • Ovarian varicosities associated with pelvic congestion syndrome are the cause of chronic pelvic pain for women. This form of venous insufficiency is often accompanied by prominent varicose veins elsewhere in the lower quadrant (buttocks, thighs, calves). Men may have similar varicosities of the scrotum (not shown).

Symptoms of ovarian varicosities reflect the vascular incompetence associated with venous insufficiency. These symptoms include pelvic pain that worsens toward the end of the day or after standing for a long time, pain after intercourse, sensation of heaviness in the pelvis, and prominent varicose veins elsewhere on the body, especially the buttocks and thighs.[39,42]

Clinical Signs and Symptoms of

Pelvic Congestion Syndrome (Ovarian varicosities)

- Lower abdominal/pelvic pain (intermittent or continuous, described as "dull aching" but can be sharp and severe)
- Unilateral or bilateral
- Pain that worsens with prolonged standing or at the end of the day
- Pain that is worse before or during menses
- Pain or "aching" that occurs after intercourse (dyspareunia)
- Presence of varicose veins in the buttocks, thighs, or lower extremities
- Low backache is a common feature, made worse by standing
- Other associated signs and symptoms (these vary; see text below)

Other associated symptoms may vary and include vaginal discharge, headache, emotional distress, GI distress, constipation, and urinary frequency and urgency. An undetermined number of women also have endometriosis, but the relationship is unknown.[43] Varicosities may be large enough to compress the ureter, leading to these urologic symptoms. Fatigue (loss of energy) and insomnia are common in women who experience headache with PCS (Case Example 15-3).

Medical treatment for pelvic congestion syndrome is under investigation. To date, analgesics, hormone therapy, and ovarian vein ligation or embolization have been used with some success.

Screening for Cancer as a Cause of Pelvic Pain

The female pelvis is a depository for malignant tissue after incomplete removal of a primary carcinoma within the pelvis, for recurrence of cancer after surgical resection or radiotherapy of a pelvic neoplasm, or for metastatic deposits from a primary lesion elsewhere in the abdominal cavity.

Metastatic spread can occur from any primary tumor in the abdominal or pelvic cavity (see Fig. 13-2). For example, colon cancer can metastasize to the pelvic cavity by direct extension through the bowel wall to the musculoskeletal walls of the pelvic cavity or to surrounding organs. This may produce fistulas into the small intestine, bladder, or vagina. Advanced rectal tumors can become "fixed" to the sacral hollow. Deep pain within the

---

pelvis may indicate spread of neoplasm into the sacral nerve plexuses.

Cancer recurrence can also occur after radiotherapy or surgery to the abdominal or pelvic cavity. This happens most often when incomplete removal of the primary carcinoma has occurred.

Using the Screening Model for Cancer

In the case of cancer as a cause of pelvic pain, a *past history* of cancer is usually present, most commonly, cancer within the pelvic or abdominal cavity (e.g., GI, renal, reproductive). A history of cancer with recent surgical removal of tumor tissue followed by back, hip, sacral, or pelvic pain within the next 6 months is a major red flag. Even if it appears to be a clear neuromuscular or musculoskeletal problem, referral is warranted for medical evaluation.

A common *clinical presentation* of pelvic or abdominal cancer referred to the soma is one of back, sacral, or pelvic pain described as one or more of the following: deep aching, colicky, constant with crescendo waves of pain that come and go, or diffuse pain. Usually, the client cannot point to it with one finger (i.e., pain does not localize).

The therapist must remember to ask whether the client is having any symptoms of any kind anywhere else in the body. This is vitally important! Signs and symptoms associated with pelvic pain can range from constitutional symptoms to symptoms more common with the GI, GU, or reproductive system.

The therapist must ask about blood in the urine or stools. Once the physical therapy examination has been completed, including the history, risk factor assessment, pain patterns, and any associated signs and symptoms, it is time to step back and conduct a Review of Systems (see Chapters 1 and 4).

The *Review of Systems* is part of the evaluation described in the Guide's Elements of Patient/Client Management that leads to optimal outcomes (see Fig. 1-4). It is part of the dynamic process in which the therapist makes clinical judgments on the basis of data gathered during the examination.

In the screening process, the therapist reviews the following:

- Do any red flags in the history or clinical presentation suggest a systemic origin of symptoms?
- Are any red flags associated signs and symptoms?
- What additional screening tests or questions are needed (if any)?

- Is referral to another health care provider needed, or is the therapist clear to proceed with a planned intervention (Case Example 15-4)?

Keep in mind the Clues Suggesting Systemic Pelvic Pain, which are listed at the end of this chapter. If hip or groin pain is an accompanying feature with pelvic pain, review Clues Suggesting Systemic Hip and Groin Pain (see Chapter 16); likewise for anyone with pelvic and back pain (see Clues Suggesting Systemic Back Pain [Chapter 14]).

The therapist can use the Special Questions to Ask at the end of Chapter 14. It may not be necessary to ask all these questions. The therapist can use the overall clues gathered from the *history, risk factor assessment, clinical presentation, and associated signs and symptoms*, while reviewing the list of special questions to see whether there is anything appropriate to ask the individual client.

Gynecologic Cancers

Cancers of the female genital tract account for about 12% of all new cancers diagnosed in women. Although gynecologic cancers are the fourth leading cause of death from cancer in women in the United States, most of these cancers are highly curable when detected early. The most common cancers of the female genital tract are uterine endometrial cancer, ovarian cancer, and cervical cancer.[44]

ENDOMETRIAL (UTERINE) CANCER

Cancer of the uterine endometrium, or lining of the uterus, is the most common gynecologic cancer, usually occurring in postmenopausal women between the ages of 50 and 70 years. Its occurrence is associated with obesity, endometrial hyperplasia, prolonged unopposed estrogen therapy (hormone replacement therapy without progesterone), and, more recently, tamoxifen used in the treatment of breast cancer.[45,46]

Clinical Signs and Symptoms Seventy-five percent of all cases of endometrial cancer occur in postmenopausal women. The most common symptom is abnormal vaginal bleeding or discharge at presentation. However, 25% of these cancers occur in premenopausal women, and 5% occur in women younger than 40 years.

In a physical therapy practice, the most common presenting compliant is pelvic pain without abnormal vaginal bleeding. Abdominal pain, weight loss, and fatigue may occur but remain unreported. Unexpected or unexplained vaginal bleeding in a woman taking tamoxifen (chemoprevention for breast cancer) is a red flag sign. Tamoxifen

CASE EXAMPLE 15-4 Peripheral Neuropathy of the Pelvic Floor

A 57-year-old woman presented with an unusual triad of symptoms. She reported numbness and tingling of the feet, urinary incontinence, and migrating arthralgias and myalgias of the lower body (e.g., low back or hip, sometimes hip adductor spasm or aching, a "heavy" sensation in the pelvic region).

Past Medical History: Significant previous medical history included a hysterectomy 10 years ago for uncontrolled bleeding, and oophorectomy 2 years ago followed by pelvic radiation for ovarian cancer.

She is a nonsmoker and a nondrinker and is in apparent good health after cancer treatment. She is not taking any medications or using any drugs or supplements. All follow-up checks have detected no signs of cancer recurrence. She is active in a women's cancer support group and exercises 4 or 5 times a week.

She has kept a journal of activities, foods, and symptoms but cannot find a pattern to explain any of her symptoms. Urinary incontinence is present continually with constant dripping and leaking. It is not made worse by exercise, the sound or feel of running water, putting the key in the door, or other triggers of urge or stress incontinence.

Bowel function is reportedly "normal." The client is a widow and is not currently sexually active.

Where do you go from here? What are the red flags? What questions do you ask? What tests do you perform? Is medical referral needed?

Red Flags

- Age
- Previous history of cancer
- Bilateral symptoms (numbness and tingling in both feet)

Screening Questions

Menstrual history, including pregnancies, miscarriages or abortions, births; current menstrual status (perimenopausal, postmenopausal, hormone replacement therapy)
Any symptoms or other problems anywhere else in the body?

Screening Tests

Can you reproduce any of the muscle or joint pain?

Neurologic screen: Besides the usual manual muscle testing, deep tendon reflexes, and sensation, the therapist should test for lower extremity proprioception and assess feet more closely to identify the level of peripheral nerve dysfunction.

- Ask about the presence of other neurologic symptoms such as headache, muscle weakness, confusion, depression, irritability, blurred vision, balance/coordination problems, memory changes, and sleepiness.
- Some of these are more likely when the central nervous system is impaired; for now it looks as though we are looking at a problem in the peripheral nervous system, but paraneoplastic syndrome or metastases to the central nervous system can occur.

Assess for signs of skin or soft tissues, including the presence of lymphedema
Palpate the lymph nodes
Assess vital signs

Medical Referral

Immediate medical referral is warranted if the patient has not been evaluated recently. It is impossible to tell whether her symptoms are radiation induced or are signs of cancer recurrence. A phone conversation between therapist and the oncologist may be all that is needed. Information gathered during the interview and examination should be summarized for the physician.

Result: The client had peripheral neuropathies that affected the bladder, pelvic floor muscles, and feet because the same nerves innervate these two areas. Physical therapy intervention remained appropriate, and cancer recurrence was ruled out.

Radiation therapy is well known to cause significant delayed, chronic effects on connective tissue and nervous system. Fibrosis of connective tissue can result in impairment of the soft tissues such as pelvic adhesions with subsequent functional limitations.

The incidence of plexopathy after radiation therapy has been reduced significantly with improved treatment, but it still occurs in a small number of cases. Younger women seem more vulnerable to radiation-induced peripheral neuropathy.

is a well-known risk factor for endometrial carcinoma.[47]

Clinical Signs and Symptoms of Endometrial (Uterine) Cancer

- Unexpected or unexplained vaginal bleeding or vaginal discharge after menopause (extremely significant sign)
- Persistent irregular or heavy bleeding between menstrual periods, especially in obese women
- Watery pink, white, brown, or bloody discharge from the vagina
- Abdominal or pelvic pain (more advanced disease)
- Weight loss, fatigue

OVARIAN CANCER

Ovarian cancer is the second most common reproductive cancer in women and the leading cause of death from gynecologic malignancies, accounting for more than half of all gynecologic cancer deaths in the Western world.[48]

Risk Factors Risk increases with advancing age, and the incidence of ovarian cancer peaks between the ages of 40 and 70 years. Other factors that may influence the development of ovarian cancer include the following:

- Nulliparity (never being pregnant), giving birth to fewer than two children, giving birth for the first time when over age 35
- Personal or family history of breast, endometrial, or colorectal cancer
- Family history of ovarian cancer (mother, sister, daughter; especially at a young age); carrying the *BRCA1* or *BRCA2* gene
- Infertility
- Early menopause
- Exposure to talc, or asbestos (remains under investigation)[49-51]

Identification of the *BRCA1* or *BRCA2* gene and subsequent evidence for a family of genes that may play a role in the breast–ovarian syndrome and familial ovarian cancer offer the possibility of identifying women truly at risk for this disease.[52]

No reliable screening test can detect ovarian cancer in its early, most curable stages. Two diagnostic tests are used, but both lack sensitivity and specificity. The CA-125 blood test (carcinoembryonic antigen, a biologic marker) shows elevation in about half of women with early-stage disease and about 80% of those with advanced disease. Transvaginal ultrasonography helps determine whether an existing ovarian growth is benign or cancerous.

Because early-stage symptoms are nonspecific, most women do not seek medical attention until the disease is advanced.

The ovaries begin in utero, where the kidneys are located in the fully developed human, and then migrate along the pathways of the ureters. Following the viscerosomatic referral patterns discussed in Chapter 3, ovarian cancer can cause back pain at the level of the kidneys. Murphy's percussion test (see Chapter 10) would be negative; other symptoms of ovarian cancer might be present but remain unreported if the woman does not recognize their significance.

Clinical Signs and Symptoms of Ovarian or Primary Peritoneal Cancer

Retrospective studies indicate that more than 70% of women with ovarian cancer have symptoms for 3 months or longer before diagnosis.[53] Early symptoms are often vague, nonspecific, and easily overlooked:

- Persistent vague GI complaints
- Abdominal discomfort, bloating, increase in abdominal or waist size (ascites)
- Indigestion, belching
- Early satiety
- Mild anorexia in a woman age 40 or older
- Vaginal bleeding
- Changes in bowel or bladder habits, especially urinary frequency or severe urinary urgency
- Pelvic discomfort or pressure; back pain
- Ascites, pain, and pelvic mass (advanced disease)

Rarely, a woman with ovarian carcinoma will present first with a paraneoplastic syndrome such as polyarthritis syndrome, carpal tunnel syndrome, myopathy, plantar fasciitis, or palmar fasciitis (swelling, digital stiffness or contractures, palmar erythema). The condition may be misdiagnosed as chronic regional pain syndrome (formerly reflex sympathetic pain syndrome (formerly reflex sympathetic dystrophy), Dupuytren's contracture, or a rheumatologic disorder.[54]

Hand and upper extremity manifestations often appear before the tumor is clinically evident. Treatment of the symptoms will have little effect on these conditions. Only successful treatment of the underlying neoplasm will affect symptoms favorably.[54]

The therapist should consider it a red flag whenever someone does not improve with physical therapy intervention. Failure to respond or worsening of symptoms requires a second screening

examination. Progression of disease is often accompanied by a cluster of new signs and symptoms.

EXTRAOVARIAN PRIMARY PERITONEAL CARCINOMA

Extraovarian primary peritoneal carcinoma (EOPPC) is an abdominal cancer (peritoneal carcinomatosis) without ovarian involvement. It arises in the peritoneum and mimics the symptoms, microscopic appearance, and pattern of spread of endothelial ovarian cancer with no identifiable disease of the ovaries.

EOPPC develops only in women and accounts for most extraovarian causes of symptoms with a presumed but inaccurate diagnosis of ovarian cancer.[55] EOPPC has been reported after bilateral oophorectomy performed for benign disease or prophylaxis.[56] The occurrence of EOPPC with the same histology as neoplasms arising within the ovary may be explained by the common origin of the peritoneum and the ovaries from the coelomic epithelium.[57]

CERVICAL CANCER

Cancer of the cervix is the third most common gynecologic malignancy in the United States. It is the most common cause of death from gynecologic cancer in the world. Since the widespread introduction of the Papanicolaou (Pap) smear as a standard screening tool, the diagnosis of cervical cancer at the invasive stage has decreased significantly. Even so, nearly half of all women diagnosed with cervical cancer are diagnosed at a late stage, with locally or regionally advanced disease and a poor prognosis.[44]

At the same time that rates of invasive cervical carcinoma have been on the decline, the highly curable preinvasive carcinoma in situ (CIS) has increased. CIS is more common in women 30 to 40 years of age, and invasive carcinoma is more frequent in women over age 40 years.

Risk Factors Risk factors associated with the development of cervical cancer are many and varied and include the following:

- Early age at first sexual intercourse
- Early age at first pregnancy
- Tobacco use, including exposure to passive smoke[58]
- Low socioeconomic status (lack of screening)
- History of any sexually transmitted disease (especially HPV and human immunodeficiency virus [HIV])
- History of multiple sex partners
- History of childhood sexual abuse

- Intimate partner abuse
- Women whose mothers used the drug diethylstilbestrol (DES) during pregnancy

Research into the health effects of intimate partner abuse points to a higher risk of STD and prevention of women from seeking health care; both contribute to an increased risk of cervical cancer. Women with a past history of childhood sexual abuse may avoid regular gynecologic care because being examined triggers painful memories. A history of childhood sexual abuse also increases a woman's risk of exposure to STIs that may contribute to the development of cervical cancer.[59]

The American Cancer Society (ACS) has issued updated recommendations for the early detection of cervical cancer.[60] The ACS advises all women to start cervical cancer screening 3 years after beginning to have vaginal intercourse, but no later than age 21. Pap smears should be done regularly, usually every year. After a total hysterectomy (including removal of the cervix) or after age 70, the Pap smear is discontinued.[61]

In the normal healthy adult female age 30 years or older, after three negative annual examinations, the Pap may be performed less frequently at the advice of the physician. Women with certain risk factors for cervical cancer (e.g., HIV infection, long-term steroid use, immunocompromised status, DES exposure before birth) should be advised to have an annual Pap smear.[60,61]

Clinical Signs and Symptoms Early cervical cancer has no symptoms. Clinical symptoms related to advanced disease include painful intercourse; postcoital, coital, or intermenstrual bleeding; and a watery, foul-smelling vaginal discharge. Disease usually spreads by local extension and through the lymphatics to the retroperitoneal lymph nodes (see Table 13-5). Metastases to the central nervous system can occur hematogenously late in the course of the disease and are generally rare. Clinical presentation of brain metastases depends on the site of the metastasized lesion; hemiparesis and headache are the most commonly reported signs and symptoms.[62]

Clinical Signs and Symptoms of

Cervical Cancer

- May be asymptomatic (early stages)
- Painful intercourse or pain after intercourse
- Unexplained or unexpected bleeding
- Watery, foul-smelling vaginal discharge
- Hemiparesis, headache (cancer recurrence with brain metastases)

Screening for Gastrointestinal Causes of Pelvic Pain

Gastrointestinal conditions can cause pelvic pain. The most common causes of pelvic pain referred from the GI system are the following:

- Acute appendicitis
- Inflammatory bowel disease (IBD; Crohn's disease or regional enteritis, ulcerative colitis)
- Diverticulitis
- Irritable bowel syndrome (IBS)

The small bowel, sigmoid, and rectum can be affected by gynecologic disease; low back or pelvic pain may result from pressure or displacement of these organs. Swelling, reaction to an adjacent infection, or reaction to the spilling of blood, menstrual fluid, or infected material into the abdominal cavity can cause pressure or displacement.

Bowel function is usually altered, but sometimes, the client experiences periods of normal bowel function alternating with intermittent bowel symptoms, and the client does not see a pattern or relationship until asked about current (or recent) changes in bowel function.

For all of these conditions, the symptoms as seen or reported in a physical therapy practice are usually the same. The client may present with one or more of the following:

- GI symptoms (see Box 4-17)
- Symptoms aggravated by increased abdominal pressure (coughing, straining, lifting, bending)
- Iliopsoas abscess (see Figs. 8-3 through 8-6; a positive test is indicative of an inflammatory/infectious process)
- Positive McBurney's point (see Figs. 8-8 and 8-9; appendicitis)
- Rebound tenderness or Blumberg's sign (see Fig. 8-10; appendicitis or peritonitis)

Appendicitis can cause peritoneal inflammation with psoas abscess, resulting in referred pain to the low back, hip, pelvis, or groin area (Case Example 15-5). The position of the vermiform appendix in the abdominal cavity is variable (see Fig. 8-9). Negative tests for appendicitis that use McBurney's point may occur when the appendix is located somewhere other than at the end of the cecum. See Fig. 8-10 for an alternate test (Blumberg's sign). Clinical signs and symptoms of appendicitis are listed in Chapter 8.

Blumberg's sign, a test for rebound tenderness, is usually positive in the presence of peritonitis, appendicitis, PID, or any other infection or inflammation associated with abdominal or pelvic conditions. Acute appendicitis is rare in older adults, but half of all those who die from a ruptured appendix are over 65.[63]

The test for rebound tenderness can be very painful for the client. The therapist is advised to do this test last (the only screening test used for abdominal or pelvic inflammation or infection) and to make a medical referral immediately when it is positive.

This is really a matter of professional preference based on experience and clinical judgment. In our experience, the iliopsoas and obturator tests are useful tools. If back pain (rather than abdominal quadrant pain) is the response, the therapist is alerted to the need to assess these muscles further and to consider their role in low back pain.

If the iliopsoas test is negative for lower quadrant pain, the therapist can palpate the integrity of the iliopsoas muscle and assess for trigger points (see Fig. 8-5). If the tests are negative (i.e., they do not cause abdominal pain), then the therapist can palpate McBurney's point for the appendix. If McBurney's is negative but an infectious cause of symptoms is suspected, the test for rebound tenderness can be conducted last.

Clients with symptoms of a possible inflammatory or infectious origin usually have a history of the conditions mentioned earlier (e.g., appendicitis, IBD or IBS, other GI disease). PID is another common cause of pelvic pain that can cause psoas abscess and a subsequent positive iliopsoas or obturator test. In this case, it is most likely a young woman with multiple sexual partners who has a known or unknown case of untreated *chlamydia*.

Crohn's disease, chronic inflammation of all layers of the bowel wall (see Chapter 8), may affect the terminal ileum and cecum or the rectum and sigmoid colon in the pelvis. In addition to pelvic and low back pain, systemic manifestations of Crohn's disease may include intermittent fever with sweats, malaise, anemia, arthralgias, and bowel symptoms.

Diverticular disease of the colon (diverticulosis), an acquired condition most common in the fifth to seventh decades, appears with intermittent symptoms. Moderate to severe pain in the left lower abdomen and the left side of the pelvis may be accompanied by a feeling of bowel distention and bowel symptoms such as hard stools, alternating diarrhea and constipation, mucus in the stools, and rectal bleeding.

IBS produces persistent, colicky lower abdominal and pelvic pain associated with anorexia, belching, abdominal distention, and bowel changes. Symptoms are produced by excessive colonic motility and spasm of the bowel (spastic colon).

CASE EXAMPLE 15-5   Appendicitis

Background: A 23-year-old woman who was training for a marathon developed groin and pelvic pain—first just on the right side, but then on both sides. She reported that the symptoms came on gradually over a period of 2 weeks. She could not point to a particular spot as the source of the pain, but rather, indicated a generalized lower abdominal, pelvic, and inner thigh area.

She denied ever being sexually active and had never been diagnosed with a sexually transmitted disease. She was on a rigorous training schedule for the marathon, did not appear anorexic, and seemed in overall good health.

No signs of swelling, inflammation, or temperature change were noted in the area. Running made the pain worse, rest made it better.

Range of motion of the hip and back was full and painless. A neurologic screening examination was normal. Resisted hip abduction was "uncomfortable" but did not exactly reproduce the symptoms.

What are the red flags here? What do you ask about or do next?

Not very many red flags are present: the bilateral presentation and overall size and location of the symptoms are the first two to be considered. Aggravating and relieving factors seem consistent with a musculoskeletal problem, but objective findings to support an impairment of the movement system are significantly lacking.

What do you ask about or do next?

Take the client's vital signs, including body temperature, blood pressure, respiratory rate, and heart rate. If you are pressed for time, at least take the body temperature and blood pressure.

Perform one or more of the tests for abdominal or pelvic infection/inflammation. You can go right to the rebound (Blumberg's) test, or you can assess the soft tissues one at a time as discussed in the text. If this is negative, consider trigger points as a possible source of painful symptoms.

Ask the client about constitutional symptoms or other symptoms anywhere else in the body.

Your next step or steps in interviewing or assessing the client will depend on the results of your evaluation so far. Once you have compiled the clinical presentation, step back and conduct a Review of Systems. If a cluster of signs and symptoms is associated with a particular visceral system, look over the Special Questions to Ask at the end of the chapter that address that system.

Check the Special Questions for Men and Women. Have you left out or missed any that might be appropriate to this case?

Results: The client had normal vital signs but reported "night and day sweats" from time to time. The iliopsoas and obturator tests caused some general discomfort but were considered negative.

McBurney's point was positive, eliciting extreme pain. Blumberg's test for rebound was not performed. The client was referred to the emergency department immediately because she did not have a primary care physician.

It turned out that this client had peritonitis from a ruptured appendix. The doctors think she was in such good shape with a high pain threshold that she presented with minimal symptoms (and survived). Her white blood count was almost 100,000 at the time that laboratory work was finally ordered.

See Chapter 8 for additional details about the referred pain patterns and most common associated signs and symptoms for each of these diseases.

Screening for Urogenital Causes of Pelvic Pain

Infection of the bladder or kidney, kidney stones, renal failure (chronic kidney disease), spasm of the urethral smooth muscle, and tumors in any of the urogenital organs can refer pain to the lower lumbar and pelvic regions, mimicking musculoskeletal dysfunction. Pelvic floor tension myalgia can develop in response to these conditions and create pelvic pain. The primary pain pattern may radiate around the flanks to the lower abdominal region, the genitalia, and the anterior/medial thighs (see Figs. 10-7 to 10-10).

Usually, the most common diseases of this system appear as obvious medical problems. In the physical therapy setting, past medical history, risk factors, and associated signs and symptoms provide important red-flag clues. The therapist needs to ask the client about the presence of painful urination or changes in urination and constitutional symptoms such as fever, chills, sweats, and nausea or vomiting.

Deep, aching pelvic pain that is worse on weight-bearing or is accompanied by sciatica or numbness and tingling in the groin or lower extremity may be associated with cancer recurrence or cancer metastases.

Screening for Other Conditions as a Cause of Pelvic Pain

Psychogenic pain is often ill defined, and its anatomic distribution depends more on the person's concepts than on clinical disease processes. Pelvic pain may co-evolve with relational dysfunction.[64]

Such pain does not usually radiate; commonly, the client has multiple unrelated symptoms, and fluctuations in the course of symptoms are determined more by crises in the person's psychosocial life than by physical changes. (See also Screening for Emotional and Psychologic Overlay in Chapter 3.)

A history of sexual abuse in childhood or adulthood (men and women) may contribute to chronic pelvic pain or symptoms of a vague and diffuse nature. In some cases, the link between abuse and pelvic pain may be psychologic or neurologic, or may result from biophysical changes that heighten a person's physical sensitivity to pain. Taking a history of sexual abuse may be warranted.[65]

Occasionally, a woman has been told there is no organic cause for her distressing pelvic pain. Chronic vascular pelvic congestion, enhanced by physical or emotional stress, may be the underlying problem. The therapist may be instrumental in assessing for this condition and providing some additional clues to the medical community that can lead to a medical diagnosis.

Surgery, in particular hysterectomy, is associated with varying amounts of pain from problems such as nerve damage, scar formation, or hematoma formation with infection, which can cause backache and pelvic pain. Lower abdominal discomfort, vaginal discharge, and fatigue may accompany pelvic pain or discomfort months after gynecologic surgery.

Other types of abdominal, pelvic, or tubal surgery, such as laparotomy, tubal ligation, or laminectomy, can also be followed by pelvic pain, usually associated with low back pain. During the client interview, the therapist must include questions about recent surgical procedures.

▶ PHYSICIAN REFERRAL

Guidelines for Immediate Medical Attention

Immediate medical attention is required anytime the therapist identifies signs and symptoms that point to fracture, infection, or neoplasm. For example, a positive rebound test for appendicitis or peritonitis requires immediate medical referral. Likewise, severe sacral pain in the presence of a previous history of uterine, abdominal, prostate, rectal, or anal cancer requires immediate medical referral.

Suspicion of any infection (e.g., STD, PID) requires immediate medical referral. Early medical intervention can prevent the spread of infection and septicemia and preserve fertility.

A sexually active female with shoulder or back pain of unknown cause may need to be screened for ectopic pregnancy. Onset of symptoms after a missed menstrual cycle or in association with unexplained or unexpected vaginal bleeding requires immediate medical attention. Hemorrhage from ectopic pregnancy can be a life-threatening condition.

Guidelines for Physician Referral

Blood in the toilet after a bowel movement may be a sign of anal fissures or hemorrhoids but can also signal colorectal cancer. A medical differential diagnosis is needed to make the distinction. History of an unrepaired hernia or suspected undiagnosed hernia requires medical referral. Lateral wall pelvic pain referred down the anteromedial side of the thigh to the knee can occur with femoral hernias; inguinal hernias are more likely to cause groin pain.

A history of cancer with recent surgical removal of tumor tissue followed by back, hip, sacral, or pelvic pain within 6 months of surgery is a red flag for possible cancer recurrence. Even in the presence of apparent movement system impairment, referral for medical evaluation is warranted.

All adolescent females and adult women who are sexually active or over the age of 21 should be asked when their last Pap smear was done and what the results were. The therapist can play an important part in client education and disease prevention by teaching women about the importance

- Lack of objective findings; special tests (e.g., Patrick's, Gaenslen maneuver, Yeoman test, central posterior–anterior overpressure or spring test on the sacrum) are negative. Soft tissue and contractile tissue can usually be provoked during a physical examination by palpation, resistance, overpressure, compression, distraction, or motion
- Look for other pelvic floor dysfunction

Associated Signs and Symptoms

- Presence of urologic or GI symptoms along with sacral pain (the therapist must ask to find out)

Clues to Screening the Pelvis

Frequently, pelvic and low back pain occur together or alternately. Whenever pelvic pain is listed, the reader should consider this as pelvic pain with or without low back or sacral pain.

Past Medical History/Risk Factors

- History of dysmenorrhea, ovarian cysts, inflammatory disease, STD, fibromyalgia, sexual assault/incest/trauma, chronic yeast/vaginal infection, chronic bladder or urinary tract infection, chronic IBS
- History of abdominal, pelvic, or bladder surgery
- History of pelvic or abdominal radiation
- Recent therapeutic or spontaneous abortion
- Recent IUCD in the presence of PID or in women with a history of PID
- History of previous gynecologic, colon, or breast cancer
- History of prolonged labor, use of forceps or vacuum extraction, and/or multiple births
- Obesity, chronic cough

Clinical Presentation

- Pelvic pain that is described as "achy" or "comes and goes in waves" and is poorly localized (person cannot point to one spot)
- Pelvic pain that is aggravated by walking, sexual intercourse, coughing, or straining
- Pain that is not clearly affected by position changes or specific movements, especially when accompanied by night pain unrelieved by change in position
- Pelvic pain that is not reduced or eliminated by scar tissue mobilization, soft tissue mobilization, or release of trigger points of the myofascial structures in the pelvic cavity

of an annual Pap smear and encouraging them to schedule one, if appropriate.

Women with conditions such as endometriosis, pelvic congestion syndrome, STI, and PID can be helped with medical treatment. Medical referral is advised anytime a therapist identifies signs and symptoms that suggest any of these conditions.

Failure to respond to physical therapy intervention is usually followed by reevaluation that includes a second screening and a Review of Systems. Any red flags or cluster of suspicious signs and symptoms must be reported. Depending on the therapist's findings, medical evaluation may be the next step.

Clues to Screening the Sacrum/Sacroiliac

Past Medical History

- Previous history of Crohn's disease; presence of skin rash with new onset of sacral, hip, or leg pain
- Previous history of other GI disease
- Previous history of rheumatic disease
- Previous history of conjunctivitis or venereal disease (Reiter's syndrome)
- History of heart disease or PVD; the therapist should ask about the effect of activity on symptoms
- Remember to consider unreported assaults or anal intercourse (partnered rape, teens, homosexual men with men). Please note that many of today's teens are resorting to anal intercourse and oral sex in an effort to prevent pregnancy. These forms of sexual contact do not prevent STD. In addition, they can result in sacral pain and other lesions (e.g., rectal fissures) caused by trauma.

Clinical Presentation

- Constant (usually intense) pain; pain with a "catch" or "click" (sacral fracture)
- Sacral pain occurs when the rectum is stimulated (pain occurs when passing gas or having a bowel movement)
- Pain relief occurs after passing gas or having a bowel movement
- Sacral or SI pain in the absence of a (remembered) history of trauma or overuse
- Assess for trigger points, a common musculoskeletal (not systemic) cause of sacral pain. If trigger point therapy relieves, reduces, or eliminates the pain, further screening may not be necessary

Associated Signs and Symptoms

- Pelvic pain in the presence of yellow, odorous vaginal discharge
- Positive McBurney's or iliopsoas/obturator tests (see Chapter 6)
- Pelvic pain with constitutional symptoms, especially nausea and vomiting, GI symptoms (possible enteropathic origin)
- Presence of painful urination; urinary incontinence, urgency, or frequency; nocturia; blood in the urine; or other urologic changes

Gynecologic

- Pelvic pain that is relieved by rest, placing a pillow or support under the hips and buttocks in the supine position, or "getting off your feet"
- Pelvic pain that is correlated with menses or sexual intercourse
- Pelvic pain that occurs after the first menstrual cycle is missed, especially if the woman is using an IUCD or has had a tubal ligation (see text for

other risk factors), with shoulder pain also present (ruptured ectopic pregnancy); assess for low blood pressure

- Presence of unexplained or unexpected vaginal bleeding, especially after menopause
- Presence of pregnancy

Vascular

- History of heart disease with a clinical presentation of pelvic, buttock, and leg pain that is aggravated by activity or exercise (claudication)
- Pelvic pain accompanied by buttock and leg pain with changes in skin and temperature on the affected side (arterial occlusion or venous thrombosis), especially in the presence of known heart disease or recent pelvic surgery
- Pain that worsens toward the end of the day, accompanied by pain after intercourse and in the presence of varicose veins elsewhere in the body (ovarian varicosities)

❂ KEY POINTS TO REMEMBER

Many of the Key Points to Remember in Chapter 14 also apply to the sacrum and sacroiliac joints. These will not be repeated here.

Sacrum/Sacroiliac Joint

✓ Sacral pain, in the absence of a history of trauma or overuse, that is not reproduced with anterior-posterior overpressure (spring test) on the sacrum is a red flag presentation that indicates a possible systemic cause of symptoms.

✓ Pain above the L5 spinous process is not likely from the sacrum or SI joint.

✓ Midline lumbar pain, especially if present when rising from sitting, more often comes from a discogenic source; clients with unilateral pain below L5 when rising from sitting are more likely to have a painful SI joint

✓ Insufficiency fractures of the spine are not uncommon with individuals who have osteoporosis or who are

taking corticosteroids; apparent insidious onset or minor trauma is common.

✓ The most common cause of noninfected, inflammatory sacral/SI pain is ankylosing spondylitis; other causes may include Reiter's syndrome, psoriatic arthritis, and arthritis associated with IBD.

✓ Infection can seed itself to the joints, including the SI joint. Watch for a history of recent dental surgery (endocarditis), intravenous drug use, trauma (including surgery), and chronic immunosuppression.

✓ Anyone with joint pain of unknown cause should be asked about a recent history of skin rash (delayed allergic reaction, Crohn's disease)

Pelvis

✓ Pelvic and low back pain often occur together; either may be accompanied by unreported abdominal pain, discomfort, or other symptoms. The therapist must ask about the presence of any unreported pain or symptoms.

⏱ KEY POINTS TO REMEMBER—cont'd

✓ Yellow or green discharge from the vagina or penis (with or without an odor) in the presence of low back, pelvic, or sacral pain may be a red flag. The therapist must ask additional questions to determine the need for medical evaluation.

✓ The first sign of pelvic infection in the older adult might not be an elevated temperature, but rather, confusion, increased confusion, or some other change in mental status

✓ Bilateral anterior pelvic pain may be a symptom of inflammation; the therapist can test for iliopsoas or obtu-

rator abscess, appendicitis, or peritonitis (see discussion, Chapter 8).

✓ Pelvic pain that is aggravated by exercise and starts 5 or more minutes after exercise begins may be vascularly induced

✓ A history of sexual abuse at any time in the person's past may contribute to chronic pelvic pain or nonspecific symptoms. Taking a history of sexual abuse may be needed.

SUBJECTIVE EXAMINATION

Special Questions to Ask: Sacrum, Sacroiliac, and Pelvis

See Special Questions to Ask: Back, and Special Questions to Ask Men/Women Experiencing Back, Hip, Pelvic, Groin, Sacroiliac, or Sacral Pain, Chapter 14.

Not all the special questions listed in Chapter 14 will have to be asked. Use your professional judgment to decide what to ask based on what the client has told you and what you've observed during the examination.

Sacral/SI Pain

- Have you ever been diagnosed with ulcerative colitis, Crohn's disease, IBS, or colon cancer?
- Are you taking any antibiotics? (long-term use of antibiotics can result in colitis)
- Have you ever been diagnosed or treated for cancer of any kind? **(metastases to the bone, especially common with breast, lung, or prostate cancer, but also with pelvic or abdominal cancer)**
- Do you have any abdominal pain or GI symptoms? (assess for lower abdominal or suprapubic pain at the same level as the sacral pain; if the client denies GI symptoms, follow up with a quick list: Any nausea? Vomiting? Diarrhea? Change in stool color or shape? Ever have blood in the toilet?)
- If sacral pain occurs when the rectum is stimulated:
  Is your pain relieved by passing gas or by having a bowel movement?
- Sacral or SI pain without a history of trauma or overuse

Remember to consider unreported assault, anal intercourse (partnered rape; adolescents may use anal intercourse to prevent pregnancy, homosexual men with men). Please note that many of today's teens are resorting to anal intercourse and oral sex in an effort to prevent pregnancy.

These forms of sexual contact do not prevent STD. In addition, they can result in sacral pain and other lesions (e.g., rectal fissures) resulting from trauma.

Pelvic Pain

- Have you ever been diagnosed or treated for cancer of any kind?
- Have you had recent abdominal or pelvic surgery (including hysterectomy, bladder reconstruction, prostatectomy)?
- Have you ever been told that you have (or do you have) varicose veins? **(pelvic congestion syndrome)**
- Do you ever have blood in the toilet?

For women with low back, sacral, or pelvic pain: See Special Questions to Ask: Women Experiencing Back, Hip, Pelvic, Groin, Sacroiliac (SI), or Sacral Pain, Chapter 14.

For anyone with low back, sacral, or pelvic pain of unknown cause: It may be necessary to conduct a sexual history as part of the screening process (see Chapter 14 or Appendix B-29).

For men with sciatica, pelvic, sacral, or low back pain: See Special Questions to Ask: Men Experiencing Back, Hip, Pelvic, Groin, or Sacroiliac Pain (Chapter 14 or Appendix B-21).

CASE STUDY

STEPS IN THE SCREENING PROCESS

When a client presents with pelvic pain, how do you get started with the screening process?

First, review the possible causes of pelvic pain (see Table 15-2).

- Was there anything in the history or presentation to suggest one of the categories in this table?
- From looking at the table, do additional questions come to mind?
- Review Special Questions to Ask: Sacrum, SI, or Pelvis, presented in this chapter. Are any of these questions appropriate or needed?
- Did you ask about associated signs and symptoms?
- Remember to ask the client the following:
- Is there anything else about your general health that concerns you?
- What other symptoms are you having that may or may not be connected to your current problem?

Next, review Clues Suggesting Systemic Pelvic Pain. Is there anything here to raise your suspicion of a systemic disorder?

- If necessary, conduct a general health screening examination:
- Have you had any recent infections or illnesses?
- Have you had any fevers, sweats, or chills?
- Any unusual discharge from the vagina or penis?
- Any unusual skin rashes or muscle/joint pain?
- Any unusual fatigue, irritability, or difficulty sleeping?
- Is there anything to suggest a pelvic floor dysfunction as the source of symptoms? Look for the following:
- Pain that comes and goes and changes location
- Pain that is not predictably reproducible
- Pain that is alleviated by heat to the lower abdomen, groin, or front of the upper thighs
- Pain made worse by William Flexion Exercises (WFEs; single or double knee to chest) but relieved by hamstring stretching
- Rectal pain or discomfort that is worse during intercourse or penetration
- Pain or discomfort (better or worse) before, during, or after menstrual cycle
- Mentally conduct a Review of Systems
- Did the past medical history, age, medications, or associated signs and symptoms point to anything?
- Use your Review of Systems table (see Box 4-17) to look for possible clusters of symptoms, or to remind you what to look for.
- If you identify a specific system in question, ask additional questions for that system:
- For example, if a significant past medical history or current signs and symptoms of GI involvement are reported, review the Special Questions to Ask in Chapter 8. Would any questions listed be appropriate to ask, given your client's clinical presentation? Or, if you suspected a renal/urologic cause of symptoms, look at the questions posed in Chapter 10.

Sometimes, the initial screening process does not raise any suspicious history or red flag symptoms. As discussed in Chapter 1, screening can take place anywhere in the Guide's patient/client management model (see Box 1-5).

The therapist may begin to carry out the intervention without seeing any red flags that suggest a systemic disorder and may then find that the client does not improve with physical therapy. This in itself is a red flag.

If someone is not improving with physical therapy intervention, the therapist reviews the findings (i.e., what you are doing and why you are doing it), while evaluating the need to repeat some steps in the screening process. Because systemic disease progresses over time, new signs and symptoms may have developed since the time of the first interview and client history taking.

The therapist may want to have someone else review the case. Often, this can provide some clarity and add insight to the evaluation process. Asking a few screening questions may bring to light some new information to be included in the ongoing evaluation. Now may be the time to repeat (or perform for the first time) specific and appropriate screening tests and measures.

PRACTICE QUESTIONS

1. Which of the following signs and symptoms does not describe pelvic pain of systemic origin?
   a. Pain that is made worse after 5 to 10 minutes of physical activity or exertion but goes away with rest or cessation of the activity
   b. Pain that is relieved by placing a pillow or support under the hips and buttocks
   c. Pain that is worse in the morning but decreases with movement or stretching
   d. Pain that is not reduced or eliminated by trigger point release or soft tissue mobilization

2. A positive Blumberg sign indicates:
   a. Pelvic infection
   b. Ovarian varicosities
   c. Arthritis associated with IBD
   d. Sacral neoplasm

3. A 33-year-old pharmaceutical sales representative reports pain over the mid-sacrum radiating to the right posterior superior iliac spine (PSIS). Overpressure on the sacrum does not reproduce symptoms. This signifies:
   a. Neoplasm is present
   b. Red flag sign of sacral insufficiency fracture
   c. A lack of objective findings
   d. Coccygodynia

4. A 67-year-old man was seen by a physical therapist for low back pain rated 7 out of 10 on the visual analog scale. He was evaluated, and a diagnosis was made by the physical therapist. The client attained immediate relief of symptoms, but after 3 weeks of therapy, the symptoms returned. What is the next step from a screening perspective?
   a. The client can be discharged. Maximum benefit from physical therapy has been achieved.
   b. The client should be screened for systemic disease even if you have already included screening during the initial evaluation.
   c. The client should be sent back to the physician for further medical follow-up.
   d. The client should receive an additional modality to help break the pain–spasm cycle.

5. McBurney's point for appendicitis is located:
   a. Approximately one-third the distance from the anterior superior iliac spine [ASIS] toward the umbilicus, usually on the left side
   b. Approximately one-half the distance from the ASIS toward the umbilicus, usually on the left side
   c. Approximately one-third the distance from the ASIS toward the umbilicus, usually on the right side
   d. Approximately one-half the distance from the ASIS toward the umbilicus, usually on the right side
   e. Impossible to tell because the appendix can be located anywhere in the abdomen

6. Which of the following is NOT a red flag finding?
   a. Sacral pain occurs when the client is passing gas or having a bowel movement.
   b. Sacral pain is relieved after the client passes gas or has a bowel movement.
   c. Sacral pain occurs without a history of trauma or overuse.
   d. Sacral pain is reduced or relieved by release of trigger points.

7. Cancer as a cause of sacral or pelvic pain is usually characterized by:
   a. A previous history of reproductive cancer
   b. Constant pain
   c. Blood in the urine or stools
   d. Constitutional symptoms
   e. All of the above

8. Reproduced or increased abdominal or pelvic pain when the iliopsoas muscle test is performed suggests:
   a. Iliopsoas trigger point
   b. Inflammation or abscess of the muscle from an inflamed appendix or peritoneum
   c. Abdominal aortic aneurysm
   d. Neoplasm

9. A 75-year-old woman with a known history of osteoporosis has pain over the sacrum radiating to the right posterior superior iliac spine and right buttock. How do you rule out an insufficiency fracture?
   a. Perform Blumberg's test.
   b. Conduct a sacral spring test (posterior–anterior overpressure of the sacrum).
   c. Perform Murphy's percussion test.
   d. Diagnostic imaging is the only way to know for sure.

10. What is the importance of the pelvic floor musculature in relation to the abdominal and pelvic viscera?

REFERENCES

1. Buchowski JC, Kebaish KM, Sinkov V, et al: Functional and radiographic outcome of sacroiliac arthrodesis for the disorders of the sacroiliac joint. *The Spine Journal* 5(5):520-528, 2005.

2. Haanpaa M, Paavonen J: Transient urinary retention and chronic neuropathic pain associated with genital herpes simplex virus infection. *Acta Obstet Gynecol Scand* 83(10):946-949, 2004.

3. Blake SP, Connors AM: Sacral insufficiency fracture. *Br J Radiol* 77(922):891-896, 2004.

4. Fortin J, April C, Dwyer A, et al: Sacroiliac joint: pain referral maps upon applying a new injection/arthrography technique. I: Asymptomatic volunteers. *Spine* 19(13):1475-1482, 1994.

5. Fortin JD, April CN, Ponthieux B, et al: Sacroiliac joint: pain referral maps upon applying a new injection/arthrography technique. Part II: Clinical evaluation. *Spine* 19(13):1483-1489, 1994.

6. Young S, April C, Laslett M: Correlation of clinical examination characteristics with three sources of low back pain. *The Spine Journal* 3(6):460-465, 2003.

7. Slipman CW, Patel RK, Whyte WS, et al: Diagnosing and managing sacroiliac pain. *J Musc Med* 18(6):325-332, 2001.

8. Dreyfuss P, Dreyer SJ, Cole A, et al: Sacroiliac joint pain. *J Am Acad Orthop Surg* 12(4):255-265, July/August 2004.

9. Schumacher HR Jr, Klippel JH, Koopman WJ, editors: *Primer on the rheumatic diseases*, 12th edition, Atlanta, Georgia, 2001, Arthritis Foundation.

10. Betancourt-Albrecht M, Roman F, Marcelli M: Grand rounds in endocrinology, diabetes, and metabolism from Baylor College of Medicine: a man with pain in his bones. *Medscape Diabetes Endocrinol* 5(1):2003.Available on-line (free service but requires login and password): http://www.medscape.com/viewarticle/445158. Accessed November 10, 2005.

11. White JH, Hague C, Nicolaou S, et al: Imaging of sacral fractures. *Clin Radiol* 58:914-921, 2003.

12. Lin JT, Lane JM: Sacral stress fractures. *J Womens Health (Larchmt)* 12(9):879-888, November 2003.

13. Leroux JL, Denat B, Thomas E, et al: Sacral insufficiency fractures presenting as acute low-back-pain-biomechanical aspects. *Spine* 18(16):2502-2506, 1993.

14. Boissonnault WG, Thein-Nissenbaum JM: Differential diagnosis of a sacral stress fracture. *J Orthop Sports Phys Ther* 12(32):613-621, December 2002.

15. Ahovuo JA, Kiuru MJ, Visuri T: Fatigue stress fractures of the sacrum: diagnosis with MR imaging. *Eur Radiol* 14(3):500-505, March 2004.

16. Khan MH, Smith PN, Kang JD: Sacral insufficiency fractures following multilevel instrumented spinal fusion. *Spine* 30(16):E484-488, August 15, 2005.

17. Parikh VA, Edlund JW: Sacral insufficiency fractures—rare complication of pelvic radiation for rectal carcinoma. *Dis Colon Rectum* 41(2):254-257, February 1998.

18. Zileli M, Hoscoskun C, Brastiano P, et al: Surgical treatment of primary sacral tumors: complications with sacrectomy. *Neurosurg Focus* 15(5):E9, November 15, 2003.

19. Randall RL: Giant cell tumor of the sacrum. *Neurosurg Focus* 15(2):E13, August 15, 2003.

20. Payer M: Neurological manifestation of sacral tumors. *Neurosurg Focus* 15(2):E1, August 15, 2003.

21. Perkins R, Schofferman J, Reynolds J: Coccygectomy for severe refractory sacrococcygeal joint pain. *J Spinal Disord Tech* 16(1):100-103, 2003.

22. Howard FM, El-Minawi AM, Sanchez RA: Conscious pain mapping by laparoscopy in women with chronic pelvic pain. *Obstet Gynecol* 96(6):934-939, December 2000.

23. Howard FM: Chronic pelvic pain. *Obstet Gynecol* 101(3):594-611, March 2003.

24. Stuge B, Hilde G, Vollestad N: Physical therapy for pregnancy-related low back and pelvic pain: a systematic review. *Acta Obstet Gynecol Scand* 82(11):983-990, 2003.

25. Baker PK: Musculoskeletal problems. In Steege JF, Metzger DA, Levy BS: *Chronic pelvic pain: an integrated approach*, Philadelphia, 1998, WB Saunders, pp. 215-240.

26. Simons DG, Travell JG: *Travell & Simons' myofascial pain and dysfunction: the trigger point manual*, vol 2, Baltimore, 1993, Williams & Wilkins, 1993. [Myopain Seminars: www.painpoints.com/seminars.html].

27. Bø K, Sherburn M: Evaluation of female pelvic-floor muscle function and strength. *Phys Ther* 85(3):269-282, March 2005.

28. Headley B: *When movement hurts: a self-help manual for treating trigger points*, Boulder, Colorado, 1997, Innovative Systems.

29. Kostopoulos D, Rizopoulos K: *The manual of trigger point and myofascial therapy*, Thorofare, NJ, 2001, Slack, Inc.

30. Giudice LC: Status of current research on endometriosis. *J Reprod Med* 43(3 suppl):252-262, 1998.

31. Giudice LC, Kao LC: Endometriosis. *Lancet* 364(9447):1789-1799, November 2004.

32. Jossens MOR: Risk factors associated with pelvic inflammatory disease of differing microbial etiologies. *Sexually Trans Dis* 23:239-247, 1996.

33. Kahn JA, Kaplowitz RA, Goodman E, et al: The association between impulsiveness and sexual risk behaviors in adolescent and young adult women. *J Adolesc Health* 30(4):229-232, April 2002.

34. Kahn JA, Rosenthal SL, Succop PA, et al: Mediators of the association between age of first sexual intercourse and subsequent pelvic inflammatory infection. *Pediatrics* 109(1):E5, January 2002.

35. Centers for Disease Control and Prevention (CDC): *Policy guidelines for prevention and management of pelvic inflammatory disease (PID)*, Washington, DC, 1991, U.S. Department of Health and Human Services. Available at: www.cdc.gov. Accessed November 15, 2005.

36. Centers for Disease Control and Prevention: *Sexually transmitted disease surveillance: 2004*, Washington, DC, 2005, U.S. Department of Health and Human Services.

37. Anderton JP, Valdiserri RO: Combating syphilis and HIV among users of internet chatrooms. *J Health Commun* 10(7):665-771, October-November 2005.

38. Douglas JM Jr, Peterman TA, Fenton KA: Syphilis among men who have sex with men: challenges to syphilis elimination in the United States. *Sex Transm Dis* 32(10 suppl):S80-S83, October 2005.

39. Tarazov PG, Prozorovskij KV, Ryzhkov VK: Pelvic pain syndrome caused by ovarian varices. *Acta Radiol* 38(6):1023-1025, 1997.

40. El-Minawi AM: Pelvic varicosities and pelvic congestion syndrome. In Howard FM, et al: *Pelvic pain diagnosis and management*, Philadelphia, 2000, Lippincott, Williams & Wilkins, pp. 171-183.

41. Hobbs JT: Varicose veins arising from the pelvis due to ovarian vein incompetence. *Int J Clin Pract* 59(10):1195-1203, October 2005.

42. Gasparini D, Geatti O, Orsolon PG, et al: Female "varicocele." *Clin Nucl Med* 23(7):420-422, 1998.

43. Hartung O, Grisoli D, Boufi M, et al: Endovascular stenting in the treatment of pelvic vein congestion cause nutcracker syndrome: lessons learned from the first five cases. *J Vasc Surg* 42(2):275-280, August 2005.

44. Jemal A, Murray T, Ward E, et al: Cancer statistics, 2005. *Cancer J Clin* 55(1):10-31, January/February 2005.

45. Ferguson SE, Soslow RA, Amsterdam A, et al: Comparison of uterine malignancies that develop during and following tamoxifen therapy. *Gynecol Oncol* December 9, 2005; Epub ahead of print.

46. Carter J, Pather S: An overview of uterine cancer and its management. *Expert Rev Anticancer Ther* 6(1):33-42, January 2006.

47. Varras M, Polyzos D, Akrivis C: Effects of tamoxifen on the human female genital tract: review of the literature. *Eur J Gynaecol Oncol* 24(3-4):258-268, 2003.

48. Eltabbakh GH: Recent advances in the management of women with ovarian cancer. *Minerva Ginecol* 56(1):81-89, February 2004.

49. Huncharek M, Geschwind JF, Kupelnick B: Perineal application of cosmetic talc and risk of invasive epithelial ovarian cancer: a meta-analysis of 11,933 subjects from sixteen observational studies. *Anticancer Res* 23(2C):1955-1960, March-April 2003.

50. Langseth H, Kjaerheim K: Ovarian cancer and occupational exposure among pulp and paper employees in Norway. *Scand J Work Environ Health* 30(5):356-361, 2004.

51. Mills PK, Riordan DG, Cress RD, et al: Perineal talc exposure and epithelial ovarian cancer risk in the Central Valley of California. *Int J Cancer* 112(3):458-464, November 2004.

52. Study questions ovary removal during hysterectomy: what factors affect ovarian cancer risk? *Harvard Women's Health Watch* 13(2):7, October 2005.

53. Goff BA, Mandel LS, Melancon CH, et al: Frequency of symptoms of ovarian cancer in women presenting to primary care clinics. *JAMA* 291(22):2705-2712, June 2004.

54. Martorell EA, Murray PM, Peterson JJ, et al: Palmar fasciitis and arthritis syndrome associated with metastatic ovarian carcinoma: a report of four cases. *J Hand Surg* 29A(4):654-660, 2004.

55. Roffers SD, WU XC, Johnson CH, et al: Incidence of extra-ovarian primary cancers in the United States, 1992-1997. *Cancer* 97(10 suppl):2643-2647, May 15, 2003.

56. Eltabbakh GH, Piver MS: Extraovarian primary peritoneal carcinoma. *Oncology* (Williston Park) 12(6):813-819, June 1998.

57. Kunz J, Rondez R: Correlation between serous ovarian tumors and extra-ovarian peritoneal tumors of the same histology. *Schweiz Rundsch Med Prax* 87(6):191-198, February 1998.

58. Trimble CL, Genkinger JM, Burke AE, et al: Active and passive cigarette smoking and the risk of cervical neoplasia. *Obstet Gynecol* 105(1):174-181, January 2005.

59. Shinn SE: Taking a stand against cervical cancer. *Nursing 2004* 34(5):36-42, May 2004.

60. Saslow D, Runowicz CD, Solomon D, et al: American Cancer Society guideline for the early detection of cervical neoplasia and cancer. *Cancer J Clin* 52(6):342-362, November/December 2002.

61. American Cancer Society (ACS): *ACS cancer detection guidelines*, Atlanta, Georgia. Available on-line: http://www.cancer.org. Accessed February 16, 2006.

62. Amita M, Sudeep G, Rekha W, et al: Brain metastasis from cervical carcinoma. *Medscape Gen Med* 7(1):2005.

63. Storm-Dickerson TL, Horattas MC: What have we learned over the past 20 years about appendicitis in the elderly? *Am J Surg* 185(3):198-201, March 2003.

64. Mathias SD, Kuppermann M, Liberman RF, et al: Chronic pelvic pain: prevalence, health-related quality of life, and economic correlates. *Obstet Gynecol* 87(3):321-327, 1996.

65. Hilden M, Schei B, Swahnberg K, et al: A history of sexual abuse and health: a Nordic multicentre study. *BJOG* 111(10):1121-1127, October 2004.

Screening the Lower Quadrant: Buttock, Hip, Groin, Thigh, and Leg

The causes of lower quadrant pain or dysfunction vary widely; presentation of symptoms is equally wide ranging. Vascular conditions (e.g., arterial insufficiency, abdominal aneurysm), infectious or inflammatory conditions, gastrointestinal (GI) disease, and gynecologic and male reproductive systems may cause symptoms in the lower quadrant and lower extremity, including the pelvis, buttock, hip, groin, thigh, and knee. Some overlap may occur, but unique differences exist.

Cancer may present as primary hip, groin, or leg pain or symptoms. Primary cancer can metastasize to the low back, pelvis, and sacrum, thus referring pain to the hip and groin. Primary cancer may also metastasize to the hip, causing hip or groin pain and symptoms.

Pain may be referred from other locations such as the scrotum, kidneys, abdominal wall, abdomen, peritoneum, or retroperitoneal region. Lower quadrant pain may be referred through conditions that affect nearby anatomic structures, such as the spine, spinal nerve roots or peripheral nerves, and overlying soft tissue structures (e.g., hernia, bursitis, fasciitis).

One of the keys to accurate and quick screening is knowledge of the types of conditions, illnesses, and systemic disorders that can refer pain to the lower quadrant, especially the hip and groin. Much of the information related to screening of the back (see Chapter 14), sacrum, sacroiliac (SI), and pelvis (see Chapter 15) also applies to the hip and groin.

USING THE SCREENING MODEL TO EVALUATE THE LOWER QUADRANT

When screening is called for, the therapist looks at the client's personal and family history, clinical presentation, and associated signs and symptoms. Knowledge of problems that can affect the lower quadrant, along with the likely history, pain patterns, and associated signs and symptoms, shows us the steps to follow in screening.

Most often, the screening process takes place through a series of special questions. A few special tests may be used as well. Recognition of red flag signs and symptoms of systemic or viscerogenic problems can direct the client toward the necessary medical attention early in the disease process. In many cases, early detection and treatment may result in improved outcomes.

Past Medical History

Some of the more common histories associated with lower extremity, hip, or groin pain of a visceral nature are listed in Box 16-1. A previous history of cancer such as prostate cancer (men), any reproductive cancers (women),

as a cause of hip, groin, or lower extremity pain are presented in Chapter 13.

Many conditions with overlap symptoms (e.g., back and hip pain, pelvic and groin pain) are presented throughout this third text section (Systemic Origins of Neuromusculoskeletal Pain and Dysfunction) as part of the discussion of back pain (see Chapter 14) or pelvic pain (see Chapter 15).

Awareness of risk factors for various problems can help alert the therapist early to the need for medical intervention, as well as for direct education and prevention efforts. Many risk factors for disease are modifiable. Exercise often plays a key role in prevention and treatment of pathologic conditions. Recognizing red flags in the history and clinical presentation and knowing when to refer versus when to treat are topics of focus in this chapter.

Clinical Presentation

If no neuromuscular or musculoskeletal cause of the client's symptoms can be identified, then the therapist must consider the following:

Follow-Up Questions

- Are red flags suggestive of a viscerogenic cause of pain or symptoms? (see Box 14-1); the lack of diagnostic testing or imaging studies may be an additional red flag[2]
- What kind of pain patterns do we expect to see with each of the viscerogenic causes?
- Are any associated signs and symptoms suggestive of a particular organ system?

Hip and Buttock

The physical therapist is well acquainted with hip or buttock pain (Table 16-1) as a result of regional neuromuscular or musculoskeletal disorders. The therapist must be aware that disorders affecting the organs within the pelvic and abdominal cavities can also refer pain to the hip region, mimicking a primary musculoskeletal lesion. A careful history and physical examination usually differentiate these entities from true hip disease.

PAIN PATTERN

True hip pain, whether from a neuromusculoskeletal or systemic cause (Table 16-2), is usually felt posteriorly deep within the buttock or anteriorly in the groin, sometimes with radiating pain down the anterior thigh. Pain perceived on the outer (lateral) side of the hip is usually not caused by an intra-articular problem, but more likely results from a trigger point, bursitis, SI, or back problem.

BOX 16-1 ▼ Red Flag Histories Associated With the Lower Extremity

- Previous history of cancer
- Previous history of renal or urologic disease such as kidney stones and urinary tract infections (UTIs)
- Trauma/assault (fall, blow, lifting)
- History of infectious or inflammatory condition
  - Crohn's disease (regional enteritis) or ulcerative colitis
  - Diverticulitis
  - Pelvic inflammatory disease (PID)
  - Reiter's syndrome
  - Appendicitis
- History of gynecologic condition(s):
  - Recent pregnancy, childbirth, or abortion
  - Multiple births (multiparity)
  - Other gynecologic conditions
- History of alcoholism (e.g., hip osteonecrosis)
- Long-term use of immunosuppressants (e.g., Crohn's disease, sarcoidosis, cancer treatment, organ transplant, autoimmune disorders)
- History of heart disease (e.g., arterial insufficiency, peripheral vascular disease)
- History of AIDS (acquired immunodeficiency syndrome)-related tuberculosis
- History of hematologic disease, such as sickle cells anemia or hemophilia

---

or breast cancer is a red flag as these cancers may be associated with metastases to the hip.

Past history of joint replacement (especially hip arthroplasty) combined with recent infection of any kind and new onset of hip, groin, or knee pain is suspicious. Postoperatively, orthopedic pins may migrate, referring pain from the hip to the back, tibia, or ankle. Loose components, improper implant size, muscular imbalance, and infection that occurs any time after joint arthroplasty may cause lower quadrant pain or symptoms (Case Example 16-1).[1]

Risk Factors

Each condition, illness, or disease that can cause referred pain to the buttock, hip, thigh, groin, or lower extremity has its own unique risk factors. Most known risk factors for systemically induced problems have been discussed in the individual chapters on each specific condition.

For example, arterial insufficiency as a cause of low back, hip, buttock, or leg pain is presented as part of the discussion of peripheral vascular disease in Chapter 6 and again in Chapter 14 because it relates just to low back pain. Likewise, known risk factors for bone cancer or metastases

CASE EXAMPLE 16-1 Medical Screening After Total Hip Replacement

A 74-year-old retired homemaker had a total hip replacement (THR) 2 days ago. She remains as an inpatient with complications related to congestive heart failure. She has a previous medical history of gallbladder removal 20 years ago, total hysterectomy 30 years ago, and surgically induced menopause with subsequent onset of hypertension.

Her medications include intravenous furosemide (Lasix), digoxin, and potassium replacement.

During the initial physical therapy intervention, the client reported muscle cramping and headache but was able to complete the entire exercise protocol. Blood pressure was 100/76 mm Hg (measured in the right arm while lying in bed). Systolic measurement dropped to 90 mm Hg when the client moved from supine to standing. Pulse rate was 56 bpm with a pattern of irregular beats. Pulse rate did not change with postural change. Platelet count was 98,000 cells/mm^3 when it was measured yesterday.

How Would You Screen a Client with This History and Current Comorbidities?

Neuromuscuskeletal Systemic

Assess orthopedic complications such as signs of infection, increased skin temperature, localized swelling, pain.

Observe patient's adherence to hip precautions; note surgical technique and approach used, type of implant, and location of incision.

Be aware that orthostatic hypotension can cause dizziness, loss of balance, falls—a very dangerous situation with a recent THR.

Monitor all vital signs.

Monitor platelet levels, international normalized ratio: If low, observe for bruising, joint bleeds, deep venous thrombosis; follow precautions and exercise guidelines.[1]

Watch for signs and symptoms of cardiovascular/pulmonary impairments such as:
- Fatigue and muscle weakness

Neuromuscuskeletal Systemic

This can be compounded by osteoporosis, if present as a result of surgical menopause.

- Peripheral edema; check jugular distention (see Fig. 4-42)
- Check nail beds for signs of decreased perfusion

Observe for side effects of medications or drug interactions:
- Diuresis from Lasix (loop diuretic) can result in potassium depletion and lead to increased sensitivity of myocardium to digoxin (digitalis); monitor serum electrolytes, and observe for signs/symptoms of potassium imbalance; observe for urinary frequency and headache.
- Common adverse effects of Lasix include: Dehydration, muscle cramping, fatigue, weakness, headache, paresthesias, nausea, confusion, orthostatic hypotension, blurred vision, rash
- Digoxin: Headache, drowsiness, other central nervous system disturbance, bradycardia, arrhythmia, gastrointestinal upset, blurred vision, halos
*Ask if the patient must use pillows and sit up or have the head of the bed elevated; often described as "1-pillow orthopnea" or "2-pillow orthopnea"

- Tachycardia
- Fluid migration from the legs to the lungs during the supine position
- Dyspnea, orthopnea,* spasmodic cough (check sputum)

CASE EXAMPLE 16-1 Medical Screening After Total Hip Replacement—cont'd

What Signs and Symptoms Should Be Reported to the Medical Staff?

Nurses will be closely monitoring the patient's signs and symptoms. Read the medical record to stay up with what everyone else knows or has observed about the patient. Read the physician's notes to see whether medical intervention has been ordered.

Report anything observed, but not already recorded in the chart, such as muscle cramping, headache, irregular heartbeat with bradycardia, low pulse, and orthostatic hypotension.

Bradycardia is one of the first signs of digitalis toxicity. In some hospitals, a pulse less than 60 bpm in an adult would indicate that the next dose of digoxin should be withheld and the physician contacted. The protocol may be different from institution to institution.

The therapist is advised to report the following:

- Irregular heartbeat with bradycardia (a possible sign of digoxin/digitalis toxicity)
- Muscle cramping (possible adverse effect of Lasix) and headache (possible adverse effect of digoxin)
- Charting of vital signs; her blood pressure was not too unusual and pulse rate did not change with position change (probably because of medications), so she does not have medically defined orthostatic hypotension.
- Monitor vital signs throughout intervention; record the time it takes for vital signs to return to normal after exercise or treatment for your own documentation of measurable outcomes.

TABLE 16-1 ▼ Causes of Buttock Pain

Systemic	Neuromusculoskeletal
Sciatica from tumor, infection, endometriosis (see Table 16-6)	Sciatica (nerve compression from surrounding soft tissues; see Table 16-6)
Neoplasm (primary or regional metastases via lymph nodes)	Hip joint disease
Osteomyelitis of the upper femur	Disc disease (thoracic or lumbar)
Fracture (sacrum, ilium, pubic ramus)	Bursitis (psoas, gluteal)
Septic arthritis (hip, sacroiliac)	Trigger points
Abscess from aseptic necrosis, Crohn's disease, or other retroperitoneal infection	
Ischemia (e.g., claudication from peripheral vascular disease, peripheral arterial aneurysm)	

With true hip joint disease, pain will occur with active or passive motion of the hip joint; this pain increases with weight bearing.[3] Often, an antalgic gait pattern is observed as the individual leans away from the affected hip and shortens the swing phase to avoid weight bearing.

When the underlying problem is related to soft tissue (e.g., abductor weakness) rather than to the joint as the source of symptoms, the client may lean toward the affected side to compensate for the downward rotation of the pelvis.[4] With soft tissue involvement of the bursa or tendons (e.g., gluteus medius, gluteus minimus) pain may radiate down the leg to the level of insertion of the iliotibial tract on the proximal tibia.[5]

Pain with medial rotation and decreased hip medial range of motion is associated with hip osteoarthritis.[6] Cyriax's "Sign of the Buttock" (Box 16-2) can help differentiate between hip and lumbar spine disease.[7,8]

NEUROMUSCULOSKELETAL PRESENTATION

Identifying the hip as the source of a client's symptoms may be difficult because pain originating in the hip may not localize to the hip but rather may present as low back, buttock, groin, SI, anterior thigh, or even knee or ankle pain (Fig. 16-1).

On the other hand, regional pain from the low back, SI, sacrum, or knee can be referred to the hip. SI pain that localizes to the base of the spine may

TABLE 16-2 ▼ Causes of Hip Pain

Systemic	Neuromusculoskeletal*
Cancer	Low back, sacroiliac joint, sacral, or knee dysfunction
Metastasis	Osteoarthritis
Bone tumors	Synovitis
Osteoid osteoma	Femoral or inguinal hernia
Chrondrosarcoma	Bursitis (trochanteric, iliopectineal, iliopsoas, ischial)
Giant cell tumor	Fasciitis
Ewing's sarcoma	Muscle impairment (weakness, loss of flexibility, hypertonus, hypotonus sprain/strain/tear/avulsion)
Vascular	Piriformis syndrome
Arterial insufficiency	Stress reactions/fractures
Abdominal aortic aneurysm	Peripheral nerve injury or entrapment; meralgia paresthetica
Avascular necrosis	Total hip arthroplasty
Urogenital	Acetabular labral or cartilage tear
Kidney (renal) impairment	Developmental hip dysplasia; hip dislocation
Testicular cancer	Legg-Calvé-Perthes disease
Infectious/inflammatory conditions	Slipped capital femoral epiphysis (SCFE)
Abdominal or peritoneal inflammation (psoas abscess; see Box 16-3)	Osteitis pubis (pubic pain radiates to anterior hip)
Crohn's disease; ulcerative colitis	
Diverticulitis	
Appendicitis	
Pelvic inflammatory disease	
Ankylosing spondylitis	
Reiter's syndrome	
Rheumatoid arthritis	
Tuberculosis	
Metabolic disease	
Osteoporosis	
Gaucher's disease	
Paget's disease	
Ochronosis	
Hemochromatosis	
Other	
Sickle cell anemia	
Hemophilia	
Ectopic pregnancy	

* This is not an exhaustive, all-inclusive list, but rather, it includes the most commonly encountered adult neuromuscular or musculoskeletal causes of hip pain.

BOX 16-2 ▼ Sign of the Buttock

James Cyriax, M.D., was the first to write about the "Sign of the Buttock," which is actually made up of seven signs that indicate serious disease posterior to the axis of flexion and extension of the hip. These signs of neural tension deficit suggest severe central nervous system compromise, requiring medical referral. When positive, this test may help the therapist to identify serious extracapsular hip or pelvic disease.

- Primary sign of the buttock: Passive hip flexion more limited and more painful than the straight leg raise
- Limited straight leg raise
- Trunk flexion limited to the same extent as hip flexion
- Painful weakness of hip extension
- Noncapsular pattern of restriction (hip); capsular pattern: Marked limitation of hip flexion and medial rotation with some limitation of abduction and little or no limitation of adduction and lateral rotation
- Swelling in the buttocks region
- Empty end feel with hip flexion

Data from: Cyriax J: Textbook of Orthopaedic Medicine. Diagnosis of Soft Tissue Lesions, 8th edition, Philadelphia, 1983, WB Saunders.

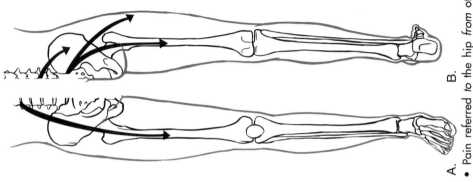

Fig. 16-1 • Pain referred *from* the hip to other structures and anatomic locations. Pain from a pathologic condition of the hip can be referred to the low back, sacroiliac or sacral area, groin, anterior thigh, knee, or ankle.

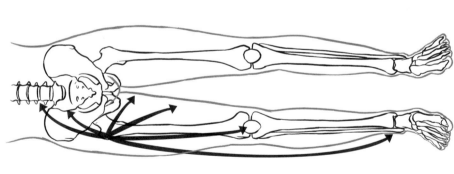

A.

B.

Fig. 16-2 • Pain referred *to* the hip *from* other structures and anatomic locations. **A,** Hip pain referred from the upper lumbar vertebrae can radiate into the anterior aspect of the thigh. **B,** Hip pain from the lower lumbar vertebrae and sacrum is usually felt in the gluteal region, with radiation down the back or outer aspect of the thigh.

be accompanied by radicular pain extending across the buttock and down the leg. It can also cross the lateral hip area. Additionally, SI joint dysfunction can cause groin pain and, with referred pain to the hip, may be accompanied by an ipsilateral decrease in hip joint internal rotation of 15 degrees or more, thereby confusing the clinical picture even further.[9]

Overlying soft tissue structure disorders such as femoral hernia, bursitis, or fasciitis; muscle impairments such as weakness, loss of flexibility, hypertonus or hypotonus, strain, sprain, or tears; and peripheral nerve injury or entrapment, including meralgia paresthetica can also cause localized hip pain.

Hip pain referred from the upper lumbar vertebrae can radiate into the anterior aspect of the thigh, whereas hip pain from the lower lumbar vertebrae and sacrum is usually felt in the gluteal

region, with radiation down the back or outer aspect of the thigh (Fig. 16-2).

The client with pain caused by component instability following total hip arthroplasty may report hip or groin pain with activity, pain at rest, or both. Clinically, a history of "start up" pain may indicate a loose component. After 5 or 10 steps, the groin pain subsides. Pain may increase again after a moderate amount of walking. Groin or thigh pain is most common with micromotion at the bone–prosthesis interface or other loose component, periosteal irritation, or an undersized femoral stem.[10-12]

The client reports a dull aching pain in the thigh with no history of systemic illness or recent trauma. Often, the pain is localized to the site of the prosthetic stem tip. The client points to a spe-

CASE EXAMPLE 16-2 Noncapsular Hip Pattern

A 46-year-old male long-distance runner developed sudden onset of right hip pain. He was given a diagnosis of trochanteric bursitis by an orthopedic physician and was referred to physical therapy.

Objective Findings

− For tenderness on palpation over the greater trochanter

− Trigger points of the hip and low back region

+ Noncapsular pattern of restriction of the hip (capsular pattern in the hip is flexion, abduction, and medial rotation); client was limited in extension and lateral rotation

+ Heel strike test

The major criteria for a medical diagnosis of trochanteric bursitis consist of marked tenderness to deep palpation of the greater trochanter and relief of pain after peritrochanteric injection with a local anesthetic and corticosteroid.

The absence of greater trochanter tenderness and the presence of a noncapsular pattern of restriction of the hip were not consistent with the given diagnosis. Local injection was not administered. If an injection had been given, trochanteric bursitis may have been eliminated from the list of possible diagnoses.

Objective findings are not consistent with trochanteric bursitis. What do you do now?

More tests, of course, and more questions! Is there any history of cancer or prostate problems? Take his vital signs. Can he squat? Clear the hip. Conduct a review of systems to look for a pattern in the past medical history, clinical presentation, and any associated signs and symptoms.

Look for a pattern of symptoms that suggests a particular visceral system. Hip pain can be caused by gastrointestinal, vascular, infectious, or cancerous causes. Ask a few screening questions directed at each of these systems. For example:

Gastrointestinal: Are you having any nausea? Vomiting? Abdominal pain? Changes in bowel function? Blood in the stool? Test for psoas abscess.

Vascular: Any throbbing pain? Presence of varicose veins? Trophic changes? History of heart disease?

Infectious: Any history of inflammatory bowel conditions such as Crohn's disease, ulcerative colitis, or diverticulitis? Ever have appendicitis? Any recent skin rashes in the legs?

Cancerous: Previous history of cancer? Bone pain at night? Night sweats? Palpate the lymph nodes in the inguinal and popliteal regions.

Result: Red flags included:

• Age

• Past history of prostate cancer at age 44

• Positive heel strike test

• Noncapsular hip pattern

• Inconsistent symptoms with diagnosis

The results of the physical therapy examination warranted further medical evaluation, and the client was returned to the physician with a recommendation for imaging studies. Magnetic resonance imaging (MRI) results indicated a nondisplaced, complete fracture of the femoral neck from prostate cancer that had metastasized to the bone.

(Case Example 16-2). The pattern of movement restriction most common with a capsular pattern for the hip is limitation of flexion, abduction, medial rotation and, sometimes, slight limitation of hip extension. Empty end feel can be an indicator of potentially serious disease such as infection or neoplasm. Empty end feel is described as limiting pain before the end range of motion is reached but with no resistance perceived by the examiner.[8] Whenever assessing hip joint pain for a systemic or viscerogenic cause, the therapist should look at

Data from Jones DL, Erhard RE: Differential diagnosis with serious pathology: A case report. *Phys Ther* 76:S89-S90, 1996.

SYSTEMIC PRESENTATION

A noncapsular pattern of restricted hip motion (e.g., limited hip extension, adduction, lateral rotation) may be a sign of serious underlying disease

cific spot along the anterolateral thigh. Pain on initiation of activity that resolves with continued activity should raise suspicion of a loose prosthesis. Persistent pain that is not relieved with rest and continues through the night suggests infection, requiring medical referral.[10]

hip rotation in the neutral position and perform the log-rolling test. With the client in the supine position, the examiner supports the client's heels in the examiner's hands and passively rolls the feet in and out. Decreased range of motion (usually accompanied by pain) is positive for an intra-articular source of symptoms. If normal hip rotation is present in this position but the motion reproduces hip pain, then an extra-articular cause should be considered.

Log-rolling of the hip back and forth is generally considered to be the most specific examination maneuver for intra-articular hip disease because it rotates the femoral head back and forth in relation to the acetabulum and capsule, not stressing any of the surrounding extra-articular structures.[13] The test does not identify the specific disease present but identifies the source of the symptoms as intra-articular.

Keep in mind that if normal rotations are present but painful, the problem may still be musculoskeletal in origin (e.g., SI, early sign of arthritic changes in the hip joint). Full motion is also possible in the early stages of avascular necrosis and sickle cell anemia. The log-rolling test should be combined with Patrick's or Faber's (flexion, abduction, and external rotation) test and the scour (quadrant) test to determine whether the hip is a possible source of symptoms.

Groin

The physical therapist may see a client with an isolated groin problem (Case Example 16-3), but more often, the individual has low back, pelvic, hip, or SI problems with a secondary complaint of groin pain. Possible systemic causes of groin pain are wide ranging, whether it appears as an isolated symptom or in combination with pelvic, hip, low back, or thigh pain (Table 16-3) (Case Example 16-4).

Palpating the groin area is usually necessary in making a differential diagnosis. This can be a sensitive issue, and the therapist is advised to have a third person in the examination area. This person should be the same gender as the client. The therapist should explain the examination procedure and obtain the client's permission.

During examination of the groin, the physical therapist may palpate enlarged lymph nodes, or the client may indicate these nodes to the examiner. Painless, progressive enlargements of lymph nodes or lymph nodes that are aberrant or suspicious for any reason, especially if present in more than one area or in the presence of a past medical history of cancer, are an indication of the need for medical referral.

Changes in lymph nodes without a previous history of cancer continue to represent a yellow or red flag. Tender, movable inguinal lymph nodes may be a sign of food intolerance or allergies or an indication that the body is fighting off an infectious process. The therapist should use his or her best clinical judgment in deciding what to do but should always err on the side of caution. When doubt arises, one should contact the physician and communicate any concerns, observations, or questions.

NEUROMUSCULOSKELETAL PRESENTATION

Neuromuscular or musculoskeletal causes of groin pain should also be considered (Case Example 16-5).[14] Groin pain is a common complaint in sports that involve kicking and rapid change of direction (e.g., soccer, hockey). The most common musculoskeletal cause of groin pain is strain of the adductor muscles, most often involving the adductor longus. The history includes a specific trauma or injury, which occurs primarily at the junction of the muscle fibers and the extended tendon of origin. Acutely, this injury causes pain with passive stretching or active contraction; eccentric activation may be even more painful. Acute injury may be followed in several days by ecchymosis.

Another common problem in the young athlete or long distance runner is acute muscle strain or stress reaction (stress fracture). Chronic, unresolved groin pain in the athletic population also has been linked with altered neuromotor control.[15] The therapist may need to evaluate groin pain from a motor control point of view.

Older adults are more likely to experience hip, buttock, or groin pain associated with arthritis, lumbar stenosis, or hip arthroplasty. Arthritis is characterized by radiating pain to the knee, but not below, with decreased hip range of motion. Gait disturbances may be seen as arthritis progresses.[11]

Hip and groin pain secondary to lumbar stenosis can manifest as low back pain that radiates to the lower extremities. The pain begins and gets worse with ambulation. Standing and walking may also increase symptoms when the lumbar spine assumes a more lordotic position and the ligamentum flavus folds in on itself, pinching the foramina closed. The client who has stenosis bends forward or sits to avoid painful symptoms. Clients who have a total hip arthroplasty for hip pain may have continued groin and buttock pain, secondary to sciatica or lumbar spinal stenosis.[11]

CASE EXAMPLE 16-3 Groin Pain in a 13-Year-Old Skateboarder

Referral: A 13-year-old boy presented with a 2-week history of left groin pain. He reported a skateboarding accident as the cause of the symptoms. He was coming down a flight of stairs, hit the last step by mistake, and caught his foot on the stair railing. His leg was forced into wide abduction and external rotation. No (heard or felt) pop or snap was perceived at the time of injury.

The client continued skateboarding but experienced increasing pain 2 hours later. At that time, he could "hardly walk" and has had trouble walking without limping ever since. He tried getting back to skateboarding but was stopped by sharp pain in the groin. No other symptoms were reported (no saddle anesthesia, no numbness and tingling, no bladder changes, no constitutional symptoms).

Clinical Presentation: An antalgic gait was observed as the boy avoided putting full weight through the hip during the stance phase. Trendelenburg gait or Trendelenburg test was not positive. He could not do a squat test because of pain. He could not put enough weight on the left leg to try heel walking or toe walking.

Generalized pain occurred along the inner thigh and was described as "tenderness." The child cannot internally rotate the hip past midline. Abduction was limited to 30 degrees with painful empty end feel. During active hip flexion, the hip automatically flexes, abducts, and externally rotates. Pain increases with active assisted or passive hip flexion when one is trying to keep the hip in neutral alignment.

Associated Signs and Symptoms: When asked about symptoms of any kind anywhere else in his body, the boy replied, "No." When offered a list of possible symptoms, these were all negative. He did admit to being slightly constipated because of the pain. Vital signs were all within normal limits.

Is medical referral indicated in the absence of any signs or symptoms of viscerogenic or systemic disease?

Some red flags are identified here, even though they do not point to a viscerogenic or systemic origin. Trauma, young age, and failure to complete a squat screening test for orthopedic clearance of the hip, knee, and ankle all suggest the need for medical referral before physical therapy intervention is initiated.

Turn to Table 16-3. As you look at the left column of Systemic Causes, what clinical presentation and signs and symptoms might be expected with each of these conditions? Does the current clinical presentation fit any of these?

Now look at the musculoskeletal causes of groin pain (right column, Table 16-3). Are past medical history, risk factors, or clinical presentation consistent for any of these problems? For example, pain in the hip or groin area in anyone who is not skeletally mature raises the suspicion of an orthopedic injury. Abduction and external rotation forces on the hip can produce a slipped capital femoral epiphysis (SCFE).

This is the case here, which required imaging studies for diagnosis. Anteroposterior x-rays were negative, but a lateral view showed slippage to confirm SCFE.

SYSTEMIC PRESENTATION

The clinical presentation of groin pain from a systemic source does not vary from musculoskeletally induced groin pain. Once again, the key is to look at the client's age (e.g., atherosclerotically induced vascular problems in the older adult), past medical history (e.g., previous history of cancer, liver disease, hemophilia), and gender (e.g., ectopic pregnancy, prostate or testicular problems).

In addition, asking about the presence of other symptoms and conducting a Review of Systems may help the therapist identify any one of the systemic causes listed in Table 16-3.

Thigh

Once again, we cannot emphasize enough the importance of conducting a thorough physical examination to rule out systemic or viscerogenic disease as the source of thigh pain; client history and lower quadrant screening examination should be performed (see Box 4-15).

Data from Learch T, Resnick D: Groin pain in a 13-year-old skateboarder: *J Musculoskel Med* 20:513-515, 2003.

TABLE 16-3 ▼ Cause of Groin Pain

Systemic causes	Neuromusculoskeletal causes
Cancer	Musculotendinous strain (adductors, hamstrings, iliopsoas, abdominals)
• Spinal cord tumors	Internal oblique avulsion
• Hodgkin's disease/lymphoma	Nerve compression (ilioinguinal, obturator, lateral femoral cutaneous, sciatic nerves)
• Leukemia	Stress reaction or fracture
• Testicular	Bursitis (iliopectineal)
• Prostate	Pubalgia
Upper urinary tract problems affecting the kidneys or ureters (inflammation, infection, obstruction)	Osteitis pubis (most common in distant runners; insidious onset of midline pain that radiates to the groin; pain reproduced by palpation of the pubis [anterior], passive hip abduction, and resisted hip adduction)
Fluid in peritoneal cavity	Trauma (physical, sexual, birth)
• Ascites (cirrhosis)	Inguinal or femoral hernia (abdominal wall abnormality)
• Congestive heart failure	Hip joint impairment
• Cancer	• Subluxation, dislocation, dysplasia
• Hyperaldosteronism	• Avascular necrosis (osteonecrosis)
Hemophilia	• Total hip arthroplasty (loosening, infection, bone loss, subsidence)
• Gastrointestinal bleeding	• Slipped capital femoral epiphysis (SCFE)
Abdominal aortic aneurysm, peripheral arterial aneurysm	• Arthritis, arthrosis
Gynecologic conditions	Sacroiliac joint (SIJ) impairment
• Cancer	Lumbar spine impairment (spinal stenosis, disc disease)
• Endometriosis	Trigger points
• Ectopic pregnancy (not common)	Thoracic disc disease (lower thoracic spine)
• Sexually transmitted infection	
• Pelvic inflammatory disease (PID)	
Infection, usually intra-abdominal or intraperitoneal infection (see Box 16-3)	
Prostate impairment (prostatitis, benign prostatic hyperplasia or BPH, prostate cancer)	

CASE EXAMPLE 16-4   Soft Tissue Sarcoma

A 38-year-old female patient was referred to physical therapy by a primary care clinic physician assistant with a diagnosis of "groin strain." The client denied any injury or trauma. Little to no pain was reported, but a feeling of "fullness" in the left proximal thigh was described. She was unable to cross her legs when sitting because of this fullness. No other constitutional symptoms or associated symptoms were noted.

When asked, "How long have you had this?" the client thought it had been present for the past 3 months. When asked, "Has it changed since you first noticed it?" she stated that she thought it was getting larger.

Examination: There was an obvious area of edema or tissue mass was identified in the proximal medial left thigh. No tenderness, bruising, erythema, or skin temperature changes were reported. The area in question had a boggy feel on palpation. Lower extremity range of motion and manual muscle testing were within normal limits.

Screening and Differential Diagnosis: Look at Table 16-3. As you review the possible systemic and musculoskeletal causes of groin pain, what additional questions and tests or measures must be asked/carried out to complete your screening examination?

CASE EXAMPLE 16-4 Soft Tissue Sarcoma—cont'd

On the Systemic Side

- **Spinal cord tumors**—no temperature changes, dermatomal changes, or associated bowel and bladder changes; no further testing required at this time

- **Hodgkin's disease/lymphoma/leukemia**—Ask about previous history of cancer, family history of cancer; palpate lymph nodes (quick screen of lymph nodes above and below the groin and careful examination of inguinal lymph nodes)

- **Urinary tract involvement**—no history of recent fever, chills, difficulty urinating, or urinary tract infection; no blood in the urine; no further questions at this time

- **Ascites**—No apparent abdominal ascites, no history of alcoholism; check for asterixis, liver palms (palmar erythema); ask about symptoms of carpal tunnel syndrome, look for spider angiomas during inspection, and observe nail beds for any changes (nails of Terry)

- **Hemophilia**—It is a long shot, but ask about personal/family history

- **Abdominal aortic aneurysm**—Ask about bounding pulse sensation in the abdomen; palpate aortic pulse width (see Fig. 4-51); ask about the presence of chest or back pain at any time, but especially with exertion

- **Gynecologic**—Ask about a history of pelvic pain, pelvic inflammatory disease, or sexually transmitted infection

- **Appendicitis**—Perform McBurney's test, Blumberg's sign, and iliopsoas and obturator tests (see Chapter 8 for descriptions)

On the Musculoskeletal Side

- **Muscle strain**—As already tested, no loss of motion or strength; no pain with resisted movement; no history of trauma or overuse; red flag: Clinical presentation is not consistent with the medical diagnosis

- **Internal oblique avulsion/stress reaction or fracture**—As above

- **Pubalgia**—As above; no painful symptoms reported, no pain on palpation

- **Sexual assault/domestic violence**—Even though the client denies trauma, consider a screening interview for nonaccidental trauma (see Chapter 2 or Appendix B-3); absence of erythema, skin bruising, or other skin changes makes this type of trauma unlikely at this time

- **Total hip arthropathy**—Negative history

- **Avascular necrosis**—Not likely, given the clinical presentation; ask about a history of long-term use of immunosuppressants (corticosteroids for Crohn's disease, sarcoidosis, autoimmune disorders)

- **Trigger points**—Atypical presentation for a trigger point; check for latent trigger points of the adductors, iliopsoas, vastus medialis, and sartorius

Special Questions to Ask: Take a final look at *Special Questions to Ask* in this chapter. Have you missed anything? Left anything out?

Result: On the basis of lack of objective findings and red flags of mass increasing in size and clinical presentation inconsistent with medical diagnosis, the therapist consulted with an orthopedic surgeon in the same health care facility. The orthopedic surgeon ordered x-rays, which were normal, and advised a short period of observation before ordering magnetic resonance imaging (MRI).

After 3 weeks, no changes were observed, and an MRI was ordered. The MRI showed a soft tissue tumor, later diagnosed on biopsy as a stage IIIB high-grade soft tissue sarcoma.

The client underwent multiple surgical procedures, including removal of the medial compartment musculature and limb salvage with an eventual hemiarthroplasty. Physical therapy included gait training, regaining safe hip active range of motion, an aquatic rehabilitation program, use of an underwater treadmill, and both open and closed kinetic chain strengthening.

Adapted from Baxter RE: Identification of neoplasm mimicking musculoskeletal pathology: A case report involving groin symptoms. Poster presented at: Combined Sections Meeting, 2004, New Orleans, LA. Used with permission.

CASE EXAMPLE 16-5 Groin Pain—Musculoskeletal Cause

A 44-year-old male patient came to physical therapy with a 7-year history of right groin pain. X-rays, bone scan, and arthrogram of the hip were negative. At the time of initial examination, the client was taking morphine for pain that was described as constant, severe, and sharp, and that was rated 8 out of 10 on the numeric rating scale (NRS; see Chapter 3). Sitting and driving made the symptoms worse, and he was unable to work as a mechanic because prolonged squatting was required. Lying supine relieved the pain.

Physical examination revealed extreme hip medial rotation associated with active hip flexion, abduction, and knee extension; each of these movements reproduced his symptoms. Passive range of motion of the right hip was painful and was limited to 95 degrees of flexion and 0 degrees of lateral rotation.

Visual inspection during movement and palpation of the greater trochanter indicated that the proximal femur had medially rotated and moved anteriorly during hip flexion. Through application of a posteroinferior glide over the proximal femur during hip flexion, groin pain was decreased and motion increased. The client was able to moderate his symptoms by avoiding hip medial rotation during hip and knee movements.

Consider: Are any red flags present? Is further screening indicated to rule out systemic origin of symptoms? If yes, what questions or tests might you consider carrying out?

Red Flags: Age (over 40); constant, intense pain

Further Screening Required: The length of time that symptoms have been present without accompanying signs and symptoms of a urologic or gastrointestinal nature (7 years) is not typical of systemic origin of musculoskeletal symptoms.

The fact that no aggravating and relieving factors are known further rules out a viscerogenic cause of pain. It would be appropriate to ask the Special Questions for Men at the end of this chapter (see also Appendix B-21).

It is always a good idea to ask one final question: *Are any other symptoms of any kind anywhere else in your body?* Special tests might include the heel strike test (fracture), translational rotation tests for stress reaction (fracture), iliopsoas and obturator tests (abscess; see Chapter 8), and trigger point assessment.

Result: The client was treated for femoral anterior glide with medial rotation (movement impairment diagnosis).[14] Training to teach the client to modify hip medial rotation during sustained postures and functional activities was a key component of the intervention. Exercises were given to strengthen the right iliopsoas muscle, hip lateral rotator muscles, and posterior gluteus medius muscle.

The client was pain-free and off pain medications 2 months later, after 6 treatment sessions. He was able to return to full-time work.

Comment: Knowledge of red flag signs and symptoms, risk factors for various systemic conditions and illnesses, associated signs and symptoms of viscerogenic pain, and typical clinical presentations for neuromuscular and musculoskeletal problems can guide the therapist in quickly sizing up a situation and deciding whether or not further screening is warranted.

In this case, the therapist can see that only a few screening questions are in order. The application of any additional special tests depends on the client's answers to screening questions. The client's immediate response to intervention is another way to verify a correct physical therapy diagnosis. Failure to progress with intervention is a red flag that indicates the need for reevaluation.

Data from Bloom NJ, Sahrmann SA: Groin pain caused by movement system impairments: A case report. Poster presented at: Combined Sections Meeting, 2004, New Orleans, LA. Submitted for publication. Used with permission.

Anterior thigh pain is more common (Table 16-4), but posterior thigh pain may occur, with ruptured abdominal aortic aneurysm. Local anterior or posterior thigh pain of systemic origin generally occurs as a deep aching generated by soft tissue irritation or bone involvement. Radicular pain is usually a sharp, stabbing pain that projects in dermatomal distributions caused by compression of the dorsal nerve roots.

NEUROMUSCULOSKELETAL PRESENTATION

The lower lumbar vertebrae and sacrum can refer pain to the gluteal and hip region, with pain radiating down the posterior or posterolateral thigh. Pain down the lateral aspect of the thigh to the knee may also be caused by inflammation of the tensor fascia lata with iliotibial band syndrome.[3]

Anterior thigh pain is commonly disc related, resulting from L3-L4 disc herniation, and occurring most often in older clients with a previous history of lumbar spine surgery. The clinical presentation varies among affected individuals, but thigh pain alone is most common (Case Example 16-6).

Back and thigh pain, a positive reverse straight leg raising test, and depressed knee reflex are described more often in clients with disc herniation at the L3-L4 level than in clients with L4-L5 and L5-S1 levels.[16,17] A positive reverse straight leg raise is defined as pain traveling down the ipsilateral leg when the person is prone and the leg is extended at the hip and the knee. A positive test is caused by tension on the femoral nerve and its roots.

Objective neurologic findings such as hyperreflexia or hyporeflexia, decreased sensation to light touch or pinprick, and decreased motor strength can occur with soft tissue problems such as bursitis. However, clients with true nerve root irritation experience pain extending into the lower leg and foot. Clients with bursitis exhibit a positive "jump" sign when pressure is applied over the greater trochanter; no jump sign is seen with nerve root irritation.[5]

A common neuromuscular cause of anterior or anterolateral thigh pain is lateral femoral cutaneous nerve (LFCN) neuralgia. Entrapment or compression of the LFCN causes pain or dysesthesia, or both, in the anterolateral thigh—a condition called meralgia paresthetica. Compression of the LFCN may occur at the level of the L2 and L3 roots through upper lumbar disc herniation or tumor in the second lumbar vertebra. LFCN neuropathy may occur after spine surgery to repair nerve damage that occurred during harvesting of the iliac bone graft or that resulted from pressure on the pelvis with use of the Relton-Hall frame.

Other causes of injury to the LFCN include abnormal posture, chronic muscle spasm, tight-fitting braces, corsets or pants, and thigh injury.[18]

TABLE 16-4 ▼ Causes of Anterior Thigh Pain

Systemic	Neuromusculoskeletal
Retroperitoneal or intra-abdominal tumor or abscess (see Box 16-3)	Musculotendinous strains (e.g., adductor, abductor, quadriceps)
Kidney stones (nephrolithiasis, ureteral or renal colic)	Iliopectineal bursitis (anterior and medial thigh pain; trochanteric bursitis (lateral thigh)
Peripheral neuropathy (bilateral, symmetric)	Peripheral neuropathy (unilateral, asymmetric)
• Diabetes mellitus	Contusions (collisions with balls, hockey pucks, the ground, other athletes)
• Neoplasm	Nerve compression (e.g., meralgia paresthetica from compression of the lateral femoral cutaneous nerve)
• Chronic alcohol use	Myositis ossificans (injury with contusion and hematoma formation)
Thrombosis (femoral artery, great saphenous vein)	Femoral shaft stress reaction or fracture; insufficiency fracture/stress reaction
Bone tumor (primary or metastases)	Hip disease (osteoarthritis, labral tear)
	Total hip arthroplasty (loose component, undersized/oversized femoral stem, periosteal irritation)
	Sacroiliac joint dysfunction
	Upper lumbar spine dysfunction; spondylolisthesis, herniated disc, previous surgery
	Trigger points
	Inguinal hernia

CASE EXAMPLE 16-6 Buttock Pain Post Prostatectomy

A 62-year-old male patient was examined by a physical therapist for a chief complaint of severe left buttock and lateral thigh pain. No injury or trauma was reported; the client noticed low back pain 3 days ago. He lifted a couple of sand bags but did not think that was the cause of his pain. He has seen the chiropractor twice this week and felt that the electrical stimulation he had on one visit "usually does it" (helped relieve the pain). Pain relief was of a very short-term nature and had no lasting effects.

Past Medical History: Prostatectomy 4 years ago for cancer followed by 36 radiation treatments. The bowel was resected, and the patient received a stoma at that time.

Current Health Report: Prostate-specific antigen has increased from 0 to 0.4 in a stepwise fashion over the past year. The patient has not seen his oncologist for any follow-up "for quite some time." At this time, the client is not taking any medications except for over-the-counter pain relievers. Supplements include calcium and fish oil.

Clinical Presentation

Pain Pattern: Pain is reported as "constant," but it "has its highs and lows." The client prefers lying on his left (involved) side. He cannot sit for longer than 1 minute without onset of radicular symptoms.

Physical Examination: Visual inspection showed flattened lumbar spine. What appeared to be atrophy was seen in the right gluteal; this was confirmed with comparative palpation. Pelvic landmarks were slightly elevated (L higher than R). Lumbar range of motion was limited in all planes with remarkably minimal flexion, which the patient said was normal for him. No centralization of pain occurred with side glides or with repeated extension in standing.

Vascular Examination: No signs of peripheral vascular disease were noted in the lower extremities. Blood pressure was not assessed.

Neurologic Screening Examination: Hyperreflexive patellar deep tendon reflexes on the right (L3); this was difficult to assess: He may have been notably hyporeflexive on the left. Achilles deep tendon reflexes (S1) appeared equal, with grading of 2/4 bilaterally. Clonus, Babinski's, and Openheim's were negative. Manual muscle testing (MMT) showed fatiguing weakness on the left at L2 (hip flexors), L3 (quadriceps), L5 (extensor hallucis longus and gluteus medius), and S1 (hamstring). No loss of light touch sensation was observed.

Associated Signs and Symptoms: No nausea or vomiting was reported. No recent significant weight loss or gain occurred. No changes in bowel or bladder function were described. The patient reported feeling chills of late, intermittently, which he says are caused by the bouts of severe pain. He showed no diaphoresis during the physical therapist's examination.

Red Flags

- Insidious onset of radicular pain in a 62-year-old with a previous history of cancer
- Constitutional symptom (chills)
- Constant, intense pain
- Notable proximal muscle weakness; multisegmental weakness on the left
- No improvement with chiropractic care or physical therapy

Result: The therapist applied some direct intervention for pain relief (positioning, Pain Reflex Release Technique™ (PRRT), trigger point release) with no immediate relief of painful symptoms. The therapist explained his concerns regarding the red flag symptoms and advised the client to make an appointment with his oncologist for further evaluation. The client was instructed to call the therapist with the name and number for the oncologist, so his findings could be relayed to her.

The client left a message on the therapist's answering machine (received the next morning) that he was "going to the ER: I've got to do something about the pain."

The client followed up midday to state that he had gone to the emergency department. Diagnostic tests were ordered, and MRI revealed a herniated nucleus pulposus (HNP) of the L3/4 disc with effacement on the L3 nerve root. The L5/S1 disc was also reportedly herniated, although this did not affect the adjacent nerve root. The client is to see a neurosurgeon next week.

For clients with hip arthroplasty, both passive and active range of motion should be evaluated to assess implant stability. X-rays are needed to look at component position, bone-prosthesis interface, and signs of fracture or infection.[10]

SYSTEMIC PRESENTATION

The pain pattern for anterior thigh pain produced by systemic causes is often the same as that presented for pain resulting from neuromusculoskeletal causes. The therapist must rely on clues from the history and the presence of associated signs and symptoms to help guide the decision-making process.

For example, obstruction, infection, inflammation, or compression of the ureters may cause a pattern of low back and flank pain that radiates anteriorly to the ipsilateral lower abdomen and upper thigh. The client usually has a past history of similar problems or additional urologic symptoms such as pain with urination, urinary frequency, low-grade fever, sweats, or blood in the urine. Murphy's percussion test (Fig. 4-51) may be positive when the kidney is involved.

The same pain pattern can occur with lower thoracic disc herniation. However, instead of urologic signs and symptoms, the therapist should look for a history of back pain and trauma, and the presence of neurologic signs and symptoms accompanying discogenic lesions.

Retroperitoneal or intra-abdominal tumor or abscess may also cause anterior thigh pain. A past history of reproductive or abdominal cancer, or the presence of any condition listed in Box 16-3 is a red flag.

Knee and Lower Leg

Pain in the lower leg is most often caused by injury, inflammation, tumor (malignant or benign), altered peripheral circulation, deep vein thrombosis (DVT), or neurologic impairment (Table 16-5). Assessment of limb pain follows the series of pain-related questions presented in Figure 3-6. The therapist can use the information in Boxes 4-12 and 4-15 to conduct a screening examination.

In addition to screening for medical problems, the therapist must remember to clear the joint above and below the area of symptoms or dysfunction. True knee pain or symptoms are often described as mechanical (local pain and tenderness with locking or giving way of the lower leg) or loading (poorly localized pain with weight bearing). Assessment of trigger points (TrPs) is also essen-

tial as pain referral to the knee from TrPs in the lower quadrant is well recognized but sometimes forgotten.[19,20]

Many therapists over the years have shared with us stories of clients treated for knee pain with a total knee replacement only to discover later (when the knee pain was unchanged) that the problem was really coming from the hip. On the flip side, it is not as likely but is still possible that hip pain can be caused by knee disease. Individual case reports of hip fracture presenting as isolated knee pain have been published[21] (Case Example 16-7).

Leg cramps, especially those occurring in the lower leg and calf, are common in the adult population. The history and physical examination are key elements in identifying the cause. The most common causes of leg cramps include dehydration, arterial occlusion from peripheral vascular disease, neurogenic claudication from spinal stenosis, neuropathy, medications, metabolic disturbances, nutritional (vitamin, calcium) deficiency, and anterior compartment syndrome from trauma, hemophilia, burns, casts, snakebites, or revascular perfusion injury.

Athletes often experience leg cramps preceded by muscle fatigue or twitching. Fractures and ligament tears can mimic a cramp. Cramping associated with severe dehydration may be a precursor to heat stroke.[22]

Burning and pain in the legs and feet at night are common in older adults. The exact cause is often unknown; many factors should be considered, including allergic response to the fabric in clothing and socks, poorly fitting shoes, long-term alcohol use, adverse effects of medications, diabetes, pernicious anemia, and restless legs syndrome.

Associated Signs and Symptoms

Asking about the presence of other signs and symptoms, conducting a review of systems, and identifying red flag symptoms will help the therapist in the clinical decision-making process. The therapist can use the Red Flags (see Appendix A-2) to guide screening questions. Always ask every client the following:

Follow-Up Questions

• Are there any other symptoms of any kind anywhere else in your body?

If the client says, "No," the therapist may want to ask some general screening questions, including questions about constitutional symptoms.

TABLE 16-5 ▲ Symptoms and Differentiation of Leg Pain

	Vascular claudication	Neurogenic claudication	Peripheral neuropathy	Restless legs syndrome
Description	Pain* is usually bilateral No burning or dysesthesia	Pain is usually bilateral but may be unilateral Burning and dysesthesia in the back, buttocks, and/or legs	Pain, aching, and numbness of feet (and hands) Motor, sensory, and autonomic changes: burning, prickling, or tingling may be present; extreme sensitivity to touch (or numbness); weakness, falling (foot drop), muscle atrophy; infection, ulcers, gangrene	Crawling, creeping sensation in legs; involuntary contractions of calf muscles, occurring especially at night Pain† can be mild to severe, lasting seconds, minutes, or hours
Associated signs and symptoms	Decreased or absent pulses Color and skin changes in feet Normal deep tendon reflexes; may be absent in people older than 60 Sciatica possible (ischemia)	Normal pulses Good skin nutrition Positive straight-leg raise Depressed or absent ankle jerks Sciatica	Pulses may be affected, depending on underlying pathologic condition (e.g., diabetes) Deep tendon reflexes diminished or absent May have positive straight-leg raise May have sciatica	Sleep disturbance, paresthesias
Location	Usually calf first but may occur in the buttock, hip, thigh, or foot	Low back, buttock, thighs, calves, feet	Feet and hands in stocking-glove pattern	Feet, calves, legs
Aggravating factors	Pain is consistent in all spinal positions; brought on by physical exertion (e.g., walking); increased by climbing stairs or walking uphill	Increased in spinal extension; increased with walking; less painful when walking uphill	Depends on underlying cause (e.g., uncontrolled glucose levels with diabetes; progressive alcoholism)	Caffeine, pregnancy, iron deficiency
Relieving factors	Relieved promptly by standing still, sitting down, or resting (1-5 minutes)	Pain decreased by sitting, lying down, bending forward, or flexion exercises (may persist for hours)	Relieved by pain medications and relaxation techniques; treatment of underlying cause	Eliminate caffeine; increase iron intake, movement, walking, moderate exercise; medications; stretching; maintain hydration; heat or cold
Ages affected	40-60+	40-60+	Varies depending on underlying cause	Variable
Cause	Atherosclerosis in peripheral arteries	Neoplasm or abscess Disc protrusion Osteophyte formation Ligamentous thickening	More than 100 causes: diabetes; medications; accidents; nerve compression; metal toxicity; nutritional deficiency; diseases such as rheumatoid arthritis, systemic lupus erythematosus, AIDS, cancer, hypothyroidism, alcoholism	Cause unknown; may be a sleep disorder, arterial disorder, or dysautonomic disorder of the autonomic nervous system; may occur with dehydration or as a side effect of many medications

* "Pain" associated with vascular claudication may also be described as an "aching," "cramping," or "tired" feeling.

† "Pain" associated with restless legs syndrome may not be painful but may be described as a "frantic," "unbearable," or "compelling" need to move the legs.

CASE EXAMPLE 16-7 Total Knee Arthroplasty

A 78-year-old woman went to the emergency department over a weekend for knee pain. She reported a knee joint replacement 6 months ago because of arthritis. X-ray examination showed that the knee implant was intact with no complications (i.e, no infection, fracture, or loose components). She was advised to contact her orthopedic surgeon the following Monday for a follow-up visit. The woman decided instead to see the physical therapist who was involved with her postoperative rehabilitation.

The physical therapist's interview and examination revealed the following information. No pain was perceived or reported anywhere except in the knee. The pain pattern was constant (always present) but was made worse by weight-bearing activities. The knee was not warm, red, or swollen. No other associated signs and symptoms or constitutional symptoms were present, and vital signs were within normal limits for her age range.

Range of motion was better than at the time of previous discharge, but painful symptoms were elicited with a gross manual muscle screening examination. After a test of muscle strength, the woman was experiencing intense pain and was unable to put any weight on the painful leg.

The physical therapist insisted that the woman contact her physician immediately and arranged by phone for an emergency appointment that same day.

Result: Orthopedic examination and pelvic and hip x-ray films showed a hip fracture that required immediate total hip replacement the same day. The knee can be a site for referred pain from other areas of the musculoskeletal system, especially when symptoms are monoarticular. Systemic origin of symptoms is more likely when multiple joints are involved or migrating arthralgias are present.

No history or accompanying signs and symptoms suggested a systemic origin of knee pain, but the pain on weight bearing made worse after muscle testing was a red flag symptom for bone involvement. Hip fractures or other hip disease can masquerade as knee pain.

Prompt diagnosis of hip fracture is important in preventing complications. This therapist chose the conservative approach with medical referral rather than proceeding with physical therapy intervention. Sometimes, the "treat-and-see" approach to symptom assessment works well, but if any identifiable red flags are identified, a physician referral is advised.

Failure to improve with physical therapy intervention may be part of the medical differential diagnosis and should be reported within a reasonable length of time, given the particular circumstances of each client.

▶ TRAUMA AS A CAUSE OF HIP, GROIN, OR LOWER QUADRANT PAIN

Trauma, including accidents, injuries, physical or sexual assault, or birth trauma, can be the underlying cause of buttock, hip, groin, or lower extremity pain.

Birth Trauma

Birth trauma is one possible cause of low back, pelvic, hip, or groin pain, with pain radiating down the leg in some cases. Multiple births, prolonged labor and delivery, forceps/vacuum delivery, and postepidural complications are just a few of the more common birth-related causes of hip, groin, and lower extremity pain. Gynecologic conditions are discussed more completely in Chapter 15.

Stress Reaction or Fracture

An undiagnosed stress reaction or stress fracture is a possible cause of hip, thigh, or groin pain. A stress reaction or fracture is a microscopic disruption, or break, in a bone that is not displaced; it is not seen initially on regular x-rays. Exercise-induced groin pain is the most common presentation.

The client is often a distance runner or military recruit (pubic ramus stress reaction) or an older adult (hip fracture). Depending on the age of the client, the therapist should look for a history of

high-energy trauma, prolonged activity, or abrupt increase in training intensity. Other risk factors include changes in running surface, use of inadequately cushioned footwear, and the presence of the female athlete triad of disordered eating, osteoporosis, and amenorrhea.[23,24]

Femoral shaft stress fractures are rare in the general population but are not uncommon among distance runners and military recruits involved in repetitive loading activities such as running and marching. Vague anterior thigh pain that radiates to the hip or knee with activity or exercise is the most common clinical presentation. The affected individual usually has full but painful active hip motion.[25] The fulcrum test (Fig. 16-3) has high clinical correlation with femoral shaft stress injury.[26]

Osteopenia or osteoporosis, especially in the postmenopausal woman or older adult with arthritis, can result in injury and fracture or fracture and injury (Case Example 16-8). The client has a small

mishap, perhaps losing her footing on a slippery surface or tripping over an object. As she tries to "catch herself," a torsional force occurs through the hip, causing a fracture and then a fall. This is a case of fracture then fall, rather than the other way around. Often, but not always, the client is unable to get up because of pain and instability of the fracture site.[27,28]

Pain on weight bearing is a red flag symptom for stress reaction or fracture in any individual. In the case of bone pain (deep pain, pain on weight bearing), the therapist can perform a heel strike test. This is done by applying a percussive force with the heel of the examiner's hand through the heel of the client's foot in a non–weight-bearing (supine) position. Reproduction of painful symptoms with axial loading is positive and highly suggestive of a bone fracture or stress reaction.[29]

The therapist can ask a physically capable client to hop on the uninvolved side and to do a full squat to clear the hip, knee, and ankle. These tests are used to screen for pubic ramus or hip stress fracture (reaction). Palpation over the injured bone may reproduce the painful symptoms, but when the stressed bone lies deep within the tissue, the therapist may be able to reproduce the pain by stressing the bone with translational (resisted active adduction) or rotational force (resisted active adduction combined with hip external rotation). Swelling is not usually evident early in the course of a stress reaction or fracture, but it does develop if the person continues athletic activity.

Look for the following clues suggestive of hip, groin, or thigh pain caused by a stress reaction or stress fracture.

Clinical Signs and Symptoms of

Stress Reaction/Stress Fracture

- Pain described as aching or deep aching
- Pain increases with activity and improves with rest
- Compensatory gluteus medius gait
- Pain localizing to a specific area of bone (localized tenderness)
- Positive Patrick's or Faber's test
- Pain reproduced by weight bearing, heel strike, or hopping test
- Pain reproduced by translational/rotational stress (exquisite pain in response to active resistance to hip adduction/hip adduction combined with external rotation)
- Thigh pain reproduced by the fulcrum test (femoral shaft fracture)

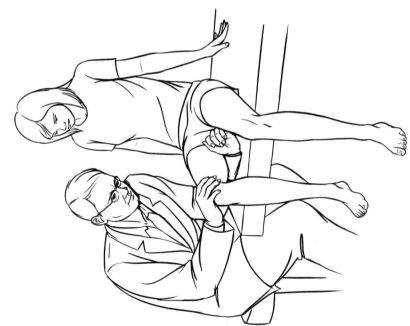

Fig. 16-3 • Fulcrum test for femoral shaft stress reaction or fracture. With the client in a sitting position, the examiner places his or her forearm under the client's thigh and applies downward pressure over the anterior aspect of the distal femur. A positive test is characterized by reproduction of thigh pain often described as "sharp," with considerable apprehension on the part of the client.[26]

- Possible local swelling
- Increased tone of hip adductor muscles; limited hip abduction
- Night pain (femoral neck stress fracture)

The therapist should keep in mind that some fractures of the intertrochanteric region do not show up on standard anteroposterior or lateral x-ray. An oblique view may be needed. If an x-ray has been ruled negative for hip fracture but the client cannot put weight on that side, and a heel strike test is positive, communication with the physician may be warranted.

Assault

The client may not report assault as the underlying cause, or he or she may not remember any specific trauma or accident. It may be necessary to take a sexual history (see Appendix B-29) that includes specific questions about sexual activity (e.g., incest, partner assault or rape) or the presence of sexually transmitted infection. Appropriate

---

CASE EXAMPLE 16-8   Insufficiency Fracture

A 50-year-old Caucasian woman was referred to physical therapy with a 4-year history of rheumatoid arthritis (RA). She had been taking prednisone (5 to 30 mg/day) and sulfasalazine (1 g twice a day).

She has a history of hypertension, smokes a pack of cigarettes a day, and drinks a six-pack of beer every night. She lives alone and no longer works outside the home. She admits to very poor nutrition and does not take a multivitamin or calcium.

Clinical Presentation: Symmetric arthritis with tenderness and swelling of bilateral metacarpophalangeal (MCP) joints, proximal interphalangeal joints (PIPs), wrists, elbows, and metatarsophalangeal joints (MTPs).

The patient reported "hip pain," which started unexpectedly 2 weeks ago in the right groin area. The pain went down her right leg to the knee but did not cross the knee. Any type of movement made it hurt more, especially on walking.

Hip range of motion was limited because of pain; formal range of motion (active, passive, accessory motions) and strength testing were not possible.

What are the red flags in this case?

- Age
- Insidious onset with no known or reported trauma
- Cigarette smoking
- Alcohol use
- Poor diet
- Corticosteroid therapy

factors for osteoporosis. Further questioning revealed that surgical menopause took place 10 years ago; this is another risk factor.

The patient was unable to stand on the right leg unsupported. She could not squat because of her arthritic symptoms. Heel strike test was negative. Patrick's (Faber's) test) could not be performed because of the acuteness of her symptoms.

The patient was referred to her rheumatologist with a request for a hip x-ray before any further physical therapy was provided. The therapist pointed out the risk factors present for osteoporosis and briefly summarized the client's current clinical presentation.

The client was given a diagnosis of insufficiency fracture of the right inferior and superior pubic rami. An insufficiency fracture differs from a stress fracture in that it occurs when a normal amount of stress is placed on abnormal bone. A stress fracture occurs when an unusual amount of stress is placed on normal bone.

Conservative treatment was recommended with physical therapy, pain medications, and treatment of the underlying osteoporosis. Weight bearing as tolerated, a general conditioning program, and an osteoporosis exercise program were prescribed by the physical therapist. Client education about managing active rheumatoid arthritis and synovitis was also included.

Result: The client was showing multiple risk

screening questions for assault or domestic violence are included in Chapter 2; see also Appendix B-3.

▶ SCREENING FOR SYSTEMIC CAUSES OF SCIATICA

Sciatica, described as pain radiating down the leg below the knee along the distribution of the sciatic nerve, is usually related to mechanical pressure or inflammation of lumbosacral nerve roots (Fig. 16-4). Sciatica is the term commonly used to describe pain in a sciatic distribution without overt signs of radiculopathy.

Radiculopathy denotes objective signs of nerve (or nerve root) irritation or dysfunction, usually resulting from involvement of the spine. Symptoms of radiculopathy may include weakness, numbness, or reflex changes. Sciatic *neuropathy* suggests damage to the peripheral nerve beyond the effects of compression, often resulting from a lesion outside the spine that affects the sciatic nerve (e.g., ischemia, direct trauma to the nerve, compression by neoplasm or piriformis muscle).

The terms radiculopathy and neuropathy are often used interchangeably, although a pathologic difference is described here. Electrodiagnostic studies, including nerve conduction studies (NCS), electromyography (EMG), and somatosensory evoked potential studies (SSEPs), are used to make the differentiation.

Sciatica has many neuromuscular causes, both discogenic and nondiscogenic; systemic or extraspinal conditions can produce or mimic sciatica (Table 16-6). Risk factors for a mechanical cause of sciatica include previous trauma to the low back, taller height, tobacco use, pregnancy, and work and occupational-related posture or movement.[30]

Risk Factors

Risk factors for systemic or extraspinal causes vary with each condition (Table 16-7). For example, clients with arterial insufficiency are more likely to be heavy smokers and to have a history of atherosclerosis. Increasing age, past history of cancer, and comorbidities such as diabetes mellitus, endometriosis, or intraperitoneal inflammatory disease (e.g., diverticulitis, Crohn's disease, pelvic inflammatory disease) are risk factors associated with sciatic-like symptoms (Case Example 16-9).

Total hip arthroplasty is a common cause of sciatica because of the proximity of the nerve to the hip joint. Possible mechanisms for nerve injury include stretching, direct trauma from retractors, infarction, hemorrhage, hip dislocation, and compression.[31] Sciatica referred to as sciatic nerve "burn" has been reported as a complication of hip arthroplasty caused by cement extrusion. The incidence of this complication has decreased with its increased recognition, but even small amounts of cement can cause heat production or direct irritation of the sciatic nerve.[32]

Propionibacterium acnes, a cause of spinal infection, has been linked to sciatica. Bacterial wound contamination during spinal surgery has been traced to this pathogen on the patient's skin. Minor trauma to the disc with a breach to the

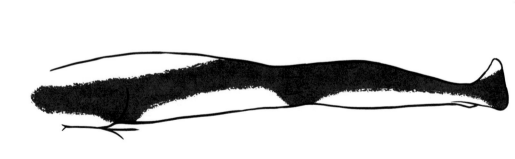

Fig. 16-4 • Sciatica pain pattern. Perceived or reported pain associated with compression, stretch, injury, entrapment, or scarring of the sciatic nerve depends on the location of the lesion in relation to the nerve root. The sciatic nerve is innervated by L4, L5, S1, S2, and sometimes S3 with several divisions (e.g., common fibular (peroneal) nerve, sural nerve, tibial nerve).

TABLE 16-6 ▼ Causes of Sciatica

Neuromuscular causes			Systemic/extraspinal causes*
Disorder	**Symptoms**	**Physical Signs**	**Disorders**
Discogenic			
Disc herniation	Low back pain with radiculopathy and paravertebral muscle spasm; Valsalva's maneuver and sciatic stretch reproduce symptoms	Restricted spinal movement; restricted spinal segment; positive Lasèque's sign or restricted straight leg raise (SLR)	Vascular • Ischemia of sciatic nerve • Peripheral vascular disease (PVD) • Intrapelvic aneurysm (internal iliac artery)
Lateral entrapment syndrome (spinal stenosis)	Buttock and leg pain with radiculopathy; pain often relieved by sitting, aggravated by extension of the spine	Similar to disc herniation	Neoplasm (primary or metastatic)
Nondiscogenic			Diabetes mellitus (diabetic neuropathy)
Sacroiliitis	Low back and buttock pain	Tender sacroiliac joint; positive lateral compression test; positive Patrick's test	Megacolon Pregnancy; vaginal delivery Infection
Trochanteric bursitis	Buttock and lateral thigh pain; worse at night and with activity	Tender greater trochanter; rule out associated leg-length discrepancy; positive "jump sign" when pressure is applied over the greater trochanter	• Bacterial endocarditis • Wound contamination[33,34] • Herpes zoster (shingles) • Psoas muscle abscess (see Box 16-3)
Iliolumbar syndrome	Pain in iliolumbar ligament area (posterior iliac crest); referred leg pain	Tender iliac crest and increased pain with lateral or side bending	• Reiter's syndrome Total hip arthroplasty Endometriosis
Piriformis syndrome	Low back and buttock pain with referred pain down the leg to the ankle or midfoot	Pain and weakness on resisted abduction/external rotation of the thigh	Deep venous thrombosis (DVT; blood clot)
Greater trochanteric pain syndrome (GTPS)	Mimics lumbar nerve root compression	Low back, buttock, or lateral thigh pain; may radiate down the leg to the iliotibial tract insertion on the proximal tibia; inability to sleep on the involved side[5]	
Ischiogluteal bursitis	Buttock and posterior thigh pain; worse with sitting	Tender ischial tuberosity; positive SLR and Patrick's tests; rule out associated leg-length discrepancy	
Posterior facet syndrome	Low back pain	Lateral bending in spinal extension increases pain; side bending and rotation to the opposite side are restricted at the involved level	
Fibromyalgia	Back pain, difficulty sleeping, anxiety, depression	Multiple tender points (see Fig. 12-2)	

Data from Namey TC, An HC: Sorting out the causes of sciatica. *Mod Med* 52:132, 1984.
* Clinical symptoms of systemic/extraspinal sciatica can be very similar to those of sciatica associated with disc protrusion.

TABLE 16-7 ▼ Risk Factors for Sciatica

Musculoskeletal or neuromuscular factors	Systemically induced factors
Previous low back injury or trauma; direct fall on buttock(s); gunshot wound	Tobacco use
	History of diabetes mellitus
Total hip arthroplasty	Atherosclerosis
Pregnancy	Previous history of cancer (metastases)
Work- or occupation-related postures or movements	Presence of intra-abdominal or peritoneal inflammatory disease (abscess):
Fibromyalgia	• Crohn's disease
Leg-length discrepancy	• Pelvic inflammatory disease
Congenital hip dysplasia; hip dislocation	• Diverticulitis
Degenerative disc disease	Endometriosis of the sciatic nerve
Piriformis syndrome	Radiation therapy (delayed effects; rare)
Spinal stenosis	Recent spinal surgery, especially with instrumentation

---

CASE EXAMPLE 16-9 Low Back Pain With Sciatica

A 52-year-old man with low back pain and sciatica on the left side has been referred to you by his family physician. He underwent discectomy and laminectomy on two separate occasions about 5 to 7 years ago. No imaging studies have been done since that time.

What follow-up questions would you ask to screen for systemic disease?

1. The first question should always be, Did you actually see your doctor? [Of course, communication with the physician is the key here in understanding the physician's intended goal with physical therapy and his or her thinking about the underlying cause of the sciatica.]

2. Assess for the presence of constitutional symptoms. For example, after paraphrasing what the client has told you, ask, "Are you having any other symptoms of any kind in your body that you haven't mentioned?" If no, ask more specifically about the presence of associated signs and symptoms; name constitutional symptoms one by one.

3. Follow-up with Special Questions for Men (see Appendix B-21). Include questions about past history of prostate health problems, cancer of any kind, and current bladder function.

4. Take a look at Table 16-6. By reviewing the possible systemic/extraspinal causes of sciatica, we can decide what additional questions might be appropriate for this man.

Vascular ischemia of the sciatic nerve can occur at any age as a result of biomechanical obstruction. It can also result from peripheral vascular disease. Check for skin changes associated with ischemia of the lower extremities. Ask about the presence of known heart disease or atherosclerosis.

Intrapelvic Aneurysm: Palpate aortic pulse width and listen for femoral bruits.

Neoplasm (primary or metastatic): Consider this more strongly if the client has a previous history of cancer, especially cancer that might metastasize to the spine. We know from Chapter 13 that the three primary sites of cancer most likely to metastasize to the bone are lung, breast, and prostate. Other cancers that metastasize to the bone include thyroid, kidney, melanoma (skin), and lymphoma. A previous history of any of these cancers is a red flag finding.

Primary bone cancer is not as likely in a middle-aged male as in a younger age group. Cancer metastasized to the bone is more likely and is most often characterized by pain on weight bearing that is deep and does not respond to treatment modalities.

Diabetes (diabetic neuropathy): Ask about a personal history of diabetes. If the client has diabetes, assess further for associated neuropathy. If not, assess for symptoms of

CASE EXAMPLE 16-9 Low Back Pain With Sciatica—cont'd

possible new-onset, but as yet undiagnosed, diabetes.

Megacolon: An unlikely cause unless the client is much older or has recently undergone major surgery of some kind.

Pregnancy: Not a consideration in this case.

Infection: Ask about a recent history of infection (most likely bacterial endocarditis, urinary tract infection, or sexually transmitted infection, but any infection can seed itself to the joints or soft tissues). Ask about any other signs or symptoms of infection (e.g., flulike symptoms such as fever and chills or skin rash in the last few weeks).

Remember from Chapter 3 to ask the following:

Follow-Up Questions

- Are you having any pain anywhere else in your body?
- Are you having symptoms of any other kind that may or may not be related to your main problem?
- Have you recently (last 6 weeks) had any of the following:
- Fractures
- Bites (human, animal)
- Antibiotics or other medications
- Infections (you may have to prompt with specific infections such as strep throat, mononucleosis, urinary tract, upper respiratory [cold or flu], gastrointestinal, hepatitis, STDs)

Total Hip Arthroplasty: Has the client had a recent (cemented) total hip replacement (e.g., cement extrusion, infection, implant fracture, loose component)?

Result: The client had testicular cancer that had already metastasized to the pelvis and femur. By asking additional questions, the physical therapist found out that the client was having swelling and hardness of the scrotum on the same side as the sciatica. He was unable to maintain an erection or to ejaculate. The physician was unaware of these symptoms because the client did not mention them during the medical examination.

Testicular carcinoma is relatively rare, especially in a man in his 50s. It is most common in the 15- to 39-year-old male group. Metastasis usually occurs via the lymphatics, with the possibility of abdominal mass, psoas invasion, lymphadenopathy, and back pain. Palpation revealed a dominant mass (hard and painless) in the ipsilateral groin area.

Sending a client back to the referring physician in a case like this may require tact and diplomacy. In this case, the therapist made telephone contact to express concerns about the reported sexual dysfunction and palpable groin lymphadenopathy.

By alerting the physician to these additional symptoms, further medical evaluation was scheduled, and the diagnosis was made quickly.

---

possible new-onset, but as yet undiagnosed, diabetes.

mechanical integrity of the disc may also allow access by low virulent microorganisms, thereby initiating or stimulating a chronic inflammatory response. These microorganisms may cause prosthetic hip infection but also may be associated with the inflammation seen in sciatica; they may even be a primary cause of sciatica.[33,34]

Anyone with pain radiating from the back down the leg as far as the ankle has a greater chance that disc herniation is the cause of low back pain. This is true with or without neurologic findings. Unremitting, severe pain and increasing neurologic deficit are red flag findings. Sciatica caused by extraspinal bone and soft tissue tumors is rare but may occur when a mass is present in the pelvis, thigh, popliteal fossa, and calf.[35]

Clinical Signs and Symptoms of
Sciatica/Sciatic Radiculopathy

Symptoms are variable and may include the following:

- Pain along the sciatic nerve anywhere from the spine to the foot (see Fig. 16-4)
- Numbness or tingling in the groin, rectum, leg, calf, foot, or toes
- Diminished or absent deep tendon reflexes
- Weakness in the L4, L5, S1, S2 (and sometimes S3) myotomes (distal motor deficits more prominent than proximal)
- Diminished or absent deep tendon reflexes (especially of the ankle)
- Ache in the calf

Continued on p. 754

Sciatic Neuropathy

- Symptoms of sciatica as described above
- Dysesthetic* pain described as constant burning or sharp, jabbing pain
- Foot drop (tibialis anterior weakness) with gait disturbance
- Flail lower leg (severe motor neuropathy)

*Dysesthesia is the distortion of any sense, especially touch; it is an unpleasant sensation produced by normal stimuli.

The therapist can conduct an examination to look for signs and symptoms associated with systemically induced sciatica. Box 4-12 offers guidelines on conducting an assessment for peripheral vascular disease. Box 4-15 provides a checklist for the therapist to use when examining the extremities. These tools can help the therapist define the clinical presentation more accurately.

The straight leg raise (SLR) and other neurodynamic tests are widely used but do not identify the underlying cause of sciatica. For example, a positive SLR test does not differentiate between discogenic disease and neoplasm.

Without a combination of imaging and laboratory studies, the clinical picture of sciatica is difficult to distinguish from that of conditions such as neoplasm and infection. Erythrocyte sedimentation rate (ESR, or sed rate) is the rate at which red blood cells settle out of unclotted blood plasma within 1 hour. A high sed rate is an indication of infection or inflammation (see Table A, inside front cover). Elevated sed rate and abnormal imaging are effective tools to use in screening for occult neoplasm and other systemic disease.[36]

Imaging studies are an essential part of the medical diagnosis, but even with these diagnostic tests, errors in conducting and interpreting imaging studies may occur. Symptoms can also result from involvement outside the area captured on computed tomography (CT) scan or magnetic resonance imaging (MRI).

10 to 20 years or more (see Table 13-10) (Case Example 16-10).

Until now, the emphasis has been on advancing age as a key red flag for cancer. Anyone older than 50 years of age may need to be screened for systemic origin of symptoms. With cancer and, specifically, musculoskeletal pain caused by primary cancer or metastases to the bone, young age is a red flag as well. Primary bone cancer occurs most often in adolescents and young adults, hence the new red flag: age younger than 20 years, or bone pain in an adolescent or young adult.

Cancer Recurrence

The therapist is far more likely to encounter clinical manifestations of metastases from cancer recurrence than from primary cancer. Breast cancer often affects the shoulder, thoracic vertebrae, and hip first, before other areas. Recurrence of colon (colorectal) cancer is possible with referred pain to the hip and/or groin area.

Beware of any client with a past history of colorectal cancer and recent (past 6 months) treatment by surgical removal. Reseeding the abdominal cavity is possible. Every effort is made to shrink the tumor with radiation or chemotherapy before attempts are made to remove the tumor. Even a small number of tumor cells left behind or introduced into a nearby (new) area can result in cancer recurrence.

Hodgkin's Disease

Hodgkin's disease arises in the lymph glands, most commonly on a single side of the neck or groin, but lymph nodes also enlarge in response to infection throughout the body. Lymph nodes in the groin area can become enlarged specifically as a result of sexually transmitted disease.

The presence of painless, hard lymph nodes that are also similarly present at other sites (e.g., popliteal space) is always a red flag symptom. As always, the therapist must question the client further regarding the onset of symptoms and the presence of any associated symptoms, such as fever, weight loss, bleeding, and skin lesions. The client must seek a medical diagnosis to be certain of the cause of enlarged lymph nodes.

Spinal Cord Tumors

Spinal cord tumors (primary or metastasized) present as dull, aching discomfort or sharp pain in the thoracolumbar area in a beltlike distribution, with pain extending to the groin or legs. Depending on the location of the lesion, symptoms may be unilateral or bilateral with or without radicular

SCREENING FOR ONCOLOGIC CAUSES OF LOWER QUADRANT PAIN

Many clients with orthopedic or neurologic problems have a previous history of cancer. The therapist must recognize signs and symptoms of cancer recurrence and those associated with cancer treatment such as radiation therapy or chemotherapy. The effects of these may be delayed by as long as

CASE EXAMPLE 16-10 Evaluating a Client for Cancer Recurrence

Referral: A 54-year-old man is self-referred to physical therapy on the recommendation of his personal trainer who is a friend of yours. He is experiencing leg weakness (greater on the right), with occasional pain radiating into the groin area on both sides.

He reports a twisting back injury 5 years ago when he was shoveling snow. At that time, he saw a physical therapist but did not get any better until he started working out at the YMCA.

Leg weakness has been present about 2 weeks. Last weekend, he went to the emergency department because his leg was numb and he could not lift his ankle. He was told to rest. The leg was better the next day.

Past Medical History: Renal calculi, surgery for parathyroid and thyroid cancer 10 years ago, pneumonia 20 years ago. Currently seeing a counselor for emotional problems.

Objective Findings:
Neurologic Screen

- Alert; oriented to time, place, person
- Pupils equal and equally reactive to light; eye movements in all directions without difficulty
- No tremor, upper extremity weakness, or changes in deep tendon reflexes (DTRs)
- Straight leg raise (SLR) was mobile and pain free to 90 degrees bilaterally
- Iliopsoas, gluteal, hamstring manual muscle testing (MMT) = 3/5 on the right side. MMT within normal limits on the left side.
- Tibialis anterior, plantar evertors and flexors: MMT = 2/5 (right); 3+ to 4 on the left
- No ankle clonus, no Babinski's, no changes in DTRs of LEs
- Increased muscle tone in both lower extremities

No pain was reported with any movements performed during the examination.

Name 3 red flag symptoms in this case.

Age is the first red flag: A man over 40 (and especially over 50 years of age) with a previous history of cancer (second red flag) and new onset of painless neurologic deficit (third red flag) is significant.

Now that we have identified three red flags, what is next? Does this signify an automatic referral to the physician? We do not think so: The need for physician referral may depend on the specific red flags that are present. For example, in the case just presented, the three red flags are pretty significant. Take a closer look, and gather as much information as possible. In this case, it appears likely that an immediate referral is warranted.

Can we tell whether this is a recurrence of his previous cancer now metastasized or the presence of prostate cancer? No, but we can ask some additional questions to look for clusters of associated signs and symptoms that might point to prostate involvement. First, ask about bladder function, urination, and finally, sexual function. Remember, you may have to explain the need to ask a few personal questions.

- Have you ever had prostate problems or been told you have prostate problems?
- Have you had any changes in urination recently?
- Can you easily start a flow of urine?
- Can you keep a steady stream without stopping and starting?
- When you are finished urinating, does it feel as though your bladder is empty? Or, do you feel like you still have to go, but you can't get any more out?
- Do you ever dribble urine?
- Do you have trouble getting an erection?
- Do you have trouble keeping an erection?
- Do you have trouble ejaculating?

Because the patient is seeing a counselor for emotional problems, you may wish to screen him for emotional overlay. You can use the three tools discussed in Chapter 3 (Symptom Magnification, McGill's Pain Questionnaire, Waddell's nonorganic tests).

After you have completed your examination, step back and put all the pieces together. Is there a cluster of signs and symptoms that point to any particular system? The answer to this question may lead you to ask some additional questions or to confirm the need for medical attention.

symptoms. The therapist should look for and ask about associated signs and symptoms (e.g., constitutional symptoms, bleeding or discharge, lymphadenopathy).

Symptoms of thoracic disc herniation can mimic spinal cord tumor. In isolated cases, thoracic disc extrusion has been reported to cause groin pain and lower extremity weakness that gets progressively worse over time. A tumor is suspected if the client has painless neurologic deficit, night pain, or pain that increases when supine.

Testing the cremasteric reflex may help the therapist identify neurologic impairment in any male with suspicious back, pelvic, groin (including testicular), or anterior thigh pain. The cremasteric reflex is elicited by stroking the thigh downward with a cotton-tipped applicator (or handle of the reflex hammer). A normal response in males is upward movement of the testicle (scrotum) on the same side. The absence of a cremasteric reflex is an indication of disruption at the T12-L1 level.

Additionally, groin pain associated with spinal cord tumor is disproportionate to that normally expected with disc disease. No change in symptoms occurs after successful surgery for herniated disc. Age is an important factor: teenagers with symptoms of disc herniation should be examined closely for tumor.[37,38]

Spinal metastases to the femur or lower pelvis may appear as hip pain. With the exception of myeloma and rare lymphoma, metastasis to the synovium is unusual. Therefore, joint motion is not compromised by these bone lesions. Although any tumor of the bone may appear at the hip, some

benign and malignant neoplasms have a propensity to occur at this location.

Bone Tumors

Osteoid osteoma, a small, benign but painful tumor, is relatively common, with 20% of lesions occurring in the proximal femur and 10% in the pelvis. The client is usually in the second decade of life and complains of chronic dull hip, thigh, or knee pain that is worse at night and is alleviated by activity and aspirin. Usually, an antalgic gait is present, along with point tenderness over the lesion with restriction of hip motion.

A great many varieties of benign and malignant tumors may appear differently, depending on the age of the client and the site and duration of the lesion (Case Example 16-11).[39,40] Malignant lesions compressing the lateral femoral cutaneous nerve can cause symptoms of meralgia paresthetica, delaying diagnosis of the underlying neoplasm. Other bone tumors that cause hip pain, such as chondroblastoma, chondrosarcoma, giant cell tumor, and Ewing's sarcoma, are discussed in greater detail in Chapter 13.

Clinical Signs and Symptoms of

Buttock, Hip, Groin, or Lower Extremity Pain Associated with Cancer

- Bone pain, especially on weight bearing; positive heel strike test
- Antalgic gait
- Local tenderness

Continued on p. 758

CASE EXAMPLE 16-11   Ischial Bursitis

Referral: A 30-year-old dentist was referred to physical therapy by an orthopedic surgeon for ischial bursitis, sometimes referred to as "Weaver's bottom." He reported left buttock pain and "soreness" that was intermittent and work related. As a dentist, he was often leaning to the left, putting pressure on the left ischium.

Background: Magnetic resonance imaging (MRI) showed local inflammation on the ischial tuberosity to confirm the medical diagnosis. He was given a steroid injection and was placed on an antiinflammatory (Celebrex) before he went to physical therapy.

The client reported a mild loss of hip motion, especially of hip flexion, but no other symptoms of any kind. The pain did not radiate down the leg. No significant past medical history and no history of tobacco use were reported; only an occasional beer in social situations was described. The client described himself as being "in good shape" and working out at the local gym 4 to 5 times/week.

Intervention/Follow-Up: Physical therapy intervention included deep friction massage, iontophoresis, and stretching. The client modified his dentist's chair with padding to take pressure off the buttock. Symptoms did not improve

CASE EXAMPLE 16-11   Ischial Bursitis—cont'd

after 10 treatment sessions over the next 6 to 8 weeks; in fact, the pain became worse and was now described as "burning."

The client went back to the orthopedic surgeon for a follow-up visit. A second MRI was done with a diagnosis of "benign inflammatory mass." He was given a second steroid injection and was sent back to physical therapy. He was seen at a different clinic location by a second physical therapist.

The physical therapist palpated a lump over the ischial tuberosity, described as "swelling"; this was the only new physical finding since his previous visits with the first physical therapist.

Treatment concentrated deep friction massage in that area. The therapist thought the lump was getting better, but it did not resolve. The client reported increased painful symptoms, including pain at work and pain at night. No position was comfortable; even lying down without pressure on the buttocks was painful. He modified every seat he used, including the one in his car.

Result: The orthopedic surgeon did a bursectomy, and the pathology report came back with a diagnosis of epithelioid sarcoma. The diagnosis was made 2½ years after the initial painful symptoms. A second surgery was required because the first excision did not have clear margins.

It is often easier to see the red flags in hindsight. As this case is presented here with the final outcome, what are the red flags?

Red Flags

- No improvement with physical therapy
- Progression of symptoms (pain went from "sore" to "burning" and intermittent to constant)
- Young age
  Clinical signs of all types of bursitis are similar and include local tenderness, warmth, and erythema. The latter two signs may not be obvious when the inflamed bursa is located deep beneath soft tissues or muscles, as in this case. The presence of a "lump" or swelling as presented in this case caused a delay in medical

referral and diagnosis because MRI findings were consistent with a diagnosis of inflammatory mass. In this case, symptoms progressed and did not fit the typical pattern for bursitis (e.g., pain at night, no position comfortable).

Other Tests

When a client is sent back a second time, the therapist's reevaluation is essential for documenting any changes from the original baseline and discharge findings. Reevaluation should include the following:

- Recheck levels above and below for possible involvement, including lumbar spine, sacroiliac joint, hip, and knee; perform range of motion and special tests, and conduct a neurologic screening examination (see Chapter 4).

- Test for the sign of the buttock to look for serious disease posterior to the axis of flexion and extension of the hip (see Box 16-2). A positive sign may be an indication of abscess, fracture, neoplasm, septic bursitis, or osteomyelitis.[8]

A noncapsular pattern is typical with bursitis and by itself is not a red flag. A capsular pattern with a diagnosis of bursitis would be more suspicious. Limited straight leg raise with no further hip flexion after bending the knee is a typical positive buttock sign seen with ischial bursitis. The absence of this sign would raise clinical suspicion that the diagnosis of bursitis was not accurate.[8]

With an ischial bursitis, expect to see equal leg length, negative Trendelenburg test, and normal sensation, reflexes, and joint movements.[40] Anything outside these parameters should be considered a yellow (caution) flag.

- Assess for trigger points that may cause buttock pain, especially quadratus lumborum, gluteus maximus, and hamstrings, but also, gluteus medius and piriformis.

- Reassess for the presence of constitutional symptoms or any associated signs and symptoms of any kind anywhere in the body.

Case Report courtesy of Jason Taitch, DDS, Spokane, Washington, 2005.

- Night pain (constant, intense; unrelieved by change in position)
- Pain relieved disproportionately by aspirin
- Fever, weight loss, bleeding, skin lesions
- Vaginal/penile discharge
- Painless, progressive enlargement of inguinal and/or popliteal lymph nodes

▶ SCREENING FOR UROLOGIC CAUSES OF BUTTOCK, HIP, GROIN, OR THIGH PAIN

Ureteral pain usually begins posteriorly in the costovertebral angle but may radiate anteriorly to the upper thigh and groin (see Fig. 16-6), or it may be felt just in the groin and genital area. These pain patterns represent the pathway that genitals take as they migrate during fetal development from their original position, where the kidneys are located in the adult, down the pathways of the ureters to their final location. Pain is referred to a site where the organ was located during fetal development. A kidney stone down the pathway of the ureters causes pain in the flank that radiates to the scrotum (male) or labia (female).

The lower thoracic and upper lumbar vertebrae and the SI joint can refer pain to the groin and anterior thigh in the same pain pattern as occurs with renal disease. Irritation of the T10-L1 sensory nerve roots (genitofemoral and ilioinguinal nerves) from any cause, but especially from discogenic disease, may cause labial (women), testicular (men), or buttock pain.[41] The therapist can evaluate these conditions by conducting a neurologic screening examination and using the medical screening model.

Referred symptoms from ureteral colic can be distinguished from musculoskeletal hip pain by the history, the presence of urologic symptoms, and the pattern of pain. Is there any history of urinary tract impairment? Is there a recent history of other infection? Are any signs and symptoms noted that are associated with the renal system?

Active trigger points along the upper rim of the pubis and the lateral half of the inguinal ligament may lie in the lower internal oblique muscle and possibly in the lower rectus abdominis. These trigger points can cause increased irritability and spasm of the detrusor and urinary sphincter muscles, producing urinary frequency, retention of urine, and groin pain.[20]

The therapist can perform Murphy's percussion test to rule out kidney involvement (see Chapter 10; see also Fig. 4-51). A positive Murphy's percussion test (pain is reproduced with percussive vibration of the kidney) points to the possibility of kidney infection or inflammation. When this test is positive, ask about a recent history of fever, chills, unexplained perspiration ("sweats"), or other constitutional symptoms.

▶ SCREENING FOR MALE REPRODUCTIVE CAUSES OF GROIN PAIN

Men can experience groin pain caused by disease of the male reproductive system such as prostate cancer, testicular cancer, benign prostatic hyperplasia (BPH), or prostatitis. Isolated groin pain is not as common as groin pain that is accompanied by low back, buttock, or pelvic pain. Risk factors, clinical presentation, and associated signs and symptoms for these conditions are discussed in Chapter 14.

▶ SCREENING FOR INFECTIOUS AND INFLAMMATORY CAUSES OF LOWER QUADRANT PAIN

Anyone with joint pain of unknown cause who presents with current (or recent, i.e., within the past 6 weeks) skin rash or recent history of infection (e.g., hepatitis, mononucleosis, urinary tract infection, upper respiratory infection, sexually transmitted infection, streptococcus, dental infection)[42,43] must be referred to a health care clinic or medical doctor for further evaluation.

Conditions affecting the entire peritoneal cavity such as pelvic inflammatory disease (PID) or appendicitis may cause hip or groin pain in the young, healthy adult. Widespread inflammation or infection may be well tolerated by athletes, sometimes for up to several weeks (Case Example 16-12).

Clinical Presentation

The clinical presentation can be deceptive in young people. The fever is not dramatic and may come and go. The athlete may dismiss excessive or unusual perspiration ("sweats") as part of a good workout. Loss of appetite associated with systemic disease is often welcomed by teenagers and young adults and is not recognized as a sign of physiologic distress.

With an infectious or inflammatory process, laboratory tests may reveal an elevated ESR. Questions about the presence of any other symptoms may reveal constitutional symptoms such as ele-

CASE EXAMPLE 16-12   Dancer With Appendicitis

A 21-year-old dance major was referred to the physical therapy clinic by the sports medicine clinic on campus with a medical diagnosis of "strained abdominal muscle."

She described her symptoms as pain with hip flexion when shifting the gears in her car. Some dance moves involving hip flexion also reproduced the pain, but this was not consistent. The pain was described as "deep," "aching," and "sometimes sharp, sometimes dull."

Past medical history was significant for Crohn's disease, but the client was having no gastrointestinal symptoms at this time. On examination, no evidence of abdominal trigger points (TrPs) or muscle involvement was found. The pain was not reproduced with superficial palpation of the abdominal muscles on the day of initial examination.

Intervention with stretching exercises did not change the clinical picture during the first week. **Result:** The client was a no-show for her Monday afternoon appointment, and the physical therapy clinic receptionist received a phone call from the campus clinic with information that the client had been hospitalized over the weekend with acute appendicitis and peritonitis.

The surgeon's report noted massive peritonitis of several weeks' duration. The client had a burst appendix that was fairly asymptomatic until peritonitis developed with subsequent symptoms. Her white blood cells were in excess of 100,000 at the time of hospitalization.

In retrospect, the client did relate some "sweats" occurring off and on during the last 2 weeks and possibly a low-grade fever.

What additional screening could have been conducted with this client?

1. Ask the client whether she is having any symptoms of any kind anywhere in her body. If she answers, "No," be prepared to offer some suggestions such as:
   - Any headaches? Fatigue?
   - Any change in vision?
   - Any fevers or sweats, day or night?
   - Any blood in your urine or stools?
   - Burning with urination?

   - Any tingling or numbness in the groin area?
   - Any trouble sleeping at night?

2. Even though she has denied having any gastrointestinal symptoms associated with her Crohn's disease, it is important to follow up with questions to confirm this:
   - Any nausea? Vomiting?
   - Diarrhea or constipation?
   - Any change in your pattern of bowel movements?
   - Any blood in your stools? Change in color of your bowel movements?
   - Any foods or smells you can't tolerate?
   - Any change in your symptoms when you eat or don't eat?
   - Unexpected weight gain or loss?
   - Is your pain any better or worse during or after a bowel movement?

3. As part of the past medical history, it is important with hip pain of unknown cause to know whether the client has had any recent infections, sexually transmitted diseases, use of antibiotics or other medications, or skin rashes.

4. In a woman of reproductive years, it may be important to take a gynecologic history:
   - Have you been examined by a gynecologist since this problem started?
   - Is there any chance you could be pregnant?
   - Are you using an IUD (or IUCD)?
   - Have you had an abortion or miscarriage in the last 6 weeks?
   - Are you having any unusual vaginal discharge?

5. Check vital signs. The presence of a fever (even low-grade) is a red flag when the cause of symptoms is unknown. With a burst appendix, she may have had altered pulse and blood pressure that could alert the therapist of a systemic cause of symptoms.

6. Test for McBurney's point (Fig. 8-9), rebound tenderness or Blumberg's sign (Fig. 8-10), and the obturator or iliopsoas sign (Figs. 8-4 to 8-6). Check for Murphy's percussion (Fig. 4-51; kidney involvement).

vated nocturnal temperature, sweats, and chills, suggestive of an inflammatory process (Case Example 16-13).

Psoas Abscess

Any infectious or inflammatory process affecting the abdominal or pelvic region can lead to psoas abscess and irritation of the psoas muscle. For example, lesions outside the ureter, such as infection, abscess, or tumor, or abdominal or peritoneal inflammation, may cause pain on movement of the adjacent iliopsoas muscle that presents as hip or groin pain. (See discussion of Psoas Abscess in Chapter 10.)

Pelvic inflammatory disease (PID) is another common cause of pelvic, groin, or hip pain that can cause psoas abscess and a subsequent positive iliopsoas or obturator test. In this case, it is most likely a young woman with multiple sexual part-

ners who has a known or unknown case of untreated *Chlamydia*.

The psoas muscle is not separated from the abdominal or pelvic cavity. Figure 8-3 shows how most of the viscera in the abdominal and pelvic cavities can come into contact with the iliopsoas muscle. Any infectious or inflammatory process (Box 16-3) can seed itself to the psoas muscle by direct extension, resulting in a psoas abscess—a localized collection of pus.

Hip pain associated with such an abscess may involve the medial aspect of the thigh and femoral triangle areas (Fig. 16-5). Soft tissue abscess may cause pain and tenderness to palpation without movement. Once the abscess has formed, muscular spasm may be provoked, producing hip flexion and even contracture. The leg also may be pulled into internal rotation. Pain that increases with passive and active motion can

---

CASE EXAMPLE 16-13 Limp After Total Hip Arthroplasty

A 70-year-old man was referred to physical therapy by his doctor 1 year after a right total hip replacement (THR) for osteoarthritis. The client reports that he is in good general health without pain. His primary problem is a persistent limp, despite completion of a THR rehabilitation protocol.

How can you tell whether this is an infectious versus biomechanical problem?

First of all, laboratory tests such as erythrocyte sedimentation rate (sed rate) and C-reactive protein level can be done to screen for infection. The therapist can request this information from the medical record.

The absence of pain usually rules out infection or implant loosening. An x-ray may be needed to rule out implant loosening. Again, check the record to see whether this was part of the medical diagnostic workup.

Besides infection, a limp after THR may have many possible causes. Loosening of the prosthesis, neurologic dysfunction, altered joint biomechanics, and muscle weakness or dysfunction (e.g., hip abductors) are a few potential causes. As always, in an orthopedic examination, check the joints above (low back, sacrum, sacroiliac) and below (knee) the level of impairment. In the

case of joint replacement, evaluate the contralateral hip as well.

Test for abdominal muscle weakness. This can be confirmed with manual muscle testing or a Trendelenburg test. An anterolateral approach to THR is more likely to cause partial or complete abductor muscle disruption than is a posterior approach.

With either approach, the superior gluteal nerve can be damaged by stretching or by cutting one of its branches. The therapist may be able to get some clues to this by looking at the incision site. Disruption of the nerve is more likely when the gluteus medius is split more than 5 cm proximal to the tip of the greater trochanter. If nerve damage has occurred, the client may not regain full strength. Electromyography (EMG) testing may be needed to document muscle denervation.

Physical therapy may be a diagnostic step for the physician. If muscle strengthening does not recondition the remaining intact muscle, a revision operation to repair the muscle may be needed. It may be helpful to communicate with the physician to see what his or her thinking is on this client.

Data from Farrell CM, Berry DJ: Persistent limping after primary total hip replacement. *J Musculoskel Med* 19:484-486, 2002.

BOX 16-3 ▼ Causes of Psoas Abscess

- Diverticulitis
- Crohn's disease
- Appendicitis
- Pelvic inflammatory disease
- Diabetes mellitus
- Any other source of infection, including dental[43]
- Renal infection
- Infective spondylitis (vertebra)
- Osteomyelitis
- Sacroiliac joint infection

- Leg pulled into internal rotation
- Positive psoas sign, i.e., pain elicited by stretching the psoas muscle by extending the hip
- Fever up and down (hectic fever pattern)
- Sweats
- Loss of appetite or other GI symptoms
- Palpable mass in the inguinal area (present with distal extension of the abscess)
- Positive iliopsoas or obturator test (see Figs. 8-4 through 8-6)

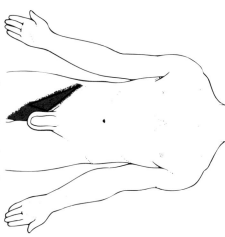

Fig. 16-5 ● Femoral triangle: referred pain pattern from psoas abscess. Hip pain associated with such an abscess may involve the medial aspect of the thigh and femoral triangle areas. The femoral triangle is the name given to the anterior aspect of the thigh formed as different muscles and ligaments cross each other, producing an inverted triangular shape.

Clinical Signs and Symptoms of Psoas Abscess

- Pain that is usually confined to the psoas fascia but that may extend to the buttock, hip, groin, upper thigh, or knee
- Pain located in the anterior hip in the area of the medial thigh or femoral triangle, often accompanied by or alternating with abdominal pain
- Psoas spasm causing functional hip flexion contracture

occur when infected tissue is irritated. Pain elicited by stretching the psoas muscle through extension of the hip, called the positive psoas sign, may be present.

A positive response for any of these tests is indicative of an infectious or inflammatory process. Direct back, pelvic, or hip pain that results from these palpations is more likely to have a musculoskeletal cause. Besides the iliopsoas and obturator tests, another test for rebound tenderness used more often by nurses is called *Blumberg's sign* (see Fig. 8-10). It may be appropriate to conduct these tests with a variety of clinical presentations involving the pelvic area, sacrum, hip, or groin.

Psoas abscess must be differentiated from trigger points of the psoas muscle, causing the psoas minor syndrome, which is easily mistaken for appendicitis. Hemorrhage within the psoas muscle, either spontaneous or associated with anticoagulation therapy for hemophilia, can cause a painful compression syndrome of the femoral nerve.

Systemic causes of hip pain from psoas abscess are usually associated with loss of appetite or other GI symptoms, fever, and sweats. Symptoms from an iliopsoas trigger point are aggravated by weight-bearing activities and are relieved by recumbency or rest. Relief is greater when the hip is flexed.[20]

SCREENING FOR GASTROINTESTINAL CAUSES OF LOWER QUADRANT PAIN

The relationship of the gut to the joint is well known but poorly understood. Intestinal bypass syndrome, inflammatory bowel disease, ankylosing spondylitis, celiac disease, postdysenteric reactive arthritis, and antibiotic-associated colitis all share the fact that some "interface" exists between the bowel and the hip articular surface. It is possible that the clinical expression of immune-mediated joint disease results from an immunologic response to an antigen that crosses the gut mucosa with an autoimmune response against self.[44-48]

For the client with hip pain of unknown cause or suspicious presentation, ask whether any

back pain or abdominal pain is ever present. Alternating abdominal pain with low back pain at the same level, or alternating abdominal pain with hip pain is a red flag that requires medical referral.

The therapist may treat a patient with joint or back pain with an underlying enteric cause before he or she realizes what the underlying problem is. Palliative intervention can make a difference in the short term but does not affect the final outcome. Symptoms that are unrelieved by physical therapy intervention are always a red flag. Symptoms that improve after physical therapy but then get worse again are also a red flag, revealing the need for further screening.

In the case of enterically induced joint pain, the client will get worse without medical intervention. Without early identification and referral, the client will eventually return to his or her gastroenterologist or primary care physician. Medical treatment for the underlying disease is essential in affecting the musculoskeletal component. Physical therapy intervention does not alter or improve the underlying enteric disease. It is better for the client if the therapist recognizes as soon as possible the need for medical intervention.

Crohn's Disease

In anyone with hip or groin pain of unknown cause, look for a known history of PID, Crohn's disease (regional enteritis), ulcerative colitis, irritable bowel syndrome, diverticulitis, or bowel obstruction.

It is possible that new onset of low back, sacral, or hip pain is merely a new symptom of an already established enteric (GI) disease. Twenty-five percent of those with inflammatory enteric disease (particularly Crohn's disease) have concomitant back or joint pain.

A skin rash that comes and goes can accompany enterically induced arthritis. A flat rash or raised skin lesion of the lower extremities is possible; it usually precedes joint or back pain. Be sure to ask the client whether he or she has had skin rashes of any kind over the past few weeks.

Several tests can be done to assess for hip pain resulting from psoas abscess caused by abdominal or intraperitoneal infection or inflammation. These were discussed in the previous section.

A positive response for each of these tests is NOT reproduction of the client's hip or groin pain, but rather, lower quadrant abdominal pain on the side of the test. This is a symptom of an infectious or inflammatory process. Hip or back pain in response to these tests is more likely muscu-

loskeletal in origin such as a trigger point of the iliopsoas or muscular tightness.

Reactive Arthritis

In the case of reactive arthritis, joint symptoms occur 1 to 4 weeks after an infection, usually GI (gastrointestinal) or GU (genitourinary). The joint is not septic (infected), but rather, it is aseptic (without infection). Affected joints often occur at a site that is remote from the primary infection. Prosthetic joints are not immune to this type of infection and may become infected years after the joint is implanted.

Whether the infection occurs in the natural joint or in the prosthetic implant, the client is unable to bear weight on the joint. An acute arthritic presentation may occur, and the client often has a fever (commonly of low grade in older adults or in anyone who is immunosuppressed). Screening questions for clients with joint pain are listed in Box 3-5 and in the Appendix B-16. These questions may be helpful for the client with joint pain of unknown cause or with an unusual presentation/history that does not fit the expected pattern for injury, overuse, or aging.

▶ SCREENING FOR VASCULAR CAUSES OF LOWER QUADRANT PAIN

Vascular pain is often throbbing in nature and exacerbated by activity. With atherosclerosis, a lag time of 5 to 10 minutes occurs between when the body asks for increased oxygenated blood and when symptoms occur because of arterial occlusion. The client is older, often with a personal or family history of heart disease. Other risk factors include hyperlipidemia, tobacco use, and diabetes.

Peripheral Vascular Disease

Peripheral vascular disease (PVD) (peripheral arterial disease (PAD); arterial insufficiency) in which the arteries are occluded by atherosclerosis can cause unilateral or bilateral low back, hip, buttock, groin, or leg pain, along with intermittent claudication and trophic changes of the affected lower extremities.

Intermittent claudication of vascular origin may begin in the calf and may gradually make its way up the lower extremity. The client may report the pain or discomfort as "burning," "cramping," or "sharp." Pain or other symptoms begin several minutes after the start of physical activity and resolve almost immediately with rest. As discussed in Chapter 14, the site of symptoms is determined

by the location of the pathology (see Fig. 14-3) (Case Example 16-14).

PVD is a rare cause of lower quadrant pain in anyone under the age of 65, but leg pain in recreational athletes caused by isolated areas of arterial stenosis have been reported.[49]

The therapist must include assessment of vital signs and must look for trophic skin changes so often present with chronic arterial insufficiency. Pulse oximetry may be helpful when thrombosis is not clinically obvious; for example, pulses can

be present in both feet with oxygen saturation (SaO$_2$) levels at 90% or less.[50] When assessing for PAD as a possible cause of back, buttock, hip, groin, or leg pain, look for other signs of PAD. See further discussion of this topic in Chapters 4, 6, and 14.

Deep venous thrombosis (DVT) as a cause of leg pain may present as swelling of the calf or ankle, with calf tenderness and erythema. Further discussion and information on assessment of DVT are presented in Chapters 4 and 6.

CASE EXAMPLE 16-14   Intermittent Claudication With Sciatica

Referral: A 41-year-old woman who was referred by her primary care physician with a medical diagnosis of sciatica reported bilateral lower extremity weakness with pain in the left buttock and left sacroiliac (SI) area. She also noted that she had numbness in her left leg after walking more than half a block.

She said both her legs felt like they were going to "collapse" after she walked a short distance and that her left would go "hot and cold" during walking. She also experienced cramping in her right calf muscle after walking more than half a block.

Symptoms are made worse by walking and better after resting or by standing still. Symptoms have been present for the last 2 months and came on suddenly without trauma or injury of any kind. No night pain was reported.

No medical tests or imaging studies have been done at this time.

Past Medical History: Significant positive for family history of heart disease (both sides of the family); smoking history: 1 pack of cigarettes/day for the past 26 years.

Clinical Presentation

Neurologic Screening Examination: Negative/within normal limits (WNL)

Neural Tissue Mobility: Tests were all negative; tissue tension WNL.

Complete Lumbar Spine Examination: Unremarkable; ruled out as a source of client's symptoms

Diminished dorsalis pedis pulse on the left side

Bike Test (reviewed in Chapter 14; this test can be used to stress the integrity of the vascular supply to the lower extremities): Cycling in a position of lumbar forward flexion reproduced leg weakness and eliminated dorsalis pedis pulse on the left; no change was noted on the right.

Associated Signs and Symptoms
None.

What are the red flags in this case?
• LE weakness without pain accompanied by "giving out" sensation
• Symptoms brought on by specific activity, relieved by rest or standing still
• Significant family history of heart disease
• No known cause; onset of symptoms without trauma or injury
• Temperature changes in lower extremities (LEs)
• Positive smoking history

Result: Given the severity of her family history of heart disease (sudden death at a young age was very common), she was sent back to the doctor immediately. The therapist briefly outlined the red flags and asked the physician to reevaluate for a possible vascular cause of symptoms.

Medical testing revealed a high-grade circumferential stenosis (narrowing) of the distal aorta at the bifurcation. The client underwent surgery for placement of a stent in the occluded artery. After the operation, the client reported complete relief from all symptoms, including buttock and SI pain.

Data from Gray JC: Diagnosis of intermittent vascular claudication in a patient with a diagnosis of sciatica: Case report. *Phys Ther* 79:582-590, 1999.

Abdominal Aortic Aneurysm

Abdominal aortic aneurysm (AAA) may be asymptomatic; discovery occurs on physical or x-ray examination of the abdomen or lower spine for some other reason. The most common symptom is awareness of a pulsating mass in the abdomen, with or without pain, followed by abdominal and back pain. Groin pain and flank pain may occur because of increasing pressure on other structures. For more detailed information, see Chapter 6.

Be aware of the client's age. The client with an AAA can be of any age because this may be a congenital condition, but usually, he or she is over age 50 and, more likely, is 65 or older. The condition remains asymptomatic until the wall of the aorta grows large enough to rupture. If that happens, blood in the abdomen causes searing pain accompanied by a sudden drop in blood pressure. Other symptoms of impending rupture or actual rupture of the aortic aneurysm include the following:

- Rapid onset of severe groin pain (usually accompanied by abdominal or back pain)
- Radiation of pain to the abdomen or to posterior thighs
- Pain not relieved by change in position
- Pain described as "tearing" or "ripping"
- Other signs, such as cold, pulseless lower extremities

An increasingly prevalent risk factor in the aging adult population is initiation of a weight-lifting program without prior medical evaluation or approval. The presence of atherosclerosis, elevated blood pressure, or an unknown aneurysm during weight training can precipitate rupture.

The therapist can palpate the aortic pulse to identify a widening pulse width, which is suggestive of an aneurysm (see Fig. 4-51). Place one hand or one finger on either side of the aorta as shown. Press firmly deep into the upper abdomen just to the left of midline. You should feel aortic pulsations. These pulsations are easier to appreciate in a thin person and are more difficult to feel in someone with a thick abdominal wall or a large anteroposterior diameter of the abdomen.

Obesity and abdominal ascites or distention make this more difficult. For therapists who are trained in auscultation, listen for bruits. Bruits are abnormal blowing or swishing sounds heard on auscultation of the arteries. Bruits with both systolic and diastolic components suggest the turbulent blood flow of partial arterial occlusion. If the renal artery is occluded as well, the client will be hypertensive.

Avascular Osteonecrosis

Avascular osteonecrosis (also known as osteonecrosis or septic necrosis) can occur without known cause but is often associated with various risk factors. Chronic use and abuse of alcohol is a common risk factor for this condition. Screening for alcohol or drug use and abuse is discussed in Chapter 2 (see also Appendices B-1 and B-2).

Osteonecrosis is also associated with many other conditions such as systemic lupus erythematosus, pancreatitis, kidney disease, blood disorders (e.g., sickle cell disease, coagulopathies), diabetes mellitus, Cushing's disease, and gout. Long-term use of corticosteroids or immunosuppressants, or any condition that causes immune deficiency, can also result in osteonecrosis. Individuals who are taking immunosuppressants include organ transplant recipients, clients with cancer, and those with rheumatoid arthritis or another chronic autoimmune disease.

The femoral head is the most common site of this disorder. Bones with limited blood supply are at enhanced risk for this condition. Hip dislocation or fracture of the neck of the femur may compromise the already precarious vascular supply to the head of the femur. Ischemia leads to poor repair processes and delayed healing. Necrosis and deformation of the bone occur next.

The client may be asymptomatic during the early stages of osteonecrosis. Hip pain is the first symptom. At first, it may be mild, lasting for weeks. As the condition progresses, symptoms become more severe, with pain on weight bearing, antalgic gait, and limited motion (especially, internal rotation, flexion, and abduction). The client may report a distinct click in the hip when moving from the sitting position and increased stiffness in the hip as time goes by.

Clinical Signs and Symptoms of Osteonecrosis

- May be asymptomatic at first
- Hip pain (mild at first, progressively worse over time)
- Groin or anteromedial thigh pain possible
- Pain worse on weight bearing
- Antalgic gait with a gluteus minimus limp
- Limited hip range of motion (internal rotation, flexion, abduction)
- Tenderness to palpation over the hip joint
- Hip joint stiffness
- Hip dislocation

SCREENING FOR OTHER CAUSES OF LOWER QUADRANT PAIN

Osteoporosis

Osteoporosis may result in hip fracture and accompanying hip pain, especially in postmenopausal women who are not taking hormone replacement. Osteoporosis accompanying the postmenopausal period—when combined with circulatory impairment, postural hypotension, or some medications—may increase a person's risk of falling and incurring hip fracture.

Transient osteoporosis of the hip can occur during pregnancy, although the incidence is fairly low. Symptoms include progressive hip pain, sometimes referred to the lateral thigh. The pain develops shortly before or during the last trimester and is aggravated by weight bearing. The pain subsides, and the x-ray appearance returns to normal within several months after delivery.[51]

Any evaluation procedures that produce significant shear through the femoral head of a pregnant woman must be performed by the physical therapist with extreme caution. The transient osteoporosis of pregnancy is not limited to the hip, and vertebral compression may also occur.

Extrapulmonary Tuberculosis

Tubercular disease of the hip or spine is rare in developed countries, but it may occur as an opportunistic disease associated with acquired immunodeficiency syndrome (AIDS) that causes hip or back pain. Usually, the diagnosis of AIDS and tuberculosis is known, which alerts the therapist about the underlying systemic cause.

With hip involvement, the client usually appears with a chronic limp and describes pain in the hip that persists at rest. Approximately 60% of affected individuals do not have constitutional symptoms, although the tuberculin skin test is usually positive, and radiographs are similar to those for septic arthritis.

Sickle Cell Anemia

Sickle cell anemia resulting in avascular necrosis (death of cells caused by lack of blood supply) of the hip and hemarthrosis (blood in the joint) associated with *hemophilia* are two of the most common hematologic diseases that cause pain in the hip, groin, knee, or leg.

Hemophilia may involve GI bleeding accompanied by low abdominal, hip, or groin pain caused by bleeding into the wall of the large intestine or the iliopsoas muscle. This retroperitoneal hemorrhage produces a muscle spasm of the iliopsoas muscle. The subsequent bleeding–spasm cycle produces increased hip pain and hip flexion spasm or contracture. Other symptoms may include melena, hematemesis, and fever.

Clinical Signs and Symptoms of
Hip Hemarthrosis

- Pain in the groin and thigh
- Fullness in the hip joint, both anterior in the groin and over the greater trochanter
- Limited motion in hip flexion, abduction, and external rotation (allows most room for the blood in the joint capsule)

Liver Disease

Ascites is an abnormal accumulation of serous (edematous) fluid in the peritoneal cavity; this fluid contains large quantities of protein and electrolytes as the result of portal backup and loss of proteins (see Fig. 9-8). This condition is associated with liver disease and alcoholism. For the physical therapist, the distended abdomen, abdominal hernias, and lumbar lordosis observed in clients with ascites may present musculoskeletal symptoms, such as groin or low back pain.

The presence of ascites as it is linked with groin pain would be physically evident. If abdominal distention is present, then the therapist should ask about a past medical history of liver impairment, chronic alcohol use, and the presence of carpal or tarsal tunnel syndrome associated with liver impairment. The therapist can carry out the four screening tests for liver impairment discussed in Chapter 9, including the following:

- Liver flap (Asterixis; see Fig. 9-7)
- Palmar erythema (Liver Palms; see Fig. 9-5)
- Scan for angiomas (Upper Body and Abdomen; see Fig. 9-3)
- Assessment of nail beds for change in color (Nail beds of Terry; see Fig. 9-6)

PHYSICIAN REFERRAL
Guidelines for Immediate Medical Attention

- Painless, progressive enlargement of lymph nodes, or lymph nodes that are suspicious for any reason and that persist or that involve more than one area (groin and popliteal areas); immediate medical referral is required for a client with a past medical history of cancer
- Hip or groin pain alternating or occurring simultaneously with abdominal pain at the same level (aneurysm, colorectal cancer)

- Hip or leg pain on weight bearing with positive tests for stress reaction or fracture

Guidelines for Physician Referral

- Hip, thigh, or buttock pain in a client with a total hip arthroplasty that is brought on by activity but resolves with continued activity (**loose prosthesis**), or who has persistent pain that is unrelieved by rest (**implant infection**)
- Sciatica accompanied by extreme motor weakness, numbness in the groin or rectum, or difficulty controlling bowel or bladder function
- One or more of Cyriax's Signs of the Buttock (see Box 16-2)
- New onset of joint pain in a client with a known history of Crohn's disease, requiring careful screening and possible referral based on examination results

Clues to Screening Lower Quadrant Pain

- See also Clues Suggesting Systemic Back Pain; general concepts from the back also apply to the hip and the groin (see especially Cardiovascular discussion)
- Client does not respond to physical therapy intervention or gets worse, especially in the presence of a past medical history of cancer or an unknown cause of symptoms

Past Medical History

- History of AIDS-related tuberculosis, sickle cell anemia, or hemophilia
- Hip or groin pain in a client who has a long-term history of use of nonsteroidal anti-inflammatory drugs (NSAIDs) or corticosteroids (**osteonecrosis**)

Clinical Presentation

- Limited passive hip range of motion with empty end feel, especially in someone with a previous history of cancer, insidious onset, or an unknown cause of painful symptoms
- Palpable soft tissue mass in the anterior hip or groin (**psoas abscess, hernia**)
- Presence of rebound tenderness, positive McBurney's, iliopsoas, or obturator test (see Chapter 8)
- Abnormal cremasteric response in male with groin or anterior thigh pain
- Hip pain in a young adult that is worse at night and is alleviated by activity and aspirin (osteoid osteoma)
- Sciatica in the presence of night pain and an atypical pattern of restricted hip range of motion[52]
- No change in symptoms of sciatica with trigger point release, neural gliding techniques, soft tissue stretching, or postural changes
- Painless neurologic deficit (**spinal cord tumor**)
- Insidious onset of groin or anterior thigh pain with a recent history of increased activity (e.g., runners who increase their mileage)

Associated Signs and Symptoms

- Hip or groin pain accompanied by or alternating with signs and symptoms associated with the GI, urologic/renal, hematologic, or cardiovascular system, or with constitutional symptoms, especially fever and night sweats
- Groin pain in the presence of fever, sweats, weight loss, bleeding, skin lesions, or vaginal/penile discharge
- Hip or groin pain, with any clues suggestive of cancer (see Chapter 13), especially anyone with a previous history of cancer and men between the ages of 18 and 24 years who experience hip or groin pain of unknown cause (**testicular cancer**)
- Buttock, hip, thigh, or groin pain accompanied by fever, weight loss, bleeding or other vaginal/penis discharge, skin lesions, or other discharge

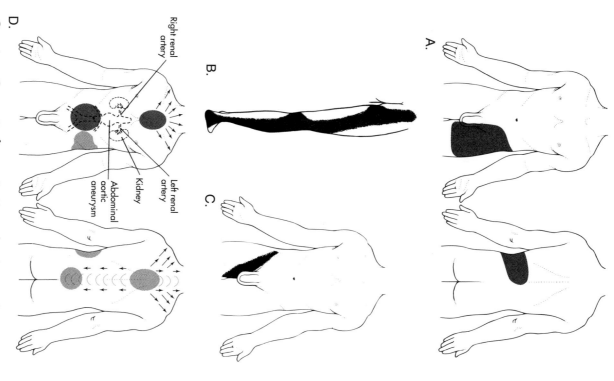

Fig. 16-6 • Overview: Composite figure. **A,** Ureteral pain may begin posteriorly in the costovertebral angle, radiating anteriorly to the ipsilateral lower abdomen, upper thigh, or groin area. Isolated anterior thigh pain is possible, but uncommon. **B,** Pain pattern associated with sciatica from any cause. **C,** Pain pattern associated with psoas abscess from any cause. **D,** Abdominal aortic aneurysm can cause low back pain that radiates into the buttock unilaterally or bilaterally (not shown), depending on the underlying location and size of the aneurysm.

KEY POINTS TO REMEMBER

✓ See also Key Points to Remember: Neck and Back Pain, Chapter 14.

✓ Identifying the hip as the source of a client's symptoms may be difficult in that pain originating in the hip may not localize to the hip, but rather, may present as low back, buttock, groin, SI, anterior thigh, or even knee or ankle pain.

✓ Hip pain can be referred from other locations, such as the scrotum, kidneys, abdominal wall, abdomen, peritoneum, or retroperitoneal region.

✓ In addition to screening for medical problems, the therapist must remember to clear the joint above and below the area of symptoms or dysfunction

✓ True hip pain from any cause is usually felt in the groin or deep buttock, sometimes with pain radiating down the anterior thigh. Pain perceived on the outer (lateral) side of the hip is usually not caused by an intra-articular problem, but likely results from a trigger point, or from bursitis, SI, or back problems.

✓ Hip pain referred from the upper lumbar vertebrae can radiate into the anterior aspect of the thigh, whereas hip pain from the lower lumbar vertebrae and sacrum is usually felt in the gluteal region, with radiation down the back or outer aspect of the thigh.

✓ Systemic or viscerogenic causes of lower quadrant pain or symptoms mimic a neuromuscular or musculoskeletal cause, but usually, a red flag history, risk factors, or associated signs and symptoms are identified during the screening process; this facilitates identification of the underlying problem.

✓ Cancer recurrence most likely to metastasize to the hip includes breast, bone, and prostate.

✓ Changes in lymph nodes with or without a previous history of cancer are a yellow or red flag.

✓ Normal but painful hip rotations (log-rolling test) present when the client is tested in the supine position with the hips in neutral extension (zero degrees of hip flexion) may be a yellow warning flag.

✓ Cyriax's "Sign of the Buttock" can help differentiate between hip and lumbar spine disease.

✓ Anyone with lower quadrant pain and a past history of hip or knee arthroplasty must be evaluated for component problems (e.g., infection, subsidence, looseness), regardless of the client's perceived cause of the problem. Watch for pain on initiation of activity that gets better with continued activity (loose prosthesis); also watch for signs of infection (recent history of infection anywhere else in the body, fever, chills, sweats, pain that is not relieved with rest, night pain, pain on weight bearing).

✓ A noncapsular pattern of restricted hip motion (e.g., limited hip extension, adduction, lateral rotation) may be a sign of serious underlying disease.

✓ Anyone with pain radiating from the back down the leg as far as the ankle has a greater chance for disc herniation to be the cause of low back pain; this is true with or without neurologic findings.

✓ The straight leg raise (SLR) and other neurodynamic tests are widely used but do not identify the underlying cause of sciatica. A positive SLR test does not differentiate between discogenic disease and neoplasm; imaging studies may be needed.

✓ Tests for the presence of hip pain caused by psoas abscess are advised whenever an infectious or inflammatory process is suspected on the basis of past medical history, clinical presentation, and associated signs and symptoms.

✓ New onset of low back or hip pain in a client with a previous history of Crohn's disease, especially in the presence of a recent history of skin rash, requires screening for GI signs and symptoms.

✓ Long-term use of corticosteroids or immunosuppressants, or any condition that causes immune deficiency may also result in hip pain from osteonecrosis. As the condition progresses, symptoms become more severe with pain on weight bearing, antalgic gait, and limited motion.

SUBJECTIVE EXAMINATION

Special Questions to Ask: Lower Quadrant

It is not necessary to ask every client every question listed. Sometimes, we ask some general screening questions because of something the client has told us. At other times, we screen because of something we saw in the clinical presentation. We may need to ask some specific questions based on gender. Finally, sometimes, the review of systems has pinpointed a particular system (e.g., GI, GU, vascular, pulmonary, gynecologic), and we go right to the end of the chapter dealing with that system and look for any screening questions that may be pertinent to the client.

The more often the therapist conducts screening interviews, the faster the process will get, and the easier it will become to remember which questions make the most sense to ask. The beginner may ask more questions than are really needed, but with practice and experience, the screening process will smooth out. Generally it takes about 3 to 5 minutes to conduct a screening interview and another 5 minutes to carry out any special tests.

Because hip pain may be caused by referred pain from disorders of the low back, abdomen, and reproductive and urologic structures, special questions should include consideration of the following:

- Special Questions for Women Experiencing Back, Hip, Pelvic, Groin, or Sacroiliac Pain (see Appendix B-32)
- Special Questions to Ask: Men Experiencing Back, Hip, Pelvic, Groin, or Sacroiliac Pain (see Appendix B-21)
- Special questions for clients (see Chapter 14; Special Questions to Ask: Neck or Back):
  - General systemic questions
  - Pain assessment
  - Gastrointestinal questions
  - Urologic questions

- For anyone with lower quadrant pain of unknown cause:

  It may be necessary to conduct a sexual history as part of the screening process. See Chapter 14 or Appendix B-29
- A quick screening interview and additional questions may include the following:

Pain Assessment

See Appendix C-4 for a complete pain assessment.

- Have you had a recent injury?

  If yes, tell me what happened.
  Did you hear any popping, snapping, or cracking when the injury occurred?
- How is the pain affected by putting weight on it?
- Does your leg "give out" on you? (or feel like it is going to give out)?
- Does your pain feel better, same, or worse after walking on it for awhile? **(With joint arthroplasty, pain improves after walking with loose components)**

Past Medical History

- Have you ever been told (or have you known) that you have a sexually transmitted infection or disease?
- Have you been treated with cortisone, prednisone, other corticosteroids, or any other drug of that type?
- Do you have a known history of Crohn's disease, diverticulitis, or pelvic inflammatory disease?
- Have you ever had cancer of any kind?

  If no, Have you ever been treated with chemotherapy or radiation therapy?
  Have you ever had a bone tumor?

Associated Signs and Symptoms

- Do you have any other symptoms anywhere else in your body?
  Any fatigue? Fever? Chills? Swollen joints?

CASE STUDY

STEPS IN THE SCREENING PROCESS

A 34-year-old woman was referred to physical therapy for pelvic pain from a nonrelaxing puborectalis muscle. She reported bilateral groin pain that was superficial and affected the skin area. She also said the area feels "warm." The pain was worse when sitting, better when standing, and had lasted longer than a month. The physician ruled out shingles and sent her to physical therapy for further evaluation.

What Are Some Steps You Can Take to Start the Screening Process?

Have the client complete a past medical history form, and review it for any clues that might help direct the screening process. Ask the usual questions about bowel and bladder function (see Appendices B-5 and B-6).

Superficial skin changes are usually a sudomotor response; messages arrive via the spinal cord, but the system has no way to know the specific source of the problem (i.e., viscerogenic vs. somatic), so it sends out a "distress" signal that something is wrong at the S2-S3 level. The therapist must consider what could be involved.

Using Table 16-3 as a guide, the therapist can assess the likelihood of each condition listed on the basis of age, gender, past medical history, and associated signs and symptoms. Screening tests may be conducted, as appropriate. For example, a neurologic screening examination may help identify discogenic disease or possible spinal cord tumor.

The client is young to have developed an AAA from atherosclerosis, but a congenital aneurysm may be present. Palpating the abdomen and the aortic pulse and listening with a stethoscope for femoral bruits may be helpful.

A stress fracture would likely have a suspicious history such as prolonged activity requiring axial loading or trauma of some kind. It may be necessary to ask about physical or sexual assault. Conduct screening tests such as heel strike, rotational/translational stress test of the pubis, hop on one leg, and full squat. Assess for trigger points.

Ureteral problems are usually accompanied by bladder changes (e.g., dysuria, hematuria, frequency) and constitutional symptoms such as fever, sweats, or chills. Take vital signs.

Gynecologic causes of low back, pelvic, groin, hip, or sacroiliac pain are usually accompanied by a significant history of gynecologic conditions or traumatic or multiple birth/delivery history. Some additional questions along these lines may be needed if the past medical history form is not sufficient. Sexually transmitted infection or ectopic pregnancy is possible, although rare causes of groin pain may occur in sexually active women.

Appendicitis or another infectious process can cause a wide range of symptoms outside of the typical or expected right lower abdominal quadrant pain, including isolated groin pain or combined hip and groin pain. McBurney's test (see Fig. 8-8) or Blumberg's sign for rebound tenderness (see Fig. 8-10) can help the therapist to recognize when medical referral is required.

PRACTICE QUESTIONS

1. The screening model used to help identify viscerogenic or systemic origins of hip, groin, and lower extremity pain and symptoms is made up of:

    a. Past medical history, risk factors, clinical presentation, and associated signs and symptoms

    b. Risk factors, risk reduction, and primary prevention

    c. Enteric disease, systemic disease, neuromusculoskeletal dysfunction

    d. Physical therapy diagnosis, review of systems, physician referral

2. When would you use the iliopsoas, obturator, or Blumberg test?

3. Hip and groin pain can be referred from

    a. Low back

    b. Abdomen

    c. Retroperitoneum

    d. All of the above

4. Screening for cancer may be necessary in anyone with hip pain who:

    a. Is younger than 20 or older than 50

    b. Has a past medical history of diabetes mellitus

    c. Reports fever and chills

    d. Has a total hip arthroplasty (THA)

5. Pain on weight bearing may be a sign of hip fracture, even when x-rays are negative. Follow-up clinical tests may include:

    a. McBurney's, Blumberg's, Murphy's test

    b. Squat test, hop test, translational/rotational tests

    c. Psoas and obturator tests

    d. Patrick's or FABER's test

6. Abscess of the iliopsoas muscles from intraabdominal infection or inflammation can cause

hip and/or groin pain. Clinical tests to differentiate the cause of hip pain resulting from psoas abscess include:

    a. McBurney's, Blumberg's, or Murphy's test

    b. Squat test, hop test, translational/rotational tests

    c. Iliopsoas and obturator tests

    d. Patrick's or FABER's test

7. Anyone with hip pain of unknown cause must be asked about:

    a. Previous history of cancer or Crohn's disease

    b. Recent infection

    c. Presence of skin rash

    d. All of the above

8. Vascular diseases that may cause referred hip pain include:

    a. Coronary artery disease

    b. Intermittent claudication

    c. Aortic aneurysm

    d. All of the above

9. True hip pain is characterized by:

    a. Testicular (male) or labial (female) pain

    b. Groin or deep buttock pain with active or passive range of motion

    c. Positive McBurney's test

    d. All of the above

10. Hip pain associated with primary or metastasized cancer is characterized by:

    a. Bone pain on weight bearing; may not be able to stand on that leg

    b. Night pain that is relieved by aspirin

    c. Positive heel strike test with palpable local tenderness

    d. All of the above

REFERENCES

1. Goodman CC, Snyder TEK: Laboratory tests and values. In Goodman CC, Boissonnault WG, Fuller K, eds: *Pathology: Implications for the Physical Therapist*, 2nd edition, Philadelphia, 2003, WB Saunders, pp. 1174-1200.

2. Browder DA, Erhard RE: Decision making for a painful hip: A case requiring referral, *J Orthop Sports Phys Ther* 35:738-744, 2005.

3. Kimpel DL: Hip pain in a 50-year-old woman with RA, *J Musculoskel Med* 16:651-652, 1999.

4. Bertot AJ, Jarmain SJ, Cosgarea AJ: Hip pain in active adults: 20 clinical pearls, *J Muscloskel Med* 20:35-55, 2003.

5. Tortolani PJ, Carbone JJ, Quartararo LG: Greater trochanteric pain syndrome in patients referred to orthopedic spine specialists, *Spine J* 2:251-254, 2002.

6. Lyle MA, Manes S, McGuinness M, et al: Relationship of physical examination findings and self-reported symptom severity and physical function in patients with degenerative lumbar conditions, *Phys Ther* 85:120-133, 2005.

7. Greenwood MJ, Erhard RE, Jones DL: Differential diagnosis of the hip vs. lumbar spine: Five case reports, *J Orthop Sports Phys Ther* 27:308-315, 1998.

8. Cyriax J: *Textbook of Orthopaedic Medicine*, 8th edition, London, UK, 1982, Bailliere Tindall.

9. Cibulka MT, Sinacore DR, Cromer GS, et al: Unilateral hip rotation range of motion asymmetry in patients with sacroiliac joint regional, *Spine* 23:1009-1015, 1998.

10. Brown TE, Larson B, Shen F, et al: Thigh pain after cementless total hip arthroplasty: Evaluation and management, *J Am Acad Orthop Surg* 10:385-392, 2002.

11. Fogel GR, Esses SI: Hip spine syndrome: Management of coexisting radiculopathy and arthritis of the lower extremity, *Spine J* 3:238-241, 2003.

12. Kim YH, Oh SH, Kim JS, et al: Contemporary total hip arthroplasty with and without cement in patients with osteonecrosis of the femoral head, *J Bone Joint Surg* 85:675-681, 2003.

13. Byrd JWT: Investigation of the symptomatic hip: Physical examination. In Byrd JWT, editor: *Operative Hip Arthroscopy*, New York, 1998, Thieme, pp. 25-41.

14. Sahrmann SA: *Diagnosis and Treatment of Movement Impairment Syndromes*, St. Louis, 2002, Mosby.

15. Cowan SM, Schache P, Brukner KL, et al: Onset of transversus abdominus in long-standing groin pain, *Med Sci Sports Exerc* 36:2040-2045, 2004.

16. Tamir E, Anekshtein Y, Melamed E, et al: Clinical presentation and anatomic position of L3-L4 disc herniation, *J Spinal Disord Tech* 17:467-469, 2004.

17. Reverse straight leg raise test. Available on-line at: http://courses.washington.edu/hubio553/glossary/reverse.html. Accessed December 24, 2005.

18. Yang SH, Wu CC, Chen PQ: Postoperative meralgia paresthetica after posterior spine surgery, *Spine* 30:E547-E550, 2005.

19. Cummings M: Referred knee pain treated with electroacupuncture to iliopsoas, *Aupunct Med* 21:32-35, 2003.

20. Travell JG, Simons DG: *Myofascial Pain and Dysfunction: The Lower Extremities*, vol 2, Baltimore, 1992, Williams and Wilkins.

21. Guss DA: Hip fracture presenting as isolated knee pain, *Ann Emerg Med* 29:418-420, 1997.

22. Steele MK: Relieving cramps in high school athletes, *J Musculoskel Med* 20:210, 2003.

23. Brukner P, Bennell KM, Matheson G: *Stress Fractures*, Australia, 1999, Blackwell Publishing.

24. Seidenberg PH, Childress MA: Managing hip pain in athletes, *J Musculoskel Med* 22:246-254, 2005.

25. Weishaar MD, McMillian DJ, Moore JH: Identification and management of 2 femoral shaft stress injuries, *J Orthop Sports Phys Ther* 35:665-673, 2005.

26. Johnson AW, Weiss CB Jr, Wheeler DL: Stress fractures of the femoral shaft in athletes—more common than expected: A new clinical test, *Am J Sports Med* 22:248-256, 1994.

27. Salter RB: *Textbook of Disorders and Injuries of the Musculoskeletal System*, 3rd edition, Baltimore, 1999, Williams and Wilkins.

28. Hoppenfeld S, Murthy VL: *Treatment and Rehabilitation of Fractures*, Philadelphia, 2000, Lippincott Williams & Wilkins.

29. Ozburn MS, Nichols JW: Pubic ramus and adductor insertion stress fractures in female basic trainees, *Milit Med* 146:332-334, 1981.

30. Jewell DV, Riddle DL: Interventions that increase or decrease the likelihood of a meaningful improvement in physical health in patients with sciatica, *Phys Ther* 85(11):1139-1150, 2005.

31. Yuen EC, So YT: Sciatic neuropathy, *Neurol Clin* 17:617-631, 1999.

32. Martin WN, Dixon JH, Sandhu H: The incidence of cement extrusion from the acetabulum in total hip arthroplasty, *J Arthroplasty* 18:338-341, 2003.

33. Stirling A, Worthington T, Rafiq M, et al: Association between sciatica and *Propionibacterium acnes*, *Lancet* 357:2024-2025, 2001.

34. McLorinn GC, Glenn JV, McMullan MG, et al: *Propionibacterium acnes* wound contamination at the time of spinal surgery, *Clin Orthop Rel Res* 437:67-73, 2005.

35. Bickels J, Kahanvitz N, Rubert CK, et al: Extraspinal bone and soft-tissue tumors as a cause of sciatica: Clinical diagnosis and recommendations: Analysis of 32 cases, *Spine* 24:1611, 1999.

36. Deyo RA, Diehl AK: Cancer as a cause of back pain: Frequency, clinical presentation, and diagnostic strategies, *J Gen Intern Med* 3:230-238, 1988.

37. Guyer RD, Collier RR, Ohnmeiss DD, et al: Extraosseous spinal lesions mimicking disc disease, *Spine* 13:328-331, 1988.

38. Bose B: Thoracic extruded disc mimicking spinal cord tumor, *Spine J* 3:82-86, 2003.

39. Arromdee E, Matteson EL: Bursitis: Common condition, uncommon challenge, *J Musculoskel Med* 18:213-224, 2001.

40. Magee DJ: *Orthopedic Physical Assessment*, 4th edition, Philadelphia, 2002, WB Saunders.

41. Doubleday KL, Kulig K, Landel R: Treatment of testicular pain using conservative management of the thoracolumbar spine: A case report, *Arch Phys Med Rehabil* 84:1903-1905, 2003.

42. Keulers BJ, Roumen RH, Keulers MJ, et al: Bilateral groin pain from a rotten molar, *The Lancet* 366:94, 2005.

43. Todkar M: Case report: Psoas abscess—Unusual etiology of groin pain, *Medscape Gen Med* 7. Available at: http://www.medscape.com/viewarticle/507610_print. Accessed on-line December 22, 2005.

44. Inman RD: Arthritis and enteritis—An interface of protean manifestations, *J Rheumatol* 14:406-410, 1987.

45. Inman RD: Antigens, the gastrointestinal tract, and arthritis, *Rheum Dis Clin North Am* 17:309-321, 1991.

46. Gran JT, Husby G: Joint manifestations in gastrointestinal diseases. 1. Pathophysiological aspects, ulcerative colitis and Crohn's disease, *Dig Dis* 10:274-294, 1992.

47. Gran JT, Husby G: Joint manifestations in gastrointestinal diseases. 2. Whipple's disease, enteric infections, intestinal bypass operations, gluten-sensitive enteropathy, pseudomembranous colitis and collagenous colitis, *Dig Dis* 10:295-312, 1992.

48. Keating RM, Vyas AS: Reactive arthritis following *Clostridium difficile* colitis, *West J Med* 162:61-63, 1995.

49. Lundgren JM, Davis BA: End artery stenosis of the popliteal artery mimicking gastrocnemius strain, *Arch Phys Med Rehabil* 85:1548-1551, 2004.

50. Brau SA, Delamarter RB, Schiffman ML, et al: Vascular injury during anterior lumbar surgery, *Spine J* 4:409-441, 2004.

51. Boissonnault WB, Boissonnault JS: Transient osteoporosis of the hip associated with pregnancy, *J Orthop Sports Phys Ther* 31:359-367, 2001.

52. Ross MD, Bayer E: Cancer as a cause of low back pain in a patient seen in a direct access physical therapy setting, *J Orthop Sports Phys Ther* 35:651-658, 2005.

Screening the Chest, Breasts, and Ribs

17

Clients do not present in a physical therapy clinic with chest or breast pain as the primary symptom very often. The therapist is more likely to see the individual with an orthopedic or neurologic impairment who experiences chest or breast pain during exercise or during other intervention by the therapist.

In other situations, the client reports chest or breast pain as an additional symptom during the screening interview. The pain may occur along with (or alternating with) the presenting symptoms of jaw, neck, upper back, shoulder, breast, or arm pain. When chest pain is the primary complaint, it is often an atypical pain pattern that has misled the client and/or the physician.

On the other hand, it is also possible for clients to have primary chest pain from a movement system impairment. Symptoms persist or recur, often with months in between when the client is free of any symptoms. Countless medical tests are performed and repeated with referral to numerous specialists before a physical therapist is consulted (see Case Example 1-7).

Finally, so many of today's aging adults with movement system impairments have multiple medical comorbidities that the therapists must be able to identify signs and symptoms of systemic disease that can mimic neuromuscular or musculoskeletal dysfunction. Systemic or viscerogenic pain or symptoms that can be referred to the chest or breast include the cardiovascular, pulmonary, and upper gastrointestinal systems, as well as other causes such as anxiety, steroid use, and cocaine use (Table 17-1). Various neuromusculoskeletal conditions such as thoracic outlet syndrome, costochondritis, trigger points, and cervical spine disorders can also affect the chest and breast.

When faced with chest pain, the therapist must know how to assess the situation quickly and decide if medical referral is required and whether medical attention is needed immediately. We must be able to differentiate neuromusculoskeletal from systemic origins of symptoms.

The therapist must especially know how and what to look for to screen for cancer, cancer recurrence, and/or the delayed effects of cancer treatment. Cancer can present as primary chest pain with or without accompanying neck, shoulder, and/or upper back pain/symptoms. Basic principles of cancer screening are presented in Chapter 13; specific clues related to the chest, breast, and ribs will be discussed in this chapter. Breast cancer is always a consideration with upper quadrant pain or dysfunction.

◆ USING THE SCREENING MODEL TO EVALUATE THE CHEST, BREASTS, OR RIBS

There are many causes of chest pain, both cardiac and noncardiac in origin (see Table 17-1). Two conditions may be present at the same time, each contributing to chest pain. For example, someone with cervicodorsal

TABLE 17-1 ▼ Causes of Chest Pain

Systemic causes	Neuromusculoskeletal causes
Cancer	Tietze's syndrome
Mediastinal tumors	Costochondritis
Cardiac	Hypersensitive xiphoid, xiphodynia
Myocardial ischemia (angina)	Slipping rib syndrome
Myocarditis	Trigger points (see Table 17-4)
Pericarditis	Myalgia
Myocardial infarct	Rib fracture, costochondral dislocations
Dissecting aortic aneurysm	Cervical spine disorders, arthritis
Aortic aneurysm	Neurologic
Aortic stenosis or regurgitation	Nerve root, intercostal neuritis
Mitral valve prolapse*	Dorsal nerve root irritation
Pleuropulmonary	Thoracic outlet syndrome
Pulmonary embolism	Thoracic disc disease
Pneumothorax	Postoperative pain
Pulmonary hypertension*	Breast
Cor pulmonale	Mastodynia
Pneumonia with pleurisy	Trigger points
Mediastinitis	Trauma (including motor vehicle accident, assault)
Epigastric/Upper Gastrointestinal	
Esophagitis*	
Esophageal spasm*	
Upper gastrointestinal ulcer	
Cholecystitis	
Pancreatitis	
Breast (see Table 17-2)	
Other	
Anemia	
Rheumatic diseases	
Anxiety, panic attack*	
Cocaine use	
Anabolic steroids	
Fibromyalgia	
Dialysis (first-use syndrome)	
Type III hypersensitivity reaction	
Herpes zoster (shingles)	
Sickle cell anemia	
Psychogenic	

* Relieved by nitroglycerin because it relaxes smooth muscle.

arthritis could also experience reflux esophagitis or coronary disease. Either or both of these conditions can contribute to chest pain.

Chest pain can be evaluated in one of two ways: cardiac versus noncardiac or systemic versus neuromusculoskeletal (NMS). Physicians and nurses assess chest pain from the first paradigm: cardiac versus noncardiac. The therapist must understand the basis for this screening method while also viewing each problem as potentially systemic versus NMS. Throughout the screening process, it is important to remember we are not medical cardiac specialists; we are just screening for sys-

temic disease masquerading as NMS symptoms or dysfunction.

Paying attention to past medical history, recognizing unusual clinical presentation for a neuromuscular or musculoskeletal condition, and keeping in mind the clues to differentiating chest pain will help the therapist evaluate difficult cases.

Additionally, the woman with chest, breast, axillary, or shoulder pain of unknown origin at presentation must be questioned regarding breast self-examinations. Any recently discovered lumps or nodules must be examined by a physician. The client may need education regarding breast self-

examination, and the physical therapist can provide this valuable information.[1,2] Techniques of breast self-examination are commonly available in written form for the physical therapist or the client who is unfamiliar with these methods (see Appendix D-6).

Past Medical History

Although the past medical history (PMH) is important, it cannot be relied upon to confirm or rule out medical causes of chest pain. PMH does alert the therapist to an increased risk of systemic conditions that can masquerade as NMS disorders. Like risk factors, PMH varies according to each system affected or condition present and is reviewed individually in each section of this chapter.

Risk Factors

Any suspicious findings should be checked by a physician, especially in the case of the client with identified risk factors for cancer or heart disease. Identifying red-flag risk factors and PMH and then correlating this information with objective findings are important steps in the screening process.

Risk for cardiac-caused symptoms increases with advancing age, tobacco use, menopause (women), family history of hypertension or premature coronary artery disease, and high cholesterol. Risk factors associated with noncardiac conditions vary with each individual condition.

Clinical Presentation

When the clinical presentation suggests further screening is needed, the therapist can follow the guide to physical assessment for the upper quadrant as presented in Table 4-13. The client's general appearance, along with vital sign assessment, will offer some idea of the severity of the condition. Watch for uneven pulses from side to side, diminished or absent pulses, elevated blood pressure, or extreme hypotension. Auscultation for breath or lung sounds and chest percussion may provide additional cardiopulmonary clues.

Chest Pain Patterns

From the previous discussion in Chapter 3, we know that there are at least three possible mechanisms for referred pain patterns to the soma from the viscera (embryologic development, multisegmental innervations, direct pressure on the diaphragm). Pain in the chest may be derived from the chest wall (dermatomes T1-12), the pleura, the trachea and main airways, the mediastinum

(including the heart and esophagus), and the abdominal viscera. From an embryologic point of view, the lungs are derived from the same tissue as the gut, so problems can occur in both areas (lung or gut), causing chest pain and other related symptoms.

Certain chest pain patterns are more likely to point to a medical rather than musculoskeletal cause. For example, pain that is positional or reproduced by palpation is not as suspicious as pain that radiates to one or both shoulders or arms or that is precipitated by exertion. Physicians agree that the chest pain history by itself is not enough to rule out cardiac or other systemic origin of symptoms. In most cases, some diagnostic testing is needed.[3]

Chest pain associated with increased activity is a red flag for possible cardiovascular involvement. In such cases, the onset of pain is not immediate but rather occurs 5 to 10 minutes after activity begins. This is referred to as the "lag time" and is a screening clue used by the physical therapist to assess when chest pain may be caused by musculoskeletal dysfunction (immediate chest pain occurs with use) or by possible vascular compromise (chest pain occurs 5 to 10 minutes after activity begins).

Parietal pain may appear as unilateral chest pain (rather than midline only) because at any given point the parietal peritoneum obtains innervation from only one side of the nervous system. It is usually not reproduced by palpation. Thoracic disc disease can also present as unilateral chest pain, requiring careful screening.[4]

The four types of pain discussed in Chapter 3 (cutaneous, deep somatic or parietal, visceral, and referred) also apply to the chest. *Parietal (somatic) chest pain* is the most common systemic chest discomfort encountered in a physical therapy practice. Parietal pain refers to pain generating from the wall of any cavity, such as the chest or pelvic cavity (see Fig. 6-5). Although the visceral pleura are insensitive to pain, the parietal pleura are well supplied with pain nerve endings. It is usually associated with infectious diseases but is also seen in pneumothorax, rib fractures, pulmonary embolism with infarction, and other systemic conditions.

Pain fibers, originating in the parietal pleura, are conveyed through the chest wall as fine twigs of the intercostal nerves. Irritation of these nerve fibers results in pain in the chest wall that is usually described as knifelike and is sharply localized close to the chest wall, occurring cutaneously (in the skin).

Pain from the thoracic viscera and true chest wall pain are both felt in the chest wall, but *visceral pain* is referred to the area supplied by the upper four thoracic nerve roots. Report of pain in the lower chest usually indicates local disease, but upper chest pain may be caused by disease located deeper in the chest.

There are few nerve endings (if any) in the visceral pleurae (linings of the various organs), such as the heart or lungs. The exception to this statement is in the area of the pericardium (sac enclosed around the entire heart), which is adjacent to the diaphragm (see Fig. 6-5). Extensive disease may develop within the body cavities without the occurrence of pain until the process extends to the parietal pleura. Neuritis (constant irritation of nerve endings) in the parietal pleura then produces the pain described in this section.

Pleural pain may be aggravated by any respiratory movement involving the diaphragm, such as sighing, deep breathing, coughing, sneezing, laughing, or the hiccups. It may be referred along the costal margins or into the upper abdominal quadrants. Palpation usually does not reproduce pleural pain; change in position does not relieve or exacerbate the pain. In some cases of pleurisy, the individual can point to the painful spot but deep breathing (not palpation) reproduces it.

Associated Signs and Symptoms

If the client has an underlying infectious or inflammatory process causing chest or breast pain or symptoms, there may be changes in vital signs and/or constitutional symptoms such as chills, night sweats, fever, upper respiratory symptoms, or gastrointestinal (GI) distress.

Signs and symptoms associated with noncardiac causes of chest pain vary according to the underlying system involved. For example, cough, sputum production, and a recent history of upper respiratory infection may point to a pleuropulmonary origin of chest or breast pain. Anyone with persistent coughing or asthma can experience chest pain related to the strain of the chest wall muscles.

Chest or breast pain associated with GI disease is often food related in the presence of a history of peptic ulcer, gastroesophageal reflux disease (GERD), or gallbladder problems. Blood in the stool or vomitus, along with a history of chronic nonsteroidal antiinflammatory drug (NSAID) use, may point to a GI problem and so on.

Many of the conditions affecting the breast are not accompanied by other systemic signs and symptoms. Risk factors, client history, and clinical presentation provide the major clues as to a viscerogenic, systemic, or cancerous origin of chest and/or breast pain or symptoms.

SCREENING FOR ONCOLOGIC CAUSES OF CHEST OR RIB PAIN

Cancer can present as primary chest, neck, shoulder, and/or upper back pain and symptoms. A previous history of cancer of any kind is a major red flag (Case Example 17-1). Primary cancer affecting the chest with referred pain to the breast is not as common as cancer metastasized to the pulmonary system with subsequent pulmonary and chest/breast symptoms.

Clinical Presentation

The most common symptoms associated with metastases to the pulmonary system are pleural pain, dyspnea, and persistent cough. As with any visceral system, symptoms may not occur until the neoplasm is quite large or invasive because the lining surrounding the lungs has no pain perception. Symptoms first appear when the tumor is large enough to press on other nearby structures or against the chest wall. The presence of any skin changes, lesions, or masses should be documented using the information presented in Box 4-10.

Skin Changes

Ask the client about any recent or current skin changes. Metastatic carcinoma can present with a cellulitic appearance on the anterior chest wall as a result of carcinoma of the lung (see Fig. 4-24). The skin lesion may be flat or raised and any color from brown to red or purple.

Liver impairment from cancer or any liver disease can also cause other skin changes, such as angiomas over the chest wall. An angioma is a benign tumor with blood (or lymph, as in lymphangioma) vessels. Spider angioma (also called spider nevus) is a form of telangiectasis, a permanently dilated group of superficial capillaries (or venules; see Fig. 9-3).

In the presence of skin lesions, ask about a recent history of infection of any kind, use of prescription drugs within the last 6 weeks, and previous history of cancer of any kind. Look for lymph node changes. Report all of these findings to the physician.

Palpable Mass

Occasionally, the therapist may palpate a painless sternal or chest wall mass when evaluating the head and neck region. Most mediastinal tumors are the result of a metastatic focus from a distant

CASE EXAMPLE 17-1 Rib Metastases Associated With Ovarian Cancer

Referral: A 53-year-old university professor came to the physical therapy clinic with complaints of severe left shoulder pain radiating across her chest and down her arm. She rated the pain a 10 on the numeric rating scale (see explanation in Chapter 3).

Past Medical History: She had a significant personal and social history, including ovarian cancer 10 years ago, death of a parent last year, filing for personal bankruptcy this year, and a divorce after 30 years of marriage.

Clinical Presentation: First Visit: During the screening examination for vital signs, the client's blood pressure was 220/125 mm Hg. Pulse was 88 beats per minute. Pulse oximeter measured 98%. Oral temperature: 98.0°F. She denied any previous history of cardiovascular problems or current feelings of stress.

Intervention: She was referred for medical attention immediately on the basis of her blood pressure readings but returned a week later with a medical diagnosis of "rib bruise." Electrocardiography (EKG) and heart catheterization ruled out a cardiac cause of symptoms. She was put on Prilosec for gastroesophageal reflux disease (GERD) and an antiinflammatory for her rib pain.

Clinical Presentation: Second Visit: The therapist was able to reproduce the symptoms described above with moderate palpation of the eighth rib on the left side and sidebending motion to the left side. The client described the symptoms as constant, sharp, burning, and intense. She had pain at night if she slept too long on either side.

Sidelying on the involved side and slump sitting did not reproduce the symptoms. There was no obvious mechanical cause for the painful symptoms (e.g., intercostal tear, costovertebral dysfunction, neuritis from nerve entrapment).

The therapist considered the possibility of a somato-visceral reflex responses (e.g., a biomechanical dysfunction of the tenth rib can cause gallbladder changes), but there were no accompanying associated signs and symptoms and the tenth rib was not painful.

Result: The therapist decided to contact the referring physician to discuss the client's clinical presentation before initiating treatment, especially given the constancy and intensity of the pain in the presence of a past medical history of cancer.

The physician directed the therapist to have the client return for further testing. A bone scan revealed metastases to the ribs and thoracic spine. Physical therapy intervention was not appropriate at this time.

---

primary tumor and remain asymptomatic unless they compress mediastinal structures or invade the chest wall.

The primary tumor is usually a lymphoma (Hodgkin's lymphoma in a young adult or non-Hodgkin's lymphoma in a child or older adult; see Fig. 4-27), multiple myeloma (primarily observed in people over 60 years of age), or carcinoma of the breast, kidney, or thyroid.

When involvement of the chest wall and nerve roots results in pain, the pattern is more diffuse, with radiation of pain to the affected nerve roots (Case Example 17-2). Irritation of an intercostal nerve from rib metastasis produces burning pain that is unilateral and segmental in distribution. Sensory loss or hyperesthesia over the affected dermatomes may be noted.

SCREENING FOR CARDIOVASCULAR CAUSES OF CHEST, BREAST, OR RIB PAIN

Cardiac-related chest pain may arise secondary to angina, myocardial infarction, pericarditis, endocarditis, mitral valve prolapse, or aortic aneurysm. Despite diagnostic advances, acute coronary syndromes and myocardial infarctions are missed in 2% to 10% of patients.[3] There is no single element of chest pain history powerful enough to predict who is or who is not having a coronary-related incident. Medical referral is advised whenever there is any doubt; medical diagnostic testing is almost always required.[3]

Cardiac-related chest pain also can occur when there is normal coronary circulation, as in the case

---

CASE EXAMPLE 17-2 Lymphoma Masquerading as Nerve Entrapment

Referral: A 72-year-old woman was referred to physical therapy for a postural exercise program and home traction by her neurologist with a diagnosis of "nerve entrapment." She was experiencing symptoms of left shoulder pain with numbness and tingling in the ulnar nerve distribution. She had a moderate forward head posture with slumped shoulders and loss of height from known osteoporosis.

Past Medical History: The woman's past medical history was significant for right breast cancer treated with a radical mastectomy and chemotherapy 20 years ago. She had a second cancer (uterine) 10 years ago that was considered separate from her previous breast cancer.

Clinical Presentation: The physical therapy examination was consistent with the physician's diagnosis of nerve entrapment in a classic presentation. There were significant postural components to account for the development of symptoms. However, the therapist palpated several large masses in the axillary and supraclavicular fossa on both the right and left sides. There was no local warmth, redness, or tenderness associated with these lesions. The therapist requested permission to palpate the client's groin and popliteal spaces for any other suspicious lymph nodes. The rest of the examination findings were within normal limits.

Associated Signs and Symptoms: Further questioning about the presence of associated signs and symptoms revealed a significant disturbance in sleep pattern over the last 6 months

with unrelenting shoulder and neck pain. There were no other reported constitutional symptoms, skin changes, or noted lumps anywhere. Vital signs were unremarkable at the time of the physical therapy evaluation.

Result: Returning this client to her referring physician was a difficult decision to make given that the therapist did not have the benefit of the medical records or results of neurologic examination and testing. Given the significant past medical history for cancer, the woman's age, presence of progressive night pain, and palpable masses, no other reasonable choice remained. When asked if the physician had seen or felt the masses, the client responded with a definite "no."

There are several ways to approach handling a situation like this one, depending on the physical therapist's relationship with the physician. In this case, the therapist had never communicated with this physician before. It is possible that the physician was aware of the masses, knew from medical testing that there was extensive cancer, and chose to treat the client palliatively.

Because there was no indication of such, the therapist notified the physician's staff of the decision to return the client to the physician. A brief (one-page) written report summarizing the findings was given to the client to hand-carry to the physician's office.

Further medical testing was performed, and a medical diagnosis of lymphoma was made.

---

of clients with pernicious anemia. Affected clients may have chest pain or angina on physical exertion because of the lack of nutrition to the myocardium.

Risk Factors

Gender and age are nonmodifiable risk factors for chest pain caused by heart disease. The rate of coronary artery disease (CAD) is rising among women and falling among men. Men develop CAD at a younger age than women, but women make up for it after menopause. Many women know about the risk of breast cancer, but in truth, they are 10 times more likely to die of cardiovascular

disease. While one in 30 women's deaths is from breast cancer, one in 2.5 deaths is from heart disease.[5]

Women do not seem to do as well as men after taking medications to dissolve blood clots or after undergoing heart-related medical procedures. Of the women who survive a heart attack, 46% will be disabled by heart failure within 6 years.[6] African-American women have a 70% higher death rate from CAD compared with Caucasian women.[5] Whenever screening individuals who have chest pain, keep in mind that older men and women, menopausal women, and African-American women are at greatest risk for cardiovascular causes.

A common treatment for CAD after heart attack is angioplasty with insertion of a stent. A stent is a wire mesh tube that props open narrowed coronary arteries. Sometimes, the stent malfunctions or gets scarred over. Cardiologists have realized that such treatments, while effective at alleviating chest pain, do not reduce the risk of heart attacks for most people with stable angina.

When the client presents with chest pain, he or she often does not think it can be from the heart because there is a stent in place, but this may not be true. Anyone with a history of stent insertion presenting with chest pain should be screened carefully. Take vital signs, and ask about associated signs and symptoms. Assess the effect of exercise on symptoms. For example, does the chest, neck, shoulder, or jaw pain start 3 to 5 minutes after exercise or activity? What is the effect on pain in the upper body when the individual is using just the lower extremities, such as walking on a treadmill or up a flight of stairs?

Other risk factors for CAD are listed in Table 6-3. The therapist can help clients assess their 10-year risk for heart attack using a risk assessment tool from the National Cholesterol Education program.[7]

Clinical Presentation

There are some well-known pain patterns specific to the heart and cardiac system. Sudden death can be the first sign of heart disease. In fact according to the American Heart Association, 63% of women who died suddenly of cardiovascular disease had no previous symptoms. Sudden death is the first symptom for half of all men who have a heart attack. Cardiac arrest strikes immediately and without warning.

Clinical Signs and Symptoms of

Cardiac Arrest

- Sudden loss of responsiveness; no response to gentle shaking
- No normal breathing; client does not take a normal breath when you check for several seconds.
- No signs of circulation; no movement or coughing

Cardiac Pain Patterns

Doctors and nurses often use "the three Ps" when screening for chest pain of a cardiac nature. The presence of any or all of these Ps suggests the client's pain or symptoms are *not* caused by a myocardial infarction (MI):

- **P**leuritic pain (exacerbation by deep breathing is more likely pulmonary in nature)
- Pain on **p**alpation (musculoskeletal cause)
- Pain with changes in **p**osition (musculoskeletal cause)

Cardiac pain patterns may differ for men and women. For many men, the most common report is a feeling of pressure or discomfort under the sternum (substernal), in the midchest region or across the entire upper chest. It can feel like uncomfortable pressure, squeezing, fullness, or pain.

Pain may occur just in the jaw, upper neck, midback, or down the arm without chest pain or discomfort. Pain may also radiate from the chest to the neck, jaw, midback, or down the arm(s). Pain down the arm(s) affects the left arm most often in the pattern of the ulnar nerve distribution. Radiating pain down both arms is also possible.

For women, symptoms can be more subtle or atypical (Box 17-1). Chest pain or discomfort is less common in women but still a key feature for some. They often have prodromal symptoms up to 1 month before having a heart attack (see Table 6-4).[8,9]

Fatigue, nausea, and lower abdominal pain may signal a heart attack. Many women pass these off

---

BOX 17-1 ▼ Signs and Symptoms of Myocardial Ischemia in Women

- Heart pain in women does not always follow classic patterns.
- Many women do not experience classic chest discomfort.
- In older women, mental status change or confusion may be common.
- Dyspnea (at rest or with exertion)
- Weakness and lethargy (unusual fatigue; fatigue that interferes with ability to perform activities of daily living)
- Indigestion or heart burn; mistakenly diagnosed or assumed to have gastroesophageal reflux disease (GERD)
- Lower abdominal pain
- Anxiety or depression
- Sleep disturbance (woman awakens with any of the symptoms listed here)
- Sensation similar to inhaling cold air; unable to talk or breathe
- Isolated midthoracic back pain
- Isolated *right* biceps aching
- Symptoms may be relieved by antacids (sometimes antacids work better than nitroglycerin).

as the flu or food poisoning. Other symptoms for women include a feeling of intense anxiety, isolated right biceps pain, or midthoracic pain. Heartburn; sudden shortness of breath or the inability to talk, move, or breathe; shoulder or arm pain; or ankle swelling or rapid weight gain are also common symptoms with MI.

Chest Pain Associated with Angina

The therapist should keep in mind that coronary disease may go unnoticed because the client has no anginal or infarct pain associated with ischemia. This situation occurs when collateral circulation is established to counteract the obstruction of the blood flow to the heart muscle. Anastomoses (connecting channels) between the branches of the right and left coronary arteries eliminate the person's perception of pain until challenged by physical exertion or exercise in the physical therapy setting.

Chest pain caused by angina is often confused with heartburn or indigestion, hiatal hernia, esophageal spasm, or gallbladder disease, but the pain of these other conditions is not described as sharp or knifelike. The client often says the pain feels like "gas" or "heartburn" or "indigestion." Referred pain from a trigger point in the external oblique abdominal muscle can cause a sensation of heartburn in the anterior chest wall (see Fig. 17-7).

Episodes of stable angina usually develop slowly and last 2 to 5 minutes. Discomfort may radiate to the neck, shoulders, or back (Case Example 17-3). Shortness of breath is common. Symptoms of angina may be similar to the pattern associated with a heart attack. One primary difference is duration. Angina lasts a limited time (a few minutes up to a half hour) and can be relieved by rest or nitroglycerin. When screening for angina, a lack of objective musculoskeletal findings is always a red flag:

• Active range of motion (AROM) such as trunk rotation, side bending; shoulder motions does not reproduce symptoms.

• Resisted motion does not reproduce symptoms (horizontal shoulder abduction/adduction).

• Heat and stretching do not reduce or eliminate symptoms.

The therapist should also watch for unstable angina in a client with known angina. Unlike stable angina, rest or nitroglycerin does not relieve symptoms associated with an MI, unless administered intravenously. Without intervention, symptoms of an MI may continue without stopping. A sudden change in the client's typical anginal pain pattern suggests unstable angina. Pain that occurs without exertion, lasts longer than 10 minutes, or is not relieved by rest or nitroglycerin signals a higher risk for a heart attack. Immediate medical referral is required under these circumstances.

▶ SCREENING FOR PLEUROPULMONARY CAUSES OF CHEST, BREAST, OR RIB PAIN

Pulmonary chest pain usually results from obstruction, restriction, dilation, or distention of the large airways or large pulmonary artery walls. Specific diagnoses include pulmonary artery hypertension, pulmonary embolism, mediastinal emphysema, pleurisy, pneumonia, and pneumothorax. Pleuropulmonary disorders are discussed in detail in Chapter 7.

Past Medical History

A previous history of cancer of any kind, recent history of pulmonary infection, or recent accident or hospitalization may be significant. Look for

---

CASE EXAMPLE 17-3   Adhesive Capsulitis

Referral: A 56-year-old man returned to the same physical therapist with his third recurrence of left shoulder adhesive capsulitis of unknown cause.

Past Medical History: There was no reported injury, trauma, or repetitive motion as a precipitating factor in this case. The client was a car salesman with a fairly sedentary job. He reported a past history of prostatitis, peptic ulcers, and a broken collarbone as a teenager.

He reported being a "social" drinker at work-related functions but did not smoke or use tobacco products. He was taking ibuprofen for his shoulder but no other over-the-counter or prescription medications or supplements.

The two previous episodes of shoulder problems resolved with physical therapy intervention. The client had a home program to follow to maintain range of motion and normal movement. At the time of his most recent discharge 6

CASE EXAMPLE 17-3   Adhesive Capsulitis—cont'd

months ago, he had attained 80% of motion available on the uninvolved side with some continued restricted glenohumeral movement and altered scapulohumeral rhythm. The client reported that he did not continue with his exercise routine at home, and "that's why I got worse again."

Clinical Presentation

Shoulder flexion and   Left: 105/100   Right: 170/165
  abduction
Shoulder medial   0-70   0-90
  (internal) rotation
Shoulder lateral   0-45   0-80
  (external) rotation

Accessory motions: Reduced inferior and anterior glide on the left; within normal limits on the right. The client reports pain during glenohumeral flexion, abduction and medial and lateral rotations.

Clinical impression: Decreased physiologic motion with capsular pattern of restriction and compensatory movements of the shoulder girdle; humeral superior glide syndrome.

Associated Signs and Symptoms: When asked if there were any symptoms of any kind anywhere else in the body, the client reported "chest tightness" whenever he tried to use his arm for more than a few minutes. Previously, he was used to "working through the pain," but he can't seem to do that anymore.

He also reported "a few bouts of nausea and sweating" when his shoulder started aching. He denied any shortness of breath or constitutional symptoms such as fever or sweats. There were no other gastrointestinal-related symptoms.

What are the red flags in this case? How would you screen further?

- Age over 50
- Nausea and sweating concomitant with shoulder pain; chest tightness
- Insidious onset
- Recurring pattern of symptoms

Screening can begin with something as simple as vital sign assessment. The therapist can consult Box 4-17 for a list of other associated signs and symptoms and look for a cluster or pattern associated with a particular system.

Given his age, sedentary lifestyle, and particular clinical presentation, a cardiovascular screening examination seems most appropriate.

The therapist can also consult the Special Questions to Ask box at the end of Chapter 6 for any additional pertinent questions based on the client's responses to questions and examination results. A short (3- to 5-minute) bike test also can be used to assess the effect of lower extremity exertion on the client's symptoms.

Result: The client's blood pressure was alarmingly high at 185/120 mm Hg. Although this is an isolated (one time) reading, he was under no apparent stress, and he revealed that he had a history of elevated blood pressure in the past. The bike test was administered while his heart rate and blood pressure were being monitored. Symptoms of chest and/or shoulder pain were not reproduced by the test, but the therapist was unwilling to stress the client without a medical evaluation first.

Referral was made to his primary care physician with a phone call, fax, and report of the therapist's findings and concerns. Although there is a known viscerosomatic effect between heart and chest and heart and shoulder, there is no reported direct cause and effect link between heart disease and adhesive capsulitis. Comorbid factors such as diabetes or heart disease have been shown to affect pain levels and function.[10]

Likewise, adhesive capsulitis is known to occur in some people following immobility associated with intensive care, coronary artery bypass graft, or pacemaker complications/revisions.

The physician considered this an emergency situation and admitted the client to the cardiology unit for immediate workup. The electrocardiogram results were abnormal during the exercise stress test. Further testing confirmed the need for a triple bypass procedure. Following the operation and phase 1 cardiac rehab in the cardiac rehab unit, the client returned to the original outpatient physical therapist for his phase 2 cardiac rehab program. Shoulder symptoms were gone, and range of motion was unimproved but regained rapidly as the rehab program progressed.

The therapist shared this information with the cardiologist, who agreed that there may have been a connection between the chest/shoulder symptoms before surgery, although he could not say for sure.

other risk factors, such as age, smoking, prolonged immobility, immune system suppression (e.g., cancer chemotherapy, corticosteroids), and eating disorders (or malnutrition from some other cause).

Clinical Presentation

Pulmonary pain patterns differ slightly depending on the underlying pathology and the location of the disease. For example, tracheobronchial pain is referred to the anterior neck or chest at the same levels as the points of irritation in the air passages. Chest pain that tends to be sharply localized or that worsens with coughing, deep breathing, other respiratory movements or motion of the chest wall and that is relieved by maneuvers that limit the expansion of a particular part of the chest (e.g., auto-splinting) is likely to be pleuritic in origin.

Symptoms that increase with deep breathing and activity or the presence of a productive cough with bloody or rust-colored sputum are red flags. The therapist should ask about new onset of wheezing at any time or difficulty breathing at night. Be careful when asking clients about changes in breathing patterns. It is not uncommon for the client to deny any shortness of breath.

Often, the reason for this is because the client has stopped doing anything that will bring on the symptoms. It may be necessary to ask what activities he or she can no longer do that were possible 6 weeks or 6 months ago. Symptoms that are relieved by sitting up are indicative of pulmonary impairment and must be evaluated more carefully.

▶ SCREENING FOR
GASTROINTESTINAL CAUSES OF
CHEST, BREAST, OR RIB PAIN

GI causes of upper thorax pain are a result of epigastric or upper GI conditions. GERD ("heartburn" or esophagitis) accounts for a significant number of

Fig. 17-1 • Chest pain caused by gastrointestinal (GI) disease with referred pain to the shoulder and back. Upper GI problems can refer pain to the anterior chest with radiating pain to the thoracic spine at the same level. Look for accompanying GI symptoms and red flag history.

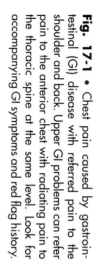
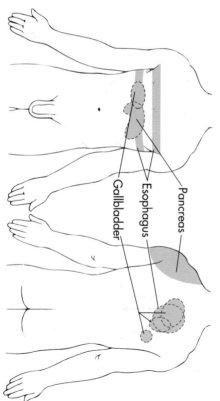

Pancreas
Esophagus
Gallbladder

cases of noncardiac chest pain. Stomach acid or gastric juices from the stomach enter the esophagus, causing irritation to the protective lining of the lower esophagus. Whether the client is experiencing GERD or some other cause of chest pain, there is usually a telltale history or associated signs and symptoms to red flag the case.

Past Medical History

Watch for a history of alcoholism, cirrhosis, esophageal varices, and esophageal cancer or peptic ulcers. Any risk factors associated with these conditions are also red flags such as long-term use of NSAIDs as a cause of peptic ulcers or chronic alcohol use associated with cirrhosis of the liver.

Clinical Presentation

The GI system has a broad range of referred pain patterns based on embryologic development and multisegmental innervations, as discussed in Chapter 3. Upper GI and pancreatic problems are more likely than lower GI disease to cause chest pain. Chest pain referred from the upper GI tract can radiate from the chest posteriorly to the upper back or interscapular or subscapular regions from T10 to L2 (Fig. 17-1).

Esophagus

Esophageal dysfunction will present with symptoms such as anterior neck and/or anterior chest pain, pain during swallowing (odynophagia), or difficulty swallowing (dysphagia) at the level of the lesion. Symptoms occur anywhere a lesion is present along the length of the esophagus. Early satiety, often with weight loss, is a common symptom with esophageal carcinoma.

Lesions of the upper esophagus may cause pain in the (anterior) neck, whereas lesions of the lower esophagus are more likely to be character-

ized by pain originating from the xiphoid process, radiating around the thorax to the middle of the back.

Chest pain with or without accompanying or alternating midthoracic back pain from an esophageal or other upper GI problem is usually red flagged by a suspicious history or cluster of associated signs and symptoms. The pain pattern associated with thoracic disc disease can be the same as for esophageal pathology. In the case of disc disease, there may be bowel and/or bladder changes and sometimes numbness and tingling in the upper extremities. The therapist should ask about a traumatic injury to the upper back region and conduct a neurologic screening examination to assess for this possibility as a cause of the symptoms.

Epigastric Pain

Epigastric pain is typically characterized by substernal or upper abdominal (just below the xiphoid process) discomfort (see Fig.17-1). This may occur with radiation posteriorly to the back secondary to long-standing duodenal ulcers. Gastric duodenal peptic ulcer may occasionally cause pain in the lower chest rather than in the upper abdomen. Antacid and food often immediately relieve pain caused by an ulcer. Ulcer pain is not produced by effort and lasts longer than angina pectoris. The therapist will not be able to provoke or eliminate the client's symptoms. Likewise, physical therapy intervention will not have any long-lasting effects unless the symptoms were caused by trigger points (TrPs).

Pain in the lower substernal area may arise as a result of reflux esophagitis (regurgitation of gastroduodenal secretions), a condition known as gastroesophageal reflux disease, or GERD. It may be gripping, squeezing, or burning, described as "heartburn" or "indigestion." Like that of angina pectoris, the discomfort of reflux esophagitis may be precipitated by recumbency or by meals; however, unlike angina, it is not precipitated by exercise and is relieved by antacids.

Hepatic and Pancreatic Systems

Epigastric pain or discomfort may occur in association with disorders of the liver, gallbladder, common bile duct, and pancreas, with referral of pain to the interscapular, subscapular, or middle/low back regions. This type of pain pattern can be mistaken for angina pectoris or myocardial infarction (e.g., hypotension occurring with pancreatitis produces a reduction of coronary blood flow with the production of angina pectoris).

Hepatic disorders may cause chest pain with radiation of pain to the shoulders and back. Cholecystitis (gallbladder inflammation) appears as discrete attacks of epigastric or right upper quadrant pain, usually associated with nausea, vomiting, and fever and chills. Dark urine and jaundice indicate that a stone has obstructed the common duct.

The pain has an abrupt onset, is either steady or intermittent, and is associated with tenderness to palpation in the right upper quadrant. The pain may be referred to the back and right scapular areas. A gallbladder problem can result in a sore tenth rib tip (right side anteriorly) as described in Chapter 9 (Case Example 17-4). Rarely, pain in the left upper quadrant and anterior chest can occur.

Acute pancreatitis causes pain in the upper part of the abdomen that radiates to the back (usually anywhere from T10 to L2) and may spread out over the lower chest. Fever and abdominal tenderness may develop.

Clinical Signs and Symptoms of
Gastrointestinal Disorders

- Chest pain (may radiate to back)
- Nausea
- Vomiting
- Blood in stools
- Pain on swallowing or associated with meals
- Jaundice
- Heartburn or indigestion
- Dark urine

▶ SCREENING FOR BREAST CONDITIONS THAT CAUSE CHEST OR BREAST PAIN

Occasionally, a client may present with breast pain as the primary complaint, but most often the description is of shoulder or arm or neck or upper back pain. When asked if any symptoms occur elsewhere in the body, the client may mention breast pain (Case Example 17-5).

During examination of the upper quadrant, the therapist may observe suspicious or aberrant changes in the integument, breast, or surrounding soft tissues. The client may report discharge from the nipple. Discharge from both nipples is more likely to be from a benign condition; discharge from one nipple can be a sign of a precancerous or malignant condition.

Asking the client about history, risk factors, and the presence of other signs and symptoms is the next step (see Box 4-16). Knowing possible causes

of breast pain can help guide the therapist during the screening interview (see Table 17-2).

Past Medical History

A past history of breast cancer, heart disease, recent birth, recent upper respiratory infection (URI), overuse, or trauma (including assault) may be significant for the client presenting with breast pain or symptoms. Any component of heart disease, such as hypertension, angina, myocardial infarction, and/or any heart procedure such as angioplasty, stent, or coronary artery bypass, is considered a red flag.

Any woman experiencing chest or breast pain should be asked about a personal history of previous breast surgeries, including mastectomy, breast reconstruction, or breast implantation or augmentation. A past history of breast cancer is a red flag even if the client has completed all treatment and has been cancer free for 5 years or more.

Breast cancer and cysts develop more frequently in individuals who have a family history of breast disease. A previous history of cancer is always cause to question the client further regarding the onset and pattern of current symptoms. This is especially true when a woman with a previous history of breast cancer or cancer of the reproductive system appears with shoulder, chest, hip, or sacroiliac pain of unknown cause.

If a client denies a previous history of cancer, the therapist should still ask whether that person has ever received chemotherapy or radiation therapy. It is surprising how often the answer to the question about a previous history of cancer is "no" but the answer to the question about prior treatment for cancer is "yes."

Clinical Presentation

For the most part, breast pain (mastalgia), tenderness, and swelling are the result of monthly hormone fluctuations. Cyclical pain may get worse during perimenopause when hormone levels change erratically. These same symptoms may continue after menopause, especially in women who

---

CASE EXAMPLE 17-4 Chest Pain During Pregnancy

Referral: A 33-year-old woman in her twenty-ninth week of gestation with her first pregnancy was referred to a physical therapist by her gynecologist. Her abdominal sonogram and lab tests were normal. A chest x-ray was read as negative.

Past Medical History: None. The client had the usual childhood illnesses but had never broken any bones and denied use of tobacco, alcohol, or substances of any kind. There was no recent history of infections, colds, viruses, coughs, trauma or accidents, and changes in gastrointestinal function and no history of cancer.

Clinical Presentation: Although there were no signs and symptom associated with the respiratory system, the client's symptoms were reproduced when she was asked to take a deep breath. Palpation of the upper chest, thorax, and ribs revealed pain on palpation of the right tenth rib (anterior).

Thinking about the role of the gallbladder causing tenth rib pain, the therapist asked further questions about past history and current gastrointestinal symptoms. The client had no red flag symptoms or history in this regard.

Knowing that transient osteoporosis can be associated with pregnancy,[11-16] the therapist gave the client the Osteoporosis Screening Evaluation (see Appendix C-3). The client replied "yes" to three questions (Caucasian or Asian, mother diagnosed with osteoporosis, physically inactive), suggesting the possibility of rib fracture.[12,14]

Result: The therapist initiated a telephone consultation with the physician to review her findings. Although the original x-ray was read as negative, the physician ordered a different view (rib series) and identified a fracture of the tenth rib.

The physician explained that the mechanical forces of the enlarging uterus on the ribs pull the lower ribs into a more horizontal position. Any downward stress from above (e.g., forceful cough or pull from the external oblique muscles) or upward force from the serratus anterior and latissimus dorsi muscles can increase the bending stress on the lower ribs.[12]

An aquatics therapy program was initiated and continued throughout the remaining weeks of this client's pregnancy.

CASE EXAMPLE 17-5 Breast Pain and Trigger Points

Referral: A 67-year-old woman came to physical therapy after seeing her primary care physician with a report of decreased functional left shoulder motion. She was unable to reach the top shelf of her kitchen cabinets or closets. She felt that at 5 feet 7 inches this is something she should be able to do.

Past Medical History: During the Past Medical History portion of the interview, she mentioned that she had had a stroke 10 years ago. Her referring physician was unaware of this information. She had recently moved here to be closer to her daughter, and no medical records have been transferred. There was no other significant history.

At the end of the interview, when asked, "Is there anything else you think I should know about your health or current situation that we haven't discussed?" she replied, "Well, actually the reason I really went to see the doctor was for pain in my left breast."

She had not reported this information to the physician.

Clinical Presentation: Examination revealed mild loss of strength in the left upper extremity accompanied by mild sensory and proprioceptive losses. Palpation of the shoulder and pectoral muscles produced breast pain. The client had been aware of this pain, but she had attributed it to a separate medical problem. She was reluctant to report her breast pain to her physician. Objectively, there were positive trigger points of the left pectoral muscles and loss of accessory motions of the left shoulder (see Fig 17-7).

- Active trigger point of the left pectoralis major with pain centered in the left breast
- Decreased left shoulder accessory motions (caudal glide, posterior glide and lateral

traction); no shoulder pain or discomfort reported
- Range of motion limited by 20% compared with the right shoulder in flexion, external rotation, and abduction
- Mild strength deficit
- Mild sensory and proprioceptive losses
- Vital signs:

Blood pressure (sitting, left arm)	142/108 mm Hg
Heart rate	72 bpm
Pulse oximeter	98%
Oral temperature	98.0 degrees

Intervention: Physical therapy treatment to eliminate trigger points and restore shoulder motion resolved the breast pain during the first week.

Should you make a medical referral for this client? If so, on what basis?

Despite this woman's positive response to physical therapy treatment, given the age of this client, her significant past medical history for cerebrovascular injury (reportedly unknown to the referring physician), current blood pressure (although an isolated measurement), report of breast pain (also unreported to her physician), and the residual paresis, medical referral was still indicated.

At the first follow-up visit, a letter was sent with the client that briefly summarized the initial objective findings, her progress to date, and the current concerns. She returned for an additional week of physical therapy to complete the home program for her shoulder. A medical evaluation ruled out breast disease, but medical treatment (medication) was indicated to address cardiovascular issues.

---

use hormone replacement therapy (HRT). Non-cyclical breast pain is not linked to menstruation or hormonal fluctuations. It is unpredictable and may be constant or intermittent, affecting one or both breasts in a small area or the entire breast.

The typical referral pattern for breast pain is around the chest into the axilla, to the back at the level of the breast, and occasionally into the neck and posterior aspect of the shoulder girdle (Fig. 17-

2). The pain may continue along the medial aspect of the ipsilateral arm to the fourth and fifth digits, mimicking pain of the ulnar nerve distribution.

Jarring or movement of the breasts and movement of the arms may aggravate this pain pattern. Pain in the upper inner arm may arise from outer quadrant breast tumors, but pain in the local chest wall may point to any pathologic condition of the breast.

Fig. 17-2 • Pain arising from the breast (mastalgia) can be referred into the axilla along the medial aspect of the arm. Referral pattern can also extend to the supraclavicular level and into the neck. Breast pain may be diffuse around the thorax through the intercostal nerves. Pain may be referred to the back and the posterior shoulder. Ask the client about the presence of lumps, nipple discharge, distended veins, or puckered or red skin (or any other skin changes).

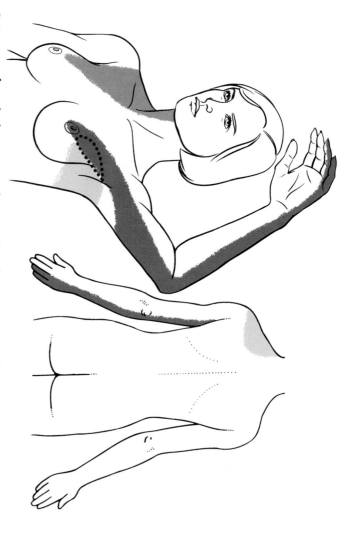

Nipple discharge in women is common, especially in pregnant or lactating women, and does not always signal a serious underlying condition. It may occur as a result of some medications (e.g., estrogen-based drugs, tricyclic antidepressants, benzodiazepines, and others).

The fluid may be thin to thick in consistency and various colors (e.g., milky white, green, yellow, brown, or bloody). Any unusual nipple discharge should be evaluated by a medical doctor. Injury, hormonal imbalance, underactive thyroid, infection or abscess, or tumors are just a few possible causes of nipple discharge.

Clinical Signs and Symptoms of Breast Pathology

- Family history of breast disease
- Palpable breast nodules or lumps and previous history of chronic mastitis
- May be painless
- Breast pain with possible radiation to inner aspect of arm(s)
- Skin surface over a tumor may be red, warm, edematous, firm, and painful.
- Firm, painful site under the skin surface

- Skin dimpling over the lesion with attachment of the mass to surrounding tissues, preventing normal mobilization of skin, fascia, and muscle
- Unusual nipple discharge or bleeding from the nipple(s)
- Pain aggravated by jarring or movement of the breasts
- Pain that is not aggravated by resistance to isometric movement of the upper extremities

Causes of Breast Pain

There is a wide range of possible causes of breast pain, including both systemic or viscerogenic and neuromusculoskeletal etiologies (Table 17-2). Not all conditions are life threatening or even require medical attention.

Although it is more typical in women, both men and women can have chest, back, scapular, and shoulder pain referred by a pathologic condition of the breast. Only those conditions most likely to be seen in a physical therapist's practice are included in this discussion.

Mastodynia

Mastodynia (irritation of the upper dorsal intercostal nerve) that causes chest pain is almost

TABLE 17-2 ▼ Causes of Breast Pain

Systemic causes	Neuromusculoskeletal causes
Infection	Pectoral myalgia or other conditions affecting the pectoralis muscles
• Mastitis (lactating women)	Trigger points (TrPs)
• Abscess	Mastodynia (mammary neuralgia)
Paget's disease	Breast implants, augmentation, reduction
Tumors, cysts, fibrocystic changes	• Scar tissue
Lymph disease	Trauma or injury (e.g., assault, breast biopsy, or surgery)
Premenstrual syndrome (PMS), menstrual or hormonal influences	Thoracic outlet syndrome
Shingles (herpes zoster)	Costochondritis
Cancer (rare cause of breast pain)	Connective tissue disorders
Pleuritis	Heavy, pendulous breasts
Gastroesophageal reflux disease (GERD)	
Medications (e.g., some hormone, cardiovascular, psychiatric drugs)	

always associated with ovulatory cycles, especially premenstrually. The association between symptoms and menses may be discovered during the physical therapist's interview when the client responds to Special Questions to Ask: Breast (see end of this chapter or Appendix B-7). The presentation is usually unilateral breast or chest pain and occurs initially at the premenstrual period and later more persistently throughout the menstrual cycle.

Mastitis

Mastitis is an inflammatory condition associated with lactation (breast feeding). Mammary duct obstruction causes the duct to become clogged. The breast becomes red, swollen, and painful. The involved breast area is often warm or even hot. Constitutional symptoms such as fever, chills, and flulike symptoms are common. Acute mastitis can occur in males (e.g., nipple chafing from jogging); the presentation is the same as for females.

Risk factors include previous history of mastitis; cracked, bleeding, painful nipples; and stress or fatigue. Bacteria can enter the breast through cracks in the nipple during trauma or nursing. Subsequent infection may lead to abscess formation. Obstructive and infectious mastitis are considered as two conditions on a continuum. Mastitis is often treated symptomatically, but the client should be encouraged to let her doctor know about any breast signs and symptoms present. Antibiotics may be needed in the case of a developing infection.

Benign Tumors and Cysts

Benign tumors and cysts were once lumped together and called "fibrocystic breast disease." With additional research over the years, scientists have come to realize that a single label is not adequate for the variety of benign conditions possible, including fibroadenomas, cysts, and calcifications that can occur in the breast.

An unchanged lump of long duration (years) is more likely to be benign. Many lumps are hormonally induced cysts and resolve within 2 or 3 menstrual cycles. Cyclical breast cysts are less common after menopause.

Other conditions can include intraductal papillomas (wartlike growth inside the breast), fat necrosis (fat breaks down and clumps together), and mammary duct ectasia (ducts near the nipple become thin-walled and accumulate secretions). Some of these breast changes are a variation of the norm, and others are pathologic but nonmalignant. A medical diagnosis is needed to differentiate between these changes.

Paget's Disease

Paget's disease of the breast is a rare form of ductal carcinoma arising in the ducts near the nipple. The woman experiences itching, redness, and flaking of the nipple with occasional bleeding (Fig. 17-3). Paget's disease of the breast is not related to Paget's disease of the bone, except that the same physician (Dr. James Paget, a contemporary of Florence Nightingale, 1877) named both conditions after himself.

TABLE 17-3 ▼ Factors Associated With Breast Cancer

Gender	Women > men
Race	White
Age	Advancing age; >60 years
	Peak incidence: 45-70
	Mean and median age: 60-61 (women)
	60-66 (men)
Genetic	BRCA1/BRCA2 gene mutations
Family history	First-degree relative with breast cancer
	Premenopausal
	Bilateral
	Mother, daughter, or sister
Previous medical history	Previous personal history of cancer
	Breast
	Uterine
	Ovarian
	Colon
	Number of previous breast biopsies
	(positive or negative)
Exposure to estrogen	Age at menarche <12
	Age at menopause >55
	Nulliparous (never pregnant)
	First live birth after age 35
	Environmental estrogens (esters)

For a more detailed guide to risk factors for breast cancer, see the American Cancer Society's document "What are the risk factors for breast cancer?" Available at http://www.cancer.org/docroot/CRI/content/CRI_2_4_2x_what_are_the_risk_factors_for_breast_cancer_5.asp

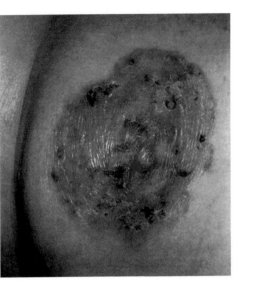

Fig. 17-3 • Paget's disease of the breast is a rare form of breast cancer affecting the nipple. It is characterized by a red (sometimes scaly) rash on the breast that often surrounds the nipple and areola, as seen in this photograph. Other presentations are possible, such as a red pimple or sore on the nipple that does not heal. Symptoms are unilateral, and the breast may be sore, itch, or burn. Diagnosis is often delayed because the symptoms seem harmless or the condition is misdiagnosed as dermatitis. (From Callen JP, Jorizzo J, Greer KE, et al: *Dermatological signs of internal disease*, Philadelphia, 1988, Saunders.)

Breast Cancer

The breast is the second most common *site* of cancer in women (the skin is first). Cancer of the breast is second only to lung cancer as a *cause of death* from cancer among women. Male breast cancer is possible but rare, accounting for 1% of all breast cancers (400 cases in 2005 compared with 30,000 for women).[17]

Although the frequency of breast cancer in men is strikingly less than that in women, the disease in both sexes is remarkably similar in epidemiology, natural history, and response to treatment. Men with breast cancer are 5 to 10 years older than women at the time of diagnosis, with mean or median ages between 60 and 66 years. This apparent difference may occur because symptoms in men are ignored for a longer period and the disease is diagnosed at a more advanced state.

RISK FACTORS

Despite the discovery of a breast cancer gene (BRCA-1 and BRCA-2), researchers estimate that only 5% to 10% of breast cancers are a result of inherited genetic susceptibility. Normally, BRCA-1 and BRCA-2 help prevent cancer by making pro-

teins that keep cells from growing abnormally. Inheriting either mutated gene from a parent increases the risk of breast cancer.[18] A large portion of cases are attributed to other factors, such as age, race, smoking, physical activity, alcohol intake, exposure to ionizing radiation, and exposure to estrogens (Table 17-3).

Women who received multiple fluoroscopies for tuberculosis or radiation treatment for mastitis during their adolescent or childbearing years are at increased risk for breast cancer as a result of exposure to ionizing radiation. In the past, irradiation was used for a variety of other medical conditions, including gynecomastia, thymic enlargement, eczema of the chest, chest burns, pulmonary tuberculosis, mediastinal lymphoma, and other cancers. Most of these clients are in their 70s now and at risk for cancer because of advancing age as well.

As a general principle, the risk of breast cancer is linked to a woman's total lifelong exposure to

estrogen. The increased incidence of estrogen-responsive tumors (tumors that are rich in estrogen receptors proliferate when exposed to estrogen) has been postulated to occur as a result of a variety of factors, such as prenatal and lifelong exposure to synthetic chemicals and environmental toxins, earlier age of menarche (first menstruation), improved nutrition in the United States, delayed and decreased childbearing, and longer average lifespan.

At the same time, it should be remembered that many women diagnosed with breast cancer have no identified risk factors. More than 70% of breast cancer cases are not explained by established risk factors.[19] There is no history of breast cancer among female relatives in more than 90% of clients with breast cancer. However, first-degree relatives (mother, daughters, or sisters) of women with breast cancer have two to three times the risk of developing breast cancer than the general female population, and relatives of women with bilateral breast cancer have five times the normal risk.[18]

Risk factors for men are similar to those for women, but at least half of all cases do not have an identifiable risk factor. Risk factors for men include heredity, obesity, infertility, late onset of puberty, frequent chest x-ray examinations, history of testicular disorders (e.g., infection, injury, or undescended testes), and increasing age. Men who have several female relatives with breast cancer and those in families who have the BRCA-2 mutation have a greater risk potential.

The presence of any of these factors may become evident during the interview with the client and should alert the physical therapist to the potential for neuromusculoskeletal complaints from a systemic origin that would require a medical referral. There are several easy-to-use screening tools available. In addition to screening for current risk, clients should be given this information for future use (Box 17-2).

CLINICAL PRESENTATION

Breast cancer may be asymptomatic in the early stages. The discovery of a breast lump with or without pain or tenderness is significant and must be investigated. Physical signs associated with advanced breast cancer have been summarized using the acronym BREAST: **B**reast mass, **R**etraction, **E**dema, **A**xillary mass, **S**caly nipple, and **T**ender breast.[20] Less common symptoms are breast pain; nipple discharge; nipple erosion, enlargement, itching, or redness; and generalized hardness, enlargement, or shrinking of the breast. Watery, serous, or bloody discharge from the nipple

---

---

is an occasional early sign but is more often associated with benign disease.

Breast cancer usually consists of a nontender, firm, or hard lump with poorly delineated margins that is caused by local infiltration. Breast cancer in women has a predilection for the outer upper quadrant of the breast and the areola (nipple) area (Fig. 17-4) involving the breast tissue overlying the pectoral muscle. During palpation, breast tissue lumps move easily over the pectoral muscle, compared with a lump within the muscle tissue itself. Later signs of malignancy include fixation of the tumor to the skin or underlying muscle fascia.

Male breast cancer begins as a painless induration, retraction of the nipple, and an attached mass progressing to include lymphadenopathy and skin and chest wall lesions. A tumor of any size in male

(CBE) and mammography. CBE alone detects 3% to 45% of diagnosed breast cancers that screening mammography misses. Studies show the sensitivity of CBE is 54% (test's ability to determine a true positive) and specificity is 94% (test's ability to determine a true negative).[21]

The previous edition of this text (*Differential Diagnosis in Physical Therapy*, ed 3) specifically stated, "breast examination is not within the scope of a physical therapist's practice." This practice is changing. As the number of cancer survivors increases in the United States, physical therapists treating postmastectomy women and clients of both genders with lymphedema are on the rise.

With direct and unrestricted access of consumers to physical therapists in many states, advanced skills have become necessary. For some clients, performing a CBE is an appropriate assessment tool in the screening process.[22] The American Cancer Society and National Cancer Institute Guidelines for CBE are provided in Appendix D-7.

Therapists who are trained to perform CBEs must make sure this examination is allowed according to the state practice act. In some states, it is allowed by exclusion, meaning it is not mentioned and therefore included. Discussion of the role of the physical therapist in primary care and cancer screening as it relates to integrating CBE into an upper quarter examination is available.[22] A form for recording findings from the CBE is provided in Fig. 4-45 and Appendix C-7.

The physical therapist does not diagnose any kind of cancer, including breast cancer; only the pathologist diagnoses cancer. The therapist can identify aberrant soft tissue and refer the client for further evaluation. Early detection and intervention can reduce morbidity and mortality.

For the therapist who is not trained in CBE, the client should be questioned about the presence of any changes in breast tissue (e.g., lumps, distended veins, skin rash, open sores or lesions, or other skin changes) and nipple (e.g., rash or other skin changes, discharge, distortion). Visual inspection is also possible and may be very important postmastectomy (Fig. 17-5). Ask the client if he or she has noticed any changes in the scar. Continue by asking:

Follow-Up Questions

- Would you have any objections if I looked at (or examined) the scar tissue?

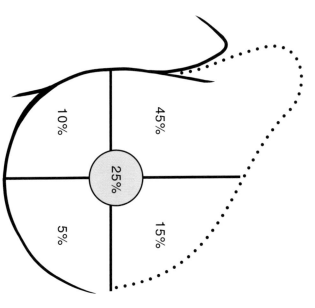

Fig. 17-4 • Most breast cancer presents in the upper outer quadrant of the breast (45%) or around the nipple (25%). Metastases occur via the lymphatic system at the axillary lymph nodes to the bones (shoulder, hip, ribs, vertebrae) or central nervous system (brain, spinal cord). Breast cancer can also metastasize hematogenously to the lungs, pleural cavity, and liver.

breast tissue is associated with skin fixation and ulceration and deep pectoral fixation more often than a tumor of similar size in female breast tissue is because of the small size of male breasts.

Clinical Signs and Symptoms of Breast Cancer

- Nontender, firm, or hard lump
- Unusual discharge from nipple
- Skin or nipple retraction dimpling; erosion, retraction, itching of nipple
- Redness or skin rash over the breast or nipple
- Generalized hardness, enlargement, shrinking, or distortion of the breast or nipple
- Unusual prominence of veins over the breast
- Enlarged rubbery lymph nodes
- Axillary mass
- Swelling of arm
- Bone or back pain
- Weight loss

CLINICAL BREAST EXAMINATION

Breast cancer mortality is reduced when women are screened by both clinical breast examination

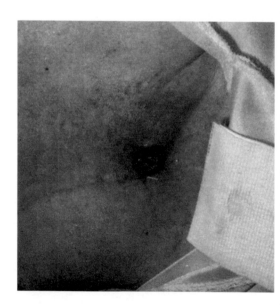

Fig. 17-5 • This photo shows the chest of a woman who has had a right radical mastectomy. There is a metastatic nodule in the mastectomy scar as a result of local cancer recurrence. Breast cancer can occur (recur) if a mastectomy has been done. A closer look at the lesion suggests that the skin changes have been present for quite some time. Even in this black and white photo, the change in skin coloration is obvious in a large patch around the nodule. Anytime a woman with a past medical history of cancer develops neck, back, upper trapezius, shoulder pain, or other symptoms, examining the site of the original cancer removal is a good idea. (From Callen JP, Jorizzo J, Greer KE, et al: *Dermatological signs of internal disease,* Philadelphia, 1988, Saunders.)

If the client declines or refuses, the therapist should follow up with counsel to perform self-inspection, emphasizing the need for continued CBEs and the importance of reporting any changes to the physician immediately.

Therapists have an important role in primary prevention and client education. The American Cancer Society offers recommendations for breast cancer screening. The therapist can encourage women (and men) to follow these guidelines (Box 17-3).

LYMPH NODE ASSESSMENT

Palpation of the underlying soft tissues (chest wall, axilla) and lymph nodes in the supraclavicular and axillary regions should be part of a screening exam in any client with chest pain (see Chapter 4 for description of lymph node palpation). Any report of palpable breast nodules, lumps, or changes in the appearance of the breast requires medical follow-up, especially when there is a personal or family history of breast disease.[24]

"Normal" lymph nodes are not palpable or visible, but not all palpable or visible lymph nodes

are a sign of cancer. Infections, viruses, bacteria, allergies, and food intolerances can cause changes in the lymph nodes. Lymph nodes that are hard, immovable, irregular, and nontender raise the suspicion of cancer, especially in the presence of a previous history of cancer. The skin surface over a tumor may be red, warm, edematous, firm, and painful. There may be skin dimpling over the lesion, with attachment of the mass to surrounding tissues preventing normal mobilization of skin, fascia, and muscle.

In the past, therapists were taught that any changes in lymph nodes present for more than 1 month in more than one region were a red flag. This has changed with the increased understanding of cancer metastases via the lymphatic system and the potential for cancer recurrence. A physician must evaluate all suspicious lymph nodes.

METASTASES

Metastases have been known to occur up to 25 years after the initial diagnosis of breast cancer. On the other hand, breast cancer can be a rapidly progressing, terminal disease. Approximately 40% of clients with stage II tumors experience relapse.

Knowledge of the usual metastatic patterns of breast cancer and the common complications can aid in early recognition and effective treatment. Because bone is the most frequent site of metastases from breast cancer in men and women, a past medical history of breast cancer is a major red flag in anyone presenting with new onset or persistent findings of NMS pain or dysfunction.

All distant visceral sites are potential sites of metastases. Other primary sites of involvement are lymph nodes, remaining breast tissue, lung, brain, central nervous system (CNS), and liver. Women with metastases to the liver or CNS have a poorer prognosis.

Spinal cord compression, usually from extradural metastases, may appear as back pain, leg weakness, and bowel/bladder symptoms. Rarely, an axillary mass, swelling of the arm, or bone pain from metastases may be the first symptom. Back or bone pain, jaundice, or weight loss may be the result of systemic metastases, but these symptoms are rarely seen on initial presentation.

Medical referral is advised before initiating treatment for anyone with a past history of cancer presenting with symptoms of unknown cause, especially without an identifiable movement system impairment.

A medical evaluation is still needed in light of new findings even if the client has been rechecked

BOX 17-3 ▼ ACS Recommendations for Breast Cancer Screening

Summary Recommendation

The American Cancer Society (ACS) recommendations for breast cancer screening are presented below in abbreviated form. Readers should refer to the original full text guideline document to see the complete recommendations, along with the rationale and summary of the evidence.

Women at Average Risk

- Begin mammography at age 40.
- For women in their 20s and 30s, it is recommended that clinical breast examination (CBE) be part of a periodic health examination, preferably at least every 3 years. Asymptomatic women aged 40 and over should continue to receive a CBE as part of a periodic health examination, preferably annually.
- Beginning in their 20s, women should be told about the benefits and limitations of breast self-examination (BSE). The importance of prompt reporting of any new breast symptoms to a health professional should be emphasized. Women who choose to perform BSE should receive instruction and have their technique reviewed on the occasion of a periodic health examination. It is acceptable for women to choose not to do BSE or to do BSE irregularly.
- Women should have an opportunity to become informed about the benefits, limitations, and potential harms associated with regular screening.

Older Women

Screening decisions in older women should be individualized by considering the potential benefits and risks of mammography in the context of current health status and estimated life expectancy. As long as a woman is in reasonably good health and would be a candidate for treatment, she should continue to be screened with mammography.

Women at Increased Risk

Women at increased risk of breast cancer might benefit from additional screening strategies beyond those offered to women of average risk, such as earlier initiation of screening, shorter screening intervals, or the addition of screening modalities other than mammography and physical examination, such as ultrasound or magnetic resonance imaging. However, the evidence currently available is insufficient to justify recommendations for any of these screening approaches.

Summary of New ACS Guidelines

- CBE every 3 years for women ages 20 to 39
- Annual CBE every year for asymptomatic women ages 40+
- SBE occasionally or not at all
- Women ages 20+ should be educated about the benefits and limitations of the SBE.
- Mammogram annually from age 40

Data from American Cancer Society: ACS News Center: Updated breast cancer screening guidelines http://www.cancer.org/docroot/NWS/content/NWS_1_1x_Updated_Breast_Cancer_Screening_Guidelines_Released.asp, May 2003. Accessed January 24, 2006.

---

by a medical oncologist recently. It is better to err on the side of caution. Failure to recognize the need for medical referral can result in possible severe and irreversible consequences of any delay in diagnosis and therapy.[25]

Clinical Signs and Symptoms of Metastasized Breast Cancer

- Palpable mass in supraclavicular, chest, or axillary regions
- Unilateral upper extremity numbness and tingling
- Back, hip, or shoulder pain
- Pain on weight bearing
- Leg weakness or paresis
- Bowel/bladder symptoms
- Jaundice

▲ **SCREENING FOR OTHER CONDITIONS AS A CAUSE OF CHEST, BREAST, OR RIB PAIN**

Breast Implants

Scar tissue or fibrosis from a previous breast surgery, such as reconstruction following mastectomy for breast cancer or augmentation or reduction mammoplasty for cosmetic reasons, is an important history to consider when assessing chest, breast, neck, or shoulder symptoms. Likewise, the client should be asked about a history of radiation to the chest, breast, or thorax.

Women who have implants for reconstruction following mastectomy for breast cancer are nearly three times more likely to have complications (e.g., pain, capsular contracture, infection, seroma) than those who receive implants for cosmetic reasons

only.[26] The rate of capsular contracture is significantly higher for irradiated breasts than for non-irradiated breasts.[27]

Clinical outcomes from the Danish Cancer Society report that ruptures are rare, but thick, tight scarring and infection occur in up to 20% of women who have breast implants after mastectomy.[28] Rates of early local complications in American women undergoing mastectomy with immediate breast implants are much higher.[29]

Other complications of breast implantation may include gel bleed, implant leaking or rupture, infection, calcifications around the implant, chronic breast pain, prolonged wound healing, and formation of granulation tissue.

Anxiety

An anxiety state or, in its extreme form, panic attack can cause chest or breast pain typical of a heart attack. The client experiences shortness of breath, perspiration, and pallor. It is the most common noncardiac cause of chest pain, accounting for half of all emergency department admissions each year for chest or breast pain (just ahead of chest pain caused by cocaine use).

Risk Factors

The first panic attack often follows a period of extreme stress, sometimes associated with being the victim of a crime or the loss of a job, partner, or close family member. The presence of another mental health disorder, such as depression or substance abuse (drugs or alcohol), increases the risk of developing panic disorder. There may be a familial component, but it is not clear if this is hereditary or environmental (learned behavior).[30]

Drugs such as over-the-counter decongestants and cold remedies can trigger panic attacks. Excessive use of caffeine and stimulants such as amphetamines and cocaine combined with a lack of sleep can also trigger an attack. Menopause, quitting smoking, or caffeine withdrawal can also bring on new onset of panic attacks in someone who has never experienced this problem before. See Chapter 3 for further discussion.

Clinical Presentation

There are several types of chest or breast discomfort caused by anxiety. The pain may be sharp, intermittent, or stabbing and located in the region of the left breast. The area of pain is usually no larger than the tip of the finger but may be as large as the client's hand. It is often associated with a local area of hyperesthesia of the chest wall. The

client can point to it with one finger. It is not reproduced with palpation or activity. It is not changed or altered by a change in position.

Anxiety-related pain may be located precordially (region over the heart and lower part of the thorax) or retrosternally (behind the sternum). It may be of variable duration, lasting no longer than a second or for hours or days. This type of pain is unrelated to effort or exercise. Distinguishing this sensation from myocardial ischemia requires medical evaluation.

Discomfort in the upper portion of the chest, neck, and left arm, again unrelated to effort, may occur. There may be a sense of persistent weakness and unpleasant awareness of the heartbeat. In the past, radiation of chest discomfort to the neck or left arm was considered to be diagnostic of atherosclerotic coronary heart disease. More recently, stress testing and coronary arteriography have shown that chest discomfort of this type can occur in clients with normal coronary arteriograms.

Some individuals with anxiety-related chest pain may have a choking sensation in the throat caused by hysteria. There may be associated hyperventilation. Palpitation, claustrophobia, and occurrence of symptoms in crowded places are common.

Hyperventilation occurs in persons with and without heart disease and may be misleading. Such clients have numbness and tingling of the hands and lips and feel as if they are going to "pass out." For a more detailed explanation of anxiety and its accompanying symptoms (e.g., hyperventilation), see Chapter 3.

Clinical Signs and Symptoms of

Chest Pain Caused by Anxiety

- Dull, aching discomfort in the substernal region and in the anterior chest
- Sinus tachycardia
- Fatigue
- Fear of closed-in places
- Diaphoresis
- Dyspnea
- Dizziness
- Choking sensation
- Hyperventilation: numbness and tingling of hands and lips

Cocaine

Cocaine use (also methamphetamine, known as crank and phencyclidine or PCP) has cardiotoxic effects, including cocaine dilated cardiomyopathy, angina, and left ventricular dysfunction, and can

precipitate myocardial infarction, cardiac arrhythmias, and even sudden cardiac death.[31]

Chronic use of cocaine or any of its derivatives is the number-one cause of stroke in young people today. The incidence of stroke associated with substance use and abuse is increasing. Use of these stimulants also has an effect on anyone with a congenital cerebral aneurysm and can lead to rupture.

The physiologic stress of cocaine use on the heart accounts for an increasing number of heart transplants. Acute effects of cocaine include increased heart rate, blood pressure, and vasomotor tone.[32] Cocaine remains the most common of illicit drug-related cause of severe chest pain bringing the person to the emergency department.[31,33] In fact, chest pain is the most common cocaine-related medical complaint.

Many people with chest pain have used cocaine within the last week but deny its use. The use of these substances is not uncommon in middle-aged and older adults of all socioeconomic backgrounds. The therapist should not neglect to ask clients about their use of substances because of preconceived ideas that only teenagers and young adults use drugs. Careful questioning (see Chapter 2; see also Appendix B-31) may assist the physical therapist in identifying a possible correlation between chest pain and cocaine use.

Always end this portion of the interview by asking:

Follow-Up Questions

- Are there any drugs or substances you take that you haven't mentioned?

Anabolic-Androgenic Steroids

Anabolic steroids are synthetic derivatives of testosterone used to enhance athletic performance or cosmetically shape the body. Used in supraphysiologic doses (more than the body produces naturally), these drugs have a potent effect on the musculoskeletal system, including the heart, potentially altering cardiac cellular and physiologic function.[34] Effects persist long after their use has been discontinued.[35]

The use of self-administered anabolic-androgenic steroids (AASs) is illegal but continues to increase dramatically among both athletes and nonathletes. It is used among preteens who do not compete in sports for cosmetic reasons. The goal is to advance to a more mature body build and enhance their looks. AASs do have medical uses and were added to prescribed controlled substances in 1990 under the control of the Drug Enforcement Administration.

In spite of stricter control of the manufacture and distribution of AASs, illegal supplies come from unlicensed sources all over the world. When dispensed without a regulating agency, the purity and processing of chemicals is unknown. The quality of black market supplies is a major concern. There is no guarantee that the products obtained are correctly labeled. Contents and dosage may be inaccurate. Some athletes are using injectable anabolic steroids intended for veterinary use only.

Clinical Presentation

Any young adult with chest pain of unknown cause, possibly accompanied by dyspnea and elevated blood pressure and without clinical evidence of NMS involvement, may have a history of anabolic steroid use. Consider anabolic steroid use as a possibility in men and women presenting with chest pain in their early 20s who have used this type of steroid since age 11 or 12.

In the pediatric population, there is a risk of decreased or delayed bone growth. Tendon and muscle strains are common and take longer than normal to heal. *Injuries that take longer than the expected physiologic time to heal are an important red flag.* Delayed healing occurs because the soft tissues are working under the added strain of extra body mass.

The alert therapist may recognize the associated signs and symptoms accompanying chronic use of these steroids. Changes in personality are the most dramatic signs of steroid use. The user may become more aggressive or experience mood swings and psychologic delusions (e.g., believe he or she is indestructible; sometimes referred to as "steroid psychosis"). "Roid rages," characterized by sudden outbursts of uncontrolled emotion, may be observed. Severe depression leading to suicide can occur with AAS withdrawal.

Clinical Signs and Symptoms of
Anabolic Steroid Use

- Chest pain
- Elevated blood pressure
- Ventricular tachycardia
- Weight gain (10 to 15 pounds in 2 to 3 weeks)
- Peripheral edema
- Acne on the face, upper back, chest
- Altered body composition with marked development of the upper torso
- Stretch marks around the back, upper arms, and chest
- Needle marks in large muscle groups (e.g., buttocks, thighs, deltoids)

Continued on p. 796

- Development of male pattern baldness
- Gynecomastia (breast tissue development in males); breast tissue atrophy in females
- Frequent hematoma or bruising
- Personality changes called "steroid psychosis" (rapid mood swings, sudden increased aggressive tendencies)
- Females: secondary male characteristics (deeper voice, breast atrophy, abnormal facial and body hair); menstrual irregularities
- Jaundice (chronic use)

The therapist who suspects a client may be using anabolic steroids should report findings to the physician or coach if one is involved. The therapist can begin by asking about the use of nutritional supplements or performance-enhancing agents. In the well-muscled male athlete, observe for common side effects of AAS such as acne, gynecomastia, and cutaneous striae in the deltopectoral region. Women who use AAS may exhibit muscular hypertrophy; male pattern baldness; excess hair growth on the face, breasts, and arms; and breast tissue atrophy.[34] Asking about the presence of common side effects of AAS and testing for elevated blood pressure may provide an opportunity to ask if the client is using these chemicals.

SCREENING FOR MUSCULOSKELETAL CAUSES OF CHEST, BREAST, OR RIB PAIN

It is estimated that 20% to 25% of noncardiac chest pain has a musculoskeletal basis.[36] Musculoskeletal causes of chest (wall) pain must be differentiated from pain of cardiac, pulmonary, epigastric, and breast origin (see Table 17-1) before physical therapy treatment begins. Careful history taking to identify red flag conditions differentiates those who require further investigation.

Movement system impairment is most often characterized by pain during specific postures, motion, or physical activities. Reproducing the pain by movement or palpation often directs the therapist in understanding the underlying problem.

Chest pain can occur as a result of cervical spine disorders because nerves originating as high as C3 and C4 can extend as far down as the nipple line. Pectoral, suprascapular, dorsal scapular, and long thoracic nerves originate in the lower cervical spine, and impingement of these nerves can cause chest pain.

Musculoskeletal disorders such as myalgia associated with muscle exertion, myofascial TrPs, cos-

tochondritis, or xiphoiditis can produce pain in the chest and arms. Compared with angina pectoris, the pain associated with these conditions may last for seconds or hours, and prompt relief does not occur with the ingestion of nitroglycerin.

Tietze's syndrome, costochondritis, a hypersensitive xiphoid, and the slipping rib syndrome must be differentiated from problems involving the thoracic viscera, particularly those of the heart, great vessels, and mediastinum, as well as from illness originating in the head, neck, or abdomen.

Rib pain (with or without neck, back, or chest pain or symptoms) must be evaluated for systemic versus musculoskeletal origins (Box 17-4). The same screening model used for all conditions can be applied.

Costochondritis

Costochondritis, also known as anterior chest wall syndrome, costosternal syndrome, and parasternal chondrodynia (pain in a cartilage), is used interchangeably with Tietze's syndrome, although these two conditions are not the same. Costochondritis is more common than Tietze's syndrome.

Although both disorders are characterized by inflammation of one or more costal cartilages (costochondral joints), costochondritis refers to pain in the costochondral articulations without swelling. This disorder can occur at almost any age but is observed most often in people older than 40. It tends to affect the second, third, fourth, and fifth costochondral joints; women are affected in 70% of all cases (Fig. 17-6). Other risk factors include trauma (e.g., driver striking steering wheel with chest during a motor vehicle accident, upper chest surgery, helmet tackle in sports, or other sports injury to the chest)[37] or repetitive motion (e.g., grocery-store clerk lifting and scanning items).

BOX 17-4 ▶ Causes of Rib Pain

Systemic

- Gallbladder disease (tenth rib)
- Shingles (herpes zoster)
- Pleurisy
- Osteoporosis
- Cancer (metastasized to the bone)

Musculoskeletal

- Trauma (e.g., bruise, fracture)
- Slipping rib syndrome
- Tietze's syndrome or costochondritis
- Trigger points
- Thoracic outlet syndrome

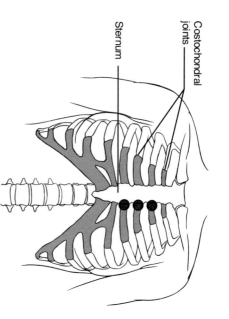

Costochondral joints

Sternum

Fig. 17-6 • Costochondritis is an inflammation of any of the costochondral joints (also called costal cartilages) where the rib joins the sternum. Sharp, stabbing, or aching pain can occur on either side of the sternum but tends to affect the left more often, even radiating down the left arm sometimes or to upper back. Many people mistake the symptoms for a heart attack. In most cases, symptoms occur at a single site involving the second or third costochondral joint, although any of the joints can be affected as shown.

Costochondritis is characterized by a sharp pain along the front edges of the sternum, especially on the left side, often misinterpreted as a heart attack. The pain may radiate widely, stimulating intrathoracic or intraabdominal disease. It differs from a myocardial infarction because during a heart attack, the initial pain is usually in the center of the chest, under the sternum, not along the edges.

Costochondritis can be similar to muscular pain and is elicited by pressure over the costochondral junctions. Occasionally, the affected individual will report a burning sensation in the breast(s) associated with this condition.

Costochondritis may follow trauma or may be associated with systemic rheumatic disease. It can come and go or persist for months. Inflammation of upper costal cartilages may cause chest pain, whereas inflammation of lower costal cartilages is more likely to cause abdominal or low back discomfort.

Tietze's Syndrome

Tietze's syndrome (inflammation of a rib and its cartilage; costal chondritis) may be one possible cause of anterior chest wall pain, manifested by painful swelling of one or more costochondral articulations.

In most cases, the cause of Tietze's syndrome is unknown. Other causes of sternal swelling may include an infectious process in the immunocom-promised person resulting from tuberculosis, aspergillosis, brucellosis, staphylococcal infection, or pseudomonal disease producing sternal osteomyelitis. Onset is usually before 40 years of age, with a predilection for the second and third decades. However, it can occur in children.

Approximately 80% of clients have only single sites of involvement, most commonly the second or third costal cartilage (costochondral joint). Anterior chest pain may begin suddenly or gradually and may be associated with increased blood pressure, increased heart rate, and pain radiating down the left arm. Pain is aggravated by sneezing, coughing, deep inspirations, twisting motions of the trunk, horizontal shoulder abduction and adduction, or the "crowing rooster" movement of the upper extremities.

These symptoms may seem similar to those of a heart attack, but the raised blood pressure, reproduction of painful symptoms with palpation or pressure, and aggravating factors differentiate Tietze's syndrome from myocardial infarction (Case Example 17-6). In rare cases, the individual has been diagnosed with Tietze's syndrome only to find out later the precipitating cause was cancer (e.g., lymphoma, squamous cell carcinoma of the mediastinum).[38,39] Tietze's syndrome can also be confused with TrPs (pectoralis major, internal intercostalis), an often overlooked cause of the same symptoms.[40]

Clinical Signs and Symptoms of
Tietze's Syndrome or Costochondritis

- Sudden or gradual onset of upper anterior chest pain
- Pain/tenderness of costochondral joint(s)
- Bulbous swelling of the involved costal cartilage (Tietze's syndrome)
- Mild-to-severe chest pain that may radiate to the left shoulder and arm
- Pain aggravated by deep breathing, sneezing, coughing, inspiration, bending, recumbency, or exertion (e.g., push-ups, lifting grocery items)

Hypersensitive Xiphoid

The hypersensitive xiphoid (xiphodynia) is tender to palpation, and local pressure may cause nausea and vomiting. This syndrome is manifested as epigastric pain, nausea, and vomiting.

Slipping Rib Syndrome

The slipping, or painful, rib syndrome (sometimes also referred to as the clicking rib syndrome)

CASE EXAMPLE 17-6 Tietze's Syndrome

Referral: A 53-year-old woman was referred by her physician with a diagnosis of left anterior chest pain. The woman is employed at a sawmill and performs repetitive tasks that require repetitive shoulder flexion and extension in using a hydraulic apparatus on a sliding track. Lifting (including overhead lifting) is required occasionally but is limited to items less than 20 pounds.

Past Medical History: Her past medical history was significant for a hysterectomy 10 years ago for prolonged bleeding. She has been a four- to five-pack/day smoker for 30 years but has cut down to one half pack/day for the last 2 months.

Clinical Presentation

Pain Pattern: The woman described the onset of her pain as sudden, crushing chest pain radiating down the left arm, occurring for the first time 6 weeks ago. She was transported to the emergency department, but tests were negative for cardiac incident. Blood pressure at the time of the emergency admittance was 195/110 mm Hg. She was released from the hospital with a diagnosis of "stress-induced chest pain."

The client experienced the same type of episode of chest pain 10 days ago but described radiating pain around the chest and under the armpit to the upper back. Today, her symptoms include extreme tenderness and pain in the left chest with deep pain described as penetrating straight through her chest to her back. There is no numbness or tingling and no pain down the arm but a residual soreness in the left arm.

The client believes that her symptoms may be "stress-induced" but expresses some doubts about this because her symptoms persist and no known cause has been found. She relates that because of divorce proceedings and child custody hearings, she is under extreme stress at this time.

Examination: The neurologic screen was negative. The deep tendon reflexes were within normal limits; strength testing was limited by pain but with a strong initial response elicited; and there were no changes in sensation, two-point discrimination, or proprioception observed.

There was exquisite pain on palpation of the left pectoral muscle with tenderness and swelling noted at the second, third, and fourth costochondral joints. Painful and radiating symptoms were reproduced with resisted shoulder horizontal adduction. Active shoulder range of motion was full but with a positive painful arc on the left. There was also painful reproduction of the radiating symptoms down the arm with palpation of the left supraspinatus and biceps tendons.

The painful chest/arm/upper back symptoms were not altered by respiratory movements (deep breathing or coughing), but the client was unable to lie down without extreme pain.

Result: The physical therapy assessment was suggestive of Tietze's syndrome secondary to repetitive motion and exacerbated by emotional stress* with concomitant shoulder dysfunction. Physical therapy intervention resulted in initial rapid improvement of symptoms with full return to work 6 weeks later.

---

* It should be noted that although the physical therapist's assessment recognized emotional stress as a factor in the client's symptoms, it may not be in the client's best interests to include this information in the documentation. Although the medical community is increasingly aware of the research surrounding the mind-body connection, worker's compensation and other third-party payers may use this information to deny payment.

---

occurs most often when there is hypermobility of the lower ribs. In this condition, inadequacy or rupture of the interchondral fibrous attachments of the anterior ribs allows the costal cartilage tips to sublux, impinging on the intercostal nerves. This condition can occur alone or can be associated with a broader phenomenon such as myofascial pain syndrome.[41]

Rib syndrome can occur at any age, including during childhood,[42] but most commonly occurs during the middle-aged years. The physical therapist is usually able to identify readily a rib syndrome as the cause of chest pain after a careful musculoskeletal examination. In some cases, persistent upper abdominal and/or low thoracic pain occurs, leaving physicians, chiropractors, and ther-

TABLE 17-4 ▼ Trigger Point Pain Guide

Location	Potential muscles involved
Front of chest pain	Pectoralis major
	Pectoralis minor
	Scaleni
	Sternocleidomastoid (sternal)
	Sternalis
	Iliocostalis cervicis
	Subclavius
	External abdominal oblique
Side of chest pain	Serratus anterior
	Lattissimus dorsi
Upper abdominal/ lower chest pain	Rectus abdominis
	Abdominal obliques
	Transversus abdominis

Modified from Travell JG, Simons DG: *Myofascial pain and dysfunction: the trigger point manual*, Baltimore, 1983, Williams & Wilkins, p 574.

apists puzzled.[43,44] A sonogram may be needed to make the diagnosis. Pain is made worse by slump sitting or side bending to the affected side. Reduction or elimination of symptoms following rib mobilization helps confirm the differential diagnosis.

Gallbladder impairment can also cause tenderness or soreness of the tip of the tenth rib on the right side. The affected individual may or may not have gallbladder symptoms. Because visceral and cutaneous fibers enter the spinal cord at the same level for the ribs and gallbladder, the nervous system may respond to the afferent input with sudomotor changes such as pruritus (itching of the skin) or a sore rib instead of gallbladder symptoms.

The clinical presentation appears as a biomechanical problem such as a rib dysfunction instead of nausea and food intolerances normally associated with gallbladder dysfunction. Symptoms will not be alleviated by physical therapy intervention, eventually sending the client back to his or her physician.

Trigger Points

The most common musculoskeletal cause of chest pain is TrPs, sometimes referred to as myofascial trigger points (MTrPs). TrPs (hypersensitive spots in the skeletal musculature or fascia) involving a variety of muscles (Table 17-4) may produce precordial pain (Fig. 17-7). Abdominal muscles have multiple referred pain patterns that may reach up into the chest or midback and produce heartburn or deep epigastric pain. Although these patterns strongly mimic cardiac pain, myofascial TrP pain shows a much wider variation in its response to daily activity than does angina pectoris to activity.[40]

In addition to mimicking pain of a cardiac nature, TrPs can occur in response to cardiac disorders. A visceral-somatic response can occur when biochemical changes associated with visceral disease affect somatic structures innervated by the same spinal nerves. In such cases, the individual has a past history of visceral disease. TrPs accompanied by symptoms such as vertigo, headache, visual changes, nausea, and syncope are yellow flags warning of autonomic involvement not usually present with TrPs strictly from a somatic origin.

Chest pain that persists long after an acute myocardial infarction may be due to myofascial TrPs. In acute myocardial infarction, pain is commonly referred from the heart to the midregion of the pectoralis major and minor muscles (see discussion of viscerosomatic sources of pain, Chapter 3). The injury to the heart muscle initiates a viscerosomatic process that activates TrPs in the pectoral muscles.[40]

After recovery from the infarction, these self-perpetuating TrPs tend to persist in the chest wall. As with all myofascial syndromes, inactivation of the TrPs eliminates the client's symptoms of chest pain. If the client's symptoms are eliminated with TrP release, medical referral may not be required. However, communication with the physician is essential; the therapist is advised to document all findings and report them to the client's primary care physician.

Past Medical History

There may be a history of upper respiratory infection with repeated forceful coughing. There is often a history of immobility (e.g., cast immobilization after fracture or injury). The therapist should also ask about muscle strain from lifting weights overhead, from pushups, and from prolonged, vigorous activity that requires forceful abdominal breathing, such as severe coughing, running a marathon, or repetitive bending and lifting.

Clinical Presentation

TrPs are reproduced with palpation or resisted motions. On examination, the physical therapist should palpate for tender points and taut bands of muscle tissue, squeeze the involved muscle, observe for increased pain with palpation, test for increased pain with resisted motion, and correlate symptoms with respiratory movements.

Chest pain from serratus anterior TrPs may occur at rest in severe cases. Clients with this

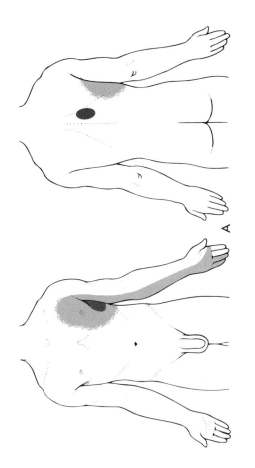

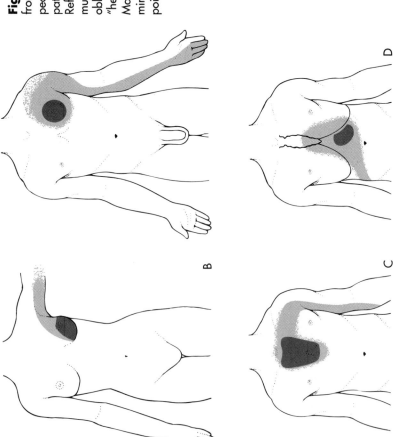

Fig. 17-7 • A, Referred pain pattern from the left serratus anterior muscle. **B,** Left pectoralis major muscle: referred pain pattern in a woman and a man. **C,** Referred pain pattern from the left sternalis muscle. **D,** Referred pain from the external oblique abdominal muscle can cause "heartburn" in the anterior chest wall. Marathon runners may report chest pain mimicking a heart attack from this trigger point.

myofascial syndrome may report that they are "short of breath" or that they are in pain when they take a deep breath. *Serratus anterior* TrPs on the left side of the chest can contribute to the pain associated with myocardial infarction. This pain is rarely aggravated by the usual tests for range of motion at the shoulder but may result from a strong effort to protract the scapula. Palpation reveals tender points that increase symptoms, and there is usually a palpable taut band present within the involved muscles.

One of the most extensive patterns of pain from irritable TrPs is the complex pattern from the *anterior scalene* muscle. This may produce ipsilateral sternal pain, anterior chest wall pain, breast pain, or pain along the vertebral border of the scapula, shoulder, and arm, radiating to the thumb and index finger.

Breast pain may be differentiated from the aching pain arising from the scalene or pectoral muscles by a history of upper extremity overuse usually associated with myalgia. Resistance to

isometric movement of the upper extremities reproduces the symptoms of a myalgia but does not usually aggravate pain associated with breast tissue. Additionally, palpation of the underlying muscle reproduces the painful symptoms.

When active TrPs occur in the left *pectoralis major* muscle, the referred pain (anterior chest to the precordium and down the inner aspect of the arm) is easily confused with that of coronary insufficiency. Pacemakers placed superficially can cause pectoral trigger points. In the case of pacemaker-induced TrPs, the physical therapist can teach the client TrP self-treatment to carry out at home.

Myalgia

Myalgia, or muscular pain, can cause chest pain separate from TrP pain but with a similar etiologic basis of prolonged or repeated movement. As mentioned earlier, the physical therapy interview must include questions about recent upper respiratory infection with repeated forceful coughing and recent activities of a repetitive nature that could cause sore muscles (e.g., painting or washing walls; calisthenics, including push-ups; or lifting heavy objects or weights).

Three tests must be used to confirm or rule out muscle as the source of symptoms: (1) palpation, (2) stretch, and (3) contraction. If the muscle is not sore or tender on palpation, stretch, or contraction, the source of the problem most likely lies somewhere else.

With true myalgia, squeezing the muscle belly will reproduce painful chest symptoms. The discomfort of myalgia is almost always described as aching and may range from mild to intense. Diaphragmatic irritation may be referred to the ipsilateral neck and shoulder, lower thorax, lumbar region, or upper abdomen as a muscular aching pain. Myalgia in the respiratory muscles is well localized, reproducible by palpation, and exacerbated by movement of the chest wall.

Rib Fractures

Periosteal (bone) pain associated with fractured ribs can cause sharp, localized pain at the level of the fracture with an increase in symptoms associated with trunk motions and respiratory movements, such as deep inspiration, laughing, sneezing, or coughing. The pain may be accompanied by a grating sensation during breathing. This localized pain pattern differs from bone pain associated with chronic disease affecting bone marrow and endosteum, which may result in poorly localized pain of varying degrees of severity.

Occult (hidden) rib fractures may occur, especially in a client with a chronic cough or someone who has had an explosive sneeze. Fractures may occur as a result of trauma (e.g., motor vehicle accident, assault), but painful symptoms may not be perceived at first if other injuries are more significant.

A history of long-term steroid use in the presence of rib pain of unknown cause should raise a red flag. Rib fractures must be confirmed by x-ray diagnosis. Rib pain without fracture may indicate bone tumor or disease affecting bone, such as multiple myeloma.

Cervical Spine Disorders

Cervicodorsal arthritis may produce chest pain that is seldom similar to that of angina pectoris. It is usually sharp and piercing but may be described as a deep, boring, dull discomfort. There is usually unilateral or bilateral chest pain with flexion or hyperextension of the upper spine or neck. The chest pain may radiate to the shoulder girdle and down the arms and is not related to exertion or exercise. Rest may not alleviate the symptoms, and prolonged recumbency makes the pain worse.

Discogenic disease can also cause referred pain to the chest, but there is usually evidence of disc involvement observed with diagnostic imaging and the presence of neurologic symptoms.

SCREENING FOR NEUROMUSCULAR OR NEUROLOGIC CAUSES OF CHEST, BREAST, OR RIB PAIN

There are several possible neurologic disorders that can cause chest and/or breast pain, including nerve root impingement or inflammation, herpes zoster (shingles), thoracic disc disease, postoperative neuralgia, and thoracic outlet syndrome (TOS; see Table 17-1).

Neurologic disorders such as intercostal neuritis and dorsal nerve root radiculitis or a neurovascular disorder such as thoracic outlet syndrome also can cause chest pain. The two most commonly recognized noncardiac causes of chest pain seen in the physical therapy clinic are herpes zoster (shingles) and TOS.

Intercostal Neuritis

Intercostal neuritis, such as herpes zoster or shingles produced by a viral infection of a dorsal nerve root, can cause neuritic chest wall pain, which can be differentiated from coronary pain.

Risk Factors

Shingles may occur or recur at any age, but there has been a recent increase in the number of cases in two distinct age groups: college-aged young adults and older adults (over 70 years). Health care experts suggest that stress is the key factor in the first group, and immune system failure is the key factor in the second group.

Anyone who is immunocompromised as a result of advancing age, underlying malignancy, organ transplantation, or AIDS is at risk for shingles. There is an increased incidence of herpes zoster in clients with lymphoma, tuberculosis, and leukemia, but it can be triggered by trauma or injection drugs or occur with no known cause.

Anyone in good health who had the chickenpox as a child is not at great risk for shingles. The risk of developing shingles increases for anyone who is immunocompromised for any reason or who has never had the chicken pox.

Herpes zoster is a communicable disease and requires some type of isolation. Anyone in contact with the client before the outbreak of the skin lesions has already been exposed. Specific precautions depend on whether the disease is localized or disseminated and the condition of the client. Persons susceptible to chickenpox should avoid contact with the affected client and stay out of the client's room.

Clinical Presentation

Herpes zoster is characterized by raised fluid-filled clusters of grouped vesicles that appear unilaterally along cranial or spinal nerve dermatomes 3 to 5 days after transmission of the virus (see Figs. 4-21 and 4-22). The affected individual experiences 1 to 2 days of pain, itching, and hyperesthesia before the outbreak of skin lesions.

The skin changes are referred to as "shingles" and are easily recognizable as they follow a dermatome anywhere on the body. The lesions do not cross the body midline as they follow nerve pathways, although nerves of both sides may be involved. The skin eruptions evolve into crusts on the skin and clear in about 2 weeks, unless the period between the pain and the eruption is longer than 2 days. Postherpetic neuralgia, with its burning and paroxysmal stabbing pain, may persist for long periods.

Neuritic pain occurs unrelated to effort and lasts longer (weeks, months, or years) than angina. The pain may be constant or intermittent and can vary from light burning to a deep visceral sensation. It may be associated with chills, fever, headache, and malaise. Symptoms are confined to the somatic distribution of the involved spinal nerve(s).

Clinical Signs and Symptoms of
Herpes Zoster (Shingles)

- Fever, chills
- Headache and malaise
- 1 to 2 days of pain, itching, and hyperesthesia before skin lesions develop
- Skin eruptions (vesicles) that appear along dermatomes 4 or 5 days after the other symptoms

Dorsal Nerve Root Irritation

Dorsal nerve root irritation of the thoracic spine is another neuritic condition that can refer pain to the chest wall. This condition can be caused by infectious processes (e.g., radiculitis or inflammation of the spinal nerve root dural sheath; shingles can also fit in this category). However, the pain is more likely to be the result of mechanical irritation caused by spinal disease or deformity (e.g., bone spurs secondary to osteoarthritis or the presence of cervical ribs placing pressure on the brachial plexus).

The pain of dorsal nerve root irritation can appear as lateral or anterior chest wall pain with referral to one or both arms through the brachial plexus. Although it mimics the pain pattern of coronary heart disease, such pain is more superficial than cardiac pain. Like cardiac pain, dorsal nerve root irritation can be aggravated by exertion of only the upper extremities. However, unlike cardiac pain, exertion of the lower extremities has no exacerbating effect. It is usually accompanied by other neurologic signs, such as muscle atrophy and numbness or tingling.

Clinical Signs and Symptoms of
Dorsal Nerve Root Irritation

- Lateral or anterior chest wall pain
- History of back pain
- Pain that is aggravated by exertion of only the upper body
- May be accompanied by neurologic signs
  - Numbness
  - Tingling
  - Muscle atrophy

Thoracic Outlet Syndrome

Thoracic outlet syndrome (TOS) refers to compression of the neural and/or vascular structures that leave or pass over the superior rim of the thoracic cage (see Fig. 17-10). Various names have been

given to this condition according to the presumed site of major neurovascular compression: first thoracic rib, cervical rib, scalenus anticus, costoclavicular, and hyperabduction syndromes.

Past Medical History

History of associated back pain may be the only significant past medical history. The presence of anatomic anomalies such as an extra rib or unusual sternoclavicular and/or acromioclavicular angle may be the only known history linked to the development of TOS.

Risk Factors

Symptoms may be related to occupational activities (e.g., carrying heavy loads, working with arms overhead), poor posture, sleeping with arms elevated over the head, or acute injuries such as cervical flexion/extension (whiplash). Athletes such as swimmers, volleyball players, tennis players, and baseball pitchers are also at increased risk for compression of the neurovascular structures. Most people become symptomatic in the third or fourth decade, and women (especially during pregnancy) are affected three times more often than are men.

Clinical Presentation

Chest/breast pain can occur (and may be the only symptom of TOS) as a result of cervical spine disorders, an underlying etiology in TOS. This is because spinal nerves originating as high as C34 can extend down as low as the nipple line.

The compressive forces associated with this problem usually affect the upper extremities in the ulnar nerve distribution but can result in episodic chest pain mimicking coronary heart disease. Neu-

rogenic pain associated with TOS may be described as stabbing, cutting, burning, or electric. The pain is often unrelated to effort and lasts hours to days.

There may be radiating pain to the neck, shoulder, scapula, or axilla, but usually the superficial nature of the pain and associated changes in sensation and neurologic findings point to chest pain with an underlying neurologic cause (Table 17-5). Paresthesias (burning, pricking sensation) and hypoesthesia (abnormal decrease in sensitivity to stimulation) are common. Anesthesia and motor weakness are reported in about 10% of the cases.

When a vascular compressive component is involved, there may be more diffuse pain in the limb, with associated fatigue and weakness. With more severe arterial compromise, the client may describe coolness, pallor, cyanosis, or symptoms of Raynaud's phenomenon. Although vascular in origin, these symptoms are differentiated from CAD by the local or regional presentation, affecting only a single extremity or only the upper extremities.

Palpation of the supraclavicular space may elicit tenderness or may define a prominence indicative of a cervical rib. The effect on pulse of the Adson or Halstead maneuvers (Fig. 17-8), the hyperabduction or Wright test (Fig. 17-9), and the costoclavicular test (exaggerated military attention posture) should be compared in both arms.

Despite the widespread use of these tests, the reliability remains unknown. Specificity reported ranges from 18% to 87%, but sensitivity has been documented at 94%.[45] During assessment for vascular origin of symptoms, a change in pulse rate or rhythm is a positive test; however, because more than 50% of normal, asymptomatic individuals

TABLE 17-5 ▼ Assessing Symptoms of Thoracic Outlet Syndrome*

Vascular component	Neural	
	Upper plexus	Lower plexus
3-minute elevated test	Point tenderness of C5-C6	Pressure above clavicle elicits pain.
Adson's test	Pressure over lateral neck elicits pain and/or numbness.	Ulnar nerve tenderness when palpated under axilla or along inner arm
Swelling (arm/hand)	Pain with head turned and/or tilted to opposite side	Tinel's sign for ulnar nerve in axilla
Discoloration of hand	Weak biceps	Hypoesthesia in ulnar nerve distribution
Costoclavicular test	Weak triceps	Serratus anterior weakness
Hyperabduction test	Weak wrist	Weak hand grip
Upper extremity claudication	Hypoesthesia in radial nerve distribution	
Differences in blood pressure	3-minute abduction stress test	
Skin temperature changes		
Cold intolerance		

* With the use of special tests, patterns of positive objective findings may help characterize thoracic outlet syndrome.

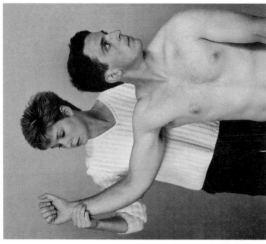

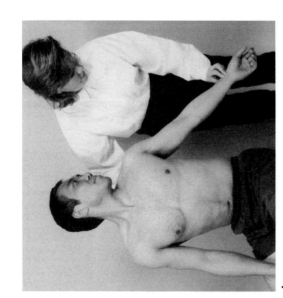

A

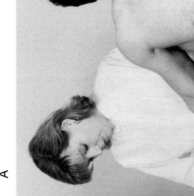

B

Fig. 17-8 • Adson maneuver. The client begins in the sitting position with arms at his or her sides and face forward. The examiner takes a baseline, resting radial pulse rate for 1 minute. **A,** The client then turns his or her head toward the test arm. The head and neck are extended slightly while the examiner laterally rotates and extends the shoulder. The client is asked to take a deep breath and hold it. Reproduction of the symptoms is the best indication of TOS, but a disappearance of the pulse is considered a positive test. **B,** Halstead maneuver. Baseline radial pulse is obtained before the client hyperextends and rotates his head to the opposite side. The examiner applies a downward, traction force on the involved side. Once again, the test is considered positive for a vascular component of a TOS when there is an change in pulse rate or rhythm. (From Magee D: *Orthopedic physical assessment,* ed 4, Philadelphia, 2002, Saunders.)

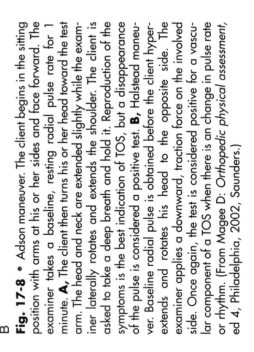

Fig. 17-9 • Modified Wright test, also known as the Allen test or maneuver. The hyperabduction test can help screen for vascular compromise in TOS. Start with the client's arm resting at his or her side. Take the client's resting radial pulse for a full minute. Make note of any irregular or skipped beats. Raise the client's arm as shown with the client's face turned away, and recheck the pulse. This test is used to detect compression in the costoclavicular space. Diminished or thready pulse or absence of the pulse is a positive sign for (vascular) TOS. In the standard test, the examiner waits up to 3 minutes before palpating to give time for an accurate assessment. In our experience, clients with a positive hyperabduction test almost always demonstrate early changes in symptoms, skin color, and skin temperature. Having the client take a breath and hold it may have an additional effect. Tests for other aspects of neurologic or vascular compromise are available.[45,47] (From Magee D: *Orthopedic physical assessment,* ed 4, Philadelphia, 2002, Saunders.)

have pulse rate changes, it is better to reproduce the client's symptoms as a true indicator of TOS.[45,46]

Other tests are described in orthopedic assessment texts.[45,47] With the use of special tests, patterns of positive objective findings may help characterize TOS as vascular, neural, or a combination of both (neurovascular). Knowing what the tests are and how they function is very helpful in guiding intervention. For example, Fig. 17-10 gives a visual representation of the effect of the hyperabduction test. A positive hyperabduction test may point to the need to restore normal function and movement of the pectoralis minor muscle. Likewise, if there is a neural component, assess for location (upper plexus versus lower plexus). Table 17-5 will help guide the therapist.

TOS should be considered when persistent chest pain occurs in the presence of a normal coronary angiogram and normal esophageal function tests.

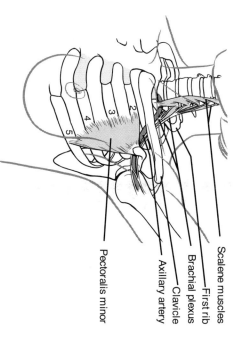

Scalene muscles
First rib
Brachial plexus
Clavicle
Axillary artery

Pectoralis minor

Fig. 17-10 • The neurovascular bundle associated with TOS can become compressed by nearby soft tissue structures such as the pectoralis minor. This illustration shows why the hyperabduction test can alter the client's pulse or reproduce symptoms. Effecting a change in the pectoralis minor may result in a change in the client's symptoms and can be measured by a return of the normal pulse rate and rhythm in the hyperabducted position.

Clinical Signs and Symptoms of Thoracic Outlet Syndrome

Vascular

- Swelling, sometimes described as "puffiness," of the supraclavicular fossa, axilla, arm and/or hand
- Cyanotic (blue or white) appearance of the hand; especially notable when the arm is elevated over head; sometimes referred to as the white hand sign
- Subjective report of "heaviness" in arm or hand
- Chest, neck, and/or arm pain described as "throbbing" or deep aching
- Upper extremity fatigue and weakness
- Difference in blood pressure from side to side (more than 10-mm Hg difference in diastolic)

Neurologic

- Numbness and/or tingling, usually ulnar nerve distribution
- Atrophy of the hand; difficulty with fine motor skills
- Pain in the upper extremity (proximal to distal); described as stabbing, cutting, burning, or electric
- Numbness and tingling down the inner aspect of the arm (ulnar nerve distribution)

A vascular component to TOS may present with significant differences in blood pressure from side to side (a change of 10mm Hg or more in diastolic is most likely). This does not mean that a medical referral is required immediately. Assess client age, past medical history, and presence of comorbidities (e.g., known hypertension), and ask about any associated signs and symptoms that might point to heart disease as a cause of the underlying symptoms.

Physical therapy intervention can bring about a change in the soft tissue structures, putting pressure on the blood vessels in this area. In fact, blood pressure can be used as an outcome measure to document the effectiveness of the intervention. If blood pressure does not normalize and equalize from side to side, then medical referral may be required.

If there is a cluster of cardiac symptoms, especially in the presence of a significant history of hypertension or heart disease, medical referral may be required before initiating treatment. If the Review of Systems does not provide cause for concern, documentation and communication with the physician are still important while initiating a plan of care.

PHYSICIAN REFERRAL

Postoperative Pain

Postoperative chest pain following cardiac transplantation or other open heart procedures is usually due to the sternal incision and musculoskeletal manipulation during surgery. Coronary insufficiency does not appear as chest pain because of cardiac denervation.

Never dismiss chest pain as insignificant. Chest pain that falls into any of the categories in Table 6-5 requires medical evaluation. This table offers some helpful clues in matching client's clinical presentation with the need for medical referral.

It may be impossible for a physician to differentiate anxiety from myocardial ischemia without further testing; such a differentiation is outside the scope of a physical therapist's practice. The therapist must confine himself or herself to a medical screening process before conducting a differential diagnosis of movement system impairments.

The therapist is not making the differential diagnosis between angina, MI, mitral valve prolapse, or pericarditis. The therapist is screening for systemic or viscerogenic causes of chest, breast, shoulder or arm, jaw, or neck or upper back symptoms.

Knowing the chest and breast pain patterns and associated signs and symptoms of conditions that masquerade as NMS dysfunction will help the therapist recognize a condition requiring medical attention. Likewise, quickly recognizing red flag signs and symptoms is important in providing early medical referral and intervention, preferably with improved outcomes for the client.

Guidelines for Immediate Medical Attention

- Sudden onset of acute chest pain with sudden dyspnea could be a life-threatening condition (e.g., pulmonary embolism, myocardial infarction, ruptured abdominal aneurysm), especially in the presence of red flag risk factors, personal medical history, and vital signs.

- A sudden change in the client's typical anginal pain pattern suggests unstable angina. For the client with known angina, pain that occurs without exertion, lasts longer than 10 minutes, or is not relieved by rest or nitroglycerin signals a higher risk for a heart attack.

- The woman with chest, breast, axillary, or shoulder pain of unknown origin at presentation must be questioned regarding breast self-examinations. Any recently discovered breast lumps or nodules or lymph node changes must be examined by a physician.

Guidelines for Physician Referral

- No change is noted in uneven blood pressure from one arm to the other after intervention for a vascular TOS component.

- The therapist who suspects a client may be using anabolic steroids should report findings to the physician or coach if one is involved.

- Symptoms are unrelieved or unchanged by physical therapy intervention.

- Medical referral is advised before initiating treatment for anyone with a past history of cancer presenting with symptoms of unknown cause, especially without an identifiable movement system impairment.

Clues to Screening Chest, Breast, or Rib Pain

Past Medical History

- History of repetitive motion; overuse; prolonged activity (e.g., marathon); long-term use of steroids, assault, or other trauma

- History of flu, trauma, upper respiratory infection, shingles (herpes zoster), recurrent pneumonia, chronic bronchitis, or emphysema

- History of breast cancer or any other cancer; history of chemotherapy or radiation therapy

- History of heart disease, hypertension, previous myocardial infarction, heart transplantation, bypass surgery, or any other procedure affecting the chest/thorax (including breast reconstruction, implantation, or reduction)

- Prolonged use of cocaine or anabolic steroids

- Nocturnal pain, pain without precise movement aggravation, or pain that fails to respond to treatment

- Weight loss in the presence of immobility when weight gain would otherwise be expected

- Recent childbirth and/or lactation (breast feeding) (**pectoral myalgia, mastitis**)

Risk Factors (see also Table 6-3)

- Age
- Tobacco use
- Obesity
- Sedentary lifestyle, prolonged immobilization

Clinical Presentation

- Range of motion (e.g., trunk rotation of side bending, shoulder motions) does not reproduce symptoms; resisted motion (e.g., horizontal shoulder abduction or adduction) does not reproduce symptoms; heat and stretching do not reduce or eliminate the symptoms; pain or symptoms are not altered or eliminated with TrP therapy or other physical therapy intervention.

- There is a lack of musculoskeletal objective findings; squeezing the underlying pectoral muscles does not reproduce symptoms (exception: intercostal tear caused by forceful coughing associated with diaphragmatic pleurisy).

- Chest pain relieved by antacid (**reflux esophagitis**), rest from exertion or taking nitroglycerin (**angina**), recumbency (**mitral valve prolapse**), squatting (**hypertrophic cardiomyopathy**), passing gas (**gas entrapment syndrome**)

- Presence of painless sternal or chest wall mass or painless, hard lymph nodes

- Unusual vital signs; changes in breathing

CARDIOVASCULAR

- Timing of symptoms in relation to physical or sexual activity (immediate, 5 to 10 minutes after engaging in activity, after activity ends (**lag time is associated with angina; symptoms occurring immediately or after an activity may be a sign of TOS, asthma, myalgias, or TrPs**)

- Assess the effect of exertion; reproduction of chest, shoulder, or neck symptoms with exertion of only the lower extremities may be cardiovascular.
- Chest, neck, or shoulder pain that is aggravated by physical exertion, exposure to temperature changes, strong emotional reactions, or a large meal (coronary artery disease)
- Atypical chest pain associated with dyspnea, arrhythmias, and light-headedness or syncope
- Other signs and symptoms such as pallor, unexplained profuse perspiration, inability to talk, nausea, vomiting, sense of impending doom, or extreme anxiety
- Symptoms can be precipitated by working with arms overhead; the client becomes weak or short of breath 3 to 5 minutes after raising the arms above the heart.

PLEUROPULMONARY (see also Clues to Screening in Chapter 7)

- Autosplinting (lying on the involved side) quiets chest wall movements and reduces or eliminates chest or rib pain; symptoms are worse with recumbency (supine position).
- Pain is not reproduced by palpation.
- Assess for the three *p*s: pleural pain, palpation, position (**pleuritic** pain exacerbated by respiratory movements, pain on **palpation** associated with musculoskeletal condition, pain with changes in neck, trunk, or shoulder **position** indicating musculoskeletal origin).
- Musculoskeletal: Symptoms do not increase with pulmonary movements (unless there is an intercostal tear or rib dysfunction associated with forceful coughing from a concomitant pulmonary problem) but can be reproduced with palpation.
- Pleuropulmonary: Symptoms increase with pulmonary movements and cannot be reproduced with palpation (unless there is an intercostal tear or rib dysfunction associated with forceful coughing).
- Increased symptoms occur with recumbency (abdominal contents push up against diaphragm and in turn push against the parietal pleura).
- Increased chest pain with exercise or increased movement can also be a sign of asthma; ask about a personal or family history of asthma or allergies.
- Presence of associated signs and symptoms such as persistent cough, dyspnea (rest or exertional), or constitutional symptoms
- Chest pain with sudden drop in blood pressure or symptoms such as dizziness, dyspnea, vomiting, or unexplained sweating while standing or ambulating for the first time after surgery, an invasive medical procedure, assault, or accident involving the chest or thorax (**pneumothorax**)

GASTROINTESTINAL (Upper GI/Epigastric; see also Clues to Screening in Chapter 8)

- Effect of food on symptoms (better or worse); presence of GI symptoms, simultaneously or alternately with somatic symptoms
- Pain on swallowing
- Symptoms are relieved by antacids, food, passing gas, or assuming the upright position.
- Supine position aggravates symptoms (**upper GI problem**); symptoms are relieved by assuming an upright position.
- Symptoms radiate from the chest posteriorly to the upper back, interscapular, subscapular, or T10 to L2 areas.
- Symptoms are not reproduced or aggravated by effort or exertion.
- Presence of associated signs and symptoms such as nausea, vomiting, dark urine, jaundice, flatulence, indigestion, abdominal fullness or bloating; blood in stool, pain on swallowing

BREAST (Alone or In Combination with Chest, Neck, or Shoulder Symptoms)

- Appearance (or report) of lump, nodule, discharge, skin puckering, or distended veins
- Jarring or movement of the breast tissue increases or reproduces the pain.
- Pain is palpable within the breast tissue.
- Assess for TrPs (sternalis, serratus anterior, pectoralis major; see Fig. 17-7); breast pain in the absence of TrPs or failure to respond to TrP therapy must be investigated further.
- Resisted isometric shoulder horizontal adduction or abduction does *not* reproduce breast pain.
- Breast pain is reproduced by exertion of the lower extremities (**cardiac**).
- Association between painful symptoms and menstrual cycle (**ovulation or menses**)
- Presence of aberrant or suspicious axillary or supraclavicular lymph nodes (e.g., large, firm, hard, or fixed)
- Skin dimpling especially with adherence of underlying tissue; ask about or visually inspect for:
  - Lump or nodule
  - Red, warm, edematous, firm, and painful area over or under skin
  - Changes in size or shape or color of either breast or surrounding area
  - Unusual rash or other skin changes (e.g., puckering, dimpling, peau d'orange)

- Distended veins
- Unusual sensations in nipple or breast
- Unusual nipple ulceration or discharge

ANXIETY (see Table 3-9)

- Pain Pattern:
  - Sharp, stabbing pain: left breast region
  - Dull aching: substernal
  - Discomfort: upper chest, neck, left arm
  - Fingertip size; does not radiate
  - Unable to palpate locally
  - Lasts seconds to hours to days
  - Not aggravated by respiratory or other (shoulder, arm, back) movements
  - Unchanged by rest or change in position
  - Unrelated to effort or exertion
- Associated Signs and Symptoms
  - Local hyperesthesia of chest wall
  - Choking sensation (hysteria/panic)
  - Claustrophobia
  - Sense of persistent weakness
  - Unpleasant awareness of heartbeat
  - Hyperventilation (can also occur with heart attack; watch for sighing respirations and numbness/tingling of face and fingertips)

NEUROMUSCULOSKELETAL

- Symptoms described using words typical of NMS origin (e.g., aching, burning, hot, scalding, searing, cutting, electric shock)
- Pain is superficial compared with pain of a cardiac or pleuropulmonary origin.
- Symptoms are confined to somatic or spinal nerve root distribution.

- History of associated back pain
- Positive hyperabduction test or other tests for TOS
- Presence of TrPs; elimination of TrP(s) reduces or eliminates symptoms (see Table 17-4 and Fig. 17-7)
- Symptoms are elicited easily by palpation (e.g., squeezing the pectoral muscle belly, palpating the chest wall, intercostal spaces, or costochondral junction).
- Symptoms are reproduced by resisted horizontal shoulder abduction, adduction, or other shoulder movements.
- Symptoms are relieved by heat and stretching.
- Soft tissues (tendon and muscle) take longer than the expected time to heal (**anabolic steroids**).
- Costochondritis or Tietze's syndrome may be accompanied by an increase in blood pressure but is usually palpable and aggravated by trunk movements.
- Presence of neurologic involvement (e.g., numbness, tingling, muscle atrophy); consider age and history of trauma or injury (**degenerative disc disease**)
- Pain referred along peripheral nerve pathway (dorsal nerve root irritation)
- Pain is unrelated to effort and lasts hours or weeks to months.
- Associated signs and symptoms: numbness and tingling, muscle atrophy (**neurologic**); rash, fever, chills, headache, malaise (**constitutional symptoms; neuritis or shingles**)

OVERVIEW   REFERRED CHEST, BREAST, RIB PAIN PATTERNS

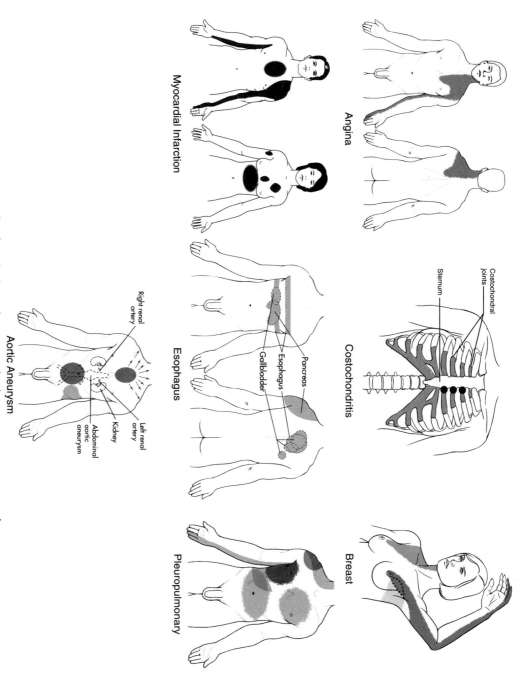

Angina

Myocardial Infarction

Costochondritis

Costochondral joints

Sternum

Esophagus

Pancreas

Esophagus

Gallbladder

Breast

Pleuropulmonary

Aortic Aneurysm

Right renal artery

Left renal artery

Kidney

Abdominal aortic aneurysm

Fig. 17-11 • Composite picture of referred chest, breast, and rib pain patterns. Not shown: trigger point patterns (see Fig. 17-7).

⚡ KEY POINTS TO REMEMBER

✓ When faced with chest pain, the therapist must know how to assess the situation quickly and decide if medical referral is required and whether medical attention is needed immediately. Therapists must be able to differentiate neuromusculoskeletal from systemic origins of symptoms.

✓ Although the past medical history (PMH) is important, it cannot be relied upon to confirm or rule out medical causes of chest pain. PMH does alert the therapist to an increased risk of systemic conditions that can masquerade as neuromusculoskeletal disorders.

✓ Likewise, chest pain history by itself is not enough to rule out cardiac or other systemic origin of symptoms; in most cases, some diagnostic testing is needed. The physical therapist can offer valuable information from the screening process to aid in the medical differential diagnosis.

✓ Chest pain associated with increased activity is a red flag for possible cardiovascular involvement. The physical therapist can assess when chest pain may be caused by musculoskeletal dysfunction (immediate chest pain occurs with use) or by possible vascular compromise (chest pain occurs 5 to 10 minutes after activity begins).

✓ Anyone with a history of stent insertion presenting with chest pain should be screened carefully. The stent can get scarred over and/or malfunction. Stents are effective at alleviating chest pain but do not reduce the risk of heart attacks for most people with stable angina.

✓ Cardiac pain patterns may differ for men and women; the therapist should be familiar with known pain patterns for both genders.

✓ Trigger points can cause chest, breast, or rib pain, even mimicking cardiac pain patterns; a visceral-somatic response can also occur following a myocardial infarction, causing persisting symptoms of myocardial ischemia (angina); releasing the trigger point relieves the symptoms.

✓ The therapist must especially know how and what to look for to screen for cancer, cancer recurrence, and/or the delayed effects of cancer treatment. Cancer can present

as primary chest pain with or without accompanying neck, shoulder, and/or upper back pain/symptoms.

✓ When a woman with a PMH of cancer develops neck, back, upper trapezius or shoulder pain, or other symptoms, examining the site of the original cancer removal is a good idea.

✓ The American Cancer Society (ACS) and the National Cancer Institute (NCI) support breast cancer screening by qualified health care specialists. With adequate training, the physical therapist can incorporate clinical breast examination (CBE) as a screening tool in the upper quarter examination for appropriate clients (e.g., individuals with neck, shoulder, upper back, chest, and/or breast signs or symptoms of unknown cause or insidious onset).[2]

✓ A physical therapist conducting a CBE could miss a lump (false negative), but this will most certainly happen if the therapist does not conduct a CBE at all to assess skin integrity and surrounding soft tissues of the breast or axilla.[2]

✓ The physical therapist does not diagnose any kind of cancer, including breast cancer; only the pathologist diagnoses cancer. The therapist can identify aberrant soft tissue and refer the client for further evaluation. Early detection and intervention can reduce morbidity and mortality.

✓ Thoracic disc disease can also present as unilateral chest pain and requires careful screening.

✓ Chest pain of unknown cause in the adolescent or young adult athlete may be the result of anabolic steroid use. Watch for injuries that take longer than expected to heal, personality changes, and any of the physical signs listed in the text.

✓ A history of long-term steroid use in the presence of rib pain of unknown cause raises a red flag for rib fracture.

✓ Many people with chest pain have used cocaine within the last week but deny its use; the therapist should not neglect asking clients of all ages about their use of substances.

SUBJECTIVE EXAMINATION

Special Questions to Ask: Chest/Thorax

Musculoskeletal

• Have you strained a muscle from (repeated, forceful) coughing?

• Have you ever injured your chest?

• Does it hurt to touch your chest or to take a deep breath (e.g., coughing, sneezing, sighing, or laughing)? **(Myalgia, fractured rib, costochondritis, myofascial trigger point)**

• Do you have frequent attacks of heartburn, or do you take antacids to relieve heartburn or acid indigestion? **(Noncardiac cause of chest pain, abdominal muscle trigger point, gastrointestinal disorder)**

• Does chest movement or body/arm position make the pain better or worse?

Neurologic

• Do you have any trouble taking a deep breath? **(Weak chest muscles secondary to polymyositis, dermatomyositis, myasthenia gravis)**

• Does your chest pain ever travel into your armpit, arm, neck, or wing bone (scapula)? **(Thoracic outlet syndrome, trigger points)**

—If yes, do you ever feel burning, prickling, numbness, or any other unusual sensation in any of these areas?

Pulmonary

• Have you ever been treated for a lung problem?

—If yes, describe what this problem was, when it occurred, and how it was treated.

• Do you think your chest or thoracic pain is caused by a lung problem?

• Have you ever had trouble with breathing?

• Are you having difficulty with breathing now?

• Do you ever have shortness of breath, breathlessness, or can't quite catch your breath?

—If yes, does this happen when you rest, lie flat, walk on level ground, walk up stairs, or when you are under stress or tension?

—How long does it last?

—What do you do to get your breathing back to normal?

• How far can you walk before you feel breathless?

• What symptom stops your walking (e.g., shortness of breath, heart pounding, or weak legs)?

• Do you have any breathing aids (e.g., oxygen, nebulizer, humidifier, or ventilation devices)?

• Do you have a cough? (Note whether the person smokes, for how long, and how much.) Do you have a smoker's hack?

—If yes to having a cough, distinguish it from a smoker's cough. Ask when it started.

—Does coughing increase or bring on your symptoms?

—Do you cough anything up? If yes, please describe the color, amount, and frequency.

—Are you taking anything for this cough? If yes, does it seem to help?

• Do you have periods when you can't seem to stop coughing?

• Do you ever cough up blood?

—If yes, what color is it? (Bright red: fresh; brown or black: older)

• Have you ever had a blood clot in your lungs? If yes, has this been treated?

—If yes, when and how was it treated?

• Have you had a chest x-ray film taken during the last 5 years? If yes, when and where did it occur? What were the results?

• Do you work around asbestos, coal, dust, chemicals, or fumes? If yes, describe.

—Do you wear a mask at work? If yes, approximately how much of the time do you wear a mask?

• If the person is a farmer, ask what kind of farming (because some agricultural products may cause respiratory irritation).

• Have you ever had tuberculosis or a positive skin test for tuberculosis?

—If yes, when did it occur and how was it treated? What is your current status?

• When was your last test for tuberculosis? Was the result normal?

Cardiac

• Has a physician ever told you that you have heart trouble?

• Have you recently (or ever) had a heart attack? If yes, when? Describe.

—If yes, to either question: Do you think your current symptoms are related to your heart problems?

—Do you have angina (pectoris)?

—If yes, describe the symptoms, and tell me when it occurs.

—If no, pursue further with the following questions.

• Do you ever have discomfort or tightness in your chest? **(Angina)**

• Have you ever had a crushing sensation in your chest with or without pain down your left arm?

SUBJECTIVE EXAMINATION—cont'd

- Do you have pain in your jaw, either alone or in combination with chest pain?
- If you climb a few flights of stairs fairly rapidly, do you have tightness or pressing pain in your chest?
- Do you get pressure or pain or tightness in the chest if you walk in the cold wind or face a cold blast of air?
- Have you ever had pain or pressure or a squeezing feeling in the chest that occurred during exercise, walking, or any other physical or sexual activity?
- Do you ever have bouts of rapid heart action, irregular heartbeats, or palpitations of your heart?
  —*If yes*, did this occur after a visit to the dentist? **(Endocarditis)**
- Have you noticed any skin rash or dots under the skin on your chest in the last 3 weeks? **(Rheumatic fever, endocarditis)**
- Have you noticed any other symptoms (e.g., shortness of breath, sudden and unexplained perspiration, nausea, vomiting, dizziness or fainting)?
- Have you used cocaine, crack, or any other recreational drug in the last 6 weeks?
- Does your pain wake you up at night? (Therapist: distinguish between awakening *from* pain and awakening *with* pain; awakening from pain is more likely with **cardiac ischemia,** whereas awakening with pain is characteristic of sleep disturbances and more common with **psychogenic or stress-induced** chest pain; this information will help in deciding whether referral is needed immediately or at the next follow-up appointment)

Epigastric

- Have you ever been told that you have an ulcer?
- Does the pain under your breast bone radiate (travel) around to your back, or do you ever have back pain at the same time that your chest hurts?
- Have you ever had heartburn or acid indigestion?
  —*If yes*, how is this pain different?
  —*If no*, have you noticed any association between when you eat and when this pain starts?

Special Questions to Ask: Breast

- Have you ever had any breast surgery (implants, lumpectomy, mastectomy, reconstructive surgery, or augmentation)?
  If yes, has there been any change in the incision line, nipple, or breast tissue?
  May I look at the incision during my exam?
- Do you have a history of cystic or lumpy breasts?
  If yes, do the lumps come and go or change with your periods?
- Is there a family history of breast disease? *If yes*, ask about type of disease, age of onset, treatment, and outcome.
- Have you ever had a mammogram or ultrasound?
  If yes, when was your last test? What were the results?
- Have you ever had a lump or cyst drained or biopsied?
  If yes, what was the diagnosis?
- Have you ever been treated for cancer of any kind? *If yes*, when? What?
- Have you examined yourself for any lumps or nodules and found any thickening or lump in the breast or armpit area?
  If yes, has your physician examined/treated this?
  If no, do you examine your own breasts? (Follow-up questions regarding last breast examination by self or other health care professional)
- Do you have any discharge from your breasts or nipples?
  If yes, do you know what is causing this discharge? Have you received medical treatment for this problem?
- Are you nursing or breastfeeding an infant (lactating)?
  If yes, are your nipples sore or cracked?
  Is your breast painful or hot? Are there any areas of redness?
  Have you had a fever? **(Mastitis)**
- Have you noticed any other changes in your breast(s)? For example, are there any noticeable bulging or distended veins, puckering, swelling, tenderness, rash, or any other skin changes?
- Do you have any pain in your breasts?
  If yes, does the pain come and go with your period? **(Hormone-related)**

SUBJECTIVE EXAMINATION—cont'd

Does squeezing the breast tissue cause the pain? Does using your arms in any way cause the pain?

- Have you been involved in any activities of a repetitive nature that could cause sore muscles (e.g., painting, washing walls, push-ups or other calisthenics, heavy lifting or pushing, over-head movements, prolonged running, or fast walking)?

- Have you recently been coughing excessively? **(Pectoral myalgia)**

- Have you ever had angina (chest pain) or a heart attack? **(Residual trigger points)**

- Have you been in a fight or hit, punched, or pushed against any object that injured your chest or breast? **(Assault)**

Special Questions to Ask: Lymph Nodes

Use the lymph node assessment form (Fig. 4-45) to record and report baseline findings.

- [General screening question:] Have you exam-ined yourself for any lumps or nodules and found any thickening or lump? *If yes*, has your physician examined/treated this?

If any suspicious or aberrant lymph nodes are observed during palpation, ask the following questions.

- Have you recently had any skin rashes any-where on your face or body?

- Have you recently had a cold, upper respira-tory infection, the flu, or other illness? (Enlarged lymph nodes)

- Have you ever had:
  Cancer of any kind?
  If no, have you ever been treated with radi-ation or chemotherapy for any reason?
  Breast implants

Mastectomy or prostatectomy
Mononucleosis
Chronic fatigue syndrome
Allergic rhinitis
Food intolerances, food allergies, or celiac sprue
Recent dental work
Infection of any kind
Recent cut, insect bite, or infection in the hand or arm
A sexually transmitted disease of any kind
Sores or lesions of any kind anywhere on the body (including genitals)

Special Questions to Ask: Soft Tissue Lumps or Skin Lesions

- How long have you had this?

- Has it changed in the last 6 weeks to 6 months?

- Has your doctor seen it?

- Does it itch, hurt, feel sore, or burn?

- Does anyone else in your household have any-thing like this?

- Have you taken any new medications (pre-scribed or over-the-counter) in the last 6 weeks?

- Have you traveled somewhere new in the last month?

- Have you been exposed to anything in the last month that could cause this? (consider exposure due to occupational, environmental, and hobby interests)

- Do you have any other skin changes anywhere else on your body?

- Have you had a fever or sweats in the last 2 weeks?

- Are you having any trouble breathing or swal-lowing?

- Have you had any other symptoms of any kind anywhere else in your body?

CASE STUDY

STEPS IN THE SCREENING PROCESS

If a client comes to you with chest pain, breast pain, or rib pain (either alone or in combination with neck, back, or shoulder pain), start by looking at Tables 17-1 and 17-2 and Box 17-4. As you look down these lists, does your client have any red flag histories, unusual clinical presentation, or associated signs and symptoms to point to any particular category? Just by looking at these lists, you may be prompted to ask some additional questions that have not been asked yet.

Could It Be Cancer?

The therapist does not make a determination as to whether or not a client has cancer; only the pathologist makes this kind of determination. The therapist's assessment determines whether the client has a true neuromuscular or musculoskeletal problem that is within the scope of our practice.

However, knowing red flags for the possibility of cancer helps the therapist know what questions to ask and what red flags to look for. Early detection often means reduced morbidity and mortality for many people. Watch for the following:

- Previous history of cancer (any kind, but especially breast or lung cancer).
- Be sure to assess for trigger points (TrPs). Reassess after trigger point therapy (e.g., Were the symptoms alleviated? Did the movement pattern change?).
- Conduct a neurologic screening exam.
- Look for skin changes or other trophic changes, and ask about recent rashes or lesions (see Examining a Skin Lesion or Mass in Box 4-10).

Could It Be Vascular?

- Consider the client's age, menopausal status (women), past medical history, and the presence of any cardiac risk factors. Do any of these components suggest the need to screen further for a vascular cause?
- Are there any reported associated signs and symptoms (e.g., unexplained perspiration without physical activity, nausea, pallor, unexplained fatigue, palpitations; see Box 4-17)?
- Is there a significant difference in blood pressure from one arm to the other? Have you checked? Do the symptoms suggest the need to conduct this assessment?
- Have you assessed for the 3 Ps? (pleuritic pain, palpation, position)

Could It Be Pulmonary?

- Consider the age of the client and any recent history of pneumonia or other upper respiratory infections. Again, consider the 3 Ps.
- Have you observed or heard any reports from the client to suggest changes in the breathing pattern? Are there other pulmonary symptoms present (e.g., dry or productive cough, symptoms aggravated by respiratory movements)?
- Are the symptoms made better by sitting up, worse by lying down, or better in sidelying on the affected side (autosplinting)? *If yes*, further screening may be warranted.

Could It Be Upper GI?

- Follow the same line of thinking in terms of mentally reviewing the client's past medical history (e.g., chronic NSAID use, GERD, gallbladder, or liver problems) and the presence of any GI signs or symptoms. Is there anything here to suggest a potential GI cause of the current symptoms? If yes, then review the Special Questions to Ask box for any further screening questions.
- Have you asked the client about the effect of eating or drinking on the symptoms? It is a quick and simple screening question to help identify any GI component.
- Be sure and assess for trigger points as a potential cause of what might appear to be GI-induced symptoms.

Could It Be Breast Pathology?

- Consider red flag histories, risk factors, and pain pattern for men and women when considering breast tissue as a possible cause of upper quadrant pain.
- Is there any cyclical aspect to the symptoms linked to menstruation or hormonal fluctuations?
- Ask if jarring or squeezing the breast reproduces the pain.
- Ask if there have been any obvious changes in the breast tissue or nipple.
- Have you palpated the axillary or supraclavicular lymph nodes? This is a quick and easy screening test that can easily be incorporated into your examination.

Could It Be Trauma or Other Causes?

- Remember to consider trauma (including assault) as a possible cause of symptoms.

CASE STUDY—cont'd

- Is there any reason to suspect drug use (e.g., cocaine, anabolic steroids)?

- Should you consider screening for emotional overlay or psychogenic source of symptoms (see Chapter 3; see Appendix B-28)?

- Consider anemia as a possible cause; without a laboratory test, this is impossible to know for certain. In the screening process, the therapist can ask some questions to help formulate a referral decision. For example, has the client complained of fatigue, a hallmark finding in anemia?

Some additional questions may include the following:

- Have you experienced any unusual or prolonged bleeding from any part of your body?

- Have you noticed any blood in your urine or stools? Have you noticed any changes in the color of your stools? (Dark, tarry, sticky stools may signal melena from blood loss in the GI tract.)

- Have you been taking any over-the-counter or prescribed antiinflammatory drugs (NSAIDs and peptic ulcer with GI bleeding)?

- Have you ever been told you have rheumatoid arthritis, lupus, HIV/AIDs, or anemia?

- Rheumatoid arthritis is a systemic condition that can cause chest pain; osteoarthritis of the cervical spine, fibromyalgia, and anxiety can also cause chest pain. When completing the Review of Systems, look for a cluster of associated signs and symptoms that might suggest any of these conditions.

- Do not forget to consider screening for anabolic steroid use, cocaine or other substance use, and domestic violence or assault.

Finally, review the clues to differentiating chest, breast, or rib pain, and then scan the Special Questions to Ask: Chest/Thorax or Special Questions to Ask: Breast in this chapter (depending on the chief complaint and presenting symptoms). Have you left anything out?

PRACTICE QUESTIONS

1. Chest pain can be caused by trigger points of the:
   a. Sternocleidomastoid
   b. Rectus abdominis
   c. Upper trapezius
   d. Iliocostalis thoracis

2. During examination of a 42-year-old woman's right axilla, you palpate a lump. Which characteristics most suggest the lump may be malignant?
   a. Soft, mobile, tender
   b. Hard, immovable, tender
   c. Soft, mobile, nontender
   d. Hard, immovable, nontender

3. A client complains of throbbing pain at the base of the anterior neck that radiates into the chest and interscapular areas and increases with exertion. What should you do first?

   a. Monitor vital signs, and palpate pulses
   b. Call the physician or 911 immediately
   c. Continue with the exam; find out what relieves the pain
   d. Ask about past medical history and associated signs and symptoms

4. A 55-year old grocery store manager reports becoming extremely weak and breathless whenever stocking groceries on overhead shelves. What is the possible significance of this complaint?
   a. Thoracic outlet syndrome
   b. Myocardial ischemia
   c. Trigger Point
   d. All of the above

PRACTICE QUESTIONS—cont'd

5. Chest pain of a pleuritic nature can be distinguished by:
   a. Increases with autosplinting (lying on the involved side)
   b. Reproduced with palpation
   c. Exacerbated by deep breathing
   d. All of the above

6. A 66-year-old woman has been referred to you by her physiatrist for preprosthetic training after an above-knee amputation. Her past medical history is significant for chronic diabetes mellitus (insulin dependent), coronary artery disease, and peripheral vascular disease. About 6 weeks ago, she had an angioplasty with stent placement. During the physical therapy examination, the client reported anterior neck pain radiating down the left arm. Which test will help you differentiate a musculoskeletal cause from a cardiac cause of neck and arm pain?
   a. Stair climbing or stationary bike test
   b. Using arms overhead for 3 to 5 minutes
   c. Trigger point assessment
   d. All of the above

7. You are evaluating a 30-year-old woman with left chest pain that starts just below the clavicle and extends down to the nipple line. The majority of test results point to thoracic outlet syndrome. Her blood pressure is 120/78 mm Hg on the right (sitting) and 125/100 on the left (sitting). She is in apparent good health with no history of surgeries or significant health problems. What plan of action would you recommend?
   a. Refer her to a physician before initiating treatment.
   b. Carry out a plan of care, and reassess after three sessions or 1 week, whichever comes first.
   c. Document your findings, and contact the physician by phone or by fax while initiating treatment.
   d. Eliminate trigger points, and then reassess symptoms.

8. A 60-year-old woman with a history of left breast cancer (10 years postmastectomy) presents with pain in her midback. The pain is described as "sharp" and radiates around her chest to the sternum. She gets some relief from her pain by lying down. Her vital signs are normal, and there are no palpable or aberrant lymph nodes. She denies any changes in breast tissue on the right or the scar and soft tissue on the left. You do not have adequate training to perform a clinical breast examination, but the client agrees to visual inspection, which reveals nothing unusual. All other findings are within normal limits; you are unable to provoke or aggravate her symptoms. Neurologic screening examination is within normal limits. The client denies any history of trauma. What plan of action would you recommend?
   a. Refer her to a physician before initiating treatment
   b. Carry out a plan of care, and reassess after three sessions or 1 week, whichever comes first
   c. Document your findings, and contact the physician by phone or by fax while initiating treatment.
   d. Eliminate trigger points, and then reassess symptoms.

9. You are working with a client in his home who had a total hip replacement 2 weeks ago. He describes chest pain with increased activity. Knowing what could cause this symptom will help guide you in asking appropriate screening questions. Is this a symptom of:
   a. Asthma
   b. Angina
   c. Pleuritis or pleurisy
   d. All of the above

10. Cardiac pain in women does not always follow classic patterns. Watch for this group of symptoms in women at risk:
   a. Indigestion, food poisoning, jaw pain
   b. Nausea, tinnitus, night sweats
   c. Confusion, left biceps pain, dyspnea
   d. Unusual fatigue, shortness of breath, weakness, or sleep disturbance

REFERENCES

1. Lovelace-Chandler V, Bassar M, Dow D, et al: The role of physical therapists assisting women in skill development in performing breast self-examination. Poster presentation. Combined Sections Meeting, New Orleans, February 2005.

2. Goodman CC, McGarvey CL: The role of the physical therapist in primary care and cancer screening: integrating clinical breast examination (CBE) in the upper quarter examination, *Rehabilitation Oncology* 21(2):4-11, 2003.

3. Swap C, Nagurney JT: Value and limitations of chest pain history in the evaluation of patients with suspected acute coronary symptoms, *JAMA* 294(20):2623-2629, 2005.

4. Bruckner FE, Greco A, Leung AW: Benign thoracic pain syndrome: role of magnetic resonance imaging in the detection and localization of thoracic disc disease, *J R Soc Med* 82:81-83, 1989.

5. American Heart Association: Heart News. Available on-line at http://www.americanheart.org. Accessed January 31, 2006.

6. Harvard Women's Health Watch: Gender matters: heart disease risk in women, 11(9):1-3, 2004.

7. National Heart, Lung, and Blood Institute: National Cholesterol Education Program (NCEP). Available on-line at http://hin.nhlbi.nih.gov/atpiii/calculator.asp?sertype=prof. Accessed January 31, 2006.

8. Marrugat J et al: Mortality differences between men and women following first myocardial infarction, *JAMA* 280:1405-1409, 1998.

9. McSweeney JC: Women's early warning symptoms of acute myocardial infarction, *Circulation* 108(21):2619-2623, 2003.

10. Wolf JM, Green A: Influence of comorbidity on self-assessment instrument scores of patients with idiopathic adhesive capsulitis, *J Bone Joint Surg Am* 84-A(7):1167-1173, 2002.

11. Smith R, Athanasou NA, Ostlere SJ, et al: Pregnancy-associated osteoporosis, *QJM* 88:865-878, 1995.

12. Baitner AC, Bernstein AD, Jazrawi AJ: Spontaneous rib fracture during pregnancy: a case report and review of the literature, *Bull Hosp Jt Dis* 59(3):163-165, 2000.

13. Boissonnault WG, Boissonnault JS: Transient osteoporosis of the hip associated with pregnancy, *JOSPT* 31(7):359-367, 2001.

14. Amagada JO, Joels L, Catling S: Stress fracture of rib in pregnancy: what analgesia? *J Obstet Gynaecol* 22(5):559, 2002.

15. Kovacs CS: Calcium and bone metabolism during pregnancy and lactation, *J Mammary Gland Gland Biol Neoplasia* 10(2):105-118, 2005.

16. Debnah UK, Kishore R, Black RJ: Isolated acetabular osteoporosis in TOH in pregnancy: a case report, *South Med J* 98(11):1146-1148, 2005.

17. Jemal A, Murray T, Ward E, Samuels A, et al: Cancer statistics 2005, *CA Cancer J Clin* 55(1):10-30, 2005.

18. American Cancer Society (ACS): What are the risk factors for breast cancer? Available at: http://www.cancer.org/docroot/CRI/content/CRI_2_4_2X_What_are_the_risk_factors_for_breast_cancer_5.asp. Accessed January 26, 2006.

19. Garfinkel L: Current trends in breast cancer, *CA Cancer J Clin* 43(1):5-6, 1993.

20. Coleman EA, Heard JK: Clinical breast examination: an illustrated educational review and update, *Clin Excell Nurse Pract* 5:197-204, 2001.

21. Barton MB, Harris R, Fletcher SW: Does this patient have breast cancer? The screening clinical breast examination: should it be done? How? *JAMA* 282:1270, 1999.

22. Goodman CC, McGarvey CL: An introductory course to breast cancer and clinical breast examination for the physical therapist is available. (Charlie McGarvey, PT, MS and Catherine Goodman, MBA, PT present the course in various sites around the U.S. and upon request.)

23. A certified training program is also available through *MammaCare Specialist*. The program isoffered to health care professionals at training centers in the United States. The course teaches proficient breast examination skills. For more information, contact: http://www.manmacare.com/ professional_training.htm.

24. Cady B, Steele GD, Morrow M, et al: Evaluation of common breast problems: guidance for primary care providers, *CA Cancer J Clin* 48(1):49-63, 1998.

25. Rubin RN: Woman with sharp back pain, *Consultant* 39(11):3065-3066, 1999.

26. Gabriel SE, Woods JE, O'Fallon WM, et al: Complications leading to surgery after breast implantation, *NEJM* 336(10):718-719, 1997.

27. Benediktsson K, Perback L: Capsular contracture around saline-filled and textured subcutaneously-placed implants in irradiated and non-irradiated breast cancer patients: five years of monitoring of a prospective trial, *J Plast Reconstr Aesthet Surg* 59(1):27-34, 2006.

28. Henriksen TF, Fryzek JP, Holmich LR, et al: Reconstructive breast implantation after mastectomy for breast cancer: clinical outcomes in young adults: the Coronary Artery Risk Development in Young Adults (CARDIA) study, *Arch Surg* 140(12):1152-1159, 2005.

29. Zuckerman D: Associated Press interview (December 20, 2005). National Research Center for Women and Families, Washington, D.C., 2005.

30. National Institute of Mental Health: Health Information—Anxiety Disorders. Available at: http://www.nimh.nih.gov/. Updated 1/27/06. Accessed January 27, 2006.

31. Velasquez EM, Anand RC, Newman WP, et al: Cardiovascular complications associated with cocaine use, *J La State Med Soc* 156(6):302-310, 2004.

32. Pletcher MJ, Kiefe CI, Sidney S, et al: Cocaine and coronary calcification in young adults: the Coronary Artery Risk Development in Young Adults, *Am Heart J* 150(5):921-926, 2005.

33. Pozner CN, Levine M, Zane R: The cardiovascular effects of cocaine, *J Emerg Med* 29(2):173-178, 2005.

34. Evans NA: Anabolic steroids: answers to the bigger questions, *J Musculo Med* 21(3):166-178, 2004.

35. Sullivan ML, Martinez CM, Gennis P et al: The cardiac toxicity of anabolic steroids, *Prog Cardiovasc Dis* 41(1):1-15, 1998.

36. Jensen S: Musculoskeletal causes of chest pain, *Aust Fam Phys* 30(9):834-839, September 2001.

37. Peterson LL, Cavanaugh DG: Two years of debilitating pain in a football spearing victim: slipping rib syndrome, *Med Sci Sports Exerc* 35(10):1634-1637, 2003.

38. Thongngarm T, Lemos LB, Lawhon N, et al: Malignant tumor with chest pain mimicking Tietze's syndrome, *Clin Rheumatol* 20(4):276-278, 2001.

39. Fioravanti A, Tofi C, Volterrani L, et al: Malignant lymphoma presenting as Tietze's syndrome, *Arthritis Rheum* 49(5):737, 2003.

40. Simons DG, Travell JG, Simons LS: *Travell & Simons' myofascial pain and dysfunction: the trigger point manual. Volume 1: Upper half of body*, ed 2, Baltimore, 1999, Williams & Wilkins.

41. Hughes KH: Painful rib syndrome: a variant of myofascial pain syndrome, *AAOHN* 46(3):115-120, 1998.

42. Saltzman DA, Schmitz ML, Smith SD, et al: The slipping rib syndrome in children, *Paediatr Anaesth* 11(6):740-743, 2001.

43. Meuwly JY, Wicky S, Schnyder P, et al: Slipping rib syndromes: a place for sonography in the diagnosis of a frequently overlooked cause of abdominal or low thoracic pain, *J Ultrasound Med* 21(3):339-343, 2002.

44. Udermann BE, Cavanaugh DG, Gibson MH, et al: Slipping rib syndrome in a collegiate swimmer: a case report, *J Athl Train* 40(2):120-122, 2005.
45. Dutton M: *Orthopaedic examination, evaluation, and intervention*, New York, 2004, McGraw-Hill.
46. Selke FW, Kelly TR: Thoracic outlet syndrome, *Am J Surg* 156:54-57, 1988.
47. Magee D: *Orthopedic physical assessment*, ed 4, Philadelphia, Saunders, 2002.

Screening the Shoulder and Upper Extremity

The therapist is well aware that many primary neuromuscular and musculoskeletal conditions in the neck, cervical spine, axilla, thorax, thoracic spine, and chest wall can refer pain to the shoulder and arm. For this reason, the physical therapist's examination usually includes assessment above and below the involved joint for referred musculoskeletal pain (Case Example 18-1).

In this chapter we explore systemic and viscerogenic causes of shoulder and arm pain and take a look at each system that can refer pain or symptoms to the shoulder. This will include vascular, pulmonary, renal, gastrointestinal (GI), and gynecologic causes of shoulder and upper extremity pain and dysfunction. Primary or metastatic cancer as an underlying cause of shoulder pain also is included. The therapist must know how and what to look for to screen for cancer.

Systemic diseases affecting the neck, breast, and any organs in the chest or abdomen can present clinically as shoulder pain (Table 18-1). Peptic ulcers, heart disease, ectopic pregnancy and myocardial ischemia are only a few examples of systemic diseases that can cause shoulder pain and movement dysfunction. Each disorder listed can present clinically as a shoulder problem before ever demonstrating systemic signs and symptoms.

► USING THE SCREENING MODEL TO EVALUATE SHOULDER AND UPPER EXTREMITY

Past Medical History

As you look over the various potential systemic causes of shoulder pain listed in Table 18-1, think about the most common risk factors and red flag histories you might see with each of these conditions. For example, a history of any kind of cancer is always a red flag. Breast and lung cancer are the two most common types of cancer to metastasize to the shoulder.

Heart disease can cause shoulder pain, but it usually occurs in an age specific population. Anyone over 50 years old, postmenopausal women, and anyone with a positive first generation family history is at increased risk for symptomatic heart disease.

Alternately, although atherosclerosis has been demonstrated in the blood vessels of children, teens, and young adults, they are rarely symptomatic unless some other heart anomaly is present.

Hypertension, diabetes, and hyperlipidemia are other red flag histories associated with cardiac related shoulder pain. Of course, a history of angina, heart attack, angiography, stent placement, and coronary artery bypass graft (CABG), or other cardiac procedure is also a yellow (caution) flag to alert the therapist of the potential need for further medical screening.

CASE EXAMPLE 18-1   Evaluation of a Professional Golfer

Referral: A 38-year-old male, professional golfer presented to physical therapy with a diagnosis of shoulder impingement syndrome, with partial thickness tears of the supraspinatus tendon.

Prior to the physical therapy intervention, x-rays taken were reported as negative for fracture or tumor. An MRI was reported as positive for bursitis and supraspinatus tendinitis with some partial tears. The shoulder specialist also provided the client with one corticosteroid injection, which gave him some relief of his shoulder pain.

Past Medical History: Past medical history and review of systems were negative for any systemic issues. He was on no medication at the time of evaluation.

Clinical Presentation: Functional deficits were reported as pain with the take-away phase of the golf swing and with the adduction motion of the shoulder in follow through. He also reported a loss of distance associated with his drive by 20 to 30 yards. He had trouble sleeping and reported pain would wake him up if his head were turned into left rotation. He also had pain when turning his head to the left (e.g., when driving a car).

UPPER QUARTER SCREEN
Shoulder ROM

Active ROM:

Left			Right
160°	Flex		170°
165°	Abd		170°
T9	I.R.		T7
T1	E.R.		T3

Passive ROM:

Left			Right
170°	Flex		175°
170°	Abd		175°
55°	I.R.		60°
60°	E.R.		75°

Isometric Muscle Testing of Rotator Cuff:

Abduction	Painful/strong
Abduction with internal rotation	Painful/strong
Internal Rotation	Painless/strong
External Rotation	Painless/strong

Special Tests:

Hawkins/Kennedy +
Neer +
Speeds +
External Rotation Lag Test –
Internal Rotation Lag Test –

Cervical ROM

Flexion 40°	
Extension 20°	Report of left scapular pain
[L] side bend 20°	Report of left scapular pain
[R] side bend 25°	No report of pain
[L] rotation 45°	Report of left scapular pain
[R] rotation 70°	No report of pain
Quadrant position	Right and left: Reproduced left posterior scapular pain with radicular pain to the thumb and second finger area

Deep Tendon Reflexes

Left	DTR	Right
2+	Biceps	2+
0	Triceps	2+
2+	Brachioradialis	2+

Strength

Left		Right
5/5	Shoulder flexion	5/5
4/5	Shoulder abduction	5/5
5/5	Elbow flexion	5/5
2/5	Elbow extension	5/5
3/5	Wrist extension	5/5
5/5	Wrist flexion	5/5
5/5	Thumb extension	5/5
5/5	Finger abduction	5/5

He did have intact sensation to light touch and proprioceptive sense. Strength testing on the Cybex weight lifting machines showed he was able to do 10 triceps extensions on the right with four plates while on the left, he was only able to do one repetition with one plate.

Result: With the data obtained in the examination, the conclusion was made that he did have an impingement syndrome as described by Neer, with involvement of the bursa and rotator cuff tendons.[1] Cyriax muscle testing revealed some musculotendon involvement with the strong/painful tests.[2]

The cervical findings required consultation with the referring physician. A provisional medical diagnosis was made of cervical radiculopathy with a C5-C6 herniated disc. The client

---

CASE EXAMPLE 18-1   Evaluation of a Professional Golfer—cont'd

was referred to a neurosurgeon for evaluation. An MRI confirmed the diagnosis and the client underwent an anterior cervical fusion with disectomy.

Summary: This case example helps highlight the importance of a complete examination process, even if a physician specialist refers a client for physical therapy services. The therapist must "clear" or examine the joints above and below the region thought to be the cause of the dysfunction. The major reason for the symptoms or a secondary diagnosis may be missed if the screening step is left out because of a lack of time or assuming someone else checked out the entire client.

Voshell S: Case report presented in fulfillment of DPT 910, Institute for Physical Therapy Education, Widener University, Chester, Pennsylvania, 2005. Used with permission.

Knowledge of pathologic conditions, illnesses, and diseases helps the therapist navigate the screening process. For example, pulmonary tuberculosis (TB) is a possible cause of shoulder pain. Who is most likely to develop TB? Risk factors include

- Health care workers
- Homeless population
- Prison inmates
- Immunocompromised individuals (e.g., transplant recipients, long-term use of immunosuppressants, anyone treated for long-term rheumatoid arthritis, anyone treated with chemotherapy for cancer)
- Older adult (over 65 years)
- Immigrants from areas where TB is endemic
- Injection drug users
- Malnourished (e.g., eating disorders, alcoholism, drug users, cachexia)

In a case like tuberculosis, there will usually be other associated signs and symptoms such as fever, sweats, and cough. When completing a screening examination for a client with shoulder pain of unknown origin or an unusual clinical presentation, the therapist might look at vital signs, auscultate the client, and see what effect increased respiratory movements have on shoulder symptoms (Case Example 18-2).

Clinical Presentation

Differential diagnosis of shoulder pain is sometimes especially difficult because any pain that is felt in the shoulder often affects the joint as though the pain were originating in the joint.[3] Shoulder pain with any of the components listed in this chapter should be approached as a manifestation of systemic visceral illness, even if shoulder

movements exacerbate the pain or if there are objective findings at the shoulder.

Many visceral diseases present as unilateral shoulder pain (Table 18-2). Esophageal, pericardial (or other myocardial diseases), aortic dissection, and diaphragmatic irritation from thoracic or abdominal diseases (e.g., renal, hepatic/biliary) all can appear as unilateral pain.

"Frozen shoulder," or adhesive capsulitis, a condition in which both active and passive glenohumeral motions are restricted, can be associated with diabetes mellitus, hyperthyroidism, ischemic heart disease, infection, and lung diseases (tuberculosis, emphysema, chronic bronchitis, Pancoast's tumors) (Case Example 18-3).[4]

Shoulder pain (unilateral or bilateral) progressing to adhesive capsulitis can occur 6 to 9 months after a coronary artery bypass graft (CABG). Similarly, anyone immobile in the intensive care unit (ICU) or coronary care unit (CCU) can experience loss of shoulder motion resulting in adhesive capsulitis (Case Example 18-4). Clients with pacemakers who have complications and revisions that result in prolonged shoulder immobilization can also develop adhesive capsulitis.

The Shoulder is Unique

It has been stressed throughout this text that the basic clues and approach to screening are similar, if not the same, from system to system and anatomic part to anatomic part.

So, for example, much of what was said about screening the neck and back (Chapter 14) applied to the sacrum, SI, pelvis (Chapter 15), buttock, hip, groin (Chapter 16), and chest, breast, and rib (Chapter 17). Presenting the shoulder last in this text is by design. These principles do apply to the shoulder, but beyond that:

Text continued

TABLE 18-1 ▼ Systemic Causes of Shoulder Pain

	Neck	Chest	Abdomen

Cancer	Metastases (leukemia, Hodgkin's disease)
	Cervical cord tumors
	Bone tumors
		Metastases to nodes in axilla or mediastinum
		Metastases to lungs from:
		  Bone
		  Breast
		  Kidney
		  Colorectal
		  Pancreas
		  Uterus
		Bone metastases to thoracic spine:
		  Breast
		  Lung
		  Thyroid
		Breast cancer
		Lung cancer
			Pancreatic cancer
			Spinal metastases
			  Kidney
			  Testicle
			  Prostate

Cardiovascular/ Vascular	Thoracic Outlet syndrome	Angina/myocardial infarct Post-coronary artery bypass graft (ICU/CABG) Pacemaker (complications) Bacterial endocarditis Pericarditis Aortic aneurysm Empyema and lung abscess Collagen vascular disease	Dissecting aortic aneurysm
Pulmonary	Pulmonary tuberculosis	Pulmonary embolism Pulmonary tuberculosis Spontaneous pneumothorax Pancoast's tumor Pneumonia	
Renal/Urologic			Kidney stones Obstruction, inflammation, or infection of upper urinary tract
Gastrointestinal /Hepatic		Hiatal hernia	Peptic/duodenal ulcer (perforated) Ruptured spleen Liver disease Gallbladder disease Pancreatic disease
Gynecologic			Ectopic pregnancy (rupture)

Other		Mastodynia (breast)
		Infection:
		  Mononucleosis
		  Osteomyelitis
		  Syphilis/gonorrhea
		  Herpes zoster (shingles)
		  Pneumonia
		Diabetes mellitus (adhesive capsulitis)
		Sickle cell anemia
		Hemophilia
			Subphrenic abscess
			Diaphragmatic hernia
			Anterior spinal surgery (post-operative hemorrhage)

Referral: A 36-year-old man was referred to physical therapy as an in-patient for a short-term hospitalization. He was a homeless man brought to the hospital by the police and admitted with an extensive medical problem list including

Malnutrition
Alcoholism
Depression
Hepatitis A
Broken wrist
Shoulder pain
Dehydration

There was no past medical history of cancer. The client was a smoker when he could get cigarettes. He would like to support a one-pack-a-day habit.

Medical service requested an evaluation of the client's shoulder pain. X-rays were not taken because the man had full active range of motion, no history of trauma, and no insurance to cover additional testing.

Clinical Presentation: The therapist was unable to reproduce the shoulder pain with palpation, position, or provocation testing. There was no sign of rotator cuff dysfunction, adhesive capsulitis, tendinitis, or trigger points in the upper quadrant. There was a noticeable stiffening of the neck with very limited cervical range of motion in all planes and directions.

Vital signs were unremarkable, but the client was perspiring heavily despite being in threadbare clothing and at rest. He reported getting the "sweats" everyday around this same time.

The therapist asked the client to take a deep breath and cough. He went into a paroxysm of coughing, which he said caused his shoulder to start aching. The cough was productive, but the client swallowed the sputum. Auscultation of lung sounds revealed rales (crackles) in the right upper lung lobe. Supraclavicular lymph nodes were palpable, tender, and moveable on both sides.

The therapist contacted the charge nurse and reported the following concerns:

- Constitutional symptoms of sweats and fatigue (although fatigue could be caused by his extreme malnutrition)
- Pulmonary impairment with reproduction of symptoms with respiratory movements
- Suspicious (aberrant) lymph nodes (bilateral)
- Cervical spine involvement with no apparent cause or recognizable musculoskeletal pattern

Result: Consult with the physician on call resulted in a medical evaluation and x-ray. Client was diagnosed with pulmonary tuberculosis, which was confirmed by a skin test. Shoulder and neck pain and dysfunction were attributed to a pulmonary source and not considered appropriate for physical therapy intervention.

The client was sent to a halfway house where he could receive adequate nutrition and medical services to treat his tuberculosis.

TABLE 18-2 ▼ Location of Shoulder Pain

Systemic origin	Right shoulder location	Systemic origin	Left shoulder location
Peptic ulcer	Lateral border, R scapula	Ruptured spleen	L shoulder (Kehr's sign)
Myocardial ischemia	R shoulder, down arm	Myocardial ischemia	L pectoral/L shoulder
Hepatic/biliary:		Pancreas	L shoulder
Acute cholecystitis	R shoulder; between scapulae;	Ectopic pregnancy	L shoulder (Kehr's sign)
	R subscapular area	(rupture)	
Liver abscess	R shoulder		
Gallbladder	R upper trapezius, R shoulder	Infectious mononucleosis	L shoulder/L upper trapezius
Liver disease	R shoulder, R subscapula	(hepatomegaly;	
(hepatitis, cirrhosis,		splenomegaly)	
metastatic tumors)			
Pulmonary:	Ipsilateral shoulder; upper	Pulmonary:	Ipsilateral shoulder; upper
Pleurisy	trapezius	Pleurisy	trapezius
Pneumothorax		Pneumothorax	
Pancoast's tumor		Pancoast's tumor	
Pneumonia		Pneumonia	
Kidney	Ipsilateral shoulder	Kidney	Ipsilateral shoulder
		Postoperative laparoscopy	L shoulder (Kehr's sign)

CASE EXAMPLE 18-3   Cardiac Cause of Shoulder Pain

A 65-year-old retired railroad engineer has come to you with a left "frozen shoulder." During the course of the subjective examination, he tells you he is taking two cardiac medications.

What questions would you ask that might help you relate these two problems or rule out cardiac as a possible cause? (shoulder/cardiac)

Try to organize your thoughts using these categories:

- Onset/History of shoulder involvement
- Medical Testing
- Clinical Presentation
- Past Medical History

Physical Therapy Screening Interview

Onset / History

- What do you think is the cause of your shoulder problem?
- When did it occur, or how long have you had this problem (sudden or gradual onset)?
- Can you recall any specific incident when you injured your shoulder, for example, by falling, being hit by someone or something, automobile accident?
- Did you ever have a snapping or popping sensation just before your shoulder started to hurt? **(ligamentous or cartilagenous lesion)**
- Did you injure your neck in any way before your shoulder developed these problems?
- Have you had a recent heart attack? Have you had nausea, fatigue, sweating, chest pain, or pressure? Any pain in your neck, jaw, left shoulder, or down your left arm?
- Has your left hand ever been stiff or swollen? **(Complex Regional Pain Syndrome after myocardial infarction)**
- Do you think your shoulder pain is related to your heart problems?
- Shortly before you first noticed difficulty with your shoulder were you involved in any kind of activities that would require repetitive movements, such as painting, gardening, playing tennis or golf?

Medical Testing

- Have you had any recent x-rays taken of the shoulder or your neck?
- Have you received medical or physical therapy treatment for shoulder problems before?

If yes, where, when, why, who, and what (see Chapter 2 for specific questions)?

- Have you had any (extensive) medical testing during the past year?

Clinical Presentation

Pain / Symptoms

Follow the usual line of questioning regarding the pattern, frequency, intensity, and duration outlined in Fig. 3-6 to establish necessary information regarding pain.

- Is your shoulder painful?

If yes, how long has the shoulder been painful?

Aggravating / Relieving Activities

- How does rest affect your shoulder symptoms? **(True muscular lesions are relieved with prolonged rest [i.e., more than 1 hour], whereas angina is usually relieved more immediately by cessation of activity or rest [i.e., usually within 2 to 5 minutes, up to 15 minutes.])**
- Does your shoulder pain occur during exercise (e.g., walking, climbing stairs, mowing the lawn or any other physical or sexual activity? **(Evaluate the difference between total body exertion causing shoulder symptoms versus movements of the upper extremities only reproducing symptoms. Total body exertion causing shoulder pain may be secondary to angina or myocardial infarction, whereas movements of just the upper extremities causing shoulder pain are indicative of a primary musculoskeletal lesion.)**

Past Medical History

- Have you had any surgery during the past year?
- How has your general health been? **(Shoulder pain is a frequent site of referred pain from other internal medical problems; see Fig. 18-2)**
- Did you ever have rheumatic fever when you were a child?
- What is your typical pattern of chest pain or angina?
- Has this pattern changed in any way since your shoulder started to hurt? For example, does the chest pain last longer, come on with less exertion, and feel more intense?
- What medications are you taking?
- Do your heart medications relieve your shoulder symptoms, even briefly?

CASE EXAMPLE 18-3 Cardiac Cause of Shoulder Pain—cont'd

If yes, how long after you take the medications do you notice a difference?

Does this occur every time that you take your medications?

Evaluating subacute/acute/chronic musculoskeletal lesion versus systemic pain pattern (see Chapter 3, Night Pain, for specific meaning to the client's answers to these questions):

- Can you lie on that side?
- Does the shoulder pain awaken you at night? *If yes,* is this because you have rolled onto that side?
- Do you notice any chest pain, night sweats, fever, or heart palpitations when you wake up at night?
- Have you ever noticed these symptoms (e.g., chest pain, heart palpitations) with your shoulder pain during the day?

- Do these symptoms wake you up separately from your shoulder pain, or does your shoulder pain wake you up and you have these additional symptoms? (As always when asking questions about sleep patterns, the person may be unsure of the answers to the questions. In such cases the physical therapist is advised to ask the client to pay attention to what happens related to sleep during the next few days up to 1 week and report back with more information.)

Other Clinical Tests: In addition to an orthopedic screening examination, the therapist should review potential side effects and interactions of cardiac medications, take vital signs, auscultate (including femoral bruits), and palpate for the aortic pulse (see Fig. 4-52).

Shoulder pain is difficult to diagnose because any pain felt in the shoulder will affect the joint as though the pain was originating in the joint.

John Mennell[6]

... even when there is a known cause, especially in the older adult.

Catherine Goodman

It is not uncommon for the older adult to attribute "overdoing" it to the appearance of physical pain or neuromusculoskeletal dysfunction. Any adult over age 65 presenting with shoulder pain and/or dysfunction must be screened for systemic or viscerogenic origin of symptoms, even when there is a known (or attributed) cause or injury.

In Chapter 2 it was stressed that clients who present with no known cause or insidious onset must be screened along with anyone who has a known or assumed cause of symptoms. Whether the client presents with an unknown etiology of injury or impairment or with an assigned cause, always ask yourself these questions.

Follow-Up Questions

- Is it really insidious?
- Is it really caused by such and such (whatever the client told you)?

The client may wrongly attribute onset of symptoms to an activity. The alert therapist may recognize a true causative factor.

Shoulder Pain Patterns

In Chapter 3 (Pain Types and Viscerogenic Pain Patterns) we presented three possible mechanisms for referred pain patterns from the viscera to the soma (embryologic development, multisegmental innervations, and direct pressure on the diaphragm). Multisegmental innervations (see Fig. 3-3) and direct pressure on the diaphragm (see Figs. 3-4 and 3-5) are two key mechanisms for referred shoulder pain.

MULTISEGMENTAL INNERVATIONS

Because the shoulder is innervated by the same spinal nerves that innervate the diaphragm (C3-C5), any messages to the spinal cord from the diaphragm can result in referred shoulder pain. The nervous system can only tell what nerves delivered the message. It does not have any way to tell if the message sent along via spinal nerves C3 to C5 came from the shoulder or the diaphragm. So it takes a guess and sends a message back to one or the other.

This means that any organ in contact with the diaphragm that gets obstructed, inflamed, or infected can refer pain to the shoulder by putting

CASE EXAMPLE 18-4   Pleural Effusion with Fibrosis, Late Complication of CABG

Referral: A 53-year-old man was referred to physical therapy by his primary care physician for left shoulder pain.

Past Medical History: The client had a recent (6 months ago) history of cardiac bypass surgery (also known as coronary artery bypass graft or CABG) and had completed Phase 1 and Phase 2 cardiac rehab programs. He was continuing to follow an exercise program (Phase 3 cardiac rehab) prescribed for him at the time of his PT referral.

Clinical Presentation: The client looked in good health and demonstrated good posture and alignment. Shoulder range of motion was equal and symmetric bilaterally but the client reported pain when the left arm was raised over 90 degrees of flexion or abduction. His position of preference was left side lying. The pain could be reduced in this position from a rated level of 6 to 2 on a scale from 0 (no pain) to 10 (worst pain).

Scapulohumeral motion on the left was altered compared to the right. Medial and lateral rotations were WNL with the upper arm against the chest. Lateral rotation reproduced painful symptoms when performed with the shoulder in 90 degrees of abduction. Physiologic motions were fully present in all directions on the left but seemed "sluggish" compared to the right.

Neuro screen–negative

Vital signs:
Blood pressure: 122/68 mm Hg
Resting pulse: 60 bpm
Body temperature: 98.6° F
Cardiopulmonary screening exam:
Diminished basilar (lower lobes) breath sounds on the left compared to the right
Decreased chest wall excursion on the left; increased shoulder pain with deep inspiration
Dyspnea was not observed at rest
When asked if there were any symptoms of any kind anywhere else in the body, the client reported ongoing but intermittent chest pain and shortness of breath for the last 3 months. The client had not reported these "new" symptoms to the physician.

What are the red flags (if any)? Is an immediate medical referral indicated?
Red Flags
- Age over 40
- Previous (recent) history of cardiac surgery
- Unequal basilar breath sounds
- Unreported symptoms of chest pain and dyspnea
- Autosplinting (lying on the affected side diminishes lung movement, reducing shoulder pain)

Medical Consultation: Shoulder problems are not uncommon following CABGs but the number and type of red flags present caught the therapist's attention. The client was not in any apparent physiologic distress and vital signs were within normal limits (although he was on antihypertensive medications). Since he was referred by his primary care physician, the therapist made telephone contact with the physician's office and faxed a summary of findings immediately.

A program of physical therapy intervention was determined but the therapist insisted on speaking with the physician first before proceeding with the program. The physician approved the therapist's treatment plan but requested immediate follow up with the client who was seen the next day.

Result: The client was diagnosed with pleural effusion causing pleural fibrosis, a rare long term complication of cardiac bypass surgery. The physician noted that the left lower lobe was adhered to the chest wall.

There is a high risk of post-operative effusion early on after bilateral internal mammary artery harvests for bypass surgery. Early effusions (less than 30 days after CABG) occur in up to two-thirds of all patients; late effusions (30 days after CABG) develop in one-third of all patients.[5]

The client was treated medically but also continued in physical therapy to restore full and normal motion of the shoulder complex. The physician also asked the therapist to review the client's cardiac rehab program and modify it accordingly due to the pulmonary complications.

pressure on the diaphragm, stimulating afferent nerve signals, and telling the nervous system that there is a problem.

DIAPHRAGMATIC IRRITATION

Irritation of the peritoneal (outside) or pleural (inside) surface of the central diaphragm refers sharp pain to the ipsilateral upper trapezius, neck and/or supraclavicular fossa (Fig. 18-1). Shoulder pain from diaphragmatic irritation usually does not cause anterior shoulder pain. Pain is confined to the suprascapular, upper trapezius, and posterior portions of the shoulder.

If the irritation crosses the midline of the diaphragm, then it is possible to have bilateral shoulder pain. This does not happen very often and is most common with cardiac ischemia or pulmonary pathology affecting the lower lobes of the lungs on both sides. Irritation of the peripheral portion of the diaphragm is more likely to refer pain to the costal margins and lumbar region on the same side.

As you review Fig. 3-4, note how the heart, spleen, kidneys, pancreas (both the body and the tail), and the lungs can put pressure on the diaphragm. This illustration is key to remembering which shoulder can be involved based on organ pathology. For example, the spleen is on the left side of the body so pain from spleen rupture or injury is referred to the left shoulder (called Kehr's sign) (Case Example 18-5).

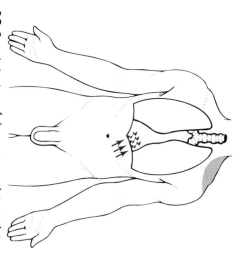

Fig. 18-1 • Irritation of the peritoneal (outside) or pleural (inside) surface of the *central* area of the diaphragm refers sharp pain to the upper trapezius muscle, neck, and supraclavicular fossa. The pain pattern is ipsilateral to the area of irritation. Irritation to the *peripheral* portion of the diaphragm refers sharp pain to the costal margins and lumbar region (not shown).

Either shoulder can be involved with renal colic, but it is usually an ipsilateral referred pain pattern depending on which kidney is impaired (see Fig. 10-7). Bilateral shoulder pain from renal disease would only occur if and when both kidneys are compromised at the same time.

The body of the pancreas lies along the midline of the diaphragm. When the body of the pancreas is enlarged, inflamed, obstructed or otherwise impinging on the diaphragm, back pain is a possible referred pain pattern. Pain felt in the left shoulder may result from activation of pain fibers in the left diaphragm by an adjacent inflammatory process in the tail of the pancreas.

Keep in mind that shoulder pain can also occur from diaphragmatic dysfunction. For anyone with shoulder pain of an unknown origin or which does not improve with intervention, palpate the diaphragm and assess its excursion and timing during respiration. Reproduction of shoulder symptoms with direct palpation of the diaphragm and the presence of altered diaphragmatic movement with breathing offer clues to the possibility of diaphragmatic (muscular) involvement.

Fig. 18-2 reminds us that shoulder pain can be referred from the neck, chest, abdomen, and elbow. During orthopedic assessment, the therapist always checks "above and below" the impaired level for a possible source of referred pain. With this guideline in mind, we know to look for potential musculoskeletal or neuromuscular causes from the cervical spine and elbow.

Associated Signs and Symptoms

One of the most basic clues in screening for a viscerogenic or systemic cause of shoulder pain is to look for shoulder pain accompanied by any of the following features:

- Pleuritic component
- Exacerbation by recumbency
- Coincident diaphoresis (cardiac)
- Associated gastrointestinal (GI) signs and symptoms
- Exacerbation by exertion unrelated to shoulder movement (cardiac)
- Associated urologic signs and symptoms

Shoulder pain with any of these present should be approached as a manifestation of systemic visceral illness. This is true even if the pain is exacerbated by shoulder movement or if there are objective findings at the shoulder.[7]

Using the past medical history and assessing for the presence of associated signs and symptoms will alert the therapist to any red flags suggesting a systemic origin of shoulder symptoms. For

CASE EXAMPLE 18-5   Rugby injury: Kehr's Sign

Referral: A 27-year-old male accountant who has an office in the same complex with a physical therapy practice stopped by early Monday morning complaining of left shoulder pain.

When asked about repetitive motions or recent trauma or injuries, he reported playing in a rugby tournament over the weekend. "I got banged up quite a few times, but I had so much beer in me, I didn't feel a thing."

Clinical Presentation: Pain was described as a deep, sharp aching over the upper trapezius and shoulder area on the left side. There were no visual bruises or signs of bleeding in the upper left quadrant.

Vital signs were taken and recorded:

Pulse:	89 bpm
Respirations:	12 per minute
Blood pressure:	90/48 mm Hg (recorded sitting, left arm)
Temperature:	97° (reported as the client's "normal" morning temperature)
Pain:	Rated as a 5 on a scale from 0 to 10

Range of motion was full in all planes and movements. No particular movement increased or decreased the pain. Gross manual muscle test of the upper extremities was normal (5/5 for flexion, abduction, extension, rotations).

Neurologic screen was negative. All special shoulder tests (e.g., impingement, anterior and posterior instability, quadrant position) were unremarkable.

What are the red flags here? What are your next questions, steps, or screening tests?
Red Flags:
• Hypotension
• Left shoulder pain within 24 hours of possible trauma or injury
• Unable to alter, provoke, or palpate painful symptoms
• Clinical presentation is not consistent with expected picture for a shoulder problem; lack of objective findings

What are your next questions, steps, or screening tests?
Repeat blood pressure measurements, bilaterally. Perform percussive tests for the spleen (see Fig. 4-50).

Depending on the results of these clinical tests, referral might be needed immediately. In this case, the percussive test for enlarged spleen was inconclusive, but there was an observable and palpable "fullness" in the left flank compared to the right.

Result: This client was told:

Mr. Smith, your exam does not look like what I would expect from a typical shoulder injury. Since I cannot find any way to make your pain better or worse and I cannot palpate or feel any areas of tenderness, there may be some other cause for your symptoms.

Given your history of playing rugby over the weekend, it is possible you have some internal injuries. I am not comfortable treating you until a medical doctor examines you first. Bleeding from the spleen can cause left shoulder pain.

When I tapped over the area of your spleen, it did not sound quite like I expected it to, and it seems like there is some fullness along your left side that I am not seeing or feeling on the right.

I do not want to alarm you, but it may be best to go over to the emergency department of the hospital and see what they have to say. You can also call your regular doctor and see if you can get in right away. You can do that right from our clinic phone.

Final Result: This accountant had clients already scheduled starting in 10 minutes. He did not feel he had the time to go check this out until his lunch hour. About 45 minutes later an ambulance was called to the building. Mr. Smith had collapsed and his co-workers called 9-1-1.

He was rushed to the hospital and diagnosed with a torn and bleeding spleen, which the doctor called a "slow leak." It eventually ruptured, leaving him unconscious from blood loss.

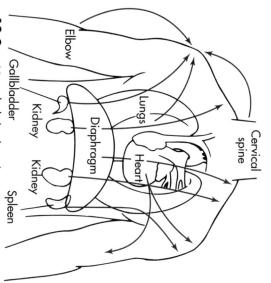

Fig. 18-2 • Musculoskeletal and systemic structures referring pain to the shoulder. (Modified from Magee DJ: *Orthopedic physical assessment*, ed 2, Philadelphia, 1992, WB Saunders; p 125.)

Elbow

Cervical spine

Lungs

Gallbladder

Kidney

Diaphragm

Heart

Kidney

Spleen

example, a ruptured ectopic pregnancy with abdominal hemorrhage can produce left shoulder pain in a woman of childbearing age. The woman is sexually active and there is usually a history of missed menses or recent unexplained/unexpected bleeding.

Another example is the left shoulder pain lasting several days that can occur after laparoscopy. During the procedure air is introduced into the peritoneum to expand the area and move the abdominal contents out of the way. Residual gas present postoperatively can put pressure on the diaphragm and refer pain to the shoulder.

Likewise distention of the renal cap from kidney disorders can cause pain to the ipsilateral shoulder (again, via pressure on the diaphragm). In the first case a recent surgery would be part of the past medical history. In the case of a kidney disorder causing shoulder pain, accompanying urologic symptoms are usually present.

The client may not recognize the connection between painful urination and shoulder pain or the link between gallbladder removal by laparoscopy and subsequent shoulder pain. It is the therapist's responsibility to assess musculoskeletal symptoms, making a diagnosis that includes ruling out the possibility of systemic disease.

Review of Systems

Associated signs and symptoms feature heavily in the Review of Systems as we step back and look to see if a cluster of any particular organ-dependent signs and symptoms is present. Based on the results of this review we formulate our final screening questions, tests, and measures. Always remember to end each client interview with the following (or similar) question:

Follow-Up Questions

• Do you have any symptoms of any kind anywhere else in your body that we haven't talked about yet?

SCREENING FOR PULMONARY CAUSES OF SHOULDER PAIN

Extensive disease may occur in the periphery of the lung without pain until the process extends to the parietal pleura. Pleural irritation then results in sharp, localized pain that is aggravated by any respiratory movement.

Clients usually note that the pain is alleviated by lying on the affected side, which diminishes the movement of that side of the chest (called "autosplinting") whereas shoulder pain of musculoskeletal origin is usually aggravated by lying on the symptomatic shoulder.

Shoulder symptoms made worse by recumbence is a yellow flag for pulmonary involvement. Lying down increases the venous return from the lower extremities. A compromised cardiopulmonary system may not be able to accommodate the increase in fluid volume. Referred shoulder pain from the taxed and overworked pulmonary system may result.

At the same time, recumbency or the supine position causes a slight shift of the abdominal contents in the cephalic direction. This shift may put pressure on the diaphragm, which in turn presses up against the lower lung lobes. The combination of increased venous return and diaphragmatic pressure may be enough to reproduce the musculoskeletal symptoms.

Pneumonia in the older adult may appear as shoulder pain when the affected lung presses on the diaphragm; usually there are accompanying pulmonary symptoms, but in older adults, confusion (or increased confusion) may be the only other associated sign.

The therapist should look for the presence of a pleuritic component such as a persistent or productive cough and/or chest pain. Look for tachypnea, dyspnea, wheezing, hyperventilation, or other noticeable changes. Chest auscultation is a valuable tool when screening for pulmonary involvement.

▼ SCREENING FOR CARDIAC CAUSES OF SHOULDER PAIN

Pain of cardiac and diaphragmatic origin is often experienced in the shoulder because the heart and diaphragm are supplied by the C5 to C6 spinal segment, and the visceral pain is referred to the corresponding somatic area (see Fig. 3-3).

Exacerbation of the shoulder symptoms from a cardiac cause occurs when the client increases activity that does not necessarily involve the arm or shoulder. For example, walking up stairs or riding a stationary bicycle can bring on cardiac induced shoulder pain.

In cases like this, the therapist should ask about the presence of nausea, unexplained sweating, jaw pain or toothache, back pain, or chest discomfort or pressure. For the client with known heart disease, ask about the effect of taking nitroglycerin (men) or antacids/acid-relieving drugs (women) on their shoulder symptoms.

Vital sign and physical assessment including chest auscultation are important screening tools. See Chapter 4 for details.

Angina or Myocardial Infarction

Angina and/or myocardial infarction can appear as arm and shoulder pain that can be misdiagnosed as arthritis or other musculoskeletal pathologic conditions (see complete discussion, Chapter 6; see Figs. 6-8 and 6-9).

Look for shoulder pain that starts 3 to 5 minutes after the start of activity, including shoulder pain with isolated lower extremity motion (e.g., shoulder pain starts after the client climbs a flight of stairs or rides a stationary bicycle). If the client has known angina and takes nitroglycerin, ask about the influence of the nitroglycerin on shoulder pain.

Shoulder pain associated with myocardial infarction is unaffected by position, breathing, or movement. Because of the well-known association between shoulder pain and angina, cardiac related shoulder pain may be medically diagnosed without ruling out other causes, such as adhesive capsulitis or supraspinatus tendinitis when, in fact, the client may have both a cardiac and a musculoskeletal problem (Case Example 18-6).

Using a review of symptoms approach and a specific musculoskeletal shoulder examination, the physical therapist can screen to differentiate between a medical pathologic condition and mechanical dysfunction[8] (Case Example 18-7).

Complex Regional Pain Syndrome (CRPS)

Complex regional pain syndrome (CRPS, types I and II) characterized by chronic extremity pain following trauma is sometimes still referred to by the outdated term shoulder-hand syndrome (see Case Example, Chapter 1). Type I was formerly known as reflex sympathetic dystrophy or RSD. Type II was referred to as causalgia.

CRPS was first recognized in the 1800s as causalgia or burning pain in wounded soldiers. Similar presentations after lesser injuries were labeled as RSD.[9] Shoulder-hand syndrome was a condition that occurred after a myocardial infarct (heart attack), usually after prolonged bedrest. This condition (as it was known then) has been significantly reduced in incidence by more up-to-date and aggressive cardiac rehabilitation programs.

Today CRPS-I, primarily affecting the limbs, develops after bone fracture or other injury (even slight or minor trauma, venipuncture, or an insect bite) or surgery to the upper extremity (including shoulder arthroplasty) or lower extremity. Type I is not associated with nerve lesion, whereas Type II develops after trauma with nerve lesion.[10] CRPS-I is still associated with cerebrovascular accident (CVA), heart attack, or diseases of the thoracic or abdominal viscera that can refer pain to the shoulder and arm.

This syndrome occurs with equal frequency in either or both shoulders and, except when caused by coronary occlusion, is most common in women. The shoulder is generally involved first, but the painful hand may precede the painful shoulder.

When this condition occurs after a myocardial infarction, the shoulder initially may demonstrate pericapsulitis. Tenderness around the shoulder is diffuse and not localized to a specific tendon or bursal area. The duration of the initial shoulder stage before the hand component begins is extremely variable. The shoulder may be "stiff" for several months before the hand becomes involved, or both may become stiff simultaneously. Other accompanying signs and symptoms are usually present, such as edema, skin (trophic) changes, and vasomotor (temperature, hydrosis) changes.

Clinical Signs and Symptoms of

Complex Regional Pain Syndrome (Type 1)

Stage I (acute, lasting several weeks)

- Pain described as burning, aching, throbbing
- Sensitivity to touch
- Swelling

Continued on p. 833

CASE EXAMPLE 18-6 Strange Case of the Flu

Referral: A 53-year-old butcher at the local grocery store stopped by the physical therapy clinic located in the same shopping complex with a complaint of unusual shoulder pain. He had been seen at this same clinic several years ago for shoulder bursitis and tendinitis from repetitive overuse (cutting and wrapping meat).

Clinical Presentation: His clinical presentation for this new episode of care was exactly as it had been during the last episode of shoulder impairment. The therapist re-instituted a program of soft tissue mobilization and stretching, joint mobilization, and postural alignment. Modalities were used during the first two sessions to help gain pain control.

At the third appointment, the client mentioned feeling "dizzy and sweaty" all day. His shoulder pain was described as a constant, deep ache that had increased in intensity from a 6 to a 10 on a scale from 0 to 10. He attributed these symptoms to having the flu.

It was not until this point that the therapist conducted a screening exam and found the following red flags:

- Age
- Recent history (past 3 weeks) of middle ear infection on the same side as the involved shoulder

- Constant, intense pain (escalating over time)
- Constitutional symptoms (dizziness, perspiration)
- Symptoms unrelieved by physical therapy treatment

Result: The therapist suggested the client get a medical check-up before continuing with physical therapy. Even though the clinical presentation supported shoulder impairment, there were enough red flags and soft signs of systemic distress to warrant further evaluation.

Taking vital signs would have been a good idea.

It turns out the client was having myocardial ischemia masquerading as shoulder pain, the flu and an ear infection. He had an angioplasty with complete resolution of all his symptoms and even reported feeling energetic for the first time in years.

This is a good example of how shoulder pain and dysfunction can exactly mimic a true musculoskeletal problem—even to the extent of reproducing symptoms from a previous condition.

This case highlights the fact that we must be careful to fully assess our clients with each episode of care.

CASE EXAMPLE 18-7 Angina vs. Shoulder Pathology

Referral: A 54-year-old man was referred to physical therapy for pre-prosthetic training after a left transtibial (TT) amputation.

Past Medical History: A right transtibial amputation was done four years ago

Coronary artery disease (CAD) with coronary artery bypass graft (CABG), myocardial infarction (heart attack), and angina

Peripheral vascular disease (PVD)

Long-standing diabetes mellitus (insulin dependent ×47 years)

Gastroesophageal reflux disease (GERD)

Clinical Presentation: At the time of the initial evaluation for the left TT amputation, the client reported substernal chest pain and left upper extremity pain with activity. Typical anginal pain pattern was described as subster-

nal chest pain. The pain occurs with exertion and is relieved by rest.

Arm pain has never been a part of his usual anginal pain pattern. He reports his arm pain began 10 months ago with intermittent pain starting in the left shoulder and radiating down the anterior-medial aspect of the arm, halfway between the shoulder and the elbow.

The pain is made worse by raising his left arm overhead, pushing his own wheelchair, and using a walker. He was not sure if the shoulder pain was caused by repetitive motions needed for mobility or by his angina. The shoulder pain is relieved by avoiding painful motions. He has not received any treatment for the shoulder problem.

CASE EXAMPLE 18-7   Angina vs. Shoulder Pathology—cont'd

Vital Signs: Heart rate   88 bpm
              Blood pressure   120/66 mm Hg
                               (position and
                               extremity, not
                               recorded)

              Respirations   WNL

Vital Signs after transfer and pregait activities:
              Heart rate   92 bpm
              Blood pressure   152/76 mm Hg
              Respirations   "Minimal
                               shortness of
                               breath"
                               recorded

Neuro screen: WNL
Special Tests: Yergason's sign: Positive
                Apprehension test: Positive
                Relocation test: Positive
                Speed's test: Positive

Palpation of the biceps and supraspinatus tendons increased the client's shoulder pain.

Active Range of Motion (Left shoulder)
                Flexion   100°
                Abduction   70°
                I/E Rotation   60°

There is a capsular pattern in the left glenohumeral joint with limitations in rotation and adduction. Significant capsular tightness is demonstrated with passive or physiologic motions (joint play) of the humerus on the glenoid.

Manual Muscle Test (gross)
                Bilateral UE   4/5 (throughout
                                 available
                                 active ROM)

Review of Systems: Dyspnea, fatigue, sweats with pain; when grouped together, these three symptoms fall under the Cardiovascular category; these do not occur at the same time as the shoulder pain.

- **How can you differentiate between medical pathology and mechanical dysfunction as the cause of this client's shoulder pain?**

- **Is a medical referral advised?**
  1. Complete special tests for shoulder impingement, tendonitis, and capsulitis as demonstrated.
  2. Assess for trigger points; eliminate trigger points and reassess symptoms.
  3. Carry out a Review of Systems to identify clusters of systemic signs and symptoms. In

this case, a small cluster of cardiovascular symptoms were identified.
  4. Correlate symptoms from Review of Systems with shoulder pain (i.e., Do the associated signs and symptoms reported occur along with the shoulder pain or do these two sets of symptoms occur separately from each other?).
  5. Assess the effect of using just the lower extremities on shoulder pain; this was difficult to assess given this client's status as a bilateral amputee without a prosthetic device on the left side.

Result: Test results point to an untreated biceps and supraspinatus tendinitis. This tendinitis combined with adhesive capsulitis most likely accounted for the left shoulder pain. This assessment was based on the decreased left glenohumeral active range of motion and decreased joint mobility.

With objective clinical findings to support a musculoskeletal dysfunction, medical referral was not required. There were no indications that the shoulder pain was a signal of a change in the client's anginal pattern.

Left shoulder impairments were limiting factors in his mobility and rehabilitation process. Shoulder intervention to alleviate pain and to improve upper extremity strength were included in the plan of care. The desired outcome was to improve transfer and gait activities.

Left shoulder pain resolved within the first week of physical therapy intervention. This gain made it possible to improve ambulation from 3 feet to 50 feet with a walker while wearing a right lower extremity prosthesis.

The client gained independence with bed mobility and supine-to-sit transfers. The client continued to make improvements in ambulation, range of motion, and functional mobility.

Physical therapy intervention for the shoulder impairments had a significant impact on the outcomes of this client's rehab program. By differentiating and treating the shoulder movement dysfunction, the intervention enabled the client to progress faster in the transfer and gait training program than he would had his left shoulder pain been attributed to angina.[8]

- Muscle spasm
- Stiffness, loss of motion and function
- Skin changes (warm, red, dry skin changes to cold (cyanotic), sweaty skin)
- Accelerated hair growth (usually dark hair in patches)

Stage II (subacute, lasting 3 to 6 months)

- Severity of pain increases
- Swelling may spread; tissue goes from soft to boggy to firm
- Muscle atrophy
- Skin becomes cool, pale, bluish, sweaty
- Nail bed changes (cracked, grooved, ridges)
- Bone demineralization (early onset of osteoporosis)

Stage III (chronic, lasting more than 6 months)

- Pain may stay same, improve, or get worse; variable
- Irreversible tissue damage
- Muscle atrophy and contractures
- Skin becomes thin and shiny
- Nails are brittle
- Osteoporosis

Thoracic Outlet Syndrome (see discussion, Chapter 17)

Compression of the neurovascular bundle consisting of the brachial plexus and subclavian artery and vein (see Fig. 17-10) can cause a variety of symptoms affecting the arm, hand, shoulder girdle, neck, and chest. Risk factors and clinical presentation are discussed more completely in Chapter 17 (Case Example 18-8).

Bacterial Endocarditis

The most common musculoskeletal symptom in clients with bacterial endocarditis is arthralgia, generally in the proximal joints. The shoulder is affected most often, followed (in declining incidence) by the knee, hip, wrist, ankle, metatarsophalangeal and metacarpophalangeal joints, and by acromioclavicular involvement.

Most clients with endocarditis related arthralgias have only one or two painful joints, although some may have pain in several joints. Painful symptoms begin suddenly in one or two joints, accompanied by warmth, tenderness, and redness. One helpful clue: as a rule, morning stiffness is not as prevalent in clients with endocarditis as in those with rheumatoid arthritis or polymyalgia rheumatica.

Pericarditis

The inflammatory process accompanying pericarditis may result in an accumulation of fluid in the pericardial sac, preventing the heart from expanding fully. The subsequent chest pain of pericarditis (see Fig. 3-9) closely mimics that of a myocardial infarction because it is substernal, is associated with cough, and may radiate to the shoulder. It can be differentiated from myocardial infarction by the pattern of relieving and aggravating factors.

For example, the pain of a myocardial infarction is unaffected by position, breathing, or movement, whereas the chest and shoulder pain associated with pericarditis may be relieved by kneeling with hands on the floor, leaning forward, or sitting upright. Pericardial pain is often made worse by deep breathing, swallowing, or belching.

Aortic Aneurysm

Aortic aneurysm appears as sudden, severe chest pain with a tearing sensation (see Fig. 3-10), and the pain may extend to the neck, shoulders, lower back, or abdomen but rarely to the joints and arms, which distinguishes it from a myocardial infarction.

Isolated shoulder pain is not associated with aortic aneurysm; shoulder pain occurs when the primary pain pattern radiates up and over the trapezius and upper arm(s) (see Fig. 6-11). The client may report a bounding or throbbing pulse (heart beat) in the abdomen. Risk factors and other associated signs and symptoms help distinguish this condition.

▲ SCREENING FOR GASTROINTESTINAL CAUSES OF SHOULDER PAIN

Upper abdominal or gastrointestinal problems with diaphragmatic irritation can refer pain to the ipsilateral shoulder. Peptic ulcer, gallbladder disease, and hiatal hernia are the most likely GI causes of shoulder pain seen in the physical therapy clinic. Usually there are associated signs and symptoms such as nausea, vomiting, anorexia, melena, or early satiety but the client may not connect the shoulder pain with GI upset. A few screening questions may be all that is needed to uncover any coincident GI symptoms.

The therapist should look for a history of previous ulcer, especially in association with the use of

Referral: A 44-year-old female referred herself to physical therapy for a two-month long history of right upper trapezius and right shoulder pain. She works as a house painter and thinks the symptoms came on after a difficult job with high ceilings.

She reports new symptoms of dizziness when getting up too fast from bed or from a chair. She is seeing a chiropractor and a naturopathic physician for a previous back injury 2 years ago when she fell off a ladder.

She wants to try physical therapy since she has reached a "plateau" with her chiropractic care.

Past Medical History: Other significant past medical history includes a total hysterectomy 4 years ago for unexplained heavy menstrual bleeding. She does not smoke or use tobacco products, but admits smoking marijuana occasionally and being a "social drinker" (wine coolers and beer on the weekends or at barbeques).

She is nulliparous (never pregnant). She is not on any medications except ibuprofen as needed for headaches. She takes a variety of nutritional supplements given to her by the naturopath. No recent history of infections or illness.

Clinical Presentation: There is no numbness or tingling anywhere in her body. No changes in vision, balance, or hearing. The client reports normal bowel and bladder function.

Postural screen:	Moderate forward head position, rounded shoulders, arms held in a position of shoulder internal rotation, minimal lumbar lordosis
Neuro screen:	WNL
TMJ screen:	Negative
Vertebral artery tests:	Negative
Upper extremity ROM:	Limited right shoulder internal rotation; all other motions in both UEs were full and pain free
Spurling's test:	Negative
Cervical spine mobility test:	Restriction of the left C45; no apparent cervical instabilities; tenderness along the entire right cervical spine with mild hypertonus
Trigger Points:	Positive for right sternocleidomastoid, right upper trapezius, and right levator scapula TrPs

Are there any red flags to suggest the need to screen for medical disease?

What other tests (if any) would you like to do before making this decision?

- Age
- Unexplained dizziness
- Failure to progress with chiropractic care
- Surgical menopause and nulliparity (both increase her risk for breast cancer; early menopause puts her at risk for osteoporosis and accelerated atherosclerosis/heart disease)

Assessment: It is likely the client's symptoms are directly related to postural overuse. Long hours with her arms overhead may be contributing factors. A more complete exam for thoracic outlet syndrome is warranted. Physical therapy intervention can be initiated, but must be reevaluated on an on-going basis. Eliminating the trigger points, improving her posture, and restoring full shoulder and neck motion will aid in the differential diagnosis.

The therapist should assess vital signs including blood pressure measurements in both arms (looking for a vascular component of thoracic outlet syndrome) and from supine to sit to stand to assess for postural orthostatic hypotension. True postural hypotension must be accompanied by both blood pressure and pulse rate changes.

Depending on the results, medical evaluation may be warranted, especially if no underlying cause can be found for the dizziness. Although there is no reported visual changes or loss of balance with the dizziness, a vestibular screening examination is warranted.

Given her age and risk factors, she should be asked when her last physical exam was done. If she has not been seen since her hysterectomy or within the last 12 months, she should be advised to see her personal physician for follow-up.

She should be encouraged to exercise on a regular basis (more education can be provided depending on her level of knowledge and the therapist's level of expertise in this area).

If baseline bone density studies have not been done, then she should pursue this now. Likewise, she should ask her doctor about baseline testing for thyroid, glucose, and lipid values if these are not already available.

In a primary care practice, risk factor assessment is a key factor in knowing when to carry out a screening evaluation. Patient education about personal health choices is also essential.

In any practice we must know what impact medical conditions can have on the neuromuscular and musculoskeletal systems and watch for any links between the visceral and the somatic systems.

nonsteroidal antiinflammatory drugs (NSAIDs). Shoulder pain that is worse 2 to 4 hours after taking the NSAID is a yellow flag. With a true musculoskeletal problem, peak NSAID dosage (usually 2 to 4 hours after ingestion; variable with each drug) should reduce or alleviate painful shoulder symptoms. Any pain increase instead of decrease may be a symptom of GI bleeding.

The therapist must also ask about the effect of eating on shoulder pain. If eating makes shoulder pain better or worse (anywhere from 30 minutes to 2 hours after eating), there may be a gastrointestinal problem. The client may not be aware of the link between these two events until the therapist asks. If the client is not sure, follow up at a future appointment and ask again if the client has noticed any unusual symptoms or connection between eating and shoulder pain.

SCREENING FOR LIVER AND BILIARY CAUSES OF SHOULDER PAIN

As with many of the organ systems in the human body, the hepatic and biliary organs (liver, gallbladder, and common bile duct) can develop diseases that mimic primary musculoskeletal lesions. The musculoskeletal symptoms associated with hepatic and biliary pathologic conditions are generally confined to the midback, scapular, and right shoulder regions. These musculoskeletal symptoms can occur alone (as the only presenting symptom) or in combination with other systemic signs and symptoms. Fortunately, in most cases of shoulder pain referred from visceral processes, shoulder motion is not compromised and local tenderness is not a prominent feature.

Diagnostic interviewing is especially helpful when clients have avoided medical treatment for so long that shoulder pain caused by hepatic and biliary diseases may in turn create biomechanical changes in muscular contractions and shoulder movement. These changes eventually create pain of a biomechanical nature.[11]

Referred shoulder pain may be the only presenting symptom of hepatic or biliary disease. Sympathetic fibers from the biliary system are connected through the celiac and splanchnic plexuses to the hepatic fibers in the region of the dorsal spine. These connections account for the intercostal and radiating interscapular pain that accompanies gallbladder disease (see Fig. 9-10). Although the innervation is bilateral, most of the biliary fibers reach the cord through the right splanchnic nerves, producing pain in the right shoulder.

SCREENING FOR RHEUMATIC CAUSES OF SHOULDER PAIN

A number of systemic rheumatic diseases can appear as shoulder pain, even as unilateral shoulder pain. The HLA-B27–associated spondyloarthropathies (diseases of the joints of the spine), such as ankylosing spondylitis, most frequently involve the sacroiliac joints and spine. Involvement of large central joints, such as the hip and shoulder, is common, however.

Rheumatoid arthritis and its variants likewise frequently involve the shoulder girdle. These systemic rheumatic diseases are suggested by the details of the shoulder examination, by coincident systemic complaints of malaise and easy fatigability, and by complaints of discomfort in other joints either coincidental with the presenting shoulder complaint or in the past.

Other systemic rheumatic diseases with major shoulder involvement include polymyalgia rheumatica and polymyositis (inflammatory disease of the muscles). Both may be somewhat asymmetric but almost always appear with bilateral involvement and impressive systemic symptoms.

SCREENING FOR INFECTIOUS CAUSES OF SHOULDER PAIN

The most likely infectious causes of shoulder pain in a physical therapy practice include infectious (septic) arthritis (see discussion, Chapter 3; see also Box 3-6), osteomyelitis, and infectious mononucleosis (mono). Immunosuppression for any reason puts people of all ages at risk for infection (Case Example 18-9).

Osteomyelitis (bone infection) is caused most commonly by Staphylococcus aureus. Children under 6 months of age are most likely to be affected by Haemophilus influenzae or Streptococcus. Hematogenous spread from a wound, abscess, or systemic infection (e.g., tuberculosis, urinary tract infection, upper respiratory infection) occurs most often. Osteomyelitis of the spine is associated with injection drug use.

Onset of clinical signs and symptoms is usually gradual in adults but may be more sudden in children with high fever, chills, and inability to bear weight through the affected joint. In all ages there is marked tenderness over the site of the infection when the affected bone is superficial (e.g., spinous

CASE EXAMPLE 18-9 Osteomyelitis

Referral: SC, an active 62-year-old cardiac nurse, was referred by her orthopedic surgeon for "PT [for] possible rotator cuff tear (RCT)," three times a week for four weeks." SC reported an "open" MRI was negative for RCT and plain films were also negative. She noted that laboratory testing was not done.

Past Medical History

Medications: Current medications included Motrin 800 mg tid for pain; Decadron 0.75 mg qid for atypical dermatitis and asthma (45-year use of corticosteroids); Avapro 75 mg qid to control hypertension; Hydrodiuril 25 mg qid to counteract fluid retention from corticosteroids; and Chlor-Trimeton 12 mg qid to suppress the high level of blood histamine resulting from the long-term comorbid condition of atypical dermatitis and asthma.

Social History: The client consumes one glass of wine per day, quit smoking in 1961, and has never done illicit drugs.

Clinical Presentation

Pain Pattern: The client presented with primary complaints of severe and limiting pain of nearly four weeks duration with any active movement at her left (L) shoulder and at rest. Her pain was rated on the visual analog scale (VAS) as 7/10 at rest and 9/10 to 10/10 with motion at glenohumeral (GH) joint. Pain onset was gradual over a 3-day period; she was not aware of injury or trauma.

She reported an inability to: (1) use her left upper extremity (UE); (2) lie on or bear weight on left side; (3) perform activities of daily living (ADLs); (4) sleep uninterrupted due to pain, awakening 4 or 5 times nightly; or (5) participate in regular weekly Yoga classes.

Vital Signs: Temperature: 37 degrees C (98.6 degrees F); Blood pressure: 120/98 mm Hg. SC reported that her medication combination of Decadron and Chlor-Trimeton had been implicated in the past by her physician as acting to suppress low-grade fevers.

Observation: Slight puffiness, minimal swelling, observed in the left supraclavicular area. SC holds left upper extremity at her side with the elbow flexed to 90 degrees and the shoulder held in internal rotation.

Standing posture: Forward head position with increased cervical spine lordosis and tho-racic spine kyphosis, with an inability to attain neutral or reverse either spinal curve.

Palpation revealed exquisite tenderness at distal clavicle and both anterior and posterior aspects of proximal humerus.

Cervical spine screen: Spurling's compression, distraction, and Quadrant testing were all negative; deep tendon reflexes at C5, C6, and C7 were symmetrically increased bilaterally; dermatomal testing was WNL; myotomes could not be reliably tested due to pain.

Special tests at the shoulder could not be performed or were unreliable due to pain limitation.

Range of Motion: Left GH joint AROM and PROM were severely limited. AROM: Unable to actively perform flexion or abduction at left shoulder. PROM lf left shoulder (measured in supine with arm at side and elbow flexed to 90 degrees):

Flexion:	35 degrees
Abduction:	35 degrees
Internal rotation:	50 degrees
External rotation:	-10 degrees

All ranges were pain limited with an "empty" end feel.

Evaluation/Assessment: SC's signs, symptoms, and examination findings were consistent with those of a severe, full-thickness RCT, including severity of pain and functional loss with empty end-feel at GH joint ROM. However, the inability to obtain results of special test results at the shoulder limited the certainty of the RCT diagnosis.

Red flags included age over 50, severe loss of motion with empty end feel, constancy and severity of pain, inability to relieve pain or obtain a comfortable position, bony tenderness, and insidious onset of the condition. Additional risk factors included long-term use of corticosteroids to treat atypical dermatitis with asthma.

Based on the objective examination findings, including swelling, bone tenderness, along with the severity and unrelenting nature of her pain, the presence of a more serious underlying systemic medical condition was considered (in addition to a possible unconfirmed RCT).

Associated Signs and Symptoms: SC denied a fever, chills, night sweats, pain in other

process, distal femur, proximal tibia). The most reliable way to recognize infection is the presence of both local and systemic symptoms.

Mononucleosis is a viral infection that affects the respiratory tract, liver, and spleen. Splenomegaly with subsequent rupture is a rare but serious cause of left shoulder pain (Kehr's sign). There is usually left upper abdominal pain and, in many cases, trauma to the enlarged spleen (e.g., sports injury) is the precipitating cause in an athlete with an unknown or undiagnosed case of mono. Palpation of the upper left abdomen may reveal an enlarged and tender spleen (Fig. 4-50).

The virus can be present 4 to 10 weeks before any symptoms develop so the person may not know mono is present. Acute symptoms can include sore throat, headache, fatigue, lymphadenopathy, fever, myalgias, and, sometimes, skin rash. Enlarged tonsils can cause noisy breathing or difficulty breathing. When asking about the presence of other associated signs and symptoms (current or recent past), the therapist may hear a report of some or all of these signs and symptoms.

▶ SCREENING FOR ONCOLOGIC CAUSES OF SHOULDER PAIN

A past medical history of cancer anywhere in the body with new onset of back or shoulder pain is a red flag finding. Brachial plexus radiculopathy can occur in either or both arms with cancer metastasized to the lymphatics (Case Example 18-10).

Questions about visceral function are relevant when the pattern for malignant invasion at the

---

CASE EXAMPLE 18-9   Osteomyelitis—cont'd

joints or bones, weight loss, abdominal pain, nausea or vomiting.

Outcomes: The client made very little progress after the prescribed physical therapy intervention. The severity of pain and functional loss remained unchanged. Numerous attempts were made by the client and the therapist to discuss this case with the referring physician. The client eventually referred herself to a second physician.

Result: The client was diagnosed with osteomyelitis as a result of a repeat MRI and a triple-phase bone scan, and laboratory test results of elevated levels of ESR and CRP values. A surgical biopsy confirmed the diagnosis. She underwent three different surgical procedures culminating in a total shoulder arthroplasty (TSA) along with repair of the full-thickness RCT.

West PR: Case report presented in fulfillment of DPT 910, Institute for Physical Therapy Education, Widener University, Chester, Pennsylvania, 2005. Used with permission.

---

shoulder emerges. Invasion of the upper humerus and glenoid area by secondary malignant deposits affects the joint and the adjacent muscles (Case Example 18-11).

Muscle wasting is greater than expected with arthritis and follows a bizarre pattern that does not conform to any one neurologic lesion or any one muscle. Localized warmth felt at any part of the scapular area may prove to be the first sign of a malignant deposit eroding bone. Within 1 or 2 weeks after this observation, a palpable tumor will have appeared, and erosion of bone will be visible on x-ray films.[2]

Primary Bone Neoplasm

Bone cancer occurs chiefly in young people, in whom a causeless limitation of movement of the shoulder leads the physician to order x-rays. If the tumor originates from the shaft of the humerus, the first symptoms may be a feeling of "pins and needles" in the hand, associated with fixation of the biceps and triceps muscles and leading to limitation of movement at the elbow (Case Example 18-12).

Pulmonary (Secondary) Neoplasm

Occasionally the client requires medical referral because shoulder pain is referred from metastatic lung cancer. When the shoulder is examined, the client is unable to lift the arm beyond the horizontal position. Muscles respond with spasm that limits joint movement.

If the neoplasm interferes with the diaphragm, diaphragmatic pain (C3, C4, C5) is often felt at the

CASE EXAMPLE 18-10   Upper Extremity Radiculopathy

Referral: A 72-year-old woman was referred to physical therapy by her neurologist with a physician's diagnosis of "nerve entrapment" for a postural exercise program and home traction. She was experiencing symptoms of left shoulder pain with numbness and tingling in the ulnar nerve distribution. She had a moderate forward head posture with slumped shoulders and loss of height from known osteoporosis.

Past Medical History: The woman's past medical history was significant for right breast cancer treated with a radical mastectomy and chemotherapy 20 years ago. She had a second cancer (uterine) 10 years ago that was considered separate from her previous breast cancer.

Clinical Presentation: The physical therapy examination was consistent with the physician's diagnosis of nerve entrapment in a classic presentation. There were significant postural components to account for the development of symptoms. However, the therapist palpated several large masses in the axillary and supraclavicular fossa on both the right and left sides. There was no local warmth, redness, or tenderness associated with these lesions. The therapist requested permission to palpate the client's groin and popliteal spaces for any other suspicious lymph nodes. The rest of the examination findings were within normal limits.

Associated Signs and Symptoms: Further questioning about the presence of associated signs and symptoms revealed a significant disturbance in sleep pattern over the last 6 months with unrelenting shoulder and neck pain. There

were no other reported constitutional symptoms, skin changes, or noted lumps anywhere. Vital signs were unremarkable at the time of the physical therapy evaluation.

Result: Returning this client to her referring physician was a difficult decision to make since the therapist did not have the benefit of the medical records or results of neurologic examination and testing. Given the significant past medical history for cancer, the woman's age, presence of progressive night pain, and palpable masses, no other reasonable choice remained. When asked if the physician had seen or felt the masses, the client responded with a definite "no."

There are several ways to approach handling a situation like this one, depending on the physical therapist's relationship with the physician. In this case the therapist had never communicated with this physician before. A telephone call was made to ask the clerical staff to check the physician's office notes (the client had provided written permission for disclosure of medical records to the therapist).

It is possible that the physician was aware of the masses, knew from medical testing that there was extensive cancer, and chose to treat the client palliatively. Since there was no indication of such, the therapist notified the physician's staff of the decision to return the client to the MD. A brief (one-page) written report summarizing the findings was given to the client to hand-carry to the physician's office.

Further medical testing was performed, and a medical diagnosis of lymphoma was made.

---

shoulder at each breath (at the fourth cervical dermatome [i.e., at the deltoid area]), in correspondence with the main embryologic derivation of the diaphragm. Pain arising from the part of the pleura that is not in contact with the diaphragm is also brought on by respiration but is felt in the chest.

Although the lung is insensitive, large tumors invading the chest wall set up local pain and cause spasm of the pectoralis major muscle, with consequent limitation of elevation of the arm. If the neoplasm encroaches on the ribs, stretching the muscle attached to the ribs leads to sympathetic spasm of the pectoralis major. By contrast, the

scapula is mobile, and a full range of passive movement is present at the shoulder joint.

Pancoast's Tumor

Pancoast's tumors of the lung apex usually do not cause symptoms while confined to the pulmonary parenchyma. Shoulder pain occurs if they extend into the surrounding structures, infiltrating the chest wall into the axilla. Occasionally, brachial plexus involvement (eighth cervical and first thoracic nerve) presents with radiculopathy.

This nerve involvement produces sharp neuritic pain in the axilla, shoulder, and subscapular area on the affected side, with eventual atrophy of the

upper extremity muscles. Bone pain is aching, is exacerbated at night, and is a cause of restlessness and musculoskeletal movement.[12]

Usually general associated systemic signs and symptoms are present (e.g., sore throat, fever, hoarseness, unexplained weight loss, productive cough with blood in the sputum). These features are not found in any regional musculoskeletal disorder, including such disorders of the shoulder.

For example, a similar pain pattern caused by trigger points of the serratus anterior can be differentiated from neoplasm by the lack of true neurologic findings (indicating trigger point) or by lack of improvement after treatment to eliminate the trigger point (indicating neoplasm).

Breast Cancer

Breast cancer or breast cancer recurrence is always a consideration with upper quadrant pain or shoulder dysfunction (Case Example 18-13). The therapist must know what to look for as red flags for cancer recurrence versus delayed effects of cancer treatment. See Chapter 13 for a complete discussion of cancer screening and prevention. Breast cancer is discussed in Chapter 17.

▶ SCREENING FOR GYNECOLOGIC CAUSES OF SHOULDER PAIN

Shoulder pain as a result of gynecologic conditions is uncommon, but still very possible. Occasionally a client may present with breast pain as the

---

CASE EXAMPLE 18-11 Shoulder and Leg Pain

Referral: A 33-year-old woman came to a physical therapy clinic located inside a large health club. She reported right shoulder and right lower leg pain that is keeping her from exercising. She could walk, but had an antalgic gait secondary to pain on weight bearing.

She linked these symptoms with heavy household chores. She could think of no other trauma or injury. She was screened for the possibility of domestic violence with negative results.

Past Medical History: There was no past history of disease, illness, trauma, or surgery. There were no other symptoms reported (e.g., no fever, nausea, fatigue, bowel or bladder changes, sleep disturbance).

Clinical Presentation: The right shoulder and right leg were visibly and palpably swollen. Any and all (global) motions of either the arm or the leg were painful. The skin was tender to light touch in a wide band of distribution around the painful sites. No redness or skin changes of any kind were noted.

Pain prevented strength testing or assessment of muscle weakness. There was no sign of scoliosis. Trendelenburg test was negative, bilaterally. Functionally, she was able to climb stairs and walk, but these and other activities (e.g., exercising, biking, household chores) were limited by pain.

How do you screen this client for systemic or medical disease?

You may have done as much screening as is possible. Pain is limiting any further testing. Assessing vital signs may provide some helpful information.

She has denied any past medical history to link with these symptoms. Her age may be a red flag in that she is young. Bone pain with these symptoms in a 33-year old is a red flag for bone pathology and needs to be investigated medically.

Immediate medical referral is advised.

Result: X-rays of the right shoulder showed complete destruction of the right humeral head consistent with a diagnosis of metastatic disease. X-rays of the right leg showed two lytic lesions. There was no sign of fracture or dislocation. CT scans showed destructive lytic lesions in the ribs and ilium.

Additional testing was performed including lab values, bone biopsy, mammography, and pelvic ultrasonography. The client was diagnosed with bone tumors secondary to hyperparathyroidism.

A large adenoma was found and removed from the left inferior parathyroid gland. Medical treatment resulted in decreased pain and increased motion and function over a period of 3 to 4 months. Physical therapy intervention was prescribed for residual muscle weakness.

Data from Insler H, et al: Shoulder and leg pain in a 33-year old woman, *Journal of Musculoskeletal Medicine* 14(6)36-37, 1997.

CASE EXAMPLE 18-12   Osteosarcoma

Referral: A 14-year-old boy presented to a physical therapist at a sports-medicine clinic with a complaint of left shoulder pain that had been present off and on for the last four months. There was no reported history of injury or trauma despite active play on the regional soccer team.

Past Medical History: He has seen his pediatrician for this on several occasions. It was diagnosed as "tendinitis" with the suggestion to see a physical therapist of the family's choice. No x-rays or other diagnostic imaging was performed to date. The client could not remember if any laboratory work (blood or urinalysis) had been done.

The client reports that his arm feels "heavy." Movement has become more difficult just in the last week. The only other symptom present was intermittent tingling in the left hand. There is no other pertinent medical history.

Clinical Presentation: Physical examination of the shoulder revealed moderate loss of active motion in shoulder flexion, abduction, and external rotation with an empty end feel and pain during passive range of motion. There was no pain with palpation or isometric resistance of the rotator cuff tendons. Gross strength of the upper extremity was 4/5 for all motions.

There was a palpable firm, soft, but fixed mass along the lateral proximal humerus. The client reported it was "tender" when the therapist applied moderate palpatory pressure. The client was not previously aware of this lump.

Upper extremity pulses, deep tendon reflexes, and sensation were all intact. There were no observed skin changes or palpable temperature changes. Since this was an active athlete with left shoulder pain, screening for Kehr's sign was carried out but was apparently negative.

What are the red flags?

- Age
- Suspicious palpable lesion (likely not present at previous medical evaluation)
- Lack of medical diagnostics
- Unusual clinical presentation for tendinitis with loss of motion and empty end feel but intact rotator cuff

Result: The therapist telephoned the physician's office to report possible changes since the physician's last examination. The family was advised by the doctor's office staff to bring him to the clinic as a walk-in the same day. X-rays showed an irregular bony mass of the humeral head and surrounding soft tissues. The biopsy confirmed a diagnosis of osteogenic sarcoma. The cancer had already metastasized to the lungs and liver.

CASE EXAMPLE 18-13   Breast Cancer

Referral: A 53-year-old woman with severe adhesive capsulitis was referred to a physical therapist by an orthopedic surgeon. A physical therapy program was initiated. When the client's shoulder flexion and abduction allowed for sufficient movement to place the client's hand under her head in the supine position, ultrasound to the area of capsular redundancy before joint mobilization was added to the treatment protocol.

During the treatment procedure the client was dressed in a hospital gown wrapped under the axilla on the involved side. With the client in the supine position, the upper outer quadrant of breast tissue was visible and the physical therapist observed skin puckering (peau d'orange) accompanied by a reddened area.

Result: It is always necessary to approach situations like this one carefully to avoid embarrassing or alarming the client. In this case the therapist casually observed, "I noticed when we raised your arm up for the ultrasound that there is an area of your skin here that puckers a little. Have you noticed any changes in your armpit, chest, or breast areas?"

Depending on the client's response, follow up questions should include asking about distended veins, discharge from the nipple, itching of the skin or nipple, and the approximate time of the client's last breast examination (self-examination and physician examination). Although not all therapists are trained to perform a clinical breast exam (CBE), palpation of lymph nodes and muscles such as the pectoral muscle groups can be performed.

There was no previous history of cancer, and further palpation did not elicit any other suspicious findings. The physical therapist recommended a physician evaluation, and a diagnosis of breast cancer was made.

primary complaint, but most often the description is of shoulder or arm, neck, or upper back pain. When asked if the client has any symptoms anywhere else in the body, breast pain may be mentioned.

Pain patterns associated with breast disease along with a discussion of various breast pathologies are included in Chapter 17. Many of the breast conditions discussed (e.g., tumors, infections, myalgias, implants, lymph disease, trauma) can refer pain to the shoulder either alone or in conjunction with chest and/or breast pain. Shoulder pain or dysfunction in the presence of any of these conditions as part of the client's current or past medical history raises a red flag.

Ectopic Pregnancy

The therapist must be aware of one other gynecologic condition commonly associated with shoulder pain: ectopic (tubal) pregnancy. This type of pregnancy occurs when the fertilized egg implants in some other part of the body besides inside the uterus. It may be inside the fallopian tube, inside the ovary, outside the uterus or even within the lining of the peritoneum (see Fig. 15-6).

If the condition goes undetected, the embryo grows too large for the confined space. A tear or rupture of the tissue around the fertilized egg will occur. An ectopic pregnancy is not a viable pregnancy and cannot result in a live birth. This condition is life threatening and requires immediate medical referral.

The most common symptom of ectopic pregnancy is a sudden, sharp or constant one-sided pain in the lower abdomen or pelvis lasting more than a few hours. The pain may be accompanied by irregular bleeding or spotting after a light or late menstrual period.

Shoulder pain does not usually occur alone without preceding or accompanying abdominal pain, but shoulder pain can be the only presenting symptom with an ectopic pregnancy. When these two symptoms occur together (either alternating or simultaneously), the woman may not realize the abdominal and shoulder pain are connected. She may think there are two separate problems. She may not see the need to tell the therapist about the pelvic or abdominal pain, especially if she thinks it is menstrual cramps or gas. In addition, ask about the presence of lightheadedness, dizziness, or fainting.

The most likely candidate for an ectopic pregnancy is a woman in the childbearing years who is sexually active. Pregnancy can occur when using any form of birth control, so do not be swayed into thinking the woman cannot be pregnant because she is on the pill or some other form of contraception. Factors that put a woman at increased risk for an ectopic pregnancy include

• History of endometriosis
• Pelvic inflammatory disease (PID)
• Previous ectopic pregnancy
• Ruptured ovarian cysts or ruptured appendix
• Tubal surgery

Many of these conditions can also cause pelvic pain and are discussed in greater detail in Chapter 15. If the therapist suspects a gynecologic basis for the client's symptoms, some additional questions about past history, missed menses, shoulder pain, and spotting or bleeding may be helpful.

▶ PHYSICIAN REFERRAL

Here in the last chapter of the text there are no new guidelines for physician referral that have not been discussed in the previous chapters. The therapist must remain alert to yellow (caution) or red (warning) flags in the history, clinical presentation, and ask about associated signs and symptoms.

When symptoms seem out of proportion to the injury, or they persist beyond the expected time of healing, medical referral may be needed. Likewise pain that is unrelieved by rest or change in position or pain/symptoms that do not fit the expected mechanical or neuromusculoskeletal pattern should serve as red flag warnings. A past medical history of cancer in the presence of any of these clinical presentation scenarios may warrant consultation with the client's physician.

Guidelines for Immediate Medical Attention

• Presence of suspicious or aberrant lymph nodes, especially hard, fixed nodes in a client with a previous history of cancer
• Clinical presentation and history suggestive of an ectopic pregnancy

Clues to Screening Shoulder/Upper Extremity Pain

• See also Clues to Differentiating Chest Pain, Chapter 17
• Simultaneous or alternating pain in other joints, especially in the presence of associated signs and symptoms such as easy fatigue, malaise, fever
• Urologic signs and symptoms

- Presence of hepatic symptoms, especially when accompanied by risk factors for jaundice
- Lack of improvement after treatment, including trigger point therapy
- Shoulder pain in a woman of childbearing age of unknown cause associated with missed menses (**rupture of ectopic pregnancy**)
- Left shoulder pain within 24 hours of abdominal surgery, injury, or trauma (**Kehr's sign, ruptured spleen**)

Past Medical History

- History of rheumatic disease
- History of diabetes mellitus (**adhesive capsulitis**)
- "Frozen" shoulder of unknown cause in anyone with coronary artery disease, recent history of hospitalization in coronary care or intensive care unit, status post-coronary artery bypass graft (**CABG**)
- Recent history (past 1-3 months) of myocardial infarction (**chronic regional pain syndrome** [CRPS]; formerly reflex sympathetic dystrophy [RSD])
- History of cancer, especially breast or lung cancer (**metastasis**)
- Recent history of pneumonia, recurrent upper respiratory infection, or influenza (**diaphragmatic pleurisy**)

Cancer

- Pectoralis major muscle spasm with no known cause; limited active shoulder flexion but with full passive shoulder motions and mobile scapula (**neoplasm**)
- Presence of localized warmth felt over the scapular area (**neoplasm**)
- Marked limitation of movement at the shoulder joint
- Severe muscular weakness and pain with resisted movements

Cardiac

- Exacerbation by exertion unrelated to shoulder movement (e.g., using only the lower extremities to climb stairs or ride a stationary bicycle)
- Excessive, unexplained coincident diaphoresis
- Shoulder pain relieved by leaning forward, kneeling with hands on the floor, sitting upright (**pericarditis**)
- Shoulder pain accompanied by dyspnea, toothache, belching, nausea, or pressure behind the sternum (**angina**)

- Shoulder pain relieved by nitroglycerin (men) or antacids/acid-relieving drugs (women) (**angina**)
- Difference of 10 mm Hg or more in blood pressure in the affected arm compared to the uninvolved or a symptomatic arm (**dissecting aortic aneurysm, vascular component of thoracic outlet syndrome**)

Pulmonary

- Presence of a pleuritic component such as a persistent, dry, hacking, or productive cough; blood-tinged sputum; chest pain; musculoskeletal symptoms are aggravated by respiratory movements
- Exacerbation by recumbency despite proper positioning of the arm in neutral alignment (**diaphragmatic or pulmonary component**)
- Presence of associated signs and symptoms (e.g., tachypnea, dyspnea, wheezing, hyperventilation)
- Shoulder pain of unknown cause in older adults with accompanying signs of confusion or increased confusion (**pneumonia**)
- Shoulder pain aggravated by the supine position may be an indication of mediastinal or pleural involvement. Shoulder or back pain alleviated by lying on the painful side may indicate autosplinting (**pleural**).

Gastrointestinal

- Coincident nausea, vomiting, dysphagia; presence of other gastrointestinal complaints such as anorexia, early satiety, epigastric pain or discomfort and fullness, melena
- Shoulder pain relieved by belching or antacids and made worse by eating
- History of previous ulcer, especially in association with the use of nonsteroidal antiinflammatory drugs

Gynecologic

- Shoulder pain preceded or accompanied by one-sided lower abdominal or pelvic pain in a sexually active woman of reproductive age may be a symptom of **ectopic pregnancy**; there may be irregular bleeding or spotting after a light or late menstrual period.
- Shoulder pain with reports of lightheadedness, dizziness, or fainting in a sexually active woman of reproductive age (**ectopic pregnancy**)

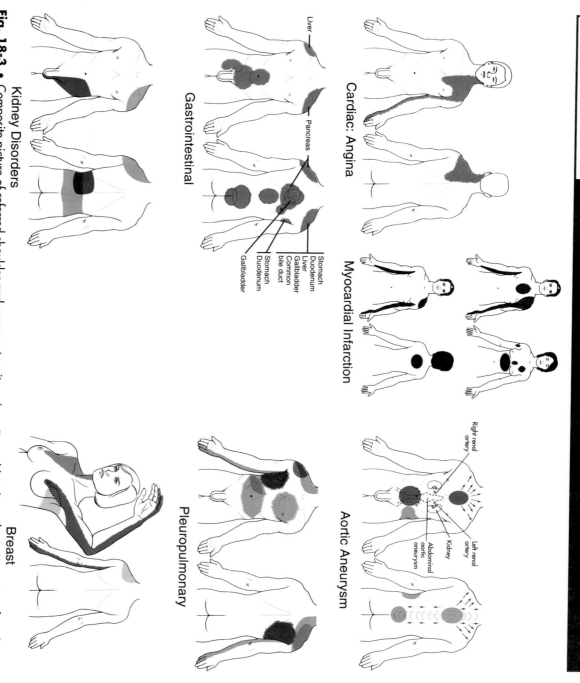

OVERVIEW **REFERRED SHOULDER AND UPPER EXTREMITY PAIN PATTERNS**

Cardiac: Angina

Myocardial Infarction

Gastrointestinal

Liver

Pancreas

Stomach
Duodenum
Liver
Gallbladder
Common
bile duct
Stomach
Duodenum

Gallbladder

Aortic Aneurysm

Right renal
artery

Left renal
artery

Abdominal
aortic
aneurysm

Kidney

Pleuropulmonary

Kidney Disorders

Breast

Fig. 18-3 • Composite picture of referred shoulder and upper extremity pain patterns. Not pictured: trigger point referred pain (see Fig. 17-7).

✓ KEY POINTS TO REMEMBER

✓ Shoulder dysfunction can look like a true neuromuscular or musculoskeletal problem and still be viscerogenic or systemic in origin.

✓ Any adult over age 65 presenting with shoulder pain and/or dysfunction must be screened for systemic or viscerogenic origin of symptoms, even when there is a known (or attributed) cause or injury.

✓ Knowing the key red flags for cancer, vascular disease, pulmonary, GI and gynecologic causes of shoulder pain and/or dysfunction will help the therapist screen quickly, efficiently, and accurately.

✓ Painless weakness of insidious onset is most likely a neurologic problem; painful, insidious weakness may be caused by cervical radiculopathy, chronic rotator cuff problems, tumors, or arthritis. A medical differential diagnosis is required.[13]

✓ As mentioned throughout this text, the therapist can collaborate with colleagues in asking questions and

reviewing findings before making a medical referral. Perhaps someone else will see the answer or a solution to the client's unusual presentation. Or perhaps another opinion will confirm the findings and give you the confidence you need to guide your professional decision making.

✓ Postoperative infection of any kind may not appear with any clinical signs/symptoms for weeks or months, especially in a client who is on corticosteroids or immunocompromised.

✓ Consider unreported trauma or assault as a possible etiologic cause of shoulder pain.

✓ Palpate the diaphragm and assess breathing patterns; shoulder pain reproduced by diaphragmatic palpation may point to a primary diaphragmatic (muscular) problem.

SUBJECTIVE EXAMINATION

Special Questions to Ask: Shoulder and Upper Extremity

General Systemic

• Does your pain ever wake you at night from a sound sleep? **(Cancer)** Can you find any way to relieve the pain and get back to sleep?

If yes, how? **(Cancer:** pain is usually intense and constant; nothing relieves it or if relief is obtained in any way, over time pain gets progressively worse)

• Have you sustained any injuries in the last week during a sports activity, car accident, etc? **(Ruptured spleen associated with pain in the left shoulder: positive Kehr's sign)**

• Since the beginning of your shoulder problem, have you had any unusual perspiration for no apparent reason, sweats, or fever?

• Have you had any unusual fatigue (more than usual with no change in lifestyle), joint pain in other joints, or general malaise? **(Rheumatic disease)**

• *For the therapist:* Has the client had a laparoscopy in the last 24 to 48 hours? **(Left shoulder pain: positive Kehr's sign)**

Cardiac

• Have you recently (ever) had a heart attack? **(Referred pain via viscerosomatic zones,** see explanation Chapter 3)

• Do you ever notice sweating, nausea, or chest pain when the pain in your shoulder occurs?

• Have you noticed your shoulder pain increasing with exertion that does not necessarily cause you to use your shoulder (e.g., climbing stairs, stationary bicycle)?

• Do(es) your mouth, jaw, or teeth ever hurt when your shoulder is bothering you? **(Angina)**

• For the client with known angina: Does your shoulder pain go away when you take nitroglycerin? (Ask about the effect of taking antacids/acid-relieving drugs for women.)

Pulmonary

• Have you been treated recently for a lung problem (or think you have any lung or respiratory problems)?

• Do you currently have a cough?
   If yes, is this a smoker's cough?
   If no, how long has this been present?

SUBJECTIVE EXAMINATION—cont'd

Is this a productive cough (can you bring up sputum), and is the sputum yellow, green, black, or tinged with blood?

Does coughing bring on your shoulder pain (or make it worse)?

- Do you ever have shortness of breath, have trouble catching your breath, or feel breathless?
- Does your shoulder pain increase when you cough, laugh, or take a deep breath?
- Do you have any chest pain?
- What effect does lying down or resting have on your shoulder pain? (In the supine or recumbent position, a pulmonary problem may be made worse, whereas a musculoskeletal problem may be relieved; on the other hand, pulmonary pain may be relieved when the client lies on the affected side, which diminishes the movement of that side of the chest.)

Gastrointestinal

- Have you ever had an ulcer?
  If yes, when? Do you still have any pain from your ulcer?
  Have you noticed any association between when you eat and when your symptoms increase or decrease?
- Does eating relieve your pain? **(Duodenal or pyloric ulcer)**
  How soon is the pain relieved after eating?
- Does eating aggravate your pain? **(Gastric ulcer, gallbladder inflammation)**
- Does your pain occur 1 to 3 hours after eating or between meals? **(Duodenal or pyloric ulcers, gallstones)**
- Fo the client taking NSAIDs: Does your shoulder pain increase 2 to 4 hours after taking your NSAIDs? If the client does not know, ask him or her to pay attention for the next few days to the response of shoulder symptoms after taking the medication.
- Have you ever had gallstones?
- Do you have a feeling of fullness after only one or two bites of food? **(Early satiety: stomach and duodenum or gallbladder)**

- Have you had any nausea, vomiting, difficulty in swallowing, loss of appetite, or heartburn since the shoulder started bothering you?

Gynecologic

- Have you ever had a breast implant, mastectomy, or other breast surgery? **(Altered lymph drainage, scar tissue)**
- Have you ever had a tubal or ectopic pregnancy?
- Have you ever been diagnosed with endometriosis?
- Have you missed your last period? **(Ectopic pregnancy, endometriosis; blood in the peritoneum irritates diaphragm causing referred pain)**
- Are you having any spotting or irregular bleeding?
- Have you had any spontaneous or induced abortions recently? **(Blood in peritoneum irritating diaphragm)**
- Have you recently had a baby? **(Excessive muscle tension during birth)**
  If yes: Are you breastfeeding with the infant supported on pillows?
  Do you have a breast discharge, or have you had mastitis?

Urologic

- Have you had any recent kidney infections, tumors, or kidney stones? **(Pressure from kidney on diaphragm referred to shoulder)**

Trauma

- Have you been in a fight or been assaulted?
- Have you ever been pulled by the arm, pushed against the wall, or thrown by the arm?
  If the answer is "Yes" and the history relates to the current episode of symptoms, then the therapist may need to conduct a more complete screening interview related to domestic violence and assault. Specific questions for this section have been discussed in Chapter 2; see also Appendix B-3.

CASE STUDY

STEPS IN THE SCREENING PROCESS

If a client comes to you with shoulder pain with any of the red flag histories and/or red flag clinical findings to suggest screening, start by asking yourself these questions:

- Which shoulder is it?
- Which organs could it be? (Use Fig. 3-4 showing the viscera in relation to the diaphragm and Tables 18-1 and 18-2 to help you.)
- What are the associated signs and symptoms of that organ? Are any of these signs or symptoms present?
- What is the history? Does anything in the history correlate with the particular shoulder involved and/or with the associated signs and symptoms? Conduct a Review of Systems as discussed in Chapter 4 (see Box 4-17).
- Can you palpate it, make it better or worse, or reproduce it in any way?

COULD IT BE CANCER?

Remember, the therapist does not make a determination as to whether or not a client has cancer. The therapist's assessment determines whether the client has a true neuromuscular or musculoskeletal problem that is within the scope of our practice. However, knowing red flags for the possibility of cancer helps the therapist know what questions to ask and what red flags to look for. Watch for

- Previous history of cancer (any kind, but especially breast or lung cancer)
- Pectoralis major muscle spasm with no known cause, but full passive ROM and a mobile scapula. Be sure to assess for trigger points (TrPs). Reassess after trigger point therapy. Were the symptoms alleviated? Did the movement pattern change?
- Conduct a neurologic screening exam.
- Shoulder flexion and abduction limited to 90° with empty end feel.
- Presence of localized warmth over scapular area. Look for other trophic changes.

COULD IT BE VASCULAR?

Watch for

- Exacerbation by exertion unrelated to shoulder movements

Does the shoulder pain and/or symptoms get worse when the client is just using the lower extremities? What is the effect of riding a stationary bike or climbing stairs without using the arms?

- Excessive, unexplained coincident diaphoresis (i.e., the client breaks out in a cold sweat just before or during an episode of shoulder pain. This may occur at rest, but is more likely with mild physical activity).
- Shoulder pain relieved by leaning forward, kneeling with hands on the floor, sitting upright (pericarditis).
- Shoulder pain accompanied by dyspnea, temporomandibular joint (TMJ) pain, toothache, belching, nausea, or pressure behind the sternum.
- Bilateral shoulder pain that comes on after using the arms overhead for 3 to 5 minutes.
- Shoulder pain relieved by nitroglycerin (men) or antacids/acid-relieving drugs (women) [angina]
- Difference of 10 mm Hg or more (at rest) in diastolic blood pressure in the affected arm (aortic aneurysm; vascular component of thoracic outlet syndrome)

Remember to correlate any of these symptoms with

- Client's past medical history (e.g., personal and/or family history of heart disease)
- Age (over 50, especially postmenopausal women)
- Characteristics of pain pattern (see Table 6-5; these characteristics of cardiac related chest pain can also apply to cardiac-related shoulder pain)

COULD IT BE PULMONARY?

- Ask about the presence of pleuritic component
  - Persistent cough (dry or productive)
  - Blood-tinged sputum; rust, green or yellow exudate
  - Chest pain
  - Musculoskeletal symptoms are aggravated by respiratory movements; ask the client to take a deep breath. Does this reproduce or increase the pain/symptoms?
- Watch for the exacerbation of symptoms by recumbence even with proper positioning of the arm. Lying down in the supine position can put the shoulder in a position of slight extension. This can put pressure on soft tissue structures in and around the shoulder, causing pain in the presence of a true neuromuscular or musculoskeletal problem.

CASE STUDY—cont'd

- For this reason, when assessing the affect of recumbence, make sure the shoulder is in a neutral position. You may have to support the upper arm with a towel roll under the elbow and/or put a pillow on the client's abdomen to give the forearms a place to rest.

- Pain is relieved or made better by side lying on the involved side. This is called autosplinting. Pressure on the rib cage prevents respiratory movement on that side thereby reducing symptoms induced by respiratory movements. This is quite the opposite of a musculoskeletal or neuromuscular cause of shoulder pain; the client often cannot lie on the involved side without increased pain.

- Ask about the presence of associated signs and symptoms. Remember to ask our final question: Are there any symptoms of any kind anywhere else in your body?

  In the older adult, listen for a self-report or family report of unknown cause of shoulder pain/dysfunction and/or any signs of confusion (confusion or increased confusion is a common first symptom of pneumonia in the older adult).

COULD IT BE GASTROINTESTINAL (GI) OR HEPATIC?

- Ask about a history of chronic (more than six months) NSAID use and history of previous ulcer, especially in association with NSAID use. This is the most common cause of medication-induced shoulder pain in all ages, but especially adults over 65.

- History of other GI disease that can refer pain to the shoulder such as:
  - Gallbladder
  - Acute pancreatitis
  - Reflex esophagitis

- Watch for coincident (or alternating) nausea, vomiting, dysphagia, anorexia, early satiety, or other GI symptoms. Clients often think they have two separate problems. The client may not think the therapist treating the shoulder needs or wants to know about their GI problems. The therapist who is not trained to screen for medical disease may not think to ask.

- Ask if shoulder pain is relieved by belching or antacids. This could signal an underlying GI problem or for women, cardiac ischemia.

- Look for shoulder pain that is changed by eating (better or worse within 30 minutes or worse 1-3 hours after eating).

  The therapist does not have to identify the specific area of the GI tract that is involved or the specific pathology present. It is important to know that true neuromusculoskeletal shoulder pain is not relieved or exacerbated by eating.

  If there is a peptic ulcer in the upper GI tract causing referred pain to the shoulder, there is often a history of NSAID use. This client will have that red flag history along with shoulder pain that gets better after eating. There may also be other GI symptoms present such as nausea, loss of appetite, or melena from oxidized blood in the upper GI tract.

  If there is liver impairment as well, there can be symptoms of carpal tunnel syndrome (CTS). For a list of possible neuromusculoskeletal and systemic causes of CTS, see Table 11-2. Again, CTS in the presence of any of these systemic conditions should be assessed carefully. Likewise, CTS may be the first symptom of some of these pathologies.

  The client with shoulder pain (GI bleed) and symptoms of CTS (liver impairment) may demonstrate other signs of liver impairment such as:
  - Liver flap (asterixis)
  - Liver palms (palmar erythema)
  - Nail bed changes (white nails of Terry)
  - Spider angiomas (over the abdomen)

  These tests along with photos and illustrations are discussed in detail in Chapter 9.

COULD IT BE BREAST PATHOLOGY?

Remember that men can have breast diseases, too although not as often as women. Red flag clinical presentation and associated signs and symptoms of breast disease referred to the shoulder may include:

- Jarring or squeezing the breast refers pain to the shoulder
- Resisted shoulder motions do not reproduce shoulder pain but do cause breast pain or discomfort
- Obvious change in breast tissue (e.g., lump(s), dimpling or peau d'orange, distended veins, nipple discharge or ulceration, erythema, change in size or shape of the breast)
- Suspicious or aberrant axillary or supraclavicular lymph nodes

PRACTICE QUESTIONS

1. A 66-year-old woman has been referred to you by her physiatrist for preprosthetic training after an above-knee amputation. Her past medical history is significant for chronic diabetes mellitus (insulin dependent), coronary artery disease with recent angioplasty and stent placement, and peripheral vascular disease. During the physical therapy evaluation, the client experienced anterior neck pain radiating down the left arm. Name (and/or describe) three tests you can do to differentiate a musculoskeletal cause from a cardiac cause of shoulder pain.

2. Which of the following would be useful information when evaluating a 57-year-old woman with shoulder pain?
   a. Influence of antacids on symptoms
   b. History of chronic NSAID use
   c. Effect of food on symptoms
   d. All of the above

3. Referred pain patterns associated with impairment of the spleen can produce musculoskeletal symptoms in:
   a. The left shoulder
   b. The right shoulder
   c. The mid- or upper back, scapular, and right shoulder areas
   d. The thorax, scapulae, right or left shoulder

4. Referred pain patterns associated with hepatic and biliary pathology can produce musculoskeletal symptoms in:
   a. The left shoulder
   b. The right shoulder
   c. The mid or upper back, scapular, and right shoulder areas
   d. The thorax, scapulae, right or left shoulder

5. The most common sites of referred pain from systemic diseases are:
   a. Neck and hip
   b. Shoulder and back
   c. Chest and back
   d. None of the above

6. A 28-year-old mechanic reports bilateral shoulder pain (right more than left) whenever he has to work on a car on a lift overhead. It goes away as soon as he puts his arms down. Sometimes he has numbness and tingling in his right elbow going down the inside of his forearm to his thumb. The most likely explanation for this pattern of symptoms is:
   a. Angina
   b. Myocardial ischemia
   c. Thoracic outlet syndrome
   d. Peptic ulcer

7. A client reports shoulder and upper trapezius pain on the right that increases with deep breathing. How can you tell if this results from a pulmonary or a musculoskeletal cause?
   a. Symptoms get worse when lying supine, but better when right sidelying when it is pulmonary
   b. Symptoms get worse when lying supine, but better when right sidelying when it is musculoskeletal

8. Organ systems that can cause simultaneous bilateral shoulder pain include:
   a. Spleen
   b. Heart
   c. Gallbladder
   d. None of the above

9. A 23-year-old woman was a walk-in to your clinic with sudden onset of left shoulder pain. She denies any history of trauma and has only a past history of a ruptured appendix three years ago. She is not having any abdominal pain or pain anywhere else in her body. How do you know if she is at risk for ectopic pregnancy?
   a. She is sexually active and is late for her period
   b. She has a history of uterine cancer
   c. She has a history of peptic ulcer
   d. None of the above

10. The most significant red flag for shoulder pain secondary to cancer is:
    a. Previous history of coronary artery disease
    b. Subscapularis trigger point alleviated with trigger point therapy
    c. Negative neurologic screening exam
    d. Previous history of breast or lung cancer

REFERENCES

1. Neer CS: Anterior acromioplasty for the chronic impingement syndrome in the shoulder: a preliminary report, *JBJS* 54(1):41-50, 1972.

2. Cyriax J: *Textbook of orthopaedic medicine*, ed 8, Baltimore, 1982, Williams and Wilkins.

3. Mennell JM: *Joint pain: diagnosis and treatment using manipulative techniques*, Boston, 1964, Little, Brown.

4. Connolly JF: Unfreezing the frozen shoulder, *J Musculoskel Med* 15(11):47-56, 1998.

5. Sadikot RT, Rogers JT, Cheng D-S, et al: Pleural fluid characteristics of patients with symptomatic pleural effusion after coronary artery bypass graft surgery, *Arch Internal Med* 160(17):2665-2668, 2000.

6. Mennell JM: *The musculoskeletal system: differential diagnosis from symptoms and physical signs*, Sudbury, MA, 1992, Jones and Bartlett.

7. Hadler NM: The patient with low back pain, *Hospital Practice*, October 30, 1987, pp 17-22.

8. Smith ML: Differentiating angina and shoulder pathology pain, *Phys Ther Case Rep* 1(4):210-212, 1998.

9. Oaklander AL, Rissmiller JG, Gelman LB, et al: Evidence of focal small-fiber axonal degeneration in complex regional pain syndrome-I (reflex sympathetic dystrophy). *Pain* 120(3):235-243, 2006.

10. Jänig W, Baron R: Is CRPS I a neuropathic pain syndrome? *Pain* 120(3):227-229, 2006.

11. Rose SJ, Rothstein JM: Muscle mutability: general concepts and adaptations to altered patterns of use, *Phys Ther* 62:1773, 1982.

12. Cailliet R: *Shoulder pain*, ed 3, Philadelphia, 1991, FA Davis.

13. McFarland EG, Sanguanjit P, Tasaki A, et al: Shoulder examination: established and evolving concepts. *J Musculoskel Med* 23(1):57-64, 2006.

Answers for Practice Test Questions

Chapter 1 Introduction to Screening for Referral in Physical Therapy

1. (b) The function of a diagnosis and diagnostic classifications is to provide information (i.e., identify as closely as possible the underlying neuromusculoskeletal [NMS] pathology) that can guide efficient treatment and effective management of the client.

2. False—See Box 1-1.

3. (b)

4. (c)

5. (b)

6. (e)

7. (a)

8. A yellow flag is a cautionary or warning symptom that signals, "Slow down, and think about the need for screening." A red flag symptom requires immediate attention, either to pursue further screening questions or tests, or to make an appropriate referral. The presence of a single yellow or red flag is not usually cause for immediate medical attention. Each cautionary or warning flag must be viewed in the context of the whole person, given his or her age, gender, past medical history, and current clinical presentation.

9. Past medical history, risk factor assessment, clinical presentation (including pain types and pain patterns), associated signs and symptoms, review of systems. Each client can be framed by these five components. Any suspicious finding or response in any of these areas warrants a closer look.

10. Check your list against Box 1-2; see also Appendix A-2.

Chapter 2 Introduction to the Interviewing Process

1. (b) Nonsteroidal antiinflammatory drugs (NSAIDs) can be potent renal vasoconstrictors that cause increased blood pressure and resultant lower extremity edema as sodium and water are conserved by the body.

2. (a) Although all details obtained from the Family/Personal History form, interview, and objective examinations provide important information, it is well documented that 80% (or more) of the information needed to determine the cause of symptoms is actually gathered during the Core Interview of the Subjective Examination.

3. Any of the following questions (or similar questions) is appropriate:

- Are any other symptoms of any kind anywhere else in your body that we haven't discussed yet?
- Is there anything else you think is important about your condition that we have not discussed yet?
- Is there anything else you think I should know?

4. (b) Antidepressants

Antidepressants are divided into three groups: tricyclics, monoamine oxidase inhibitors (MAOIs), and miscellaneous antidepressants. The tricyclics work by blocking reuptake of norepinephrine and serotonin into nerve endings and increasing the action of norepinephrine and serotonin in nerve cells. Any of the antidepressants can have gastrointestinal adverse effects, but especially, the selective serotonin uptake inhibitors (SSRIs) such as Paxil, Zoloft, Prozac, and Celexa.

5. (c)

6. (a) True

7. (d)

8. True. This includes any woman who has experienced a surgical menopause (e.g., oophorectomy for ovarian cancer) or any postmenopausal woman who is not taking hormone replacements.

9. (e)

All of these are red flags, along with previous history of cancer, symptoms that last longer than expected (beyond physiologic time period for healing), age, gender, comorbidities, bilateral symptoms, other constitutional symptoms, unexplained falls, substance use/abuse, unusual vital signs, and constant and intense pain; see also Appendix A-2.

10. The first question should always be, "Did you actually see your physician?" Then ask questions directed at assessing for the presence of constitutional symptoms. For example, after paraphrasing what the client has told you, ask, "Are you having any other symptoms of any kind in your body that you haven't mentioned?" If no, ask more specifically about the presence of associated signs and symptoms, including naming constitutional symptoms one by one. Follow up with Special Questions for Men (see Appendix B-21).

11. (d) Water retention. Look for sacral and pedal edema.

12. (c) Inform the primary care provider of both conditions; the therapist can also screen for

...potential adverse effects of NSAIDs and can monitor blood pressure.

10. (a) True. Visceral involvement can occur without preceding or prodromal symptoms, but most often, associated signs and symptoms are present. Because visceral pain can be referred to the neck, back, or shoulder, the client who experiences gastrointestinal (GI) or genitourinary (GU) symptoms does not report these additional symptoms to the therapist when providing information about the musculoskeletal condition.

11. (d) Irritation of the retroperitoneal space begins when bleeding occurs behind the stomach, most often from a posterior duodenal ulcer. Rupture of the spleen causes Kehr's sign. The pancreas and low back structures are not formed from the same embryologic tissue. Disease of the pancreas, whether it involves the head, the body, or the tail, can put pressure on the corresponding portion of the respiratory diaphragm, resulting in shoulder or low back pain according to the location of the diaphragmatic irritation. Central diaphragmatic pressure results in referred pain to the ipsilateral shoulder; peripheral involvement of the diaphragm results in low back pain. This can occur in the right shoulder when the head of the pancreas is distended far enough, but it is more likely to affect the left shoulder via disease in the tail of the pancreas.

involved side and applying pressure to that area. Gallbladder pain is sometimes relieved by leaning forward. Cardiac pain brought on by use of the upper extremities overhead may be relieved by bringing the arms back down to the sides.

13. (b) It may not be necessary to screen every client for alcohol use. You may not conduct a full screening assessment when someone appears to have been drinking, but it may still be appropriate to ask, "I smell alcohol on your breath. How many drinks have you had?" Screening questions should be asked privately and confidentially without other family and friends listening.

Chapter 3 Pain Types and Viscerogenic Pain Patterns

1. (b)

2. (a) Pain that wakes a client up as soon as he or she rolls onto that side is indicative of an acute inflammatory process. Night pain associated with neoplasm is more likely to wake the client up after he or she falls asleep, when the tumor keeps normal tissue from obtaining essential blood and nutrients, thus creating tissue ischemia and subsequent pain. With chronic musculoskeletal conditions, the client can often get to sleep with just the right positioning and may even be able to sleep on that side for up to an hour or two before pressure and ischemia develop, causing pain.

3. (a) Left shoulder pain associated with damage or injury to the spleen is called Kehr's sign.

4. (a) True. See Table 3-2.

5. (b) Throbbing, pounding, and beating are more often associated with pain of a vascular nature. Aching, heavy, and sore are words used to describe musculoskeletal pain. According to the McGill Pain Questionnaire, words like agonizing, piercing, and unbearable convey more emotional content than is communicated by actual descriptors of organic disease. See Table 3-1; see also Fig. 3-11.

6. (a) Neoplasm, in particular, primary bone cancer.

7. (e) Artificial sweeteners have come under fire, primarily by manufacturers of artificial sweeteners. Evidence supplied by two prominent board certified neurosurgeons (see text) combined with the author's own clinical experience is sufficient to include this agent as a causative factor in joint pain.

8. (a) Bone pain would be accompanied by a positive heel strike test. Symptoms of angina are sometimes relieved by antacids in women. Even if bone pain were caused by metastases from the GI tract, eating would not alleviate the symptoms.

9. (b) False. Some types of viscerogenic pain can be relieved by a change in position early in the disease process. For example, pain from an inflammatory or infectious process that affects the kidney may be reduced by leaning toward the...

Chapter 4 Physical Assessment as a Screening Tool

1. (c) Percussion and palpation can change bowel sounds. Look and listen before you palpate.

2. (a)

3. (c)

4. (c)

5. First of all, do you need to? How far out from the first medical diagnosis and final treatment is the client? Is the client still being treated? Without laboratory values, physical assessment becomes much more important. Check vital signs; observe the skin, eyes, and nailbeds, and ask about the presence of associated signs and symptoms.

6. We confess this is a bit of a "trick" question. Thoughts on this topic vary. Some therapists advocate taking each client's body temperature (answer "e") as one of the simplest and most inexpensive ways to screen for the presence of systemic problems. Others are more selective in the screening process and advise answer "d" (b and c) as the most appropriate response. The decision may depend, in part, on the type of practice or...

clinical setting in which you practice. For the new graduate, it is highly recommended that all vital signs be taken on all clients until the therapist is proficient in this skill area. With experience, each clinician will develop the decision-making skills needed to determine when additional screening, and which screening tests, should be carried out.

7. Bruits are abnormal blowing or swishing sounds heard on auscultation of narrowed or obstructed arteries. Bruits with both systolic and diastolic components suggest the turbulent blood flow of partial arterial occlusion that is possible with aneurysm or vessel constriction.

The therapist is most likely to assess for bruits when the client or patient is older than 65 years of age and describes problems (i.e., neck, back, abdominal, or flank pain) in the presence of a history of syncopal episodes, a history of cardiovascular disease (CVD), serious risk factors for CVD, or a previous history of aortic aneurysm. Look for other signs of peripheral vascular disease that may account for the client's current symptoms.

Symptoms may be described as "throbbing" and may increase with activity and decrease with rest. In the most likely candidate, neck or back pain is not affected by physical therapy intervention. The client is an older adult, a postmenopausal woman, and/or has significant risk factors for CVD or a history of CVD.

8. (d) You may decide to conduct additional tests and provide the information to the physician. This should include a review of past medical history, current medications, and any pharmaceuticals she may be taking, as well as any other symptoms present but unnoticed or unreported. Carry out a screening interview using Special Questions for Joint Pain (see Appendix B-16).

9. Yes. The therapist must be familiar with past medical history and any factors that could put the client at risk for a medical incident of any type. Health status can change for any client within a 2-week period, but especially, the aging adult. Surgery is a major event that is traumatic to the physiologic body, despite the client's previous excellent health. Surgery can trigger the onset of new health problems or may bring to fulmination something that was present only subclinically before the operation. Some postoperative complications do not develop until 10 to 14 days later. Exercise is an additional physiologic stressor. Symptoms may not be seen when the client is at rest or sedentary and may occur only after exercise has been initiated.

Time pressure and the complexities of today's health care delivery system can also result in conditions remaining unnoticed by the examining health care professional. Systemic diseases often develop slowly and gradually over time. It is not until the disease has progressed enough that the client shows any signs and symptoms of visceral or systemic involvement. What the physician, physician's assistant, nurse, or nurse practitioner observed preoperatively may not be the clinical presentation seen by the therapist postoperatively.

10. Bad breath (halitosis) can be a symptom of diabetic ketoacidosis, dental decay, lung abscess, throat or sinus infection, or gastrointestinal disturbance from food intolerance, *Helicobacter pylori* bacteria, or bowel obstruction. Keep in mind that ethnic foods and alcohol can affect breath and body odor.

After past medical history has been assessed for any of these conditions, it may be necessary for the therapist to ask directly, "I notice an unusual smell on your breath. Do you know what might be causing this?" Ask appropriate follow-up questions depending on the type of smell that you perceive. You may wish to consider screening for alcohol use at a later time, after you have established a good rapport with the client.

11. The patient's blood pressure (vasomotor) system is "untuned"; peripheral blood vessels do not constrict properly, so venous pooling may occur. The patient also may be receiving medication(s) that have the potential to reduce blood pressure directly or as an adverse effect of the drug or drugs in combination. Other factors may include dehydration, if the patient has not been on intravenous fluids and has not maintained adequate fluid intake.

Chapter 5 Screening for Hematologic Disease

1. (b)
2. (b)
3. When you live at an elevation of 3500 feet above sea level (or higher) and the client describes symptoms of unknown origin such as headache, dizziness, fatigue, and changes in sensation of the feet and hands (decreased feeling, burning, numbness, tingling, [polycythemia] or joint pain, swelling, and loss of motion [sickle cell disease])
4. (c) Platelets are affected by anticoagulant drugs, including aspirin and heparin. Platelets are important in the coagulation of blood, a necessary process during and after surgery.
5. (b)
6. Local heat applied to the involved joint(s)
7. (b)

8. (1) Trunk flexion over the hips produces severe pain in the presence of iliopsoas bleeding. Only mild pain occurs on trunk flexion over the hips for a hip hemorrhage. (2) Gently rotating the hip internally or externally causes severe pain in the presence of a hip hemorrhage but only minimal (or no) pain with iliopsoas bleeding.

9. *Nadir*, or the lowest point the white blood count reaches, usually occurs 7 to 14 days after chemotherapy or radiation therapy. At that time, the client is extremely susceptible to infection; the therapist must follow all universal precautions, especially those pertaining to good handwashing.

10. (1) Client tolerance; (2) Perceived exertion levels

Chapter 6 Screening for Cardiovascular Disease

1. (b)

2. *Myocardial ischemia* is a deficiency of blood supply to the heart muscle that is usually caused by narrowing of the coronary arteries. *Angina pectoris* is the chest pain that occurs when the heart is not receiving an adequate supply of blood, and therefore, has insufficient quantities of oxygen for the workload. *Myocardial infarction* is death of the heart tissue when blood supply to that area is interrupted.

3. Monitor vital signs, and palpate pulses. Evaluate past and current medical history for the presence of coronary artery disease. Any suspicion of thoracic aneurysm must be reported to the physician immediately. It is beyond the scope of a physical therapist's practice to suggest the possibility of an aneurysm. Rather, clinical observations should be documented and submitted to the physician. A summary comment can be made such as, "This clinical presentation is not consistent with a musculoskeletal problem. Please evaluate."

4. The three Ps include:
• Pleuritic pain (exacerbated by respiratory movement involving the diaphragm, such as sighing, deep breathing, coughing, sneezing, laughing, or the hiccups; this may be cardiac with pericarditis, or it may be pulmonary); have the client hold his or her breath, and reassess symptoms—any reduction or elimination of symptoms with breath holding or the Valsalva maneuver suggests a pulmonary or cardiac source of symptoms.
• Pain on palpation (musculoskeletal origin).
• Pain with changes in position (musculoskeletal or pulmonary origin; pain that is worse when lying down and that improves when sitting up or leaning forward is often pleuritic in origin).

5. Palpitations may be considered physiologic (i.e., "within normal limits") when they occur at a rate of less than six per minute. Palpitations lasting for hours or occurring in association with pain, shortness of breath, fainting, or severe lightheadedness require medical evaluation. Palpitations in any person with a history of unexplained sudden death in the family require medical referral. Palpitations can also occur as an adverse effect of some medications, through the use of drugs such as cocaine, as the result of an overactive thyroid, or because of caffeine sensitivity. Palpitations as a recurring symptom (even if less than six/minute) should always be reported to the physician.

6. **Past medical history/risk factors**—Personal or family history of coronary artery disease, heart disease, angina, myocardial infarction, or risk factors associated with these (see Table 6-3). Assess menstrual history: A menopausal or postmenopausal woman with a high risk for heart disease may develop symptomatic coronary artery disease.

Clinical presentation—Objective findings from the clinical evaluation do not seem consistent with temporomandibular dysfunction; assess the effect of using a stationary bicycle or treadmill (stairs or walking will also work) without upper extremity exertion on jaw pain. Increased pain or symptoms with increased lower body exertion may be a sign of cardiac involvement and should be reported to the referring dentist.

Associated signs and symptoms—Assess for coincident nausea, diaphoresis, pallor, or dyspnea during painful or symptomatic periods. Look for recent history (last 6 weeks to 6 months in onset) of shortness of breath at night, extreme fatigue, lethargy, and weakness. Ask about the presence of other body aches and pains (be alert for "heartburn" unrelieved by antacids, isolated right biceps muscle aching, and breast or chest pain). Measure vital signs for any unusual findings, and assess changes in vital signs with changes in workload during exercise.

7. The onset of myocardial infarction can be precipitated by working with the arms extended over the head. Ischemia or infarction may be the cause of this client's symptoms. Assess for history of heart disease and the presence of known hypertension, angina, past episodes of heart attack, or congestive heart failure. Assess vital signs and changes in vital signs with increased workload and assess the effect of increasing the workload of the lower extremities only.

Evaluate for thoracic outlet syndrome (TOS), especially with a cardiovascular component (see Table 17-5). Evaluate for and treat trigger

points of the chest, upper abdomen, and upper extremity.

This client should be evaluated by his physician; the therapist's information gathered from the assessment will be helpful in the medical differential diagnosis.

8. Examine this client for the presence of cyanosis, orthopnea, and tachycardia; for changes in renal function (decreased urination during the day but frequent urination at night); and for a spasmodic cough triggered by lying down or at night. These may be indicators of congestive heart failure and must be reported to the physician. Take note of whether this client is taking NSAIDs and digitalis together; this combination of medications can cause ankle swelling—a symptom that must also be reported to the physician.

9. (d) Arterial and occlusive diseases are synonymous for the same thing: Occlusion of the arteries produces arterial disease; occlusion of the veins produces venous disorders. Arteries and veins constitute the major peripheral blood vessels; therefore, any diseases or disorders of the arteries and/or veins are included in peripheral vascular disorders.

10. (c) Pain from arterial disease is relieved by dangling (not elevating) the extremity to help blood flow distally; the feet are cold and demonstrate pallor from loss of blood flow.

11. (a)

12. (c)

Chapter 7 Screening for Pulmonary Disease

1. As always, look at past medical history, risk factors, clinical presentation, and associated signs and symptoms. Ask about a past medical history (within the last 6 to 8 weeks) of upper respiratory infection, pneumonia, pleurisy, or traumatic injury.

Evaluate whether the symptoms can be reproduced with palpation or movement. Pulmonary symptoms may be exacerbated or increased by the supine position and alleviated or decreased when the patient is lying on the involved side (autosplinting).

Look for associated signs and symptoms such as fever, chills, night sweats, digital clubbing, persistent cough, or dyspnea. Examine the client for trigger points; reexamine after any trigger points have been eliminated.

2. (c)

3. In accordance with our screening model, we always take a look at past medical history, risk factors, clinical presentation, and associated signs and symptoms. This patient's age, history of tobacco use, and previous history of breast cancer are red flags and risk factors for cancer recurrence and other systemic disorders.

The following tests and measures can help the therapist to differentiate musculoskeletal from systemic origin of symptoms in this case:
• Vital signs and pulmonary auscultation
• Palpation (Can symptoms be reproduced with palpation? [Bone mets are not usually painful to palpation, whereas trigger points or impaired soft tissue structures may be painful upon palpation.]). Are the intercostal spaces symmetric? Asymmetry may be noted with rib dysfunction.
• Active and passive spinal motion (Can symptoms be reproduced, alleviated, or changed in any way with active spinal movement? Are the accessory motions within normal limits?)
• Ask about the presence of other pulmonary signs and symptoms.
• Is the pattern of symptoms consistent with a musculoskeletal disorder?

Because breast cancer can metastasize to the bone, and especially, to the thoracic spine, a neurologic screening examination may be in order, depending on the client's response to previous questions and tests.

4. (f) Pain can also radiate to the costal margins or upper abdomen (see Figs. 7-9 and 7-10).

5. False. However, medical referral is usually not considered necessary when a client presents with a singular systemic sign or symptom, especially in the presence of a clear clinical presentation of a musculoskeletal pattern.

6. (e)

7. Autosplinting occurs when lying on the involved side quiets respiratory movement and reduces or eliminates symptoms. Most musculoskeletal problems are made worse by placing this kind of pressure on the symptomatic shoulder, neck, or thoracic spine. The therapist must also evaluate the presence of associated signs and symptoms, the effect of increased respiratory movements on symptoms, and the effect of the supine position (recumbency) on shoulder/upper trapezius pain.

8. These have equal significance when viewed as part of a continuum; dyspnea that has progressed from exertional to rest is a red flag symptom. The usual progression of dyspnea is for a client to first notice shortness of breath after a specific length of time or intensity while engaging in an activity such as walking or climbing stairs. Progression to dyspnea at rest usually occurs after the client notices shortness of breath sooner and with less intensity in the activity.

Exertional dyspnea may be the result of deconditioning alone without a specific pulmonary disease. In addition, early, mild congestive heart failure may be characterized by shortness of breath at rest that is not present with exertion. In such a case, increased activity may improve results from increased activity may improve venous return enough to alleviate dyspnea with exertion. Over time, as the congestion progresses, dyspnea will increase with less provocation and will occur at rest as well as with exertion.

Either exertional dyspnea or dyspnea at rest that is out of proportion to the situation should be considered a red flag. Progression to dyspnea at rest usually occurs after the client notices shortness of breath that occurs sooner and with less intensity in the activity.

9. (b)
10. (d)

Chapter 8 Screening for Gastrointestinal Disease

1. (b) Melena
2. (a) Kehr's sign (left shoulder pain) can occur as the result of blood (e.g., following trauma to the spleen, ruptured ectopic pregnancy) or air (laparoscopy) in the abdomen. Kehr's sign following a laparoscopy will resolve within 24 to 48 hours as the gas bubble is absorbed or passed. The physician must be notified of shoulder pain associated with traumatic injury, nonsteroidal antiinflammatory drug (NSAID)-associated gastrointestinal bleeding, or possible ectopic pregnancy for possible medical evaluation (even if the clinical presentation is consistent with musculoskeletal dysfunction) (see Shoulder, Chapter 18).

3. (d)
4. (d)
5. (b)
6. Infection of the peritoneum (e.g., peritonitis, appendicitis) can cause abscess formation of the psoas (or obturator) muscle, resulting in right lower quadrant (abdominal or pelvic) pain in association with specific movements of the right leg (see Iliopsoas Muscle Test, Fig. 8-3, and Obturator Muscle Test, Fig. 8-6).

7. (b)
8. (d) Psoas abscess can affect the hip, buttock, groin, and parts distal but does not cause sacral pain; hemorrhoids and rectal fissures may cause rectal or anal pain, but not sacral pain; Crohn's disease can be accompanied by sacroiliitis, but this client does not have a reported history of Crohn's disease; narcotics are well known for constipation as a common adverse effect, especially in the older adult.

9. Using Special Questions to Ask for possible GI involvement, carefully screen for any other associated signs and symptoms. Have the client pay close attention to digestion and bowel habit patterns over the next 24 to 48 hours. Ask her to report any gastrointestinal symptoms and any changes in bowel odor, color, or consistency. Provide her with a home program to improve strength, balance, and coordination, and observe or test for functional improvement.

If she reports any additional gastrointestinal signs and symptoms, especially if no improvement in her physical status is observed, immediate medical referral is required. Otherwise, send the physician a brief note outlining your findings, your program, and any progress (or lack of progress), and include a question such as:

Dr. Smith, Mrs. Jones has had several episodes of lightheadedness. At the same time, she says her legs feel "rubbery and weak." This is not a typical musculoskeletal pattern. Is there any connection between her use of NSAIDs (she is taking a prescription NSAID and an over-the-counter NSAID daily) and this pattern of weakness?

Always remember to relay information and ask questions that demonstrate that you are practicing within the scope of physical therapy practice.

10. (a) or (d) Some physicians and physical therapists advocate taking the body temperature as part of a vital sign assessment in all clients (answer [a]). Others suggest that this may not be necessary in cases in which a clear musculoskeletal cause is noted for the clinical presentation, as well as an absence of any systemically associated signs and symptoms.

As a general guideline, vital sign assessment can provide valuable screening and overall health information. For the student and inexperienced clinician, we highly recommend this practice. For further discussion of this topic, see Chapter 4.

Chapter 9 Screening for Hepatic and Biliary Disease

1. (c) Technically, answer (b) is also correct because referred shoulder pain may be the only presenting symptom of hepatic or biliary disease. However, when the overall referral pattern is viewed, answer (b) leaves out the upper back and scapulae; answer (d) refers to the part of the body between the neck and the abdomen and includes the primary pain pattern present in the right upper quadrant but not the mid or upper back associated with the referred pain pattern. Kehr's sign—left shoulder pain associated with blood or

air in the abdominal cavity—is not part of the hepatic/biliary system.

2. Radiating pain to the mid back, scapula, and right shoulder occurs as the result of splanchnic fibers (a network of nerves innervating the viscera of the abdomen) that synapse with adjacent phrenic nerve fibers—the branch of the celiac plexus (also known as the solar plexus) that innervates the diaphragm.

The liver is innervated by the hepatic plexus, also a part of the celiac plexus (see Fig. 3-3). Interconnecting nerve fibers between the phrenic nerves and the brachial plexus then refer pain to the right shoulder. These connections occur bilaterally, but most biliary fibers reach the dorsal spinal cord through the right splanchnic nerve to produce pain primarily in the right shoulder.

3. Normally, the breakdown of protein in the gut (whether derived from food or blood in the stomach) produces ammonia that is transformed by the liver to urea, glutamine, and asparagine. These substances are then excreted by the renal system. When the liver is diseased and unable to detoxify ammonia, ammonia is transported to the brain, where it reacts with glutamate, an excitatory neurotransmitter, thus producing glutamine. Reduction in brain glutamate impairs neurotransmission, leading to altered nervous system metabolism and function. Additionally, ammonia may cause the brain to produce false neurotransmitters. The result of this ammonia abnormality is peripheral nerve disease with numbness and tingling of the hands and/or feet that can be misinterpreted as carpal/tarsal tunnel syndrome. Check also for asterixis.

4. Ask about numbness and tingling in the feet. Tarsal tunnel symptoms do not always occur with upper extremity numbness and tingling, but when both are present, a medical evaluation is required.

Ask the client about any associated signs and symptoms, especially constitutional symptoms (see Systemic Signs and Symptoms Requiring Physician Referral at the end of this chapter). Look for liver flap, liver palms, and other skin and nailbed changes.

Look for risk factors associated with liver impairment (e.g., alcohol use, hepatotoxic medications, previous history of any type of cancer).

If subjective and objective examinations do not reveal any red flags, treatment may be initiated. If treatment does not result in objective or subjective improvement, ask the client again about the development of any new symptoms, especially constitutional symptoms or other associated symptoms discussed here.

Failure to progress in treatment should result in physician evaluation or reevaluation. The development of any new systemic symptoms requires medical evaluation as well.

5. Jaundice is first noted as a yellowing of the sclerae of the eyes. The skin may take on a yellow hue as well, but this is not as easily observed as the change in the eye. This change in eye and skin color can also occur with pernicious anemia, a condition that may be accompanied by peripheral neuropathy as well.

6. Given most people's concern about their physical appearance, it is best not to point out the change in eye color directly, but rather, ask some questions that may provide you with the information needed. For example,
- Mrs. Jackson, have you ever been given a diagnosis of jaundice, hepatitis, or anemia?
- Are you experiencing any new symptoms or problems that we haven't discussed?
- Have you noticed any smells or foods that you cannot tolerate?
- Have you (or your husband) noticed any changes in your skin or eyes?
- At this point, if nothing comes to light, you may broach your observation by saying, "I have noticed some yellowing of the white part of your eye. Is this something you have noticed or discussed with your physician?"

7. (d)

8. (c) Answer (a) (decreased serum albumin) is not a good laboratory measure because serum albumin has to be severely decreased for tissue damage to occur; coagulation times is a much better indicator of potential tissue injury in a clinical setting.

9. (d)

10. (b)

11. (b) Albumin is a protein that is formed in the liver and that helps to maintain normal distribution of water in the body.

Chapter 10 Screening for Urogenital Disease

1. (d)

2. (e)

3. (d)

4. Anyone with back pain or shoulder pain of unknown origin, especially when accompanied by changes in urination, blood in the urine, or constitutional symptoms.

5. Dyspareunia—Difficult or painful sexual intercourse in women

Dysuria—Painful or difficult urination

Hematuria—Blood in the urine

Urgency—A sudden, compelling desire to urinate

6. Urge incontinence—Inability to hold back urination when one is feeling the urge to void (putting the key in the door or passing by a bathroom may trigger urine to leak)

   Stress incontinence—Involuntary escape of urine due to strain on the bladder (e.g., cough, sneeze, standing up, lifting, exercising)

7. "Skin pain" may be a sign of referred pain from the upper urinary tract because visceral sensory fibers via the autonomic nervous system and cutaneous sensory fibers via the peripheral nervous system (dermatomes) enter the spinal cord in close proximity and even converge on some of the same neurons. When visceral pain fibers are stimulated, concurrent stimulation of cutaneous fibers also occurs that is then perceived as "skin pain."

8. A physical therapist who is screening for prostate involvement must ask direct questions. A medical evaluation is necessary to identify actual prostate disease. Questions may include the following (see also Appendix B-27):

   • Are you experiencing any other symptoms of any kind? (If no, you may have to prompt with specifics: Have you had any fever or chills? Muscle or joint aches?)
   • Have you ever had any problems with your prostate in the past?
   • When you urinate, do you have trouble starting or continuing the flow of urine?
   • (Alternate questions): Has your urine stream changed in size? Do you urinate in a steady stream, or does the flow of urine start and stop?
   • Are you getting up to urinate at night? (If the answer is "yes," make sure this is something new or unusual for the client.)
   • Have you noticed any blood in your urine (or change in the color of your urine)?

9. Visceral pain is not well differentiated because innervation of the viscera is *multisegmental* with few nerve endings (see Fig. 3-3). As was previously discussed in question (7), renal/urologic pain enters the spinal cord at the same level and in close proximity to cutaneous nerves in these multiple segments (from T10 to L1). Stimulation of these renal/urologic fibers can lead to stimulation of cutaneous fibers. As a result, renal and urethral visceral pain may be felt as skin pain throughout the T10-L1 dermatomes.

10. If the diaphragm becomes irritated as the result of pressure from a distended kidney (caused by tumor, cyst, inflammation), pain can be referred via interconnections between the phrenic nerve (innervating the diaphragm) and the cervical plexus (innervating the shoulder).

Chapter 11 Screening for Endocrine and Metabolic Disease

1. Proximal muscle weakness, myalgia, carpal tunnel syndrome, periarthritis, adhesive capsulitis (shoulder) (see Table 11-1)

2. Endocrine disorders, infectious diseases, collagen disorders, cancer, liver disease (see Table 11-2).

3. Depends on the underlying disease process. For example, thickening of the transverse carpal ligament is associated with acromegaly and myxedema. Increased volume of the contents of the carpal tunnel occurs with pregnancy, neoplasm, gouty tophi deposits, and lipids in diabetes mellitus. Hormonal changes (e.g., menopause, pregnancy) can also result in carpal tunnel syndrome (CTS). See also liver-related causes in Chapter 9.

4. (f)

5. Polydipsia, polyuria, polyphagia

6. The major differentiating factor between diabetic ketoacidosis (DKA) and hyperosmolar hyperglycemic state (HHS) is the absence of ketosis in HHS.

7. Yes. If their glucose levels are high, you will not endanger them any further with a small amount of sugar, and you may help someone who is experiencing hypoglycemia associated with diabetes mellitus.

8. (a)

9. (d)

10. (d)

11. (b)

12. (a) The American Diabetes Association recommends that people with diabetes maintain a level of 7% or below on the A1C; this reflects average blood-sugar levels over a period of 2 to 3 months.

13. (d)

Chapter 12 Screening for Immunologic Disease

1. (c) Although the muscles and connective tissues are involved, the underlying cause is thought to be dysregulation of the autonomic nervous system as it interfaces with the neurohormonal system.

2. (a) Answers (b) and (c) are more characteristic of osteoarthritis (OA); rheumatoid arthritis (RA) is rarely accompanied by night pain, and advanced

structural damage is more typical of OA because RA has a tendency to "burn itself out"; answer (d) describes pain of vascular insufficiency.

3. (a) Psoriatic arthritis
   (b) Systemic lupus erythematosus (subcutaneous nodules may also occur with SLE)
   (e) HIV infection
   (d) Scleroderma
   (h) Rheumatoid arthritis
   (g) Allergic reaction (see Table 12-1)
   (f) Lyme disease
   (c) Thrombocytopenia

4. Many red flag clues must be considered. The therapist may observe or hear reports of any one or combination of the following:
   • Previous history of allergies, especially if the client has received medications over the past 6 weeks (even if the client is no longer taking the medications)
   • Recent history or presence of burning or urinary frequency (urethritis)
   • Recent history or presence of conjunctivitis or eye crusting, redness, burning, or tearing that lasts only a few days
   • Recent report or presence of skin rash, especially combined with a report of exposure to ticks
   • Positive family history for arthritis, spondyloarthropathy, psoriasis
   • Recent report of dry mouth or sore throat
   • Recent history of operative procedure
   • Other extra-articular signs or symptoms, such as diarrhea, constitutional symptoms, or other symptoms already mentioned
   • Enlarged lymph nodes

5. (c)

6. An electric shock sensation down the spine and radiating to the extremities when the neck is flexed; this is a fairly common sign in multiple sclerosis but may also accompany disc protrusion against the spinal cord.

7. (f)
8. (b)
9. (d)
10. (b) Symptoms of hives, itching, periorbital edema, and gastrointestinal involvement may occur with allergic reactions, but these do not usually require immediate medical treatment. The possible exception may include facial hives accompanied by constriction of the throat or upper respiratory symptoms (listed in answer [b]), leading to an inability to breathe.

Chapter 13 Screening for Cancer

1. Previous personal history of cancer; age in correlation with a personal or family history of cancer; age and gender in correlation with incidence of certain cancers; exposure to environmental and occupational toxins; geographic location; lifestyle (e.g., consumption of alcohol, smoking cigarettes, poor diet)

2. In any patient or client who is undergoing cancer treatment (especially chemotherapy), laboratory values offer a guide for determining appropriate frequency, intensity, and duration of exercise. In an outpatient setting, laboratory values may be unavailable or outdated. Without the benefit of laboratory values (and even when laboratory values are available), the therapist can and should monitor vital signs and rate of perceived exertion (RPE), and should look for associated signs and symptoms (e.g., pallor, dyspnea, unexplained or excessive diaphoresis, heart palpitations, visual changes, dizziness). Anything out of the ordinary should be considered a yellow (cautionary) flag that requires careful observation, further evaluation, and possibly medical referral.

3. (a)

4. In any individual, any neurologic sign may be the presentation of a silent lung tumor.

5. • Changes in bowel or bladder habits
   • A sore that does not heal within 6 weeks
   • Unusual bleeding or discharge
   • Thickening or lump in the breast or elsewhere
   • Indigestion or difficulty in swallowing
   • Obvious change in a wart or mole
   • Nagging cough or hoarseness

6. • How long have you had this area of skin discoloration/mole/spot/lump?
   • Has it changed over the past 6 weeks to 6 months?
   • Has your physician examined this area? (Alternate question: Has your physician seen this?)

7. This is a medical decision and is not within the scope of physical therapist practice. If the clinician has any doubt, the physician should be contacted. The therapist can certainly take vital signs, ask about the presence of constitutional symptoms such as fever, weight loss, nausea, vomiting, and look for and document associated signs and symptoms. All of these findings can be submitted to the physician for consideration.

8. Space-occupying lesions (whether discogenic, bony spurs in the foraminal spaces, or tumor cells invading and occupying the spaces next to nerve roots) may cause an increase in deep tendon reflexes when compression irritates the nerve but

does not obstruct the reflex arc. When any anatomic obstruction is large enough to compress the nerve and interfere with the reflex arc, the deep tendon reflex is diminished or absent.

9. Pain, movement dysfunction, and disability usually result in weight gain due to inactivity. When someone is experiencing back pain, for example, and reports a significant weight loss, this may be a red flag for systemic origin of the problem.

10. c—When tumors produce signs and symptoms at a site distant from the tumor or its metastasized sites, these "remote effects" of malignancy are collectively referred to as paraneoplastic syndromes. Paraneoplastic syndromes with musculoskeletal manifestations are of clinical importance for physical therapy because they may accompany relatively limited neoplastic growth and may provide an early clue to the presence of certain types of cancer.

11. (d) See discussion of Leukopenia in Chapter 5.

12. (b)

13. (a) See Fig. 4-31 and discussion of Beau's lines, Chapter 4.

14. (d)

15. (c)

16. (b)

17. (a)

18. (a) A history of chronic immunosuppression (e.g., antirejection drugs for organ transplants, long-term use of immunosuppressant drugs for inflammatory or autoimmune disease, cancer treatment) in the presence of this clinical presentation is a major red flag.

A painless, enlarged lymph node or skin lesion of this type, when associated with immunosuppression from organ transplantation, may be caused by lymphoma, in which case, it is followed by weakness, fever, and weight loss.

19. (d)

Chapter 14 Screening the Head, Neck, and Back

1. (b)

2. (d)

3. Back pain can be examined and classified in many ways. We have presented Sources of Back Pain (e.g., visceral, neurogenic, vasculogenic, spondylogenic, psychogenic, neoplasm; see Table 3-3) and Location of Back Pain (e.g., cervical spine, scapula, thoracic spine, lumbar spine, sacrum, sacroiliac; see Table 14-1).

4. (c) Answer (a) is not correct because pain from arterial disease is not relieved by elevating the extremity; (b) is not correct for the same reason; (d) is not correct because arterial disease is characterized by cold skin temperature and pallor caused by the lack of oxygen and blood flow to the lower extremities; venous disease is characterized by redness or warmth caused by blood that gets pooled in the lower extremities and cannot return centrally because of valve insufficiency.

5. (e) Pain associated with pulmonary disorders can occur anywhere over the lung fields (see Fig. 7-1), with the possibility of additional referral to the neck and shoulder on the involved side(s).

6. (b) Temporomandibular joint (TMJ) pain is possible with cardiac involvement but not likely with gastrointestinal disease; pain alleviated by a bowel movement usually occurs with disease of the colon, which does not refer pain to the shoulder unless massive retroperitoneal bleeding occurs, in which case, earlier symptoms of pain, bowel distention, and blood in the stools would prevail.

7. (d) A positive Murphy's percussion test for renal disease is suspected; Murphy's percussion should be negative in the presence of pain and symptoms caused by radiculitis or pseudorenal pain from any cause.

8. (d) Vascular pain is often described as "throbbing"; vascular claudication may be described as "aching" or "cramping" or "tired," but this could be caused by the aggravating factors (increases with physical exertion, promptly relieved by resting); remains unchanged regardless of the position of the spine.

Neurogenic pain may be described as hot or burning; stabbing, shooting, or tingling. Look for other neurologic changes; perform the bicycle test. Pain increased by spinal extension and relieved by spinal flexion is a positive sign of neurologic involvement.

Muscular pain is often described as dull, sore, aching, and hurting; palpate for myalgia and trigger points, and perform resistive muscle testing.

9. (a) Joint pain affects the hips, sacrum, and sacroiliac most often and may be preceded or accompanied by skin lesions or rash.

10. (a)

11. (b) Autosplinting refers to lying on one side to decrease respiratory movements; the client will use autosplinting when pain is induced by lung excursion.

12. (a) Pancreatic disease can also refer pain to the shoulder, depending on which portion of the pancreas is affected.

13. Red flags include age (over 50), previous history of cancer, and lack of pain relief with recumbency. Screening should follow the decision-making model presented in Chapter 1. Conduct a careful history of symptoms, and ask about symptoms anywhere else in the body.

Find out when the last medical follow-up was done by the oncologist and when the patient had her last clinical breast examination and mammogram. Clinical assessment should include vital signs, lymph node palpation, skin inspection that includes the mastectomy site, and a neurologic screening examination. Palpate the painful area, and perform a percussive Tap test.

Chapter 15 Screening the Sacrum, Sacroiliac, and Pelvis

1. (c) Answer (a) describes a vascular pattern; (b) describes response to vascular congestion.

2. (a)

3. (c)

4. (b) Reevaluate findings and prescribed intervention, including a screening or rescreening examination; medical referral may be the final decision after this step is taken. Answer (c) may not be the best answer because reevaluation and screening/rescreening may provide additional information that may be helpful to the physician.

5. (d) When present, McBurney's point is found approximately one-half the distance from the anterior superior iliac spine (ASIS), moving toward the umbilicus (see Fig. 8-8); if the appendix is located somewhere else, McBurney's point is likely to be negative. Blumberg's sign for rebound tenderness (see Fig. 8-10) can be used to assess for appendicitis when generalized peritonitis is present, or when the appendix is located somewhere in the abdomen other than at the end of the cecum.

6. (d)

7. (e)

8. (b)

9. (d) The sacral spring test or overpressure is contraindicated in the presence of osteoporosis; even minor trauma can result in fracture.

10. See Figs. 15-2 and 15-3.

Chapter 16 Screening the Lower Quadrant: Buttock, Hip, Groin, Thigh, and Leg

1. (a)

2. Any time you suspect an infectious or inflammatory cause of hip, groin, or pelvic symptoms. Abdominal or intraperitoneal inflammation leads to irritation and/or abscess formation of the psoas muscle, causing musculoskeletal pain. These tests are especially appropriate for the client who has a history of Crohn's disease, diverticulitis, pelvic inflammatory disease, or *Chlamydia* with a new onset of hip and/or groin pain. Combined with findings of Blumberg's rebound test and McBurney's point, the information gained can help the clinician to identify signs and symptoms of possible appendicitis.

3. (d)

4. (a)

5. (b)

6. (c)

7. (d)

8. (c) Coronary artery disease does not cause referred hip pain (it is a disease of the heart that causes angina with chest, neck, or upper extremity pain or discomfort); intermittent claudication is a symptom, not a disease; aortic aneurysm may cause low back pain that radiates into the buttock and hip.

9. (b)

10. (d)

Chapter 17 Screening the Chest, Breasts, and Ribs

1. (a) Sternocleidomastoid

2. (b) Hard, immovable, nontender

3. (a) Monitor vital signs and palpate pulses.

4. (b) Myocardial ischemia

5. (c) Exacerbated by deep breathing

6. (d) Although you can use all three of these tests, answer (a) Stair climbing or stationary bike test, is likely the most definitive of the tests listed for cardiac causes of symptoms.

7. (c) Document your findings, and contact the physician by phone or by fax while initiating treatment.

8. (a) Refer her to a physician before initiating treatment.

9. (d) All of the above

10. (d) Unusual fatigue, shortness of breath, weakness, or sleep disturbance.

Chapter 18 Screening the Shoulder and Upper Extremity

1. Orthopedic evaluation: Palpate structures of the shoulder, including trigger point assessment; perform special orthopedic tests such as Yergason's, apprehension test, relocation test, and Speed's test; perform neurologic screening

examination, including reflex testing, coordination, manual muscle testing, and sensory testing; screen for mechanical dysfunction above and below (temporomandibular joint, cervical spine, elbow).

Systemic evaluation: Assess the effects of stair climbing or stationary bicycle riding (using only the lower extremities) on shoulder pain; assess for associated signs and symptoms (e.g., dyspnea, fatigue, palpitations, diaphoresis, cough, dizziness), and perform a systems review; measure vital signs on both sides.

2. (d)

3. (a) Kehr's sign

4. (c)

5. (b)

6. (c) Thoracic outlet syndrome (TOS) is discussed more completely in Chapter 17.

7. (a)

8. (b)

9. (a)

10. (d)

Appendices

This textbook provides a step-by-step approach to client evaluation. The following appendices contain examples of forms, questionnaires, and checklists that can be used in client evaluation. The more streamlined your paperwork process is, the more time you will have to treat your clients. These appendices will provide you with some of the tools needed to screen for systemic diseases and medical conditions that can mimic neuromuscular or musculoskeletal problems.

We have also included all appendices on our Evolve web site, which will be updated on a regular basis, as well as a CD that provides MS Word and PDF documents for your use. You may customize them to suit your needs or print them on your letterhead. For the clinic, it may be beneficial for you to print several copies at one time for ease of use.

APPENDIX A SCREENING SUMMARY

The following appendices are also provided for you on the enclosed CD and can also be found on the EVOLVE website.

863

APPENDIX A-1 Quick Screen Checklist

Remember that this is not a physical therapy assessment of neuromusculoskeletal function; it is a quick screening examination as part of the overall physical therapy evaluation. Using the screening model presented in Chapter 1, include each of the following components:

- Past Medical History
- Risk Factor Assessment
- Clinical Presentation
- Associated Signs and Symptoms
- Review of Systems

The first step in making a diagnosis is to confirm (or rule out) the need for physical therapy intervention. Use this screening checklist to answer these questions:

Follow-Up Questions

- Is this an appropriate physical therapy referral?
- Is there a problem that does not fall into one of the four categories of conditions outlined by the *Guide?*
- Are there any red flag histories, red flag risk factors, or cluster of red flag signs and/or symptoms?
- And always ask: Were you examined by a (your) doctor?

▶ PAST MEDICAL HISTORY

- Previous history of (for a complete list, use Family/Personal History form; see Fig. 2–2):

Cardiovascular	Pulmonary disease
Cancer	Recent surgery
Diabetes	Trauma
Infection (any kind)	Tuberculosis

For women: pregnancy, birth, miscarriage, abortion, and other reproductive history
- Psychosocial Screen
  - Orientation (person, place, time)
  - Anxiety, depression, panic disorder
  - Recent travel overseas
  - Occupational/environmental exposure
- Medications

▶ RISK FACTORS (PARTIAL LIST)

Substance use/abuse	Alcohol use/abuse
Age	Occupation
Body mass index (BMI)	Domestic violence
Gender	Hysterectomy/ oophorectomy

Race/ethnicity	Sedentary lifestyle
Tobacco use	Exposure to radiation
Overseas travel	Multiple sexual partners

▶ CLINICAL PRESENTATION

See Guide to Physical Assessment: Appendix D-1
See Extremity Examination Checklist: Appendix D-2
See Hand and Nail Bed Assessment: Appendix D-3
See Peripheral Vascular Assessment: Appendix D-4
- General Survey
- Upper and Lower Quadrant Exam
  - Integument
  - Musculoskeletal
  - Neuromuscular
  - Cardiopulmonary
  - Genitourinary

▶ ASSOCIATED SIGNS AND SYMPTOMS

Always ask: Are there any symptoms of any kind anywhere else in your body? If no, follow-up with:

Have you had any (check all that apply):
- ☐ Blood in urine, stool, vomit, mucus
- ☐ Changes in bowel or bladder
- ☐ Confusion
- ☐ Cough
- ☐ Difficulty chewing/swallowing/speaking
- ☐ Dizziness, fainting, blackouts
- ☐ Dribbling or leaking urine
- ☐ Fever, chills, sweats (day or night)
- ☐ Headaches
- ☐ Heart palpitations or fluttering
- ☐ Joint pain
- ☐ Memory loss
- ☐ Nausea, vomiting, loss of appetite
- ☐ Numbness or tingling
- ☐ Problems seeing or hearing
- ☐ Skin rash or other changes
- ☐ Sudden weakness
- ☐ Swelling or lumps anywhere
- ☐ Trouble breathing
- ☐ Trouble sleeping
- ☐ Throbbing sensation/pain in belly or anywhere else
- ☐ Unusual fatigue, drowsiness

▼ OTHER TESTS AND MEASURES

Emotional overlay (McGill Pain Questionnaire, Symptom Magnification, Waddell's nonorganic signs); see Chapter 4

Special tests (e.g., Murphy's percussion, Obturator or Iliopsoas tests for abscess, abdominal aortic pulse, visceral palpation, auscultation of femoral bruits, Blumberg sign, clinical breast exam, or other as appropriate)

▼ FINAL STEP: PERFORM A REVIEW OF SYSTEMS

See Appendix D-5: Review of Systems

This form may be duplicated for use in clinical practice. From Goodman CC, Snyder TE: *Differential diagnosis for physical therapists: screening for referral*, ed 4, Philadelphia, Saunders, 2007.

APPENDIX A-2 Red Flags

The presence of any one of these symptoms is not cause for extreme concern, but it should raise a red flag for the alert therapist. The therapist is looking for a pattern that suggests a viscerogenic or systemic origin of pain and/or symptoms. Often, the next step is to look for associated signs and symptoms. The therapist will proceed with the screening process depending on which symptoms are grouped together.

▶ PAST MEDICAL HISTORY (PERSONAL OR FAMILY)

- Personal or family history of cancer
- Recent (last 6 weeks) infection (e.g., mononucleosis, upper respiratory infection [URI], urinary tract infection [UTI], bacterial infection such as streptococcal or staphylococcal; viral infection such as measles, hepatitis), especially when followed by neurologic symptoms 1 to 3 weeks later (Guillain-Barré syndrome), joint pain, or back pain
- Recurrent colds/flu with a cyclical pattern (i.e., the client reports that s/he just cannot shake this cold or the flu; it keeps coming back over and over)
- Recent history of trauma such as motor vehicle accident or fall (fracture; any age) or minor trauma in older adult with osteopenia/osteoporosis
- History of immunosuppression (e.g., steroids, organ transplant, HIV)
- History of injection drug use (infection)

▶ RISK FACTORS

Risk factors vary depending on family history, previous personal history, and disease, illness, or condition present. For example, risk factors for heart disease will be different from risk factors for osteoporosis or vestibular/balance problems. As with all decision-making variables, a single risk factor may or may not be significant and must be viewed in the context of the whole patient/client presentation.

Substance use/abuse   Alcohol use/abuse
Age   Occupation
Body mass index (BMI)   Domestic violence
Gender   Hysterectomy/
Race/ethnicity   oophorectomy
Tobacco use   Sedentary lifestyle

Overseas travel   Exposure to radiation
   Multiple sexual partners

▶ CLINICAL PRESENTATION

- No known cause, unknown etiology, insidious onset
- Presence of symptoms that are unrelieved by physical therapy intervention is a red flag.
- Physical therapy intervention does not change the clinical picture; client may get worse!
- Presence of symptoms that get better after physical therapy but then get worse again is also a red flag indicating the need to screen further.
- Significant weight loss/gain without effort (more than 10% of the client's body weight in 10–21 days)
- Gradual, progressive, or cyclical presentation of symptoms (worse/better/worse)
- Unrelieved by rest or change in position (no position is comfortable)
- If relieved by rest, positional change, or application of heat, these relieving factors no longer reduce symptoms in time.
- Symptoms seem out of proportion to the injury.
- Symptoms persist beyond the expected time for that condition.
- Unable to alter (provoke, reproduce, alleviate, eliminate, aggravate) the symptoms during exam
- Does not fit the expected mechanical or neuromusculoskeletal pattern
- No discernible pattern of symptoms
- A growing mass (painless or painful) is a tumor until proved otherwise; a hematoma should decrease (not increase) in size with time.
- Postmenopausal vaginal bleeding (bleeding that occurs a year or more after the last period [significance depends on whether the woman is on hormone replacement therapy and which regimen is used])
- Bilateral symptoms (see Chapter 1)
  Numbness/tingling   Burning
  Edema   Clubbing or other nail
  Weakness   bed changes
  Skin rash, lesions, or pigmentation changes
- Change in muscle tone or range of motion for individuals with neurologic conditions (e.g., cerebral palsy, spinal cord injury, traumatic brain injury, multiple sclerosis)

Pain Pattern

- Pain of unknown cause
- Back or shoulder pain (most common location of referred pain; other areas can be affected as well, but these two areas signal a particular need to take a second look)
- Pain accompanied by full and painless range of motion (see Table 3-1)
- Pain that is not consistent with emotional or psychologic overlay (e.g., Waddell's test is negative or insignificant; ways to measure this are discussed in Chapter 3; screening tests for emotional overlay are negative
- Night pain (constant and intense; see complete description in Chapter 3)
- Symptoms (especially pain) are constant and intense [Remember to ask anyone with "constant" pain: Are you having this pain right now?]
- Pain made worse by activity and relieved by rest (e.g., intermittent claudication, cardiac: upper quadrant pain with the use of the lower extremities while upper extremities are inactive)
- Pain described as throbbing (vascular), knife-like, boring, or deep aching
- Pain that is poorly localized
- Pattern of coming and going like spasms, colicky
- Pain accompanied by signs and symptoms associated with a specific viscera or system (e.g., gastrointestinal, genitourinary, gynecologic, cardiac, pulmonary, endocrine)
- Change in musculoskeletal symptoms with food intake or increased pain with medication use (immediately up to several hours later)

Neurologic Signs and Symptoms

General

- Confusion/increased confusion (most common in older adults)
- Depression
- Irritability
- Drowsiness/lethargy/sleepiness
- Blurred vision
- Headache
- Balance/coordination problems
- Weakness
- Change in memory
- Change in muscle tone for individual with previously diagnosed neurologic condition

Cauda Equina Syndrome

Cauda equina syndrome is defined as compression of the lumbar nerves in the central canal causing sensory and motor deficit, saddle anesthesia, and bowel and bladder dysfunction.

- Low back pain
- Loss of sensation in the lower extremities
- Muscle weakness and atrophy
- Bowel and/or bladder changes
  - Urinary retention
  - Difficulty starting a flow of urine
  - Decreased urethral sensation
  - Fecal incontinence
  - Constipation
  - Loss of anal tone and sensation
- Perineal pain
- Saddle and perineal hypoesthesia or anesthesia
- Unilateral or bilateral sciatica
- Change in deep tendon reflexes (reduced or absent in lower extremities)

Cervical Myelopathy

- Wide-based spastic gait
- Clumsy hands
- Visible change in handwriting
- Difficulty manipulating buttons or handling coins
- Hyperreflexia
- Positive Babinski test
- Positive Hoffman sign
- Lhermitte's sign
- Urinary retention followed by overflow incontinence (severe myelopathy)

ASSOCIATED SIGNS AND SYMPTOMS

- Recent report of confusion (or increased confusion); this could be a neurologic sign; it could be drug-induced (e.g., NSAIDs); usually it is a family member who takes the therapist aside to report this concern
- Presence of constitutional symptoms (see Box 1-3) or unusual vital signs (see Chapter 4); body temperature of 100° F (37.8° C) usually indicates a serious illness
- Proximal muscle weakness, especially if accompanied by change in deep tendon reflexes (DTRs) (see Fig. 13-3)
- Joint pain with skin rashes, nodules (see discussion of systemic causes of joint pain, Chapter 3; see Table 3-6)
- Any cluster of signs and symptoms observed during the Review of Systems that are characteristic of a particular organ system (see Box 4-17)

It is imperative at the end of each interview that the therapist ask the client a question such as the following:

Follow-Up Questions

- Are there any other symptoms or problems anywhere else in your body that may not seem related to your current problem?

This form may be duplicated for use in clinical practice. From Goodman CC, Snyder TE: *Differential diagnosis for physical therapists: screening for referral*, ed 4, Philadelphia, Saunders, 2007.

APPENDIX A-3 Systemic Causes of Joint Pain

When assessing joint pain, consider the following infectious and noninfectious systemic causes of joint pain. Look for history, risk factors, and associated signs and symptoms that might point to any of the following:

- Allergic reactions (e.g., medications such as antibiotics)
- Side effect of other medications such as statins, prolonged use of corticosteroids
- Delayed reaction to chemicals or environmental factors
- Sexually transmitted infections (STIs; e.g., HIV, syphilis, chlamydia, gonorrhea)
- Infectious arthritis
- Infective endocarditis
- Lyme disease
- Rheumatoid arthritis

- Other autoimmune disorders (e.g., systemic lupus erythematosus, mixed connective tissue disease, scleroderma, polymyositis)
- Leukemia
- Tuberculosis
- Acute rheumatic fever
- Chronic liver disease (hepatic osteodystrophy affecting wrists and ankles; hepatitis causing arthralgias)
- Inflammatory bowel disease (e.g., Crohn's disease or regional enteritis)
- Anxiety or depression (major depressive disorder)
- Fibromyalgia
- Artificial sweeteners

See Appendix B-16: Special Questions to Ask: Screening Joint Pain

APPENDIX A-4 The Referral Process

As a general rule, try to send the client back to the referring physician or other health care provider if there is one. If this does not seem appropriate, call and ask the physician how he or she wants to handle the situation. Describe the problem and ask:

Follow-Up Questions

- Do you want Mr. S. to check with his family doctor or do you prefer to see him yourself?

For example, if a client with an orthopedic medical diagnosis demonstrates signs and symptoms of depression, it could be a side effect from medications prescribed by another physician. List the observed cluster of signs and symptoms, and offer the physician an open-ended question such as:

Follow-Up Questions

- How do you want to handle this? Or How do you want me to handle this?

Do not suggest a medical diagnosis. When providing written documentation, a short summary of the physical therapist's evaluation is followed by a list of concerns or red flag signs and symptoms with the following comment:

These do not seem consistent with a neuromuscular (or musculoskeletal or movement system) problem (choose the most appropriate phrase to describe the client's impairment or dysfunction, or name the medical diagnosis [e.g., total hip replacement]). Then, follow up with one of the following:

Follow-Up Questions

- What do you think?
- Please advise.

Sometimes, it may seem like a good idea to suggest a second opinion. You may want to ask the client:

Follow-Up Questions

- Have you ever thought about getting a second opinion?

Take care not to tell the client what to do. If the client asks you what she or he should do, pose one of these questions:

Follow-Up Questions

- What do you think your options are?

Or

- What are your options?

After asking a question like this, you can always follow up with the suggestion that the client think about it for a day or two, consult with family and friends, and get back to you with his or her decision.

This form may be duplicated for use in clinical practice. From Goodman CC, Snyder TE: *Differential diagnosis for physical therapists: screening for referral*, ed 4, Philadelphia, Saunders, 2007

APPENDIX **B** SPECIAL QUESTIONS TO ASK

The appendices listed here are provided for you on the enclosed CD and can also be found on the EVOLVE website.

APPENDIX **C** SPECIAL FORMS TO USE

The appendices listed here are provided for you on the enclosed CD and can also be found on the EVOLVE website.

APPENDIX **C-1** Family/Personal History

APPENDIX **C-2** Wells' Clinical Decision Rule for DVT

APPENDIX **C-3** Osteoporosis Screening Evaluation

APPENDIX **C-4** Pain Assessment Record Form

APPENDIX **C-5** Risk Factor Assessment for Skin Cancer

APPENDIX **C-6** Examining a Skin Lesion or Mass

APPENDIX **C-7** Breast and Lymph Node Examination

APPENDIX D SPECIAL TESTS TO PERFORM

The appendices listed here are provided for you on the enclosed CD and can also be found on the EVOLVE website.

APPENDIX **D-1** Guide to Physical Assessment in a Screening Examination

APPENDIX **D-2** Extremity Examination Checklist

APPENDIX **D-3** Hand and Nail Bed Assessment

APPENDIX **D-4** Peripheral Vascular Assessment

APPENDIX **D-5** Review of Systems

APPENDIX **D-6** Self-Breast Examination (SBE)

APPENDIX **D-7** Clinical Breast Examination: Recommended Procedures

APPENDIX **D-8** Testicular Self-Examination

Index

Page references followed by "f" indicate figures, by "b" indicate boxes,
and by "t" indicate tables

875

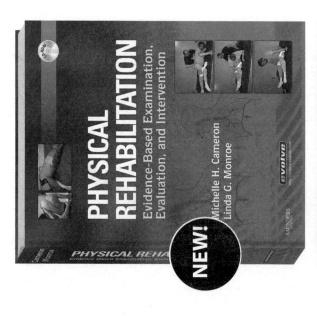
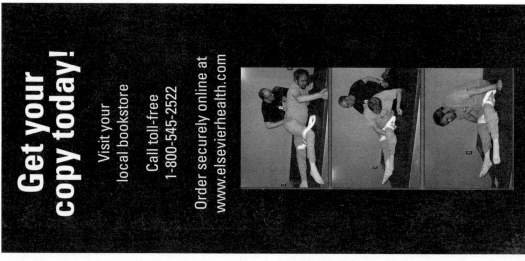